Critical
Care
Nursing

A Holistic Approach

J. B. Lippincott Company

Philadelphia

London

Mexico City

New York

St. Louis

São Paulo

Sydney

Carolyn M. Hudak, R.N., Ph.D.

Adult Nurse Practitioner
Formerly Associate Professor of Nursing and
Assistant Professor of Medicine
University of Colorado Health Sciences Center
Denver, Colorado

Barbara M. Gallo, R.N., M.S.

Assistant Director
Visiting Nurse And Home Care, Inc.
Hartford, Connecticut

Thelma "Skip" Lohr, R.N., M.S.

Instructor, Psychiatric Nursing
Bloomsburg University of Pennsylvania
Bloomsburg, Pennsylvania

Critical
Care
Nursing

A Holistic Approach

Fourth Edition

4th Edition

Copyright © 1986 by J. B. Lippincott Company
Copyright © 1982, 1977, 1973 by J. B. Lippincott Company
All rights reserved. No part of this book may be used or
reproduced in any manner whatsoever without written
permission except for brief quotations embodied in critical
articles and reviews. Printed in the United States of America.
For information write J. B. Lippincott Company, East
Washington Square, Philadelphia, Pennsylvania 19105.

6   5   4   3   2   1

Library of Congress Cataloging in Publication Data
Main entry under title:

Critical care nursing.

   Includes bibliographies and index.
   1. Intensive care nursing.   2. Holistic medicine.
I. Hudak, Carolyn M.   II. Gallo, Barbara M.   III. Lohr,
Thelma. [DNLM: 1. Critical Care — nurses' instruction.
2. Intensive Care Units — nurses' instruction.
WY 154 C9328]
RT120.I5C74   1986   610.73'61   85-4520
ISBN 0-397-54507-X

The authors and publisher have exerted every effort to ensure
that drug selection and dosage set forth in this text are in
accord with current recommendations and practice at the
time of publication. However, in view of ongoing research,
changes in government regulations, and the constant flow of
information relating to drug therapy and drug reactions, the
reader is urged to check the package insert for each drug for
any change in indications and dosage and for added warnings
and precautions. This is particularly important when the
recommended agent is a new or infrequently employed drug.

Sponsoring Editor: Diana Intenzo
Manuscript Editor: Linda Fitzpatrick
Indexer: Julia Schwager
Design Director: Tracy Baldwin
Designer: Arlene Putterman
Production Supervisor: J. Corey Gray
Compositor: Progressive Typographers Inc.
Printer/Binder: The Murray Printing Company

To Ann, who encouraged my first publishing efforts over fifteen years ago,
Carolyn

To patients, families, and the critical care nurses who care for them,
Bobbie

Contributors

Patricia D. Barry, R.N., M.S.N.
Psychiatric Liaison Nursing Consultant
West Hartford, Connecticut

Julie J. Benz, R.N., M.S.
Assistant Director of Nursing
Critical Care
Denver General Hospital
Denver, Colorado

H. L. Brammell, M.D.
Associate Professor of Physical Medicine and
    Rehabilitation
University of Colorado Health Sciences Center
Denver, Colorado

Patricia K. Brannin, R.N., M.S.N., R.R.T., A.N.P.
Formerly Associate Director of Nursing, Adult
    Medicine Units, National Jewish Hospital and
    Research Center
Clinical Coordinator, Institute for Transtracheal
    Oxygen Therapy
Presbyterian Denver Hospital, a Division of
    Presbyterian/St. Luke's Medical Center
Denver, Colorado

Eileen A. Brent-Hemman, R.N., M.S., C.C.R.N.
Respiratory Nurse Specialist
San Francisco, California

Barbara F. Brockway-Fuller, R.N., Ph.D.
Professor of Nursing
University of Colorado
School of Nursing
Denver, Colorado

Joseph O. Broughton, M.D., F.A.C.C.P.
Pulmonary Specialist
Denver, Colorado

Helen C. Busby, R.N., B.S.N., C.C.P.
Instructor, Critical Care, Mesa College; and
Staff Nurse, Critical Care, St. Mary's Hospital and
    Medical Center
Grand Junction, Colorado

Karen D. Busch, R.N., Ph.D.
Assistant Professor of Nursing
University of Utah College of Nursing
Salt Lake City, Utah

Donald E. Butkus, M.D.
Colonel, Medical Corps, Director, Division of Medicine
Department of the Army, Walter Reed Army Institute
    of Research, Walter Reed Army Medical Center
Washington, D.C.

Christine M. Ceccarelli, R.N., M.S.
Head Nurse, Dialysis Unit
Mt. Sinai Hospital
Hartford, Connecticut

Jacquelyn M. Clement, R.N., Ph.D.
Assistant Professor of Nursing
Southern Illinois University at Edwardsville
Edwardsville, Illinois

Sarah Dillian Cohn, M.S.N., J.D.
Risk Management
Yale New Haven Hospital
New Haven, Connecticut

Lane D. Craddock, M.D.
Associate Clinical Professor of Medicine
University of Colorado School of Medicine; and
Associate Director of Abe Ravin Division of
    Cardiovascular Medicine
Rose Medical Center
Denver, Colorado

Cynthia Johnson Dahlberg, M.A., C.C.C.-Sp.
Director, Department of Speech and Language
  Pathology
Craig Hospital
Englewood, Colorado

Frank Davidoff, M.D.
Chief of Medicine, New Britain General Hospital, New
  Britain, Connecticut
Professor of Medicine
University of Connecticut School of Medicine
Farmington, Connecticut

Carole K. Hahn, M.A., C.C.C.-Sp.
Speech Pathologist
Craig Hospital
Englewood, Colorado

Robert W. Hendee, Jr., M.D.
Associate Clinical Professor, Neurosurgery
University of Colorado Health Sciences Center; and
Chief of Neurosurgery Service, Children's Hospital
Denver, Colorado

Shirley J. Hoffman, R.N., B.S.N.
Patient Care Manager, Critical Care Departments
St. Luke's Hospital, a Division of Presbyterian/St.
  Luke's Medical Center
Denver, Colorado

Betty C. Irwin, R.N., M.S.
Clinical Nurse Specialist, Renal Transplantation
Johns Hopkins Hospital
Baltimore, Maryland

Judith L. Ives, R.N., M.S.
Denver, Colorado

Daniel Liberthson, Ph.D.
Palo Alto, California

Margaret A. Marcinek, R.N., M.S.N., Ed.D.
Nurse Consultant
Point Marion, Pennsylvania

Dorothy Murphy Mayer, R.N., B.S.N., C.C.R.N.
Stress Test Specialist
Stanford University Hospital
Stanford, California

Naomi Domer Medearis, R.N., M.A., M.B.A.
Program Specialist, Wellness Lifestyles
Jefferson County Adult and Continuing Education
Wheat Ridge, Colorado

Joan Mersch, R.N., M.S.
Clinical Nursing Coordinator, CCU
Stanford Medical Center
Palo Alto, California

Marilynn Mitchell, R.N., M.S.N., C.N.R.N.
Head Nurse, Neuro ICU and Intermediate Units
Denver General Hospital
Denver, Colorado

Deborah Moisan, R.N., B.S.N.
Staff Nurse, Poison Control Lab
Denver General Hospital
Denver, Colorado

Ann Marie Powers, R.N., M.S.
Clinical Nurse Specialist, Renal Transplantation
Chester, New Hampshire

Suzanne Provenzano, R.N., B.S.N., C.C.R.N.,
  C.N.R.N.
Critical Care Instructor
Swedish Medical Center
Englewood, Colorado

Karen Robbins, R.N., M.S.
Clinical Nurse Specialist, Renal Transplantation
West Hartford, Connecticut

William A. Seiffert, M.D.
Internal Medicine
West Nebraska General Hospital
Scottsbluff, Nebraska

Julie A. Shinn, R.N., M.A., C.C.R.N.
Educational Coordinator, Critical Care Units
Stanford University Hospital
Stanford, California

John B. Simpson, M.D.
Cardiologist, Sequoia Hospital
Redwood City, California

Janice S. Smith, R.N., M.S.
Professor of Nursing
Front Range Community College, Community College
  of Denver Systems
Denver, Colorado

Rae Nadine Smith, R.N., M.S.
Clinical Nursing Specialist
Medical Communicators and Associates
Los Angeles, California

Phillip S. Wolf, M.D.
Clinical Professor of Medicine
University of Colorado; and Director, Coronary Care
  Unit
Rose Medical Center
Denver, Colorado

Sally V. Zouras, R.N., B.S.N.
Cardiac Catheterization Lab
Sequoia Hospital
Redwood City, California

Preface

Critical care nursing continues to be a unique and challenging specialty. The critical care nurse must of necessity be well versed in both professionally oriented matters and pathophysiologically based material. The challenge for us has been to combine these two aspects successfully to arrive at a broader perspective of critical care nursing.

Previous editions of *Critical Care Nursing* have always been dedicated to the theory of holism. This edition, we feel, achieves an expanded synthesis of technical and professional issues. It provides a unique blend of all aspects of care related to the critically ill person. Machinery, technology, patient, family, nurse, and professional issues all are addressed in theory and in practical application. This edition emphasizes the delivery of care to patients and their families based on environmental and human care knowledge.

With respect to holistic issues, the nurse will find material related to the patient's response to stages of illness, concepts on extending critical care nursing to the patient's family, patient responses to the critical care environment, and some fascinating ideas on caring and touching as nursing interventions. Addressing professional concerns are a chapter on the effects of the critical care unit on the nurse, a chapter on applied legal principles related to critical care nursing practice, and a special chapter on training and development of the critical care nursing staff.

In this edition, there is a new focus on the nursing process, and nursing diagnoses have been integrated as appropriate to specific patient problems.

One goal has been to integrate concepts, skills, and applications within each core body system. A unit on the metabolic system has been added and includes chapters on the gastrointestinal and endocrine systems. The section on core body systems now includes discussions of more specific disease entities with an emphasis on assessment, intervention, and evaluation for each pathological condition. For example, the unit on the cardiovascular system includes chapters on heart failure, acute myocardial infarction, and disseminated intravascular coagulation. Material on new technologies such as intracoronary streptokinase, percutaneous transluminal coronary angioplasty, and high-frequency jet ventilation, on the latest in drug therapies, on the state of the art in diagnostic procedures, and on the newly recognized role of nutritional support in the critically ill patient has been added. In addition, the unit on the nervous system has been extensively reorganized and revised, and the chapter on common neurologic problems has been significantly expanded.

We are grateful to our contributors, both old and new, whose expertise is dedicated to improving professional nursing practice. A special thank you to Susie Peterson for typing most of the manuscript and for her commitment to perfection.

Carolyn M. Hudak, R.N., Ph.D.

Barbara M. Gallo, R.N., M.S.

Thelma "Skip" Lohr, R.N., M.S.

Contents

Section I
Holistic Framework for
Critical Care Nursing

Section II
Core Body Systems

Unit One
Cardiovascular System

Unit Two
Respiratory System

Unit Three
Renal System

Unit Four
Nervous System

Unit Five
Metabolic System: Gastrointestinal
and Endocrine Systems

Section III
Professional Practice Issues
in the Critical Care Unit

Section I

Holistic Framework for Critical Care Nursing

1
The Nursing Process Applied to Critical Care Nursing

Greg Sherry

688-5693

Carolyn M. Hudak
Barbara M. Gallo
Thelma L. Lohr

CRISIS CARE COMPARED WITH CRITICAL CARE

Critical and *crisis* are two static terms that have had a close association. They are so frequently interchanged in nursing discussions that many practitioners are cognizant only of the similarities, not of the differences. Webster defines each of these terms as follows:

> Crisis—an emotionally significant event or radical change of status in a person's life . . . an unstable state of affairs in which a decisive change is impending.
> Critical—exercising or involving careful judgment or judicious evaluation; discriminating, careful, exact . . . indispensable for the weathering, the solution, or the overcoming of a crisis . . . of doubtful issue: attended by risk or uncertainty.

Although both these terms broaden nursing activities to include more of the nurse's intellect and decision-making processes, the essence of the difference begins with the purpose and the way it is achieved—that is, through the steps of the nursing process. Table 1-1 delineates the differences between crisis care and critical care as related to purpose, orientation, focus, and the essential steps of the nursing process.

THE BASIS OF CRITICAL CARE NURSING

The essence of critical care nursing lies not in special environments or amid special equipment but in the nurse's decision-making process and willingness to act on decisions made.

The critical care nurse is the person who sees beyond the patient's blood pressure, pulse, and respiration. She feels a pulse and notes its quality, makes a mental note of the temperature of the skin and its state of hydration, compares the pulse rate with the temperature and blood pressure, and, if the anticipated correlation is not there, she asks herself "Why?" In short, she functions according to her intellect.

The critical care nurse anticipates events on the basis of her knowledge of normal physiology and the patient's condition. If findings other than the expected ones materialize, the critical care nurse proceeds to gather additional clinical data to determine the nature and cause of the deviations. She attempts to seek the rational basis for all interpretations and responses to clinical cues.

THE NURSING PROCESS IN CRITICAL CARE

The steps that a nurse follows in the decision-making process are as follows:

1. Appropriate information is collected.
2. An assessment is made based on the data collected.
3. A plan of action is decided on and implemented.
4. The results of these actions are evaluated.

This nursing process serves as a framework for decision-making and administering nursing care.

Data collection includes the accumulation of two types of information: subjective (interviewing and history-taking) and objective (physical examination and testing). An assessment is made on the basis of all available information. It may be described in terms of

3

TABLE 1-1
CRISIS CARE VERSUS CRITICAL CARE WITHIN A NURSING PROCESS FRAMEWORK

Crisis Care	Critical Care
Purpose	
Lifesaving	Life-maintaining
Data Collection	
On body systems in failure—to reverse the failure or maintain the system	On all body systems—to support those in trouble and to maintain those in health
Assessment	
Discriminating for presenting signs and symptoms	Discriminating, exact, careful for subtle signs and symptoms before they become grossly presenting
Planning	
Established protocol and procedures	Constant adjustment and adaptation of established protocol and procedures to patient's individuality and frequently changing status (days/weeks)
Intervention	
Treatment of the presenting crisis symptoms and stabilization of patient	Treatment of the first presenting symptoms and prevention of a crisis
Continuous until life is stabilized for transportation to a unit or until death occurs (hours)	Continuous with a wider range, until adaptation to a higher level of wellness is attained or until death occurs
Evaluation	
Immediate for effectiveness of treatment	Immediate and long-term for effectiveness of each therapy procedure, planned and frequent assessment of each body system with a variety of tools, continuous adjustment of short-term and long-range goals as the patient's status changes

---

Nursing Process

• Data collection
• Assessment
• Care planning and intervention
• Evaluation

---

one or more factors, including patient problem and nursing diagnosis. In any case, the assessment paves the way for the next step in the process, planning care. The more specific the plan of care, the easier it is to evaluate. Expected outcomes also are used to evaluate the care plan. If the interventions were effective and restored equilibrium, the problem is resolved and the process is complete. If not, the nurse must repeat the process beginning with data collection and continuing with reassessment, further planning, and reevaluation. For example, a postoperative patient has a blood pressure of 88/60, pulse 100, respirations 28, and diaphoresis. Perhaps these symptoms are the result of pain . . . or hemorrhage. *Further information* about the patient and his symptoms is needed to support either premise.

• Does he complain of pain?
• Does he "splint" the area when he moves?
• Is his dressing wet?
• Is urine output diminished?
• Is there any evidence of bleeding into the incisional area?
• What is the pulse quality?
• Does the CVP lend any clues?

After analyzing these findings, the nurse makes an assessment. An assessment that indicates that the patient is in pain may be stated as a nursing diagnosis, such as alteration in comfort or acute pain. If the assessment indicates that pain control is necessary, the plan will be to medicate the patient for pain. Next, the outcome of the intervention is evaluated. For example, after medicating the postoperative patient, the nurse will anticipate a given outcome. The patient should be able to relate that he feels more comfortable after treatment for pain. If the vital sign parameters noted previously are due to pain, the nurse will anticipate that the patient's vital signs will return to baseline if pain is relieved. If this anticipated outcome does not occur, the nurse then asks "Why?" and proceeds to gather additional data to answer that question. This leads to reassessment, further planning, and reevaluation. *The process is continuous until the problem is resolved.*

We stated previously that the essence of critical care nursing is a decision-making process that is based on a sound understanding of physiological and psychological entities. It requires the ability to deal with critical situations with a rapidity and precision not usually necessary in other health-care settings. It requires adeptness at integrating information and establishing priorities because, when illness strikes one body system, other systems become involved in the effort to cope with the disequilibrium.

The patient admitted to a critical care unit needs excellent care directed not only at the pathophysiological problems but also at the psychosocial, environmental, and family issues that become intimately intertwined with the physical illness. Within the framework of the nursing process, the concepts of the hierarchy of human needs, adaptation, and patient advocacy assume special relevance to critical care nursing.

HIERARCHY OF HUMAN NEEDS

Individuals seek to preserve their lives by directing all their energies toward the most basic unmet needs. For example, all the compensatory mechanisms of a person with inadequate cardiac output will work to maintain the circulation of oxygen, thus meeting the most basic requirement for life. In this situation, energy is directed away from subsystems such as the gastrointestinal, skin, and kidney functions. This phenomenon can be described as *physiological amputation.* Energy is directed away from less critical functions in order to help the organism through the physiological crisis. If the crisis is not stabilized, the subsystems eventually move from a compensatory state (physiological amputation) to a decompensatory one.

Fundamental needs, although closely interrelated, are arranged in order of dominance. The most basic needs are physiological, aimed at self-preservation. Upper-level needs are security, belonging, self-esteem, and self-actualization.

The need for a sense of security to allay anxiety is always present, but it is not the most basic need at, for

example, the time of inadequate cardiac output. Later, when needs for air, cellular nutrition, and elimination are met, the efforts of the individual are directed toward seeking security, a sense of belonging, and self-esteem (Fig. 1-1).

Although each of us has physiological and psychological mechanisms that compensate for disequilibrium, there are situations in which we cannot adapt without outside intervention. It is in these situations that the critical care nurse becomes the patient's advocate and fosters adaptation.

NURSING INTERVENTION AND ADAPTATION

The individual's attempts to cope with the environment include *avoidance,* in which one flees from the situation; *counteraction,* in which body defenses try to destroy the stressor, often at the expense of other systems; and *adaptation,* in which one seeks to estab-

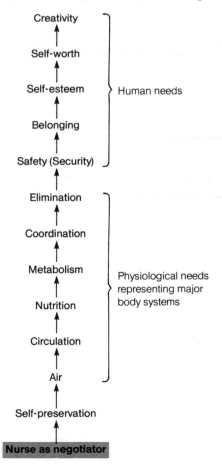

FIGURE 1-1
Hierarchy of human needs for critical care nursing.

Creativity

Self-worth

Self-esteem ⎫
           ⎬ Human needs
Belonging |

Safety (Security) ⎭

Elimination ⎫

Coordination |

Metabolism ⎬ Physiological needs
           | representing major
Nutrition | body systems

Circulation |

Air   ⎭

Self-preservation

Nurse as negotiator

lish a compatible response to the stress and still retain a steady state.

Although all mechanisms foster self-preservation, nursing intervention is aimed at adaptation. By fostering responses that encourage both physiologically and emotionally useful functioning, nurses enhance adaptation and aid the patient in reducing stress and conserving energy. Conversely, when nursing intervention or lack of it does not foster adaptation, the patient's energy is wasted, and a state of increased tension exists; that is, the patient will have a diminished capacity to deal with a changing situation. Thus, stress is increased when a patient's energy is devoted to maladaptive functioning that perpetuates the disequilibrium, and stress is minimized when the patient expends energy that fosters adaptation to the disequilibrium (see Fig. 3-1).

An example of maladaptation versus adaptation is seen in a patient with restrictive lung disease who develops a lung infection resulting in ↑ PCO_2 and ↓ PO_2. This patient cannot compensate because of his restrictive lung disease; thus, his established pattern of breathing is maladaptive, perpetuating the problem of gas exchange. Adaptive nursing intervention involves helping the patient breathe more deeply and fostering the drainage of secretion either by having him do breathing exercises or by using mechanical aids. Although the energy is still expended, it is spent usefully. This concept of minimizing tension and stress is consistent with the ultimate goal of health care: to restore the person to a steady state with minimal stress to the rest of the body.

ADVOCACY

Fostering adaptive functioning means that the nurse negotiates for the patient. Because the critically ill patient often cannot effectively cope with both the physiological problem and the rest of his environment, it becomes necessary for the nurse to do for the patient what he is unable to do for himself so that his energy is conserved. As patient advocate, the nurse must refrain from adding burdens that increase the patient's need to interact when such interaction will not foster adaptation. For example, patient energy spent in fearful suspense about the equipment nearby is not as helpful as energy spent in asking about it and then listening to a reply. Likewise, energy expended in persistently requesting a loved one to be present may not be as helpful as energy spent interacting with that person.

Fostering security in the critically ill patient involves decreasing his vulnerability both physiologically and emotionally. The feeling of security is lost or at least significantly decreased whenever there is a decrease in one's control of body functions. Loss of control may vary from fatigue and weakness to paralysis. It may result from pathology, the environment (*e.g.,* restraint by IV tubing or machinery), or both; from fatigue and sleeplessness caused by physical discomfort; or from physiological fatigue (*e.g.,* dyspnea and sensory overload). Regardless of the decrease or loss of control, the nurse intervenes in order to increase the patient's feeling of safety. She may accomplish this by using technical skill, tools, medication, and interaction; by providing assisted breathing with a respirator; by encouraging breathing exercises; or by staying with the patient during a time of anxiety or loneliness. Recognition of a patient's safety needs is an important element in the holistic approach to patient care. In addition, it is this very consideration of the "whole" patient that allows us to establish priorities as patient negotiators.

Negotiating for the patient is not without its hazards. This kind of caring and giving requires our energies in place of those that the patient is temporarily lacking. Therefore, to maintain our own emotional reserves, we also need to support one another as colleagues in the critical care unit and to enhance one another's feelings of belonging and self-esteem. Other hazards involve speaking on behalf of the patient, often as a minority voice and in the face of administrative, physician, or peer pressure. Acting as patient advocate means experiencing the joy of patients who recover as well as the sadness and anger of those who do not.

This philosophy of nursing need not and should not be confined to critical care areas. It is every patient's right to expect this type of intelligent care; it is the nurse's responsibility and challenge to provide it.

2
Sociometric Impact on the Patient

Thelma "Skip" Lohr

Since the 1950s, researchers from many health fields have been investigating the role of psychosocial factors in the pathogenesis and prognosis of physical illness. Now, it is commonly accepted that these factors indeed play an important role. Investigators, realizing the uniqueness of life-events data, have developed scales that measure stress associated with specific situations. One premise of these scales is that some life events are inherently more stressful than others and thus will have a greater impact. According to one study of patients suffering from myocardial infarctions, it is not only the event but also how the person perceives it and, thus, his emotional response to it that determine the impact.[1] Measurement scales can help predict who is at risk for developing psychological and physiological disequilibrium as the result of high levels of stress.

Moreno postulated another framework that examines psychosocial factors.[2] Following is a discussion of Moreno's concept of a psychosocial model that is as old as mankind and as contemporary as this moment: an exciting, viable theory that allows us to "see" the invisible structures of our everyday lives that foster health and creativity. It also reinforces the fact that critical care nurses are in pivotal positions to aid both patients and families in maintaining or building these invisible structures of life and health.

Early in the 1900s, Jacob Moreno moved from the traditional sociometry of *macro*scopic study of social structures to become the creator of a new system of sociometry. He began to study the *micro*scopic dynamics of people within groups. His work resulted in a new framework of sociometry based on two positive aspects of people and groups—spontaneity and creativity. Hollander concludes, ". . . sociometry is

based on the concept that individuals must have a specific number of people with whom they can meaningfully relate or feel close to in order to experience their creativity and power: i.e., self-confidence."[3]

Within Moreno's framework, a new language emerged, a language with energy words such as *social atom, tele,* and *social equilibrium.*

THE SOCIAL ATOM

The word *atom* suggests an awesome source of powerful energy—a suggestion that holds true for the social atom. The social atom is a powerful energy source of each individual's life. It is also a fact of life that we *live.* Moreno defined it as "the smallest functional unit within our social group." This social unit, which exists at birth and continues and expands into adulthood, is formed by numerous relationships that Moreno called *tele* structures. Originating from a Greek concept, *tele* is a term he used to describe the far-reaching transmission of a feeling, positive or negative, from one person to another—the instinctive ability that allows one to know another intuitively. Tele is always mutual; one-way intuitive understanding of another is called *empathy.* People have given this phenomenon mystical and magical qualities, and teenagers who recognize their ability to "feel another" call it "picking-up vibes."

The Psychological Social Atom

This atom is the smallest number of people each person requires to maintain social equilibrium and, thus, a healthy and creative life. The number each person requires usually varies from two to five. Generally, these people are family members or friends, or both, who are vital to the person's life.(Interestingly, there are some individuals who have replaced people with plants, animals, or objects.) Although these relationships seem to "just happen," they are the result of mutual tele selection by both individuals. They allow for the expression of human feelings (*e.g.*, warmth, love, anger, joy, sorrow, sexuality) and endure over long periods of time.

When the psychological social atom drops below the required number because of events of separation, social disequilibrium results, and the person experiences shock and grief. This effect is evidenced in inappropriate behaviors (*i.e.*, forgetfulness, thoughtlessness, disorganization) or symptoms of ill health (*i.e.*, colds, headaches, angina, cancer). The person *must* regain social equilibrium and will search to fill the void. The void, however, cannot truly be filled until grieving is complete.

Many elderly people in the United States have social atoms that are either below or at the edge of a safe level needed for affiliation, socialization, and physical help with activities of daily living. When significant others are in short supply, the potential for disequilibrium is high. In these situations, *one* event that interferes with *one* person in the social atom can cause the unit to collapse. When the person's atom is composed of only one, all energy will be directed toward maintaining this member. An example of this situation is described in the following case study.

CASE STUDY: RICHARD AND ANN

Richard and Ann were two elderly people living in a nursing home. They had become very good friends and were inseparable. Ann broke her hip in a fall, and following surgery she remained in a coma for several weeks. When Ann was taken to the hospital, Richard wanted to follow, but nursing home personnel thought it would be inappropriate and so detained him. He feigned sleep and waited until 2 A.M. to leave "out the back way." He came to the hospital to "be with her!" He was so unobtrusive that several shifts passed before people began to mention the old man in the room. Then the staff became aware of Richard's presence and concerned for his health and hygiene. He had neither eaten (Ann was on IVs and receiving no trays) nor bathed. He absolutely refused to return to the nursing home for anything. The unit's staff quietly and spontaneously began caring for Richard, too. He joined them in the dining room (he had very little vision) and shared their trays, which always seemed to have "too much food." Although he beamed from the attention, he remained quietly content just to be in Ann's room. When physicians and nurses were finished with their cares, he could be found gently stroking Ann's arm or forehead softly reminiscing about their life and his love for her—very private and intimate moments that caused the staff members' eyes to tear as they appreciated this gift of caring. Staff, well-aware that it

was against unit visiting policies, found nonverbal consensus through others' behaviors.

This situation continued for 3 to 4 weeks, and as the social worker began plans to prepare Richard for Ann's seemingly imminent death and the elderly man's return to the nursing home, Ann came out of the coma. She became progressively stronger and walked with a walker, and together Richard and Ann returned to the home.

Richard's behaviors were most understandable and appropriate because Ann was the last significant person in his life. His social atom was near zero, with his own survival at stake. In a psychological social atom of two, it is not uncommon that when one dies, the other follows within a short period of time.[4]

The Collective Social Atom

This collective is one's cultural atom, consisting of the smallest number of groups or affiliations in which a person must have membership. Collectives are the tele structures in which people assume roles and counterroles of their culture for the expression of their creativity and productivity. They provide one's identity (*e.g.*, mother or child, husband or wife, teacher or student, nurse or patient). Collectives that are common for most people are familial, work, social, recreational, educational, and religious groups.

The relationships within a collective begin the sociometric network that links the collective to other social groups and the community. One example is the critical care nurse who designs and presents cardiopulmonary resuscitation (CPR) learning experiences for her husband's realtor group and then is asked by other realtor groups to do the same for them. Another network pattern is the collective of hospital nurses who have membership in the district nurse's association, which is part of the state's association, which is part of the national organization.

Although a person may belong to numerous collectives, only one or two will be vital for homeostasis. If membership is terminated in one of these, the person will again experience shock and grief and will begin a search to replace the collective.

The Individual Social Atom

This atom is the smallest number of people within a collective that one needs to feel a sense of belonging. These are the people who respond positively, negatively, or indifferently to our many needs — from sharing our creativity to supporting our efforts or comforting our hurts. These people are a source for our motivation and energy, and, although many are important, only a few are vital to our survival within a collective.

As in the previous two atoms, should the number drop below what is required, a sociometric crisis develops for the person. He will "look" in crisis and may not be able to function. Soon his energies will be directed toward searching for replacements. If people are not available, death within the collective occurs, and the person will then terminate his position and search for a new collective as well. All critical care units have staff members who stand out—"stars." Should one of these people resign, it will not be long before statements such as, "It just isn't the same," "I feel burned-out," and "I'd like to try something different" are heard. Either someone moves in to fill the void, or the statement-makers resign also. The new staff members, given time and opportunity, will change the undercurrent of turmoil to one of belonging by building their own telic structure of relationships.

The psychological, collective, and individual social units, three distinct atoms within one, are not separate and isolated entities in one's life. What happens in one atom affects the total. For example: Tony lost his job. He was very upset and irritable—with his children, his wife, and his friends—until he found employment and replaced his work collective with another.

Patients in critical care units who are under stress because of specific life events may also be in a socio-metric crisis. This can further compromise their vulnerable physiological state. For example, if Tony, who lost his job, also became critically ill, his irritability and other symptoms of being upset would affect not only those in his new social atom (the critical care unit staff) but also his ability to cope with his illness. Life events that are known to produce high levels of stress also affect an individual's social atom. Examples include divorce, death of a loved one, geographical relocation, or a change in a job (even one involving a promotion). *Nursing diagnoses* that may result when individual social atoms are in flux include grief, social isolation, powerlessness, anxiety, depression, and ineffective coping.

Richard's Social Atom

A diagram of Richard's sociometric network may best portray the social atom concept. Prior to moving to the nursing home, Richard's social atom had been diminishing gradually, and his physical and emotional energy waned with each loss. Figure 2-1 starkly illustrates that Richard's collective of friends, which included Ann, was his only remaining network for living. He was literally dying from without—moving toward social atom death.

Together, Richard and Ann chose to move into the

FIGURE 2-1
Richard's social atom prior to the nursing home. Dotted circles and lines indicate what had been and were now memories.

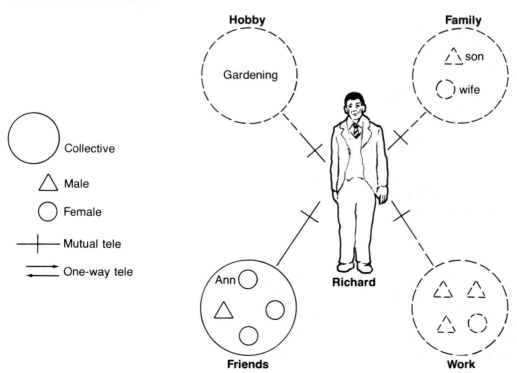

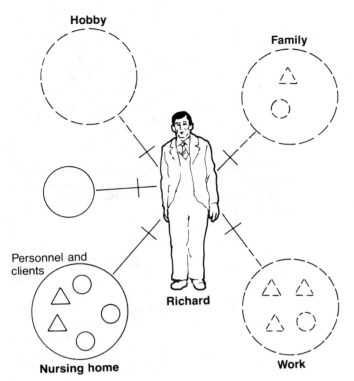

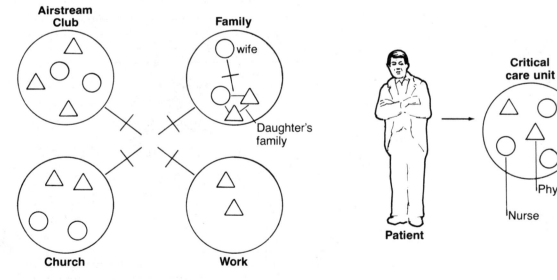

FIGURE 2-2
Richard's social atom in the nursing home.

FIGURE 2-3
A diagram of a social atom upon hospitalization.

nursing home, for Ann had grown to be a close companion who lovingly cared for him. Figure 2-2 indicates that the nursing home residents replaced his collective of friends. There, Richard developed many individual relationships while Ann grew stronger as his psychological and individual atom.

APPLYING SOCIOMETRY TO CRITICAL CARE

Examining one's social atom helps answer these vital questions:

1. Who am I?

2. Where do I fit?
3. How well am I functioning?

These three questions become paramount when a person is removed from the uniqueness of his social atom for hospitalization. The effect is momentary termination of one's usual life processes and sensory deprivation of familiar sounds, sights, and experiences—*plus* the addition of a new collective with its unique individuals and environment. Figure 2-3 illustrates such a move. The staff members who care for the patient upon admission do in fact become his individual atom within his new collective. The primary nurse becomes one of the required few people necessary to maintain homeostasis within the collective.

Individuals from within his atom, also at loose ends, follow him to the hospital, seeking to keep their connections. One of two of these people, usually family members or close friends, become extensions of the patient and have a vital role in establishing and maintaining the patient's relationships (and theirs) within the unit. The most common behaviors that accomplish this are demonstrated by family members who ask the questions the patient cannot, seek the explanations the patient cannot, and contribute information when the patient does not.

The nurse has a hospital collective that she maintains with the required number of people for belonging and homeostasis. She also has (as does everyone) an expansiveness for accommodating others, including the critical care patients. The patients are usually short-term and frequently leave without notice—by transfer or death. For the nurse to invest in each new patient means that she must constantly cope with pain and loss of relationships. Continually investing in new patients without completing terminations with the previous patients is exhausting. The nurse's social atom overexpands, resulting in disequilibrium. When this occurs, the nurse will seek a return to homeostasis, frequently by making a token investment in the patient while more completely focusing on her own work relationships and activities.

It helps to be aware of this phenomenon so that steps can be taken to reestablish one's homeostasis. Nurses can be alert for the signs of disequilibrium, such as behavior that becomes more mechanical or task-oriented.

The concept of sociometry can be applied to a variety of situations throughout this text and serves as a framework on which to build concepts in the next three chapters of this unit.

It has long been accepted that critical care environments can precipitate a wide variety of feelings and mental states, including isolation, confinement, boredom, relief, fear, confusion, hallucinations, and paranoia. For the patient, the cause is paradoxical—sensory overload from the new environment's persistent lights, sounds, and noises and sensory deprivation from loss of familiar sensory stimuli and periods of time that keep the person oriented (see Chap. 6). Human stimuli in the form of family, friends, and nurses are discovered most times to be the solution, for people need to feel connected to avoid feeling "crazy."

Many critical care nurses also experience isolation, confinement, boredom, and fear. The unit is not part of mainstream traffic; the patient's room is small and compact; patient assignments absorb hours of time; unresponsive, unchallenging patients provoke nursing by habit. The intensity and duration of these feelings are of a lesser degree for the nurse than for the patient. The nurses seek relief through the people in their collective atom with comments such as, "Relieve me for a moment, will you? I've got to get out of there before I go crazy." Another remark that might be heard is, "I'm so bored—do you (nurse) need any help?" These solutions are extremely important because when the nurse has minimized the environment's effects on her own self, she is then available to do the same for the patient.

Transfer from critical care is another paradox for the patient. The stress and fears of going into a new collective can be overwhelming; at the same time, the knowledge of getting better is reassuring. Linkage to this new collective is through the nurse and physician. A vital connection is the nurse who accompanies the patient to the next unit and introduces him to the people in the new environment. To start with, the new collective of individuals will at least know his name and that he now belongs to them. Yet in that same moment the patient experiences a great loss, and again the need for and importance of family members increase.

Many nurses are indeed searching for ways to minimize their unit's impact and are finding solutions. I believe the answers are in both what the patient and the nurse experience. When staff must constantly rotate shifts and units, their individual and collective atoms will be in constant crisis. Their emotional energies will go toward making and renewing relationships, and they will have very little energy available for the patient. However, in a unit in which the staff is stable and its members have had time to develop high cohesion, the nurse is free to be emotionally available to her patients. In this unit, the patient will be able to find a powerful energy source in his primary nurse and nurse advocate.

REFERENCES

1. Byrne DG, Whyte HM: Life events and myocardial infarctions revisited: The role of measures of individual impact. J Human Stress 42, No. 1:1–9, 1980

2. Moreno JL: Who Shall Survive, 3rd ed. Beacon, Beacon House, 1978
3. Hollander CE: Psychodrama, role playing, and sociometry: Living and learning processes. In Kurpous D (ed): Learning: Making Learning Environments More Effective, p 220. Muncie, Accelerated Development, 1978
4. Cottingham E et al: Environmental events preceding sudden death in women. Psychosom Med 42, No. 6:569–573, 1980

BIBLIOGRAPHY

Weeks JR, Cuellas JB: Role of family members in helping networks of older people. Gerontologist 21:388–394, 1981
Wells L, Macdonald G: Interpersonal networks and post relocation adjustment of the institutionalized elderly. Gerontologist 21:177–183, 1981

3
Stages of Illness: The Patient's Response*

Karen D. Busch

When people develop symptoms that deviate from their usual feeling of well-being, they typically perceive themselves to be sick. If severe illness impinges on the person's dynamic stability and anxiety is extreme, routine coping mechanisms may not even be employed; if they are, they may not be effective enough to allow the patient to deal with the crisis. A large portion of this textbook is focused on supporting and implementing the patient's response to the threat of illness through physiological maintenance and adjustments. It is the purpose of this chapter to consider the intimate relationship between one's emotional response to illness and the effect of this response on adaptation to temporary or permanent limitations. Concepts of stress, anxiety, dependency, grief, adaptation and transference will be presented so that the nurse may develop related interventions based on sound theory and knowledge about the interdependent relationships between physical and emotional well-being. Patient teaching and learning and transfer from the critical care unit also are addressed. The framework and concepts provided in this chapter can be applied and adapted to specific illnesses and patient situations presented throughout the book.

In order to facilitate healing and the maintenance of the personal integrity of the patient, the nurse must plan patient care so that both emotional and physical needs are met in an optimal way. An understanding of the intricate relationship among mind, body, and the healing process will help the critical care nurse value and provide emotional support to the patient.

*Barbara Gallo helped write and revise this chapter in the first three editions of *Critical Care Nursing*. In this edition, overall editing of the text took precedence.

STRESS AND ILLNESS

The stresses of illness and the patient role are likely to reintroduce childhood conflicts regarding autonomy and dependency. These conflicts together with the stress of illness are likely to arouse a state of tension in the patient. In order to deal with the discomfort of the tension state, the patient will attempt to employ coping behaviors, such as denial, anger, passivity, or aggression. These attempts at coping may be adaptive or maladaptive in handling the stress and its resultant anxiety. When the coping behaviors are adaptive, energy is freed and may be directed toward healing. When coping attempts fail or are maladaptive, however, the tension state is increased; accordingly, there is an increased demand for energy. Thus, the original stress of illness looms larger (Fig. 3-1).

The relationship among stress, anxiety, and coping is a complex one that manifests itself continuously in any critical care setting. Stress has been defined as any stimulus that results in a disequilibrium of psychological functioning. In turn, this disequilibrium initiates attempts to restore the original state of dynamic equilibrium.

Anxiety

Anxiety can be viewed as a state of disequilibrium or tension that prompts attempts at coping. Coping can then be viewed as a transaction between the person and his environment. Successful transactions reduce tension and promote a sense of well-being.

Any stress that threatens one's sense of wholeness, containment, security, and control will cause anxiety. Illness is one such stress. The physiological responses

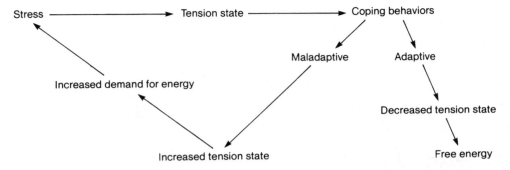

FIGURE 3-1
Stress and coping behaviors.

of rapid pulse rate, increased blood pressure, increased respirations, dilated pupils, dry mouth, and peripheral vasoconstriction may go undetected in a seemingly cool, calm, self-contained patient. These autonomic responses to anxiety are frequently the most reliable index of the degree of anxiety when behavioral responses do not confirm the nurse's expectations.

Behavioral responses indicative of anxiety are often family-based and culturally learned. They vary from quiet composure in the face of disaster to panic in the presence of an innocuous insect. Such extremes of control and panic use valuable energy. When this energy is not directed toward eliminating the stressor, it serves only to perpetuate the discomfort of the tension state. The goal of nursing care is always to promote physiological and emotional equilibrium.

Whenever possible, the threat of stress is reduced or eliminated. When this is accomplished, the problem is quickly resolved and the patient is returned to a state of equilibrium. Usually, however, the stress is not eliminated so easily because many other stresses (secondary stresses) are introduced by attempts to remedy the original problem. For most people, hospitalization is an example of secondary stress. To find oneself in a critical care unit as a patient is tangible proof that one's life is in jeopardy. For most patients, fears that life is being threatened are justified, as is the feeling of being wholly at the mercy of strangers. A sense of inadequacy or inferiority results because the patient is unable to understand what is happening to his body and whether or not the personnel and surrounding machinery will return him to his previous state of health.

Nursing Assessment and Intervention

Helping The Patient Cope

It often is not possible for the nurse simply to remove the noxious stimulus that evokes anxiety. In these circumstances, the nurse must assess the effectiveness of the patient's coping behaviors and either support them, help the patient modify them, or teach new coping behaviors. Frequently, levels of anxiety are so high that the anxious state becomes the stimulus that demands additional coping responses.

Assess coping behaviors and either

- support them
- help patient modify them
- teach new ones

Coping behaviors may be directed toward eliminating the stress either of illness or of the anxiety state itself. The nurse must evaluate each behavior in light of whether or not it functions to restore a steady state. Those behaviors that are consistent with movement toward a steady state can then be supported and encouraged. More likely, the nurse may need to help the patient modify or find substitutes for those coping devices that are disruptive or threatening to homeostasis. At times, it may be necessary for the nurse to teach or introduce new coping behaviors to facilitate movement toward the overall primary goal of homeostatic equilibrium.

In a critical period, patients may be more capable of experiencing concern and worry over the variety of equipment that engulfs them than of focusing on the threat to life. This activity may allow some necessary denial of the reality of the crisis, but the worry itself may drain needed resources of energy. Information and explanation of the machinery may reduce secondary anxiety, and expert nursing care may reassure the patient nonverbally of his security without stripping away the defense of denial.

Anxiety commonly is experienced when there is a threat of helplessness or lack of control. Nursing measures that reinforce a sense of control help increase the patient's sense of autonomy and reduce the overpowering sense of loss of control. Providing order and predictability allows the patient to anticipate and prepare for what is to follow. Perhaps it creates only a mirage of control, but anticipatory guidance keeps the patient from being caught off-guard and allows the mustering of those coping mechanisms that can be brought to bear.

Allowing small choices when the patient is willing and ready decreases the patient's feeling that he has no control over the environment. Would he prefer to lie on his right or left side? In which arm would he like his IV? How high does he want the head of his bed? Does he want to cough now or in 20 minutes following pain medication? All permit the patient to participate in ways that allow a certain amount of control and predictability. They also may help the patient accept lack of control of procedures that involve little choice. Minute decisions allow the patient to exercise some self-governance in a way designed to help reduce the anxiety-provoking sense of helplessness.

Help increase patient's sense of control.

• Provide order and predictability
• Use anticipatory guidance.
• Allow choices whenever possible.

A second common cause of anxiety is a sense of isolation. Rarely is one lonelier than when in the midst of a socializing crowd of strangers. In such a situation, people attempt to either include themselves, remove themselves, or emotionally distance themselves. The sick person surrounded by active and busy persons is in a similar situation but with few resources available to reduce the sense of isolation. Serious illness and the fear of dying separate the patient from his family. The reassuring cliche "You'll be all right" reinforces the sense of distance that the patient is experiencing. It shuts off expression of fears and questions of what is to come next. The efficiency and activity that surround the patient increase the sense of separateness.

A third category of anxiety-provoking stimuli includes those that threaten the individual's security. Admittance to the critical care unit dramatically confirms for the family and patient that their security on all levels is being severely threatened. For most people, the critical care unit is related to a life-and-death crises. Many associate it with the deaths of relatives and friends.

To the nurse, the unit may represent a closer and safer vigilance of life, with attention directed more toward the preservation of life than toward the fears of dying that may be occupying the minds of the patient and his family. When the patient is admitted to the unit, his initial insecurity undoubtedly concerns life itself. Later, questions regarding such issues as length of hospitalization, return to work, well-being of the family, and permanent limitations arise, so the patient's insecurity is continuously present.

Cognitive Techniques that Deal with Anxiety
Techniques that have evolved from cognitive theories of learning may help anxious patients and their families. These techniques are promising because they can be initiated by the patient and do not depend on complex insight or understanding of one's own psychological makeup. They can also be employed to reduce anxiety in a way that avoids probing into the patient's personal life. Furthermore, the patient's friends and family members can be taught these techniques to help them and the patient reduce tension.

Positive Thinking. Highly anxious people are most likely giving themselves messages that increase or perpetuate their anxiety. These messages are conveyed in one's continuously running "self-talk," or internal dialogue. The patient in the critical care unit may be silently saying things such as, "I can't stand it in here. I've got to get out." Another unexpressed thought might be, "I can't handle this pain." By asking the patient to share aloud what is going on in his internal dialogue, the nurse can bring to his attention those messages that are distracting him from rest and relaxation. Substitute messages should be suggested to the patient. It is important to ask the patient to substitute rather than delete messages because the internal dialogue is continuously operating and will not turn off, even if the patient wills it to do so. Therefore, asking the patient to substitute constructive, assuring comments is more likely to help him reduce significantly the level of tension. Comments such as "I'll handle this pain just one day at a time" or "I've been in tough spots before, and I am capable of making it through this one!" will automatically reduce anxiety as well as help the patient shape coping behaviors accordingly. Any message that enhances the patient's confidence and puts the individual in an active role rather than in the passive role of a victim will increase a sense of coping and well-being.

Help patient develop self-dialogue messages that increase

• confidence
• sense of control
• ability to cope

A similar method can be applied to the patient's external conversation with other people. By simply requiring the individual to speak accurately about himself to others, the same goals can be accomplished. For example, the patient who exclaims, "I can't do anything for myself!" should be asked to identify the things that he is able to do, such as lifting his own body, turning to one side, making a nurse feel good with a rewarding smile, or helping his family understand what is happening. Even the smallest movement in the weakest of patients should be acknowledged and claimed by the patient. This technique is useful in helping patients correct their own misconceptions of themselves and the way others see them. In this way, a patient's sense of helplessness and therefore his anxiety are reduced.

Mental Imagery and Relaxation. These are two other useful techniques that can be taught to the patient to help him reduce tension. The nurse can encourage the patient to imagine either being in a very pleasant place in which he has been before or taking part in a very pleasant experience that he has had or would like to have. The patient should be instructed to focus and linger on the sensations that are experienced. For example, asking the patient "What colors do you see?" "What sounds are present?" "How does the air smell?" "How does your skin feel?" "Is there a breeze in the air?" helps increase the intensity of the fantasy and thereby promote relaxation through mental escape.

Guided mental imagery also can be used to help reduce unpleasant feelings of depression, anxiety, and hostility. Patients who must relearn life-sustaining tasks such as walking and feeding themselves can use imagery to prepare themselves mentally to meet the challenge successfully. In these instances, patients should be taught to visualize themselves moving through the task and successfully completing it. If this method seems trivial or silly to the patient, he can be reminded that this is a method commonly used by athletes to improve their performance and to prepare themselves mentally before an important event.

Techniques that induce deep muscle relaxation also can be used by the nurse to help the patient decrease anxiety and avoid the use of tranquilizing and sedating drugs when they are contraindicated. The patient is first directed to find as comfortable a position as possible and then to take several deep breaths and let them out slowly. Next, the patient is asked to clench his fist or curl his toes as tightly as possible, to hold the position for a few seconds, and then to let go while focusing on the sensations of the releasing muscles. The patient should practice this technique, beginning with the toes and moving upward through other parts of the body—the feet, calves, thighs, abdomen, chest, and so on. This procedure is done slowly while the patient gives nonverbal signals (*e.g.,* lifting a finger) to indicate when each new muscle mass has reached a state of relaxation. Special attention should be given to the back, shoulders, neck, scalp, and forehead because these are the areas in which many people experience physical tension.

Once the patient has achieved a state of relaxation, the nurse can suggest that he fantasize or sleep as deeply as he chooses. A moderately dark room and a soft voice will facilitate relaxation. Asking the patient to relax is frequently nonproductive compared with directing him to release a muscle mass, to let go of tension, or to imagine his tension draining through his body and sinking deeply into the mattress.

Unfortunately, anxiety-reducing methods are often of limited value to many patients in critical care units who are confronted with especially intense problems relating to dependency conflicts and to loss of health, body parts, and physiological functions. These problems will be discussed subsequently.

Dependency

Critical care patients commonly demonstrate unresolved dependency conflicts, often by either craving or denying a dependent position when they move into the role of a sick person. Those who crave dependence will more readily adjust to the protective environment of an intensive care unit. They also are more likely to have difficulty in withdrawing from it. These patients may attempt to develop overly dependent relationships with nurses and may make many demands on their time and attention. Some nurses may view them to be somewhat hypochondriacal. The convalescence of these patients tends to be drawn out, characterized by frequent requests for pain-relieving and tranquilizing medications.

Patients who crave dependency can be especially frustrating for busy nurses. These patients seem to wait for the nurse to leave and then request or demand a service that could have been provided earlier. The manipulation to keep the nurse present is obvious and annoying, especially when the nurse has sicker patients waiting for care. The nurse senses the ever-present bind: If she is brisk, the patient's feelings are hurt; if she is yielding, other patients are neglected.

In the patient's view, however, being dependent is equivalent to being cared about and perhaps even prescribed by the patient role. Moreover, the patient must find congruent role behaviors with a variety of personalities. Some nurses reinforce dependency in patients by their own behavior, whereas others are intolerant of patients whom they believe are demanding services that they could accomplish themselves.

Patients who deny their dependency needs demonstrate more difficulty in assuming the patient role. Although they also long for their dependency needs to be satisfied, their unresolved childhood conflict between being an adult and a dependent, cared-for child arouses a good deal of anxiety. They are less likely to ask for help when needed and make demands on themselves instead of others. These patients are both afraid and ashamed of dependency. Like their counterparts who crave dependency, they also are likely to have a more protracted convalescence than those who have learned to balance their need for dependency with that for independence.

Overly independent patients will not wait for a nurse's help. They attempt to get out of bed by themselves, they hesitate to request pain medication when needed, or they fear that they will be viewed as helpless or childish by others. All these patients are likely to lack confidence in themselves and ultimately resent their dependence on others.

Nursing Assessment and Intervention

For most nurses, coping with and providing optimal care to the overly dependent or overly independent patient are a challenge both emotionally and physically. The reaction of nurses to these frustrating patients can be as much a problem as the patients' behavior. A first approach is for the nurse to determine which type of patient is easier to accept and like. It is this personality type with which the nurse is most likely to identify. The nurse will probably avoid the patient of whom she feels less accepting. Since both overly dependent and overly independent patients are dealing with conflicts of dependence, the nurse's avoidance of either type of patient is likely to increase the undesirable behavior.

Again, order and predictability are likely to help the patient control anxiety that is associated with his dependent role. The nurse should inform the patient of how much time she has to spend with him and then let him know when there are only 5 or 6 minutes left for the visit. The nurse should also tell the patient when her next visit will be and then make every effort to return as scheduled. The patient should have a clock so that he can keep track of time.

Allowing the patient to impose order on the routine of care and to establish priorities of how to use the nurse's time may help reduce less important requests. By encouraging the patient to identify and talk about feelings of weakness, disability, and helplessness, the nurse helps him begin to distinguish feelings and fears from what is potential and what is real. Patients often have so little understanding about what is occurring within their bodies and what events in the environment mean that they can only guess and therefore frequently distort what is happening to them. Their behavior is likely to reveal their misunderstandings. It is important to clarify in as simple a way as possible what is occurring and why.

When nurse–patient encounters are short by necessity, they also must be frequent. Touching the patient physically in a gentle, warm way can help compensate for unspent time and unspoken conversations. It often will convey feelings that some nurses are unable to verbalize.

Although it is not likely that the nurse will alter dependency conflicts in her patients, she can help alleviate their anxiety and promote their physical and emotional health by offering them constructive dependency experiences.

RESPONSES TO LOSS

The threat of illness precipitates the coping behaviors associated with loss. Dying patients must adapt to the loss of life; other patients must adjust to the loss of health or loss of a limb, a blow to self-concept, or a necessary change in life-style. All these events require a change—a loss of the familiar self-image and its replacement with an altered one. Regardless of the nature of loss, the dynamics of grief present themselves in some form.

The response to loss can be described in the following four phases:

1. Shock and disbelief
2. Development of awareness
3. Restitution
4. Resolution

Each phase involves characteristic and predictable behaviors that fluctuate among the various phases in an unpredictable way. Through recognition and assessment of the behaviors and an understanding of their underlying dynamics, the nurse can plan interventions to support the healing process.

Shock and Disbelief

In the first stage of response to loss, the patient demonstrates the behaviors characteristic of denial. He fails to comprehend and experience the emotional impact and rational meaning of his diagnosis. Because the diagnosis has no emotional meaning, the patient often fails to cooperate with precautionary measures. For example, he may attempt to get out of bed against the physician's advice, deviate from the prescribed diet, and assert that he is there for a rest! Denial may go so far as to allow the patient to project difficulties onto what is perceived as ill-functioning equipment, mistaken lab reports, or—more likely—the sheer incompetence of physicians and nurses.

When such blatant denial occurs, it is apparent that

the problem is so anxiety-provoking to the patient that it cannot be handled by the more sophisticated mechanisms of rational problem-solving. Thus, the stressor is temporarily obliterated. This phase of denial also may serve as the period during which the patient's resources, briefly blocked by the shock, can be regrouped for the battle ahead.

Nursing Intervention.   *The principle of intervention consists not in stripping away the defense of denial but in supporting the patient and acknowledging the situation through nursing care.*

The nurse recognizes and accepts the patient's illness by watching the monitor or changing the dressings. She communicates acceptance of the patient through tone of voice, facial expression, and touch. She can reflect to the patient statements of denial in a way that allows the patient to hear them—and eventually to examine their incongruity and apply reality—by saying something such as, "In some ways you believe that having a heart attack will be helpful to you?" The nurse can also acknowledge the patient's difficulty in accepting restrictions by making comments such as, "It seems hard for you to stay in bed." By verbalizing what the patient is expressing, the nurse gently confronts behavior but does not cause anxiety and anger by reprimanding and judging. Thus, in this phase the nurse supports denial by allowing for it, but she does not perpetuate it. Instead, she acknowledges, accepts, and reflects the patient's new circumstance.

Advantages of Denial.   It is interesting that although denial of illness can prevent adaptation at a new level, it also has its advantages. High deniers with myocardial infarctions have been shown to have a higher survival rate than moderate or low deniers.[1] They also often return to work sooner and reach higher levels of rehabilitation. This finding illustrates the effectiveness of denial as a coping mechanism as well as the hazards of stripping it away before the patient is ready.

Development of Awareness

In this stage of grief, the patient's behavior is characteristically associated with anger and guilt. The anger may be expressed overtly and may be directed at the staff for oversights, tardiness, and minor insensitivities. In this phase, the ugliness of reality has made its impact. Displacement of the anger on others helps soften the impact on the patient. The expression of anger itself gives the patient a sense of power in a seemingly helpless state. A demanding manner and a whining tone often characterize this stage and represent the patient's attempts to regain the control that appears to have been lost. However, such behavior often alienates the nurse and other personnel. The pa-

tient who does not demand or whine has probably withdrawn into depression because he is directing his anger toward himself rather than toward others. This patient will demonstrate verbal and motor retardation, will likely have difficulty sleeping, and may prefer to be left alone.

During this phase, the nurse is likely to hear irrational expressions of guilt. Patients seek to answer, "Why me?" They will attempt to isolate their human imperfections and attribute the cause of the malady to themselves. Both patients and their families may look for a person or object to blame.

Guilt feelings concerning one's own illness are difficult to understand unless one examines the basic dynamic of guilt. Guilt arises when there is a decrease in the feeling of self-worth or when the self-concept has been violated. In this light, the nurse can understand that what is behind an expression of guilt is a negatively altered self-concept. Blame thus becomes nothing more than projection of the unbearable feeling of guilt.

Nursing Intervention.   During the patient's development of awareness, nursing intervention must be directed toward supporting the patient's basic sense of self-worth and allowing and encouraging the direct expression of anger. Nursing measures that support a patient's sense of self-worth are numerous and include calling the patient by name; introducing strangers, particularly when they are to examine the patient; talking to, rather than about, the patient; and, most important, providing and respecting the patient's need for privacy and modesty. The nurse needs to guard against verbal and nonverbal expressions of pity. It is more constructive to empathize with the patient's specific feelings of anger, sadness, and guilt rather than with a condition.

The nurse can create outlets for anger by listening and by refraining from defending either herself, the physician, or the hospital. A nondefensive, accepting attitude will decrease the patient's sense of guilt, and the expression of anger will avert some of the depression. Later, when the patient apologizes for an irrational outburst, the nurse can interpret the patient's need to make this kind of verbalization as a step toward rehabilitation and health.

Restitution

In this stage, the griever puts aside anger and resistance and begins to cope constructively with the loss. The patient tries new behaviors that are consistent with the new limitations. The emotional level is one of sadness, and much time may be spent crying. As the patient adapts himself to a new image, considerable time is spent going over and over significant memories relevant to the loss. Behaviors in this stage include the verbalization of fears regarding the future. Often these go undetected because they are unbearable for the family to hear. After severe trauma, which may have resulted in scarring or removal of a body part or loss of sensation, patients may question their sexual adequacy. They worry about the future response of their mates to their changed bodies. The patient probably also questions his new role in the family. Most likely, the patient has a variety of concerns that are specific to his own life-style.

Thus, in the mourning process such manifestations as reminiscing, crying, questioning, expressing fears, and trying out new behaviors help the patient modify the old self-concept and begin working with and experiencing a revised concept.

Nursing Intervention. During restitution, nursing care should again be supportive so that adaptation can occur. Listening to the patient for lengthy periods of time will be necessary. If the patient is able to verbalize fears and questions about the future, he will be better able to define the anxiety and to solve new problems. Furthermore, hearing oneself talk about fears will help put them into a more rational perspective. The patient may require privacy, acceptance, and encouragement to cry so that he can find respite from sadness.

During this stage, the nurse might have the patient consider meeting someone who has successfully adapted to similar trauma. This measure would provide the patient with a role model as he begins to assume a new identity, which often occurs after the crisis period.

Additionally, the patient, with appropriate support from the nurse, will begin to identify and acknowledge changes that are arising from adaptation to illness. Relationships can and do change. Because the way that friends respond to the patient who has suffered a permanent disability is different from their response to a healthy person, the patient will not feel or believe that he is being treated in the same way.

During this time the family has also been going through a similar process. They too have experienced shock, disbelief, anger, and sadness. When they are ready to try to solve their problems, their energies will be directed toward wondering how the changes in the patient will affect their mutual relationship and their life-style. They, too, will experience the pain of turmoil and uncertainty. Nurses must also help the family. By allowing the family to ventilate their repulsion and fear and by showing acceptance of these feelings, the nurse can help the family be more useful to, and accepting of, the patient. Through intensive listening, the nurse provides a sounding board and then redirects the members of the family back to each other so that they can give and receive support.

Resolution

Resolution is the stage of identity change. At first the patient can be observed to be overidentifying himself as an invalid. The patient may discriminate against himself and make derogatory remarks about his body. Another method that the patient may use is to detach himself emotionally from the source of trauma (*e.g.,* a stoma, prosthesis, scar, or paralyzed limb) by naming it and referring to it in a simultaneously alienated and affectionate way. Patients are alert to the ways in which health-care workers respond to their bodies. A patient will make negative remarks to test the acceptance of the nurse. Chiding or telling the patient that many others share the problem will be less helpful than acknowledging feelings and indicating acceptance by continuing to care for, and talk with, the patient.

As time passes and the patient adapts, the sting of the endured hurt abates, and the patient moves toward identifying himself as an individual who has certain limitations due to illness rather than as a "cripple" or an "invalid." The patient no longer uses a defect as the basis of identity. As the resolution is reached, the patient is able to depend on others when necessary and should not need to push beyond his endurance or to overcompensate for an inadequacy or limitation. Often, the individual will reflect on the crisis as a growing period. Hopefully, the patient will have achieved a sense of pride at accomplishing the difficult adaptation and is able to look back realistically on successes and disappointments without discomfort. At this time, the patient may find it useful and gratifying to help others by serving as a role model for those people in the stage of restitution who are experiencing their own identity crises.

Unfortunately, the critical care nurse is rarely in a position to observe the successful outcome. It is useful to know the process in order that the nurse may work with and communicate an attitude of hope, especially when the patient is most self-disparaging.

Nursing Intervention. The goal of nursing care during the resolution stage is to help the patient attach a sense of self-esteem to a rectified identity. Nursing intervention revolves around helping the patient find the degree of dependence that is needed and can be accepted. The nurse must accept and recognize with the patient that periods of vacillation between independence and dependence will occur. The nurse should encourage a positive emotional response to a new state of modified dependence. Certainly, the nurse can support and reinforce the patient's growing sense of pride in his rehabilitation. For those nurses who have had the experience of successfully working through the process with one individual, the problem will be to stand back and allow the patient to move away from them.

ADAPTATION TO ILLNESS

Another method of understanding the characteristic problems of adapting to limitations enforced by illness is to understand the relationship between emotional regression and physical disability or illness. There is an observable lag between the emotional acknowledgement of illness and its physical onset; that is, the individual experiences illness and disability physically before he can acknowledge it fully on an emotional level. Denial is an example of this lag. Likewise, when physical health has been reestablished or stabilized, the patient is still experiencing concerns and fears related to acute illness. At this point, the patient is likely to resist independence and be reluctant to cooperate with increased expectations for activity and self-care. Preparation for return to health, acknowledgment of concerns about increased activity, and the reassurance of watchful eyes will help alleviate anxiety as the patient progresses.

Figure 3-2 demonstrates one pattern of adapting to various stages of illness. The shaded area represents transition into illness and shows the disparity between a person's actual health and his perception of his health. In this situation there is denial. The acceptance phase demonstrates that physical well-being and mental well-being are congruent, whereas the convalescent phase shows that an emotional lag exists between physical and emotional well-being.

One principle that greatly affects understanding the patient's response is the fact that during stress the patient will regress in an attempt to conserve energy. During times of acute exacerbation or heightened expectations or during any significant change, the initial response will be regression to an earlier emotional position of safety. Weaning from a respirator, removal of monitor leads, and increased activity and reduction in medication often trigger anxiety and regression. This regression may even include a retreat into increased dependency, depression, and anger. At such times, the patient may find comfort in regressing to a state that he has already discovered can be coped with

or mastered. The regression is usually temporary and brief and pinpoints the cause of anxiety. At this point, nurses may become disappointed, anxious, or angry with the patient's regression and may wish to retreat from him. It is more helpful, however, to acknowledge that regression is inevitable and to support the patient with intervention appropriate to earlier stages. Helping the patient understand what is happening by explaining the emotional lag phenomenon may also allow him to share in understanding the relationship between what he is experiencing emotionally and what is occurring physiologically.

If different patients' responses to illness could be plotted on a graph, they would show both common and unique points, just as electrocardiograms from different people show common characteristics as well as individual differences. There will be variations in time and in the congruence between physical and sociopsychological responses, but the stages will occur predictably. Like the electrical events of the heart, responses to illness, both adaptive and maladaptive, can be anticipated and, it is hoped minimized.

The prevalence of anxiety and depression as part of the response to illness has been documented in a classic research study by Cassem and Hackett.[2] In this study, any patient whose outlook or behavior endangered his physical or emotional well-being was referred for psychiatric consultation. Of 441 patients who were admitted to the coronary care unit because of myocardial infarction, 145 (32.7%) were referred because of anxiety, depression, or behavioral problems. Referrals due to anxiety were highest on the patients' first and second days in the unit, with referrals for depression peaking on the third and fourth days. Behavioral problems were the third most common reason for consultation. The greatest number of patients with behavioral problems were referred on day 2, with a fewer number of referrals occurring on day 4. Patients demonstrated behaviors, such as denying illness by threatening to leave the hospital, euphoria, sexually suggestive comments, and conflicts about hospital or treatment restrictions. This study documented the premise that anxiety accompanies transition into illness and that depression emerges as people recognize the impact of the illness.

Although these responses occurred in patients who

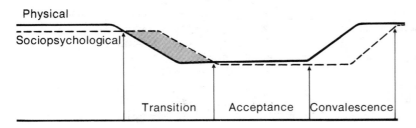

Physical

Sociopsychological

Transition   Acceptance   Convalescence

FIGURE 3-2
The solid line represents a normal level of physical well-being, the broken line a corresponding degree of sociopsychological integration.

had had myocardial infarctions, they may be generalized to include other persons who have a sudden onset of illness and who need intensive care. Moreover, the researchers noted that the interventions that helped patients deal with their situation did not have to be carried out by psychiatrists alone.[3]

Both physicians and nurses were invited to make referrals. Not only did nurses make more referrals than physicians, but also those patients referred by physicians had already been referred earlier by nurses. This finding indicates that nurses make early and astute observations about coping mechanisms. Because of their expertise and proximity to the patient, nurses should continue to both intervene and make referrals.

TEACHING AND LEARNING

Recognizing the patient's response to illness helps the nurse predict when teaching will be best absorbed and most useful to the patient. Learning is most likely to occur during quiet stages, when the patient's emotional outlook corresponds to his physical condition. This means that the patient feels just about as sick or as well as he actually is. Providing information in this phase of illness will help the patient move on to the next phase of recovery. When there is less congruence between the patient's physical condition and his emotional acknowledgement of it, motivation for learning will be impaired and teaching will less likely be effective.

Nursing Assessment and Intervention

To enhance teaching effectiveness, the nurse can employ the following seven-step plan for assessment and intervention (Fig. 3-3).

1. Motivation. Motivation for learning should be assessed in two areas. Intrinsic motivation considers the learner's attitudes, values, personality, and life-style. The teaching method as well as what is taught must be adjusted for these aspects of the patient's life. Extrinsic motivation includes the learning climate, physical environment, time of teaching, possible reinforcers, interpersonal relationship with the teacher, and skill of the instructor. The nurse has far more control over the extrinsic sources of motivation. Does the patient respond best when alone or with others? Does he prefer the solarium to his bedroom? Do touching, smiling, and encouraging enhance learning? Does the patient like to spend time with the nurse? Has the nurse developed teaching skills and methods for this particular type of learner? Trial-and-error attempts at teaching each patient can be shared with other nurses to increase extrinsic motivation skills.

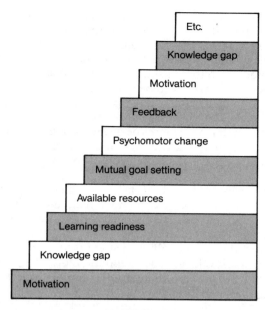

FIGURE 3-3
Staircase of patient teaching and learning.

2. Knowledge Gap. Assessing the knowledge gap is recognizing what needs to be taught and learned to effect behavior change. A knowledge gap can also be assessed in terms of "what is" compared with "what could be." An honest, accurate assessment will lead to realistic, achievable goals rather than unrealistic ones that, if attempted, will result in the patient's experiencing failure. In this phase of the plan, it is important for the patient and family to recognize the advantages inherent in learning the new knowledge, skills, and attitudes. As this phase is completed, the patient should become aware that he has a better basis for a choice concerning whether or not he will learn and change. The patient's right to make this choice should be acknowledged and accepted by the nurse.

3. Learning Readiness. The step of learning readiness deals with the patient's level of adaptation to illness, anxiety level, developmental level, opportunities for immediate application of new knowledge and skill, and a safe learning environment.

As the patient adjusts to the sick role, he will become more receptive to learning about his illness. Because progress heightens anxiety, teaching is usually more effective during the period of emotional acceptance than during the times when the patient is moving either into or out of the sick role. Whenever there is movement forward or backward on the health–illness continuum, there is likely to be an emotional response of anxiety, worry, or depression that will interfere with concentration and learning. Therefore, admission, transfer, or readmission to the critical care unit, as well as hospital discharge, are poor times for learning to occur. During periods of anxiety, it is useful for the nurse to ascertain the patient's perceptions of what is happening so that misunderstandings that may cause unnecessary worry can be corrected.

Informal teaching and the provision of information that enhances equilibrium are best woven into the other nursing procedures occuring throughout the patient's stay in the critical care unit. For effective learning to take place, the high levels of anxiety commonly found in critical care units must be decreased to no more than mild anxiety states in which the patient demonstrates alertness without fear, motivation to learn, and interest. The more facts there are to absorb and the more behavior change is implied by the information, the more likely the patient is to respond with increased levels of anxiety, and therefore, the greater the need to teach during periods of mild anxiety.

Anxiety levels, physiological function, and the patient's own priorities must be assessed when the readiness of the patient-learner is evaluated. Worry, pain, and some medications also will interfere with the patient's ability to learn.

The patient's developmental stage must also be considered in the plan. Young adolescents will not deal as well with philosophical issues regarding their care and life choices as will older adolescents and adults.

Because adults in the later stages of life are likely to have trouble remembering details, it is especially important that they be provided with written material so that they can review what they need to learn. Pamphlets, booklets, and individualized lists and directions will be useful to everyone.

It is also important to have immediate opportunities for the learner to try on or try out new skills and behaviors. Early successful application of new knowledge is a reinforcer that cannot be replaced effectively by anything else. Often, anticipation of hospital discharge and return to home can be a powerful motivator and increase readiness for learning and carrying out new skills.

Owing to the trend of early hospital discharge, individualized teaching in the home is usually necessary to complete instruction that was begun in the hospital. At home, in their own surroundings and with their own routines, the patient and his family can be evaluated in terms of their knowledge and their ability to apply it by community health nurses.

Informal teaching and rehabilitation programs that may involve structure and extended periods of time should occur after the crisis, when the patient has reached a fairly stable period of adjustment. Often, this stage of readiness does not occur until after discharge. Therefore, in order to provide this type of essential health teaching, hospital-based personnel can conduct programs for patients to return to after hospital discharge. In addition, community-based classes can be conducted, and teaching can be done in the home. Follow-up learning sessions are necessary, regardless of where they take place.

Most of the learning required of patients who are recovering from critical illness involves a change in behavior that will alter their life-style. Dietary changes that restrict calories, sodium, cholesterol, or carbohydrates are common. A change in activity level may be imposed, exercise may be prescribed, and a decrease in smoking may be imperative. None of these changes is easy to make. Providing information is rarely sufficient to alter behavior.

Group teaching is a technique that is well-suited to learning that involves life-style changes. Group process can provide support, offer encouragement and motivation, and reinforce information and accomplishments.

An effective approach to learning includes a combination of informal teaching, group instruction, and individualized learning and evaluation at home. Teaching can be begun in the hospital, but it can rarely be completed there.

Providing a safe environment conducive to learning is included in this phase. Learning occurs more easily when security, a sense of belonging, and self-esteem are high. Often, learning about illness means that the patient and family not only must learn facts and techniques but also must apply and adapt to their own lives what is taught. This will be difficult when there are high degress of anxiety, depression, or acute physical dysfunction. It will be impossible for patients to respond creatively when they are struggling to maintain basic physiological needs.

When the teachable moment appears, the following reminders will help keep communication open:

• Find out about the patient's concerns before teaching.
• Ask for the patient's ideas and perceptions of what is happening.
• Avoid judgmental statements.
• Ask yourself, "Is what the patient wants to learn what I want to teach?"

The nursing process will help you answer the last question. This process can be used to determine the teaching plan in the same way that it is used to determine any other nursing action.

4. Available Resources. A careful assessment of the availability of resources will have an important effect on the outcome of patient learning. Without a realistic appraisal of resources, the nurse may spend valuable time teaching the patient activities that he has no way of implementing once he is discharged. Equipment, appropriate finances, values and cultural influences, family involvements, and community support all are resources that are likely to need careful appraisal to ensure a successfully implemented teaching plan. For example, when the nurse is teaching the patient how to reduce carbohydrate or sodium intake, she should find out the types of foods eaten (a sample meal plan) and the ways they are prepared. This information should be used to help the patient and family tailor the diet regimen to their meals. The combination of the patient's learning style and the appropriate teaching media is evaluated in this phase. Audio and video tapes are increasingly available to nurses for teaching. These media are especially valuable because they can be repeated continually without embarrassing the patient or frustrating the nurse. Despite the availability of new forms of media, nothing can replace a warm, encouraging, supportive relationship between the patient and a skilled and knowledgeable nurse. Even when mechanical media are frequently used, the nurse should offer time for questions, support, and encouragement.

5. Mutual Goal Setting. During the phase of mutual goal setting, the nurse and patient formulate a contract about what is to be learned and how they will know that the specified material has been learned. An understanding is developed about what the nurse will do to help the patient learn and what the patient will do. The actual goals, or objectives, to be accomplished will provide direction about the content to be taught and prescribe behaviors for teacher and learner. Words that define or specify behaviors are more useful and less ambiguous than words that make vague statements about what the patient is to accomplish. For example, "The patient will list ten common foods that are high in sodium (or salt)" is better than "The patient will develop an understanding regarding high-sodium foods to be avoided." Return demonstrations of how to care for equipment and appliances or of how to perform exercises also are specific objectives likely to lead to success. For example, "After 1 week of practice, the patient will be able to make three bed-to-chair or chair-to-bed transfers within 2 hours" is a useful goal-oriented objective. It tells the nurse and patient how much time is available for learning, the exact behavior expected, and how many times it should be accomplished within a specified period of time.

Goals can and should be renegotiated as the situation or circumstance changes, but, most importantly, they should be formulated so that success is achievable. Therefore, goals should be written in increments and for short periods of time. After one goal is achieved, it can be increased or modified. If it does not appear to be attainable, it should be modified downward so that the patient who makes a reasonable effort does not fail and give up.

6. Psychomotor Change (Compliance). Achieving actual psychomotor change or compliance in patients is one of the most difficult aspects of patient teaching and learning. In most seriously ill patients, compliance typically demands a difficult long-term life-style change. For example, a nurse who is trying to lose 6 pounds that she gained on a vacation may feel frustrated, but her situation is in no way comparable to that of a patient who, having experienced the threat of severe illness, must lose and keep off 50 pounds. Most likely, the patient's physical and emotional energies have been compromised by the illness and hospitalization. Now, medical personnel demand extensive life-style changes that seem necessary and logical to them for restoring the patient's health. However, the patient more likely experiences the demand for change as deprivation, following the emotional and physical depletion caused by illness.

Giving up smoking, deleting salt from the diet, and losing weight are difficult objectives, even for the most knowledgeable and motivated health professional. Finding ways to help patients comply with life-style changes is a nursing problem that deserves intensive attention and extensive research. Adequate teaching plans, reinforcement, support, and encouragement, even when there is regression, constitute a beginning. Involving the patient as well as his family in mutual goal-setting and connecting them with community support systems are likely to enhance and sustain the necessary life-style changes.

Sometimes, serendipitous changes occur that can be utilized to encourage behavior modification. For example, a patient who loses 20 of a prescribed 50 pounds may be more reinforced by his improved self-image than by health improvement. This kind of change in self-image motivates the patient to lose more weight. Nurses can observe these changes that improve attitude and use them to increase reinforcement and enhance motivation.

7. Feedback. Feedback is useful for evaluation of gains and modification of goals. It must be descriptive rather than judgmental and specific rather than general. Thus, "You've lost 3 pounds!" is more constructive than "You're doing well!" Timely feedback is more reinforcing than delayed feedback and is more useful in helping the patient resist temptations to transgress objectives for change.

Helpful negative feedback promotes choices rather than guilt. The observation, "You've smoked more cigarettes today than yesterday" provides the patient with more support to modify or control behavior than the statement, "You're ruining your health," a judgment of self-destruction that will fill the patient with guilt.

Positive feedback reinforces successes and extends the previously established motivation. As the teaching plan continues, new areas of knowledge gaps will be recognized and a new plan can be established according to the alterations that have been experienced.

Although most of the preceding discussion has focused on the individual, each of these learning steps and concepts should also be applied to the instruction of family members or significant others who will be involved with the patient in his daily activities. Most of the time it is necessary and valuable for significant others to acquire the same knowledge and skills as the patient, especially when they are involved in life-style changes, such as performing a procedure (*e.g.,* injection, irrigation, dressing), shopping or cooking for a special diet, offering support, and sometimes even participating with the patient in certain activities (*e.g.,* accompanying him on a walking regimen).

TRANSFERENCE AND COUNTERTRANSFERENCE

There are some types of irrational behavior directed toward nurses that cannot be explained by adaptation or grieving. The phenomenon of *transference* may be used to explain some reactions patients have toward nurses that are inappropriate in intensity and, sometimes, attitude. *Transference* can be thought of as an unconscious response that represents feelings and attitudes that originated in early childhood. Transference reduces the patient's anxiety by allowing him to experience current anxiety-provoking situations in terms of previous situations. Transference reactions are usually marked by an expression of intense feelings that seem inappropriate for the event that has triggered them. Exhibitionism, extreme dependency, and irrational demands are some behaviors that can often be accounted for by transference.

It may be that in times of crisis and regression, reality-testing is impaired, and the patient is more likely to act and react to the irrational fears and feelings that originated when he was a helpless child. In such instances, the patient must be treated and addressed as an adult and helped to test reality in the current environment. For example, if a patient fears that the nurses do not care about him, he can be encouraged to ask specific nurses how they feel, or he can be helped to identify what it is about the nurses that suggests to him that they do not care for him. At that time, specific explanations can be given about nurses' behavior. This type of intervention satisfies the patient's need to be cared about far better than global reassurance that the nurses do care.

Critical care nurses must be ready to be subjected to powerful positive and negative feelings. An understanding of the regressive nature of these inappropriate and intense expressions and the dynamics involved can help the nurse retain composure and respond con-structively rather than react impulsively with rejection or withdrawal.

Countertransference is the same phenomenon as transference when it occurs in the helper or nurse. Intensity of positive or negative feelings directed toward the patient should suggest to the nurse that this reaction is a product of countertransference rather than objective observation of, and response to, patient behaviors. Clues that suggest countertransference include an inability to empathize with the patient, spending unusually short or long periods with certain patients, feelings of anger and discouragement at the patient for not responding to care, personal and social involvement, as well as dreaming and preoccupation about the patient. The desire to argue with a patient or extreme protectiveness of a particular patient are common ways that nurses display countertransference.

In general, countertransference is viewed as destructive to patient care and the nurse–patient relationship because it is likely to interfere with accurate appraisals of the patient's condition. Countertransferences will occur in nurses and other personnel. Nurses need to be supportive of each other in confronting and dealing with these reactions. When countertransference occurs, it is helpful for nurses to recognize the dynamics of transference and countertransference and work together to achieve an accurate appraisal of nurses' and patients' responses with the objective of providing nursing care that will potentiate reality-testing and constructive interactions.

TRANSFER FROM THE CRITICAL CARE UNIT

Regression is often elicited when the patient is told that he is ready to be transferred to the general unit. The stage of illness greatly influences the patient's response to transfer. If the patient is transferred while he is denying his illness, the move will be accomplished with ease because it further fortifies his feeling that he isn't very sick. On the other hand, if the patient is transferred when improving physically more than he acknowledges emotionally, anxiety will be heightened. The patient is saying, "I'm sick, and being transferred means you think I'm improving when I'm not." In trying to cope with the anxiety generated by the move, the patient will regress and become more dependent. Transferring a patient when he first acknowledges the severity of his illness may create discomfort for nurses because the patient is likely to be frightened, angry, uncooperative, and demanding.

Preparing the Transfer

Regardless of the timing, in preparing for transfer both the nurse and the patient need to accept the fact that their relationship with each other will be ending. They may accomplish this by reminiscing about an initial meeting or a special moment and by talking about the move.

If the patient is feeling dependent, more time may be needed to talk about what it will be like to leave. Often, because of discomfort associated with saying goodbye, nurses withdraw under the guise that it is easier for the patient when the nurse ignores the termination process. This unexplained withdrawal may be interpreted by the patient as a lack of interest or as anger over earlier unresolved outbursts when a change in body image and lowered self-esteem were being experienced.

The news of transfer often comes without warning or preparation. Even though the patient may be pleased with his progress, he will be at the same time concerned about losing the reassurance of special equipment, close surveillance, and the presence of familiar faces. It has long been advocated that continuity of care be provided by thoughtful preparation. Introduction to the new nurses who will take over care of the patient, as well as follow-up visits by the critical care nurses, will increase familiarity, enhance security, and let the patient know that he is important. Disconnecting equipment and monitors before the time of transfer will lessen the strain of having to give up his room, equipment, and nurse all at the same time.

Schwartz and Brenner[4] demonstrated that family members can provide valuable support during the transfer process when they know what will happen and when they have had their questions answered and their concerns addressed. Family members who either accompany patients during the transfer or meet them at the new room and then stay with them during the remainder of the day can lessen the stress associated with the change.

In Schwartz and Brenner's study, 30 patients hospitalized for acute myocardial infarctions in coronary care units were randomly assigned to one of three groups: two experimental and one control. In one experimental group, nurses provided families with information about transfer and encouraged them to maintain contact with the patient similar to that already described. In the second experimental group, the patient met and developed a relationship with the nurse to whom he would be transferred. The usual transfer procedure was used for the control group. The researchers' hypothesis that the two experimental groups in which nursing interventions were applied would demonstrate reduced amounts of stress associated with transfer, when compared with the control group, was supported. Additionally, the patients in the experimental groups experienced fewer cardiovascular complications during the 72 hours following transfer. However, there were no differences among groups regarding the number of physical complaints

reported during the evening of the transfer. Furthermore, the investigators noted that patients in both experimental groups were more likely to comply with physician orders, had fewer readmissions to the coronary care unit, and spent fewer days hospitalized on the nursing unit.

In an earlier investigation reported by Klein and co-workers,[5] urine catecholamine studies on patients transferred to a general unit from a coronary care unit indicated that increased stress with transfer occurred in five of seven patients. All five of these patients had a cardiovascular complication such as arrhythmia. In a follow-up study, however, seven patients were prepared for transfer from the beginning of their stay. They had follow-up visits by the nurse and care by the same physician. No cardiovascular complications occurred, and only two had a rise in urine catechols at the time of transfer.

These studies provide nurses with the rationale for using their time to make patient transfers an important aspect of nursing care. Even when the patient is prepared for transfer, regression and anxiety may occur; however, if the nurse acknowledges his concerns and offers him support, the patient will again mobilize his energy. Because these processes have proved predictable, they give the nurse a basis for her care and provide rationale for appropriate intervention. Despite the predictability of these responses in human behavior, they will have an impact on the individual and are unique. By the time they are modified by personality and by sociocultural and economic variables, they have become a significant part of life and are indeed made unique as they become a historical and living part of one's identity.

REFERENCES

1. Hackett T. Cassem NH, Wishnie H: The coronary care unit: An appraisal of its psychological hazards. N Engl J Med 279, No. 25:1365–1370, 1968
2. Cassem NH, Hackett TP: Psychiatric consultation in a coronary care unit. Ann Intern Med 75, No. 1:9–11, 1971
3. *Ibid.*
4. Schwartz LP, Brenner ZR: Critical care unit transfers: Reducing patient stress through nursing interventions. Heart Lung 8:540–546, 1979
5. Klein F et al: Transfer from a coronary care unit: Some adverse responses. Arch Intern Med 122:104–108, 1968

BIBLIOGRAPHY

Kaplan HI, Sadock BJ: Modern Synopsis of Comprehensive Textbook of Psychiatry/III, 3rd ed. Baltimore, Williams & Wilkins, 1981
Rankin SH, Duffy K: Patient Education: Issues, Principles and Guidelines. Philadelphia, JB Lippincott, 1983
Stuart GR, Sundeen J: Principles and Practice of Psychiatric Nursing, 2nd ed. St Louis, CV Mosby, 1983

4
Extending Critical Care Nursing to the Patient's Family

Karen D. Busch

A holistic approach to critical care nursing must include the patient's family. For the purposes of this chapter, *family* means any persons who share intimate and routine day-to-day living with the critical care patient—in other words, those persons whose social homeostasis is altered by the patient's entrance into the arena of critical illness or injury, and who are a significant part of the patient's normal life-style and therefore must be a part of holistic care.

STRESS AND FAMILY ADAPTATION

The patient's entrance into a life-death sick role threatens and alters the family's homeostasis for many reasons. The patient's responsibilities will now have to be added to the responsibilities of others and therefore will demand an alteration in their schedules and activities. When these responses are left undone, the members experience various degrees of discomfort and annoyance. Financial concerns are usually major; also, daily activities that previously were of little consequence to family members now become important and often difficult to manage. Such activities as packing school lunches for children, keeping the family car filled with gasoline, taking out the garbage, and balancing the checkbook can, when unfulfilled, all become critical incidents with the right timing.

In addition to the responsibilities the patient normally carries, the social role that the patient plays in the family will be missing. Disciplinarian, provider of affection, lover, humorist, time-keeper, motivator, comforter, and so on are all important roles; when they

are missing, considerable havoc and even grief in the family may ensue.

The family enters into a crisis situation under the following conditions:

- A stressful event occurs, which threatens lasting changes for the family.
- Usual problem-solving activities are inadequate and therefore do not lead rapidly to the previous state of balance.
- The present state of family disequilibrium cannot be maintained and will lead either to improved family health and adaptation or to decreased family adaptability and increased proneness to crisis events.

By using these conditions to identify and define families in crisis, one can appreciate the stress of normal maturational events of family life such as marriage, pregnancy, enrollment in school, and retirement in a different light. Scales have been developed that score these stressful life events and thus help predict who is at risk for developing illness. These life events all require readjustment and include such things as marital reconciliation, change in finances, and trouble with in-laws or the boss. Thus, not only situations of disease and injury propel families into crisis. A family who has been coping adequately with unemployment may not be able to deal with the added stress of a critically ill family member. What appears to be a family's overreaction to a small stress may be explained as having a "last straw" effect added onto a maturational crisis.

Some families experience many more crises than others. Often the challenges and demands that face these families are similar to the ones that present themselves to all families. There appears to be an additional factor of *cognitive appraisal* that must be considered. Some persons or families appear to assign catastrophic meaning to some events that others would not. If family members appraise a situation by giving it the proportions and labels of crisis events, the emotions, stress, and anxiety associated with a crisis, as well as attempts to cope, will follow. This phenomenon implies that crises based on cognitive appraisal are individual and unique—that is, a crisis for one family is not necessarily a crisis for another. The wide range of family behaviors and reactions observed by critical care nurses can in large part be explained by this concept. Cultural and age variables can also be accounted for in this way.

There are four important generalizations about crises that can form a basis for nursing care of families dealing with them:

1. Whether a person emerges stronger or weaker as a result of a crisis is not based so much on his previous character as on the kind of help he receives during the actual crisis.
2. People become more amenable to suggestions and open to help during actual crises.
3. With the onset of a crisis situation, old memories of past crises may be evoked. If maladaptive behavior was used to deal with previous situations, the same type of behavior may be repeated in the face of a new crisis.
4. The only way to survive a crisis is to be aware of it.

Families try to maintain a steady state. When a family member is in a critical care unit, the rest of the family may accomplish this at first by either minimizing the significance of the illness or being overprotective.

The family member in the critical care unit is primarily in a biological crisis, whereas the rest of the family is experiencing an emotional crisis. At first, this coping mechanism may seem to work, and the family system may appear to improve in spite of increasing stress. However, as stress continues, the family system is likely to disintegrate unless there is intervention.

Reactions to crisis situations are difficult to categorize because they depend on individual responses to stress, and within a family, several mechanisms for handling stress and anxiety will be employed. In general, the nurse may observe behaviors that indicate emotions signifying helplessness and urgency. An inability to make decisions and mobilize resources can be noted. A sense of fear and panic pervades. Irrational acts, demanding behavior, withdrawal, perseveration, and fainting all have been observed by critical care nurses. Just as the patient is experiencing shock and disbelief about his illness, so too is the family. A nurse must perceive the feeling that a crisis victim is experiencing, particularly when that person cannot identify the problem or feeling to himself or others.

Nursing Assessment

The critical care nurse can expect to deal with large numbers of persons who can be defined as being in a crisis. Almost all patients and their families who populate the waiting room will fit the aforementioned crisis conditions. The problem will be to assess the immediate events causing the disruption and then to help the families assign priorities to their needs so that they can act accordingly.

The nurse will need to identify current methods of coping and to evaluate them in terms of adaptation (see Chap. 3). The nurse will need to determine, and sometimes point out to the clients, chronic problems resulting from the threatening crisis. When the situational crisis seems inconsequential or obscure to the nurse, she must attempt to discern and understand the meaning that the clients have attributed to the event. Furthermore, it will help to evaluate current maturational problems with which the family may be attempting to cope. Understanding the parameters of the crisis may give the direction for action.

Nursing Intervention

Nursing intervention must be designed to help families do the following:

- Reach a higher level of adaptation by learning from the crisis experience
- Regain a state of equilibrium
- Experience the feelings involved in the crisis to avoid delayed depressions and allow for future emotional growth

The Use of the Relationship

Establishing an emotionally meaningful relationship with people in crisis tends to be easier than at any other time. Persons in crisis are highly receptive to an interested and empathic helper. In the first meeting with the patient's family, the nurse must demonstrate an ability to help.

The family must be prepared for their experience in the critical care unit. The patient's condition, alertness, and appearance should be described in terms suitable to the family's level of understanding. Any equipment should be explained before the family views the patient. At the bedside further explanation can be made.

Other specific help can be given at this time to demonstrate the nurse's interest. Looking up telephone numbers can be extremely difficult for the highly anxious family member. Even deciding who is to be notified of the patient's status can be an overwhelming decision at these times.

With this kind of timely intervention, the family will begin to trust and depend on the nurse's judgment. This process then allows family members to believe the nurse when she conveys a feeling of hope and confidence in their ability to deal with whatever is ahead of them in the days to come. It is important to avoid giving false reassurance; rather, the reality of the situation can be expressed in statements like, "This is a complicated problem; together we can work on it."

Defining the Problem

As the relationship develops from one interaction to another, the nurse can formulate the dynamics of the problem. The formulations would include such items as the following:

- The meaning the family has attached to the event
- Other crises with which the family may be already coping
- The coping mechanisms previously used in times of stress, with an idea of why these behaviors are or are not working at this time
- The normal resources of the family, which may include friends, neighbors, relations, colleagues, and so forth. The nurse, having identified these areas, will best use them with the family to help them deal with their predicament.

A vital part of the problem-solving process is to help the family clearly state what their immediate problem is. Often people feel overwhelmed and immobilized by the free-floating anxiety or panic caused by acute stress. Stating the problem in words helps the client achieve a degree of *cognitive mastery*. Regardless of the difficulty or threat the problem implies, being able to state it as such reduces anxiety by helping the family feel that they have achieved some sort of understanding of what is happening.

Defining and redefining the problem or problems must occur many times before resolution of the crisis occurs. Stating the problem clearly automatically helps the family assign priorities and direct the needed actions. For example, finding a babysitter may become the number-one priority, superseding notification of close relatives of a tragic accident. Goal-directed activity will further help decrease anxiety and the irrational acts that sometimes go with it.

In high levels of stress, some people expect themselves to react differently. Rather than turning to the resources they use daily, they become reluctant to involve them. Simply asking people who it is that they usually turn to when they are upset and finding out what has gotten in the way of turning to these people now helps direct the client back to the normal mecha-

nisms that he uses to maintain homeostasis. When the client is reluctant to call on a friend, the nurse can help resolve the indecision by asking, "Wouldn't you want to help her if she were in your place?" Most families are truly not without resources; they have only failed to recognize and call on them.

Defining and redefining the problem may also help put the problem in a different light. It is possible in time to view a tragedy as a challenge and the unknown as an adventure.

The nurse can also help the family call on their own strengths. How have they handled stress before? Have they used humor, escape, exercise, or friendship? Do they telephone close friends and relatives who are far away? Even though the family may be threatened financially at this time, some expenditures of this sort may be well worth the money.

Problem Solving

A problem-solving technique that emphasizes choices and alternatives will help the family achieve a sense of control over part of their lives. It will also remind them, as well as clarify for them, that they are ultimately responsible for dealing with the event and that it is they who must live with the consequences of their decisions.

Helping the family focus on feelings is extremely important in order to avoid delayed grief reactions and protracted depressions later on. The nurse can give direction to the family to help each other cry and to share their fear and sadness. Reflection of feelings or active listening will be necessary throughout the crisis. If the nurse can start a statement by saying, "You feel . . . ," she will be reflecting a feeling. If she says, "You feel *that* . . . ," she will be reflecting a judgment instead of a feeling. Describing and recognizing one's feelings will decrease the need to look for someone to blame. Valuing the expression of feelings may help the clients avoid the use of tranquilizers, sedatives, and excessive sleep to escape painful feelings. In sad and depressing times, the nurse can authentically promise the family that they will feel better with time. Depression is self-limiting.

During the difficult days that a person is critically ill, the family may become very dependent on the judgment of professionals. It may be difficult for them to identify the appropriate areas in which to accept others' judgments. The nurse can best handle inappropriate expectations like, "Tell me what I should do?" by acknowledging the feelings involved in an accepting manner and stating the reality of the situation; for example, "You wish I could make that difficult decision for you, but I can't, because you are the ones who will have to live with the consequences." This type of statement acknowledges the clients' feelings and recognizes the complexity of the problem while emphasizing each individual's responsibility for his own feelings, actions, and decisions.

Once the problem has been defined and the family begins goal-directed activity, the nurse may help further by asking them to identify the steps they must take. This anticipatory guidance will help reduce anxiety and make things go more smoothly.

Crisis victims must always be left with a specific plan of action. This plan may be as simple as, "Call me tomorrow at 2:00 P.M."; regardless of its simplicity, it implies hope, responsibility, and a reason to get through the night.

The critical care nurse's time with families is often limited owing to the nature of her work, so it is important to make every interaction as useful to the family as possible. The nurse will have to take responsibility for directing the conversation and focusing on the here and now. She will need to avoid the temptation of giving useless advice in favor of emphasizing a problem-solving approach. However, the nurse must use her judgment and recognize those moments when direction is vital to health and safety. It is often necessary to direct families to return home to rest. This can be explained by saying that by maintaining their own health they will be more helpful to the patient at a later time. To make each interaction meaningful, the nurse must focus on the crisis situation and avoid getting involved in long-term chronic problems and complaints. For example, she would help the family of the overdose patient deal with the events immediately preceding the suicide attempt rather than with longstanding family problems.

Referral

Regardless of the nurse's ability in this area, there will be some families who will profit most by referral to a mental health nurse clinician, a social worker, a psychologist, or a psychiatrist. A nurse can best encourage the client to accept help from others by emphatically acknowledging the difficulty of the problem and providing a choice of names and phone numbers. At times, it even may be appropriate for the nurse to set up the first meeting; however, the chances of follow-through are greater when the client makes his own arrangements. Many hospitals have skilled mental health nurses and social workers who can help the nurse intervene with very short notice.

WHEN THE PATIENT IS DYING

For the most part, the goals of the critical care nurse are to preserve life and facilitate healing. Too often nurses experience a sense of disappointment and failure—

even anger with the patient—when the patient does not recover. When a patient dies, whether unexpectedly or as the inevitable end of a tragic and painful illness, the family of the patient becomes intimately involved in a crises that will shape their memories, feelings, and attitudes about death for the rest of their lives.

The challenge for nurses working with the dying patient and the family is to turn an often painful and traumatic experience into one that is also constructive and positive. When there is time, the last days of life can be a time of resolution, reconciliation, and termination.

An attitude of mutual trust among the staff, the patient, and the patient's family is essential to meeting this challenge. To promote trust, the nurse must develop the courage to answer the questions of the patient and the family honestly but with a sensitivity that allows the family members to maintain hope and integrity. Cassem identifies nine treatment recommendations for the care and management of the dying patient.[1] These areas of recommendation, described in the following pages, contribute to nursing strategies directed toward establishing an atmosphere in which trust and communication among the staff, the patient, and the family are most likely to occur.

Competence

Critical care nurses will be quick to recognize the amount of comfort and care that is conveyed through absolute technical competence. Even though extreme lifesaving measures may be withheld, competence brings emotional as well as physiological benefits to the patient. Being lifted and handled by competent hands is reassuring to both patient and family. Likewise, sloppy and shortcut techniques will be interpreted by the family as a devaluing of life because it is ending.

Concern

Concern or compassion is conveyed to the family when the staff is actively involved with them. Often nurses attempt to defend themselves against the pain of involvement by trying to hide or cover their sensitivity. The problem with this defense is that it is interpreted as callousness by the patient and his family. For some nurses, lack of involvement is a way of protecting themselves from becoming overly involved. Overinvolvement occurs for most nurses from time to time and, in fact, can threaten their competence and judgment. However, it can be managed with understanding supervision, good listening, and personal insight. Perhaps a greater problem for many nurses is that other nurses and colleagues may interpret the signs of compassion and healthy involvement as indications of overinvolvement. A nurse whose eyes become filled with tears at a sensitive moment conveys a sense of empathy to clients, not a loss of control. The major goal for many nurses is to learn to demonstrate comfortably the concern and compassion that are already an integral part of their emotional makeup.

Comfort

The aggressive pursuit of comfort is a primary nursing goal for the dying patient. This is especially important when a decision has been made to discontinue treatments and the goal changes from curing to supporting and comforting.

Pain relief is an important part of providing comfort for many critical care patients. The nurse must communicate closely with the patient and the physician to create a regimen in which the patient's integrity and peace of mind are not reduced by pain or the need to beg for medication. When a patient is in continuous pain, it is more appropriate to give medication on a predetermined schedule (*e.g.,* q3h) rather than as needed (*e.g.,* prn). Furthermore, Cassem, referring to the work of Marks and Sachar, states, "Fewer than 1% of hospitalized medical patients given narcotics for pain develop a serious problem of addiction.[2] In the terminal patient, concern for comfort supersedes concern for the problems of addiction. Knowing the patient's concern and desires about his pain experience is of utmost importance. For example, some patients will elect not to trade alertness for pain reduction. Many nurses will want to medicate these patients because working with people in excruciating pain is trying and frustrating. It also increases the nurse's feelings of helplessness and, therefore, anxiety.

In addition, nurses should be made aware that staff attitudes appear to have much to do with the ordering and giving of analgesic medication. In general, patients who are young and female tend to receive more powerful analgesics than others. Age, rather than physical condition, degree of pain, or other variables, may be the determining factor relating to the nurses' implementation of prn medication orders for patients with pain. This points out that nurses must be careful to assess the individual's need and capacity for pain medication and separate this assessment from other factors that are not relevant to the individual.

Finally, *every possible comfort measure* that can be employed without greatly increasing discomfort should automatically be taken. Mouth care can be easily overlooked in a patient who is not eating. Dryness, drooling, odor, and poor nutrition may cause pain and discomfort. The family can be involved in applying lip balm to the patient's lips and washing saliva from the skin. Positioning, skin care, and massage are all useful measures in promoting comfort. Some family members will choose to participate in this type of care, whereas others may be uncomfortable or fear that they will hurt the patient. Sometimes, the family's participation means more work for the nurse; however, this participation in care can be a highly significant and useful experience for the grieving family.

Promoting comfort for the dying requires constant and judicious decision-making. Should a febrile patient be covered when he is cold? Should someone with depressed respirations be sedated when he is restless and anxious? Comfort measures that break the usual protocol of the critical care unit may be required. Honest and direct communication with the patient and the family will help guide the actions of nurses and physicians on complicated matters.

Communication

Listening, and listening well, is the cornerstone of effective communication. Some patients do not wish to talk about dying. To do so will strip them of whatever hope they are holding. Others will deal with death in a symbolic way. They will speak of autumns and winters and other subjects that may symbolize endings. This is an effective way of terminating one's life, and no interpretation is necessary.

Family members may elect to use the time to go over special memories, reconcile past misunderstandings, and forgive each other for past transgressions. It is hoped that they will have the time and atmosphere to say the things they need to say.

The nurse's responsibility to establish an atmosphere in which this type of communication can occur. What does the family need to be comfortable on the unit—a cup of coffee, a pillow, a place to sit, permission to leave? Does the family wish to be present at the time of death? How can they be reached? All these questions require sensitive timing and a straightforward approach on the part of the nurse. When words escape the nurse, as they often may in difficult moments, or if words seem inadequate, much can be conveyed by touching a shoulder or an arm.

Children

Allowing children to visit a critical care unit may require special arrangements on the part of the staff. If the patient wishes to see his child or grandchild and if the child wishes to see the patient in a critical care unit, the child should be offered short, simple explanations concerning the patient's condition. Answering the child's questions in terms that the child will understand will help reduce possible fears. The person who is taking care of the child should be made aware that invasive procedures and equipment such as nasogastric tubes will most likely upset children. If a visit from the child is not possible, arrangements for a telephone visit should be made.

Family Cohesion and Integration

The family in crisis is vulnerable to all types of other stresses. As has been stated previously, helping family members provide support for one another is of paramount importance. If they wish to have some member of the family stay with the patient, they can support one another by providing meal and rest breaks. Being together and being available to one another will be sufficient for many families. The nurse may choose to say to some family members that even though it seems that they are not doing anything for the patient, their presence seems to relax or comfort the patient or the patient's spouse.

Cheerfulness

Not even dying people like a sad and grumpy nurse. Keeping one's sense of humor and expressing it appropriately offer relief in a difficult situation. Generous smiles and a sense of humor will also help the family relax and share themselves in their usual ways. A good joke can also be appreciated by a dying patient.

Sensitivity to the patient's mood and a sense of timing are useful in assessing a patient's receptivity to light-heartedness. Talking to the patient in one's typical fashion will help the family relax and communicate more easily with one another and the patient. In turn, the patient should feel less isolated and alone in this final crisis.

Consistency and Perseverance

During times of crisis, complaints and criticisms are frequently directed toward the nurse. A nondefensive, tolerant attitude and a willingness to continue working with the patient and family are the most effective ways of conveying compassion and understanding. Continued interest in a patient and family demonstrates a sense of worth and respect to those involved.

As patients get closer to death, nurses are likely to spend less time with them.[3] This decreased contact may evoke feelings of abandonment, sadness, and hopelessness in both patients and family. Moreover, changes in staff shifts increase the patient's sense of isolation and cause him to use up his energy adjusting to new people. Providing consistent staff who do not withdraw helps the patient and family develop trust

and a sense of belonging that can become a rewarding experience for everyone involved.

Equanimity

Cassem describes equanimity as the "capacity to be comfortable with the dying patient."[4] For many nurses, being comfortable about death depends on the ability to modify goals that are aimed at preserving life with goals that are designed to preserve personal integrity and family stability when a patient is dying. Rather than considering death as a symbol of failure, nurses can view it as a life-enriching and professionally gratifying experience.

The Critical Care Nurse

The nature of critical care nursing is such that the nurse is exposed to repeated losses. When the nurse has experienced this type of loss as a result of death in her personal life, then dealing with dying patients may at times reactivate feelings and memories associated with these personal losses. Therefore, it is essential that the nursing staff support one another, especially by listening in a tolerant way when a colleague is expressing what is generally considered to be unacceptable feelings. As Quint implies, a supportive relationship is necessary to acquire the ability to communicate with dying patients.[5]

Few nurses come to the critical care unit with these abilities. It will be necessary for most nurses to request specific educational experiences, as well as consultation and supervision from appropriate resources. The intensity of emotion and involvement demanded by a nursing role in critical care makes these nurses particularly vulnerable to the "burnout" syndrome (see Chap. 37).

Crisis intervention for families undergoing acute stress is an important preventive mental health function that nurses can provide. Their knowledge of and proximity to the problem allow them to be first-line resource professionals. As patient advocates, their role will be to realize and point out that dealing with a psychological crisis in the family greatly affects the recovery and well-being of the patient and decreases the chances for further disequilibrium in the family unit.

REFERENCES

1. Cassem N: The dying patient. In Hackett TP, Cassem N (eds): Handbook of General Hospital Psychiatry, pp 300–318. St Louis, CV Mosby, 1978
2. *Ibid,* p 306
3. Glaser B, Strauss A: Awareness of Dying, p 227. Chicago, Aldine, 1965

4. Cassem: The dying patient, p 310
5. Quint JC: The Nurse and the Dying Patient, p 199. New York, Macmillan, 1967

BIBLIOGRAPHY

Calus KE, Baily JT (eds): Living with Stress and Promoting Well-Being. St. Louis, CV Mosby, 1980

Freidman MM: Family Nursing. New York, Appleton-Century-Crofts, 1981

Northhouse L: The Impact of Cancer on the Family: An Overview. Int J Psychiatry Med 14, No 3: 215–242, 1984

Peric-Knowlton W: The Understanding and Management of Acute Pain in Adults: The Nursing Contribution. Int J Nurs Stud 21, No 2: 131–143, 1984

Sedqwick R: Family Mental Health. St Louis, CV Mosby, 1981

Wells N: Responses to Acute Pain and the Nursing Implications. J Adv Nurs 9, No 1: 51–58, 1984

5
Caring and Touching as Nursing Interventions

Jacquelyn M. Clement

Since the 1960s, there has been a prolific growth of critical care units in general hospital settings. Along with this growth and progress there have been previously unimagined developments in technology, highly modern facilities, and increasingly available invasive and noninvasive devices for measuring, monitoring, and regulating body systems.

Being a patient in a critical care setting has the potential for being more frightening, more lonely, more confusing, and, in many ways, more dehumanizing than ever before. The dimensions of the nursing role in the setting have similarly changed. This new role is more technological, more physiologically oriented, more intense, and more intellectually demanding than in previous years. Because of these changes, the aspect of caring as the major dimension of nursing has become more important and increasingly threatened.

The nurse can express care for a patient in a number of ways. There are descriptions in the nursing literature of mechanisms of providing emotional, social, spiritual, and physical support in the care setting. One behavior that permeates all these endeavors is that of touch. By using touch in a meaningful, genuine, sincere way, the nurse can clearly convey caring and support to patients and families. By understanding the power of touch in interactions, the nurse can more successfully plan it into her care and develop her own skills by including it into communication processes.

CARING AND TOUCHING: A REVIEW OF THE LITERATURE

Caring

There is little dispute among nursing authorities that caring is the central focus of nursing. Leininger expresses a firm belief in the importance of caring behaviors in nursing. She describes a strong link between curing (the major focus of health care) and caring by health care practitioners. In her own words, "caring acts and decisions make the crucial difference in effecting curing consequences . . . there can be no curing without the elements and processes of caring."[1] It is nursing that primarily should be concerned with "caring behaviors, caring lifestyles, caring processes and caring consequences."[1]

Hyde describes the process of caring as "part of the healing process for the patient."[2] The caring process is a phenomenon of interaction between the caregiver and the person receiving care. It is the decision of each nurse as to whether this process is part of her professional role. The inclusion of this phenomenon into the professional role can significantly improve the quality of nursing care.

Other authors address the notion of caring from a slightly different perspective. Marsh suggests that the caring aspect of nursing is related to the nurse's efforts to meet individual patient needs. The needs of particular consideration include the following: (1) the need to retain a feeling of self-worth, (2) the need for companionship, and (3) the need to feel supported by the caregiver.[3]

Cohn describes nursing behaviors that express caring from a slightly different perspective. She describes these behaviors as humanistic attributes of patient care that cannot be replaced by technology: listening, caring, humor, involvement, and sharing. Cowper-Smith suggests the preservation of courtesy, compassion, respect, dignity, and genuineness as essentials in caring for patients. Kalisch describes high-level empathy as the major ingredient in the caring process.[4,5,6]

Sidney Jourard very vividly describes his feelings about the nurse–patient relationship, caring, and the influence that they have on patient recovery. According to Jourard, the recovery of the patient depends, to a great extent, on the understanding that someone cares for him. Caring by the nurse increases patient comfort, identity, and integrity. The lack of caring can actually cause detrimental effects on the health and recovery of a patient. Human warmth, love, and responsive care are among the essentials in any recovery situation. The nurse is the professional who is most likely and able to provide these humane aspects of care.[7]

Communicating Caring Through Touch

Meaningful communication can be the vehicle for the caring process utilized in meeting psychosocial needs of the patient. One form of communication that is of particular importance in any health care setting is that of touch. The need for tactile contact is present in everyone at birth and continues throughout life. It is a need that, when met, adds richness and growth to human potential and is basic to the healthy development of the individual. The need for touch is thought to intensify during episodes of high stress and cannot be totally met by other forms of communication. Nurses, when using touch, are usually trying to convey understanding, support, warmth, concern, and closeness to the patient. This communication is an activation of the caring process. Touching not only improves the sense of well-being of the patient but also promotes physical recovery from disease.

The role of touch in nursing care can be viewed from many perspectives. It serves a multitude of purposes within nurse–patient interactions. Communication with touch is simple, straightforward, and direct. Touch is basically a positive behavior that produces a satisfying effect on the individual and is among the elementary needs for healthy mental and physical development. It is one of the most important senses. Touch confirms the reality perceived through other senses and is a central part of human communication processes. It has a positive effect on perceptual and cognitive abilities and can influence physiological pa-

rameters such as respiration and blood flow. In summary, touch represents a positive, therapeutic element of human interaction.

The act of touching or being touched involves the stimulation of receptors in the skin that transmit messages to the brain that are then interpreted by the person. A large segment of the brain is devoted to touch. Undoubtedly, touch contributes greatly to many aspects of communication, learning, and understanding.

Touch alone is a frequently used form of interpersonal communication done with little space or distance between individuals. Intimate space is considered to be approximately the area of 6 to 18 inches from a person's body. Touching invades this intimate space and becomes of great significance to the message being sent.

There is an increased importance for touch in the critical care unit, where machines and technology contribute so vividly to depersonalization of the patient. Before these modern developments, the greatest things that a nurse could offer a patient were the comfort and caring of her presence and touch, and these accomplished so much. Nurses may be tempted to think that touching seems too simple to be effective. However, few medical advances can supercede the benefits of "a good backrub, a clasp and squeeze of hands, and a warm smile".[8]

Touch that is non–task-related (affective touch) is a powerful therapeutic intervention that communicates caring. Nursing authorities generally believe that an increase in meaningful affective touch in conjunction with treatment-related touch can significantly improve the nurse–patient communication process.[9]

Other Effects of Nursing Touch

The effects of touch in the clinical environment may be far-reaching. Touch has played a major part in promoting and maintaining reality orientation in patients prone to confusion about time, place, and personal identification.[10] The use of touch may be most helpful in situations in which individuals are experiencing fear, anxiety, or depression. It may also be beneficial for patients who have a need for encouragement or nurturing, who have difficulty verbalizing needs, or who are disoriented, unconscious, or terminally ill.

The age of the patient can greatly affect his perception of touch. According to Day's study, the younger patient felt that touch should be used as an everyday positive component in nursing care, whereas the elderly patient felt that it should be used for therapeutic purposes in episodes of pain, loneliness, and depression. Patients also felt that the desire for touch increased with the seriousness of the illness and decreased with increased closeness of the family.[11]

Even though touching can greatly improve older

people's quality of communication as well as the over-all quality of their lives, it has been found that the elderly and the sickest patients are touched least frequently by nurses.[12] Because the elderly's sensory abilities are often diminished, it is recommended that nurses practice a "well-defined" touch when working with them. Elderly patients' desire and need for touch greatly surpass their need for verbal communication, and fulfillment of this need reassures them of their wholeness and worth.[13]

According to another study, the use of touch by nurses in critical care units does not vary according to the age or sex of the patient.[14] Unfortunately, the most ill individuals — those who probably need and desire touch the most — seem to be touched the least. A study of touching habits and behaviors of nurses in a geriatric home suggested that people with little or no evidence of physical impairment were touched the most. Men and those who were physically impaired received little touching.[15]

These findings point out the need to include touch as a nursing intervention in the patient care plan. When efforts are coordinated by nurses, the use of touch may be more relaxing to a patient than sedatives or tranquilizers.

Nurses convey a wide variety of messages through the use of touch in nursing care, including security, understanding, sincerity, respect, support, warmth, concern, reassurance, interest, empathy, comfort, closeness, encouragement, acceptance, willingness to help, and willingness to become involved. Despite the convictions of nurses concerning these messages, approximately one third of them consciously utilize touch in their practice only in conjunction with verbal communication because of possible misinterpretation by patients.

The Messages of Touch

Touch can be interpreted in a variety of ways depending on the following characteristics: duration, location, frequency, action, intensity, and sensation.

Duration of touch is the total time over which the touch episode occurs. Generally, longer durations of touch allow for an increased opportunity for the patient to identify and integrate the touch. Longer durations also allow for more realization of body parts and details and boundaries as well as higher self-esteem.[16]

Location of touch pertains to the areas and parts of the body being touched. The location of touch gives messages concerning the specific body parts and the integration of these parts into the whole. Touching the trunk (referred to as *centripetality*) more than the limbs can often convey a message of closeness and

intimacy with the toucher. The number of locations touched in relationship to those available to be touched can transmit a positive message of self-evaluation to the person who is being touched.

Frequency of touch, or the total amount of touching experienced, has the most potential for affecting self-esteem, closeness with others, cognitive and emotive ability, and sexual identity.

Action of touch "represents the rate of approach to a body surface" along with the energy used in the initiation of touch.[17] A rapid-approach action of touch increases the self-perception of the person who is being touched, allowing him to see himself as an independent sexual being.

Intensity of touch refers to the pressure used on the body surface during touch. Intensity is measured by degree of skin indentation. Moderate intensity of touch has been reported to produce the least therapeutic effects, whereas a variation of strong and weak touching has the highest potential for positive effects.

Sensation is the body interpretation of touch as being either pleasurable or painful. Painful sensations distort the body image by impairing normal use of the body's perceptual abilities. Pleasurable touch is more apt to provide a feeling that one's body is worthwhile and valuable.

Although these symbols of touch provide us with measurable components to look for in our behaviors, the messages sent and received and the context in which the message occurs will be individual. It is helpful to remember, however, that touching is a "language" that can be a powerful part of nurse–patient interaction.

TAXONOMY OF TOUCHING

Heslin developed a very graphic taxonomy based on research findings on touch as a widely used nonverbal form of communication. The taxonomy illustrates an informal set of relationships that exist to regulate the kinds of touch allowed by society. Within the context of this taxonomy, the intensity of the relationship between the toucher and the recipient increases as they progress through the levels.[18]

Level I: Functional/Professional

In this level of relationship, touching is done in order to accomplish a professional task. Often the touching is intimate; however, it remains appropriate within the functional/professional relationship. Examples of this level of relationship are nurse–patient, nurse–patient's family, respiratory therapist–patient, and physician–patient.

Level II: Social/Polite

This level of relationship is typical of touching behaviors that are indicative of cultural restraints and prescriptions. The handshake is an example of a touch behavior typical of this level that functions as a neutralizing act between two individuals.

Level III: Friendship/Warmth

This level of a relationship is often thought of with the most uneasiness. Because it is less formal than the social polite level, it is often misinterpreted as a representation of a higher level of love or sexual attraction. It carries with it a message of caring and affection but often is misunderstood for more intense feelings. The messages that some people sense concerning sexuality with people of the same sex or opposite sex cause them to shun touch at this level. A very common touch behavior at this level is the hug.

Level IV: Love/Intimacy

This level of touching conveys the message of deep caring and commitment. Discomfort with gestures on this level often reflect ambivalence in the commitment to a relationship. People will be more comfortable with the touch gesture when the level of the relationship is appropriate for the message that is being sent.

Level V: Sexual Arousal

This is the level of intensity in relationships in which touch conveys sexual meaning and stimulation. This message may include or exclude love and commitment.

Heslin hypothesizes that there are two possible ways in which this taxonomy provides a score of intensity for personalizing and humanizing another person. One model predicts that the level of humanizing and individualizing increases in correlation to the levels of the taxonomy, from levels I to V. In this situation, an individual becomes less of an object and more of a person as the level of the relationship increases.

An alternate model is one in which the most appreciation of another individual occurs at the friendship/warmth level. Within this level of a relationship, there is more open acceptance of another person and greater tolerance of his idiosyncrasies. It would be ideal if this

same acceptance always occurred at levels IV and V in this taxonomy.

Nurse–Patient Bond

From Heslin's work the question arises, "Where does the nurse–patient relationship fit within this taxonomy?" It is certainly appropriate that many of our task-related interactions correlate with the functional/professional level, which allows for numerous care activities requiring touch (*e.g.,* physical assessment, repositioning the patient, bathing, changing a dressing, or attaching cardiac monitor electrodes). But what about "affective touch?" The acceptance, concern, caring, and support transmitted by these behaviors are more indicative of interaction at the friendship/warmth level. It is possible that the nurse has the capacity for moving between those two levels in a way that maintains her professional role while also relating on a very human level with genuine caring for each patient as an individual. It is this combination that makes the nurse–patient relationship unique and powerful.

The caring, trust, and support that develop between the nurse and the patient constitute the foundation of the nurse–patient bond. No other health care professional has the consistent and frequent opportunities to interact with the patient within this same framework. No other framework of interaction can offer the patient a more powerful source of support: a professional, knowledgeable foundation and a caring, human acceptance as an individual of worth and dignity.

Hypohugganemia

The concept of "hypohugganemia" is being introduced to signify a state of touch deficiency in a patient. Because touch is a basic need from birth through adulthood, every person strives to meet his need as it varies with life experiences. Being ill or hospitalized, losing a loved one, or experiencing a crisis can increase a person's need or desire for touch. When such events occur and the need is not sufficiently met, the person is in a state of "hypohugganemia." Even though other forms of stimuli may reduce the immediacy of this need, only human touch can satisfy it.

HIGH-RISK PATIENTS AND FAMILIES

Although any patient admitted to a critical care unit will probably experience some threats of touch deficiency, there are particular experiences that signal the high-risk patient or family. Conscious, well-planned touch may be an effective strategy for alleviating the state of touch deficiency that may occur in these situations.

Sensory Deprivation. Because of impaired use of the senses or inadequate quality and quantity of sensory input, an ICU patient may experience altered abilities to relate to his environment meaningfully. This patient may benefit from planned, individualized touch by the nurse. Tactile stimulation can be used to convey meaningful messages to the patient about himself, his body boundary perception, his self-esteem, his wholeness, and his contact with reality. Touching can be very effective when used alone or in conjunction with other forms of verbal or nonverbal communication.

Body Boundary Threats. The critical care setting offers a particular challenge to a patient to maintain a clear understanding of the boundaries of his own body. The increasing use of machinery and technology at the bedside as well as invasive monitoring and treatment techniques can frighten and confuse the critically ill patient. Tubes, catheters, and wires extend beyond the body surface to connect with intravenous feedings, monitoring equipment, and mechanical devices to support life. It can become difficult for a patient to know where his body ends and the machinery begins. This difficulty can increase when the nurse spends much time at the bedside touching and manipulating the equipment. In this situation, the nurse may find it helpful to make the effort to touch the patient while at the bedside. It is believed that touching a large number of the body areas available is consistent with the patient's ability to perceive the form and shape of his body accurately and to integrate information about his body parts and body as a whole.

Fear, Anxiety, and Loss of Control. The critical care setting is an environment that makes it difficult for even the strongest and bravest patient to feel fearless, calm, and content. The nurse must give attention to the patient's psychological processes if optimal progress is to be made in the care regimen. One goal for care must always be that the patient be allowed to participate as much as possible. His participation depends to a great extent on the communication and support processes used to build trust, decrease fear, reduce anxiety, and maintain dignity. This process can be greatly enhanced by the nurse's conveyance of genuine caring, warmth, support, and understanding through the use of touch. The messages transmitted through touch can be vivid and profound, even during a crisis situation. When used in conjunction with a calm and clear verbal message, eye contact, or effective listening, the communication of caring becomes more vivid.

Separation From Family. Even the most liberal visiting policies in a critical care unit cannot totally accommodate family and other loved ones so that they are sure to be nearby when a patient is in crisis. A crisis need not be an abrupt physiological change or even a life-threatening event. It may be a sudden episode of feeling alone, awakening in an unfamiliar environment, the fear of dying, or simply a lack of physical contact with loved ones. The nurse has the opportunity to assist a patient through episodes like these by being with the patient and touching him in therapeutic ways to give him contact with his environment, the feeling of closeness with another person, and the belief that someone near him cares about his well-being.

Communication Barriers. Patients need to experience communication with their caregivers in order to maintain perceptions of themselves as worthwhile individuals who have contact with reality and who can interact with other people. The challenge of communicating increases when patients are deaf, are unable to speak or understand the language of the nurse, or are unable to communicate verbally owing to intubation or a physical disorder of illness. The paralyzed patient who is also unable to move his hands, arms, or facial muscles is even more restricted in his options for communication strategies. Using touch to enhance verbal communication, to get a patient's attention, or to convey a message can be very effective. Allowing the patient to touch the nurse may also give him an acceptable way to communicate with her. Patients can convey many emotions and messages using touch. Fear, pain, understanding, calmness, and joy might be among the messages transmitted by a patient who can hold the nurse's hand, touch her face, or grasp her arm. This can be a very productive and useful vehicle for patients who offer unusual challenges with regard to communication.

The Family of a Critical Care Patient. The family is an extension of the patient, and, when we care for a patient, we also need to care for his loved ones. In numerous ways, families experience many of the same crises as patients in critical care. They are often anxious and fearful and feel very helpless in their abilities to intervene and help the patient. Like the patient, they have to some extent surrendered control to the health care team. They find themselves separated from their loved ones and become victims of visiting policies, a strange and fearful environment, and the unknown. Aside from the time actually spent with the patient, the most meaningful and supportive communication for the family often comes from the nursing staff. Nurses can decrease "communication barriers" for families by using clear, understandable terminology, taking the time to listen to questions and concerns, and using touch with the family members. By touching an arm or shoulder or holding hands, the nurse can enhance genuine listening and give support while sharing information with the family. Frequently, the nurse may be in situations in which she feels unable to offer verbal support or understanding. Touching alone can be a very powerful silent transmission of support during these episodes.

Family's Fear of Touching the Patient. The family often feels helpless and fearful at the bedside of a critically ill patient. The tubes, dressings, wires, and machinery that the nurse is so accustomed to are frightening to family members. They see this equipment attached to their loved one and may be reluctant to reach out and touch him for fear of causing harm to the patient or the equipment. They are often startled and shocked at the sight of someone they love who now appears so ill.

The nurse has the opportunity at this time to offer support to the family and patient in a unique way. <u>By explaining and describing the equipment and patient's appearance to the family before they go to the bedside, the nurse can prepare them for this often difficult experience.</u> During this explanation, the nurse can use touch to develop a feeling of trust and support with the family. Again, touching a family member's arm or shoulders or putting an arm around him while he is approaching the bedside can convey understanding, caring, and support. At the bedside, the nurse can touch the patient while talking with him and a family member to demonstrate that tactile contact is safe. By taking a family member's hand and touching the arm, face, shoulders, or hand of the patient, the nurse can help initiate the touching behavior as well as assist in alleviating the fear of harming the patient or the equipment. This process of acting as a role model for the family can be an excellent way of decreasing the anxiety of the family and patient and helping them feel more comfortable in a strange environment.

NURSING ASSESSMENT GUIDELINES OF NEEDS FOR TOUCH BY PATIENT AND FAMILY

Individual assessment of touching needs is a very important step for the nurse. Because so many factors affect desire for touch, the nurse must keep in mind that everyone's need and reaction to touch will be individualized. There is no absolute formula for quantifying and qualifying these aspects of each person because of the complexity of factors that contribute to one's beliefs and feelings about touch. Individual fam-

Assessment Guide

T **T**otal amount of touching is now by family and health team members.

O **O**lder patient.
Orientation problems.

U **U**nusual threats to body image or body boundary.

C **C**onsciousness level?
Communication problems? Intubated? Tracheostomy?
Crisis situation?

H **H**igh technology at bedside?
High stress period?
Helplessness and **H**opelessness? Signs of depression?

I **I**CU psychosis? Confused: Restless?
Initiation of touch by patient?

N **N**ormal use of senses?

G **G**iving behavior cues? Verbally? Nonverbally?

FIGURE 5-1
Assessment guide.

ily practice, cultural practices, and coping styles are other powerful influences on desire for—and interpretation of—touch by another person. Nurses must use information available in the care setting as well as their subjective instincts and interpretations of family interaction patterns to determine their strategies for meeting the touch needs of their patients and families.

Assessment Guidelines

There are some key questions that the nurse must consider when assessing the touch needs of the patient and family (Fig. 5-1). Some of the *major signals of increased need for touch* include the following:

T *Total amount of touching is low* by family and health team members. The patient may require little physical care, may be in isolation, or may be using a kinetic bed. This could also be a patient who is relatively stable and situated in an area in the unit in which there is little traffic. Thus, few people go near the bedside unless it becomes necessary to implement a procedure or treatment. Often, this patient has few or no visitors or the family members are very hesitant to touch the patient. When with the patient, they remain distant from the bed and appear fearful or uncomfortable with touching or displays of affection and caring.

O *O*lder patients often have an increased need for meaningful touch during episodes of crisis. The aging process may also make them more prone to sensory deprivation, confusion, and communication difficulties that can sometimes be decreased by the meaningful use of touch in care. Having few visitors and little verbal interaction may intensify their touching needs.

U *U*nusual threats to body image and body boundary occur when patients experience discomfort and confusion about their body parts and the integration of those parts into the whole body. They also may experience difficulty with differentiating their bodies from the mechanical equipment used in their care. Patients who have undergone surgery or other invasive procedures or who have experienced side effects from medications, weight loss or gain from the illness or treatments, and dependency on life support equipment all are likely to have body perception problems. Patients who have received organ transplants may also experience some confusion about their body perceptions. Transplantation of other people's organs into their bodies may create mixed feelings about wholeness, self-identity, and self-image.

C *C*onsciousness level of the patient may render clues about touching needs. There may be less tendency to touch alert patients if they are stable and able to participate in their own care. This tendency, if prolonged, may actually contribute to an unmet need for touch.

Patients who are less alert, lethargic, stuporous, semicomatose, and comatose may need more touching by the nurse. Because their modes of communication are limited by altered levels of consciousness, touching may be an avenue of communication that is very therapeutic. Using touch with these patients may convey all the messages of caring and support and provide them with some meaningful contact with the environment. The comfort and security transmitted through touch may be extremely meaningful to these patients.

Communication difficulties are common challenges to the ICU nurse. Patients who are intubated, who have tracheostomies, or who are physically unable to communicate verbally because of their illness or disability have always posed a communication challenge for the ICU nurse. Patients who cannot speak or understand the language of the nurse are equally disabled in an ICU setting. All these patients experience an increased need for meaningful communication. The importance of effective touch may be increased with these patients.

Crisis can trigger an increased need for support, closeness with others, and clear communication. Often, there is little opportunity for the nurse to provide prolonged verbal support during a crisis situation, even though the need for support and caring may be intense. Patients experiencing a crisis episode may have an increased need for supportive touch.

H *H*igh technology has contributed greatly to the intensive care regimen. It may also, however, contribute to the dehumanization process that can occur in the ICU setting. Attention to machinery and equipment may make ICU patients feel very insignificant and invisible among the tubes, wires, computers, and so forth. These patients may need human touch as a reassurance of their humanness, dignity, and self-worth in a setting that is frightening, awesome, and highly technological.

*H*igh-stress episodes in the ICU need not always be physiological crises. Whenever a patient experiences feelings of fear, increased anxiety, or loss of control there may be a need for increased communication of support and caring. Some routine care activities, such as repositioning a patient, feeding a patient, or even moving a pillow, may remind the patient that he is unable to do these things for himself. The nurse who recognizes that these "routine" interventions may be psychologically threatening to the patient's self-esteem can use touch to convey understanding, closeness, and caring.

*H*elplessness and *h*opelessness are feelings that patients may experience when they perceive that they are unable to improve their situations to an acceptable level. These feelings may leave them devastated and depressed. They may exhibit these feelings by appearing apathetic about their conditions or care, by being withdrawn and uncommunicative, or by weeping and looking hurt. Feelings of being alone in their crises only make them feel more hopeless. These patients may be very open to supportive and caring touch by the nurse as a sign that someone cares and is with them.

I *I*CU psychosis, confusion, and restlessness all may be side effects of the environment in which the patient is cared for in combination with his individual stress level. Lack of restful sleep, altered nutritional status, and use of medications also contribute to the psychological disequilibrium that the patient experiences. Careful and planned touch may assist the patient through such episodes.

    Initiation of touch by the patient may be a cue to his need for tactile contact by another person. Patients who reach out to the nurse or who cling tightly to the nurse's hand or arm may be signaling their need for closeness and contact with another human being.

N Normal use of the five senses and a normal amount and quality of sensory input enhance a person's ability to cope with anxiety, a strange environment, and crisis. Unfortunately, critical illness, aging, and the critical care setting often distort sensory input and its utilization. The nurse can attempt to increase the patient's use of sensory input by evaluating each individual in an attempt to identify behaviors of touch that can reinforce a balanced sensory process. Giving sensitive attention to a patient's behavior is the first step in achieving this balance. The second step involves using meaningful touch in an attempt to communicate caring and the patient's connection with reality, dignity, and esteem. The third step requires the nurse to watch for the patient response in order to evaluate her intervention on an individual level.

G Giving behavior cues about touching needs may be a subconscious phenomenon for a patient. Facial expression, eye contact, verbalization, initiation of touch, and frequent calling for the nurse may signal that the patient needs to have someone near. Sometimes, the desire for touch is transmitted so subtly that it is difficult to identify the exact characteristics of the message. Whether the messages are overt or subtle and whether the nursing assessment is objective or intuitive make no difference. The nurse who is sensitive to the touch needs of the patient will be able to identify messages and cues much of the time. The nurse who spontaneously and genuinely uses touch with patients to convey caring may already be processing patients' subtle cues.

MOVING FROM "KNOWING" TO "DOING"

It is always very interesting to be enlightened by new information or to gain a new perspective on a frequently observed phenomenon. However, new insight does not always give a person the practical means by which he can transform new awareness into useful strategies. It is with this in mind that the following case study is presented. This is one example of how a criti-

cal care nursing staff made some relatively simple but very meaningful and effective changes in their care on the basis of their increased awareness of patient–nurse interactions using touch.

CASE STUDY

Mrs. B was admitted to a large medical center critical care unit approximately 10 days ago. She is a 79-year-old married woman who was transferred from a small community hospital, approximately 100 miles away, after having undergone a bowel resection for cancer. Following her difficult surgery, Mrs. B exhibited signs of acute renal failure and congestive heart failure. She suffered from severe fluid and electrolyte imbalance and was found to have toxic levels of gentamicin in her blood. Her major treatment since transfer has been hemodialysis.

Mrs. B's condition has remained stable throughout the week, yet she has shown signs of continued confusion and disorientation. It is suspected at this point that she has suffered a severe hearing loss as a result of her toxic drug levels. She has a very anxious facial expression and appears very restless. She has been using her nurse call light every 10 to 15 minutes and has great difficulty communicating her needs when the nurse arrives.

Nancy Smith, R.N., has been taking care of Mrs. B for several days. She suspected that along with other necessary aspects of care, Mrs. B could benefit from some planned touch interaction by the nurses. She scheduled a nursing care conference for the purpose of assessing Mrs. B's touch needs and developing some strategies for care in which all the nursing staff would participate.

The conference was productive and thought-provoking. The staff rapidly identified the high-risk factors for touch deficiency and the symptoms that may be associated with decreased tactile stimulation. They include the following:

• Mrs. B is elderly and may have less effective use of available sensory stimuli because of the effects of the aging process.
• This is a crisis experience for the patient.
• There is increased use of highly technical equipment at the bedside that may be frightening and awesome.
• The patient is experiencing increased separation from family and loved ones owing to the increased distance from home and limited visiting times available in the critical care unit.
• Mrs. B, because she has suffered some hearing loss, is having extreme difficulty in interpreting her new surroundings and communicating effectively with other people.
• The sensory stimuli available to Mrs. B are strange to her and add to her confusion about her surroundings. Her bed is located on the end of the unit, where there is no window and little traffic flow by the staff. The head of her bed has been in low Fowler's position much of the time, limiting her visual access to her immediate surroundings.
• Mrs. B has experienced a variety of threats to her body image. She has a long incision on her abdomen, intravenous needles and tubes in her arms, an oxygen mask on her face, and an unfamiliar hospital gown covering her body. Her heart rhythm is on display on a cardiac monitor next to her bed.

• Lastly, the body that for so long was strong and agile is now weak and helpless. She cannot turn from side to side by herself, comb her own hair, or use the toilet. These all represent significant alterations in how she now sees herself.

Based on the assessment phase of the nursing care conference, the staff developed the following plans, which were to be recorded on the Kardex care plan and implemented in daily care.

• Relocate Mrs. B in the ICU so that she has a clear view of the main nursing area. The nurses agreed to make planned and frequent visits to her bedside, where they would use a number of communication techniques: a chalk board for writing messages and eye contact and variations of moderately firm and gentle touches while communicating.

• Have a nurse stay with Mrs. B during any treatments or procedures for the specific purpose of providing support and reassurance through touch. Because audible messages would be ineffective, it would be very difficult for the nurse who is performing a procedure to be able to provide adequate communication of support when the patient is confused or frightened or both.

• Make special arrangements so that the family, who is traveling a great distance, can be with the patient as much as possible. Be flexible with visiting policies and consult with the family as to the best times.

• Be a role model of touch for the family members. Use touch in interactions with them to build trust. Greet them with a handshake and accompany them to the bedside. Touch the patient to show them that they will not harm the patient or equipment. Take their hands and touch the patient and equipment with them to help put them at ease. In talking with them, encourage them to use touch alone or with verbal interaction with the patient. Tell them what areas they need to avoid touching.

• Incorporate planned, meaningful touch into nursing care activities. During physical assessment, use reasonably long periods of touch to extremities to support Mrs. B's perception of her body boundaries. Use opportunities to touch the body trunk whenever possible. Touch the shoulder while ausculating the heart or lungs. Massage the back when assessing for sacral edema. Use eye contact generously to reinforce the communication process that occurs during touch.

• Be alert to patient response to touch and cues for more or less touch. Observe facial expression, body movement, visible responses to touch, or any attempts to initiate touch. Watch for changes in behavior, restlessness, anxiety reduction, heart rate changes, and so forth.

At the conclusion of the conference, the nurses agreed to document the implementation of their touch behaviors and evaluate the responses by the patient. They planned to have a follow-up conference in 2 days to evaluate the results.

Follow-up Conference

Two days later, the nursing staff met to discuss the progress with Mrs. B and the reevaluation of their strategies. They identified the following changes in the patient and family status that they felt were associated with their planned uses of touch:

• Mrs. B appeared less restless and anxious. She rarely used the call light, and, when she did, she was calmer and could communicate her needs more clearly. The nurses noted that her sleep habits were more clearly delineated. She slept more soundly at night and seemed to be more alert during the day.

• Mrs. B appeared to communicate more effectively using the chalk board to read the messages from the nurse. She still seemed to have difficulty speaking clearly because her hearing was diminished, but she was noticeably improved. She occasionally reached for the nurse and touched her during the verbal and written exchange.

• Mrs. B exhibited symptoms of confusion only rarely. She began to address one nurse by her name and asked about her family. Mrs. B frequently reached for the nurse at the bedside.

• Mrs. B's family visited regularly at times that best met their schedules. They seemed more comfortable at the bedside, hugged and kissed Mrs. B upon arriving and leaving, and used a lot of touching and handholding while there. They also approached the nurses more freely, asked questions, talked about Mrs. B's condition, and seemed more relaxed.

Interestingly, the nurses in the conference described feeling closer to Mrs. B and her family than to some other patients. They agreed that their feelings and the patient changes that they identified were difficult to measure objectively. However, they did feel that their plans had a positive effect on the patient's progress. They agreed to continue to give attention to their strategies with the goal of refining their abilities in using more effective touch in patient care.

Conclusion

The dynamics of patient–nurse interaction are rapidly changing along with the evolution of health care in general. The patient is not the same as he was many years ago. Likewise, the health care environment has undergone massive changes, with technology and science guiding the way. It is eminent that nurses' respond to patients' needs, which have evolved with, and as a result of, modern health care. It is vital that the patient remain the central focus of care and that nurses develop new insights and skills to assure individualized patient care. Perhaps a revitalization of the basic caring acts, such as the use of touch, can bring new life and humanization into care as nurses face the challenges of the future.

REFERENCES

1. Leininger M: The phenomenon of caring, part V: Caring, the essence and central focus of nursing. Nurse Res Rep 12:2, 14, 1977
2. Hyde A: The phenomenon of caring, part VI. Nurse Res Rep 12:2, 1977
3. Marsh N: Teaching care to the carers. Nurs Mirror 147, No. 18:20–22, 1978
4. Cohn L: Barriers and values in the nurse/client relationship. J Assoc Rehab Nurs III, No. 6:3–8, 1978
5. Cowper-Smith F: Nurse could you care more? Nurs Times 74, No. 46:1882–1883, 1978
6. Kalish BJ: An experiment in the development of empathy in nursing students. Nurs Res 20, No. 3:202–211, 1971
7. Jourard S: The Transparent Self: Self-Disclosure and Well-Being. Princeton, D Van Nostrand Co, 1964
8. Goodykoontz L: Touch: Dynamic aspect of nursing care. J Nurs Care 13:16–18, 1980
9. Burnside I (ed): Nursing and the Aged, 2nd ed, p 511. New York, McGraw-Hill, 1981
10. Cashar L, Dixson B: The therapeutic use of touch. J Psych Nurs 5:442–451, 1967
11. Day F: The patient's perception of touch. In Anderson E et al (eds): Current Concepts in Clinical Nursing. St Louis, CV Mosby, 1973
12. Barnett K: A survey of the current utilization of touch by health team personnel with hospitalized patients. Int J Nurs Stud 9:195–208, 1972
13. Goodykoontz L: Touch: Attitudes and practice. Nurs Forum 18, No. 1.1:1–17, 1979
14. Clement JM: A Descriptive Study of the Use of Touch by Nurses with Patients in Critical Care. Doctoral dissertation, The University of Texas at Austin, Austin, Texas, 1983
15. Watson W: The meaning of touch: Geriatric nursing. J Commun 25:104–111, 1975
16. Weiss S: Familial Tactile Correlates of Body Image in Children. Unpublished doctoral dissertation, San Francisco, University of California, 1975
17. Weiss S: The language of touch. Nurs Res 28, No. 2:76–80, 1979
18. Heslin R: Steps toward a taxonomy of touching. Paper presented to the Midwestern Psychological Association, May, 1974

BIBLIOGRAPHY

Ball T, Edgar C: The effectiveness of sensorimotor training in promoting generalized body image development. J Spec Educ 1:387–395, 1967
Brady S: Patterns of Mothering. New York, International Universities Press, 1956
Broderman A et al: Touch me, like me: Testing an encounter group assumption. J Appl Behav Sci 8:527–533, 1972
Burnside I: Touching is talking. Am J Nurs 73:2060–2063, 1973
Burton A, Heller L: The touching of the body. Psychoanal Rev 51:127–133, 1964
Casler L: Effects of extra tactile stimulation on a group of institutionalized infants. Genet Psychol Monogr 71:137–175, 1965
Cratty BJ: Motor Activity and the Education of Retardates, 2nd ed. Philadelphia, Lea and Febiger, 1974
Farrah S: The nurse—the patient—and touch. In Duffy M (ed): Current Concepts in Clinical Nursing. St Louis, CV Mosby, 1971
Forer B: The taboo against touching in psychotherapy. Psychother Theor, Res, Pract 6:229–231, 1969
Geldard F: Some neglected possibilities of communication. Science 131:1583–1588, 1960
Jourard S: An exploratory study of body accessibility. Br J Soc Clin Psychol 5:221–231, 1966
Kenshalo D: Intensive and extensive aspects of tactile sensitivity as a function of body part, sex, and laterality. In Skin Senses, pp 195–218. Proceedings of the First International Symposium on the Skin Senses, Florida State University. Springfield, IL, Charles C Thomas, 1968
Lowen A: Language of the Body. New York, Collier Books, 1958
Mintz E: On the rationale of touch in psychotherapy. Psychother Theor, Res, Pract 6, No. 4:232–234, 1969
Mongagu A: Touching. New York, Harper & Row, 1971
Pluckhan ML: Human Communications: The Matrix for Nursing. New York, McGraw-Hill, 1978
Ribble MA: The Rights of Infants. New York, Columbia University Press, 1943
Rubin R: Maternal touch. Nurs Outlook 11:828–831, 1963
Seaman L: Affective nursing touch. Geriatric Nurs 3:162–164, 1982

6
Patient Responses to the Critical Care Setting

Janice S. Smith

There are many factors affecting patients in critical care units in addition to the illness or injury for which they are admitted. This chapter will discuss the following factors affecting patients and ways in which nurses can avoid or minimize factors that cause adverse affects:

- Sensory input (deprivation, overload, hospital phenomenon)
- Nursing assessment and intervention including, special consideration for the unresponsive patient
- Periodicity and sleep
- Special considerations for the elderly, including sensory deficit, acute brain syndrome, privacy needs, facing death.

Patients in today's critical care units are surrounded by advanced technology that, on one hand, is essential to saving their lives but, on the other hand, may create a totally alien and life-threatening environment for them. Critical care unit personnel must possess expertise in the use of this equipment while remaining aware that fear of equipment may create serious stress reactions in patients. If life-preserving measures are to have any value for the patient, the nurse must be aware of aspects of care beyond the patient's physical needs and the mechanical workings of the ever-increasing array of machines that medical technology is producing.

The psychosocial support needed by the patient in the critical care unit demands more than assistance in dealing with a critical illness. The sounds and activities of the unit are bombarding the patient 24 hours a day; in addition, the patient must cope with the effects of fear concerning illness. Normal defense mechanisms that allow us to cope with threatening situations are diminished in all patients and probably absent in the unresponsive patient. The ability to run from a frightening or painful stimulus is gone, as is the ability to analyze a situation objectively and take action to control it.

To appreciate how devastating confinement to a critical care unit can be, the nurse needs only to think of her own feelings about reversing roles with a patient. When asked if they would volunteer to spend 24 hours in the patient role in the crisis care unit, nurses respond readily with a definite "No!" Because of awareness of the environmental threats of such units, the nurse, as primary caretaker, can function as the negotiator for the patient. The following concepts may help the nurse be an effective negotiator.

SENSORY INPUT

The broad concept of sensory input deals with stimulation of all of the five senses: visual, auditory, olfactory, tactile, and gustatory. Stimuli to all the senses may be perceived in a qualitative manner as pleasant or unpleasant, acceptable or unacceptable, desirable or undesirable, soothing or painful. Individual perceptions of stimuli may vary drastically. Some individuals may consider the sounds and smells of a metropolitan business section to be pleasant, acceptable, and desirable, whereas others may find it painful.

Everyday activities, including the choice of food or drink, are based on the individual's perception of what is liked or disliked. Thus, people tend to choose, whenever possible, the environment or stimuli from the environment most acceptable to them. Patients in the critical care unit, however, have no control over the choice of their environment or most of its stimuli.

In addition to the *quality* of a stimulus, the nurse must also consider the *quantity*. Too much of a desirable stimulus can become as unacceptable as too little stimulation. For example, gorging oneself with a favorite food to the point of revulsion is "too much of a good thing." In the critical care unit, too much undesirable stimuli such as excessive and constant noise, bright light, and hyperactivity can be as distorting and bothersome as too little stimuli such as gloom, silence, and inactivity.

In trying to control environmental stimuli in a critical care unit, the nurse must therefore be aware of both the type and the amount of sensory input. If sensory stimuli are diminished too drastically, the patient is exposed to *sensory deprivation,* which can cause severe disorganization of normal psychological defenses. When sensory stimuli occur in excessive quantity, the phenomenon of *sensory overload* will create an equally undesirable response to the environment, including confusion and withdrawal.

Sensory Deprivation

Sensory deprivation is a general term used to identify a variety of symptoms that occur following a reduction in the quantity or the degree of structure or quality of sensory input. Other terms used to denote sensory deprivation or some form of it include *isolation, confinement, informational underload, perceptual deprivation,* and *sensory restriction.* A variety of symptoms or changes in behavior have been noted in normal adults following exposure to sensory deprivation for varying lengths of time. These include loss of sense of time; presence of delusions, illusions, and hallucinations; restlessness; and any of the types of behavior or symptoms present in psychoses.

Sensory deprivation need not be present for a period of days or weeks for psychopathologic reactions to occur. For example, in one study conducted on a normal young male subject, an 8-hour period of sensory deprivation elicited an acute psychotic reaction followed by continuation of delusions for several days and severe depression and anxiety for a period of several weeks.[1]

The degree of sensory deprivation possible in a laboratory setting is greater than that likely in a critical care unit. We must remember, however, that laboratory subjects are aware of the time involved in the experiment and have the ability to stop anytime they wish. They also possess clinically normal defense mechanisms and total control of the situation. Hospital patients do not have these advantages.

Sensory Overload

The area of sensory overload has not received as much attention as that of sensory deprivation, but some of its effects on humans are known. One of the best-documented adverse effects is that of decreased hearing following long-term exposure to high noise levels. It is also recognized that tension and anxiety increase when an individual is exposed to noise for continuous periods of time without quiet periods of rest. Edgar Allan Poe capitalized on such knowledge in horror stories dealing with the effect of continuous rhythmic sounds such as the dripping of water or the whirring of machinery, as in "The Pit and the Pendulum." In more modern settings we have heard of the use of continuous noise as a means of torturing prisoners of war. Nurses must capitalize on such information. For example, when patients become increasingly anxious or restless, nurses must consider environmental causes such as noise as well as physiological reasons such as hypercarbia in trying to determine the cause of such behavior.

Many years ago Florence Nightingale expressed her awareness of the effects of noise on patients: "Unnecessary noise is the most cruel absence of care which can be inflicted on either sick or well."[2]

Clues about the significance of both the quantity and quality of noise are offered by a study conducted in a recovery room. It was found that high levels of noise increased the need for pain medication. It is interesting to note, however, that the most pronounced reaction on the part of the recovery room patient was that of resentment of the sound of occasional laughter from the recovery room personnel.[3]

The normal egocentricity of persons facing an illness crisis must be recognized by the nurse. With this knowledge it is easy to understand that transient paranoia will cause the patient to interpret all action around him as pertaining to him. The laughter of the staff is laughter at him. The patient who overhears a discussion by staff members may interpret it as meaning, "I am dying, but they won't tell me." Hospital personnel should be certain that all talking and laughing in the patient care areas is intended to be heard by the patients. If patients do not have soundproof areas, the staff must modify their behavior and go to another area to socialize.

The Hospital Phenomenon. The ideal environment for anyone who is ill is one that is conducive to rest and recuperation from illness. No one would describe the hospital critical care units in such terms. A bitter joke frequently heard from patients is that a luxury hotel room is cheaper, has better food and service, and provides a better chance to get a rest.

The fact is that the hospital environment is one that

deprives the patient of normal sensory stimuli while it bombards him with continuous strange sensory stimuli not found in the average home environment. This situation is a combination of sensory deprivation and sensory overload that will be referred to as the *hospital phenomenon.*

Normal sounds at home include voices of loved ones and friends; barking of neighborhood dogs; automobile, bus, and train traffic and horns; the television or radio on a familiar station; children at play; the washing machine or dishwasher; daytime telephone calls; and many other sounds and sights that diminish when night comes. Sounds in critical care units, however, include voices of strangers in large numbers; movement of bed rails; beeping of cardiac monitors; paging systems calling strange names; suctioning of tracheostomies; telephones ringing at all hours; whispers, laughter, and muffled voices. These are accompanied by continuous lighting, strange views of equipment, fear, and pain.

Stress. Signs of high psychological stress occur in from 30% to 70% of all patients in critical care units.[4] This finding indicates that the surroundings must be controlled as much as possible so that environmentally induced stress can be minimized.

It is possible that nurses in critical care units like the noisy, hectic environment and inadvertently may encourage rather than control it. Whether or not that is so, over 25 years of evidence suggest that psychotic behavior can result when sensory deprivation occurs. More recent evidence from the 1970s and 1980s indicates that sensory overload has similar effects.

Nursing Assessment of Sensory Input

Because both sensory deprivation and sensory overload can adversely affect patients, the environment should be assessed for sensory stimuli (sounds, lights, touch, interruptions) throughout the entire day and night. The nurse should note the type of stimuli as well as their source, location, duration, and frequency. The nurse must also evaluate the quality and quantity of stimuli and how they affect the patient.

Excessive stimuli in the environment are significant causes of psychological problems in patients in critical care units. When environmental stimuli exceed the limits to which the human organism can comfortably adapt, the coping system fails. When this occurs, behaviors such as anxiety, panic, confusion, delusions, illusions, or hallucinations may occur (Table 6-1).

The combination of the loss of familiar stimuli and the continuous exposure to strange stimuli elicits different types of defensive responses from patients. Withdrawal is a common coping mechanism and may cause a patient to be labeled erroneously as confused or disoriented unless a complete assessment is done. Some degree of withdrawal from the frightening reality of the situation is common. Table 6-2 lists additional responses to sensory overload.

TABLE 6-1
NURSING DIAGNOSES AND SYMPTOMS RELATED TO HIGH NOISE LEVELS

Diagnoses	Symptoms
Alterations in comfort (pain)	Increased need for pain medication
Sleep pattern disturbance	Inability to sleep
Anxiety	Feelings of fear, helplessness, forgetfullness, withdrawal
Sensory-perceptual alterations	Reaction that talk, laughter, and so forth is aimed at him
Alterations in thought processes	Confusion, delusions, illusions, or hallucinations

---

TABLE 6-2
INFORMATION OVERLOAD RESPONSES

No processing of information
Incorrect processing of information
Selective processing of information
Escape from the flow of information

Nursing Intervention for Sensory Input

Using the Nursing History to Plan Sensory Stimulation

A nursing history included in the initial phase of planning can help make nursing intervention an effective part of the total care. Such a history requires that individualized questions be asked of both patient and family members. A brief outline of a normal 24-hour period of activity and sleep habits gives the nurse a good starting point in compiling data. A simple rule to use in collecting a nursing history is to determine what is significant or familiar to the patient and expose him to it, if possible.

Additional information that may be included in the nursing history can be anything from food likes and dislikes to favorite type of music or TV programs. It would be desirable to provide exposure to familiar stimuli such as playing a favorite record from home or finding the right radio station to listen to or requesting a taped message sent from a loved one who cannot visit. Such action will offer meaningful sensory stimulation to the patient in an otherwise unfamiliar environment. The family and friends should be involved in planning and providing such sensory input, especially for unresponsive patients. The potential value of a familiar voice in giving information or encouragement to a patient is made clear in the following case study.

CASE STUDY

A young woman was admitted to a critical care unit shortly after Christmas. She had a diagnosis of viral encephalopathy and a guarded prognosis. She became unresponsive within a few hours, and her husband was told that she was not expected to live. In spite of this she held on to life for 2 months, during which the hopeless prognosis remained. Twice more, the husband was told that death was imminent.

Finally, after the last message from the hospital that his wife was dying, the young husband told his 2½-year-old son that his mother was dying. The child repeatedly told his father not to worry because his mommy wouldn't die. The father took the boy to the critical care unit to see his mother for the last time.

While there the boy said, "I love you, Mommy." To the shock of all except the boy, his mother opened her eyes for the first time. The young woman later told everyone, "I had forgotten everything until I heard his voice say 'I love you, Mommy.'" She is well on the road to recovery now.

Reality Testing

For reality testing to occur, there must be continuous input of familiar, meaningful information from the person's outside world. When this does not occur, such as under experimental conditions of sensory deprivation, the person's internal mental events can be mistaken for external ones.[5] This could easily explain why some critical care patients appear to have hallucinations, and it points out the need to provide familiar and *meaningful* information to all patients in such a threatening setting.

The sounds of the critical care unit cannot be said to be familiar, however, to more than a few medical and nursing personnel who spend long periods of their working life in such an environment. Therefore, the nurse in the critical care unit should be certain that the environment offers the patient appropriate stimuli to provide for reality testing.

As human beings we take our physical environment for granted, but if we suddenly awoke in a world without grass or sunlight or the sounds of traffic or human speech, we would not have the necessary stimuli to keep our minds in contact with reality. We would try to interpret the unknown stimuli on the basis of that with which we have always been familiar. In reality, however, our interpretations may be wrong. This is especially true of patients who suffer temporary loss of any of the senses, particularly vision or hearing, because people normally employ a combination of senses to interpret their environment.

This lack of reality testing may offer at least partial explanation for the high incidence of psychosis in patients commonly assigned to critical care units for long-term care due to an "unconscious state." The fact that no physical reason has ever been identified to explain posttraumatic psychosis offers additional support for such an assumption.

Nursing has been influenced by authorities in the field who perpetuate the concept that unconscious patients are insensitive to their environment and have perceptual disturbances that affect their responses to the environment. In view of the necessity of reality testing and the lack of meaningful information to allow such testing in the critical care unit, it is reasonable to explain some of the reactions of patients, even those of the unconscious patient, as being caused by the lack of meaningful input, which can be referred to as *sensory deprivation*. There is more empirical data to support this assumption than there is evidence for believing that posttraumatic psychosis is due to physical phenomena.

One example of sensory deprivation in the critical care unit involved an unresponsive patient assumed to be unconscious by both the medical and nursing team members. This situation is described in the following case study.

CASE STUDY

Carol was a 20-year-old college student with severe basal skull trauma and multiple injuries. She was unresponsive throughout the 8-day period she spent in a critical care unit.

When Carol began responding verbally, her first words to her mother were, "Am I free now? I was in the hands of the Soviet Union!" An immediate interpretation of such a statement could reasonably be that she was totally out of contact with reality owing to the injury and had dreamed such an episode. It is just as reasonable to assume that she could have perceived that the actions in the unit and the treatments she received were related to torture and that she was the victim for some unknown reason.

Carol had no noticeable motor control of her facial muscles, so she was "blind." She had a tracheostomy that required frequent suctioning. She was almost immobile because of fractures and spasticity necessitating plaster casts or cloth restraints on all extremities. Because she had no means of interpreting her experience realistically from meaningful cues in the environment, it is reasonable to assume that such a situation could cause her to believe that she was being tortured.

Although all patients are susceptible to sensory deprivation and overload, those who are at highest risk and most likely to be seriously affected are the following groups:

• The very young
• The very old
• The postoperative
• The unconscious (unresponsive)

Special Consideration: The Unresponsive Patient
The patient who can communicate is likely to seek out relevant and meaningful information by questioning visitors and those involved in his care. However, the nurse in the critical care unit must be the eyes, ears, and voice for those at risk, specifically the unresponsive patient.

Because the unresponsive patient may be most likely to suffer the greatest psychological trauma related to the effects of the environment, his psychosocial needs require the greatest concern. One barrier to providing this attention may be the attitude of hopelessness fostered by the patient's being referred to as "unconscious" rather than "unresponsive." "Unconscious" denotes a lack of sensory awareness that cannot currently be measured in the absence of concurrent motor response, whereas "unresponsive" means that motor- and sensory-coordinated responses cannot be elicited.

Replacing the label "unconscious" with the term "unresponsive" can help remove the connotation of lack of awareness that is usually associated with the first word. It is very likely that some unresponsive patients are also unconscious. However, because it is currently impossible to validate such an assessment, the best approach is to assume that *no patient is unconscious.* This attitude paves the way for providing sensory input to unresponsive patients.

Intervention for the Unresponsive Patient. This involves provision of total physical care and a structured environment that includes intentional, meaning-

ful, sensory stimulation. To accomplish this, the nurse must collect data from any person who knows the patient and who is available to give information. For example, the nurse can ask about the patient's musical tastes, his favorite radio station, his hobbies, and his activities during a typical week. Answers to the last question make it possible for the nurse to provide familiar activities that can help keep the patient oriented to time. The nurse must always be on the lookout for clues that will help her provide information that may make it easier for the patient to keep in contact with his world. Other ways of creating a structured and familiar environment include having as much care given by the same person as is possible on each shift. Encouraging family and friends to visit and to communicate will result in further meaningful sensory stimulation.

Family and friends may need instruction and encouragement about approaching the unresponsive patient. The nurse should let them know that they can speak to and then touch the patient. She should communicate to them that it is not only alright but also very desirable for them to touch the patient's hand, arm, or face or to kiss him if it is part of their usual relationship (and does not interfere with any equipment attached to the patient). Do not assume that loved ones standing at the bedside know that they can touch the unresponsive person. Most visitors must be given permission as well as instruction.

One of the most agonizing feelings is that of uselessness on the part of a family member or friend at the bedside of an unresponsive loved one. The scene of a mother, father, husband, wife, or other close relative standing at the bedside and staring with a variety of emotions at the unresponsive patient is the opportunity for intervention. A simple direction or, in some cases, encouragement to touch the patient's hand and talk to him may bring a look of relief and gratitude to their faces. With further assistance on what to say to the patient, visitors can be very effective in diminishing sensory deprivation by discussing familiar people or subjects and topics of interest to the patient.

The value of simple conversation about everyday activities is underestimated in the care of the unresponsive patient in critical care units. This is pointed out vividly in the following case study.*

CASE STUDY
While caring for a patient in her late fifties who was comatose as a result of metastatic carcinoma of the brain, I carried on a one-sided conversation about many things, including a daily introduction of myself, explanations of care to be given, and discussion of the day and the weather. There was no percepti-

*Smith JS: *A Study of Sensory Response in the Unconscious Patient.* Thesis submitted to the faculty of the Graduate School of the University of Colorado in partial fulfillment of the requirements for the degree of Master of Science, School of Nursing, 1970

ble response from the patient. Her condition appeared to be slowly deteriorating. I lost contact with her after 4 days because of an assignment change.

While boarding a train about 2 months later, I was approached by a woman on crutches who called me by name and asked if I were a nurse. I answered yes and eventually recognized the patient. Our discussion revealed much about our initial relationship. The patient expressed how she had felt during the days she lay in the hospital bed, totally defenseless and at the mercy of those on the nursing team. She said it was very important to her that I had identified myself and talked to her each day.

Of particular interest to the patient was information about when I would leave and when I would return. When I said I would be leaving for another assignment she said she cried because she anticipated receiving no further information about the outside world. The patient recalled much more about the interaction than I did.

Such experiences indicate that even in today's modern nursing world the little things, such as consideration of the patient as an individual deserving common courtesies, are very important to patients. It cannot be taken for granted that such behavior is automatic; nurses are conditioned to be comfortable around the hectic environment of a critical care unit and quickly forget the sense of awe or fear that was present the first time they saw the unit.

It might be helpful for the nurses in the critical care unit to stop for a moment each day and project themselves mentally into the patient's role to determine what information or activity might be desirable. This can help nurses maintain human dignity in their patients, even those who have been subjected to the regressive procedures of being bathed, fed, and forced to meet toileting needs in bed, shielded from other patients only by a cloth curtain with wide openings at top and bottom.

Many other situations and case histories can be reported to stress the importance of planning for and providing meaningful sensory stimulation for the patients cared for in all hospital units, especially the ones in critical care units. Nurses can play a significant role in alleviating the unnecessary stress caused by sensory deprivation by recognizing the need for the structuring of sensory input.

The use of auditory stimuli such as the explanation of any treatment or procedure to be performed on a patient is a basic requirement and must not be overlooked as insignificant. But explanation alone is not adequate to prevent adverse effects of sensory deprivation. This type of communication can be considered a minimal requirement in a broader area of communication called *security information.*

Providing for Security Information

Security information helps prevent unnecessary anxiety and disorientation regarding date, time, and place. It also includes explanation of treatment and proce-

dures. This is particularly important for patients with deviations in levels of consciousness due to trauma, drugs, or toxicity. Nurses can encourage orientation to date and time not only by including the information in conversation but also by providing large-faced clocks that are readily visible to the patient and large calendars that display the day, month, and year in large figures. The simplicity of such information sometimes causes it to be overlooked, but the nurse can increase the patient's comfort by providing information that we take for granted. In addition, it is necessary to provide this information because an assessment of the patient's state of orientation is often based on his answers to questions concerning time and place.

Because many patients cope by withdrawing, nurses should anticipate a delayed response when calling the patient's name and should provide extra environmental objects and planned repetition to orient the patient to time, date, and place. In addition to the voices of the nursing staff, a familiar person's voice can be very helpful in providing such information.

Controlling Noise

The nursing staff can control the general environmental stimuli, with the exception of some equipment essential to life support systems. Nurses can determine the amount of lighting needed and may be able to control various sounds used on some monitors that have light alarms instead of sound alarms. Cardiac monitors should not be kept in areas in which patients are exposed to their continuous beeping. The physical planning for units must provide facilities in which patients on continuous respirators are not in the same open area as other patients. However, methods have not yet been devised for protecting patients on respirators from the machine's incessant cycling noise. Other patients in the unit also should be protected from the respirator's noise. If individual soundproofed patient units are not provided, at least one unit should be available for use by all patients who are on noisy life-support systems.

Preventing Exhaustion

The continual high level of environmental stimuli in critical care units *must be minimized at planned periods* of time during every 24-hour period. Critical care personnel must form a definite plan to accomplish this goal rather than simply allowing it to happen. Only a major crisis should prevent each patient from having a "quiet time" in each 24-hour period. The optimal plan allows for up to 8 hours of sleep; the minimal plan provides for at least some full 2-hour periods of uninterrupted sleep. Current monitoring systems usually allow for a safe 2-hour undisturbed period for most patients because they permit vital signs to be obtained without direct patient contact.

Sleep is essential to both physical well-being and

mental well-being. The human organism must have normal, uninterrupted periods of sleep that are long enough to allow all stages of sleep to occur. Normally, a minimal period of 2 to 3 hours is required, but even that is probably not adequate for most people for longer than a day or two (see discussion of sleep, further on).

Providing for sleep seems simple until one realizes what is necessary to meet such a need. A darkened room makes it impossible to observe the critically ill patient visually, but few people can sleep in a lighted room even if the lighting level is low or soft. Normal practice is to sedate patients in such a unit, but the nurse must realize that drug-induced or interrupted sleep is not adequate for any significant period of time.

PERIODICITY/SLEEP

Another area of knowledge necessary for the nurse in the critical care unit involves the broad concept of *periodicity*. Other terms include *circadian rhythm, biological clock, internal clock,* and *physiological clock.* It has been recognized for a number of years that all living creatures have not only an identifiable life cycle but also short-term cycles that are rhythmical in nature; disruption of that rhythm can cause deviations from the norm or cessation of life.

Daily Cycle. The human organism possesses a 24-hour cycle that is resistant to change, and long-term disruption can be fatal. Many of the biochemical and biophysical processes of the human body have rhythms, with peaks of function or activity that occur in consistent patterns within the normal, customary 24-hour day.

Physiological Variations. Knowledge of when physiological functions are at their lowest level would allow for more intelligent assessment of the significance of vital-sign fluctuation. For example, normal variations in the quantity of urine output should be expected, because the kidneys possess their own unique rhythm as demanded by sleep and activity patterns.

In the future, health care personnel may schedule drug dosage, sleep periods, and stressful procedures such as surgery on the basis of their knowledge of individual circadian rhythms, thus avoiding further stress in the most vulnerable part of the cycle and capitalizing on the strongest parts of the cycle.

Sleep. The human organism functions on a 24-hour cycle and cannot adapt to any other one. There are both physiological and psychological necessities for sleep that affect humans' potential for maximal recovery from illness in minimal time. Probably the most significant sleep deprivation is in the area of rapid eye

movement (REM) sleep because it occurs later in the sleep cycle. REM sleep is necessary for mental restoration and occurs mainly in the last cycles of an uninterrupted night of sleep. The normal person experiences four or five cycles of sleep, with each lasting about 90 minutes. Disrupting the continuity of sleep cycles in the critical care unit probably causes most deprivation in the REM stage. This further threatens the psychological well-being of the patient.

Adverse side effects are numerous in people who are deprived of the stages of deep sleep and REM sleep for even a few days. The adverse effects include irritability and anxiety, physical exhaustion and fatigue, and even disruption of metabolic functions, including adrenal hormone production.

Such adverse effects indicate the necessity for providing an environment that is conducive to all stages of sleep, including the REM stage. Because a cycle of sleep measured from REM stage to REM stage requires from 90 to 100 minutes, it is important to provide periods of a minimum of 2 hours of uninterrupted sleep during the night. More frequent arousal can cause enough disruption to deprive the patient of essential cyclic rest and activity periods and create a situation incompatible with life.

Nursing Assessment and Intervention That Consider Periodicity

When assessing the patient's condition, the nurse should consider whether or not there have been adequate uninterrupted time periods for all stages of sleep to occur. The plan must provide such periods as early as possible following the patient's admission to the unit. The necessity of taking vital signs every 1 or 2 hours during the night must be weighed against the damage caused to the human organism when it is deprived of sleep. Physiological functions reach their lowest levels in the middle of the night, whereas in the early morning hours functions are beginning to reach a maximum level. Therefore, normal fluctuations in vital signs should be expected and patients should not be subjected to activity or stressful procedures in the early morning hours (see preceding discussion of preventing exhaustion).

The night hours must be treated in such a way that the human organism is provided with essential rest at the optimal time. Only absolutely essential life-preserving activities should be allowed to disturb the patient at night. For example, critically ill patients should not be bathed between 2:00 and 5:00 A.M. only because the staff has time available.

Visiting hours should be adjusted to allow for longer periods of rest. For example, the potentially harmful and unnecessarily rigid policy of allowing visitors 5 minutes with the patient every hour should be seriously reconsidered. For the patient to be disturbed every hour is certainly more harmful than using knowledge of sleep research and periodicity in planning visiting times and nursing care activities. Longer periods of time with the patient could be provided during the nonsleeping hours as one way of individualizing visiting policies.

In addition, such visiting restrictions often produce hostility from family members as they struggle to have some time with the patient. Sharing knowledge of sleep research and periodicity with family members in a proper manner will probably elicit a willingness to work out an acceptable arrangement for sharing time with the patient. Nursing care measures should not always take priority over time for relatives or significant others.

Rest periods for the patient should be provided with the same emphasis as that given to assessment of cardiac status and other aggressive physical measures of care. Commitment to controlling the activity of the environment can diminish the constant level of noise, but additional measures may be necessary. If the patient is receptive to wearing darkened eyeshades and ear plugs to shut out light and sound, he may be able to tolerate the environment with less stress. This is the least we can offer a patient to minimize the adverse effects of the environment until units can be developed that consider rest and sleep for the critically ill patient. No patient needs such consideration more, but the irony of the situation is that the critically ill patient is placed in the least desirable environment for meeting such needs. Perhaps our intense efforts to improve care through the development of special critical care units is in some ways causing us to endanger the well-being of the patients.

SPECIAL CONSIDERATIONS FOR THE ELDERLY IN CRITICAL CARE

Because of the large number of elderly people who require intensive care, critical care nurses need to be knowledgeable about the special problems of the elderly. Because the elderly often experience some deterioration of their senses, they are at higher risk for developing psychological problems as a result of altered sensory input.

In order to diminish the potentially adverse effects of the critical care environment for the elderly, the nurse must do the following:

- Assess the senses and build in nursing interventions for sensory deficits.
- Assess for the symptoms of acute brain syndrome
- Use reality orientation therapeutically.
- Use touch in a therapeutic way.
- Apply the concept of territoriality as it relates to aging.

- Know the view on death and dying commonly held by elderly people.

Nursing Assessment and Intervention for Sensory Deficits

It is necessary to assess fully the senses of each elderly person, particularly for a history of visual and auditory deficits. If the elderly patient is unable to filter out environmental sounds in order to hear soft-spoken words, talking louder or asking the patient to use a hearing aid may help. It will not help, however, to talk loudly (or yell) at the elderly person whose hearing is intact but whose motor responses are diminished or blocked by injury, such as that caused by a cerebral vascular accident. The nurse should always speak within the patient's line of vision because lip reading is used (often unconsciously) by many people who have a slowly developing hearing loss.

If an elderly patient wears glasses, it is important to provide a clean pair even if he does not request them. Clean glasses will enable the patient to familiarize himself with the environment and see what is going on around him. Also, if the patient must rely on lip reading to understand what is being said to him, glasses will enhance his ability to communicate.

Older people may also require more time to respond to verbal requests because motor responses tend to slow with age. This, along with the tendency to withdraw from the hyperactivity of the critical care unit, may further delay the response time. Because of these factors, it may be necessary when asking questions to allow a longer period of time for any motor or vocal response. It is reasonable to wait a full minute before repeating a request.

Nursing Assessment of Acute Brain Syndrome

Actions that appear to denote disorientation of a pathologic nature may be prematurely labeled *chronic brain syndrome* when they may actually be *acute brain syndrome*. In view of the grave consequences of hopelessness projected on the patient with chronic brain syndrome, it is imperative that adequate historic data be collected to differentiate between the two conditions. The primary difference between acute and chronic brain syndromes is that acute brain syndrome has a rapid onset but is considered reversible, whereas chronic brain syndrome is slow in onset and is irreversible. The significance of such differences has a great impact upon nursing care.

To begin, the nurse should obtain a concise but complete nursing history, including as much recent information about normal functioning of the individual patient as can be obtained. If the patient is unable to provide the information, every effort must be made to contact the person or persons who have lived most closely with the patient. A telephone call to the home may provide much information and improve the quality of care for the patient while he is in the highly stressfull environment. If the patient's functioning has been adequate for self-care prior to admission to the critical care unit, it should be assumed that any confusion or mental malfunctioning is potentially reversible.

The patient who is admitted to a CCU will have either a serious trauma or sudden illness that automatically places him at risk for developing acute brain syndrome. Assessing for acute brain syndrome is not always easy, but the nurse may anticipate some symptoms, such as the following:

• Fluctuation in the level of awareness
• Visual hallucinations (auditory hallucinations are not present)
• Misidentification of persons (usually in the form of thinking a nurse is some close relative such as a sister or daughter)
• Severe restlessness
• Memory impairment

Table 6-3 lists other symptoms of acute brain syndrome.

It must be recognized that the environmental stresses of the CCU coupled with the psychosocial impact of illness can be enough to cause mental impairment that may be labeled acute brain syndrome.

A sudden change in the elderly person's life, such as removal from familiar surroundings or administration of certain sedative and tranquilizing drugs, can precipitate these symptoms. The following situation reported by Kiely illustrates these points.[6]

CASE STUDY

A 78-year-old retired schoolteacher was knocked down by a purse snatcher while on her way to a neighborhood grocery store. There was no physical injury evident, but the event triggered an episode of paroxysmal tachyarrhythmia accompanied by vascular collapse with a blood pressure of 79/30 mm Hg.

At the emergency room she was able to recount her experience coherently and seemed more upset by the loss of her eyeglasses than her purse. She seemed mildly disoriented about time and place. A comprehensive physical and laboratory examination revealed only a low blood pressure and atrial flutter. With treatment, both returned to normal.

The patient's mental status, however, continued to deteriorate. She became increasingly disoriented and demanded that nursing personnel explain their presence in her "apartment." She became restless, climbed over the bedrails, and, when soft restraints were applied, became even more restless. Then she heard voices and screamed that people were trying to kill her. Amytal (amobarbital sodium), 500 mg IM, initially sedated her but later heightened her arousal.

TABLE 6-3
SYMPTOMS OF ACUTE BRAIN SYNDROME

Disorders of Cognition

Impairment in perception, memory, and thinking
Behavior includes
1 = disorientation for location and time
2 = confusion of unknown persons with familiar ones
3 = delusions that food is poisoned
4 = memory impairment (makes it difficult to learn instructions about own care, such as when to take medications)

Abnormal Sleep – Waking Cycle

Disorders of attention, vigilance, and sleep dysfunction
Behavior includes
1 = insomnia
2 = vivid night dreams
3 = agitation as darkness occurs ("sundown syndrome")
4 = reduced attention time
5 = under-alertness or over-alertness
6 = fluctuation of awareness from drowsiness to lucidity

Disorders of Psychomotor Behavior

Generally nonspecific
Behavior includes
1 = wandering
2 = fluctuation from intense agitation to somnolence
3 = combative behavior, usually due to fear

(Compiled in part from Granacher RP Jr: Agitation in the elderly: An often-treatable manifestation of acute brain syndrome. Postgrad Med 72, No. 6:83–96, 1982)

The shock of these events and the changes that they created for this elderly woman were further aggravated by the following:

• Decreased sensory input (due to loss of her glasses)
• Misinterpreted sensory input
• Use of restraints
• Use of drugs

It is easy to see how situations like this one escalate. One can even imagine that these events could lead to institutionalization in an extended care facility if thoughtful assessment, planning, and care did not short-circuit or eventually help reverse the symptoms. Table 6-4 shows additional causes of acute brain syndrome.

Nursing Intervention in Acute Brain Syndrome

While a comprehensive and exhaustive evaluation is made to determine a possible causative factor that can be corrected, the nurse must use all knowledge available to make the environment a therapeutic tool rather than a stressor for the patient. A concerted effort by the nursing staff to help the patient achieve reality orientation must be started immediately as a primary treatment, regardless of the cause of symptoms (Table 6-5).

Need for Reality Orientation

Reality orientation requires a rigid, repetitive regimen of giving security information at predetermined times around the clock. The monotony of the procedure may make nurses want to give up the regimen when there is no positive response after a few days. For the benefit of the patient, however, the regimen must continue until the patient can repeat the information on request (or until the patient's death releases the nurse from the responsibility). After a few days, repetition is more comfortable if the nurse prefaces the information with a statement to the patient that she knows the information has been stated many times but that it is important to repeat it until the patient is able to say it to her. Such repetition should continue until the patient recovers or dies.

Nursing interventions include the following:

TABLE 6-4
POSSIBLE REVERSIBLE CAUSES OF ACUTE BRAIN SYNDROME: SELECTED FACTORS

Pharmacological factors	Narcotics, sedatives, digitalis, tranquilizers, steroids, antihypertensives, antidepressants, diuretics, chemotherapeutic agents, bronchodilators, anticholinergics
Environmental factors	Abrupt change in environment, sensory deprivation, sensory overload, isolation
Psychosocial factors	Depression, loss, grief
Nutritional imbalances	Vitamin deficiencies (B$_{12}$, folic acid, niacin), starvation
Elimination imbalances	Fecal impaction, urinary retention
Trauma	Fractures, surgery, concussion/contusion, subdural hematoma, cerebral hemorrhage
Alcohol abuse	Alcohol withdrawal when hospitalized may be overlooked
Pain	Due to trauma of external or internal origin
Fluid and/or electrolyte imbalances	Sodium excess of depletion, dehydration, acid–base imbalance
Metabolic factors	Hypo- or hyperthyroidism, renal impairment, liver malfunction
Cardiovascular factors	Anemia, hypotension, congestive heart failure, myocardial infarction, arrhythmias
Bacteriologic factors	Infection (*e.g.,* pneumonia)
Body temperature	Hyperthermia, hypothermia

(Compiled from LaPorte HJ: Reversible causes of dementia: A nursing challenge. J Gerontol Nurs 8, No. 2:74–80, 1982; Doran O: Are you listening? Crit Care Nurse Sept. 2, No. 5:12, 15, 18, 1982; Chisholm E et al: Prevalence of confusion in elderly hospitalized patients. J Gerontol Nurs 8, No. 2:87–96, 1982.

TABLE 6-5
NURSING CARE PLAN: ACUTE BRAIN SYNDROME

Nursing Diagnosis/Needs	*Nursing Intervention*
Thought Processes, Alterations in	
Need for reality orientation	1:1 Give security information at predetermined times around the clock.
	1:2 <u>Repeat this information until patient is able to say it to you.</u>
Sensory Perception Alteration (Tactile)	
Need for therapeutic touch	2:1 Gently touch the patient's hand or arm frequently.
	2:2 Speak to patients with impaired sight before touching them.
Powerless	
Need for Privacy and Personal space	3:1 Ask permission to look at dressing or to perform a procedure.
	3:2 Knock before entering the patient's room.
	3:3 Use covers and curtains to provide some privacy.
	3:4 Preface intrusion into the personal territory of the patient with an explanation of the reason for invading the space.
Sleep Pattern Disturbance	
Need for sleep and rest	4:1 Provide periods of a minimum of 2 hours of uninterrupted sleep during the night.
	4:2 <u>Plan nursing care so activity and stressful procedures will not be done in the early morning hours.</u>
	4:3 When possible provide sleep time during patient's usual sleeping hours.
Anxiety/Fear; Grieving	
Facing the reality of death	5:1 Listen to the patient's feelings about dying.
	5:2 Include the family in discussions and decisions.
	5:3 DO NOT allow hospital policy to remove humanistic values from nursing care.
	5:4 Consider the right to die with human dignity.

- Answering questions repeatedly in short simple sentences
- Demonstrating things concretely and nonverbally
- Telling the patient when you do not understand him
- Not supporting his disorientation
- Orienting him as frequently as possible with vocal repetition of time and use of clocks, calendars, lights, and so forth.

Need for Therapeutic Touch

Touch is a highly therapeutic tool that the nurse should use to alleviate the intense fear that patients often feel when faced with a crisis. Even the person who normally rejects touching may feel the need for such contact at this time.

It is possible that the only comforting contact with reality for some patients is touch. The warm, firm, human touch provided by a caring nurse may be the one thing that keeps a patient hoping for life to con-

tinue. Touch accompanied by verbal communication may be the most significant factor in helping a patient maintain consciousness in a life-threatening situation.

Elderly patients who have verbal or sensory impairment may benefit greatly from supportive touch. The nurse can easily determine the patient's receptiveness by gently touching his hand or arm. If the arm is not withdrawn, it is a cue of acceptance. The nurse should take care to speak to patients who have impaired sight before touching them to avoid startling them unnecessarily (see Chap. 5).

Need for Personal Space (Territoriality)

All people have an unconsciously marked territory around them that is known as personal space. The actual size of this space is generally thought to be flexible and is thought to provide a margin of safety and security. Factors that influence the size of the space include the social situation, the physical area, the person's cultural background, and the relationship to others who are present.

Invasion of one's personal space may cause the person to experience discomfort, anger, and anxiety. It is normal for the person to defend against such a threat in order to maintain control of their personal space. In a hospital setting such space is severely limited and is often invaded by the nursing staff.

Nurses can provide the patient with some control over their personal space by practicing some common courtesies, such as knocking on the door before entering and asking permission to perform a procedure or observe a dressing. Using covers and curtains to provide some privacy also diminishes the invasion of personal space.

At a time in life when adapting to change becomes increasingly difficult and painful, the elderly patient is confronted with an extreme limitation of territory. Even the patient coming from a long-term care facility has had more space to claim and greater freedom to organize it in the manner so desired. The historically diminishing size of the territory possessed and controlled by the elderly patient creates psychological pain and a decrease in self-esteem. The nurse in a critical care unit can show sensitivity to this by avoiding unnecessary intrusion into the patient's now further diminished territory.

A visit to the home or room of an elderly person characteristically reveals the presence of multiple treasures on walls, tables, and shelves, including pictures, books, glass items, and so forth. No matter how poverty-stricken the person is, there will be some highly prized items. These objects develop increased value for the elderly as the years pass, and the nurse must protect such possessions brought to the unit and allow the patients to position them wherever they wish within the pathetically small territory allotted to them.

Further intrusions also occur in the form of impersonal equipment kept at the bedside (*e.g.,* suction machines, monitors, oxygen equipment, and IV equipment). This creates a situation in which territory is further limited to the confines of the bed and possibly a bedside stand. For this reason, the patient usually clusters all personal possessions in the bed or on the small stand.

Further limits occur because extensions of territoriality are usually not available in this setting. Examples of extensions include radio, television, and telephones. Both televisions and telephones are normally denied to the patients in the CCUs. However, the availability of small television sets with earplugs for sound control and telephones with wall jacks makes it more feasible to use both items in a critical care unit. Nursing assessment can determine the patient's ability to benefit from their use without harmful effects.

It is possible that a telephone call from a special person will do more than any medication to help a patient relax. Certainly the judicious use of ear phones to enjoy a favorite radio program will help counteract the adverse effects of the strange sounds of the critical care unit. The nurse who recognizes the potentially great therapeutic effect of such territorial extensions will incorporate them into the humanistic plan of care for all patients, with special awareness of the unique needs of the elderly.

Facing the Reality of Death

The inevitability of death must be accepted at times in the critical care unit. Being aware that many elderly people accept dying as the final stage and natural outcome of life may help the staff when it has been decided that the patient should be allowed to die without further intervention. Although this question of when to withhold further intervention is certainly not unique to the elderly, there are certain aspects of the problem that are generally more common in older people. Certainly a healthy 80-year-old patient with a history of a CVA will have dealt more directly with his feelings of dying (and his family with their feelings of losing him to death) than will have an 18-year-old patient and his family. No implication is intended, however, that age alone is the criterion for determining the extent of the heroic effort to sustain life. Age is, however, a highly significant factor to be considered along with factors such as previous state of health and current cause of illness.

It is important that whenever possible the patient's feelings about dying be listened to, and the family must be included in discussions and decisions (see Chap. 4). Enforcement of restrictive visiting rules should be ignored in such a situation to prevent further adverse effects of isolation on the patient and to assist the family in dealing with the common feelings of guilt at such a time. The family also suffers from adverse effects caused by the critical care environment. Hospital policy must not be allowed to remove humanistic values from nursing care.

Roberts has expressed an opinion that perhaps we ignore the patient's wishes and prolong the process of dying rather than the process of living.[7] She also reminds us that many aged patients have control over their lives until they lose control when admitted to the critical care unit. The role of the nurse becomes vital, and she must resolve her own feelings about death as she works with the patient and family in an advocacy role. Perhaps the elderly see what we cannot when they plead with us to let them die. It is wrong to project our personal fear of death on the patient who repeatedly pleads with us to stop our heroic efforts to sustain a poor quality of life manifested many times by constant pain and exhaustion. The right to die while human dignity is still present must be considered seriously.

REFERENCES

1. Curtis GC et al: A psychopathological reaction precipitated by sensory deprivation. Am J Psychiatry 125:255–260, 1968
2. Hurst TW: Is noise important in hospitals? Int J Nurs Stud 3:125–131, 1966
3. Minckley B: A study of noise and its relationship to patient discomfort in the recovery room. Nurs Res 17, No. 3:247–250, 1968
4. Noble MA (ed): The ICU Environment: Directions for Nursing. Reston, Virginia, Reston Publishing, 1982
5. Leff JP: Perceptual phenomena and personality in sensory deprivation. Br J Psychiatry 114:1499–1508, 1968
6. Kiely WF: Critical care psychiatric syndrome. Heart Lung 2, No. 1:54–55, 1973
7. Roberts SL: To die or not to die: Plight of the aged patient in ICU. In Burnside IM (ed): Psychosocial Nursing Care of the Aged, pp 96–106. New York, McGraw-Hill, 1973

BIBLIOGRAPHY

Adams M et al: The confused patient: Psychological responses in critical care units. Am J Nurs 78, No. 9:1504–1512, 1978
Baker CF: Sensory overload and noise in the ICU: Sources of environmental stress. Crit Care Q March, 1984, pp 66–80
Ballard KS: Identification of environmental stressors for patients in a surgical intensive care unit. Issues Mental Health Nurs 3, No. 1–2:89–108, 1981
Barry MJ: Sensory alterations, overload, and underload: Making a nursing diagnosis. In Kennedy M and Pfeifer G (eds): Current Practice in Nursing Care of the Adult, Vol 1, pp 33–45. St Louis, CV Mosby, 1979
Brigman C et al: The agitated-aggressive patient. Am J Nurs 83, No. 10:1408–1412, 1983
Bullock-Loughran P: Territoriality in critical care. Focus AACN 9, No. 5:19–21, 1982
Burnside IM: Nursing and the Aged, 2nd ed. New York, McGraw-Hill, 1981
Chisholm SE et al: Prevalence of confusion in elderly hospitalized patients. J Gerontol Nurs 8, No. 2:87–96, 1982
Doran MO: Are you listening? (Delirium). Crit Care Nurse 2, No. 5:12,15,18 1982
Falk S, Wood NF: Hospital noise-levels and potential health hazards. N Eng J Med 289:774–781, 1973
Flaherty MJ: Care of the comatose: complex problems faced alone. Nurs Manage 13, No. 10:44–46, 1982
Fulmer TT: Termination of life support systems in the elderly. Discussion: The registered nurses's role. J Geriatric Psychiatry 14, No. 1:23–30, 1981
Gorrell K: A recovery. Am J Nurs 83, No. 12:1672–1673, 1983
Gowan NJ. The perceptual world of the intensive care unit: An overview of some environmental considerations in the helping relationship. Heart Lung 8, No. 2:340–344, 1979
Granacher RP Jr: Agitation in the elderly: an often-treatable manifestation of acute brain syndrome. Postgrad Med 72, No. 6:83–95, 1982
Griffin J: Forced dependency in the critically ill. Dimens Crit Care Nurs 1, No. 6:350–352, 1982
Hamner ML, Lalor LJ: The aged patient in the critical care setting. Focus Crit Care 10, No. 6:22–29, 1983
Harris JS: Home study program. Stressors and stress in critical care. Crit Care Nurse 4, No. 1:72–76, 1984
Hayter J: The rhythm of sleep. Am J Nurs 80, No. 3:457–461, 1980
Hayter J: Sleep behaviors of older persons. Nurs Research 32, No. 4:242–246, 1983
Helton MC et al: The correlation between sleep deprivation and the intensive care unit syndrome. Heart Lung 9, No. 3:464–468, 1980
Keep P et al: Windows in the intensive therapy unit. Anaesthesia 35, No. 3:257–262, 1980
Kleck HG: ICU syndrome: onset, manifestations, treatment, stressors, and prevention. Crit Care Q 21–28, 1984
LaPorte, HJ: Reversible causes of dementia: A nursing challenge. J Gerontol Nurs 8, No. 2:74–80, 1982
Lindenmuth JE et al: Sensory overload. Am J Nurs 80, No. 8:1456–1458, 1980
Luce GG, Body time: Psychological rhythms and social stress, p 86. New York, Pantheon, 1971
MacKinnon-Kessler S: Maximizing your ICU patient's sensory and perceptual environment. Can Nurse 79, No. 5:41–45, 1983
Mappes TA, Zembaty JS: Biomedical Ethics. New York, McGraw-Hill, 1981
Mauss-Clum N: Bringing the unconscious patient back safely: nursing makes the critical difference. Nursing (Horsham) 12, No. 8:34–42, 1982
McGuire MA: A touch in the dark. Crit Care Nurse 3, No. 5:53–56, 1983
Meisenhelder JB: Boundaries of personal space: An abstract. Image 14, No. 1:16–19, 1982
Mukheibir SC: Man's inhumanity to man: Intensive care may threaten the human life. Curationis 1:9–11, 1978
Palmer MH: Alzheimer's disease and critical care. Interactions, implications, interventions. J Gerontol Nurs 9, No. 2:87–90, 116, 1983
Parsons LC and VerBack D: Sleep-awake patterns following cerebral concussion. Nurs Research 31, No. 5:260–264, 1982
Richardson K: Hope and flexibility—your keys to helping OBS patients. Nursing (Horsham) 12, No. 6:64–69, 1982
Robertson S: Them lot won't let me go. Nurs Times 74:34, 1978
Shragg TA, Albertson TE: Moral, ethical, and legal dilemmas in the intensive care unit. Crit Care Med 12, No. 1:62–68, 1984
Sime AM, Kelly JW: Lessening patient stress in the CCU. Nurs Manage 14, No. 10:24–26, 1983
Tobiason SJB: Touching is for everyone. Am J Nurs 81, No. 4:728–730, 1981
Vanson SR et al: Stress effects on patients in critical care units from procedures performed on others. Heart Lung 9, No. 3:494–497, 1980

Section II

Core Body Systems

Unit One

Cardiovascular System

7
Normal Structure and Function of the Cardiovascular System

Barbara Brockway-Fuller

During the 70 years in the life of the average person, the heart will pump approximately 5 quarts of blood per minute, 75 gallons per hour, 57 barrels a day, and 1.5 million barrels in a lifetime. The work accomplished by this organ is completely out of proportion to its size, but the surprising thing is that for most people the heart presents no illness problem. It functions normally throughout their life spans. For the person who does develop a cardiac problem, however, the result is much different. When a pathologic condition manifests itself in this vital organ, the effects may be extremely dramatic and the outcome often drastic.

This chapter will deal with the following:

• Cardiac microstructure
• Anatomical and physiological basis for contraction
• Physiological basis for events of the cardiac cycle
• Factors influencing cardiac output and perfusion.

MICROSTRUCTURE

Microscopically, cardiac muscle contains visible striations similar to those found in skeletal muscle. The ultrastructural pattern also resembles that of striated muscle. The cells branch and anastomose freely, as can be seen in Figure 7-1B, and they form a three-dimensional complex network. The elongated nuclei, like those of smooth muscle, are found deep in the interior of the cells and not adjacent to the sarcolemma, as they are in striated muscle.

Unlike skeletal muscle, which is a morphologic syncytium, cardiac muscle fibers are completely surrounded by a cell membrane. At the point where two fibers meet, the two membranes become elaborately folded into a structure known as an *intercalated disc.* These intercalated discs provide strong connections among all the fibers of the cardiac muscle.

Although cardiac muscle is not a morphologic syncytium, it functions as one. Because of the presence of the intercalated discs, whose electrical potentials are extremely low, the rapid spread of excitation from cell to cell is possible. With each contractile impulse generated at the pacemaker, the spread of excitation is so rapid that there is essentially simultaneous contraction of the entire muscle.

Yet another difference (perhaps the most important difference between cardiac muscle and skeletal muscle cells) is that of *automaticity*, whereby cardiac muscle cells are capable of initiating rhythmic action potentials, and thus waves of contraction, without any outside humoral or nervous intervention.

CONTRACTION

Within each cell lay the thousands of contractile elements: overlapping actin and myosin filaments. Figure 7-2 illustrates these elements and the changes seen during diastole and systole. Not shown in the illustration are the many cross bridges that extend like rows of oars from the surface of the thicker myosin filaments. During diastole these bridges are unattached to other filaments.

Before contraction, the action potential causes a release of *calcium ions* from their sites on the sarcoplasmic reticulum of the myocardial cell. These ions then travel to the sarcomere (the basic contractile unit) where they attach to binding sites that are located at

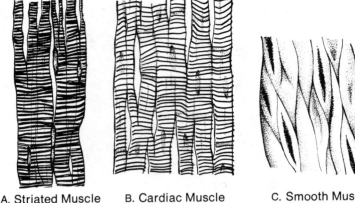

A. Striated Muscle   B. Cardiac Muscle   C. Smooth Muscle

FIGURE 7-1
Histologic features of the three types of contractile tissue.

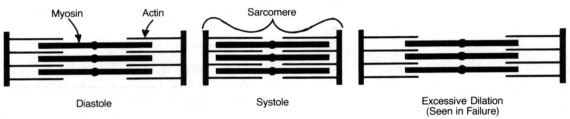

Myosin   Actin   Sarcomere

Diastole   Systole   Excessive Dilation
(Seen in Failure)

FIGURE 7-2
Contractile elements lying inside a single sarcomere of a myocardial cell.

regular intervals along the length of each actin filament. This action of calcium uncovers the myosin cross-bridge binding sites on the actin filaments. The myosin cross bridges (oars) then can attach to these binding sites or actin. With a release of energy stored in adenosine triphosphate (ATP), these cross bridges move unidirectionally in a folding manner (like an oar stroke). This movement slides the actin and myosin filaments past each other, thereby increasing their interdigitation. Rapid, successive uncoupling of cross bridges and their reattachment to new actin binding sites serve to increase the interdigitation of these filaments even more.

The moving of the actin and myosin filaments past each other causes the sarcomere to shorten (see Fig. 7-2). This shortening is the essence of myocardial contraction (systole). Contraction ceases when the calcium ions return to their storage sites on the sarcoplasmic reticulum, thereby causing the binding sites on the actin filaments to be covered again. The separated actin and myosin filaments then slip past each other in the reverse direction, decreasing their interdigitation and thereby again lengthening the sarcomere to its relaxed state.

As can be seen, contraction requires both calcium and energy. Calcium that is loose in the sarcoplasm (cytoplasm of muscle cells) can cause contraction. Hence, calcium in excess of sarcoplasmic reticular storage sites could cause "perpetual contraction" or calcium rigor of the heart. Insufficient intracellular calcium can potentially weaken contractions.

ELECTRICAL CHANGES AND CONTRACTION

Membranes of all the cells in the human body are charged—that is, they are polarized and therefore have electrical potentials. This means simply that there is a separation of charges at the membrane. In humans, all cell membranes regardless of type are positively charged, there being more positively charged particles at the outer surface of the cell membrane than at the inner surface.

Figure 7-3A illustrates this "resting stage." This does not mean that there is a lack of negatively charged particles at the outer surface, nor that there is a lack of positively charged particles at the inner surface. It merely means that there is a net difference in the number and kind of charged particles at the outer surface as compared with the inner surface.

Cardiac muscle membranes are polarized, and the

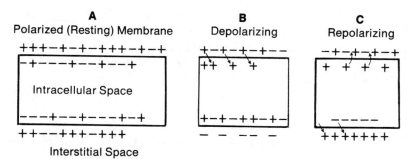

FIGURE 7-3
Electrical events at rest (diastole) and preceding contraction (systole).

electrical potential can be measured, as it can in any of the cells in the human body. The potential results from the difference of intracellular and extracellular concentrations of electrolytes. When compounds of salts of the elements are dissolved in aqueous solutions, they dissociate into their charged particles called *ions*.

In the resting myocardial cell, there are more potassium ions inside than outside the cell and more sodium and unbound calcium ions outside than inside the cell. All three of these positively charged ions (cations) may diffuse through pores, or channels, in the cell membrane. However, if each ion freely obeyed the law of diffusion, potassium would diffuse out of the cell, whereas sodium and calcium would diffuse into it. Soon there would be equal concentrations of each ion between the intra- and extracellular fluids, however, and no resting potention would exist. It is through the selective regulation of the concentrations of these ions on either side of the membrane that the resting membrane potential is maintained. Several factors contribute to this regulation. The first is the sodium–potassium "pumps" within the cell membrane. They move sodium out of the cell and potassium into the cell, with both movements occurring against the concentration gradients for each of these ions. The second factor is the coupled diffusion of sodium and calcium wherein the passive diffusion of sodium into the cell in line with its concentration gradient triggers the active movement of calcium out of the cell against its concentration gradient. The third is the closure of membrane channels whereby calcium ions can enter the resting myocardial cell. The fourth factor is the presence of intracellular anions (negatively charged particles) that are too large to exit from the cell. Keeping these factors in mind, let us now look at the physiological events underlying both the resting potential and the action potential.

Physiological Basis of the Resting Potential

The cardiac cell contains large anions that cannot exit the cell. These anions attract sodium and potassium cations, which diffuse through membrane channels

into the cell. The anions would attract the cation calcium also, except that the membrane channels for the entry of this ion are closed when the cell is at rest. The potassium ions remain within the cell, but the sodium ions are pumped out of the cell almost as fast as they enter by an active transport enzyme carrier system (the sodium–potassium "pumps") located within the cell membrane. While forcing sodium out of the cell, these pumps actively transport potassium ions into the cell, against its concentration gradients. This increase in intracellular potassium is still insufficient to offset all the intracellular anions. Thus, the inside of the myocardial cell remains negative with respect to the outside — as long as the pumps are operative. This produces the *resting potential,* which is approximately −80 mV. For each molecule of an ion "pumped" from the cell, one molecule of ATP is required to provide the energy necessary to effect the chemical bond between ion and carrier. Maintaining a resting potential thus requires energy.

Physiological Basis of the Action Potential

When a stimulus is applied to the polarized cell membrane, the membrane that ordinarily is only slightly permeable to sodium permits sodium ions to diffuse rapidly into the cell. This occurs because of inactivation of the sodium active transport enzymes ("pumps"). The result is a reversal of net charges. The outer surface is now more negative than positive, and the membrane is said to be *depolarized* (Fig. 7-3B).

When the sodium influx reduces the polarity from −80 mV to approximately −35 mV, the electrical change opens the previously closed "calcium channels" in the myocardial cell membrane. Once opened, these channels permit the influx of calcium. The entry of this cation, together with the continued entry of sodium, is responsible for the remainder of the depolarization, which continues until the extracellular side (approximately +30 mV). Such a maximal depolarization inactivates sodium–potassium pumps in nearby membranes. This can cause depolarization in these areas. When the original depolarization becomes self-propagating in this way, it is termed an *action poten-*

tial. In a myocardial cell, an action potential also triggers the release of intracellular calcium from its storage sites on the sarcoplasmic reticulum. This plus the calcium influx elevates intracellular calcium levels, thereby initiating muscular contraction, as previously described.

If the depolarization remains below a certain critical (threshold) point, it will die out without having opened any calcium channels or inactivated any adjacent sodium–potassium pumps. Because it does not become self-propagating and remains localized, such a depolarization is termed a *local depolarization*.

During depolarization, the elevated intracellular sodium concentration frees potassium ions to diffuse out of the cell in accordance with their concentration gradient. Just as this potassium efflux gains some momentum, however, the sodium–potassium pumps automatically reactivate (they can be only temporarily inactivated). Once reactivated, they begin to restore the original resting potential. This is termed *repolarization* (Fig. 7-3,*C*). During the initial phase of repolarization, the efflux of both potassium and sodium ions exceeds their influx, but as the intracellular sodium ions are removed from the cell potassium ions remain as the major cation to be electrostatically held within the cell by the intracellular anions. This halts the potassium efflux. The remainder of repolarization consists of "pump" activity that increases intracellular potassium and decreases intracellular sodium. Thus, the resting potential is reestablished. The electrical events at the start of repolarization also reclose the calcium entry channels, thereby halting calcium influx. Intracellular calcium levels are reduced via the "coupled diffusion" of sodium and calcium, wherein the diffusion of sodium into the cell causes a movement of calcium out of the cell against the latter's concentration gradient.

MACROSTRUCTURE AND CONDUCTION

The heart chambers and specialized tissues are diagrammed in Figure 7-4. In the wall of the right atrium is the sinoatrial *(SA) node.* This specialized tissue acts as normal cardiac pacemaker. In the lower right portion of the interatrial septum is the *atrioventricular (AV) node.* This tissue acts to conduct, yet delay, the atrial action potential before it travels to the ventricles. Such a delay is necessary to allow separate atrial and ventricular contractions.

Although the myocardium is syncytial in nature, the atria are physically discontinuous from the ventricles. A specialized conduction system exists to conduct the action potential into and throughout the ventricles. From the AV node, the impulse travels down the *bundle of His* in the interventricular septum into either a right or left bundle branch and then through one of many *Purkinje fibers* to the ventricular myocardial tissue itself. An action potential can traverse this conducting tissue three to seven times more rapidly than it can travel through the ventricular myocardium. Thus the bundle, branches, and Purkinje fibers enable a near

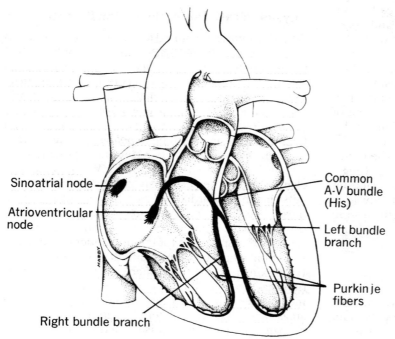

FIGURE 7-4
Distribution of the Purkinje system and the location of the sinoatrial node in the human heart.

Sinoatrial node

Atrioventricular node

Right bundle branch

Common A-V bundle (His)

Left bundle branch

Purkinje fibers

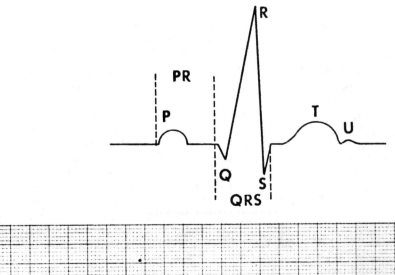

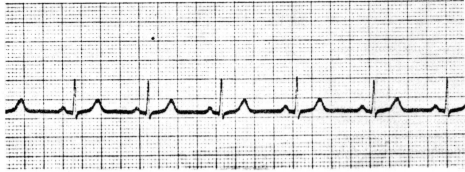

FIGURE 7-5
Normal electrocardiogram tracing.

simultaneous contraction of all portions of the ventricle, thereby allowing the maximal unified pump action to occur.

Electrocardiograms

Let us now examine these events as they are depicted by an electrocardiogram (ECG) (Fig. 7-5). ECGs will be extensively covered in a later chapter, so discussion here will be brief:

- The P wave represents the atrial depolarization that occurs with atrial systole.
- The P–Q interval represents the duration required for the impulse to reach the ventricular myocardium.
- The QRS complex denotes the electrical events concurrent with ventricular systole. This wave hides the electrical representation of atrial repolarization.
- The Q–T interval represents the length of time taken by ventricular depolarization and repolarization.
- The T wave represents repolarization and is caused in part by a reentry of potassium ions.

- The U wave depicts a supernormal phase that occurs during the beginning of ventricular recovery.

Rhythmicity and Pacing

An inherent property of myocardial cells is a spontaneous and rhythmic inactivation of their sodium pumps. Thus, any portion of atrial or ventricular cells can produce their own rhythmic series of action potentials and, thus, their own stimulus for contraction. However, if there were no coordination of these activities, the heart could not function as a pump.

Fortunately, rates of spontaneous discharge vary throughout the heart. The sinoatrial node, a specialized piece of cardiac tissue located between the openings of the inferior and superior venae cavae in the wall of the right atrium, discharges at a resting rate of 90 to 100 times per minute. Regular atrial myocardial cells have a discharge rate of about 60 to 70 per minute. The remainder of the conduction system and ventricles have progressively slower rates of discharge culminating in an idioventricular rhythm of about 40 per minute. If the actions of the various parts of the heart were independent and uncoordinated, effective pumping could never occur. This does not happen because the fastest area paces the remainder—provided intact conduction pathways exist between them. Normally, the SA node will act as the pacemaker. Without modification, however, this would result in an *unregulated* heart rate of 100 beats per minute because that is the rhythmic discharge rate of SA nodal time. However, in the healthy person, continued parasympathetic influences lower this spontaneous nodal rhythm to about 70 to 80 beats per minute. (This will be discussed further in the section on regulation of cardiac output.)

Should the normal conduction pathways be interrupted, the fastest pacemaker tissue on both sides of this interruption will govern their respective areas, and the ECG may evidence two independent such rhythms. Atrial systole is not needed in order for the ventricle to fill with blood. The important rhythm, clinically, is that of the ventricles. They are the chambers that supply the lungs and the rest of the body with blood. Their systolic rate helps determine true perfusion. The slower the rate, the less able are the ventricles to meet the perfusion needs of the body during exercise or activities of daily living. A very rapid ventricular rhythm also can compromise perfusion needs, because the shorter the diastole, the less time for filling of the chambers. Decreased ventricular filling can reduce cardiac output.

THE CARDIAC CYCLE

In the foregoing sections, the more subtle and less typically measurable features of cardiac function have been discussed. Pulse, blood pressure, and heart sounds are very important indicators of cardiac function and will now be discussed in light of the characteristics that have just been presented. Figure 7-6 summarizes the events during this cycle.

During diastole, blood enters the relaxed atria and flows passively into the relaxed ventricles. Diastole typically lasts 0.4 second (in a heart rate of 70 beats/minute). Then the SA node discharges and atrial systole occurs, with a duration of 0.1 second. This atrial contraction is not responsible for most of ventricular filling. It squeezes only a small amount of remaining blood into the ventricles. Then the ventricles contract (the delay is due to the time needed for the action potential to traverse the AV node and conduction system). Ventricular systole elevates the pressure within the chambers, forcing both (1) the blood out into the pulmonary artery and aorta, and (2) the tricuspid and bicuspid valves shut. The slamming shut of these valves creates the *lub heart sound.*

At the same time as the lub sound there is a surge of fluid pressure against the walls of the major arteries as a result of increased volume of blood pumped from the ventricles. This surge is felt in the peripheral circulation and is known as the *pulse.* The contractile phase or period is known as *systole,* and thus the blood pressure of this period of ventricular systole is called the *systolic pressure.*

Ventricular systole lasts about 0.3 second. After this, the ventricles relax, which causes the arterial pressure to exceed the intraventricular pressure, closing the semilunar valves. The closing of these valves (pulmonary and aortic) is heard as the *dub cardiac sound,* denoting the onset of ventricular diastole.

Because there is no pushing of blood into the arteries during ventricular diastole, blood pressure falls, and the diastolic blood pressure is lower than the systolic blood pressure.

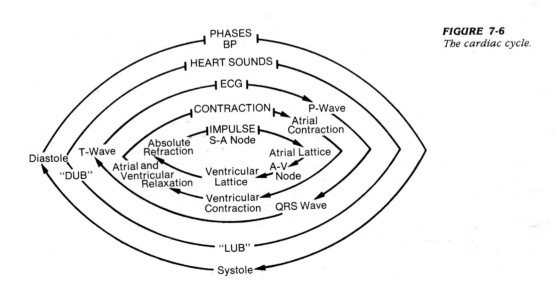

FIGURE 7-6
The cardiac cycle.

CARDIAC OUTPUT

Cardiac output (CO) is a traditional measure of cardiac function. It equals the product of heart rate (HR) and stroke volume (SV):

$$CO = (HR) \times (SV)$$

Although it is approximately 4.8 liters per minute at rest, cardiac output can be altered to meet changing bodily demands for tissue perfusion. Because the latter is a function of body size, a newer and more accurate measure of cardiac function is the *cardiac index,* which equals the cardiac output divided by the surface area of the body. It typically averages 3.0 ± 0.2 liters per minute.

$$cardiac\ index = \frac{CO}{surface\ area\ (M^2)}$$

Because of the relationship of stroke volume and heart rate on cardiac index, we will examine these further.

Regulation of Heart Rate

Although the heart has the ability to beat independently of any extrinsic influence, cardiac rate is under autonomic and adrenal catecholamine influence. Both parasympathetic and sympathetic fibers innervate the SA and AV nodes. In addition, there are sympathetic fibers that terminate in myocardial tissue. Figure 7-7 illustrates this innervation.

Parasympathetic stimulation releases acetylcholine near the nodal cells. This decreases their rate of depolarization, thereby slowing cardiac rate. Stimulation of sympathetic fibers causes them to release norepinephrine (NE). This chemical increases the rate of nodal depolarization. It also has ionotropic effects on myocardial fibers, which will be discussed later. Thus, sympathetic stimulation increases heart rate. The adrenal medulla also releases norepinephrine and epinephrine into the bloodstream. These catecholamines act on the heart in the same way as sympathetic stimulation.

There are two reflexes that adjust heart rate to blood pressure: the *aortic reflex* and the *Bainbridge reflex.* In the aortic reflex, a rise in arterial blood pressure stimulates aortic and carotid sinus baroreceptors to fire sensory impulses to the cardioregulatory center in the medulla. This causes an increase in parasympathetic stimulation or a decrease in sympathetic stimulation to the heart. Thus, a rise in arterial blood pressure reflexively causes a slowing of cardiac rate. That results in a decrease in cardiac output which, in turn, can decrease arterial blood pressure. Conversely, a fall in arterial blood pressure, such as in shock, will reflexively increase heart rate. This aortic reflex is an ongoing regulatory mechanism for homeostasis of arterial blood pressure.

The Bainbridge reflex utilizes receptors in the venae cavae. An increase in venous return stimulates these receptors, which then fire sensory impulses that travel to the cardioregulatory center. These reflexively cause a decrease in parasympathetic cardiac stimulation and an increase in sympathetic cardiac stimulation, thereby increasing cardiac rate. A fall in venous return

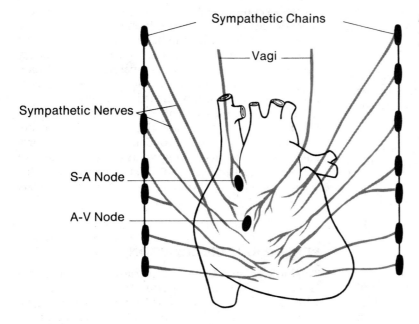

Sympathetic Chains

Vagi

Sympathetic Nerves

S-A Node

A-V Node

FIGURE 7-7
Distribution of autonomic nerve fibers to the human heart.

causes a decrease in heart rate. Thus, the Bainbridge reflex adjusts cardiac rate to handle venous return.

Regulation of Stroke Volume

Three factors are involved in stroke volume: (1) preload, (2) afterload (or wall tension), and (3) inherent ionotropic myocardial contractility. We will examine each in turn.

Preload. This refers to *Starling's law of the heart.* The more a myocardial fiber is stretched immediately prior to contraction, the stronger it will contract. Stretch is determined by the volume of blood in a heart chamber at the end of diastole, referred to as *end diastolic volume (EDV).* Hence, increased venous return will increase the EDV, which will result in a more forceful systole (within normal limits). In this way, ventricular emptying (cardiac output) is automatically adjusted to venous return. Generally, the most clinically important EDV is that of the left ventricle, and by convention EDV is ventricular unless otherwise specified.

Anatomically, stretch decreases the overlap between actin and myosin filaments. This increases the number of "empty" or potential cross-bridge binding sites that can be involved per contraction (see Fig. 7-2). Overstretch caused by ventricular dilation in heart failure is thought to decrease contractile force by decreasing overlap too much. As a result, there are too few actual binding sites (so that only a few cross bridges can operate) to produce much of an initial contractile force. By the time the filaments interdigitate sufficiently, so that more myosin cross-bridges can be induced, contraction is almost over. Thus, overstretch reduces the force of systole and can actually decrease ventricular emptying, thereby exacerbating the problem.

Afterload or Wall Tension. This is the second factor affecting stroke volume. It is the *force* required by the ventricles in order to open the aortic and pulmonary valves during systole (systolic ejection force). The higher the arterial pressure, the more force required (to push against this) by the ventricles. Also, the larger the ventricular diameter, the greater the required force. These relationships are described by the following equation:

$$AL = VEF = AP \times VA$$

Where

AL	represents	*afterload*
VEF	represents	*ventricular ejection force* (wall-tension)
AP	represents	*arterial pressure*
VA	represents	*ventricular cross-sectional area*

Some sources equate afterload with diastolic blood pressure. As can be seen from this equation, this is not strictly the case. Diastolic blood pressure can provide only a rough index of afterload. Afterload increases the work that the heart must perform. In cases in which the heart cannot meet the necessary wall tension (force) requirements, afterload will then reduce stroke volume. This is most often seen in the failing heart.

Inherent (Ionotropic) Capabilities. This last factor involves intracellular processes that may act to increase or decrease contraction. These processes operate independently of Starling's law or extrinsic stimuli. Cellular stores of calcium and norepinephrine can be such factors. Also, sympathetic stimulation or β-adrenergic drugs may increase inherent contractility. Much remains to be learned about these capabilities.

CORONARY CIRCULATION

Blood supply to the myocardium is derived from the two main coronary arteries that originate from the aorta, immediately above the aortic valve. The left coronary artery supplies the major portion of the left ventricle, and the right coronary artery supplies the major portion of the right ventricle.

Shortly after its origin, the left coronary vessel branches into the anterior descending artery, which traverses the groove between the two ventricles on the anterior surface of the heart, and the circumflex artery, which passes to the left and posteriorly in the groove between the left atrium and the left ventricle. The circumflex branch may terminate before reaching the posterior side of the heart, or it may continue into the posterior groove between the left and right ventricles. The coronary circulation is referred to as *dominant left* if this branch of the left coronary artery supplies the posterior aspect of the heart, including the septum.

Eighty percent of human hearts are *dominant right*. When this situation prevails, the right coronary artery passes posteriorly and is responsible for the blood supply to the posterior side of the heart and the posterior portion of the interventricular septum.

Because of their anatomic deviation from the aorta (above the aortic valve) and the fact that they lay between myocardial fibers, blood flow through the coronary arteries occurs during ventricular diastole, not systole. Therefore, anything that decreases the diastolic time (*e.g.,* tachycardia) will decrease coronary perfusion.

PERIPHERAL CIRCULATION

The biologic significance of the cardiovascular system is tissue perfusion. Such perfusion supplies the cells with oxygen and nutrients while carrying away metabolic wastes, including carbon dioxide. Tissue perfusion is indirectly proportional to the rate of blood flow, which, in turn, depends on several factors. One such factor is the difference between the mean arterial blood pressure and right atrial pressure (usually represented by the central venous pressure). The greater this difference, the faster the flow rate (all else being unchanged). Conversely, if the arterial pressure falls or the central venous pressure rises, flow rate and, thus, tissue perfusion will be decreased.

Another factor affecting flow rate is vessel resistance. This resistance is due in part to the friction of the fluid along the sides of the vessel. As such, it is inversely proportional to the fourth power of the radius of the vessel. The equation is

$$\text{vessel resistance} = \frac{1}{\text{vessel radius}^4}$$

Thus, the more constricted or narrower the vessel lumen, the greater the resistance. Vessel dilation decreases resistance and, as a result, increases the rate of blood flow. The relationship between vessel radius and blood flow has two general applications. One is to describe the flow rate through vessels of differing diameters (*e.g.*, arteries, capillaries). The other application concerns the ongoing regulation of blood flow by means of adjustments in arteriole diameters (*i.e.*, constriction and dilation). Arteriole constriction reduces the radius, thereby increasing resistance and thus decreasing the flow rate. Arteriole dilation, conversely, increases the flow rate.

The other two factors that can affect the flow rate are normally held constant. They are (1) the sum of all vessel lengths and (2) blood viscosity. Because they do not normally change significantly, they are usually omitted from flow rate considerations. Their relationships are obvious, however. The greater the length of a vessel, the more resistance, and thus the slower the flow rate. Also, the more viscous the blood, the slower the rate of its flow. Blood viscosity is determined by the proportion of solvent (water) to solute and other particles, including blood cells and platelets. The less of the former and the more of the latter, the more viscous the blood. The complete equation that describes all four factors is as follows:

$$\text{flow rate} = \frac{\text{mean arterial pressure} - \text{central venous pressure}}{\text{resistance} \times \text{viscosity} \times \text{vessel length}}$$

Because blood volume and pressure have such an important influence on tissue perfusion, we will examine the factors that alter and regulate these.

Blood Volume. Urinary output and fluid input are the major normal mechanisms for regulating volume. The greater the output or the less the fluid input, the less the volume—if all else is held constant. Factors that alter the volume of urine excreted every 24 hours include those that alter the glomerular filtration rate and the tubular reabsorption of water, with or without electrolytes. (For a more detailed explanation of these factors, see Chapter 18, specifically the discussion of normal endocrine physiology that considers the hormone ADH.) Pathological conditions that promote any type of fluid loss (*e.g.,* burns, severe diarrhea, osmotic diuresis) or a shift of water from the vascular to the interstitial compartment have the potential for reducing blood volume.

Blood Pressure. Because the *difference* between arterial and venous pressures is the driving force for blood circulation and tissue perfusion, we will examine first those factors that influence central venous pressure, then the factors that regulate arterial blood pressure. Central venous pressure is, strictly speaking, the pressure of blood in the venae cavae just prior to its entry into the right atrium. It can be increased by either an increase in blood volume (*e.g.,* IV fluid overload) or a decrease in the pumping ability of the heart (*e.g.,* cardiac failure).

Arterial blood pressure is regulated by the vasomotor tone of the arteries and arterioles, the amount of blood entering the arteries per systole (*i.e.,* cardiac output) and blood volume *per se*. The greater the volume or cardiac output, the greater would be the blood pressure and *vice versa*—if vasomotor tone were held constant. Factors influencing blood volume have been previously presented. Adjustment of cardiac output to regulate arterial blood pressure is effected by the aortic reflex, also discussed earlier. The normal regulation of systemic arterial pressure involves both neural and hormonal mechanisms. In addition, other factors may affect arterial blood pressure.

Neural regulation is mediated by the vasomotor center of the medulla oblongata. This center consists of vasopressor and depressor subdivisions. It receives neural input from (1) baroreceptors in the carotid sinuses and aorta, (2) atrial diastolic stretch receptors, (3) limbic system and hypothalamus, (4) midbrain, and (5) pulmonary stretch receptors. Additionally, it is directly responsive to local hypoxia or hypercapnia. Neural outputs from this center travel from the medulla down the cord to various thoracic and lumbar levels, where they synapse with internuncials, which in turn synapse with the nerve cell bodies of sympathetic neurons lying in the lateral horns of the gray matter. Stimulation of the pressure area results in increased sympathetic stimulation to arterial smooth muscle cells. This causes them to contract, causing arterial constriction and a rise in arterial blood pressure. Stimulation of the depressor area decreases such sympathetic stimulation.

Rapid adjustments in arterial blood pressure are primarily effected by the baroreceptor reflexes. Here, an increase in the pressure on these receptors (directly by elevated blood pressure or manual compression and indirectly by increased blood volume) reflexly stimulates the depressor area. This results in decreased sympathetic stimulation to major arteries and the aorta, which causes a fall in arterial blood pressure. Decreased baroreceptor stimulation by a fall in arterial blood pressure reflexly stimulates the pressor area and results in increased sympathetic stimulation to arterial muscles, causing a rise in arterial blood pressure. Thus, homeostasis of arterial pressure is maintained.

The baroreceptor reflex is also involved both in the valsalva maneuver and in orthostatic (postural) hypotension. The valsalva maneuver causes tachycardia and elevated arterial pressure by compressing the thoracic vena cava, leading to a decreased venous return and cardiac output. The fall in cardiac output decreases pressure on the baroreceptors, thereby triggering vasoconstriction. This outweighs any increase that this maneuver might place directly on the baroreceptors by increased intrathoracic pressure. The decreased venous return simultaneously prompts reflex tachycardia. The sudden change from a recumbent or stooped posture to a sitting or erect position causes a decrease in the stimulation of baroreceptors as the result of the effects of gravity on blood distribution. Decreased baroreceptor stimulation causes a prompt reflex vasoconstriction that elevates arterial blood pressure. This increases brain perfusion, thereby preventing lightheadedness or syncope. In orthostatic hypotension, the baroreceptor reflex is sluggish. Arterial pressure is not elevated rapidly enough, so the postural change results in a temporary decrease in brain perfusion that leads, in extreme cases, to syncope. (The walls of the atria contain receptors that are stimulated by the stretch of atrial walls during diastolic filling. Increases in venous return will stimulate these receptors, which, reflexly via the vasomotor center, cause arterial vasodilation and a fall in arterial pressure. Thus, the arteries can relax a bit, so that an increase in cardiac output does not unduly elevate arterial pressure.)

Various factors may reflexly alter arterial blood pressure by their influences on the vasomotor center. Nerve fibers from the limbic system and hypothalamus are believed to mediate emotionally produced alterations in blood pressure. Neural inputs from the midbrain and possibly from ascending spinothalamic fibers in the medulla result in both the elevation in arterial pressure that initially accompanies severe pain and in the later fall in arterial pressure that occurs when severe pain is prolonged. Lung inflation stimulates pulmonary stretch receptors. Their input to the vasomotor center reflexly decreases arterial pressure. Hypercapnia and, to a lesser extent, hypoxia of vasomotor neurons stimulate the pressor area, reflexly causing a rise in arterial pressure. Such stimuli ob-

viously are not part of a normal daily regulatory mechanism but can operate as a normal compensatory mechanism in certain pathological situations. Elevated intracranial pressure can promote medullary hypercapnia and hypoxia. This increase in arterial pressure reflexly produced by these stimuli (Cushing's reflex) increases medullary perfusion and tends to ameliorate the medullary hypoxia or hypercapnia or both. Hormonal regulation of arterial blood pressure is effected by adrenal medulla catecholamines or the renin-angiotensin system. In the former, adrenal medullary catecholamines mimic the action of sympathetic fibers innervating the tunica media, elevating arterial pressure. The renin-angiotensin system is discussed in Chapter 18. Briefly, a decreased glomerular filtration rate, which can result, for example, from a fall in blood volume or renal perfusion, stimulates the secretion of renin from the juxtaglomerular apparatus. This leads to the production of the angiotensin II, which acts directly on tunica media muscles to promote vasoconstriction. Thus, renin elevates arterial pressure, which, in turn, increases renal perfusion and glomerular filtration.

Finally, arterial blood pressure can be influenced by alterations in the level of unbound calcium within tunica media muscle cells. Such levels are, in turn, influenced by factors that open or close calcium channels in the membranes of these muscle cells. Drugs that block calcium channels ("calcium blockers") inhibit the entry of calcium into cells. Such decreased calcium influx can lower intracellular calcium levels sufficiently to decrease muscle contractility, thereby promoting a degree of vasodilatation and lowering the arterial pressure. Dietary sodium intake in "renally predisposed" individuals may decrease the exit of calcium from tunica media cells, thereby promoting vasoconstriction and an elevation in arterial blood pressure. It is thought to do so through its influence on natriuretic hormone secretion. This hormone inhibits the renal distal cation exchange system (see Chapter 18). While the source of natriuretic hormone has not been discovered, it is known to be secreted in response to increases in extracellular fluid volume. Excess salt intake can, in certain individuals, lead to fluid retention and increase in extracellular fluid volume. In such "renally predisposed" persons this increase in extracellular fluid volume stimulates natriuretic hormone secretion. Secretion of this hormone, in turn, inhibits sodium and water reabsorption. The increased water and sodium excretion then restores the normal quantity of extracellular fluid. By itself, this normal homeostatic mechanism would not influence blood pressure appreciably, but natriuretic hormone also seems to inhibit the sodium–potassium pumps in smooth muscle cells. A decrease in sodium–potassium pump activity will lead to increased intracellular levels of sodium that can be below those needed to trigger the polarization. Yet, this increased intracellular level of sodium will decrease the passive diffusion of sodium into the cell. This decreased sodium influx will lead to a decreased calcium efflux (see earlier discussion of the coupled sodium calcium diffusion mechanism). Thus, decreased pump activity will lead to elevated intracellular calcium levels and increased vascular muscle contractility, thereby elevating arterial blood pressure.

BIBLIOGRAPHY

Ganong WF: Review of Medical Physiology, 11th ed. Los Altos, Lange Medical Publications, 1983

Guyton AC: Textbook of Medical Physiology, 5th ed. Philadelphia, WB Saunders, 1976

Levine HJ (ed): Clinical Cardiovascular Physiology. New York, Grune & Stratton, 1976

Price SA, Wilson LM: Pathophysiology: Clinical Concepts of Disease Processes. New York, McGraw-Hill, 1978

Ross WS: You Can Quit Smoking in 14 Days. California, Berkeley, 1976

Stephens G: Pathophysiology for Health Practitioners. New York, Macmillan, 1980

8
Assessment: Cardiovascular System

Auscultation of the Heart

Joan Mersch

Nurses throughout the United States have played an instrumental role in terminating and preventing lethal arrhythmias. With the development of ECG monitoring and the education of nurses in interpreting arrhythmias and initiating emergency treatment, the mortality incidence among patients with myocardial infarction has decreased. However, nurses need to improve their care of patients who develop heart failure. Of the patients who develop blatantly obvious left ventricular failure, many still die.

One of the earliest and frequently the only cardiac sign of congestive heart failure in the adult is the development of a third heart sound. By detecting the third heart sound and realizing its clinical significance, nurses help decrease the incidence of heart failure in patients.

THE CHARACTERISTICS OF SOUND

Sound is a series of disturbances in matter to which the human ear is sensitive. Sound is a wave motion that has four characteristics—intensity, pitch, duration, and timbre.

Intensity is the force of the amplitude of the vibrations. It is a physical aspect of sound, whereas loudness is a subjective aspect that depends on (1) intensity of the sound and (2) sensitivity of the ear.

Pitch is the frequency of the vibrations per unit of time. The human ear is most sensitive to vibrations of 500 to 5,000 per second. Vibrations of less than 20 per second cannot be heard by the human ear.

Duration is the length of time that the sound persists.

Timbre is a quality that depends on overtones that accompany the fundamental tone. In other words, most fundamental vibrations have higher frequency vibrations called *overtones*. Overtones account for the difference in sound between the same note played on a piano and on a flute.

Heart Sounds. Sound waves are initiated by vibrations. The heart sounds are produced by vascular walls, flowing blood, heart muscle, and heart valves. Sudden changes in intra-arterial pressures cause the vascular walls to vibrate, resulting in sound production. Turbulence of blood flow is produced when rapidly moving blood passes through chambers of irregular size, such as the chambers of the heart and the great vessels. When the heart muscles contract, sound waves are initiated by the contracting fibers. Sound waves are produced when the heart valves open as the blood flows through or when they close, especially with a sudden snapping of the chordae tendineae. Of the previously mentioned causes of heart sounds, closing of the heart valves accounts for most of the sound production.

Systole is defined as the time during which the ventricles contract. Systole begins with the beginning of the first heart sound and ends with the beginning of the second heart sound.

Diastole is defined as the time during which the ventricles relax. Diastole begins with the beginning of the second heart sound and ends with the beginning of the next first heart sound. The cardiac cycle is determined by the cycle of the ventricles. In other words, cardiac systole and ventricular systole are synonymous.

Transmission of Heart Sounds. The transmission of the heart sounds depends on the position of the heart, the nature of the surrounding structures, and the position of the stethoscope in relation to the origin of the sound. The stethoscope is a tool used to transmit sounds produced by the body to the ear. Sound waves that travel a shorter distance are of greater intensity; likewise, the shorter the distance the less the possibility for distortion to occur. It then follows that the shorter the tube of the stethoscope, the better the transmission of sound. Convenience and comfort as well as maximum sound production must be considered.

In order to facilitate accurate auscultation, one must ensure that the patient is comfortable, in a quiet room, and in a recumbent position. The bell of the stethoscope transmits low-pitched sounds best when there is an airtight seal and when the instrument is applied lightly to the chest wall. An airtight seal helps occlude extraneous sounds. The diaphragm of the stethoscope best transmits the high-pitched sounds when it is applied with firm pressure to the chest wall.

CLASSIFICATION OF HEART SOUNDS

The First Heart Sound

The first heart sound is produced by the asynchronous closure of the mitral and tricuspid valves. Mitral closure precedes tricuspid closure by 0.02 to 0.03 second. Such narrow splitting is generally not audible.

The first heart sound is therefore composed of two separate components. The first component of the first heart sound is the closure of the mitral valve. The second component of the first heart sound is the closure of the tricuspid valve.

The first heart sound is generally best heard at the apex. It represents the beginning of ventricular systole.

The Second Heart Sound

The second heart sound is produced by the vibrations initiated by the closure of the aortic and pulmonary semilunar valves.

The second heart sound, like the first heart sound, consists of two separate components. The first component of the second heart sound is closure of the aortic valve. The second component of the second heart sound is the closure of the pulmonic valve.

With inspiration, systole of the right ventricle is slightly prolonged owing to increased filling of the right ventricle. With increased right ventricular filling, the pulmonary valve closes later than the aortic valve.

FIGURE 8-1
Normal heart sounds.

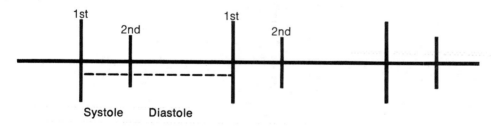

FIGURE 8-2
Third heart sound.

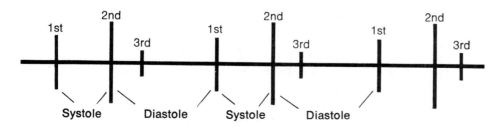

Aortic valve sounds are generally best heard in the second intercostal space to the right of the sternum, whereas the sound produced by the pulmonary valve is generally best heard in the second left intercostal space.

Splitting of the second heart sound is best heard upon inspiration with the stethoscope placed in the second intercostal space to the left of the sternum. The second heart sound represents the beginning of ventricular diastole. See Figure 8-1 for a graphic representation of the normal first and second heart sounds.

The Third Heart Sound

A third heart sound represents pathology in the adult. The third heart sound is believed to be produced by the rapid inrush of blood into a nonpliable ventricle. During ventricular diastole, the apex extends downward and the mitral valve extends upward. As the ventricle fills, the chordae tendineae become tense and partially close the mitral valve. This, along with the increasing resistance of diastole, causes a sudden decrease in blood flow. The cardiac muscle, chordae tendineae, heart valves, and blood are set into motion and are responsible for the production of sound.

The third heart sound is heard after the closure of the semilunar valves, early in diastole, and best at the apex. Most third heart sounds are of relatively low pitch, between 25 and 35 vibrations per second. They are best heard with the bell of the stethoscope applied lightly to the chest wall (Fig. 8-2).

The Fourth Heart Sound

The fourth heart sound, also called an atrial sound, is believed to be produced by atrial contraction that is more forceful than normal. At the end of atrial contraction, more blood is forced from the atria into the ventricle, which causes a sudden increase in ventricular pressure. This increased pressure produces vibrations that cause the fourth heart sound. The fourth heart sound is therefore believed to be produced by atrial contraction and the consequent impact of the rapid inflow of blood on the ventricle.

The fourth heart sound is of low pitch, heard best at the lower end of the sternum and sometimes at the apex. It has a short duration and a low frequency. It is best heard with the bell of the stethoscope. Figure 8-3 shows the timing of the fourth heart sound.

Gallop Rhythms

Gallop rhythm is the name given to the heart sounds when they are grouped so as to mimic the cadence of galloping horses. There are three types of gallop rhythms: the ventricular gallop, the atrial gallop, and the summation gallop.

The protodiastolic, or early diastolic, gallop rhythm, also known as the *ventricular gallop rhythm,* is believed to be due to an exaggerated third heart sound. This rhythm is commonly heard in congestive heart failure. It is frequently the earliest sign of heart failure, and its presence signifies the loss of ventricular distensibility.

The ventricular gallop is generally believed to result from the rapid inflow of blood into a dilated ventricle early in diastole. The third heart sound occurs between 0.12 and 0.18 second after the second heart sound. It is of low pitch and heard best at the apex with the bell of the stethoscope.

A *presystolic gallop* rhythm exists when the gallop sound occurs late in diastole or immediately preceding systole. The sound occurs with atrial systole and is believed to represent an accentuated atrial sound. It occurs with systolic overloading, notably in hypertension, myocardial infarction, aortic stenosis, pulmonary hypertension, pulmonary stenosis, and various cardiomyopathies. It is often unaccompanied by heart failure. The presystolic or atrial gallop rhythm is low-pitched and is heard best with the bell of the stethoscope. A left atrial sound is heard best on expiration at the apex, whereas a right atrial sound is best heard on inspiration at the left border of the sternum.

A *summation gallop* occurs because of a tachycardia so rapid that the third and fourth heart sounds combine and are heard as one (Fig. 8-4).

FIGURE 8-3
Fourth heart sound.

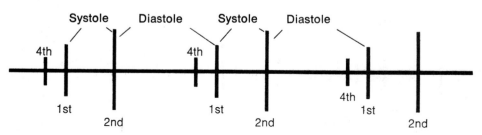

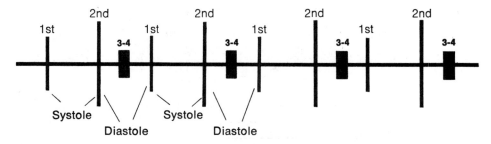

FIGURE 8-4
Summation gallop.

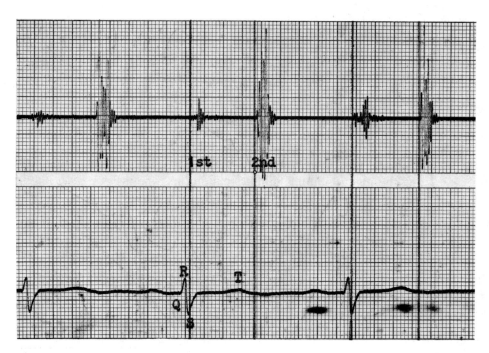

FIGURE 8-5
*Simultaneous recording of a
phonocardiogram and an
electrocardiogram.*

COMPARISION OF ECG AND PHONOCARDIOGRAM

To facilitate understanding of the phonocardiogram, we will compare it with the ECG. The ECG is a graphic representation of the electrical activity of the heart, whereas the phonocardiogram is a recording of the sound vibrations produced by the heart.

When the sinoatrial (SA) node fires, the electrical current travels through the atrial muscle to the atrioventricular (AV) node. The P wave is then written on the ECG. The electrical current then travels down the common bundle of His, right and left bundle branches, Purkinje fibers, and throughout the ventricular muscle. Following electrical stimulation of the ventricles, the latter contract. Early in ventricular systole the mitral and tricuspid valves close. This is the reason the first heart sound occurs during oɪ following ventricular depolarization, which is represented on the ECG by the QRS complex (Fig. 8-5).

During ventricular systole, the blood is forced from the right and left ventricles into the pulmonary and aortic arteries. When the ventricles relax, the aortic and pulmonary semilunar valves close. The second heart sound represents the beginning of ventricular diastole. The second heart sound occurs after the repolarization of the ventricular muscle, which is represented by the T wave on the ECG.

HEART MURMURS

Mechanisms

In order to understand the heart murmurs, one must comprehend both the mechanism responsible for the sound production and the principles of *turbulence of blood flow.* Blood flows most rapidly in the center of a vessel, less rapidly nearer the wall, and least rapidly immediately along the internal surface of the vessel. In other words, as blood flows through a vessel the friction along the wall of the vessel tends to slow the rate of blood flow nearest the wall. The smoother the internal surface of the vessel, the less turbulence in blood flow. The slower the rate of blood flow, the less chance there is for turbulence.

Any irregularity in the inner surface of the vessel or change in the size of the lumen results in turbulence of blood flow and sound production. The narrower the opening, the more rapid the rate of blood flow and the greater the possibility for turbulence and murmur formation.

The murmurs of mitral stenosis, mitral insufficiency, aortic stenosis, and aortic insufficiency will be discussed. With the knowledge of the mechanisms that produce these murmurs, we can deduce the mechanisms responsible for the other murmurs not discussed.

The mechanisms responsible for the murmurs of mitral stenosis and mitral insufficiency are also responsible for the murmurs of tricuspid stenosis and tricuspid insufficiency. The only difference is that the latter murmurs occur on the right side of the heart. Likewise, the mechanisms responsible for the murmurs of aortic stenosis and aortic insufficiency are also responsible for the murmurs of pulmonary stenosis and pulmonary insufficiency. The difference is that the latter murmurs occur on the right side of the heart.

While it might not be necessary to distinguish the specific heart murmur, it is important to recognize the difference between the extra heart sounds and the murmurs. The key diagnostic sign of early congestive heart failure is the development of the third heart sound.

The Murmur of Mitral Stenosis

In mitral stenosis, the mitral orifice can be narrowed by inflammation or fibrosis of the mitral valve because of rheumatic heart disease or arteriosclerosis. A stenotic mitral valve causes an increased left atrial pressure during ventricular diastole. In ventricular diastole the left atrium contracts, forcing blood through the narrowed opening. This produces turbulence of blood flow and a diastolic murmur. The murmur is low-pitched and rumbling.

The murmur of mitral stenosis may be a crescendo or decrescendo in configuration. It may be a crescendo in shape because the left atrium contracts progressively, the rate of blood flow increases, and the mitral valve becomes narrower. It may be a decrescendo in shape because as the ventricle fills, the left atrium empties, and the amount of blood passing through the stenotic valve decreases. The murmur therefore decreases in intensity and is a decrescendo in shape (Fig. 8-6).

The Murmur of Mitral Insufficiency

The murmur of mitral insufficiency is heard in systole. Mitral insufficiency occurs when the mitral valve is incompetent, and the valve leaflets fail to approximate. During ventricular systole, intraventricular pressure exceeds intra-atrial pressure. With an incompetent mitral valve, the blood regurgitates through the valve opening into the left atrium. This results in turbulence of blood flow and a high-pitched, blowing murmur. The murmur is systolic, heard best at the apex, and is transmitted laterally to the axillary line when the heart is enlarged. As a rule, a murmur is transmitted in the direction of the blood flow that is responsible for the turbulence. The murmur of mitral insufficiency is generally pansystolic or holosystolic (lasting all of systole) (Fig. 8-7).

The murmur of mitral insufficiency is the murmur of myocardial infarction. In myocardial infarction, dilatation of the left ventricle occurs because of ischemia or necrosis. When the left ventricle is dilated, the papillary muscle tends to move away from the valve leaflets. The chordae tendineae are unable to lengthen, and the mitral leaflets are held open, preventing complete approximation. With dilatation of the left ventricle, the mitral ring dilates. The leaflets remain the same size

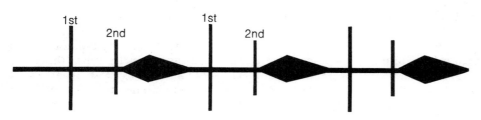

FIGURE 8-6
Murmur of mitral stenosis.

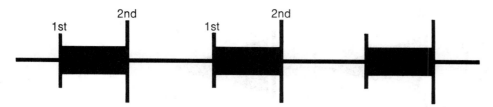

FIGURE 8-7
Murmur of mitral insufficiency.

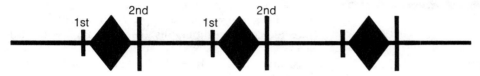

FIGURE 8-8
Murmur of aortic stenosis.

and are unable to close the enlarged opening. When the left ventricle dilates, it loses its ability to contract and there is an associated papillary muscle dysfunction.

The Murmur of Aortic Stenosis

The murmur of aortic stenosis is heard during systole. Aortic stenosis is the result of narrowing of the aortic cusps. During ventricular systole, the pressure within the ventricle exceeds the pressure of the aorta, and the blood flows out of the ventricle into the aorta. If there is thickening of the aortic cusps or narrowing of the aortic valve, the rapidly flowing blood passes through the constricted valve and causes turbulence of blood flow.

The murmur is of medium pitch and has a rough or harsh sound. It is heard best over the aortic valve area, the second right intercostal space. The murmur of aortic stenosis is transmitted into the arteries of the neck because the blood flow responsible for the turbulence is moving in that direction. It can also be transmitted to the apex, where it may be confused with the murmur of mitral insufficiency—also a systolic murmur. The murmur of aortic stenosis occurs in systole, and it is a diamond shape. It is composed of a crescendo and a decrescendo (Fig. 8-8).

The Murmur of Aortic Insufficiency

The murmur of aortic insufficiency is diastolic in time. In ventricular diastole, the intraventricular pressure is lower than the intra-aortic pressure. The aortic cusps fail to support the blood and it regurgitates into the ventricle. Turbulence of blood flow results in the formation of a high-pitched, blowing murmur. It is usually best heard in the third left intercostal space. As the pressure in the ventricle increases and the aortic pressure decreases, the turbulence of blood flow decreases. The murmur is therefore a decrescendo in shape (Fig. 8-9).

BIBLIOGRAPHY

Braunwald E: Determinants and assessment of cardiac function. N Engl J Med 296:86–89, 1977
DeGowin EL, DeGowin RL: Bedside Diagnostic Examination, 3rd ed. New York, Macmillan, 1977
Hurst J, Schlant R: Auscultation of the heart. In Hurst J, Logue R (eds): The Heart, 4th ed. New York, McGraw-Hill, 1978
Mason DT (ed): Advances in Heart Disease. New York, Grune & Stratton, 1977
Prior JA, Silberstein JS: Physical Diagnosis: The History and Examination of the Patient, 5th ed. St. Louis, CV Mosby, 1977
Thorn GW et al (eds): Harrison's Principles of Internal Medicine, 8th ed. New York, McGraw-Hill, 1977

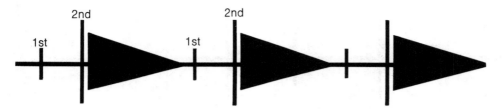

FIGURE 8-9
*Murmur of aortic insuffi-
ciency.*

Arrhythmias and Conduction Disturbances

Phillip S. Wolf

Disorders of the heartbeat occur in the majority of patients with acute myocardial infarction. Acute respiratory failure is a frequent cause of arrhythmias as well. The importance of rhythm disturbances in these situations differs; some lack clinical significance, whereas others are lethal.

Arrhythmias commonly encountered in monitored patients can be recognized with a little practice. The types that occur most frequently are discussed in the following section. In dealing with these disturbances of rhythm, the nurse must appraise the patient's total clinical situation.

Understanding of arrhythmias is helped by knowledge of the conduction system. Before beginning your study of this section, you might find it helpful to review the conduction system (see pp. 64–65) and the principles of electrocardiography (see also Figs. 8-10 and 8-11).

An arrhythmia will result when any of the following three situations exists:

- The *rate* is too slow or too fast (the rhythm may be regular or irregular).
- The *site* of the impulse formation is abnormal (atrial fibers, fibers of the AV junction, the His bundle or its branches, or the Purkinje fibers).
- The *conduction* of impulses is abnormal at any point within the conduction system.

To analyze arrhythmias, one must understand some of the terms commonly used. A partial list of definitions can be found in the accompanying chart.

Sinus Tachycardia

Definition. Sinus tachycardia is defined as a rapid heart rate (100 to 180 beats/min). The rhythm is regular but usually varies from minute to minute. The rapid rate decreases diastole more than systole (Fig. 8-12).

ECG TERMS ASSOCIATED WITH ARRHYTHMIAS

Tachycardia—A heart rate in excess of 100/min.

Bradycardia—A heart rate under 60/min.

Isoelectric Line—The straight line seen when no electrical activity is occurring. The baseline of the tracing.

P Wave—A deflection from the baseline produced by *depolarization* of the atria.

P–R Interval—The time required for the impulse to travel through the atria into the first portion of the conduction system, the AV junction. Normal limits are 0.12 to 0.2 sec. The interval is measured from the beginning of the P wave to the start of the QRS complex.

QRS Complex—A deflection from the baseline produced by depolarization of the ventricles. Normal duration is 0.06 to 0.08 sec.

S–T Segment—The segment between the *end* of the QRS complex and the *beginning* of the T wave.

Q–T Interval—The time required for the ventricles to depolarize and repolarize. Usual duration is 0.32 to 0.40 sec. The interval is from the *beginning* of the QRS complex to the *end* of the T wave.

T Wave—A deflection from the baseline produced by ventricular *repolarization* and normally of the same deflection as the QRS complex.

U Wave—A small, usually positive deflection following the T wave. Its significance is uncertain, but it is typically seen with hypokalemia.

FIGURE 8-10
Schematic representation of the electrical impulse as it traverses the conduction system, resulting in depolarization and repolarization of the myocardium.

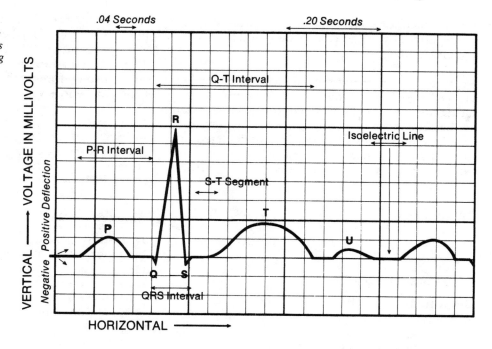

FIGURE 8-11
Normal sinus rhythm. (Rate = 60 to 100 beats per minute.)

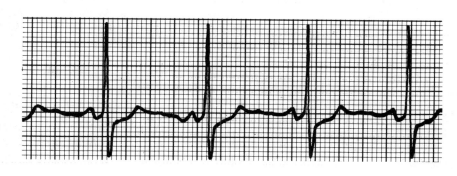

FIGURE 8-12
Sinus tachycardia.

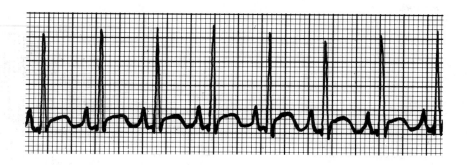

Etiology. Sinus tachycardia may be a physiological response to any form of stress and is found in all age groups. It occurs in such diverse conditions as excitement, physical exertion, fever, anemia, hyperthyroidism, and hypoxia, and with the administration of some drugs, such as atropine, isoproterenol, and epinephrine. Sinus tachycardia may also occur with heart disease and is often present with congestive heart failure.

Sinus tachycardia results from decreased vagal tone or increased sympathetic nervous system activity and the release of catecholamines (epinephrine and norepinephrine) by the adrenal medulla and from nerve endings in the heart.

Symptoms. Ordinarily, the only symptom described is a sense of "racing of the heart." The cause of sinus tachycardia determines its prognosis not the duration of the arrhythmia, which in and of itself is usually harmless. In persons who already have depleted cardiac reserve, ischemia, or congestive heart failure, the persistence of a fast rate may worsen the underlying condition.

Treatment. Specific measures may include sedation, digitalis (only if heart failure is present), or propranolol, if the tachycardia is due to thyrotoxicosis.

Sinus Bradycardia

Definitions. Sinus bradycardia is defined as a heart rate of fewer than 60 beats per minute with impulses originating in the SA node. Rhythm is regular but may vary from minute to minute. The duration of diastole is lengthened (Fig. 8-13).

Etiology. Sinus bradycardia is common among all age groups and is present in both normal and diseased hearts. It is also seen in highly trained athletes, patients with severe pain, myxedema, or acute myocardial infarction, and as the result of medication (digitalis, reserpine, verapermil, or diltiazem).
Sinus bradycardia results from excessive parasympathetic activity. Slow rates are tolerated well in persons with healthy hearts. With severe heart disease, however, the heart may not be able to compensate for a slow rate by increasing the volume of blood ejected per beat as is true of the healthy heart. In this situation, sinus bradycardia will lead to a low cardiac output. This in turn may lead to weakness (resulting from inadequate blood flow to the muscles), congestive heart failure, or serious ventricular arrhythmias.

Treatment. No treatment is usually indicated unless symptoms are present. If the pulse is very slow and symptoms are present, appropriate measures include atropine to block the vagal effect, isoproterenol, or transvenous pacing.

Sinus Arrhythmia

Definition. All impulses originate in the SA node, but the rate of discharge varies. Some occur prematurely, whereas others are delayed, which causes the rate to increase and decrease alternately. In young persons, the heart rate usually varies with respiration, increasing with inspiration and slowing with expiration (Fig. 8-14).

Etiology. Sinus arrhythmia is usually a physiological variation in young people. It may indicate disease of the SA node in the elderly (see section on sick sinus syndrome).

Treatment. Usually no treatment is necessary.

Atrial Premature Contraction (APC)

Definition. During the normal cardiac rhythm, a contraction occurs earlier than expected. The stimulus for this contraction arises not in the SA node but in

FIGURE 8-13
Sinus bradycardia.

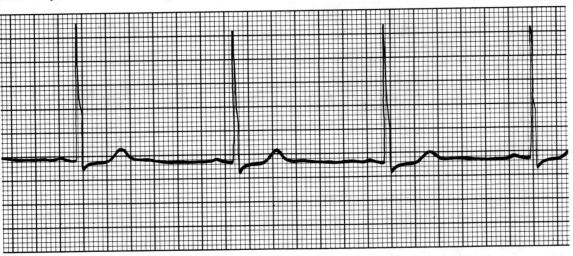

FIGURE 8-14
Sinus arrhythmia.

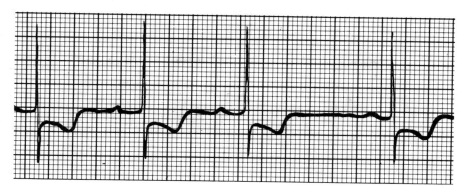

FIGURE 8-15
Atrial premature contraction.

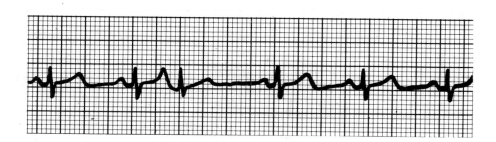

another area of the atrium. The P wave is usually visible and typically has a somewhat different form than the P wave of the sinus impulse. The QRS complex is usually of normal configuration but may appear distorted when the APC is conducted aberrantly, or the QRS may not occur at all (APC is blocked). A short pause, usually less than "compensatory," is present (see definition of VPC, further on) (Fig. 8-15).

Etiology. This is a common arrhythmia seen in all groups. It may occur in normal individuals and in patients with rheumatic heart disease, ischemic heart disease, or hyperthyroidism.

An impulse arises in the atrial musculature from an ectopic focus, producing an atrial contraction. Usually the stimulus travels through the AV junction and continues its normal course through the ventricles. If an APC occurs too early, it may be blocked because the AV junction is refractory from the previous stimulus and is unable to receive the current one. In most instances, the atrial ectopic beat is followed by an incomplete compensatory pause. The patient may have the sensation of a "pause" or "skip" in rhythm.

Treatment. In many cases, no treatment is necessary. Mild sedation or removal of the exciting cause is indicated if the APCs are symptomatic. If they occur as a result of underlying heart disease, specific drugs such as quinidine, digitalis, or propranolol may be in order.

Supraventricular Tachycardia

Definition. These tachycardias are rapid, regular rhythms. They may originate in an ectopic atrial focus (paroxysmal atrial tachycardia) or in the AV junction (paroxysmal nodal tachycardia). These ectopic rhythms are similar in all respects except their site of origin. In almost all instances recorded, the tachycardia begins with a premature atrial or junctional beat (Fig. 8-16).

Significant ECG Changes

Rate. The range is 140 to 220 beats per minute. The rhythm is regular, and the paroxysms may last from a few seconds to several hours or even days.

P Waves. These waves are usually upright with atrial tachycardia and may be inverted in leads II, III, and aVF when the tachycardia is of junctional origin. If the rate is very rapid, the P wave may merge with the QRS complex superimposed on the T wave (Fig. 8-17).

P–R Interval. If seen, the P–R interval is usually shortened with junctional tachycardia and normal, shortened, or, rarely, lengthened with atrial tachycardia.

QRS Complex. This is usually of normal configuration but may be distorted if aberrant conduction is present.

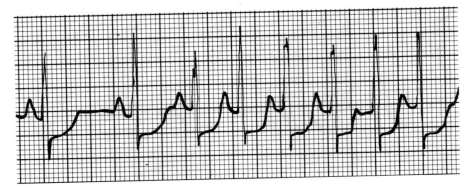

FIGURE 8-16
Supraventricular tachycardia.

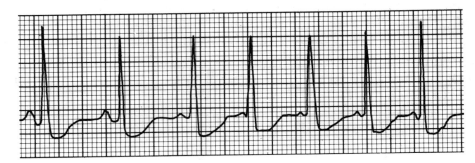

FIGURE 8-17
A-V junctional tachycardia.

Etiology. These arrhythmias occur often in adults with normal hearts and for the same reasons as APCs. When heart disease is present, such abnormalities as rheumatic heart disease, acute myocardial infarction, and digitalis intoxication may serve as the background for these arrhythmias.

Atrial tachycardia is typically preceded by an APC. The ectopic pacemaker discharges impulses to which the atrium or AV junction responds, firing so rapidly that the SA node is suppressed. Extreme regularity (in a given person the rate stays constant) is one of the hallmarks.

Symptoms. Early symptoms are palpitations and lightheadedness. With underlying heart disease, dyspnea, angina pectoris, and congestive heart failure may occur.

Differential Diagnosis. A supraventricular tachycardia must be differentiated from sinus tachycardia. The following points favor the diagnosis of ectopic atrial tachycardia:

- An atrial premature beat often initiates the rhythm.
- It begins and terminates abruptly.
- The rate is often faster than a sinus tachycardia and tends to be more regular from minute to minute.
- In response to a vagal maneuver, such as carotid sinus massage, the ectopic tachycardia will either be unaffected or revert to a normal sinus rhythm. Sinus tachycardia, however, will slow slightly in response to increased vagal tone.

Treatment. Stimulation of the vagal reflex will often terminate the paroxysms. This reflex may be elicited by brief massage on the carotid sinus (unilaterally) or by the Valsalva maneuver. Verapamil, given intravenously, is now considered the drug of choice for terminating supraventricular tachycardia and is successful in the majority of instances. The usual IV dose is 5 to 10 mg given over 3 minutes.

Atrial Flutter

Definition. Atrial flutter is defined as an ectopic atrial rhythm occurring at a rate of 250 to 350 beats per minute. The ventricular rate is usually one half the atrial rate at the beginning of the attack. With treatment, the degree of AV block increases and the ventricular rate slows further. The rapid and regular atrial rate produces a "saw tooth," or "picket fence," appearance on the ECG. It is usual for a flutter wave to be partially concealed within the QRS complex or T wave. The QRS complex exhibits a normal configuration except when aberrant conduction is present. The QRS complexes do not follow each flutter wave because the ventricles cannot respond this rapidly (Fig. 8-18).

FIGURE 8-18
Atrial flutter.

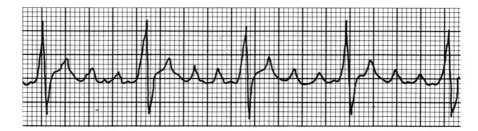

FIGURE 8-19
Atrial fibrillation.

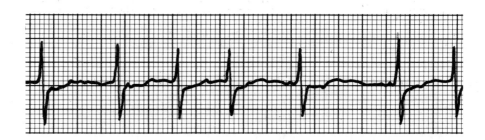

Etiology. In the patient with atrial flutter, underlying cardiac disease is usually present, including coronary artery disease, cor pulmonale, and rheumatic heart disease. The ectopic focus becomes the dominant pacemaker and is conducted through the AV junction into the ventricles in normal fashion. Two theories are currently favored as to the mechanism of atrial flutter:

- A continuous impulse travels through the atrium, causing a "circus" movement at a very rapid but coordinated rate, or
- A single ectopic focus discharges rapidly.

At the onset of the arrhythmia, the ventricles respond once to every two atrial impulses. Further AV block may develop if the arrhythmia persists, and the ventricles usually respond irregularly every two to six beats. If the ventricular rate is within normal limits, the cardiac output will remain adequate. If the rate is so rapid that the chambers cannot fill adequately, hemodynamic changes occur as described in the section on supraventricular tachycardia.

When the ventricular rate is rapid, the diagnosis of atrial flutter may be difficult. Vagal maneuvers such as carotid sinus massage will often increase the degree of AV block and allow recognition of flutter waves.

Treatment. If flutter is associated with a high degree of AV block so that the ventricular rate remains within normal limits, no treatment is necessary. When the ventricular rate is rapid, prompt treatment to control the rate or revert the rhythm to a sinus mechanism is indicated. Digitalis is the initial drug of choice. It increases the degree of AV block and thus controls the

ventricular rate, or it may produce atrial fibrillation. Reversion to a sinus mechanism often follows. If complications occur suddenly and more immediate action is required, countershock is indicated.

Atrial Fibrillation

Definition. Atrial fibrillation is defined as an atrial arrhythmia occurring at an extremely rapid atrial rate (400 to 600 per minute), lacking coordinated activity. The AV junction is able to respond only partially to the rapid rate of discharge from the atria; thus, the ventricular rate is slower, irregular, and usually 140 to 170 beats per minute at the onset of the arrhythmia.

Significant ECG Changes (Fig. 8-19)

P Waves. These waves are absent; irregular "fibrillary" waves (an uneven pattern in the baseline of the tracing) are usually seen.

QRS Complex. Complexes may appear normal or show aberrant conduction.

Etiology. Although atrial fibrillation may occur as a transient arrhythmia in healthy young people, the presence of permanent atrial fibrillation is almost always associated with underlying heart disease. One or both of the following are present in patients with permanent atrial fibrillation: atrial muscle disease and atrial distention together with disease of the SA node. Atrial fibrillation is usually initiated by APCs. Once established, it is sustained by multiple small circulating wave fronts within the atrium. This is also known as microreentry.

In patients with heart disease, atrial fibrillation causes the cardiac output to fall because of (1) a rapid rate that allows less time for the ventricles to fill, and (2) loss of effective atrial contractions. Signs of another complication may arise from atrial fibrillation, that of peripheral arterial emboli. Because of the passive dilated state of the atria, thrombi can form on the atrial wall and dislodge, producing embolization. The incidence of embolization can be reduced by anticoagulation.

The nurse will note a pulse deficit with atrial fibrillation. The radial pulse is slower than the apical pulse because some systolic contractions are feeble and not palpable in the peripheral arteries.

Treatment. If complications develop rapidly, countershock is indicated immediately. If cardiac output remains sufficient and the patient is not hypotensive or in significant heart failure, drug therapy is usually tried first. Digitalis is specifically useful because it increases AV block and allows more time for diastolic filling of the ventricles. This produces more volume per stroke.

FIGURE 8-20
Multifocal atrial tachycardia.

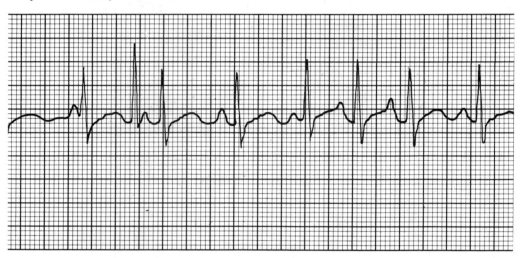

FIGURE 8-21
Sick sinus syndrome. Atrial fibrillation is followed by atrial standstill. A sinus escape beat is seen at the end of the strip.

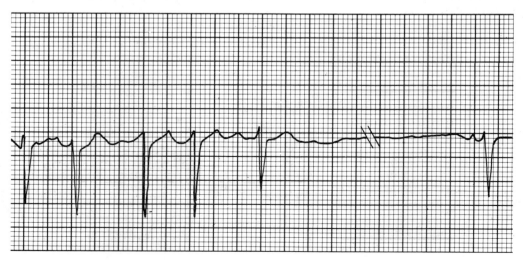

The rhythm may also convert with digitalis to a normal sinus mechanism. Quinidine aids in maintenance of normal sinus rhythm.

Multifocal Atrial Tachycardia

Definition. This rhythm characteristically occurs in patients with severe pulmonary disease. Often such patients exhibit hypoxemia, hypokalemia, alterations in serum pH, or pulmonary hypertension. In the example shown in Figure 8-20, note the rapid rate and the variable morphology of the P waves.

Sick Sinus Syndrome

Definition. Sick sinus syndrome refers to the condition in patients exhibiting severe degrees of sinus node depression including marked sinus bradycardia, SA block, and SA node arrest. Often, rapid atrial arrhythmias coexist, such as atrial flutter or fibrillation (the "tachycardia-bradycardia syndrome"), which alternate with periods of sinus node depression (Fig. 8-21).

Treatment. Management of this condition requires control of the rapid atrial arrhythmias with drug ther-

apy and, in selected cases, control of very slow heart rates as well (a permanent transvenous pacemaker).

Atrial Standstill

Definition. In atrial standstill, complete cessation of the SA node occurs. The pacemaker shifts to a lower focus, either in the atrium, in the AV junction, or within the Purkinje system (Fig. 8-22).

Etiology. As with sick sinus syndrome, this arrhythmia may occur in the elderly patient with disease of the SA node. It is also the result of intoxication from quinidine, digitalis, or potassium. Acute myocardial infarction may also produce atrial standstill.

Symptoms. Lightheadedness or fainting will occur depending on the duration of standstill. Sudden death, of course, is inevitable if a lower pacemaker does not take over.

Treatment. Intravenous atropine or isoproterenol is sometimes of value. Drugs that depress SA node function such as digitalis and quinidine should be discontinued, and hyperkalemia, if present, should be managed with intravenous sodium bicarbonate or glucose

FIGURE 8-22
Atrial standstill (lower pacemaker does not take over).

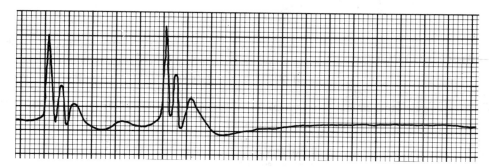

FIGURE 8-23
AV junctional premature beats.

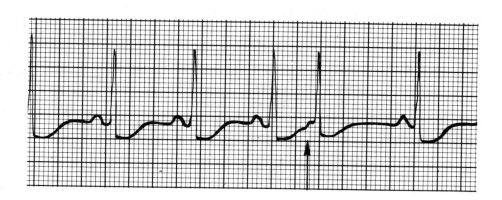

and insulin mixtures. If the arrhythmia is recurrent, an artificial pacemaker is the preferred management.

AV Junctional Premature Beats

Definition. An AV junctional premature beat is defined as an impulse from an ectopic focus in the AV junction or His bundle occurring earlier than the normal sinus impulse. The P waves are inverted in leads II, III, and aVF and may occur before, during, or after the QRS complex (Fig. 8-23).

Etiology. As with APCs, junctional premature beats may occur in normal persons or in those with underlying heart disease. The AV junction or His bundle acts as pacemaker. The impulses pass normally through the conduction system into the ventricles, producing a normal QRS. Aberrant conduction, however, may occur and lead to confusion with a ventricular premature contraction (VPC). It is helpful to obtain a long rhythm strip to find prematurities that are normally conducted. This may establish that the abnormal-appearing beats with wide QRS complexes are atrial with aberrant conduction.

An inverted P wave is produced when the AV junction stimulates the atria and causes the impulse to travel upward through the atrial fibers in retrograde fashion.

Treatment. Management is identical with that for APCs.

Ventricular Premature Contraction (VPC)

Definition. A ventricular contraction originating from an ectopic focus in the Purkinje network of the ventricles, occurring earlier than the expected sinus beat. In contrast to an APC with aberrant conduction, there is no P wave before the QRS complex. An inverted P wave may follow the VPC due to retrograde depolarization of the atria (see Fig. 8-24).

The QRS complex cannot be missed. It is not only premature, but it is bizarre, widened, and notched, and it may be of greater amplitude. The T wave of the VPC is opposite in deflection to the QRS complex. A compensatory pause often follows the premature beat as the heart awaits the next stimulus from the SA node. The pause is considered fully compensatory if the cycles of the normal and premature beats equal the time of two normal heart cycles.

Etiology. VPCs are the most common of all arrhythmias and can occur in any age group, with or without heart disease. They are especially common in a person with myocardial disease (ischemia, myocardial infarc-

tion, or following cardiac surgery) or with myocardial irritability (hypokalemia or digitalis intoxication).

If VPCs occur after each sinus beat, a bigeminal rhythm is present (Fig. 8-25). Trigeminy is a VPC occurring after two consecutive sinus beats. When VPCs originate from different ectopic foci, they are known as *multifocal*.

Symptoms. Often VPCs are asymptomatic, but some people may experience a "thump" or "skipping" sensation. VPCs may be the earliest sign of heart disease, and when they are especially frequent or approach the apex of the T wave, they may be the forerunner of more serious arrhythmias such as ventricular tachycardia or fibrillation.

Treatment. If infrequent, isolated VPCs require no treatment. Multiple, "back to back" VPCs, or VPCs falling on the apex of the T wave of the previous beat, are managed with antiarrhythmic agents, including lidocaine, procainamide, quinidine, and propranolol. If the serum potassium is low, potassium replacement may correct the arrhythmia. If the arrhythmia is due to digitalis toxicity, withdrawal of the drug may correct it.

Ventricular Tachycardia

Definition. The ventricular ectopic focus emits a series of rapid and regular impulses, and the ventricular contractions are dissociated from the atrial contractions.

The ventricular rate ranges from 100 to 220 beats per minute. P waves are rarely seen to superimpose on the rapid, bizarre QRS–T complexes. The QRS complex resembles that of VPCs, and the T wave, when visible, is opposite in deflection to the QRS complex. In the example shown, ventricular tachycardia terminates spontaneously, resulting in sinus rhythm. An "R on T" VPC is present in the next to last beat (Fig. 8-26).

Etiology. Ventricular tachycardia is rare in adults with normal hearts but is common (20% to 30%) as a complication of myocardial infarction or digitalis intoxication.

Ventricular tachycardia is thought to arise within the Purkinje network. A reentrant mechanism is usually present, causing a circulating wave front. Each completion of the wave front causes a ventricular contraction appearing as a series of VPCs. The atria continue to respond to the SA node, but the atria and ventricles beat independently. The rapid rate without a properly timed atrial contraction leads to decreased cardiac output.

Symptoms. Palpitations, angina pectoris, weakness, and fainting are frequent symptoms. Hypotension or

FIGURE 8-24
Ventricular premature contraction.

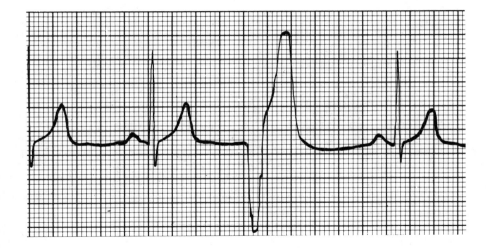

FIGURE 8-25
Bigeminal rhythm.

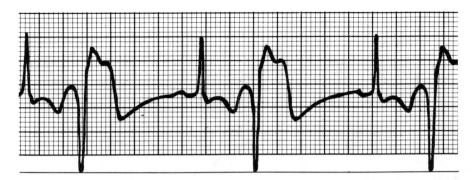

congestive heart failure may follow as the result of decreased stroke volume.

Treatment. Lidocaine, procainamide, propranolol, quinidine or disopyromide, and occasionally potassium chloride may terminate the arrhythmia. Electrical countershock is almost always effective. If the arrhythmia is due to digitalis intoxication, digitalis should be stopped, and potassium should be given.

Accelerated Ventricular Rhythm

Definition. This ectopic ventricular rhythm resembles ventricular tachycardia except that the rate is slower. The ventricular rate is between 60 and 100 beats per minute, and the characteristically wide QRS complexes are identified as being of ventricular origin. Often the ventricular rate closely parallels the sinus rate (see Fig. 8-27).

Etiology. Typically, this rhythm occurs in patients with acute myocardial infarction. Less commonly, it may occur as a result of ischemia or digitalis intoxication.

Treatment. In most cases, no treatment is necessary because the arrhythmia terminates spontaneously in less than 30 seconds.

Torsades de Pointes

Torsades de pointes ("twisting of the points") is a specific variety of ventricular tachycardia. The term refers to the polarity of the QRS complex, which swings from positive to negative and *vice versa* (Fig. 8-28). This form of ventricular tachycardia is most likely to develop with severe myocardial disease when the Q–T interval has been prolonged. The rhythm is highly unstable. It may terminate in ventricular fibrillation, or it may revert to sinus rhythm.

Etiology. Torsades de pointes is favored by conditions that prolong the Q–T interval. Examples include hypokalemia, hypomagnesiemia, and antiarrhythmic agents such as quinidine, procainamide, and disopyramide. It has also been reported with tricyclic and phenothiazine psychoactive agents.

Treatment. Treatment consists of correcting the electrolyte deficiency or stopping the offending phar-

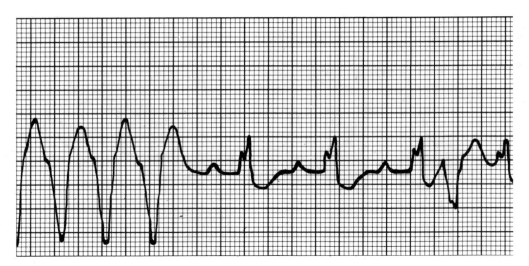

FIGURE 8-26
Ventricular tachycardia.

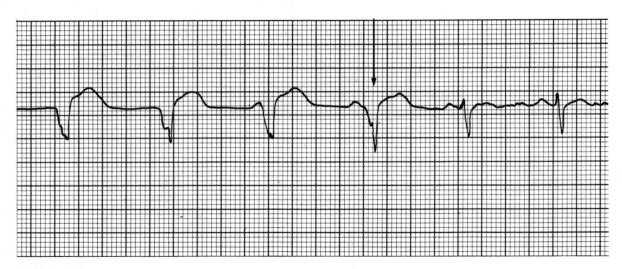

FIGURE 8-27
Accelerated ventricular rhythm. The first three beats are of ventricular origin. The fourth beat
(arrow) *represents a fusion beat. The subsequent two beats are of sinus origin.*

macologic agent. Intravenous isoproterenol and dopamine have been used with success.

Ventricular Fibrillation

Definition. Ventricular fibrillation is defined as rapid, irregular, and ineffectual contractions of the ventricle. The ECG shows a wavering baseline and bizarre waveforms.

Etiology. Ventricular fibrillation is favored by several causes. These include myocardial infarction, VPCs oc-

curring at the apex of the preceding T wave, and drugs such as digitalis and quinidine in toxic doses (Fig. 8-29).

Symptoms. With ventricular fibrillation, the ventricles immediately cease to expel blood, and death will occur rapidly in untreated cases. Loss of consciousness occurs within 8 to 10 seconds, and a seizure may occur. No pulse is elicited, and the pupils become dilated. Clinical death is present, and biologic death follows in a few moments. Ventricular fibrillation is the most common basis of sudden death and is nearly always fatal if resuscitation is not immediately instituted.

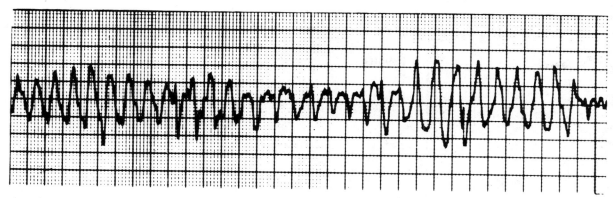

FIGURE 8-28
Torsades de pointes.

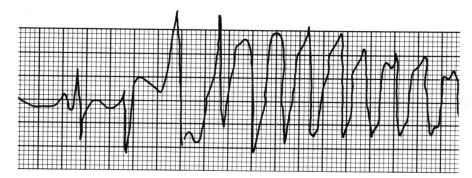

FIGURE 8-29
Ventricular fibrillation.

Rarely, ventricular fibrillation will terminate spontaneously within seconds.

Treatment. The best treatment is prevention. In monitored patients with multiple, consecutive, or encroaching VPCs, immediate treatment with lidocaine or procainamide will often prevent more serious ventricular rhythms. If fibrillation occurs, rapid defibrillation with DC countershock performed by the nurse in attendance is the management of choice (see the discussion of cardiopulmonary resuscitation in Chap. 9).

First Degree AV Block

Definition. A delay in conduction through the AV junction. The P–R interval exceeds the upper limit of 0.20 second in duration. In the example shown, the P–R interval is 0.30 second (Fig. 8-30).

Etiology. This finding occurs in all ages and in both normal and diseased hearts. Drugs such as digitalis, quinidine, and procainamide may prolong the P–R interval into the abnormal range.

The impulse originates normally in the SA node and travels through the atria in normal sequence. The AV junction delays the conduction for a longer than normal interval. When the impulse does pass through the AV junction, the ventricles respond normally. This conduction disturbance is of no significance except when it is a precursor of second or third degree AV block.

Treatment. No treatment is needed.

Second Degree Block — Mobitz I (Wenckebach)

Definition. With each beat, the delay of conduction through the AV junction is progressively increased. Eventually, the sinus impulse is completely blocked, and no QRS complex occurs.

Significant ECG Changes (Fig. 8-31.)

P–R Interval. The P–R interval progressively lengthens with each beat.

QRS Complex. The QRS complex has a normal configuration, but is progressively delayed after each P wave until one is dropped. The interval between suc-

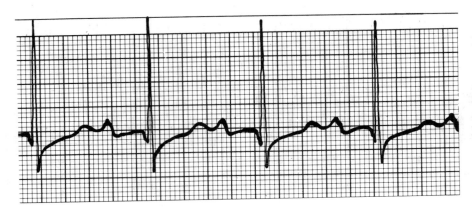

FIGURE 8-30
First-degree AV block.

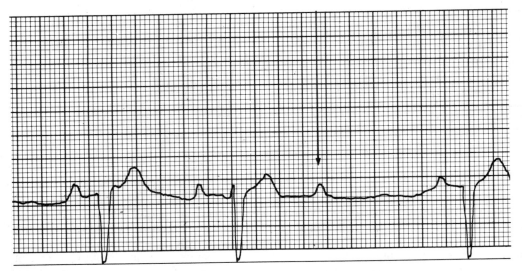

FIGURE 8-31
Second-degree block—Mobitz I (Wenckebach). The arrow indicates the nonconducted P wave in this sequence.

cessive QRS complexes shortens until a dropped beat occurs.

Etiology. Of the two types of second degree block, the Wenckebach phenomenon is the more common. Inferior myocardial infarction and digitalis toxicity may cause this type of second degree block.

Treatment. No treatment is required except to discontinue digitalis when it is the offending agent.

Second Degree Block — Mobitz II

Definition. With this rhythm, some sinus impulses are conducted through the AV junction with a constant P–R interval. Other sinus impulses are blocked completely. The ventricular rate is a fraction (1:2, 1:3, 1:4, *etc.*) of the atrial rate. In the strip shown, note the blocked P waves (Fig. 8-32, *arrows*).

Etiology. Mobitz II AV block indicates more severe impairment of AV conduction. It is seen, for example, with acute anterior myocardial infarction, and its presence implies extensive destruction of the ventricular septum. Digitalis toxicity is not a cause.

Atrial contractions result from regular SA impulses. Only those impulses that penetrate the AV junction cause ventricular contractions. No symptoms occur unless the ventricular rate is so slow that cardiac output falls. This type of arrhythmia is potentially dangerous because it may progress to third degree block or ventricular standstill.

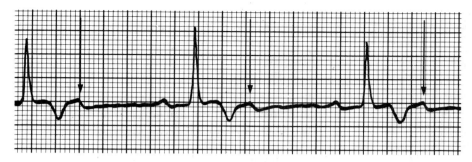

FIGURE 8-32
Second degree block — Mobitz II. Arrows denote blocked P waves.

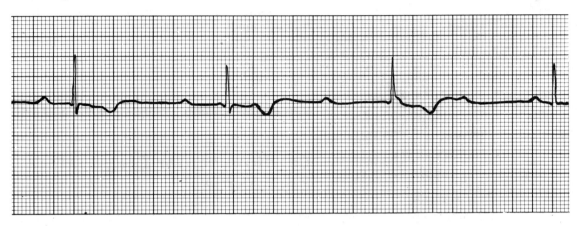

FIGURE 8-33
Third degree block (complete AV block).

Treatment. Constant monitoring and observation for progressive degrees of AV block are required. Medications used include isoproterenol and epinephrine. Transvenous pacing is often indicated.

Third Degree Block (Complete AV Block)

Definition. None of the sinus impulses are conducted through the AV junction. The atrial rate is faster than the ventricular rate, and it is usually normal and regular. The ventricular rate is regular but slower, averaging 30 to 45 beats per minute. The P–R interval is variable, as in the example shown. The QRS complex is of normal configuration if it originates in the His bundle and becomes widened if it originates from below this point (Fig. 8-33).

Etiology. Occasionally, complete heart block is congenital. In acquired cases, causes include degeneration of the conduction system due to advanced age, acute myocardial infarction, myocarditis, cardiac surgery, and digitalis intoxication.

With complete AV block, the SA node continues to pace in normal fashion, but the impulse is blocked at the AV junction. A lower cardiac pacemaker initiates the rhythm from a point distal to the AV junction.

Symptoms. If the ventricular rate is adequate to allow a normal cardiac output, the person is asymptomatic. When the rate is slow and cardiac contraction impaired from underlying heart disease, the cardiac output will fall. In the latter instance, heart failure may result and the patient may develop Adams-Stokes seizures (episodes of ventricular tachycardia, fibrillation, or cardiac standstill resulting in syncope, hypoxic seizures, coma, or death). Untreated patients with symptoms have a poor prognosis, and many such patients die within the year.

Treatment. Isoproterenol is the drug of choice. Temporary or permanent pacing is usually indicated. The nurse should familiarize herself with the benefits and hazards of electrical pacing (see Chap. 9).

Bundle Branch Block (BBB)

Definition. A delay of conduction through the right or left bundle.

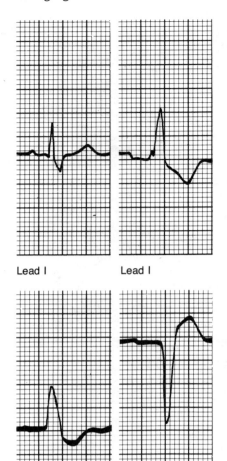

Lead I   Lead I

Lead V₁   Lead V₁
RBBB   LBBB

FIGURE 8-34
Bundle branch block.

It may also result from medications, including procainamide and quinidine, and from hyperkalemia.

When conduction through one bundle is blocked, the impulse travels along the unaffected bundle and eventually reaches the other blocked area by way of the ventricular musculature. Transmission by this route is slower, and right and left ventricular contractions do not occur simultaneously. The abnormal contraction produces a wide QRS complex.

Symptoms. Cardiac output is not decreased, and thus the arrhythmia itself does not produce symptoms.

Treatment. The underlying heart disease determines treatment and prognosis.

Cardiovascular Diagnostic Techniques

Dorothy Murphy Mayer*

Cardiovascular diagnostic techniques represent a rapidly expanding area of cardiology. As the technology expands, the diagnostic value of these procedures also expands. Some of these procedures are used alone, whereas others are used together. For example, the electrocardiogram provides information about the heart in a resting state. When this is combined with an exercise stress test, valuable information about the status of myocardial oxygen supply and demand is obtained. When the stress test is used in conjunction with a radioisotope, as in an exercise thallium study, even more specific information about myocardial perfusion is obtained.

The critical care nurse often cares for patients who undergo one or more of these procedures. Understanding the principles behind the procedure enables the nurse to answer questions, incorporate diagnostic findings into the patient's care plan, and provide high-level nursing care. The critical care nurse can also decrease anxiety for the patient's family by providing them with a brief, simple explanation of the procedure that the patient is to experience.

Significant ECG Changes

QRS Complex. The QRS complex is prolonged to 0.12 second or longer. Typically, the QRS complex is notched or slurred with a widening of the QRS complex. With right BBB, the S wave in lead I is broadened, and an R^1 is present in V_1. Left BBB produces a positive broad deflection in lead I and a broad negative deflection in lead V_1. The T wave is wide and of opposite direction to the QRS complex (Fig. 8-34).

Etiology. The most common causes of BBB are myocardial infarction, hypertension, and cardiomyopathy.

* The author wishes to thank Julie Shinn, R.N., M.A., CCRN for her support and encouragement during the preparation of this material.

STANDARD 12-LEAD ELECTROCARDIOGRAM

Because the electrocardiogram displays electrical impulses of the heart, it is possible to obtain a tracing of the electrical cardiac activity by placing electrodes at different areas of the body and connecting these electrodes to a recorder. A resting ECG is a valuable adjunct to any cardiovascular assessment. Information is obtained to evaluate heart rate and rhythm, the position of the heart in the thorax, enlarged heart chambers, ischemia or infarction patterns, and the effects of drugs and electrolytes on the conduction system.

The ECG is a simple, noninvasive test. It takes only a few minutes to record the tracing, and there are no restrictions before or after the procedure. There are no contraindications for performing an ECG, although patient cooperation is helpful.

Test Procedure

For comparison, it is important that each resting ECG be taken in a consistent manner. The position of each electrode is standardized, and any deviations from the standard should be noted on the tracing. Deviations might be required owing to the presence of surgical dressings or an amputation. Patients are placed in a supine position, with arms and legs straight and uncrossed. Standardized lead position is illustrated in Figure 8-35.

Limb leads are attached to the forearms and calves via straps, with a small amount of conduction gel placed under a small metal plate. This allows three limb leads (I, II, and III) and three augmented leads (aVR, aVL, and aVF) to be recorded. Chest precordial lead placement is secured by applying a small amount of conduction gel over the six V lead positions (V_1, V_2, V_3, V_4, V_5, and V_6) with a suction cup or electrode applied over the gel. Exact chest lead placement is outlined in Table 8-1. A tracing is recorded with the patient lying as still as possible. A sample from each of the 12 leads and a 10-second rhythm strip of three leads is obtained. Any motion or tremor on the part of the patient can cause artifact in the tracing. Artifact can also be caused by electrical interference or poor electrode contact with the skin. If artifact occurs, the electrical connections should be checked for tightness. Electrodes should be securely positioned on the chest. If possible, the tracing should be repeated until it is free of artifact.

Nursing Assessment and Intervention

Critical care nurses often record an ECG in the event of a change in patient status. This change in status in-

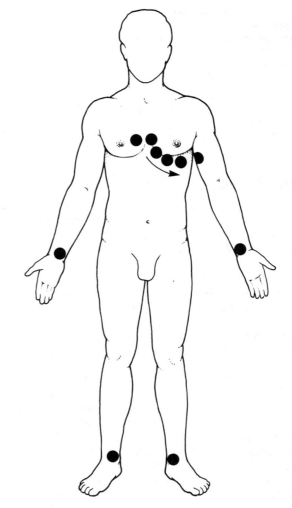

FIGURE 8-35
Standardized 12-lead ECG positions. (Adapted from King E et al: Illustrated Manual of Nursing Techniques, 2nd ed. Philadelphia, JB Lippincott, 1981.)

cludes the development of arrhythmias such as atrial fibrillation or flutter, supraventricular tachycardia, bundle branch blocks, and ventricular tachycardia. Often, an ECG is obtained during episodes of chest pain prior to the administration of sublingual nitroglycerin. The ECG provides documentation of ST changes associated with the pain. If the anginal attack is the result of coronary artery spasm, the ECG will show S–T segment elevation. If ischemia is the cause of the angina, S–T depression will be demonstrated.

Some patients fear that they will receive an electrical shock from the ECG recorder, so preparatory instruction for the patient should include an explanation of the manner in which the electrical impulses of the heart are recorded.

TABLE 8-1
PROPER PRECORDIAL LEAD POSITION

V_1: 4th intercostal space at the right sternal border
V_2: 4th intercostal space at the left sternal border
V_3: midway between V_2 and V_4
V_4: 5th intercostal space at the midclavicular line
V_5: directly lateral to V_4 at the anterior axillary line
V_6: directly lateral to V_4 at the midaxillary line

CHEST ROENTGENOGRAM

A chest roentgenogram, or x-ray film, is a valuable diagnostic test that is used in conjunction with other tests to assess cardiac size, isolated chamber size, and pulmonary blood flow. An x-ray film is a crude but effective tool used to evaluate the difference in density between the heart and its surrounding structures. Bone is the densest structure in the thorax.

It allows almost all the x-rays through and appears as a darkened area on the film. Soft tissues and blood are mainly water and absorb more x-rays than air but less than bone. Therefore, their appearance on the film is gray. It is the contrast between the densities that allows the structures in the thorax to be outlined.

Indications for an x-ray film of the chest include base line evaluation, pre- and postoperative evaluation, and the assessment of therapeutic interventions. Often, a portable x-ray film of the chest is obtained in the critical care unit to confirm appropriate placement of an endotracheal tube, of a central intravenous line, or of a chest tube. There are no contraindications for thoracic x-ray films in the critically ill patient.

Test Procedure

In many instances, the patient is too ill to be transported to the radiology department, and a portable x-ray film of the chest is obtained at the bedside. Portable films are different from standard films in several aspects. First, the x-ray beam is sent from the front of the chest to the x-ray plate behind the patient's back, resulting in an anterior-posterior (AP) view. This places the heart further away from the x-ray film than in a standard posteroanterior (PA) film. This causes greater magnification and a less distinct outline of the structures in the thorax. Second, the patient is usually lying supine in bed or sitting up as erectly as possible. This alternates the position of the diaphragm and heart in relation to the size of the chest cavity. Third, the distance between the origin of the x-ray beam and the film is shorter than in a standard PA film, so the amount of x-ray scatter is decreased. This also causes greater magnification of the thoracic structures. Although an AP film is not as accurate as a PA film, it provides valuable diagnostic information.

Nursing Assessment and Intervention

The critical care nurse's role in obtaining diagnostic thoracic x-ray films is often limited to the critical care unit, where portable x-ray films are made. With unstable patients, the nurse must decide when the film can be taken. It is important that intravenous lines not become tangled or loosened while one is trying to place the x-ray plate in the proper position. Because of x-ray scatter, it is wise for the nurse to leave the room momentarily during filming. If the nurse is unable to leave because of the patient's instability, she should wear a lead apron.

The nurse should explain the procedure to the patient, noting that the x-ray plate will be cold and hard. If possible, the patient should take a deep breath so that a good film can be obtained. This may be painful if the patient has undergone recent surgery.

LONG-TERM AMBULATORY MONITORING

An ambulatory monitor (also known as the Holter monitor) is a noninvasive, diagnostic test that is used to assess known or suspected arrhythmias. Monitoring might also be used to evaluate the treatment of known arrhythmias (*e.g.,* atrial and ventricular arrhythmias), heart blocks, and preexcitation syndromes and to assess pacemakers. This technique can also be used to verify the efficacy of medical or surgical control of known arrhythmias. In addition, Holter monitoring is used to evaluate the presence of arrhythmias during sleep apnea research and during investigational antiarrhythmic drug studies to assess the suppression of known arrhythmias.

There are no major contraindications to ambulatory monitoring, although patient cooperation is essential to the procurement of reliable diagnostic information. This procedure is used more frequently in telemetry units than in critical care areas.

Test Procedure

The patient is connected by three to five electrodes to a small portable recorder that is worn for 12 to 24 hours. The recorder is the size of a radio and is carried with a shoulder strap or on a belt clip. During the continuous recording, the patient accounts for his daily activities and any symptoms in a diary. When the monitoring period is completed, the patient returns the recorder to the lab to be analyzed. Patient symptoms such as dizziness and syncope are recorded in the diary and are correlated with any arrhythmias noted on the recorder.

Nursing Assessment and Intervention

It is important for the nurse to explain the patient's role in this procedure. For example, the patient should be encouraged to maintain normal activities while wearing the monitor. The only restriction is that the patient should avoid showering or tub-bathing until the monitoring time is completed. Often, the skin under and around the electrodes becomes irritated, and the patient must be cautioned to avoid pulling at the electrodes because loss of electrical contact can mimic sinus pauses or heart block, making the diagnostic interpretation of the test difficult.

The patient should be told that it is desirable to record an entry in his diary at least every 2 hours. The nurse might be required to do the recording if the patient's condition precludes his participation.

EXERCISE ELECTROCARDIOGRAPHY

Exercise electrocardiography is a diagnostic test that expands the use of the ECG in the diagnosis of cardiovascular abnormalities. A resting ECG can be normal even in the presence of critical coronary stenoses. An exercise test can document ECG changes during increased cardiac demand for myocardial oxygen. The presence of coronary artery disease may limit coronary blood flow. This imbalance between myocardial oxygen supply and demand causes changes in the S–T segment of the ECG that can be detected during an exercise test.

In the original exercise test developed by Masters, patients were required to walk up and over steps. An ECG was recorded as soon as possible after a certain number of repetitions was completed. Often, this exercise was submaximal or not strenuous enough to cause an imbalance between myocardial oxygen supply and demand. It may still be used in outlying areas, but it is generally considered out of date by current exercise testing standards.

Currently, multilevel exercise tolerance tests utilizing a stationary bicycle or a treadmill with continuous ECG monitoring are available. The advantages and disadvantages of these exercise tools are outlined in Table 8-2.

Indications for exercise testing as defined by the American Heart Association Committee on Exercise include establishment of a diagnosis of overt or latent disease, evaluation of cardiovascular functional capacity, evaluation of responses to conditioning and pre-ventive programs, and a need to provide individual motivation for entering and adhering to exercise programs.

Contraindications for exercise testing include severe left ventricular dysfunction, acute myocardial infarction within 10 days, unstable angina, uncompensated aortic stenosis, and cardiomyopathy. Other contraindications that may be waived with caution include complex ventricular arrhythmias, resting arterial hypertension, uncompensated valvular disease, and an uncontrolled systemic disease. Sound clinical judgment should be used in evaluating all patients prior to an exercise test.

Test Procedure

Baseline ECG, heart rate, and blood pressure are recorded in several positions (lying, sitting, standing) prior to beginning exercise. Three to 12 ECG leads are monitored throughout the test. The patient is instructed on how to walk on the treadmill and what symptoms to report during the exercise. Reportable symptoms include the onset of chest pain or pressure, fatigue, shortness of breath, leg cramps, and dizziness. The speed of walking and the percent of grade are increased every 3 minutes.

Ideally, the patient exercises to a target heart rate determined for his age. This target heart rate can be obtained from one of several formulas. An example is the following formula:

$$(220 - age) \times 85\% = \text{target heart rate}.$$

Thus, for a 50-year-old patient, the target heart rate would be 144 bpm. This is the minimum heart rate that the patient must achieve without S–T changes for a negative treadmill test. Normally, the target heart rate is easily achieved unless the patient is taking medication, such as a beta-blocker.

Generally, the patient exercises to the point of fatigue unless signs or symptoms of decreasing exercise tolerance develop. These signs and symptoms include cyanosis or pallor, ataxia, hypotension, severe S–T segment changes, rapid atrial or ventricular arrhythmias, heart block, dizziness, lightheadedness, confusion, leg pain or claudication, dyspnea, and fatigue. Often, the patient is asked to continue the exercise after the onset of angina in order to document any ECG changes associated with the pain. If the angina increases with continued exercise or causes patient anxiety, exercise should be stopped. The patient is monitored for 5 to 10 minutes after exercise or until all signs or symptoms return to baseline.

In any exercise test, the areas of concern are the heart rate and blood pressure response, the ECG rhythm, the patient's status, and exercise tolerance and

TABLE 8-2
ADVANTAGES AND DISADVANTAGES OF EXERCISE INSTRUMENTS

	Advantages	*Disadvantages*
Treadmill	☐ Best means of achieving maximum response ☐ Automatic pacing	☐ May cause static and electromagnetic interference ☐ Cable moves, potentially causing artifact ☐ Patients may have balancing difficulties ☐ Periodic recalibration required ☐ Expensive
Bicycle Ergometer	☐ Less expensive ☐ Little upper body movement ☐ Easier for patients with balancing difficulties	☐ Patient controls pacing ☐ Localized leg fatigue ☐ Difficult to attain maximal stress ☐ Tension belts can break
Steps	☐ Simplest test ☐ Least expensive	☐ Limited to submaximal testing ☐ Work loads are generally too low to show moderate heart disease ☐ Single level work load

(From Hewlett-Packard, Andover, MA)

functional classification. The heart rate should rise with increasing workloads. If the heart rate rises slowly during exercise and drops within 3 minutes to under 100 beats per minute it is a sign of aerobic conditioning. Conversely, a heart rate that rises quickly and takes considerable time to return to less than 100 beats per minute is a deconditioned response.

The blood pressure should also rise with exercise. A systolic drop of 10 mm Hg or greater is a sign of decreasing left ventricular function, and exercise should be stopped. A hypertensive blood pressure (generally 250 to 260 mm Hg/110 to 120 mm Hg) is another indication that exercise should cease.

The ECG is continuously observed for arrhythmias. Exercise should be terminated for the development of ventricular tachycardia, second- or third-degree heart block, or an atrial or supraventricular tachycardia. The ECG is also observed for signs of ischemia (*i.e.,* S–T segment depression or elevation). Most testers will stop exercise when S–T segment changes are greater than 2 to 3 mm from the baseline. The patient is questioned about symptoms of angina, fatigue, dyspnea, or lightheadedness and is observed for signs of pallor, clamminess, or ataxia.

Exercise tolerance and functional classification are based on the maximal workload completed. The workload is measured in METS, which are resting multiples of oxygen consumption. Oxygen consumption during testing is estimated to be 3.5 cc/kg of body weight. Therefore, 1 MET equals 3.5 cc O_2/kg, 5 METS equal 17.5 cc O_2/kg, 10 METS equal 35 CC O_2/kg and so on. Based on the maximal workload completed, the patient's MET level and functional classification are determined from a chart similar to that shown in Table 8-3. For example, a patient who completes stage 3 of

the Naughton protocol (2.0 miles/hr at a 3.5% grade) achieves a workload of 3 METS and is in functional class III of the New York Heart Classification.

Many exercise testing protocols exist, but the most commonly used is the Bruce protocol. The Naughton protocol is used when submaximal exercise is needed for low-level, postinfarction testing. Other available protocols are listed in Table 8-3. In any exercise test, the amount and type of exercise must be individualized for each patient, and it is sometimes necessary to switch from one protocol to another.

Nursing Assessment and Intervention

The critical care nurse may be responsible for explaining the general format of an exercise test to the patient and family. It is important that the patient understand why the test is indicated and what will be expected of him. It is reassuring for the patient to know that someone will be observing him closely throughout the test and that he is encouraged to express all concerns before, during, and after the procedure. The patient should also understand that he may have to continue exercising after the development of angina but that he will not be expected to do more exercise than is safe.

TABLE 8-3
COMPARISON OF TREADMILL PROTOCOLS, MET LEVELS, OXYGEN CONSUMPTION, AND FUNCTION CLASS*

Conditions Associated With False-Positive Exercise Stress Tests		METS	1.6	2	3	4	5	6	7	8	9	10	11	12	13	14	15	16
		Ellestad					1.7	3.0			4.0						5.0	
Organic heart disease (noncoronary)								10% Grade										
1. Left ventricular hypertrophy	Treadmill Tests	Bruce	1.2 0	1.7 5		1.7 10		2.5 12		3.4 14			4.2 16					
a. Rheumatic and other valvular diseases																		
b. Cardiomyopathies		Balke							3.4 Miles/hr									
c. Hypertension					2	4	6	8	10	12	14	16	18	20	22	24	26
2. Intraventricular conduction abnormalities		Balke					3.0 Miles/hr											
a. Left bundle-branch block				0	2.5	5	7.5	10	12.5	15	17.5	20	22.5				
b. Wolff-Parkinson-White syndrome		Naughton	1.0		2.0 Miles/hr												
c. Right bundle-branch block			0	0	3.5	7	10.5	14	17.5								
Functional cardiac conditions		METS	1.6	2	3	4	5	6	7	8	9	10	11	12	13	14	15	16
1. Syndrome of angina pectoris with normal coronary angiogram		O_2,ml/kg/min	5.6	7		14		21		28		35		42		49		56
2. Midsystolic click, late systolic murmur syndrome		Clinical Status	Symptomatic Patients															
3. Hyperventilation				Diseased, Recovered														
4. Drug and electrolyte effects: digitalis, quinidine, procainamide, hypokalemia					Sedentary Healthy												
						Physically Active Subjects											
		Functional Class	IV		III		II		I and Normal								

* Unlabeled numbers refer to treadmill speed (*top*) and percentage grade (*bottom*). See text for complete description. (From DeBusk R: The value of exercise stress testing. JAMA 232:956, 1975)

Generally, the procedure takes from 1 to 2 hours, and the patient usually abstains from eating for 2 hours prior to the test to prevent abdominal cramps or nausea from developing at maximal exercise. If possible, the patient should also avoid stimulants such as coffee, tea, and tobacco for several hours prior to the test because these may increase the excitability of the conduction system. Routine medication may or may not be discontinued prior to the test.

In some centers, nurses with extensive training in exercise testing are supervising these studies. Advanced cardiac life support certification is mandatory, and physician backup must be immediately available in the event of an emergency.

PHONOCARDIOGRAPHY

In phonocardiography, heart sounds are recorded by a microphone and converted to electrical activity that is recorded. This procedure may be used to obtain precise measurements of the timing of events of the cardiac cycle, to determine the characteristics and timing of murmurs and abnormal heart sounds, to measure systolic time intervals, and to teach cardiac auscultation. There are no contraindications or risks associated with this procedure.

Test Procedure

For a phonocardiogram, the patient is brought to a quiet room, where he is asked to lie on a comfortable table or bed. Microphones are applied to the chest wall over areas where the heart sounds and murmurs are best auscultated. The microphones pick up the sound of the heart beat and convert it to an electrical impulse that is then amplified, filtered, and recorded. Some of the microphones are allowed to lie free on the chest; others are attached by straps or ace bandages. A recording of sound waves is obtained, usually in conjunction with an ECG and a carotid pulse wave recording. These accessory recordings provide a reference point for the timing of cardiac events.

Special maneuvers or the use of pharmacologic agents may accentuate certain heart sounds and murmurs. These include the inhalation of amyl nitrate, injection of intravenous isoproterenol or vasopressors, changes in position (sitting or squatting), variations in breathing (deep inspiration and expiration), and the performance of a Valsalva maneuver.

Nursing Assessment and Intervention

Generally, phonocardiography takes 1 to 2 hours. The patient should be told beforehand that he may be asked to perform certain maneuvers or may be administered certain agents to facilitate the diagnostic value of the test.

ECHOCARDIOGRAPHY

Improvements in the technology of diagnostic echocardiography have expanded the ability of this noninvasive procedure to provide valuable information about cardiac function. Echocardiography utilizes high-frequency ultrasound waves that are inaudible to the human ear. A transducer placed on the chest wall pulses these sound waves at short intervals and then awaits their reflection. The reflected sound waves are referred to as "echos." Based on the varying density of myocardial structures, more or less sound is reflected back. More specifically, the interface between tissues of different densities causes the echo to be reflected. These echos are graphically displayed in a characteristic pattern.

The graphic display of the echo recording varies with the recording technique that is utilized. The most frequently used methods of recording are two-dimensional and M-mode echocardiography. The M-mode technique records both the motion and the amplitude of the returned echos. These lines are displayed simultaneously with the electrocardiogram. This type of recording provides a narrow, segmental view of the heart known as the "ice pick" view of M-mode echocardiography (Fig. 8-36).

Two-dimensional echocardiography provides a more accurate assessment of cardiac motion than the M-mode technique. In this procedure, the sound waves are emitted in a fanlike fashion rather than in the ice pick fashion of the M-mode technique. The two-dimensional technique shows cardiac motion in real time, making it easier to determine the spatial relationship of the various structures. Instead of being observed through a narrow path, the heart is examined through slices, or planes.

Uses for echocardiography include assessment of valvular function, evaluation of congenital defects, diagnosis of myocardial tumors or effusions, measurement of cardiac chamber size, evaluation of ventricular function, and serial evaluation of disease progression. The mitral and aortic valves can be assessed for the presence of stenosis or regurgitation, and mitral valve function during systole can be observed for the presence of mitral valve prolapse. The tricuspid and pulmonary valves are slightly more difficult to visualize, but they can also be observed. The functioning of prosthetic valves can be evaluated, and congenital defects and the chamber abnormalities that result from these defects can be assessed. The presence of intracardiac shunts also can be evaluated.

A pericardial effusion can easily be detected with

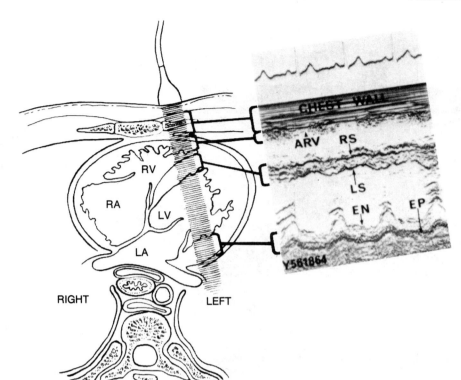

FIGURE 8-36
Diagram and echocardiogram illustrating how the M-mode technique obtains an "ice-pick" view of the heart. ARV = anterior right ventricular wall; RS = right septum; LS = left septum; EN = endocardium; EP = epicardium. (From Feigenbaum H: Echocardiography. Philadelphia, Lea and Febiger, 1981.)

echocardiography. The pericardial sac is a potential space; if fluid accumulates in this area, the echocardiogram will show a space between the ventricles and their surrounding structures that is usually not visible. In the critical care unit, a portable echocardiogram can be used to assess ventricular function or papillary muscle function in the patient with an acute infarction.

Because of the noninvasive nature of echocardiography, there are no associated contraindications. The risks associated with ultrasonography are the subject of current debate.

Test Procedures

Generally, the patient lies in a supine position with the chest partially bared. ECG limb leads are applied for simultaneous recording of the ECG with the echocardiogram to allow determination of the systolic and diastolic portions of the cardiac cycle. Conducting gel is applied over a small area on the chest; the transducer is applied over the gel and is angled against the chest wall. In M-mode echocardiography, the standard initial transducer position is in the third to fifth intercostal space at the left sternal border. The oscilloscope is observed for the appearance of the anterior leaflet of the mitral valve. Once this landmark is identified, the transducer is angled to allow the ultrasonic beam to pass through different cardiac structures. See Figure

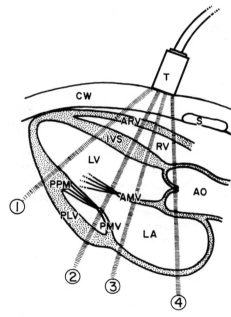

FIGURE 8-37
A cross-section of the heart showing the structures through which the ultrasonic beam passes as it is directed from the apex (1) toward the base (4) of the heart. CW = chest wall; T = transducer; S = sternum; ARV = anterior right ventricular wall; RV = right ventricular cavity; IVS = interventricular septum; LV = left ventricle; PPM = posterior papillary muscle; PLV = posterior left ventricular wall; AMV = anterior mitral valve; PMV = posterior mitral valve; AO = aorta; LA = left atrium. (From Feigenbaum H: Clinical applications of echocardiography. Prog Cardiovasc Dis 14: 535, 1972.)

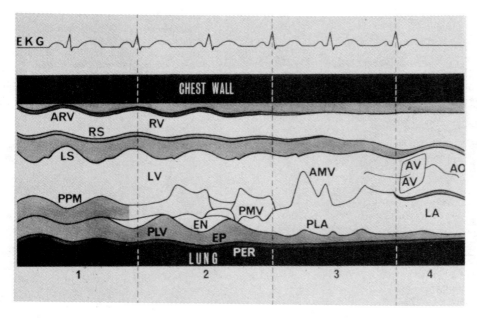

FIGURE 8-38
Diagrammatic presentation of the M-mode echocardiogram as the transducer is directed from the apex (1) to the base of the heart (4). The areas between the dotted lines correspond to the transducer positions as shown in Figure 8-37. RS = right septum; LS = left septum; EN = endocardium of the left ventricle; EP = epicardium of the left ventricle; PLA = posterior left atrial wall; PER = pericardium. Other abbreviations are as in Figure 8-37. (From Feigenbaum H: Clinical applications of echocardiography. Prog Cardiovasc Dis 14: 536, 1972.)

8-37 for a cross-section of the heart showing the structures the ultrasonic beam transects as it is angled from the apex toward the base of the heart. Figure 8-38 shows the M-mode tracing that corresponds with Figure 8-38.

The transducer location and imaging planes used in two-dimensional echocardiography have been standardized by the American Society of Echocardiography. The imaging planes used are the long-axis plane, the short-axis plane, and the four-chamber plane. The long-axis plane transects the heart perpendicular to the dorsal and ventral surfaces of the body and parallel to the long axis of the heart. The short-axis plane also transects the heart perpendicular to the dorsal and ventral surfaces of the body, but it is perpendicular to the long axis of the heart. The four-chamber plane transects the heart parallel to the dorsal and ventral surfaces of the heart.

Nursing Assessment and Intervention

Echocardiography should be explained to the patient and family in simple terms. The length of testing will vary from 30 minutes to 2 hours, depending on the ease of visualization of the cardiac structures. Pharmacologic agents or isotonic or supine exercise may be used to obtain expanded diagnostic information.

Echocardiography might be performed at the bedside of the critically ill patient, and the critical care nurse will need to coordinate this procedure with the patient's care plan.

RADIOISOTOPE STUDIES

With radioisotopes and a scintillation gamma camera, a relatively simple and noninvasive assessment of myocardial perfusion can be accomplished. Although many different radioisotopes have been tried, the two commonly employed are thallium-201 (^{201}tl) and technetium (^{99m}Tc) pyrophosphate (Table 8-4). Radioisotope studies are based on the fact that normal myocardial cells accept an isotope in a similar manner. Only in abnormal myocardial cells will there be an increased or decreased uptake of the isotope. An area of increased uptake is known as a "hot spot"; an area of decreased uptake is referred to as a "cold spot."

"Hot Spot" Imaging

In "hot spot" imaging, technetium pyrophosphate is used to identify areas of the myocardium that take up an increased amount of the isotope. Indications for hot spot imaging include a suspected acute myocardial in-

TABLE 8-4
COMPARISON OF RADIOISOTOPE STUDIES

	"Hot Spot" Imaging	*"Cold Spot" Imaging*
Isotope	Technetium 99m	Thallium 201
Method	Areas of damaged myocardium appear as a "hot spot" of increased radioactivity.	Areas of ischemia or infarction appear as a "cold spot" of decreased radioactivity. "Cold spots" that reperfuse with rest indicate reversiable ischemia; fixed "cold spots" indicate infarction.
Advantages	Can identify infarction that occurred from 12 hours to 6 days previously.	Can identify infarction before ECG or enzyme changes. Can identify stress-induced ischemia.
Disadvantages	Not accurate when infarction is nontransmural or in the presence of ventricular aneurysm or lung neoplasm.	Not able to assess accurately the age of the infarction without a second scan.

farction that is confused by an atypical or inconsistent history, an abnormal ECG, or a borderline enzyme elevation. If a delay occurs between the onset of symptoms and when the patient presents for medical assistance, valuable ECG and enzyme changes may be missed. Technetium scanning can be used to identify infarctions that occurred as recently as 12 hours ago or as long as 6 days previously. It is important to remember that the accuracy of hot spot imaging decreases when the infarction is nontransmural.

In patients with an abnormal resting ECG, such as a left bundle branch block, an ECG yields no information about the presence of ischemia or infarction. A cardiac enzyme evaluation is not reliable in patients who have experienced recent chest massage, defibrillation, intramuscular injections, or cardiac surgery. These situations cause an enzyme elevation that results from cardiac muscle trauma, not infarction. Technetium pyrophosphate imaging is useful in the aforementioned settings and may also be used to confirm the suspicion of an intraoperative myocardial infarction when the patient presents postoperatively with an abnormal ECG and an enzyme elevation. A false-positive may result in the patient with a ventricular aneurysm or neoplasm.

There are no contraindications for hot spot imaging, there are no risks associated with this procedure for either the patient or the nurse because only a small dose of radiation is involved.

Test Procedures
The procedure involves an injection of the isotope, followed by scanning approximately 2 to 3 hours later. The delay between injection and scanning allows the isotope to be cleared from the bloodstream. The infarcted myocardium will appear as an area of increased

radioactivity, or a "hot spot." Several scans with the patient in different positions are obtained, including an anteroposterior view, a right anterior oblique view, a left anterior oblique view, and a left lateral view. Each scan requires approximately 5 minutes, and these multiple views enable all areas of ventricular perfusion to be evaluated.

Nursing Assessment and Intervention
The nurse should explain the procedure and answer questions asked by the patient and his family. The patient needs to understand that he will receive an injection followed by scanning 2 to 3 hours later. During scanning, the patient is required to lie quietly under the camera. Total scanning time is generally 30 minutes. Patients are often anxious about the radiation involved and the appearance of the equipment; the nurse plays an important role in allaying these patient anxieties.

"Cold Spot" Imaging

In "cold spot" imaging, thallium is the isotope used to assess myocardial perfusion. An area of decreased uptake (a "cold spot" indicates an area of decreased perfusion that could be secondary to coronary stenosis or a previous infarction.

This modality might be used in the critical care unit to confirm the presence of a myocardial infarction before ECG and enzyme changes have occurred. Thallium scanning can also be used to identify the area and extent of an infarction. One limitation is that the age of the infarct (old versus acute) cannot be easily determined. To accurately confirm an acute infarction, one must obtain a second scan several days after the first scan. The acuteness of the infarction is confirmed if the ischemic zone around the infarction has resolved. The accuracy of thallium scanning in the acute setting is greatest when performed within 6 to 12 hours after symptoms develop.

More frequently, thallium scanning is used in conjunction with an exercise ECG to assess myocardial perfusion after exercise. An exercise thallium study involves maximal exercise on a treadmill and an injection of thallium through a previously placed intravenous heparin lock 30 to 60 seconds prior to the discontinuation of the exercise. Two scans, are obtained, one immediately after exercise and one approximately 4 hours later. Any areas of decreased uptake, or "cold spots," immediately after exercise that reperfuse, or "fill in," over the 4-hour period suggest reversible ischemia secondary to coronary artery disease. This contrasts with the cold spot that persists on the delay scan and suggests a previous infarction. Again, the scanning time is generally 30 to 45 minutes. Three scans are obtained, the anterior view, the 45° to 55° left anterior oblique (LAO) view, and the 65° to 70° LAO view. One needs to obtain the two LAO views to view the intraventricular septum adequately.

Indications for exercise thallium studies include an abnormal resting ECG, digitalis therapy, atypical angina, and an abnormal exercise test in an otherwise asymptomatic patient. In patients with abnormal ECG changes (*e.g.,* left bundle branch block or left ventricular hypertrophy), the resting S–T abnormalities may mask ischemic changes. If the electrocardiogram is inconclusive, the thallium scan provides an accurate assessment of the presence of ischemia. Digitalis causes false S–T depression, and patients receiving digitalis may have inconclusive stress ECG's because it is difficult to distinguish S–T changes that result from digitalis from those that result from ischemia.

Patients with atypical angina present another dilemma. If the exercise ECG is negative for ischemia but chest pain occurs, there is a chance that coronary artery disease is present. An exercise thallium study may save the patient from undergoing cardiac catheterization if it demonstrates that cardiac perfusion is normal. In asymptomatic patients with abnormal exercise tests, an exercise thallium study provides information about the extent of ischemia. In patients with known coronary artery disease, an exercise thallium study is used to assess reperfusion prior to coronary artery bypass surgery.

There are no contraindications for "cold spot" thallium imaging. The dosage of radioactivity is minimal and has no known side effects. When an exercise thallium study is performed, all the risks and contraindications associated with exercise testing apply. Full emergency equipment and trained personnel must be present.

Nursing Assessment and Intervention

The critical care nurse's responsibilities in providing care for patients who are undergoing this diagnostic procedure include an appropriate explanation of the test. There are eating restrictions for 2 to 4 hours prior to the injection of the thallium because the increased blood flow that aids in digestion diverts thallium away from cardiac muscle. During scanning, the patient must lie quietly under the camera. After the procedure is completed, there are no restrictions.

CARDIAC CATHETERIZATION

Cardiac catheterization refers to the introduction of a catheter into the cardiac chambers. At the time of catheterization, evaluation of intracardiac pressures, intracardiac blood oxygen levels, cardiac output, and coronary circulation may be performed. Valvular function and ventricular function can be evaluated, and congenital heart disease can be confirmed.

Uses for cardiac catheterization include confirmation of suspected coronary artery disease and determination of the location and severity of coronary artery disease and any associated symptoms. In many instances, cardiac catheterization is the definitive procedure in the patient with a confusing clinical picture, such as the person with physically limiting chest pain of unknown etiology and the asymptomatic patient with an abnormal stress test.

Contraindications include acute myocardial infarction, acute heart failure, severe or uncontrolled hypertension, acute infection or febrile illness, digitalis toxicity, hypokalemia, uncontrolled or irretractable ventricular arrhythmias, cardiogenic shock, and irreversible anticoagulation. Contraindications that can be controlled or corrected may be treated prior to catheterization.

Complications that may occur as a result of catheterization include stroke, embolization, conduction disturbances, cardiac perforation, phlebitis, infection, allergic reactions, myocardial infarction, and death. In 1979, the Coronary Artery Surgery Study (CASS) reported complications of coronary arteriography based on investigations of 7533 patients.[1] The mortality rate was 2 deaths/1000 patients, with the presence of congestive heart failure, hypertension, and multiple VPCs increasing the risk of death. The presence of a left main coronary artery stenosis greater than 50% and an ejection fraction less than 30 also increased risk of death. The rate of myocardial infarction was 2.5/1000 patients; the presence of unstable angina increased this risk. The CASS also reported a higher mortality with the brachial approach compared than with the femoral approach, except in laboratories using 80% or more brachial approaches. Vascular complications occurred more frequently with the brachial approach.

Test Procedure

Introduction of the catheters into the cardiac chambers can be accomplished in one of two ways. In the direct approach, using local anesthesia, the brachial artery or brachial or basilic vein is surgically exposed. This approach is used when there is known disease in the descending aorta or in the iliac or femoral vasculature and when an increased risk of bleeding exists, as in the patient who is receiving anticoagulation therapy. Upon removal of the catheters, the artery and vein must be surgically repaired.

Two disadvantages of this approach are an increased risk of thrombosis and the length of time involved with the exposure and suturing processes.

Percutaneous femoral puncture is the second catheterization approach. Under local anesthesia, the femoral artery and/or vein is cannulated through a small skin incision. A guide wire is advanced through a needle to the appropriate cardiac chamber. The needle is then removed, and the selected catheter is advanced over the guide wire. The guide wire is removed during the catheterization. One advantage of this approach is the ease with which the guide wire can be reinserted to change catheters. Also, this procedure is not as time-consuming as the direct approach. Once the catheters are removed, pressure is applied to the insertion site to prevent bleeding.

If the right side of the heart is catheterized, the appropriate catheter is inserted through the venous system and advanced into the vena cava, then into the right atrium, and through the tricuspid valve into the right ventricle. The advancement of the catheter is monitored by fluoroscopy and pressure wave forms. Pressure measurements or blood samples are obtained in both chambers. The catheter can then be advanced into the pulmonary artery and on into a pulmonary capillary, where the pulmonary artery wedge pressure is measured.

In catheterization of the left side of the heart, the catheter is advanced retrograde through the arterial system into the ascending aorta, to just above the aortic valve. The advancement of the catheter is once again observed by fluoroscopy and pressure wave forms. Arterial pressure measurements are recorded above the aortic valve. The catheter is then advanced across the valve into the left ventricle.

Generally, it is difficult to reach the left atrium by this retrograde approach. When left atrial pressures are required, a transseptal approach is employed. This necessitates a right-sided heart catheterization, and, once in the right atrium, a puncture is made through the atrial septum at the fossa ovalis. This transseptal technique is contraindicated in patients who are receiving anticoagulants. Associated risks are cardiac perforation and hemorrhage.

The last approach for left-sided heart catheterization is direct ventricular puncture through the chest wall. This technique is rarely employed, and then it is used only when other approaches have been unsuccessful or when severe aortic stenosis makes the retrograde approach too risky.

Systemic heparinization is employed during left-sided heart catheterization to decrease the possibility of clot formation at the tip of the catheter or guide wire. Heparinization is reversed with protamine sulfate once the procedure is completed. Direct pressure is applied to all arterial puncture sites for at least 15 minutes after the catheters are removed.

At the time of cardiac catheterization, coronary arteriography is performed to evaluate the patency of the coronary circulation. In the indirect approach, a single catheter is advanced to the aortic root, contrast material is injected, and its passage through the coronary circulation is recorded. The major disadvantage of this method is the large amount of contrast material (up to 40 ml under pressure) that is needed for adequate visualization.

More frequently, the direct approach is used. In the Sones technique, which requires one catheter, first the right coronary artery is studied, then the left coronary artery. With the catheter in the ostium of the coronary vessel, 5 to 10 ml of contrast material is hand-injected, and the passage of the contrast material is recorded by cinefluoroscopy. Patients often experience a hot flash or a sensation of nausea with the injection of the contrast material. Coughing after the injection assists in clearing the contrast material from the coronary arteries.

Ergonovine may be administered during coronary arteriography to provoke underlying coronary artery spasm. The spasm is immediately reversed with the administration of intravenous nitroglycerine. Also, intracoronary streptokinase can be given to the patient with an acute myocardial infarction to limit clot formation and permit reperfusion of ischemic myocardial tissue.

Nursing Assessment and Intervention

Physical assessment should include inspection of the catheterization site for bleeding, swelling, or hematoma formation. Arterial pulses distal to the insertion site should be palpated and checked frequently. If the femoral approach was used, the affected leg should be kept straight for several hours. A sandbag or pressure dressing may be used to assist in clot formation and to remind the patient not to hyperextend the affected limb. Usually, the patient is confined to bed for 12 to 24 hours.

When the brachial approach is used, a pressure dressing is applied instead of a sandbag. The affected arm should not be flexed for several hours. Bed rest is generally required for a short period of time. Suture removal occurs approximately 1 week later.

Vital signs should be assessed frequently for the first few hours after catheterization. Because the contrast medium acts as an osmotic diuretic, patients may easily become volume-depleted. This volume depletion may initially cause an increased heart rate and a decreased blood pressure. Fluids need to be replaced either orally or intravenously.

ELECTROPHYSIOLOGY STUDIES

An electrophysiology study enables the physician to evaluate the mechanism of cardiac arrhythmias and to evaluate pharmacologic or surgical control of these arrhythmias.

Indications for electrophysiology studies include arrhythmias, cardiac conduction system disease, sinus node dysfunction, and syncope of unknown etiology.

Owing to the invasive nature of both cardiac catherization and electrophysiology studies, the contraindications and complications associated with these procedures are similar. Because a recent myocardial infarction will limit the ability of the heart to tolerate the rapid pacing required during the procedure, an electrophysiology study should be avoided in the acute infarction setting.

Test Procedure

From one to six catheters are inserted percutaneously into the heart. The three most common positions for the catheters are the high right atrium, the His bundle, and the right ventricular apex. A catheter in the high right atrium position is located at the junction of the inferior vena cava and the right atrium. In this position, the catheter records the atrial activity and stimulates the atria. A catheter in the His bundle position is located just across the tricuspid valve at the septum. Here, the catheter records the electrical activity of the His bundle. The right ventricular apex catheter is used to record ventricular activity and to stimulate the ventricle. When the appropriate catheter positioning is confirmed by fluoroscopy, baseline recordings are obtained in conjunction with a surface ECG. Then, either rapid pacing or extra stimuli are used to stress the conduction system. If arrhythmias are induced, their origin is distinguished as atrial, supraventricular, or ventricular. Pharmacologic agents may then be used to control these arrhythmias. Sometimes, cardioversion or defibrillation is necessary to convert life-threatening arrhythmias.

Nursing Assessment and Intervention

Generally, an electrophysiology study is a long procedure, often 4 to 6 hours in length. The physical assessment includes frequent monitoring of vital signs and assessment of pulses on the affected limb. The catheter insertion site is checked frequently for bleeding or swelling. The emotional assessment is extremely important after an electrophysiology study because the patient is kept awake throughout the procedure and may remember being cardioverted or losing consciousness prior to being defibrillated.

In patients with life-threatening arrhythmias, electrophysiologic testing often must be repeated several times. This frequent testing enables the appropriate antiarrhythmic drug to be prescribed. Finding the correct antiarrhythmic drug or drug combinations is sometimes a time-consuming process. A drug that initially controls the arrhythmia may cause untolerable side effects or later fail to control the arrhythmia. Occasionally, a drug will exacerbate the underlying arrhythmia instead of suppressing it. Nursing assessment is crucial for the recognition and prevention of serious side effects associated with antiarrhythmic medications.

If a pharmacologic agent cannot control the arrhythmia, surgical therapy may be considered. This includes coronary artery bypass grafting if ischemia is responsible for the arrhythmia. An ectopic focus may develop in the area of a ventricular aneurysm, in which case a ventricular aneurysmectomy may be indicated. Surgical ablation of an ectopic focus or reentrant pathway may be necessary.

New Techniques

Digital subtraction angiography (DSA) and nuclear magnetic resonance (NMR) are noninvasive imaging methods that appear very promising in their application to diagnostic cardiology. Digital subtraction angiography utilizes a computer and a television camera to record cardiovascular structures after an intravenous injection of contrast material. A preinjection image obtained by the computer is subtracted from later images containing the contrast material. This enables the cardiovascular structures outlined by the contrast material to be visualized free of background. With DSA, it is possible to obtain consistent cardiovascular images with lower doses of contrast material.

Currently, DSA is used for the analysis of ventricular wall motion, calculation of ejection fraction, and evaluation of coronary artery bypass grafting. At present, DSA is not applicable to the assessment of coronary arteries, but it is hoped that this use will become possible in the future.

Nuclear magnetic resonance is a technique that

chemists have used to determine the structure of molecules. It is only recently that this technique has been applied to imaging parts of the body.

Nuclei of certain isotopes produce a magnetic field when moved. These nuclei line up when placed in an external magnetic field. When a short radiofrequency is applied, the nuclei become tilted from their aligned position. As they realign themselves with the external magnetic field, they emit a radiofrequency that can be detected by an antenna. These reemitted radiofrequency waves contain spatial information. A computer reconstructs this spatial information into a three-dimensional image. The application of NMR to diagnostic cardiology has great promise because it may be used to differentiate between healthy and ischemic tissue.

REFERENCE

1. Davis K et al: Complications of Coronary Arteriography from the Collaborative Study of Coronary Artery Surgery Study (CASS). Circulation, June, 1979, pp 1105–1111

BIBLIOGRAPHY

Ellestad MH: Stress Testing Principles and Practice. Philadelphia, FA Davis, 1980

Feigenbaum H: Echocardiography, 3rd ed. Philadelphia, Lea & Febiger, 1981

Goldman MR et al: Nuclear magnetic resonance imaging: potential cardiac applications. Am J Cardiol, December 18, 1980, pp 1278–1283

Grossman W: Cardiac catherization and angiography, 2nd ed. Philadelphia, Lea & Febiger, 1980

Henry WL et al: Report of the American Society of Echocardiography Committee on Nomenclature and Standards in two-dimensional echocardiography. Circulation, August 1980, pp 212–217

King E, Wieck L, Dyer M: Illustrated Manual of Nursing Techniques, 2nd ed. Philadelphia, JB Lippincott, 1981

Morganroth J, Parisi AF, Pohost GM: Noninvasive Cardiac Imaging. Chicago, Year Book Medical Publishers, 1983

Sanderson RG, Kurth CL: The Cardiac Patient: A Comprehensive Approach, 2nd ed. Philadelphia, WB Saunders, 1983

Selzer A: Principles and Practice of Clinical Cardiology, 2nd ed. Philadelphia, WB Saunders, 1983

Underhill SL et al: Cardiac Nursing. Philadelphia, JB Lippincott, 1982

Winkle RA: Cardiac Arrhythmias: Current Diagnosis and Practical Management. Menlo Park, CA, Addison-Wesley Publishing Co, 1983

Serum Electrolyte Abnormalities and the Electrocardiogram

Shirley J. Hoffman

The maintenance of adequate fluid and electrolyte balance assumes high priority in the care of patients in any medical, surgical, or coronary intensive care unit. Patients being treated for renal or cardiovascular diseases are especially vulnerable to electrolyte imbalances. The cure may well be worse than the disease if electrolyte abnormalities go undetected or ignored because they frequently are caused by the treatment rather than by the disease itself.

Dialysis can very quickly cause major shifts in electrolytes. Certainly, the often insidious drop of serum potassium levels in the digitalized cardiac patient who received diuretics is well known. Diuretics are also frequently used as part of the medical regimen for the control of hypertension. Any addition, deletion, or change in diuretic therapy warrants close following of serum electrolytes.

A history of any of the aforementioned problems should alert the nurse to check the patient's serum electrolytes on an ongoing basis.

Potassium and calcium are probably the two most important electrolytes that are concerned with proper function of the heart. They help produce normal contraction of cardiac muscle. They are also important in the propagation of the electrical impulse in the heart. Because of the latter function, excess or insufficiency of either electrolyte frequently causes changes in the ECG. The nurse who is aware of and is able to recognize these changes may well suspect electrolyte abnormalities before clinical symptoms appear or hazardous arrhythmias occur.

Potassium

Hypokalemia (hypopotassemia) is probably the most frequently encountered electrolyte abnormality. It is commonly associated with vomiting, diarrhea, prolonged digitalis and diuretic therapy, and prolonged nasogastric suctioning. The alkalotic patient may also be hypokalemic. Hypokalemia may also accompany excessive steroid administration.

In general, a rise of 0.1 in the pH will account for a fall of 0.5 mEq per liter in serum potassium. In most laboratories, normal serum potassium levels are about 3.5 to 5.0 mEq per liter. The ECG that exhibits U waves

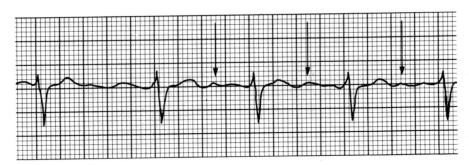

FIGURE 8-39
Presence of U waves (hypokalemia).

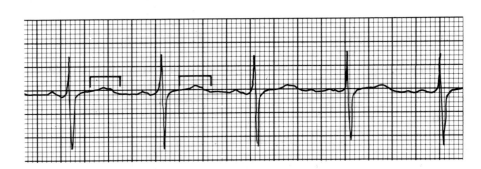

FIGURE 8-40
Fusion of T and U waves (hypoka-lemia).

should immediately alert the nurse to the possibility of hypokalemia in that patient (Fig. 8-39). Although the U wave is normal for many people, it is worthwhile to obtain a serum potassium level because it may be an early sign of hypokalemia. The normal U wave is often seen best in lead V_3. It is usually easily recognized, but it may encroach on the preceding T wave and go unnoticed (Fig. 8-40). The T wave may look notched or prolonged when it is hiding the U wave, giving the appearance of a prolonged Q–T interval.

As potassium depletion increases, the U wave may become more prominent as the T wave becomes less so. The T wave becomes flattened and may even invert. The S–T segment tends to become depressed, somewhat resembling the effects of digitalis on the ECG. These ECG changes are not particularly well correlated with the severity of hypokalemia; however, they are good indicators of this abnormality and can be recognized by the nurse who has basic knowledge of ECG complexes.

Untreated hypokalemia can produce ventricular premature contractions (VPCs), atrial or junctional tachycardias, and eventually ventricular tachycardia, ventricular fibrillation, and death. The severity of the arrhythmias resulting from hypokalemia certainly points out the need for early recognition of this problem.

The U wave may also be accentuated in association with digitalis, quinidine, epinephrine, hypercalcemia, thyrotoxicosis, and exercise. The normal U wave

should be upright in all leads that have upright T waves, and its polarity may be reversed in the presence of myocardial ischemia and left ventricular strain.

Hyperkalemia (hyperpotassemia) is often the result of overenthusiastic or poorly supervised treatment of hypokalemia. Sometimes, early detection of hypokalemia is accomplished, treatment is instituted, and the problem is considered solved. However, if potassium supplements are not stopped or reduced when normal serum potassium levels are reached, hyperkalemia will result.

Other causes of hyperkalemia include Addison's disease, acute renal failure, and acidosis. Tissue breakdown following trauma may cause the release of large amounts of potassium into the bloodstream.

Another not infrequently seen cause of high potassium levels is the use of potassium-sparing diuretics. Triamterene (Dyrenium) is an example of this type of drug that is currently in common usage as an adjunct to the more potent diuretics. It must be remembered that these drugs not only spare potassium but also may increase the potassium level of the serum.

The earliest sign of hyperkalemia on the ECG is a change in the T wave. It is usually described as tall, narrow, and "peaked" or "tenting" in appearance (Fig. 8-41). The T wave height is normally not more than 5 mm in any standard lead and not more than 10 mm in any precordial lead. T waves may be abnormally tall in myocardial infarction and may also be

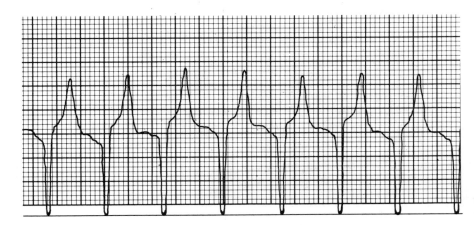

FIGURE 8-41
Hyperkalemia.

found in ventricular overloading and in patients with cerebrovascular accidents.

As potassium levels rise, changes occur first in the atrial portion of the ECG complex, then in the ventricular portion. The P wave flattens and becomes wider as the result of intra-atrial block. Further potassium elevation causes progression to AV nodal block and a prolonged P–R interval. The P wave may disappear entirely. With even higher potassium levels, the QRS begins to widen, indicating intraventricular block.

If untreated, severe hyperkalemia will progress to increased widening of the QRS until ventricular fibrillation occurs at serum potassium levels of 8 to 10 mEq per liter. In terms of arrhythmias, the patient may progress from sinus bradycardia to first degree block, through junctional rhythm, idioventricular rhythm, and ventricular tachycardia and fibrillation. Hyperkalemic changes on ECG correlate well with serum potassium levels. The described changes in T waves begin to appear at serum levels of 6 to 7 mEq/liter; the QRS widens at 8 to 9 mEq/liter. Vigorous treatment must be instituted to reverse the condition at this point because sudden death may occur at any time after these levels are reached.

Calcium

Calcium is the second electrolyte important to normal functioning of the heart. It is thought to have an effect on linking the electrical impulse to myocardial contraction. Calcium increases cardiac contractility and is often administered intravenously to the patient who has sustained cardiac arrest in an attempt to increase the force of cardiac contraction.

Hypercalcemia. Normal serum calcium is about 9 to 11 mg/dl. Hypercalcemia is often seen in patients with hyperparathyroidism, neoplastic diseases, and acute osteoporosis. It may also be seen in patients with sar-

coidosis, hyperthyroidism, adrenal insufficiency, acute immobilization, and chlorothiazide therapy.

Clinical symptoms relative to hypercalcemia are mainly neurologic. These may include somnolence or irritability, muscle weakness, or peripheral neuropathies. The patient may also exhibit gastrointestinal symptoms, such as anorexia, constipation, nausea, and vomiting. Other hypercalcemic patients may be totally asymptomatic.

Hypocalcemia may occur in patients with renal failure, hypoparathyroidism, and malabsorption syndromes.

Tetany is the most obvious manifestation of hypocalcemia, beginning with numbness and tingling of the mouth and extremities and progressing to muscle spasm and seizure. The patient with mild hypocalcemia may be asymptomatic; however, neurologic testing (Chvostek's sign and Trousseau's sign) may indicate calcium deficit.

ECG Indicators. The Q–T interval length is the most frequent ECG indicator of excess or insufficient calcium. It is somewhat shortened in hypercalcemia and lengthened in hypocalcemia (Figs. 8-42 and 8-43). In the hypercalcemic patient, the shortening of the Q–T interval takes place especially in the portion from the beginning of the QRS to the apex of the T wave, making the beginning of the T wave an abrupt slope. If this portion of the complex is less than 0.23 to 0.29 second, hypercalcemia may be suspected. U waves may also develop or be accentuated in the hypercalcemic patient. Hypocalcemia may also cause lowering and inversion of the T wave.

The Q–T interval is measured from the beginning of the QRS to the end of the T wave. The normal length of this interval varies with heart rate, sex, and age and can be determined by consulting the chart of calculated normal Q–T intervals found in most texts on electro-

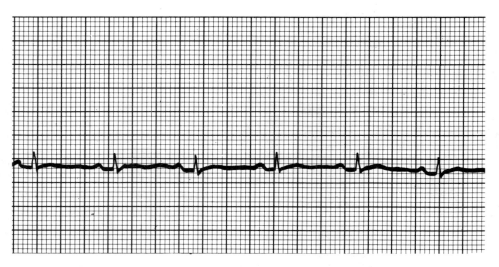

FIGURE 8-42
*Shortened Q–T interval (hypercalcemia). The normal Q–T interval for the above heart rate of
88 beats/minute is 0.28 second to 0.36 second. This patient's serum calcium level is 12.1
mg/dl, and the Q–T interval measures 0.24 second.*

cardiography. A general guideline that can be used in clinical situations is that the Q–T interval should be less than half the preceding R–R interval when the heart rate is 65 to 90 beats per minute. The interval will normally shorten during tachycardia and lengthen during bradycardia.

Calcium abnormalities are not often seen in the cardiac patient unless there is an associated noncardiac disease. The more frequent cause of Q–T interval shortening or prolongation in the cardiac patient is the administration of cardiac drugs. Digitalis may cause a *shortened* Q–T interval. Quinidine and procainamide frequently cause *prolongation* of the Q–T interval. Drugs should always be considered when the ECG is evaluated for electrolyte abnormalities.

Arrhythmias are not commonly associated with either calcium excess or calcium insufficiency; however,

too rapid intravenous infusion of calcium salts may result in ventricular fibrillation and sudden death. The digitalized patient who receives calcium salts seems especially prone to this reaction for reasons not known.

Summary

Just as the patient who sustains myocardial infarction may not have chest pain, the patient who has electrolyte abnormalities may not exhibit any of the ECG changes described (Table 8-5). Conversely, a patient with normal serum electrolytes may show some of these ECG changes for other reasons. None of the ECG manifestations described here even approaches being diagnostic. They are of value primarily in alerting one to suspect electrolyte abnormalities. It is appropriate

FIGURE 8-43
*Prolonged Q–T interval (hypocalcemia). For this heart rate of 70 beats per minute, the Q–T
interval should be between 0.31 and 0.38 seconds. This patient's Q–T interval measures 0.50
seconds because his serum calcium level is 5.4 mg/dl. (Normal serum calcium is 8.5 to 10.5
mg/dl.)*

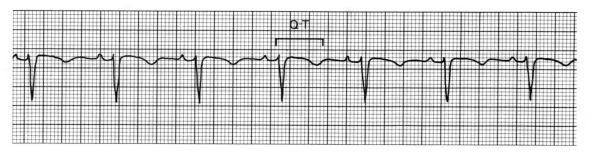

TABLE 8-5
ECG CHANGES ASSOCIATED WITH ELECTROLYTE IMBALANCES

Electrolyte Imbalance	ECG Changes	Arrhythmias
Hypokalemia	Abnormal U Waves	Ventricular ectopic beats; supraventricular tachycardias; ventricular tachycardias; ventricular fibrillation
Hyperkalemia	Tall, narrow, peaked T waves; flat, wide P waves; widening QRS	Sinus bradycardia; first-degree block; junctional rhythm; idioventricular rhythm; ventricular tachycardia; ventricular fibrillation
Hypercalcemia	Shortened Q – T interval; abnormal U waves	Rare
Hypocalcemia	Lengthened Q – T interval; T wave lowering and inversion	Rare

for the nurse, especially one who cares for the critically ill patient, to be alert to ECG changes and to interpret what is seen in the context of what is already known about that patient.

BIBLIOGRAPHY

Goldman JM: Priciples of Clinical Electrocardiography, 11th ed. Los Altos, Lange, 1982
Mangiola S: Self-Assessment in Electrocardiography. Philadelphia, JB Lippincott, 1977
Marriott JH: Practical Electrocardiography, 7th ed. Baltimore, Williams & Wilkins, 1983
Ritota MC: Diagnostic Electrocardiography, 2nd ed. Philadelphia, Lippincott, 1977

Serum Enzyme Studies

Shirley J. Hoffman

As the role of the nurse has expanded, there is a need for more knowledge on which to base the judgments necessary to assume new responsibilities. Knowledge of the purpose, functions, and significance of laboratory values in relation to the diagnosis and prognosis of acute myocardial infarction can enhance the quality of nursing care available to patients. Armed with a basic understanding of serum enzyme determinations, the nurse can exercise judgment in interpreting them in relation to other information known about the patient. The ability to use this kind of judgment may well affect the clinical course or prognosis of the patient. It is certainly as important to the physical and mental well-being of these patients to rule out the presence of acute myocardial infarction as it is to confirm its existence.

ENZYME FUNCTION

Enzymes are proteins that are found in all living cells. Different enzymes are found in different kinds of cells and in varying concentrations. The function of enzymes is to serve as accelerating agents or catalysts for chemical reactions. They temporarily combine with one substance to form an enzyme substrate complex, which then breaks down to form the end products of the chemical reaction. When the enzyme has completed this task, it is liberated, unchanged, to continue functioning as a chemical catalyst.

Enzymes are produced in the cells and are released into the plasma. Overactive, diseased, or injured cells increase the release of their particular enzymes into the serum. The difference in composition and concentration of various enzymes from one kind of tissue to another (cardiac, liver, skeletal muscle, and the like) determines which serum enzyme elevations reflect damage to specific tissues. Thus, serum enzyme determinations can be used to detect cell damage and to suggest where the damage has occurred.

SERUM ENZYME DETERMINATIONS

Many studies have been done in relation to the diagnostic value of serum enzyme determinations. As sometimes happens in research, the results vary and are debated by clinical diagnosticians and pathologists alike. To further cloud the issue, enzymes are evaluated by a variety of laboratory methods, and the determinations are reported in different quantitative units. This results in different "normal" ranges, which vary according to the procedures used by the particular laboratory. The nurse must become familiar with the range of normals for each enzyme as it is reported by the laboratory where she works.

Serum enzyme determinations have been helpful in the diagnosis of cardiac, hepatic, pancreatic, muscular, bone, and malignant diseases. Each of these kinds of tissue releases a particular enzyme or enzymes when diseased or damaged. Because each kind of cell contains and releases more than one enzyme, there is overlapping of enzymes from one tissue source to another. For this reason there is no one serum enzyme elevation that is diagnostic of any one disease.

CARDIAC ENZYMES

The term *cardiac enzyme* refers to those enzymes that occur in, and are released in proportionately larger amounts from, cardiac tissue. These include creatine kinase, or CK (formerly creatine phosphokinase, or CPK), hydroxybutyric dehydrogenase (HBD), serum glutamic-oxalacetic transaminase (SGOT), and lactic dehydrogenase (LDH). Serum glutamic-pyruvic transaminase (SGPT) may show a slight increase in the presence of massive myocardial infarction, but it is more specific for liver disease.

Each of these enzymes varies in its degree of specificity for myocardial disease. The relationship between acute myocardial infarction and elevated SGOT and LDH was established in the mid-1950s. CK was added to the list of diagnostic acids in the mid-1960s. Controversy regarding their usefulness continues.

LDH

Total LDH is probably the lease specific for cardiac disease of the cardiac enzymes. It is abundant in kidney, cardiac, liver, and muscle tissues and in red cells (Table 8-6). The onset of LDH elevation occurs 12 to 24 hours after tissue damage, and peak elevation, averaging about three times upper normal, is at 72 hours. Return to normal is not complete for 7 to 11 days. The fact that LDH elevation is prolonged for a week or more after myocardial infarction is often helpful in late diagnosis. Some patients do not come to the hospital until several days after their initial symptoms, so early blood specimens cannot be obtained.

LDH Isoenzymes. Because LDH has widespread distribution in body tissues, its serum level is elevated in a variety of diseases. In 1957 it was found that LDH could be subjected to certain procedures that separate the enzyme into five components, or isoenzymes, that demonstrate five zones of activity of the enzyme. Because enzyme activity is measured by its rate of acceleration of chemical reactions, these five zones range from fastest-acting to slowest-acting.

The two fastest-acting isoenzymes are found in cardiac muscle, the renal cortex, erythrocytes, and the cerebrum and reflect disease or damage in these tissues. Thus, if these isoenzymes are elevated in the serum of a patient who presents with chest pain but who has no evidence of renal, hemolytic, or cerebral disease, myocardial infarction is the likely diagnosis.

The two slowest-acting LDH isoenzymes are found in the liver, skeletal muscle, and skin. These reflect acute liver disease or hepatic congestion, muscle injuries, or dermatologic disease or trauma. The intermediate isoenzyme is found in lymph nodes, spleen, leukocytes, pancrease, and lung tissue. It in turn reflects disease or damage to these tissues.

TABLE 8-6
ENZYME DISTRIBUTION IN CELLS

	SGOT	CK	LDH (Isoenzymes)
Fast-acting	Heart Kidney Red cells Brain	Brain	Heart Kidney Red cells Brain
Intermediate	Lung Pancreas	Heart	Lymph nodes Spleen Leukocytes Pancreas Lung
Slow-acting	Liver Skeletal muscle	Skeletal muscle	Liver Skeletal muscle Skin

These five isoenzymes, also called *fractions* of LDH, are numbered 1 through 5. Many laboratories report LDH_1 and LDH_2 as the fastest isoenzymes and LDH_4 and LDH_5 as the slowest, whereas others report them in reverse order. Care must be taken in reading the literature on serum enzymes to avoid the confusion caused by various methods of reporting. LDH_1 will henceforth be referred to as fastest-acting and LDH_5 as slowest-acting. Here again the nurse must be aware of how LDH isoenzymes are reported in her hospital laboratory.

The introduction of isoenzyme separation has made determination of the LDH isoenzymes one of the most specific tests for the diagnosis of myocardial infarction. Most diagnosticians consider myocardial infarction the problem when LDH_1 activity is greater than LDH_2. If LDH_2 is greater than LDH_1, the patient may have experienced a severe ischemic episode or only minimal heart damage. Both these isoenzymes have been found in the serum up to 2 weeks or more after infarction, even though total LDH has returned to normal. LDH isoenzymes should be determined, even when total LDH is normal, because the LDH_1 fraction may be elevated in the presence of normal total LDH.

When blood specimens for LDH determinations are collected, it is essential to avoid hemolysis of the sample. Because LDH is found in erythrocytes, even slightly hemolyzed blood will show an elevation of the serum LDH. It is for this same reason that hemolysis caused by an artificial valve or by use of the cardiopulmonary bypass pump results in elevation of serum LDH. When LDH_1 is greater than LDH_2 on admission and the cardiac isoenzyme CK is not present, a serum haptoglobin level should be determined to exclude hemolysis.

HBD

The enzyme HBD may possibly be the same as the fast-moving cardiac isoenzyme of LDH. It correlates with the LDH fractions and therefore is frequently omitted from the commonly used series of enzymes. HBD activity is always assocaited with LDH activity. The serum evaluation of both enzymes after myocardial infarction is about the same, both in quantity and in duration of elevation, with only a slight time lag in HBD. In laboratories that do not have the necessary equipment for fractionating LDH isoenzymes, HBD determination can serve as an alternate for this study, although it is felt to be less specific.

CK

CK is the fastes-rising and fastest-falling of all the cardiac enzymes. Onset of serum elevation is about 4 to 6 hours after infarction, with a peak elevation of five to twelve times normal, or more, by 12 to 20 hours. Serum levels may return to normal by the second or third day. This transient nature of CK elevation following myocardial infarction can be a distinct aid to diagnosis if the patient is reached early in the acute episode. However, this frequently is not the case; the CK rise may be missed entirely by the time the patient enters the hospital and is seen by a physician and a tentative diagnosis made. About 90% of patients with myocardial infarction show the early rise in serum CK.

The CK enzyme is second only to LDH isoenzymes in specificity for cardiac damage. CK is found in skeletal and cardiac muscle and in brain tissue. Since red cells contain almost no CK, slight hemolysis does not interfere with the accuracy of its determination. It is of particular value in diagnosing cardiac disease because it is not found in liver tissue as are LDH and SGOT. Hepatic congestion or disease, which frequently accompanies cardiac disease, will therefore not affect CK values. CK determination is also helpful in differentiating myocardial infarction from pulmonary embolism, which often present very similar clinical pictures. Because of the proportionately smaller amount of CK in lung tissue, any rise with pulmonary embolism will be much smaller than the very high elevation associated with myocardial infarction. CK values are normal in pericarditis, but an elevation occurs in myocarditis because of the cardiac muscle involvement.

Recall that overactivity as well as disease or damage of tissue cells will cause release of enzymes into the serum. This should be kept in mind when CK elevation is found in the patient who collapsed on the golf course or while skiing. Severe or prolonged exercise of the untrained "social athlete" can result in CK elevation for up to 48 hours.

Other conditions causing a rise in CK levels include acute cerebrovascular disease, muscular dystrophy, and other muscle trauma. Elevations are sometimes found following peripheral arterial embolism, repeated intramuscular injections, and operative procedures. Even minor trauma to muscle cells near the sampling site may distort the results. It has been reported that morphine sulfate injected intramuscularly causes a significant increase in CK values in 25% of patients. This should be considered by ambulance and emergency department personnel who treat patients with chest pain. A single intramuscular injection may be responsible for causing major problems in interpretation of cardiac enzymes and misdiagnosis of myocardial infarction.

High concentrations of barbiturates, diazepam (Valium, morphine sulfate, and anesthetic agents have been shown to decrease the disappearance of CK from the circulation in experimental animals. Acute alcohol intoxication, seizures, and even undue prolonged pressure on muscle masses may result in elevation of total CK. An elderly patient who has been found lying on the floor in an empty apartment may have an elevated CK because of pressure on large muscle masses due to prolonged unchanged position.

CK Isoenzymes. The discovery that CK can be fractionated into isoenzymes is seen by many to be a great boon to the diagnosis of myocardial infarction. CK isoenzymes are again measured by their rate of chemical reaction acceleration. They are designated as BB, the slow-acting isoenzyme found in brain tissue; MB, the intermediate-acting myocardial isoenzyme; and MM, the fast-acting isoenzyme found in skeletal muscle.

Because there are so many causes for total CK release, especially from injured skeletal muscle tissue, the ability to differentiate muscle, myocardial, or brain tissue as the source of the CK elevation can be extremely helpful. CK–MB is reported to be up to 94% sensitive and 100% specific for myocardial infarction. CK–MB may be elevated after acute myocardial infarction, even though total CK is not.

The CK–MB isoenzyme is elevated in the serum for only 24 to 72 hours after its initial appearance. It is obvious that proper timing of the blood specimen is extremely important. The peak rise of CK–MB is 12 to 20 hours after initial elevation. If the patient is not seen until 24 to 48 hours after the onset of symptoms of myocardial injury, one must rely more on the LDH isoenzymes.

The rapid appearance and disappearance of the CK–MB isoenzyme may be a positive factor in its usefulness in diagnosing the extension of an acute myocardial infarction. This can be a very difficult diganosis to make when the resolved chest pain of myocardial infarction recurs and the initial total enzyme elevations have not yet returned to normal. Determination of CK–MB may be especially helpful in the coronary care unit patient when there are additional causes for total enzyme elevations, such as cardioversion or defibrillation, multiple intramuscular injections for pain or vomiting, trauma due to falls secondary to arrhythmias, prolonged use of rotating tourniquets, and hypotension.

CK–MB may also be helpful in diagnosing acute myocardial infarction in the postoperative patient. The muscle trauma incurred during surgical procedures will cause all three of the total cardiac enzymes to rise. In these patients, one should be able to determine whether total CK elevation is entirely due to surgical trauma or partially due to myocardial infarction by employing CK isoenzymes as a specific test. Unfortunately, CK isoenzymes are not very helpful in diagnosing myocardial infarction in the postoperative cardiac patient. Some rise in CK–MB will occur after open heart surgery owing to cardiac manipulation and cannulation.

SGOT

SGOT is the last of the cardiac enzymes to be discussed. Its tissue distribution is quite widespread, with large SGOT concentrations in red cells and cardiac, liver, skeletal muscle, and renal tissue. Lesser amounts are found in brain, pancreas, and lung tissue. Because SGOT is prevalent in so many kinds of tissue and because of the current capabilities to fractionate LDH and CK, many physicians no longer feel the need to include SGOT as a routine cardiac enzyme determination. Its widespread distribution makes it one of the least specific enzymes, second only to total LDH. Over 95% of patients with myocardial infarction have SGOT elevation; an infarction as little as 5% can cause a serum rise.

SGOT falls between CK and LDH in both degree and duration of elevation. SGOT rise begins about 6 to 8 hours after onset of an acute myocardial episode, reaches its peak in 18 to 36 hours, and returns to normal at the end of 4 to 6 days. Average elevation following myocardial infarction is five times normal but may go much higher with an extensive infarct.

SGOT may become elevated with tachyarrhythmias with or without myocardial infarction, probably reflecting liver decompensation due to decreased perfusion. Liver damage resulting from congestive heart failure or shock due to myocardial infarction can also cause an increase in SGOT. It has been reported that about 25% of cardioverted patients have elevation of SGOT up to three times normal, probably because of muscle release of the enzyme.

Other causes of SGOT elevation include acute liver damage after alcohol ingestion, tachyarrhythmias with a ventricular rate of over 160 per minute, shock, pericarditis, dissecting aortic aneurysm, unaccustomed vigorous exercise, trauma, cerebral infarction, acute cholecystitis, pancreatitis, and certain drugs such as narcotics and anticoagulants. SGOT rises several days after pulmonary infarction. This may help differentiate this problem from acute myocardial infarction when the time of onset of symptoms of pulmonary infarction can be determined.

SGPT

As mentioned previously, the SGPT enzyme is more specific for liver disease and does not usually rise with cardiac damage. However, both SGOT and SGPT will rise if myocardial infarction is accompanied by prolonged or profound shock or severe congeestive heart failure that results in liver congestion or damage.

SGOT evaluation may be of particular value in the early diagnosis of reinfarction. A second infarction often cannot be read on ECG because of the changes already incurred by the first infarction. A rise in SGOT within 6 to 8 hours after an episode of chest pain will help establish the diagnosis.

COMPARATIVE ENZYME PEAK AND DURATION

One can almost always be assured that myocardial infarction has not occurred if serum enzyme levels remain normal for 24 hours after onset of symptoms. Transfer from the coronary care unit at this time can be justified because there is only a remote possibility of missing myocardial injury. If infarct has occurred, all the enzymes should be elevated by 24 hours after symptom occurrence (Fig. 8-44). In comparing enzyme elevations, one may note that CK rises first and highest and falls to normal first, followed by SGOT, with LDH rising last. LDH elevation is the lowest but the most prolonged. In comparing the specificity of each enzyme as an indicator of myocardial necrosis, CK isoenzymes are most specific, followed by LDH isoenzymes, total CK, SGOT, and total LDH (least specific).

In general, it can be said that the size of a myocardial infarction correlates fairly well with the height of the enzyme peaks and the duration of enzyme elevation as well as with patient mortality. Some studies show that CK elevation of ten times normal is accompanied by 50% mortality, whereas a mortality rate of 6% is shown with CK rises of less than five times normal. It has been reported that (1) 81% of ventricular arrhythmias occur in patients whose enzyme levels are more than four times normal; (2) the incidence of congestive heart failure is significantly increased in those with enzyme levels of four to five times normal; (3) patients with cardiogenic shock have enzyme increases of more than five times normal. Research is being done in an effort to use CK–MB to estimate infarct size in terms of grams of necrotic tissue. Currently it is not of sufficient reliability and accuracy to be of clinical use.

If enzyme peak levels do indeed correlate with infarct size, they should be helpful to the nurse in anticipating those complications that are related to infarct size, as well as prognosis and ultimate rehabilitation.

Interferring Factors

There are a number of "red herrings" to be kept in mind when elevated serum enzymes are evaluated. Severe or *prolonged exercise* has been mentioned. *Defibrillation* with large amounts of voltage or repeated defibrillation may cause enzymes to rise because of the sudden severe contraction of all muscle tissues. Even one defibrillation with 400 watt-seconds may result in enzyme rise sufficient to mimic myocardial infarction. HBD, which is thought to be much like the cardiac isoenzymes of LDH and CK, sometimes rises with *liver disease*.

The extent of *surgical trauma* during operative

FIGURE 8-44
Peak elevation and duration of serum enzymes after myocardial injury.

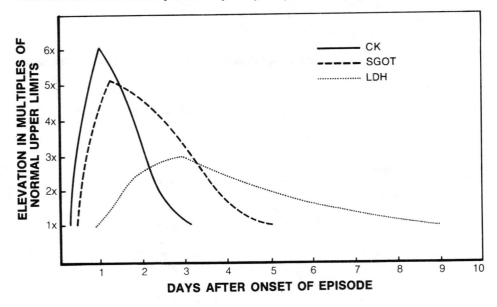

procedures should be considered when enzyme elevations are evaluated postoperatively. Tissue damage from frequent *intramuscular injections* must also be remembered as a source of enzyme rises. CK elevations of more than eight times normal have been seen after frequent injections. It is also possible to produce elevation of SGOT and SGPT with administration of salicylates, sodium warfarin (Coumadin), and other *drugs* that are detoxified in the liver.

There may be minimal enzyme elevations after *cardiac catheterization* and coronary *angiography,* but these are mainly caused by the injection of intramuscular premedications. The introduction of catheters of arteriotomy or percutaneous routes alone does not cause significant rise of enzymes.

Diagnostic Limitations

It is apparent from the discussion of these four enzyme studies used in diagnosing myocardial infarction that none are actually diagnostic. Many areas still remain unclear or unknown. No enzyme or enzyme fraction has yet been found to exist in cardiac muscle alone. There is much disagreement about the normal range of CK activity. Some studies indicate that the upper limit of normal in females is about two-thirds that of males, and that blacks may have higher normals than whites. Other enzymes have been found to rise with myocardial necrosis, but they are either no more specific than the ones currently used or are technically difficult and time-consuming to measure.

As yet, enzyme determinations can serve only as an adjunct to diagnosis by ECG and the patient's clinical picture. In order to be of most value they should be ordered with discretion. Consideration must be given to the length of time that has passed since the onset of symptoms, as each enzyme rises and returns to normal at different time intervals. One often finds an order for "stat" enzymes upon admission of the patient with suspected myocardial infarction to the critical care unit. The results will be useless if only an hour or two has passed since the onset of symptoms. If the patient suffered only moderate symptoms and did not come to the hospital until several days later, CK determination is useless because the enzyme will already have returned to normal. Usually, two enzyme determinations are considered more valid than one, but the gamut of enzyme tests may not be necessary.

Enzyme determinations have been of greatest value in the patient whose ECG and clinical picture are equivocal for diagnosis of myocardial infarction. Enzyme elevation may well confirm a suspected diagnosis in this case. Sometimes it is difficult or impossible to interpret infarction on ECG because of previous infarction changes, the effects of certain drugs or electrolyte imbalances, conduction defects such as bundle branch block or Wolff-Parkinson-White syndrome, arrhythmias, or a functioning pacemaker. Enzyme determination may be a distinct advantage here. If a definite diagnosis can be made by ECG, there may be no need for enzyme tests, except for academic interest.

It must be stressed that serum elevations are nonspecific in the diagnosis of myocardial infarction, and they must be considered in view of the total clinical picture. We are in a highly technical age of nursing and must not forget to look at and listen to the patient before making judgments and decisions.

BIBLIOGRAPHY

Baillie EE: CK isoenzymes: Part I. Clinical aspects. Lab Med 10:267–270, 1979

Baillie EE: CK isoenzymes: Part II. Technical aspects. Lab Med 10:339–340, 1979

Galen R: Editorial: Enzymes in the diagnosis of myocardial infarction. Heart Lung 10:484–485, 1981

Lott JA, Stang JM: Serum enzymes and isoenzymes in the diagnosis and differential diagnosis of myocardial infarction. Arch Intern Med 140:317, 1980

Roberts R: Can we clinically measure infarction size? JAMA 242:183–185, 1979

Seager SB: Cardiac enzymes in the evaluation of chest pain. Ann Emergency Med 9, No. 7:346–349, 1980

Thompson PL et al: Enzymatic indices of myocardial necrosis: Influence on short- and long-term prognosis after myocardial infarction. Circulation 59, No. 1:113–119, 1979

Vijayan VK et al: Correlation of ST–segment elevation in 12–lead electrocardiogram with serum CPK in acute myocardial infarction. Ind Heart J 31, No. L:31–33, 1979

Wagner GS: Optimal use of serum enzyme levels in the diagnosis of acute myocardial infarction. Arch Intern Med 140:317, 1980

Walter P: The role of cardiac enzymes in the diagnosis of myocardial infarction. Primary Care 8:371–377, 1981

Central Venous Pressure

Carolyn M. Hudak

Central venous pressure (CVP) refers to the pressure of blood in the right atrium or vena cava. It provides information about three parameters—blood volume, the effectiveness of the heart as a pump, and vascular tone. CVP is to be differentiated from a peripheral venous pressure, which may reflect only a local pressure. Although isolated CVP recordings have generally been replaced by more sophisticated hemodynamic monitoring techniques, an understanding of the physiologic principles of central venous pressure is valuable in the critical care setting.

CVP is measured in centimeters or millimeters of water pressure, and considerable variation exists in the range of normal values cited. Usually, pressure in the right atrium is 0 to 4 cm H_2O, and pressure in the vena cava is approximately 6 to 12 cm H_2O.

More important, it is the trend of the readings that is most significant regardless of the baseline value. The upward or downward trend of the CVP, combined with clinical assessment of the patient, will determine appropriate interventions.

For example, a patient's CVP may gradually rise from 6 cm H_2O to 8 cm and then to 10 cm. Although this may still be in the range of "normal," other parameters may indicate ensuing complications. Auscultation of breath sounds may reveal basilar rales, a third heart sound may be audible, or the pulse and respiratory rate may be increasing insidiously. In this context, the trend of a gradual rise in CVP is more significant than the actual isolated value.

When interpreting CVP data in conjunction with other clinical observations, the nurse has a better understanding of their significance for that particular patient and recognizes the outcome to which nursing interventions must be aimed. In the example cited in the previous paragraph, the nurse is aware that too much fluid administration would further compromise the patient's circulatory status, and she would act accordingly to reduce this risk.

Sometimes, rate of fluid administration is titrated according to the patient's CVP and urinary output. As long as the urinary output remains adequate and the CVP does not change significantly, this is an indication that the heart can accommodate the amount of fluid

being administered. If the CVP begins to rise and the urine output drops, indicating a decreased cardiac output to perfuse the kidneys, circulatory overload must be suspected and either ruled out or validated in view of other clinical symptomatology.

The patient who is started on a vasopressor agent will show a rise in CVP that is due to the vasoconstriction produced. In this situation, the blood volume is unchanged, but the vascular bed has become smaller. Again, this change must be interpreted in conjunction with other assessments that the nurse makes about the patient. Alone, a CVP value can be meaningless, but used in conjunction with other clinical data, it is a valuable aid in managing and predicting the patient's clinical course.

CVP Measurement. For CVP recordings, a long intravenous catheter is inserted into an arm or a leg vein or the subclavian vein and threaded into position in the vena cava close to the right atrium. Occasionally, the catheter may be advanced into the right atrium as indicated by rhythmic fluctuations in the pressure manometer corresponding to the patient's heartbeat. In this situation, the catheter may simply be withdrawn to the point at which the pulsations cease.

Figure 8-45 illustrates a typical set-up for measuring the CVP. A manometer with a three-way stopcock is introduced between the fluid source and the patient's intravenous catheter. In this way, three separate systems can be created by manipulating the stopcock.

System 1 connects the fluid source with the patient and can be used for routine administration of intravenous fluids or as an avenue to keep the system patent.

System 2 runs from the fluid source to the CVP manometer and is opened in order to raise the fluid col-

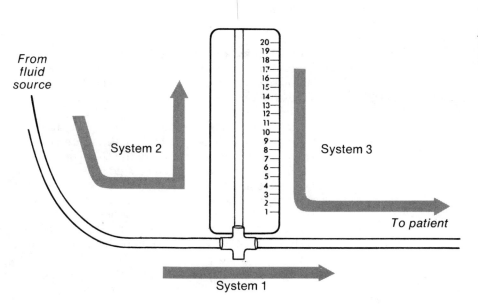

FIGURE 8-45
Central venous pressure set-up.
(See text for description.)

umn in the manometer prior to measurement of the venous pressure.

System 3 connects the patient's intravenous catheter with the manometer, and it is this pathway that must be open to record the CVP. Pressure in the vena cava displaces or equilibrates with the pressure exerted by the column of fluid in the manometer, and the point at which the fluid level settles is recorded as the CVP.

To obtain an accurate measurement, the nurse should make sure that the patient is flat, with the zero point of the manometer at the same level as the right atrium. This level corresponds to the midaxillary line of the patient or can be determined by measuring approximately 5 cm below the sternum. However, consistency is the important detail, and all readings should be taken with the patient in the same position and the zero point calculated in the same manner. If deviations from the routine procedure must be made, as when the patient cannot tolerate being flat and the reading must be taken with the patient in a semi-Fowler's position, it is valuable to note this on the patient's chart or care plan to provide for consistency in future readings.

A patent system is assured when the fluid column falls freely and slight fluctuation of the fluid column is apparent. This fluctuation follows the patient's respiratory pattern and will fall on inspiration and rise on expiration owing to changes in interpulmonary pressure. If the patient is being ventilated on a respirator, a falsely high reading will result. If possible, the respirator should be discontinued momentarily for maximum accuracy. If the patient cannot tolerate being off the respirator for even this short period, significant trends in the CVP can still be determined if consistency in taking the readings is followed.

Variations in CVP. As noted earlier, changes in CVP must be interpreted in terms of the clinical picture of the patient. There are, however, some situations that commonly produce an *elevated CVP*. These include congestive heart failure when the heart can no longer effectively handle the venous return, cardiac tamponade, a vasoconstrictive state, or states of increased blood volume such as overtransfusion or overhydration.

A *low CVP* usually accompanies a hypovolemic state due to blood or fluid loss or drug-induced vasodilation. Increasing the rate of fluid administration or replacing blood loss is indicated in this situation.

Hemodynamic Pressure Monitoring

Joan Mersch

The concept of pressure is a key parameter in patient assessment. Mathematically, pressure is defined as the product of flow and resistance:

$$\text{pressure} = \text{flow} \times \text{resistance}$$

Blood pressure is one of the "vital signs" routinely obtained, reported, and recorded.

For the critical care nurse to make important clinical decisions, the knowledge of pressure concepts must be incorporated into patient evaluation. The purposes of this section are to describe a current method of measuring heart and blood pressures, to discuss normal and abnormal hemodynamic pressures, and to assist the nurse in determining the physiological importance of these pressures.

METHOD OF MEASURING HEART AND BLOOD PRESSURES

Advances in medical technology have made it possible to measure pressures directly within the chambers of the heart and great vessels. Essential to direct measurement of hemodynamic pressures are catheters, a transducer, and a pressure module.

Essentials

Catheters

Flow-Directed (Swan-Ganz). The development of the flow-directed catheter has made possible the measurement of pulmonary artery wedge (PAW) pressure at the bedside. This pressure is an index of left ventricular function.

The catheter has two lumens, one for intravenous fluid to assure catheter patency and the second for the balloon (Fig. 8-46). At the tip of the radiopaque catheter is a balloon, which when inflated causes the tip of the catheter to become buoyant. If then advanced, the catheter will float in the diretion of blood flow. Introduced into either a brachial or a femoral vein, it can be passed into the superior or inferior vena cava respectively. It then can be passed to the right atrium, through the tricuspid valve into the right ventricle, through the pulmonary valve, and into the pulmonary

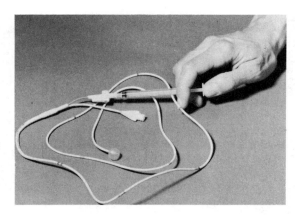

FIGURE 8-46
Flow-directed catheter.

artery. If advanced further, the catheter will obstruct forward blood flow, which allows *left* heart pressures to be reflected through the catheter tip. Because of the catheter size, it obstructs forward flow in a small pulmonary artery.

Right atrial (RA), right ventricular (RV), and pulmonary artery (PA) pressures give precise information on heart valve function and circulatory volume. The value of the flow-directed catheter is that left ventricular function can be determined by inserting a catheter into the right side of the heart. This procedure has fewer risks and is simpler to perform than measuring left ventricular pressures directly.

Arterial. Direct measurement of arterial pressures has been available for a longer time than the flow-directed procedure. A simple catheter inserted into an artery suffices. Directly measuring arterial pressure affords the nurse precise blood pressure readings and easy access to arterial blood samples. In addition, it saves the patient from numerous arterial punctures.

Transducer

The transducer is the second essential component for measuring pressure. It is an electrical device that converts one form of energy into another. Specifically, it senses mechanical energy (pressure) and converts it into electrical energy (the waveform). The pressures generated by myocardial contraction and relaxation are reflected through the lumen of the catheter to the transducer, where the pressure is converted to an electrical waveform. For the wareform to have meaning, two conditions must be met, a zeroing condition and a calibrating condition.

For accurate pressure measurement, the transducer must be placed at a standard level in relation to patient position — midchest suffices as a reference level.

1. To meet the *zeroing condition,* the transducer must be set at an arbitrarily assigned zero value pressure. This can be done by opening the transducer to room air or atmospheric pressure (760 mm Hg at sea level) and assigning that pressure zero value in millimeters Hg (0 mm Hg).

2. The second necessary condition for the transducer is the *calibrating condition.* That is, the amplitude of the electrical signal (height of the waveform) must be assigned a value in millimeters of mercury pressure. The transducer is calibrated when a numerical value in mm Hg pressure is assigned to each centimeter of waveform amplitude. For instance, 1 cm = 4 mm Hg or 1 cm = 20 mm Hg.

Pressure Module

The pressure module allows the transducer to be zeroed and calibrated and allows the pressure waveform to be displayed on an oscilloscope or paper tracing. Different pressure modules and transducers require varying techniques for zeroing and calibrating. Although the technical procedure changes according to specific equipment, the principles for zeroing and calibrating are the same.

Preparation for Pressure Measurement

Prepare for pressure measurement by (A) gathering supplies and (B) assembling supplies.

A. Gather supplies
  1. Intravenous (IV) fluid in a plastic bag
  2. Heparin (1 ml/l000 units) and syringe
  3. Pressure bag
  4. IV tubing (15 gtt/ml)
  5. Pressure valve (C.S.F. ®Intraflo, Continuous Flush System)*
  6. Three 3-way stopcocks (2 plain, 1 with Luer-Lok)
  7. IV extension tubing
  8. Transducer
  9. Pressure module
B. Assemble supplies
  1. Heparinize the IV solution in the plastic bag by adding 1 unit of heparin per ml IV fluid. Label solution.
  2. Connect the IV tubing to the IV solution in the plastic bag (Fig. 8-47).
  3. Place the IV solution bag in the pressure bag and inflate to 300 mm Hg pressure.
  4. Connect the IV tubing to the IV port of the pressure valve.

* Sorenson Research Company, Salt Lake City, Utah.

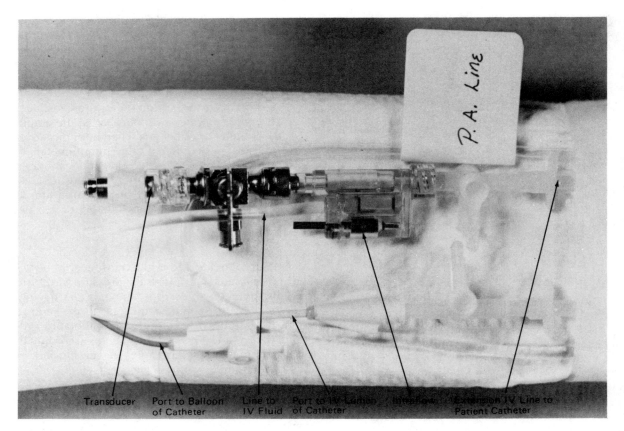

P. A. Line

Transducer   Port to Balloon   Line to   Port to IV Lumen   Interflow   Extension IV Line to
of Catheter   IV Fluid   of Catheter   Patient Catheter

FIGURE 8-47
Arterial line set-up.

5. Connect the 3-way stopcock with Luer-Lok to the pressure valve port, which is at the same end as the IV port.
6. Attach transducer to stopcock, step 5.
7. Fill dome of transducer with IV fluid (fluid without air bubbles must fill dome for accurate pressure measurement).
8. Attach a 3-way stopcock to the distal port of the pressure valve.
9. Connect IV extension tubing to the stopcock, step 8.
10. Attach a 3-way stopcock to the other end of the IV extension tubing.
11. Flush the line with IV fluid and connect it to the patient's flow-directed or arterial catheter. The assembled setup is shown in Figure 8-48.

Pressure Measurement

Following are the steps for pressure measurement:

1. Flush line with IV fluid.
2. Open stopcock attached to transducer to room air.
  a. Zero transducer.
  b. Calibrate transducer.
3. Open stopcock attached to transducer to patient pressure.
4. Assess quality of waveform.
5. Measure and record pressures.
6. Flush line with IV fluid.
7. Adjust treatment according to pressure values.

NORMAL PRESSURE VALUES

The nurse must have an understanding of the physiological mechanisms producing normal pressure to care knowledgeably for the patient who requires invasive pressure monitoring. A systematic approach to waveform analysis is essential. One such approach consists of the following steps:

1. Review the mechanical events of the heart and the normal pressures.
2. Learn the normal waveform characteristics.
3. Correlate the electrical and mechanical events of the heart.

In the following section, this approach will be em-

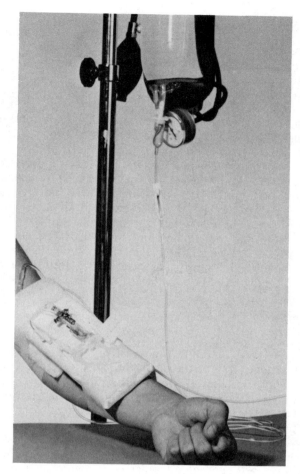

FIGURE 8-48
Assembled set-up for monitoring hemodynamic pressures.

Although the most frequently monitored pressures in the critical care setting are pulmonary artery, pulmonary artery wedge, and arterial, this section will discuss normal pressure values within all chambers of the heart and great vessels, emphasizing the process of waveform analysis.

Right Atrial Pressure

Visualize the catheter tip in the right atrium. The pressure created during RA systole, contraction, is greater than during RA diastole, relaxation. During RA systole, the tricuspid valve will open when RA pressure exceeds RV pressure. When the RV contracts, the tricuspid valve will be closed. The pulmonary artery cusps will open when the RV pressure exceeds the pressure in the pulmonary artery.

An RA pressure tracing appears as shown in Figure 8-49.

Waveform Interpretation

The right atrial waveform has three positive waves: *a, c,* and *v.* The *a* wave represents RA systole. The *v* wave represents RA diastole. Following RA systole, the tricuspid valve closes. The RA is filling with blood, and the RV is beginning to contract. At this point, the pressure within the RA briefly increases because the force of RV contraction causes the tricuspid valve to balloon into the RA, producing the *c* wave. Thus, the *c* wave is caused by the closed tricuspid valve's pushing into the RA during RA diastole. Sometimes, the *c* wave is superimposed on the *a* wave and is not distinguishable, or it appears as a notch in the *a* wave.

The RA pressure tracing has three negative waves or descents: x, x^1, and y. The descents are of less significance and will be briefly mentioned here. The x descent follows the *a* wave and represents right atrial relaxation. The x^1 descent follows the *c* wave and represents atrioventricular movement during ventricular contraction. The y descent follows the *v* wave and represents passive right atrial emptying immediately after opening of the tricuspid valve just before right atrial systole.

The right atrium is a low-pressure chamber; the significant RA pressure is the mean, or midpoint, between the systolic and diastolic pressures. Normal right atrial mean ($\overline{RA}$) pressure is <6 torr.

Comparison of ECG with Waveform

The electrical energy of the heart is demonstrated by the ECG; the mechanical energy is demonstrated by the pressure waveform. The electrical events precede and cause the mechanical events. On the ECG, the P wave represents the discharge of electrical current from the SA node (Fig. 8-49). Following electrical activation, the atria contract. In comparing the ECG

ployed to analyze normal pressure tracings. Under the subheading "Waveform Interpretation," the mechanical events, waveform characteristics, and normal pressure values will be discussed. The correlation between electrical and mechanical events will be discussed under the subheading "Comparison of ECG with Waveform." The following abbreviations will be used throughout when referring to pressures:

• Right atrial—RA
• Right ventricular—RV
• Right ventricular end-diastolic pressure—RVEDP
• Pulmonary artery—PA
• Pulmonary artery diastolic—PAd
• Pulmonary artery wedge—PAW
• Left atrial—LA
• Left ventricular—LV
• Left ventricular end-diastolic pressure—LVEDP
• Aortic—Ao
• Mean arterial pressure—MAP

with the pressure waveform, it can be seen that the P wave on the ECG precedes the *a* wave, atrial systole, on the pressure tracing. The QRS complex represents ventricular depolarization, and it precedes ventricular systole. While the right ventricle is contracting, the right atrium is relaxing. Thus, on the ECG, the QRS complex will precede the *v* wave on the RA pressure tracing.

The *v* wave frequently extends beyond the T wave, which demonstrates ventricular repolarization on the ECG.

If the *c* wave is visible, it will occur between the *a* and *v* waves, immediately after the QRS complex. Early in ventricular systole, the pressure within the ventricle pushes the closed tricuspid valve into the right atrium, causing a slight increase in RA pressure, demonstrated by the *c* wave on the RA pressure-tracing.

Right Ventricular Pressure

Again, visualize the flow-directed catheter in the right atrium. When the balloon at the tip of the catheter is inflated, the catheter tip will become buoyant. The catheter will tend to float in the direction of blood flow. If it is advanced, the slack in the line will allow the catheter to float through the open tricuspid valve into the ventricle. Figure 8-50 shows how the right ventricular waveform would be seen on the oscilloscope at this point.

Waveform Interpretation
In order to identify in simple terms the specific mechanical events causing the right ventricular waveform

configuration, we will assign arbitrary letters *a* through *e* to each activity. The initial rapid rise in the right ventricular waveform represents isovolumetric contraction, *a*. That is, the tricuspid and pulmonary valves are closed, and the volume of blood within the right ventricle remains constant while the pressure increases. When RV pressure exceeds PA pressure, the pulmonary valve opens, *b*. Blood is then ejected from the right ventricle into the pulmonary artery. Maximum RV systolic pressure is presented by point *c* on the waveform. The pulmonary valve closes, and the RV pressure rapidly decreases. The tricuspid valve opens, and the right ventricle passively fills with blood from the right atrium. Point *d* represents right atrial contraction, with *e* representing right ventricular end diastole.

Note that the RV pressure waveform goes below baseline. It is generally characteristic of both right ventricular and left ventricular waveforms to return to or to go below baseline. Significant RV pressures are systolic and end-diastolic. RV systolic pressure is <30 torr, and RVEDP is <5 torr.

Comparison of ECG with Waveform
The P wave on the ECG generally precedes two positive deflections on the right ventricular waveform. Following electrical activation of the atrium (P wave), the tricuspid valve opens, and the right ventricle passively fills with blood, causing an increase in RV diastolic pressure. The second positive deflection is caused when the atrium contracts, *d*, emptying the right atrium more completely, which increases RV diastolic pressure. Ventricular depolarization demonstrated by the QRS complex on the ECG precedes ventricular contraction, causing a rapid increase in the RV pres-

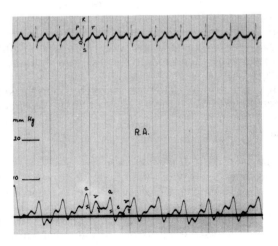

FIGURE 8-49
Right atrial pressure recording.

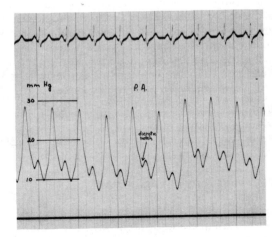

FIGURE 8-51
Pulmonary artery pressure recording.

sure wave. Following the electrical event of ventricular depolarization, the mechanical event of isovolumetric contraction occurs. During ventricular repolarization (T wave on the ECG), maximum ejection, reduced ejection, pulmonary valve closure, and rapid decrease in pressure occur.

Sometimes a slight increase in pressure can be seen following reduced ejection on the downward slope of the right ventricular tracing. Immediately after closure of the pulmonary valve, the pressure in the right ventricle increases slightly as the column of blood behind the closed valve pushes toward the ventricular chamber.

Pulmonary Artery Pressure

To float the catheter from the right ventricle into the pulmonary artery, the balloon is inflated and the catheter is advanced. The PA pressure tracing is shown in Figure 8-51.

Waveform Interpretation
The rapid rise in the pulmonary artery waveform represents right ventricular ejection. The dicrotic notch in the downward slope corresponds with pulmonary valve closure. Note that the pulmonary artery waveform always has a positive pressure; at no time does the pressure wave fall to zero or reach baseline. Normal PA pressures are systolic < 30 torr, diastolic < 10 torr, and mean < 20 torr.

Under normal conditions, the mean pulmonary artery ($\overline{PA}$) pressure will be closer to diastolic pressure than to systolic pressure. This pressure is not a true mathematic mean because systolic pressure is sus-

tained for approximately one third of the cardiac cycle, whereas diastole lasts about two thirds of the cycle. The diastolic pressure, therefore, contributes more in determining the $\overline{PA}$. As heart rate increases, systole changes little, but diastole is shortened; likewise, as heart rate slows, systole changes minimally, but diastole is prolonged. Thus, as heart rate increases, diastole contributes less to the mean value, while, as heart rate decreases, diastolic pressure contributes more to the mean pressure value.

Comparison of ECG with Waveform
Immediately after ventricular depolarization (QRS complex), ventricular ejection occurs. As the ventricle contracts, blood is ejected into the pulmonary artery, causing the rapid rise in PA pressure. Maximum PA pressure is reached during ventricular repolarization (T wave). Closure of the pulmonary valve, dicrotic notch, corresponds with the end of ventricular repolarization.

Pulmonary Artery Wedge Pressure

A flow-directed catheter in the pulmonary artery can be wedged in the pulmonary capillary bed by advancing the catheter or by inflating the balloon (Fig. 8-52). When forward blood flow is prevented, the catheter is wedged. The PAW pressure reflects left heart pres-

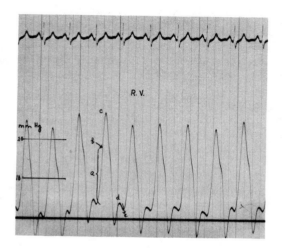

FIGURE 8-50
Right ventricular pressure recording.

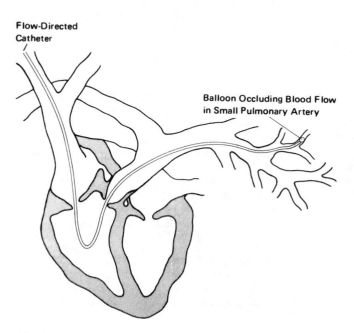

FIGURE 8-52
Diagram of catheter wedged in pulmonary capillary bed.

sures. That is, it reflects LA mean and LVEDP. When the catheter is advanced from the pulmonary artery to the pulmonary artery wedge position, the waveform configuration will change as shown in Figure 8-53.

Waveform Interpretation

The pulmonary artery wedge tracing has an *a* wave and a *v* wave. The *a* wave reflects left atrial contraction and left ventricular relaxation. The *v* wave reflects left atrial relaxation and left ventricular contraction. Mean PAW pressure is < 12 torr.

Comparison of ECG with Waveform

The P wave on the ECG will precede the *a* wave on the pulmonary artery wedge tracing. On the ECG, the QRS complex will precede the *v* wave of the pressure recording. Note that the QRS precedes both the *a* wave and the *v* wave because of delay in PAW pressure transmission (Fig. 8-53).

Left Atrial Pressure

The LA pressure is rarely measured in the critical care setting. It is, however, measured in the cardiac catheterization laboratory. A special catheter, one that can be passed transseptally from the right atrium to the left atrium, is used. The LA pressure is shown in Figure 8-54.

Waveform Interpretation

The LA pressure tracing has the same characteristics as the PAW pressure tracing. It has an *a* wave and a *v* wave. The *a* wave corresponds with left atrial contrac-tion, whereas the *v* wave corresponds with left atrial relaxation. A *c* wave is not generally seen on an LA pressure tracing; however, it may be seen as the *c* wave on the RA pressure tracing. Left atrial mean ($\overline{LA}$) pressure is < 12 torr.

Comparison of ECG with Waveform

The P wave precedes the *a* wave because the electrical events precede and cause the mechanical events; likewise, the QRS complex precedes the *v* wave.

Left Ventricular Pressure

The configuration of the LV pressure waveform is comparable to that of the right ventricular waveform. The significant difference is the pressure that each ventricle can generate. An LV pressure tracing appears in Figure 8-55.

Waveform Interpretation

Again, arbitrary letters have been assigned to various points in the waveform for ease of discussion. Interval *a* represents left ventricular isovolumetric contraction. As the pressure within the left ventricle exceeds the pressure in the aorta, the aortic valve is forced open, point *b*. Maximum ejection pressure is shown by *c*. The point at which the aortic valve closes, *d*, is followed by a rapid decrease in LV pressure. Opening of the mitral valve, *e*, allows passive left ventricular filling, and *f* demonstrates the increases in LV pressure due to left atrial contraction. Point *g* represents LVEDP.

LVEDP is an indication of function. It is not custom-

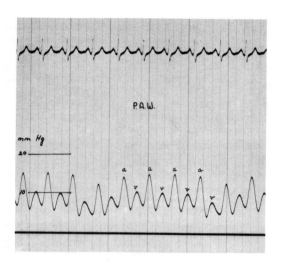

FIGURE 8-53
Pulmonary artery wedge pressure recording.

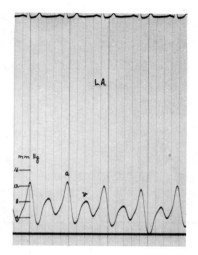

FIGURE 8-54
Left atrial pressure recording.

ary to measure LV pressures directly; therefore, the flow-directed catheter is used. The value of this catheter lies in the following relationships (≈ means "is approximately equal to")

$$\frac{PAd \approx \overline{PAW}}{\overline{PAW} \approx \overline{LA}}$$
$$\overline{LA} \approx LVEDP$$

The normal, significant LV pressures are systolic < 140 torr and end-diastolic < 12 torr.

Comparison of ECG with Waveform
Following atrial depolarization, P wave, the mitral valve opens, causing a slight increase in pressure, *e* on the pressure recording. Left atrial contraction, *f*, causes a second positive wave during ventricular diastole. The QRS complex precedes the systolic component of the left atrial waveform. As the ventricles repolarize, maximal LV pressure, *c*, is attained. The dicrotic notch represents aortic valve closure, *d*, and occurs at the end of repolarization.

Arterial Wave Pressure

Radial and femoral arteries are common sites for arterial lines. The arterial pressure waveform has the same configuration as that of the pulmonary artery. The primary difference is that the systemic arteries support greater pressures than the pulmonary artery.

Waveform Interpretation
When LV systolic pressure exceeds Ao pressure, the aortic valve opens. On the arterial pressure tracing,

this is the point at which the pressure rapidly rises. On the LV pressure tracing, it is point *b*, the end of isovolumetric contraction. The rapid rise in arterial pressure occurs after left ventricular ejection. An arterial line measuring pressure within the aorta will have a systolic pressure rise at the time of ventricular contraction; however, a line measuring radial artery pressure will have a delayed pressure rise because the artery is more distal to the left ventricle. Even though the line is in a distal artery, the dicrotic notch, which indicates aortic valve closure, can generally be seen (Fig. 8-56). Arterial pressures are systolic < 140 torr, diastolic < 90 torr, and mean 70 to 90 torr.

Comparison of ECG with Waveform
The rapid rise in arterial pressure follows electrical depolarization of the ventricles, QRS complex. The more distal the artery is to the left ventricle, the greater the delay in systolic pressure rise is. For instance, the time interval between the QRS complex and a radial artery pressure waveform will be greater than between the QRS complex and an Ao pressure tracing. The dicrotic notch occurs at the end of ventricular repolarization, T wave.

ABNORMAL PRESSURE VALUES

Before proceeding, we will emphasize the importance of understanding the normal mechanisms of hemodynamic pressures. In the previous discussion of normal pressures, the waveform components and pressures in Table 8-7 were identified as important.

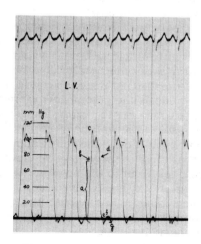

FIGURE 8-55
Left ventricular pressure recording.

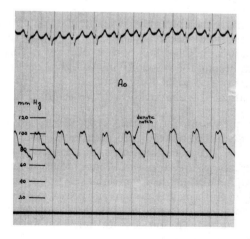

FIGURE 8-56
Aortic pressure recording.

TABLE 8-7
**SIGNIFICANT HEMODYNAMIC PRESSURES AND
WAVEFORM COMPONENTS**

Chamber or Vessel	Significant Components of Waveform	Significant Pressure
RA	*a* wave	$\overline{RA}$ (< 6 torr)
	c wave	
	v wave	
RV	systole	RV systole (< 30 torr)
	end-diastole	RVEDP (< 5 torr)
PA	systole	PA systole (< 30 torr)
	diastole	PA diastole (< 10 torr)
		$\overline{PA}$ (< 20 torr)
PAW	*a* wave	$\overline{PAW}$ (< 12 torr)
	v wave	
LA	*a* wave	$\overline{LA}$ (< 12 torr)
	v wave	
LV	systole	LV systole (< 140 torr)
	end-diastole	LVEDP (< 12 torr)
Ao	systole	systole (< 140 torr)
	diastole	diastole (< 90 torr)
		$\overline{Ao}$ or MAP (70–90 torr)

A working knowledge of the normal hemodynamic pressures is the basis for identifying and interpreting abnormal pressures. A nurse with this knowledge will feel at ease with the systematic approach to waveform analysis and will automatically consider the following:

1. The mechanical events of the heart and the normal pressures
2. The characteristics of each waveform
3. The correlation between the electrical and mechanical events of the heart

From this the nurse will be able to

1. Identify the abnormal component or components.
2. Identify the mechanical events that cause and that affect the abnormal portion of the waveform.
3. Enumerate the possible physiological reasons.
4. Review the goals of treatment.
5. Evaluate the effectiveness of treatment.

It is not within the realm of this section to address steps 4 and 5, but they are mentioned here because they, too, are necessary steps for the nurse to take in order to assure sound clinical decision. Steps 1 through 3 outline the approach used in this section to analyze abnormal hemodynamic pressures. Under the subheadings, the components of each waveform will be discussed. The process for determining abnormal pressures will be emphasized.

Right Atrial Waveform Abnormalities

Normal $\overline{RA}$ pressure is < 6 torr. $\overline{RA}$ pressure is equivalent to central venous pressure. A catheter in the right atrium reflects systemic venous pressure; in addition, it reflects pressures beyond the right atrial chamber. Problems that affect systemic venous resistance, pulmonary vascular resistance, tricuspid or pulmonary valves, or myocardial contraction or relaxation will be reflected by changes in $\overline{RA}$ pressure. Both increased vascular tone and hypervolemia elevate systemic venous pressure and, likewise, increase $\overline{RA}$ pressure, whereas loss of systemic venous tone and hypovolemia decrease $\overline{RA}$ pressure. Pulmonary vascular resistance is increased in pulmonary hypertension, and as the right ventricle fails, the $\overline{RA}$ pressure increases. Valvular problems, notable tricuspid stenosis and tricuspid insufficiency, elevate $\overline{RA}$ pressure. Problems that affect the ability of the myocardium to contract and relax include right heart failure, constrictive pericarditis, and pericardial tamponade, all of which elevate $\overline{RA}$ pressure.

a-Wave Changes

On an RA pressure tracing, the *a* wave represents right atrial contraction and follows the P wave when compared with the ECG. The electrical impulse that causes atrial depolarization, the P wave on the ECG, initiates atrial contraction. In cardiac arrhythmias such as atrial fibrillation and junctional rhythms, there are no P waves, no organized atrial contraction, and therefore no *a* wave on a right atrial tracing.

When the right atrium must generate increased systolic pressure in order to eject blood into the right ventricle, the *a* wave would be elevated. In tricuspid stenosis, the right atrioventricular valve is narrowed, and the right atrium must contract with greater force to squeeze blood through the stenotic opening. Conditions beyond the right atrial chamber that cause increased pressure will be reflected in an elevated *a* wave. For instance, right ventricular hypertrophy causes the right ventricle to contract with greater force, which in turn causes the right atrial *a* wave to have a higher pressure than normal. Such conditions include pulmonary stenosis and pulmonary hypertension.

Pathologic conditions that cause changes in myocardial tissue itself or prevent the heart muscle from relaxing completely elevate the ventricular filling pressure and thus cause the *a* wave to be elevated. When fibrotic changes occur in the myocardium, as in constrictive pericarditis, the elevated RV diastolic pressure is reflected in the RA pressure tracing by an elevated *a* wave.

Cardiac tamponade occurs when fluid collects under pressure in the cardiac sac between the visceral and parietal pericardium. With fluid filling this space, the heart muscle is restricted and prevented from filling normally. Fluid compressing the myocardium during ventricular diastole causes an elevated *a* wave on the RA pressure tracing. Severe cases of both constrictive pericarditis and pericardial tamponade cause pressure changes in all chambers of the heart. These two conditions elevate RA, LA, RVED, and LVED pressures.

v-Wave Changes

The *v* wave on an RA pressure tracing corresponds with right atrial filling and right ventricular systole. It occurs after the T wave and precedes the P wave when compared with the ECG. On an RA tracing, the *v* wave will be elevated in conditions that cause an increase in RA filling pressure. For example, in tricuspid insufficiency, the tricuspid valve is incompetent. The valve remains open, when, under normal conditions, it should be closed. With the tricuspid valve open during right ventricular contraction, blood regurgitates from the right ventricle into the right atrium, causing an increased *v* wave.

c-Wave Changes

A normal variant of the RA pressure tracing can demonstrate the absence of a *c* wave or a *c* wave superimposed on the *a* wave. Because the *c* wave occurs as a result of ballooning of the closed tricuspid valve into the right atrium during right ventricle contraction, it is not seen in the pressure tracing of a patient with tricuspid insufficiency. No *c* wave is seen because the valve leaflets do not close and cannot bulge into the right atrium, causing a slight pressure increase.

Right Ventricular Waveform Abnormalities

Normal significant RV pressure are systolic <30 torr and end-diastolic <5 torr. Abnormal RV pressures are seen in right ventricular failure, pulmonary stenosis, pulmonary insufficiency, and pulmonary hypertension. Eventually, untreated left ventricular failure will cause RV pressures to be elevated; however, other signs and symptoms will be obvious to the nurse before the RV pressures become elevated.

Right Ventricular Systolic Changes

RV systolic pressures are elevated in conditions that require greater force to eject the blood. For example, in pulmonary stenosis the right ventricle must generate enough pressure to overcome the resistance caused by the narrowed pulmonary valve. Pulmonary hypertension is a common cause of elevated RV sys-

tolic pressure and usually occurs because of left ventricular failure.

Right Ventricular End-Diastolic Changes

Under normal conditions, the pulmonary valve is closed during right ventricular diastole. The right ventricle fills with blood only from the right atrial, and the RVEDP is <5 torr. When the pulmonary valve is incompetent, blood regurgitates through the opened pulmonary cusps from the pulmonary artery into the right ventricle. In severe cases of pulmonary insufficiency, the additional blood volume due to regurgitant flow causes an elevated RVEDP.

Right Ventricular Systolic and End-Diastolic Changes

Initially, in right ventricular failure the right ventricular tracing shows a decreased systolic and an increased end-diastolic pressure. As the failure increases, systolic pressure decreases, the body's compensatory mechanisms fail, and cardiac output declines. Thus, the RV systolic pressure may be low or within normal limits, but the end-diastolic pressure remains elevated, indicating decreased right ventricular output that is due to reduced ventricular contractile force. In this situation, a larger volume of blood remains in the ventricle at the end of diastole.

Pulmonary hypertension elevates the RV systolic and end-diastolic pressures. The more severe the pulmonary hypertension, the greater the RV pressures. Eventually, the right ventricle fails, at which point the pressures vary according to the pressure changes seen in right ventricular failure.

Pulmonary Artery Waveform Abnormalities

Normal PA pressure values are systolic <30 torr, diastolic <10 torr, and mean <20 torr. The pulmonary artery diastolic (PAd) pressure is an approximation of the mean pulmonary artery wedge ($\overline{PAW}$) pressure, which reflects mean left atrial ($\overline{LA}$) pressure, which indicates left ventricular function. For this reason, the PAd is the most significant PA pressure. The exception occurs in pulmonary hypertension, which causes elevated PA systolic, diastolic, and mean pressures but a normal PAW pressure. PA pressures are elevated in pulmonary vascular disease, mitral stenosis, and left ventricular failure.

Pulmonary Artery Diastolic Changes

In the absence of pulmonary vascular disease, PAd pressures accurately reflect pressures in the left chambers of the heart. Conditions that require increased LA systolic pressures increase PA pressure values. For example, the LA systolic *a*-wave pressure would be elevated if the mitral valve were narrowed. This increase in LA *a*-wave pressure would be reflected in the pulmonary system and the PAd pressure would be abnormally high because the left atrium must contract with greater force to eject the blood through the stenotic mitral valve. Thus, in mitral stenosis, the PAd pressure would be elevated. In the presence of mitral stenosis, simultaneous PA and LV pressure tracings would demonstrate a pressure difference between the PAd and the LVEDP. Recall the following:

$$PAd \approx \overline{PAW}$$
$$\overline{PAW} \approx \overline{LA}$$
$$\overline{LA} \approx LVEDP$$

Normally, none of these pressures varies more than 1 to 3 torr. When the difference among these pressures is >1 to 3 torr, pathology exists.

Pulmonary Artery Systolic and Diastolic Changes

Left ventricular failure is reflected in the pulmonary artery tracing by an elevation of all pressures. Early in left ventricular failure, the loss of left ventricular compliance causes the LVEDP to be elevated. The heart rate increases in an attempt to compensate for the decreased force of left ventricular contraction. With the increase in heart rate, diastole is shortened, and there is less time for ventricular filling. With decreased ventricular filling time and loss of compliance, the blood volume ejected from the left ventricle is less, and cardiac output falls. LV systolic pressure decreases as the left ventricular compliance decreases. Concurrently, the LVEDP increases because the increased blood volume remains in the ventricle. This cycle is reflected in the pulmonary artery and eventually causes the PA pressures to be elevated.

Pulmonary Artery Wedge Abnormalities

PAW pressure is <12 torr. It reflects left ventricular function. The catheter is wedged in the pulmonary capillary bed, pressures from the right heart are blocked, and only pressures forward to the catheter are sensed. PAW pressures are elevated in mitral stenosis, mitral insufficiency, and left ventricular failure. When aortic stenosis and aortic insufficiency are severe, the elevated LV pressures are also reflected in the pulmonary artery wedge tracing.

a-Wave Changes

The *a* wave of the pulmonary artery wedge tracing corresponds with left atrial systole and will therefore be elevated in conditions that elevate LA systolic pres-

sure. LA systolic pressure is elevated in mitral stenosis. This increase in LA systolic pressure will cause the *a* wave of the PAW pressure to be elevated.

v-Wave Changes

The *v* wave on the PAW pressure tracing reflects left atrial filling and left ventricular contraction. Conditions that cause the LA diastolic pressure to be elevated will cause the PAW *v* wave to be elevated. In mitral regurgitation, the LA diastolic pressure is increased because of blood regurgitation from the left ventricle, through the incompetent mitral leaflets. This additional volume of blood in the left atrium during left atrial relaxation elevates the *v* wave on the pulmonary artery wedge tracing.

a-Wave and v-Wave Changes

Both *a* waves and *v* waves will be elevated on the pulmonary artery wedge tracing in left ventricular failure. The myocardium loses elasticity, compliance, and its ability to contract. In early left ventricular failure, the LVEDP is elevated. The heart rate increases to compensate for the decreased force of contraction. Diastole is shortened, less blood is ejected, more blood remains in the ventricle, and the LVEDP increases. An elevated *a* wave on the PAW tracing reflects this increase in pressure. The *v* wave pressure likewise increases, reflecting the increase in LV pressure. The $\overline{PAW}$ pressure is elevated because it is an approximation of the LVEDP.

The abnormal pressures discussed heretofore are pressures with which the critical care nurse will become familiar. These pressure abnormalities were discussed in detail so that the nurse will have the understanding necessary to make sound clinical judgments in caring for patients who require invasive monitoring. The following abnormal pressure tracings are ones seen more commonly in the cardiac catheterization laboratory rather than the critical care setting.

Left Atrial Waveform Abnormalities

Mean LA pressure is <12 torr. The *a* waves and *v* waves of the LA pressure tracing are elevated in the same pathologic conditions that cause the pulmonary artery wedge waveforms to be elevated. Because they are elevated for the same reasons that were previously discussed, the rationale will not be reiterated.

Left Ventricular and Aortic Waveform Abnormalities

The LV and Ao pressures will be discussed together because most frequently the pressures are measured simultaneously. Normal LV pressures are systolic

<140 torr and end-diastolic <12 torr. Normal Ao pressures are systolic <140 torr, diastolic <90 torr, and mean 70 to 90 torr. LV and Ao systolic pressures are equal. Differences among these pressures indicate a gradient across the aortic valve and demonstrate pathology. The diagnosis of aortic valvular problems is made by a composite patient examination that includes palpation, auscultation, phonocardiography, and catheterization.

Left Ventricular and Aortic Systolic Pressure Differences

In the presence of aortic stenosis, the left ventricle must contract with greater force to overcome resistance caused by the narrowed orifice. In this condition, LV systolic pressure is elevated; however, Ao systolic pressure is within normal limits. The mm Hg pressure difference between these two systolic values demonstrates the pressure gradient across the aortic valve. As the degree of stenosis increases, the left ventricle requires increasing pressure in order to eject blood out the aortic valve and maintain cardiac output. Simultaneous LV and Ao pressure tracings demonstrate systolic pressure differences between the left ventricle and aorta and a slowly rising initial aortic systolic upstroke. The obstructed aortic valve prevents the normal rapid ejection of blood from the left ventricle into the aorta, causing the delayed pressure rise. Study the pressure tracing shown in Figure 8-57.

Left Ventricular and Aortic Diastolic Pressure Changes

In aortic insufficiency, blood regurgitates from the aorta into the left ventricle during diastole, which elevates the LVEDP. As the aortic valve deteriorates, the Ao diastolic pressure decreases, which increases the pulse pressure. The characteristics of aortic insufficiency on a simultaneous LV and Ao pressure tracing are the following: (1) an elevated LVEDP, (2) a pulse pressure <100 torr, and (3) no dicrotic notch on the Ao pressure waveform. Because the dicrotic notch is caused by aortic valve closure, which does not occur in aortic regurgitation, no dicrotic notch is seen. Study the pressure tracing shown in Figure 8-58.

Nonphysiological Waveform Changes

When changes occur in waveform configurations, one way to identify the problem is to consider possible causes. The nurse should begin by checking with the

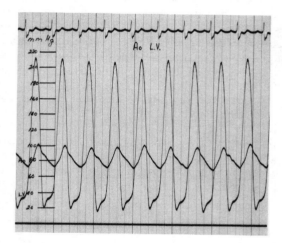

FIGURE 8-57
Simultaneous aortic and left ventricular pressure recordings from patient with aortic stenosis.

FIGURE 8-58
Left ventricular pressure recording with catheter pull-back to aorta in patient with aortic insufficiency. Note that the LVEDP is not elevated in this patient at rest.

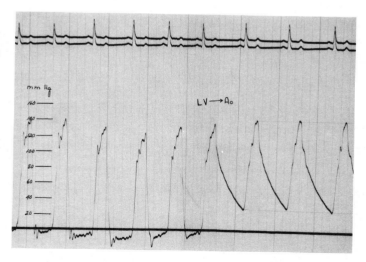

patient to ascertain whether the problem is with the hardware. Once she has confirmed that there has been no patient change in status, she should start the equipment check: Are the electrical plugs secure in the outlet? Is the power on? If she finds no problem, she then proceeds to the transducer. The transducer needs to be covered with fluid; air cannot be in the dome of the transducer. All connections must be secure. Stopcocks connecting lines must be turned correctly to zero and calibrate the transducer, measure patient pressures, and aspirate blood samples. The problem identification search must be continued until the cause is found. Then the nurse can proceed with the problem-solving process.

A waveform that becomes flattened is said to be "damped." Figure 8-59 shows a damped waveform.

Damped waveforms occur when there is air in the fluid line, when intravenous flow rate decreases and blood stasis occurs, when a fibrin clot is at the catheter tip, or when the catheter adheres to the vessel wall. A damped waveform indicates that air needs to be evacuated from the line, that the line needs to be flushed with heparinized saline, or that the line tip needs to be rotated or moved slightly. To flush the line, use the pressure valve or a bolus of 10 ml heparinized saline.

The flow-directed catheter can become wedged in the pulmonary capillary bed by inflating the balloon or by advancing the catheter into the pulmonary artery. When the catheter goes from the pulmonary artery into the pulmonary artery wedge position, the waveform on the oscilloscope changes and appears as shown in Figure 8-60.

Noting a tracing such as in Figure 8-60 or seeing a pulmonary artery wedge waveform on the oscillo-

scope, the nurse would consider first that the catheter balloon may be inflated, and second that the catheter tip may have floated into the wedge position. Pulmonary infarction has occurred when the flow-directed catheter was unintentionally in the wedge position. Because of this danger, the catheter balloon must be deflated or the catheter must be withdrawn into the pulmonary artery immediately.

Occasionally, the Swan-Ganz catheter floats from the pulmonary artery to the right ventricle. In this situation, the pattern on the oscilloscope changes from the pulmonary artery to the right ventricular waveform (Fig. 8-61).

FIGURE 8-60
Pulmonary artery and pulmonary artery wedge pressure recording.

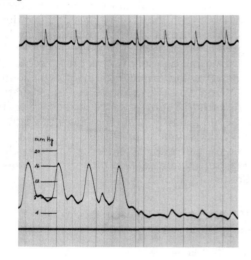

FIGURE 8-59
Damped pressure waveform.

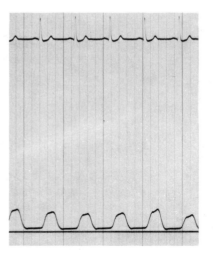

FIGURE 8-61
Pulmonary artery pressure recording with catheter pull-back to right ventricle.

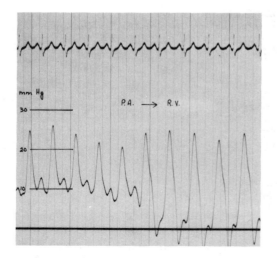

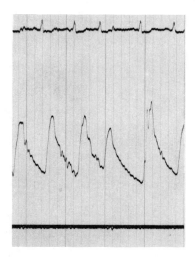

FIGURE 8-62
Aortic pressure recording demonstrating catheter fling.

To correct this situation, the nurse inflates the balloon with air and allows the catheter to float from the right ventricle into the pulmonary artery.

Catheter fling is caused when the catheter can move laterally in the vessel. The pressure tracing shown in Figure 8-62 demonstrates catheter fling. It produces spiked waves, distorting the waveform configuration and pressure values. The addition of IV extension tubing between the patient line and the pressure valve remedies this problem.

NURSING ASSESSMENT AND INTERVENTION

The Nurse – Patient Relationship

The nurse who desires to care for the patient requiring hemodynamic pressure monitoring must know normal physiology, normal pressure values, the reasons for abnormal pressures, and problem-solving procedures. It is essential to be at ease with the technical and theoretic components of invasive monitoring in order to work with each patient as an individual and to establish a therapeutic nurse–patient relationship.

Nurses have the responsibility to create an environment in which the patient is free to ask questions, express concerns, participate in patient care and decision-making, and relate to family and friends. Some patients requiring invasive monitoring are severely weakened by their cardiac problem, whereas others are stronger and more troubled by the activity restriction imposed because of the lines. These patients have individual concerns, but they also have common concerns and potential problems that the nurse can alleviate, prevent, or correct.

Patient fear and anxiety are allayed by the nurse who is confident in knowledge, skill, and problem-solving abilities. This nurse is free to listen to the patient's fears and concerns and to watch for nonverbal cues that need to be clarified. A caring attitude includes an explanation of the routines and reasons for them. Family members should be included in this education process. Both patient and family members need to realize that the nurse cares for the patient as a whole individual and that the technical equipment assists the nurse in monitoring parameters necessary for optimal care.

Prevention of Problems

Circulation and Exercise. Patients need to be instructed to exercise the extremities where the lines are inserted. Exercising the fingers and toes and contracting and relaxing arm and leg muscles will promote circulation in the extremity. Most patients requiring invasive monitoring have compromised circulation. Inactivity adds to this problem. Patients unable to exercise extremities need to have routine passive exercises done for them.

Catheter Care. The presence of a catheter in a vessel increases the likelihood of inflammation, leading to the development of *phlebitis*. The catheter site should be looked at several times daily for early signs of inflammation, such as tenderness, changes in local temperature, redness, and swelling. The dressing should be changed every 8 hours; the insertion site is cleansed with soap and water, and antiseptic ointment, sponges, and tape are applied in a secure but comfortable manner. The previously pictured method for securing the lines and transducers on a short armboard recommended for patient safety and nurse convenience is shown again in Figure 8-63.

Deep Breathing. Patients who are confined to bed for several days consciously need to take slow, deep breaths, using their abdominal muscles. The patient should be instructed to breathe in this manner ten times per hour while awake so that the alveoli will be expanded and atelectasis will be prevented. Although pressures are generally recorded with the patient in the supine position, he should be encouraged to rest on either side between pressure readings.

It is essential that the critical care nurse understand the concept of pressure because it affects all body systems. Along with basic knowledge of the body systems, the critical care nurse must possess a questioning mind and a caring spirit. An inquisitive nurse will formulate questions in a methodic, scientific manner, seek answers, and find new questions. The analytic approach to patient care fosters improved patient care. The critical care nurse is well named because a caring

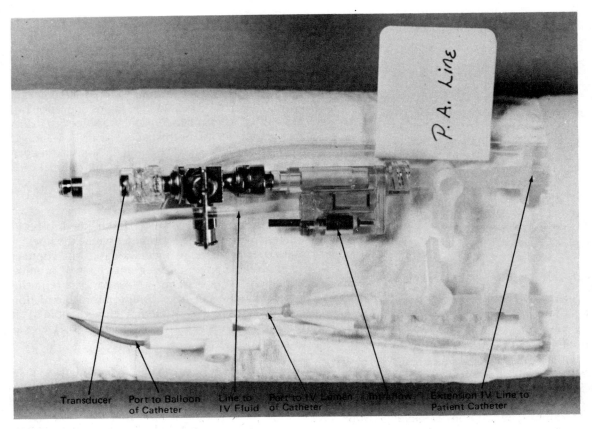

Transducer   Port to Balloon   Line to   Port to IV Lumen   Inflow   Extension IV Line to
of Catheter   IV Fluid   of Catheter   Patient Catheter

FIGURE 8-63
Pressure lines mounted on armboard.

spirit makes the nurse's efforts complete by combining the science and art of nursing intervention.

Direct Cardiac Output Measurement

Shirley J. Hoffman

Cardiac output refers to the amount of blood that is pumped out of the heart and is expressed in liters per minute. It is a function of stroke volume and heart rate. Flow is determined by the ratio of pressure to resistance; thus, cardiac output is determined by the ratio of mean arterial pressure to total peripheral resistance.

Any condition that causes uncompensated changes in arterial pressure or peripheral resistance will cause a change in cardiac output. Because many disease states, as well as their modes of therapy, affect arterial pressure, peripheral resistance, and cardiac output, it is often important that the critically ill patient's cardiac output be measured so that he can be provided with optimal medical and nursing care.

Normal Cardiac Output and Cardiac Index

Normal cardiac output at rest is considered 4 to 7 liters per minute; however, actual cardiac output is related to body size. The cardiac index is a more realistic guide for evaluating the cardiac output of any one individual. The cardiac index is obtained by dividing cardiac output by the body surface area. Body surface area can be determined with the Dubois body surface chart (Fig. 8-64). A straight line drawn between the patient's height in the left-hand column will cross the number in the middle column that represents his body surface area in square meters. Normal cardiac index is 2.5 to 4 liters per minute per square meter.

Low Cardiac Output

Many disease states may decrease the pumping effectiveness of the left ventricle, resulting in a decrease in the pressure generated within the ventricle. This in turn will cause the cardiac output to fall. Myocardial infarction is the most common cause of compromised pumping ability of the left ventricle. Other causes include valvular heart disease, congestive heart failure, myocarditis, cardiac tamponade, and some congenital anomalies. In monitoring therapy in patients who are critically ill because of these disease states, cardiac output determinations, in conjunction with various intracardiac and pulmonary pressure measurements, can be very helpful.

Venous return to the right side of the heart is a major factor in determining cardiac output. The heart can pump out only the volume presented to it. If inadequate blood volume is present, the cardiac output must, of necessity, fall. In the critical care unit, low cardiac output due to decreased venous return is commonly caused by severe hemorrhage and dehydration.

It must be remembered that any patient who receives mechanical ventilation with positive pressure breathing may have a decreased cardiac output because of increased intrathoracic pressure and decreased venous return. In the patient with acute respiratory distress syndrome who is being treated with positive end-expiratory pressure (PEEP), cardiac output monitoring may help determine the level of PEEP that will produce the optimum PO_2 with minimal decrease in cardiac output.

High Cardiac Output

Normally, the cardiac output increases with exercise as a result of increased oxygen consumption at the cellular level. The trained athlete may raise his cardiac output to several times normal during strenuous exercise. Stimulation of the sympathetic nervous system will also increase cardiac output by increasing heart rate and the contractile force of the left ventricle.

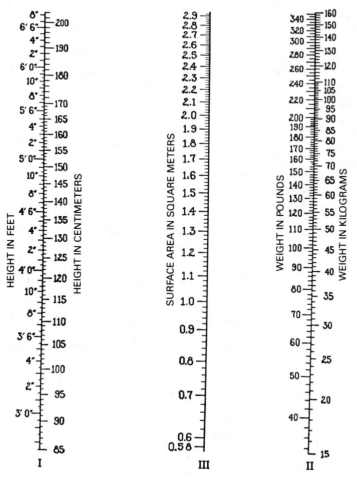

FIGURE 8-64

Dubois body surface chart (as prepared by Boothby and Sandiford of the Mayo Clinic). To find body surface of a patient, locate the height in inches (or centimeters) on scale I and the weight in pounds (or kilograms) on scale II and place a straight edge (ruler) between these two points, which will intersect scale III at the patient's surface area.

In the critical care unit, septic shock is one of the causes of abnormally high cardiac output. This occurs because of massive vasodilation, probably from the toxic substances produced by sepsis, thus decreasing peripheral resistance. The cardiac output in septic shock may increase to three or four times normal.

The thiamine deficiency associated with beriberi may also cause vasodilation and high cardiac output.

Because of their effects on peripheral resistance, many of the potent antihypertensive drugs used in the critical care unit should be titrated by monitoring the pressures obtained from a Swan-Ganz catheter and cardiac output determinations.

A high rate of metabolism as found in thyrotoxicosis, fever, and certain tumors, may also cause an increase in cardiac output because of increased oxygen consumption.

Measurement of Cardiac Output

Methods

The Fick method of measuring cardiac output involves determination of the difference in oxygen concentration of mixed venous blood and arterial blood and measurement of oxygen consumption in the lungs. The cardiac output is then calculated from a formula. To accomplish the indicator dilution method, one injects dye into a large vein or into the right side of the heart, obtains a time-concentration curve from peripheral artery sampling, and calculates cardiac output. Neither of these methods is feasible in the clinical setting.

With the advent of the four-lumen Swan-Ganz thermodilution catheter and cardiac output computers, it is now a relatively simple procedure for the critical care nurse to measure cardiac output at the patient's bedside. The thermodilution method is similar to the indicator dilution method. When thermodilution is used, the indicator is cold solution injected into the right atrium, and the sampling device is a thermistor near the end of the catheter in the pulmonary artery (Fig. 8-65). The thermistor continuously measures the temperature of the blood flowing past it. The catheter is connected to a cardiac output computer that determines the cardiac output from the time-temperature curve resulting from the rate of change in temperature of the blood that flows past the thermistor. Because of the number of variables inherent in the procedure, computation of the average of several consecutive cardiac output determinations will assure greater accuracy.

Initial Considerations

It is important for the critical care nurse to eliminate as many potential sources of error as possible in order to obtain an accurate cardiac output. The procedure

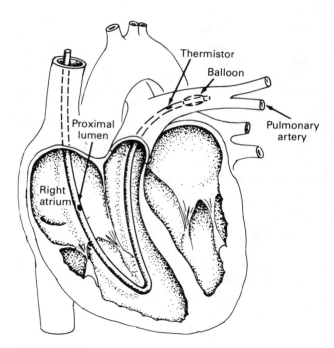

FIGURE 8-65
Swan-Ganz thermodilution catheter in place.

should be done at a time when the patient is in a quiet, steady state. Agitation increases the cardiac output, and the measurement will not be meaningful relative to the resting output or those obtained during various degrees of agitation. It is felt by some that respiratory variations may cause changes in the temperature of the blood in the pulmonary circulation and thus render the cardiac output measurement something less than accurate. This possible source of error may be avoided if the determination is done when the patient is breathing quietly.

Each cardiac output measurement should be obtained with the patient in the same position, either supine or semierect. Although accurate measurements can be obtained in either position, the actual cardiac output may significantly change with change in position, usually decreasing when the patient is semierect.

The *Swan-Ganz thermodilution catheter* should be checked for proper functioning before beginning the procedure (Fig. 8-66). If the proximal lumen of the catheter is not fully patent, the cardiac output measurement will be inaccurate. The proximal lumen should be flushed before the cold solution is injected. If the proximal lumen is being used for the administration of intravenous medications, slow flushing before injection will also preclude the administration of a bolus of the infusing medication.

The *thermistry circuit* in the catheter and the *cardiac output computer* should be checked for proper

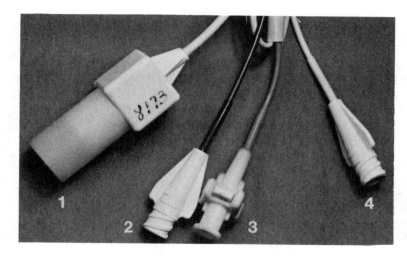

FIGURE 8-66
Entry sites for the four lumens of the Swan-Ganz thermodilution catheter. 1, Thermistor. 2, Proximal (right atrium). 3, Balloon inflation. 4, Distal (pulmonary artery).

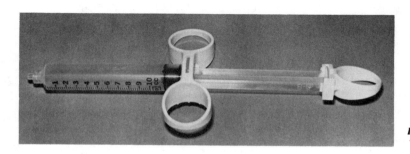

FIGURE 8-67
"Control" syringe.

functioning before each set of cardiac outputs is determined. This requires connection of the catheter thermistry circuit to the computer cable. Care must be taken to avoid damaging or breaking the relatively fragile connector mechanism. Follow the directions in the cardiac output computer operator's manual for checking the catheter and computer. This should also be done at any time a cardiac output determination that does not correlate with the patient's clinical condition is obtained.

The *computation constant* should be checked and set on the cardiac output computer to reflect the volume and temperature of the injectate being used. This number also takes into account catheter size and the rise in temperature of the injectate as it is being injected through the catheter. A table of computation constants can be found in the cardiac output computer operator's manual.

Injectate
The injectate solution used for the procedure is usually sterile 5% dextrose in water, although sterile normal saline may be used. Either 5 or 10 ml may be used, although 10 ml allows for more accuracy in the cardiac output determination.

Either glass or plastic Luer-Lok syringes may be used; "control" syringes, which have two finger rings attached to the barrel and a thumb ring at the end of the plunger, facilitate the speed of injection and also allow one to hold the syringe without handling the barrel (Fig. 8-67).

The injectate can be used at room temperature, but greatest accuracy is obtained at 0° to 4°C. The injectate can be cooled by a variety of methods. Electrical coolers manufactured for this purpose are available. An ice bath may also be used, and alcohol may be added to the ice bath for faster cooling. (One should take care when using an electric cooling plate or when adding alcohol to the ice bath that the solution in the syringes does not freeze.) Refrigeration of the injectate solution will also allow for faster cooling.

Each syringe should be filled with sterile injectate, and the sterile cap should be replaced over the tip of the syringe. The syringes can be placed in a container that is then immersed in the ice bath or placed directly into the cooler.

An extra syringe must be filled with the same amount of injectate, the sterile cap replaced, and the plunger removed from the barrel. This syringe is placed in the container with the other syringes, and the injectate temperature probe is placed into the solution in this syringe. The probe is connected to the computer, which measures the temperature of the injectate. All the syringes, including the one containing the temperature probe, should be filled from the same container of solution so that the initial temperature of the injectate in each will be the same. Because the temperature of the solution actually being injected is not measured, the solution in which the temperature *is* being measured should simulate the injectate as closely as possible. The assumption is that the temperature of the solution in all the syringes is the same.

After the cardiac output determinations have been made, it is helpful to fill a new set of syringes to cool in preparation for the next set of determinations. One should be sure to replace the temperature probe syringe along with the injectate syringes because they must all have the same initial temperature.

Injection

When the injectate solution has cooled to 0° to 4°C as indicated by the cardiac output computer, injection can be accomplished with greatest accuracy. Although automatic injectors are available, accurate measurements can be obtained with manual injection.

Because significant warming of the injectate can result from holding the syringe in the hand, one should handle the syringe using the finger and thumb rings, avoiding contact of the hands with the syringe barrel. It must be made certain that the syringe has been filled to the *exact* volume indicated by the computation constant used, usually 10 ml. Use of inaccurately measured injectate volume will result in inaccurate cardiac output measurements. One should follow the cardiac output computer manufacturer's directions when operating the computer.

The injectate syringe is attached to the proximal lumen of the Swan-Ganz catheter. A three-way stopcock between the proximal lumen and intravenous tubing allows maintenance of a closed system and facilitates rapid attachment of the syringe (Fig. 8-68). Inject the solution into the proximal line at the time the computer indicates readiness. Injection should be accomplished during the end-expiratory phase of the respiratory cycle to minimize the effects of blood temperature variations from respirations. Injection time for 10 ml of solution should be 4 seconds or less. The elapsed time from removal of syringe from the cooling mechanism until injection should be as short as possible so that environmental warming of the injectate is avoided.

The cardiac rhythm should be observed immediately after injection because the sudden bolus of cold solution into the right atrium may precipitate atrial or ventricular arrhythmias. The pulmonary artery pressure waveform should also be observed after injection for migration of the catheter into the wedge position or retrograde into the right ventricle. The empty syringe should be removed and discarded after injection.

Measurements may be repeated when the computer signifies readiness. The catheter thermistry circuit is disconnected from the computer cable after the entire procedure is completed. The protective cap is replaced over the end of the thermistry circuit "tail" of the Swan-Ganz catheter.

Some cardiac output computers are equipped with strip chart recorders, so that the thermodilution curve can be observed and recorded. The curve should have a smooth upstroke, peak, and smooth downstroke. If the curve is distorted because of poor injection technique or improper catheter positioning, that cardiac output measurement should be rejected (Fig. 8-69).

Averaging Cardiac Outputs

The average of several cardiac outputs is more accurate than one isolated determination because of the number of possible variables in the patient and procedure performance. Four consecutive determinations should be obtained if possible. If one measurement is unduly high or low relative to the others in the series, it should

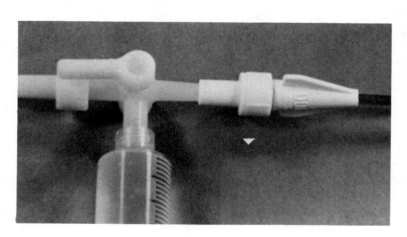

FIGURE 8-68
Attachment of injectate syringe to three-way stopcock between proximal lumen of Swan-Ganz thermodilution catheter on right and intravenous tubing on left. Handle on stopcock points to "off."

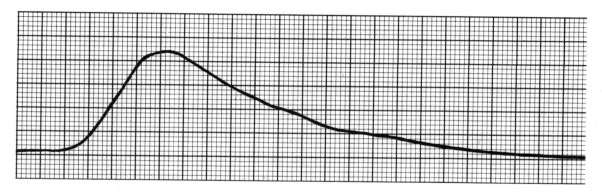

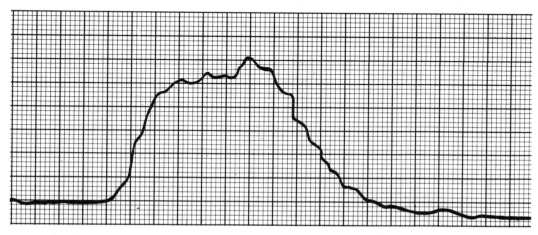

FIGURE 8-69
Examples of accurate and distorted thermodilution curves as produced on strip chart recorder.
(A) Smooth recording is accurate. (B) Irregular recording is distorted.

be discarded as inaccurate. To assure optimal accuracy, one should obtain the measurements within 0.5 liter per minute of each other. The remaining determinations are then averaged for the measurement to be recorded in the patient's chart. The cardiac index is calculated as described earlier and also recorded in the chart.

Electrical Safety

An electrically safe environment must be maintained at all times for the critical care patient. This is especially important when cardiac output determinations are being made by the Swan-Ganz catheter, which traverses the heart.

The following guidelines should be used to maintain electrical safety for the patient with a Swan-Ganz thermodilution catheter:

• The patient should be in a nonelectric bed. If an electric bed must be used, it should be unplugged from the wall outlet.

• Bed linens should be changed immediately when wet.

• The amount of electrical equipment in the immediate environment should be minimal and, when required for patient care, properly grounded.

• The cardiac output computer cable should be inspected for continuity before use.

• The protective cap should be in place over the thermistry tail on the catheter when not in use.

• The catheter should not be connected to the computer cable during insertion procedure.

• The computer should be on battery power, not AC power, when connected to the catheter.

• The electrical cooler should be disconnected from the wall outlet or the temperature probe removed from the cooler while the catheter is connected to the computer cable.

• Personnel handling the catheter should not be in simultaneous contact with any other electrical equipment.

• The computer and the cable should be kept dry and clean.

• The computer should not be operated in the presence of explosive anesthetic agents.

Evaluation of Cardiac Output and Cardiac Index

The cardiac output and index should always be evaluated in conjunction with other assessed parameters and the clinical status of the patient. For example, one would expect the patient in cardiogenic shock to have a low cardiac output and cardiac index and high pulmonary capillary wedge (PCW) and pulmonary artery diastolic (PAd) pressures. With improvement in the patient's clinical status, the cardiac output and index should rise, and the PCW and PAd pressures should decrease. If one of the preceding measurements does not reflect the trend of the others and the patient's clinical status, the nurse should suspect an error in technique or equipment malfunction and begin troubleshooting or repeating measurements. One of the reasons for determining multiple hemodynamic measurements is to use each determination to verify the others.

The gamut of measured hemodynamic parameters can be used to calculate other parameters that cannot be measured directly. Calculators that can be programmed to calculate such information as stroke volume, right and left ventricular stroke work, and systemic and pulmonary vascular resistance from measured parameters are now available. Systemic vascular resistance can be hand-calculated as follows:

$$\frac{(\text{mean arterial pressure} - \text{PCW}) \times 80}{\text{cardiac output}}$$

The patient who has a low mean arterial pressure (MAP), high cardiac index, and low systemic vascular resistance (as seen in septic shock) may be best treated with additional circulatory volume and vasoconstrictor therapy. The patient who has cardiogenic shock may demonstrate a low MAP, low cardiac index, and high systemic vascular resistance because of maximal vasoconstriction and may be best treated with circulating volume, vasodilator therapy, and inotropic agents.

In the patient with acute myocardial infarction, cardiac outputs can be evaluated in conjunction with changes in PCW pressures. By relating these two measurements, one may be able to modify therapy to obtain a PCW pressure that will result in optimal cardiac output and arterial pressure for that patient.

It is obvious that these hemodynamic parameters can be very useful in assessing the efficacy of vasodilators, vasoconstrictors, additional volume, diuretics, and inotropic agents.

It is important that the critical care nurse be adept at setting up, maintaining, and troubleshooting all types of hemodynamic and cardiac monitoring equipment in the critical care unit. Measurements of the various parameters must be made with accuracy and evaluated in conjunction with one another and with the patient's clinical status. Appropriate use of these determinations will aid in medical diagnosis, choice of therapy, monitoring of therapy, and anticipation of prognosis. The ultimate goal in the use of these hemodynamic parameters is the reduction of morbidity and mortality in critically ill patients.

BIBLIOGRAPHY

Davies H, Nelson WP: Understanding Cardiology. Boston, Butterworths, 1978

Editorial: Swan-Ganz catheters. Lancet 2, No. 8085:357–358, 1978

Guyton AC: Basic Human Physiology: Normal Function and Mechanisms of Disease. Philadelphia, WB Saunders, 1977

Hathaway R: The Swan-Ganz catheter: A review. Nurs Clin North Am 13, No. 3:389–407, 1978

Kaplan JA: Hemodynamic Monitoring and Ischemic Heart Disease. Edwards Laboratories, Division of American Hospital Supply Corp, October, 1979

Levett JM, Replogle RL: Current research review: Thermodilution cardiac output: A critical analysis and review of the literature. J Surg Res 27:392–404, 1979

Loeb H, Gunnar R: Hemodynamic monitoring in a coronary care unit. Heart Lung 11:302–305, 1982

O'Connor L: Hemodynamic Monitoring and Cardiovascular Medicine. Edwards Laboratories, Division of American Hospital Supply Corp, November, 1979

Understanding Hemodynamic Measurements Made with the Swan-Ganz Catheter. Edwards Laboratories, Division of American Hospital Supply Corp, May, 1978

9
Management Modalities: Cardiovascular System

Cardiac Monitoring

Shirley J. Hoffman

Monitoring the patient with cardiac disturbances is now accepted as routine practice. Since the first hard wire bedside monitor, modern electronics has made constant sophisticated advances in monitoring equipment. Remote display systems currently incorporate features such as *nonfade scopes,* which keep the electrocardiogram (ECG) pattern visible across the screen; *freeze* modes, which allow the ECG pattern to be held for more detailed examination; *storage capability,* either by tape loops or an electronic memory, which permits retrieval of arrhythmias from 8 to 60 seconds after their occurrence; *automatic chart documentation,* in which the ECG recorder is activated by alarms or at preset intervals; *heart rate monitors,* which display the rate either by meter or by digital display (the alarm system is incorporated into the heart-rate monitor with adjustments for both the high and low settings); *multiparameter displays,* which offer display of pressures, temperature, electroencephalogram (EEG), respirations, and so forth; and *computer systems,* which store and analyze ECG data. The information can then be retrieved at any time to aid in diagnosis and to note trends in the patient's status.

Two types of patient monitoring equipment presently in use are hard wire devices and telemetry. Hard wire monitors require an electrical cable between the patient and the ECG display device. Telemetry simply requires the patient to carry a small battery-operated transmitter. No wire connection is needed between the patient and the ECG display device. In addition to the *transmitter,* which has a frequency similar to radio stations, telemetry systems require *receivers,* which pick up and display the signal on a scope, and *antennas,* which are built into the receiver and which may be mounted in the vicinity of the receiver to widen the range of signal pick-up. Batteries are the power source for the transmitter and thus make it possible to avoid electrical hazards by isolating the monitoring system from potential current leakage and accidental shock.

Manufacturers of hard wire and telemetry monitoring systems provide operating instructions, which should be followed so that proper, safe functioning of the equipment is ensured.

ELECTRODE APPLICATION

A high-quality trace will exhibit a narrow, stable baseline, absence of distortion or "noise," and sufficient amplitude of the QRS complex to activate the rate meters and alarm systems properly and to allow for identification of P waves.

Types of Electrodes

Needle electrodes are placed under the skin and thus eliminate variations caused by skin resistance. However, they are traumatic and provide a source of infection because of the break in skin integrity, and therefore they are not appropriate for long-term use. Metal disc electrodes are cumbersome and restricting to the patient. Considerable artifact occurs because of the inability to seal the disc adequately to the skin.

Disposable silver- or nickle-plated electrodes centered in a circle of adhesive paper or foam rubber are currently used for cardiac monitoring. Most electrodes are pregelled by the manufacturer. They may have disposable wires attached to the electrodes or nondisposable wires that snap onto the electrodes. They are comfortable for the patient, but if not properly applied, undue artifact and false alarms may result.

Portable monitor-defibrillators are now available in which the defibrillator paddles can be used as electrodes for rapid institution of monitoring in emergencies. The two paddles are placed on the chest and act as positive and negative electrodes. This provides a tracing on the oscilloscope and allows for immediate treatment of arrhythmias.

Skin Preparation

Proper skin preparation and application of electrodes which are imperative to good monitoring, are managed as follows:

1. A site is selected. Bony protuberances, joints, and folds in skin are avoided. Areas in which muscle attaches to bone have the least motion artifact.
2. Excessive body hair is shaved from the site.
3. Residue from oils, lotion, and so forth used in pa-

tient care is removed from the skin. Sites must be free of any oil film or residue that could affect electrode adhesion.

It is important to follow the electrode manufacturer's directions for skin preparation because the chemical reaction between alcohol or other skin-prep materials and the adhesives used in some electrodes may cause skin irritation or nonadhesion to the skin.

The electrode manufacturer's directions should also be followed in the application of electrodes. Proper application of electrodes will ensure a good monitor trace and comfort for the patient.

SOLVING ECG MONITOR PROBLEMS

Several problems may occur in monitoring ECG, including baseline but no ECG trace, intermittent traces, wandering or irregular baseline, low amplitude complexes, 60-cycle interference, excessive triggering of heart rate alarms, and skin irritation. The steps that one should follow when such problems occur are outlined in the chart titled "ECG Monitor Problem Solving."

EXCESSIVE TRIGGERING OF HEART RATE ALARMS

- Is Hi-Low alarm set too close to patient's rate?
- Is monitor sensitivity level set too high or too low?
- Is patient cable securely inserted into monitor receptacle?

ECG Monitor Problem Solving

BASELINE BUT NO ECG TRACE

- Is the size (gain or sensitivity) control properly adjusted?
- Is appropriate lead selector being used on monitor?
- Is the patient cable fully inserted into ECG receptacle?
- Are electrode wires fully inserted into patient cable?
- Are electrode wires firmly attached to electrodes?
- Are electrode wires damaged?
- Is the patient cable damaged?
- Call for service if trace is still absent.

INTERMITTENT TRACE

- Is patient cable fully inserted into monitor receptacle?
- Are electrode wires fully inserted into patient cable?
- Are electrode wires firmly attached to electrodes?
- Are electrode wire connectors loose or worn?
- Have electrodes been applied properly?
- Are electrodes properly located and in firm skin contact?
- Is patient cable damaged?

WANDERING OR IRREGULAR BASELINE

- Is there excessive cable movement? This can be reduced by clipping to patient's clothing.

- Is the power cord on or near the monitor cable?
- Is there excessive movement by the patient? Does he have muscle tremors from anxiety or shivering?
- Is site selection correct?
- Were proper skin preparation and application followed?
- Are the electrodes still moist?

LOW AMPLITUDE COMPLEXES

- Is size control adjusted properly?
- Were the electrodes applied properly?
- Is there dried gel on the electrodes?
- Change electrode sites. Check 12-lead ECG for lead with highest amplitude and attempt to simulate that lead.
- If none of the above steps remedies the problem, the weak signal may be the patient's normal complex.

SIXTY-CYCLE INTERFERENCE

- Is the monitor size control set too high?
- Are there nearby electrical devices in use, especially poorly grounded ones?
- Were the electrodes applied properly?
- Is there dried gel on the electrodes?
- Are lead wires or connections damaged?

- Are lead wires or connections damaged?
- Has the electrode site been properly selected? A site of low amplitude may cause failure of the monitor to sense each QRS.
- Were electrodes applied properly?
- Is the baseline unstable, or is there excessive cable or lead wire movement? Check steps to remedy the problem.

SKIN IRRITATION

- Is there a residue of alcohol or acetone or skin conditioners on the skin under the electrodes?
- Was the skin dry before the electrodes were applied?
- Was skin preparation technique harsh?
- Is the patient sensitive to gels, adhesives, or prep solutions?
- Is there DC leakage from the monitor?

Monitor Leads

The numerous monitoring devices currently on the market vary from the two-electrode telemetry devices to three-, four-, and five-electrode hard wire monitors.

All monitors require use of a positive and a negative electrode that can be placed on the chest in positions that simulate the positive and negative poles of any of the three standard limb leads. Telemetry monitors utilize only these two electrodes.

Monitors that require three electrodes utilize positive, negative, and ground electrodes that are placed in the right arm, left arm, and left leg positions on the chest.

FIGURE 9-1
Positive, negative, and ground electrodes in the standard limb leads.

	Lead I	Lead II	Lead III
RA	–	–	Ground
LA	+	Ground	–
LL	Ground	+	+

Figure 9-1 indicates which electrodes are positive, negative, and ground in each standard limb lead. The electrode that is not being utilized as the positive or negative pole becomes the ground when lead selection is changed.

Four-electrode monitors require a right leg electrode that is the ground for all leads. Because only the positive, negative, and ground electrodes are being utilized for any single lead, the fourth electrode is not in use. This system is convenient when electrodes need to be replaced on a critically ill patient. One can replace all electrodes except the ground without loss of ECG visualization on the monitor by changing the "unused" electrode in each lead (Fig. 9-2).

The fifth electrode on a five-electrode monitor is a "chest" electrode that allows one to obtain a simulated 12-lead ECG. This electrode can be placed in any of the positive-pole positions for the six chest leads. It is seldom used on a continuous basis because of the inconvenience of having five electrodes in place.

The monitoring lead that is most helpful in differentiating arrhythmias is MCL_1. This is a modification of chest lead V_1, the lead in which bundle branch blocks are most easily differentiated. Because ectopic supraventricular beats with aberrant ventricular conduction often resemble right bundle branch block (RBBB) and ectopic ventricular beats almost never resemble RBBB, MCL_1 is often helpful in making this important differentiation. Bundle branch blocks can also be differentiated in MCL_6, a modification of chest lead V_6.

One can use the MCL_1 lead with any monitor system by placing the positive electrode for the lead selected *lead I, II, or III* in the V_1 position on the chest and the negative electrode below the left clavicle. One can similarly obtain MCL_6 by placing the positive electrode in the V_6 position and the negative electrode below the left clavicle. Figure 9-3 indicates electrode placements for MCL_1 and MCL_6 with capability for visualization of

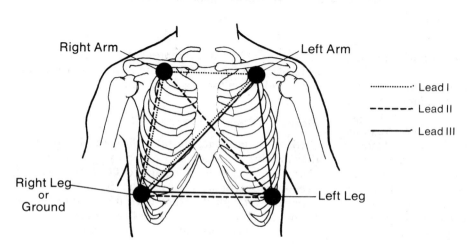

FIGURE 9-2
Four-electrode system for obtaining simulation of the standard limb leads. Some monitors utilize a "floating ground" and require only three electrodes, eliminating the right leg electrode.

············ Lead I
------- Lead II
——— Lead III

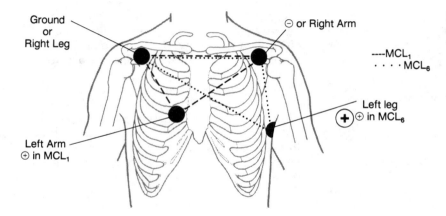

FIGURE 9-3
MCL$_1$ (use lead I selection) and
MCL$_6$ (use lead II selection).

TABLE 9-1
SUGGESTED MONITORING LEAD SELECTION

Status	Lead	Rationale
Anticipated ventricular ectopy	MCL$_1$ or MCL$_6$	The preponderance of aberrantly conducted supraventricular ectopic beats have a RBBB configuration. Because RBBB configurations are relatively standard in leads V$_1$ and V$_6$, modifications of these leads should be used when differentiation of ventricular ectopy and supraventricular ectopy with aberrant ventricular conduction might be required.
RBBB and normal axis in presence of acute anterior myocardial infarction	Lead II or III	Sinus beats have RBBB configuration, and premature supraventricular beats have RBBB configuration or are nonconducted, so "RBBB aberrations" do not exist. Change in direction of complex in lead II or III from positive to negative might indicate left-axis deviation. Twelve-lead ECG is indicated to determine onset of hemiblock.
Poor P wave visualization	Lead II	Because the normal axis of lead II is parallel to the normal P wave axis, P waves are usually visualized best in lead II. Sinus P waves are upright in this lead, and junctional P waves are usually negative.
Ventricular ectopy	MCL$_1$ or MCL$_6$	Ectopic beats originating in the left ventricle are usually more upright in MCL$_1$ and more negative in MCL$_6$. Those originating in the right ventricle are usually more negative in MCL$_1$ and more upright in MCL$_6$. Although primary ventricular fibrillation is most often precipitated by left ventricular ectopy, ectopic beats from either ventricle should probably be treated in the acutely ill patient.
Right ventricular pacemaker	MCL$_1$ or MCL$_6$	The paced QRS complex originating in the right ventricle should be negative in MCL$_1$ and positive in MCL$_6$. Reversal of these configurations may result from pacemaker catheter perforation of the ventricular apex or septum.

MCL$_1$ when lead I is selected on the monitor and MCL$_6$ when lead II is selected.

Myocardial ischemia, injury, and infarction are represented by T wave inversion, S–T segment elevation, and significant Q waves, respectively. These changes are reflected in the leads that have their positive poles geographically closest to the damage. The V leads in the 12-lead ECG reflects anterior and lateral wall changes. Standard lead I may also show lateral wall damage. Inferior wall changes are indicated in standard leads II, III, and aVF. Ischemia, injury, and infarction may be suspected when these changes occur on the monitor ECG. They must always be confirmed by 12-lead ECG because monitor leads are only simulations of comparable leads on the 12-lead ECG and cannot be relied on for diagnosis. (Table 9-1).

Monitor Observation

Cardiac monitors are useful only if the information they provide is "observed," either by computers with alarms for programmed parameters or by the human eye, and appropriately acted upon by competent, responsible individuals. Many critical care units utilize the monitor technician whose sole responsibilities are to observe monitors, obtain chart samples, and give appropriate information to the nurse regarding each patient's ECG status. Individuals who are assigned the responsibility of monitor observation must not let their attention be drawn away from the monitors. They should be given the parameters for reporting arrhythmias to the nurse for each patient. Alarms should be on the functioning mode, except when direct physical care of the patient necessitates that the alarms be turned off. The patient who is watching monitors should be notified of any interruptions in monitoring, such as those caused by changing electrodes and by changing the patient to a portable monitor in order to leave the unit for diagnostic tests in another department.

Because monitor artifact obscures the true ECG patterns, all efforts should be made to reduce or eliminate it. Occasionally, artifacts can resemble the configurations of arrhythmias. The patient vigorously brushing his teeth has been known to "produce" ventricular flutter on the monitor. Clapping the patient's back at a rapid rate as part of pulmonary hygiene may simulate atrial flutter waves. Hiccoughs may look like extrasystoles. The monitor observer should be apprised of these situations when they occur so that they may be taken into consideration in arrhythmia diagnosis.

It is not unusual for monitored patients to use their monitors to "test" their nurses in order to determine their response time. The patient with myocardial infarction in the coronary care unit may disconnect an electrode to simulate asystole. The patient who has been transferred to the telemetry unit may tap on the telemetry transmitter box, thus simulating ventricular tachycardia. These situations can be very frustrating for both the monitor observer and the busy critical care nurse. It must never be assumed that repeated episodes of this nature are not true arrhythmias. They must be reported and assessed immediately. Most often, it will be found that the patient's motivation consists of fear and insecurity. When the patient discovers that the simulated arrhythmia results in immediate response by the nurse, he will usually feel secure in this knowledge and will have no further need to test the nurse.

BIBLIOGRAPHY

Hammond C: Plain talk about cardiac monitoring. RN 42:34–43, 1979

Marriott JH: Practical Electrocardiography, 7th ed. Baltimore, Williams & Wilkins, 1983

Vinsant MO: Commonsense Approach to Coronary Care, 3rd ed. St. Louis, CV Mosby, 1981

Whley HN: Present status of monitoring in the coronary care unit. Heart Lung 7:67–68, 1978

Artificial Cardiac Pacing

Shirley J. Hoffman

Electrical stimulation of the heart was tried experimentally as early as 1819. In 1930, Hyman noted that he could inject the right atrium with a diversity of substances and restore a heartbeat. He devised an "ingenious apparatus" that he labeled an *artificial pacemaker,* which delivered a rhythmic charge to the heart. In 1952, Zoll demonstrated that patients with Stokes-Adams syndrome could be sustained by the administration of current directly to the chest wall. Lillehei in 1957 affixed electrodes directly to the ventricles during open-heart surgery. In the period ranging from 1958 to 1961, implantable pacemakers for treatment of complete heart block came into rather extensive use. Over subsequent years, various improvements and refinements have been and continue to be made for both short-term temporary pacing and long-term permanent pacing.

INDICATIONS FOR ARTIFICIAL PACING

Artificial cardiac pacing is indicated for any condition that results in failure of the heart to initiate or conduct an intrinsic electrical impulse at a rate normally adequate to maintain body perfusion. It may be used prophylactically when certain arrhythmias or conduction defects warn of such failure. Cardiac pacing may also be used to interrupt tachyarrhythmias that are unresponsive to other forms of therapy.

Bradyarrhythmias that may preclude adequate cardiac output include symptomatic sinus bradycardia, sinus arrest, sick sinus syndrome, and symptomatic second and third degree heart blocks. One must evaluate the effect on the patient and the underlying cause of each of these rhythms when considering artificial pacing as a mode of therapy or when considering the need for permanent pacing.

Heart Block. Mobitz I (Wenckebach) second degree block following inferior myocardial infarction is most often asymptomatic and transient and usually does not require pacing. Mobitz II second degree block resulting from anterior myocardial infarction is a much less stable rhythm. It may result in sudden third degree block with a slow ventricular rhythm or even ventricular standstill, and it usually requires pacing. Bifascicular block (right bundle branch block with hemiblock of the left bundle branch) following anterior myocardial infarction is considered an indication for pacing by many physicians because this can also result in symptomatic third degree block or ventricular standstill.

Third degree (complete) block may or may not be an indication for pacing, depending on the anatomic site of the block. Complete block in the atrioventricular (AV) node usually results in a junctional escape rhythm with an adequate heart rate. It is usually transient and does not require pacing. Complete block at the level of the bundle branches, however, requires an escape focus in the Purkinje fibers to stimulate the ventricles. If such a focus arises, it will usually depolarize the ventricles at a rate that is too slow to provide adequate cardiac output, and the patient will require artificial pacing.

Sick Sinus Syndrome. This is often manifested by alternating tachycardia and bradycardia (tachy-brady syndrome). It requires artificial pacing for the bradycardia and suppressive antiarrhythmic therapy to control the tachyarrhythmia.

Persistent Ventricular Tachycardia. This condition is sometimes successfully suppressed by overdriving with an artificial pacemaker. Pacing is used

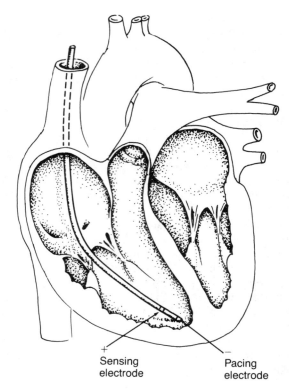

Sensing
electrode

Pacing
electrode

FIGURE 9-5
Transvenous pacing catheter in place.

FIGURE 9-4
Screw-in type electrode for permanent epicardial pacing.

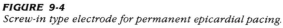

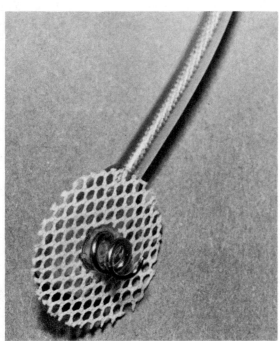

occasionally to suppress supraventricular tachyarrhythmias.

Rapid atrial pacing may be used to induce atrial fibrillation in the patient whose chronic atrial fibrillation has been converted to sinus rhythm with inadequate rate. Recently, pacing has been used successfully to prevent symptoms of severe bradycardia due to vagal reaction or hypersensitive carotid body.

The critical care nurse should anticipate any of the aforementioned arrhythmias in patients who have atherosclerotic heart disease, acute myocardial infarction, or digitalis toxicity. Myocardial fibrosis and cardiomyopathies may cause these arrhythmias; occasionally, heart block may be of congenital origin.

METHODS OF PACING

Various methods of pacing have been used over the years, including external pacing, transthoracic pacing, epicardial pacing, and endocardial pacing.

External Pacing. This method involves pacing electrodes on the chest wall and requires large amounts of electrical energy. It is used only in severe emergencies for the unconscious patient. It has been abandoned for

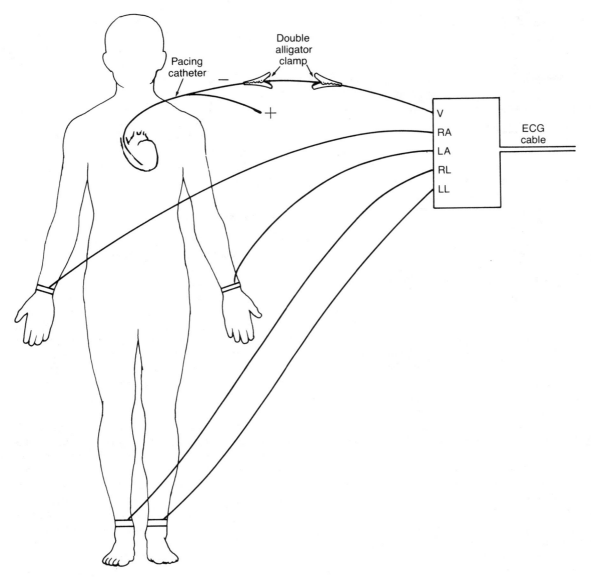

FIGURE 9-6
Set-up for using the distal (negative) pacing electrode as an "exploring" electrode during transvenous pacemaker catheter placement.

use in the conscious patient because of the severe pain and burns associated with this method.

Transthoracic Pacing. This type of pacing is occasionally used in emergency situations, but it is not suitable for long-term pacing or as prophylaxis against warning arrhythmias. This method involves introduction of a pacing wire into the heart through a needle in the anterior chest wall.

Epicardial Pacing. This method can be accomplished via thoracotomy (or occasionally through a subxyphoid incision) and the placement of pacing electrodes directly on the surface of the heart. It is often used as a temporary adjunct during and after heart surgery. The pacing wires are sutured to the epicardial surface of the heart, brought outside through the chest incision, and connected to a temporary pacemaker generator. The wires may be removed without reopening the incision after scar tissue has formed over the tips. Permanently implanted epicardial pacemakers are used in patients in whom thoracotomy is warranted, either for surgery or for the specific purpose of pacemaker implantation. Many physicians prefer to use the "screw-in" type electrodes, the tips of which can be rotated into the epicardium (Fig. 9-4).

The main advantage of epicardial pacing is the stability of the electrodes. They have a very low incidence of displacement.

Endocardial Pacing. This method, which involves a transvenous pacing catheter, is the most common type of pacing. It can be used for either temporary or permanent pacing. For temporary pacing, the catheter is introduced into a superficial vein with use of local anesthesia. The brachial, femoral, external jugular, or subclavian veins may be used. The subclavian site affords catheter stability and allows for patient mobility; however, pneumothorax may occur as a complication of catheter insertion. The femoral vein affords easy access, but use of this site markedly reduces patient mobility.

The pacing catheter is threaded through the vein, the vena cava, the right atrium, and into the right ventricle. It is lodged between the trabeculae and placed in contact with the endocardial surface of the right ventricle (Fig. 9-5). The insertion procedure may be done under fluoroscopy. An alternate guide for positioning the catheter is to attach the "V" lead of the ECG machine to the negative (pacing, distal) electrode on the catheter with an alligator clamp (Fig. 9-6). The distal catheter electrode becomes an "exploring" ECG electrode, and catheter position can be determined by analysis of ECG complex changes as the catheter is advanced. The ECG will reveal a current of injury pattern when the tip of the catheter touches the endocardium.

The experienced clinician can often accomplish "blind" insertion, utilizing only the standard ECG monitor to indicate successful pacing. Many physicians prefer to use the balloon-tipped flow-directed pacing catheter to facilitate insertion. The balloon is inflated with air in the vena cava and carries the catheter in the direction of blood flow through the right atrium, the tricuspid valve, and into the right ventricle. The balloon is then deflated and lodged against the right ventricular wall.

Some physicians place the tip of the catheter in the pulmonary outflow tract when the right ventricle is enlarged. Because the heart size often decreases after the initiation of effective pacing, this position reduces the risk of perforation of the ventricle relative to positioning in the ventricular apex.

CLASSIFICATION OF PACEMAKERS
Functional Capabilities of Pacemakers

For many years pacemaker usage has been limited to fixed-rate (asynchronous) and demand (synchronous) pacing of the ventricles. The advent of the successful use of AV sequential pacemakers and increased pacemaker programmability has greatly broadened the functional capabilities of pacemakers currently in use. The Inter-Society Commission for Heart Disease Resources (ICHD) developed a code for differentiation of the various functional capabilities of pacemakers (Table 9-2). Although this code has been in existence since 1974, it has only recently come into common usage. The three-letter ICHD code includes the paced chamber or chambers, the sensing chamber or chambers, and the mode of response to sensed electrical impulses (inhibited or triggered).

Pacemaker Pulse Generators

There are four classes of pacemaker pulse generators: temporary, permanent, fixed-rate, and demand.

Temporary Generators. These are used for short-term pacing. The proximal ends of the pacing catheter are attached to the generator, and the generator is secured to the patient, usually on the arm or abdomen. Once the catheter has been connected to the generator, the nurse must hold the generator until it has been secured to the patient. This will prevent the generator (and the catheter) from being dropped inadvertently to the floor.

Permanent Generators. As shown in Figure 9-7, permanent generators are implanted within the patient, usually in the pectoralis major muscle or overlying the abdomen. The catheter is placed by way of a central vein, and the pacing electrodes are connected subcutaneously to the implanted generator. If the electrodes remain functional at the time of generator battery failure, the electrodes are left intact and only the generator is replaced.

Presently, most permanent pulse generators are powered by lithium batteries that have an expected power life of 7 to 12 years. Although the generators now in use are much smaller than those used a few years ago, researchers are continuing their efforts to

TABLE 9-2
THE INTER-SOCIETY COMMISSION FOR HEART DISEASE RESOURCES (ICHD) CODE FOR DIFFERENTIATION OF PACEMAKER FUNCTIONAL CAPABILITIES

Paced Chamber	Sensing Chamber	Response to Sensing
V = Ventricle	V = Ventricle	I = Inhibited
A = Atrium	A = Atrium	T = Triggered
D = Dual chambers	D = Dual	D = Dual
	0 = None	0 = None

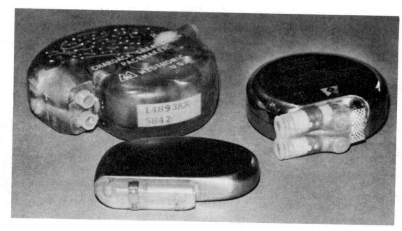

FIGURE 9-7
Permanent pulse generators, old and new. Note the decrease in size and weight that has been achieved over the years.

increase the effective life span and decrease the size of permanent generators.

Fixed-Rate (Asynchronous) Pacemakers. These pacemakers discharge an electrical stimulus at a preset interval and function independently of any other electrical activity in the heart. The VOO pacemaker discharges an electrical stimulus into the ventricle at a preset rate without sensing any other electrical activity. This mode of pacing is used only for patients who are entirely pacemaker-dependent (no spontaneous supraventricular impulses reach the ventricles) and free from ventricular depolarization by ectopic beats. If any spontaneous beats are conducted through the ventricles, there is danger of the asynchronous pacemaker initiating a stimulus during the vulnerable period (downstroke) of the T wave and precipitating dangerous ventricular arrhythmias.

The AOO pacemaker discharges an electrical stimulus into the atrium at a preset rate without sensing other electrical activity. This mode of pacing is limited to the patient who has inadequate function of the sinus node and normal conduction through the AV node.

The DOO pacemaker paces both the atrium and the ventricle at a preset rate and with a preset delay interval between atrial and ventricular pacing. This mode of pacing may be used for the patient with inadequate function of the sinus node, inadequate AV conduction, and absence of ectopic beats.

Demand (Synchronous) Pacemakers. These pacemakers initiate an impulse only when a preset R–R interval has elapsed without any spontaneous electrical activation of the ventricle. This escape interval is determined by the rate at which the pacemaker is set; that is, if the rate is set at 60 beats per minute, the escape interval is 1 second. The VVI pacemaker senses and is inhibited by ventricular depolarization. This ability to sense depolarization allows spontaneous

ventricular beats to occur without interference from the pacemaker and obviates the risk of pacemaker discharge on the T wave (if the unit is functioning properly). If the patient is entirely pacemaker-dependent, discharge will occur regularly at the preset escape interval. If the patient's spontaneous R–R intervals are shorter than the escape interval of the pacemaker, pacemaker activity is suppressed (Fig. 9-8).

Occasionally, the demand pacemaker will sense high amplitude ventricular repolarizations in addition to depolarizations, thus resetting the escape interval from the T wave on the ECG instead of the QRS (Fig. 9-9). This situation is not dangerous but results in a pacing rate that is slower than that indicated by the rate setting on the generator. Proper function can be attained by decreasing the sensitivity of the pacemaker until only depolarization is sensed.

Some pacemakers allow for a longer escape interval after a sensed spontaneous beat than the escape interval between subsequent paced beats. This lengthened escape interval, called *rate hysteresis,* provides more opportunity for normal conduction of spontaneous impulses and results in less competition between intrinsic and paced rhythms.

The atrial demand pacemaker (AAI) has a single pacemaker wire in the atrium with pacing and sensing electrodes. It senses and is inhibited by spontaneous atrial electrical impulses and may be used in the patient who has an inadequate sinus rate with normal AV conduction.

Variations. Temporary pacemakers can be operated in either the demand or fixed-rate mode. They can be made to discharge at a fixed rate by turning the sensing mechanism off. One can convert permanent demand pacemakers to fixed-rate pacemakers by applying a specially manufactured magnet over the implanted generator to turn off the sensing mechanism. This procedure can be used to assess the discharge and capture

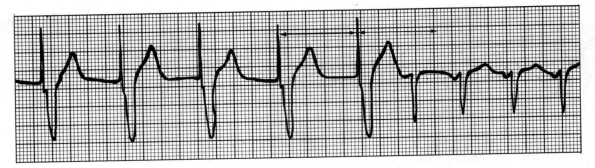

FIGURE 9-8
Demand pacing. Pacemaker is inhibited by each spontaneous beat that appears at a shorter interval than that indicated on the pacemaker rate settings.

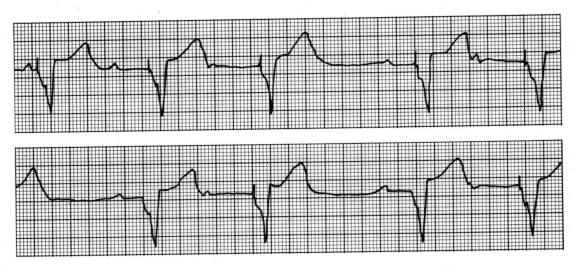

FIGURE 9-9
Ventricular-inhibited pacemaker sensing T waves.

capabilities of the demand pacemaker (ventricular depolarization by the pacemaker stimulus) that are being inhibited by a spontaneous rhythm.

Many of the newer, permanently implanted pacemakers can be externally programmed. By using a special programmer, one can accomplish changes in rate, energy output, sensitivity, mode, refractory period (period after the QRS during which the pacemaker cannot discharge an impulse), and hysteresis.

Pacemakers with Dual Chamber Leads

AV sequential pacemakers can initiate electrical impulses sequentially in the atria and in the ventricles (Fig. 9-10). Because atrial contraction contributes 15% to 20% to ventricular stroke volume, patients who have low cardiac reserve will develop hypotension or congestive heart failure without this "atrial kick." When a

ventricular pacemaker is used, either AV dissociation or retrograde atrial conduction results (Fig. 9-11). In either case, the atria and ventricles do not contract in proper sequence, and atrial kick is lost.

The AV sequential pacemaker has come into more common usage with the advent of the tined and J-shaped atrial pacing lead. This catheter has been found to be less easily displaced than those previously available (Fig. 9-12).

The DVI sequential pacemaker has both atrial and ventricular pacing electrodes that pace both chambers in sequence with a preset delay interval (Fig. 9-13). Both atrial and ventricular impulse discharges are reset by *ventricular* stimuli. The atrial electrode does *not* sense P waves (Fig. 9-14). It resets its timing from the QRS and stimulates the atria at the preset escape interval after the last QRS. The ventricular electrode senses the same QRS and stimulates the ventricles at

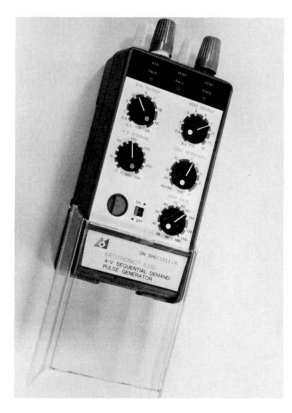

FIGURE 9-10
AV sequential temporary pulse generator.

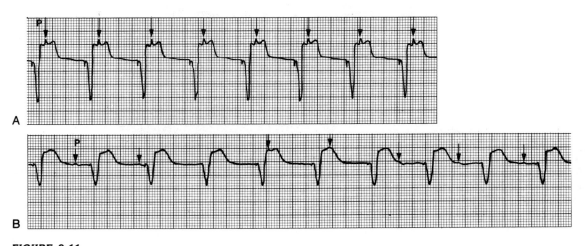

FIGURE 9-11
(A) *Pacing with retrograde conduction. Each pacemaker stimulus is conducted retrograde through the atria as well as antegrade through the ventricles. Retrograde atrial conduction produces a P wave after each paced QRS.* (B) *Pacing with AV dissociation. P waves are dissociated from paced QRSs, indicating that pacemaker stimulus is not conducted retrograde to atria.*

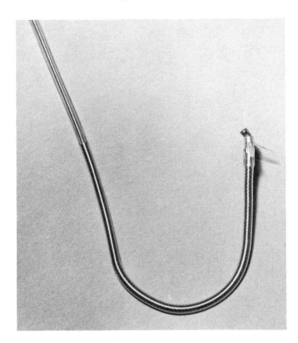

FIGURE 9-12
J-shaped, tined transvenous atrial pacing lead.

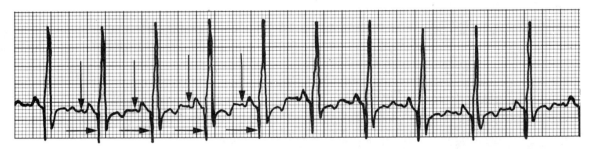

FIGURE 9-13
AV sequential pacemaker stimulating both the atria and the ventricles. Ventrical arrows
indicate atrial pacing spikes; horizontal arrows indicate ventricular pacing spikes.

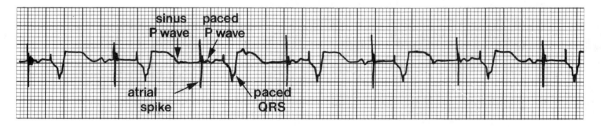

FIGURE 9-14
AV sequential (DVI) pacemaker. Because pacemaker does not sense spontaneous atrial
activity, sinus P waves may be found that are unrelated to pacemaker activity. Lack of paced
P waves in complexes 2, 5, and 7 results from atrial pacemaker discharging during the atrial
refractory period following sinus P waves.

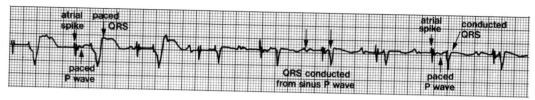

FIGURE 9-15
AV sequential (DVI) pacemaker with QRSs resulting from ventricular pacing, from conduction of sinus impulse, and from conduction of paced P waves.

an escape interval equal to the atrial escape interval plus the preset AV delay interval.

If the atrial impulse is conducted to the ventricles before the AV delay interval has elapsed, the ventricular electrode will sense this impulse and will be inhibited (Fig. 9-15). These mechanisms allow each ventricular contraction to be preceded by atrial contraction, thus approximating a normal hemodynamic situation.

The VAT pacemaker has an atrial lead that senses atrial impulses and triggers the ventricular pacing lead to stimulate the ventricle at a preset delay interval. Because ventricular pacing depends on spontaneous atrial impulses, the ventricular pacing rate varies with the patient's intrinsic sinus rate and the physiologic needs of the body. If spontaneous atrial activity fails, the pacemaker will function as a fixed rate ventricular (VOO) pacemaker. Ventricular ectopic beats and normally conducted ventricular beats are not sensed by the ventricular pacing lead, and there is risk of the pacemaker firing into the T waves of these intrinsic beats. This pacemaker should therefore be used only in the presence of permanent complete heart block without ventricular ectopic beats.

The VDD pacemaker has a pacing lead in the ventricle with sensing leads in both the atrium and the ventricle. The atrial lead senses intrinsic atrial activity and triggers ventricular pacing at a preset delay interval. If a supraventricular conducted impulse or ventricular ectopic beat occurs, the ventricular lead senses this intrinsic beat and is inhibited. This pacemaker can be programmed to pace the ventricles between limited high and low rates if atrial activity is faster than the preset high rate or slower than the preset low rate. This pacemaker is used for the patient who has normal sinus node function and complete AV block.

The DDD pacemaker is referred to as the universal pacemaker and is gaining in usage because of the multiplicity of functions it offers. This pacemaker has sensing and pacing electrodes in both the atrium and the ventricle. It functions as a combined VDD and DVI pacemaker. When intrinsic atrial activity occurs at a rate within the programmed upper and lower rate limits, ventricular pacing is triggered. When intrinsic atrial activity falls below the preset low rate, the atrium is paced. If the paced atrial impulse is not conducted to the ventricle before the preset delay interval has been reached, the ventricle is paced. Ventricular pacing is inhibited by conducted supraventricular beats and ectopic beats.

OVERDRIVE AND UNDERDRIVE PACING

Occasionally, pacing is used to interrupt tachyarrhythmias that are unresponsive to other forms of therapy. These arrhythmias may be of either ventricular or supraventricular origin. A temporary transvenous pacemaker catheter electrode is placed in the chamber of arrhythmia origin. Because most supraventricular tachycardias are of the reentry type, a pacemaker stimulus is initiated at such time as to render the reentry circuit refractory, thus interrupting completion of the circuit and terminating the arrhythmia.

The same principle can be applied to reentrant ventricular tachycardias. One may accomplish overdrive pacing by increasing the pacing rate until pacemaker capture occurs during the nonrefractory period between spontaneous beats. Once the ectopic focus has been suppressed, the pacing rate can usually be decreased gradually, and the pacing stimulus will continue to maintain control of the ventricles.

When overdrive pacing fails to terminate the ventricular arrhythmia, underdrive pacing may be attempted. The pacing rate is set at less than the ectopic discharge rate in an attempt to accomplish ventricular capture by the pacing stimulus.

The most common cause of ventricular tachyarrhythmias is acute myocardial infarction. Usually, the ectopic focus will be inherently suppressed at some point after the infarct has begun to heal. The pacemaker is then no longer needed and can be removed.

TYPES OF PACING CATHETERS

A pacing catheter is either unipolar or bipolar, having *within* it one electrode or two, respectively. All electrical circuits must have two electrodes to complete the

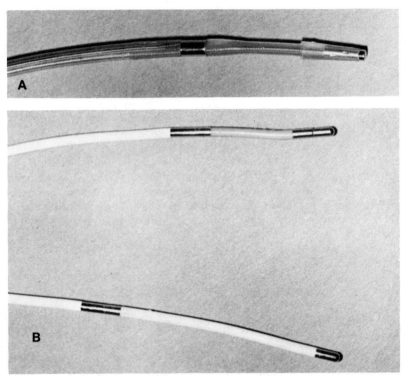

FIGURE 9-16
(A) *Permanent bipolar pacing catheter.* (B)
Temporary bipolar pacing catheters.

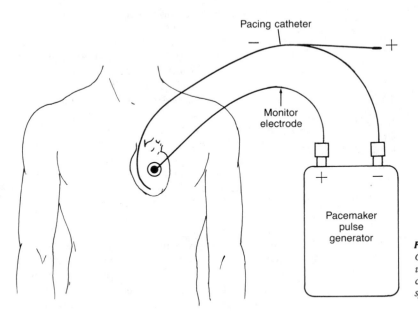

FIGURE 9-17
*Conversion of bipolar pacing system to
unipolar. The monitoring electrode on anterior
chest is used as positive pole in pacemaker
system.*

circuit. The unipolar catheter requires a second electrode outside the catheter itself.

The *bipolar catheter* has a negative pacing electrode
at the tip and a positive sensing electrode about one
centimeter proximal to the tip (Fig. 9-16). Virtually all
temporary pacemakers utilize bipolar catheters. The
negative distal electrode should be attached to the
negative terminal on the generator, and the positive
proximal electrode should be attached to the positive
terminal. Occasionally, improper sensing can be corrected by reversing the attachment of the catheter tips
at the generator terminals (reversed polarity). When

reversing the polarity of a bipolar catheter does not correct faulty sensing, conversion to a unipolar system may solve the problem. This is accomplished by disconnecting the bipolar positive electrode from the generator and replacing it with the wire from a monitoring electrode on the anterior chest (Fig. 9-17). When the chest electrode is used as part of the pacing system, it should be labeled as such so that it will not be confused with other chest electrodes that are being used for monitoring cardiac rhythm.

The *unipolar catheter* has only a negative pacing electrode at its tip. The positive pole is outside the catheter itself. In permanent pacing, the generator case is the positive pole. The majority of permanent pacemakers use the unipolar catheter.

PACING AND SENSING THRESHOLDS

The pacing electrodes should be positioned so that the generator can be set at a relatively small amount of electrical energy and low degree of sensitivity and still allow successful pacing.

The lowest level of electrical energy that is required to initiate consistent ventricular capture at the pacing electrode site is called the *pacing threshold*. This threshold level is determined after successful pacing has been established by decreasing the energy output of the generator until capture ceases, then increasing output until capture is regained. The threshold is expressed as milliamperes (MA) at this level. The generator output is then set at several MA above threshold to allow for the usual increase in threshold level that occurs over a period of a few days after pacing has been initiated. Hypokalemia may cause an increase in pacing threshold, as do β-adrenergic and mineralocorticoid drugs.

Sensing threshold is determined for permanent pacemakers. The amplitude of the intrinsic depolarization wave at the site of the sensing electrode is measured. If the amplitude is insufficient to ensure sensing, the pacing electrode is repositioned.

COMPLICATIONS OF PACING

Failure of proper function in the demand pacemaker can be determined on the cardiac monitor or ECG. The pacemaker may malfunction because of failure to discharge a stimulus, failure to capture the ventricles, or failure to sense intrinsic depolarizations.

Because stimulus discharge from the pacemaker

FIGURE 9-18
VVI pacemaker. Failure to discharge is indicated by lack of pacemaker spikes at appropriate intervals.

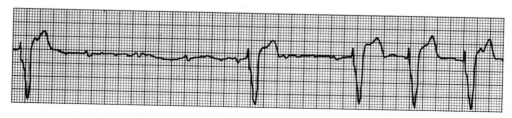

FIGURE 9-19
Ventricular demand pacemaker. Lack of QRS following each pacemaker spike indicates failure to capture. Complexes 1, 3, 4, and 5 result from a spontaneous ventricular escape focus.

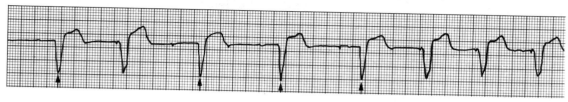

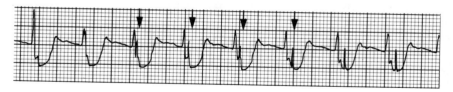

FIGURE 9-20
Ventricular demand pacemaker. Failure to sense is indicated by pacemaker spikes at inappropriate intervals following spontaneous QRSs.

causes an artifact, or "spike," to appear on the ECG, *failure to discharge* results in absence of the artifact (Fig. 9-18). This failure may be within the generator itself (either mechanism or battery failure), at the site of lead attachment to the generator, or within the lead due to fracture of wires. When failure occurs in the temporary pacemaker, check the connections at the generator terminals, replace the batteries in the generator, or replace the generator. If these efforts do not solve the problem, it must be assumed that wire fracture is the culprit. If only one wire is fractured, conversion to a unipolar system, with a chest electrode to replace the fractured wire, will provide successful pacing. When the permanent pacemaker fails to discharge a stimulus, the problem must be solved operatively. If the situation is emergent, the physician may insert a temporary transvenous pacemaker to support the patient hemodynamically until the permanent pacemaker problem can be corrected.

Failure of the pacing stimulus to capture the ventricles will be noted by the absence of the QRS immediately following the pacemaker artifact on the ECG (Fig. 9-19). If the pacing threshold has increased, the MA may need to be increased until ventricular capture occurs. Displacement of the pacing electrode may cause failure to capture. It is sometimes possible to regain capture by repositioning the patient, often in the left lateral decubitus position, until the electrode can be repositioned.

Battery failure can also cause failure to capture. If the patient is pacemaker-dependent and becomes symptomatic, drug therapy (atropine, isoproterenol) and cardiopulmonary resuscitation may be required until the cause of the problem is found and corrected.

Failure of the pacemaker to sense spontaneous beats results in inappropriately placed pacemaker artifacts on the ECG (Fig. 9-20). This may be caused by improper electrode placement, battery or component failure, or lead wire fracture. Ventricular arrhythmias caused by occurrence of the pacemaker stimulus during the vulnerable phase of the T wave are most likely to occur in the patient who has an acute cardiac disease process, electrolyte imbalance, or drug toxicity but are seldom seen in the patient who is hospitalized for battery replacement rather than acute illness. The most likely cause for sensing failure in the temporary pacemaker is electrode displacement. If nonsensing renders the pacemaker totally ineffective, it may be advantageous to turn the pacemaker off until the electrode can be repositioned.

Failure of proper function in pacemakers with dual leads is not as easily detected on the ECG as in the single lead pacemakers. The nurse must know the functional capabilities and the parameters that have been programmed into the particular pacemaker in use. The ECG strip can then be examined with consid-

eration of programmed parameters for each pacemaker function. One must examine each electrical event, both paced and intrinsic, in relation to the preceding electrical event in order to determine whether pacing, sensing and inhibition, or triggering are occurring, and whether they are occurring at the appropriate programmed intervals.

Ventricular irritability at the site of the endocardial catheter tip is a frequent occurrence after initial catheter insertion. The premature ventricular complexes usually appear similar in configuration to the pacemaker complexes (Figs. 9-21 and 9-22). Irritability from the catheter as a foreign body usually disappears after 2 or 3 days.

Perforation of the ventricular wall or septum by the transvenous catheter occurs in a small number of patients. This may or may not result in noncapture. It can be suspected on cardiac monitoring if the patient is monitored in a modified V_1 lead. Right ventricular pacing should provide a negative QRS in this lead. Often ventricular perforation results in pacing from the left ventricle, and the QRS becomes positive in polarity. Pericardial tamponade, causing a decrease in blood pressure and increase in sinus node discharge rate, must be watched for after ventricular wall perforation.

Tamponade occurs infrequently because of the ability of myocardial fibers to regain their integrity after the catheter has been pulled back into the ventricle; however, anticoagulation therapy should be discontinued after perforation.

Retrograde migration of the right ventricular pacing catheter into the right atrium may result in atrial pacing (pacing artifact followed by P wave) or inhibition of the pacemaker by atrial depolarizations. The effects on the patient depend on the ability of the AV node to conduct atrial impulses and on the ability of a lower escape focus to emerge at an adequate rate.

Abdominal twitching or hiccoughs occur occasionally as a result of electrode placement against a thin right ventricular wall and resultant electrical stimulation of the abdominal muscles or diaphragm. This is usually very uncomfortable for the patient, and the electrode should be repositioned as soon as possible.

Infection and phlebitis can occur at the temporary pacemaker insertion site, and infection or *hematoma* may occur at the site of permanent generator implantation. These sites must be inspected for swelling and inflammation and kept dry. Sterile technique must be used when dressings are being changed.

Migration of the permanent generator from its initial site of implantation may occur in patients who have very loose connective tissue. This may or may not require reimplantation. *Erosion* at the implantation site occurs rarely.

Defibrillation of the patient while the temporary pacemaker system is intact may affect various compo-

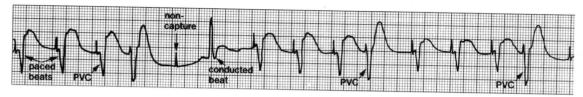

FIGURE 9-21
Ventricular demand pacemaker with PVCs. This strip also shows one noncaptured pacemaker spike followed by a spontaneous conducted beat.

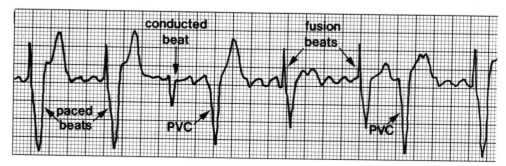

FIGURE 9-22
Ventricular demand pacemaker with PVCs and with fusion beats that result from ventricular depolarization by both the pacemaker and a spontaneous beat.

nents of the generator and cause it to malfunction. The temporary generator should be turned off *and* the catheter wires disconnected from the generator if at all possible before defibrillating.

A number of other pacemaker innovations are currently under investigation. These include a steroid-tipped pacing catheter that should reduce the fibrosis of tissue around the catheter tip. Pacemakers with built-in defibrillation capabilities are being studied, as are pacemakers capable of cardioversion of recognized bursts of tachycardia.

Swan-Ganz catheters with pacing electrodes at various intervals along the catheter for AV sequential pacing are now being studied. If successful, they would obviate the need for a separate pacing catheter for the patient who also needs hemodynamic pressure monitoring.

PACEMAKER SAFETY

Electrical safety precautions must be observed when the patient has a temporary pacemaker. Electrical equipment in the room should be kept at a minimum and must be properly grounded. Use of a nonelectric bed is preferable. If an electric bed is used, it should remain disconnected from AC current. A tap bell should be provided for the patient, and the electric call

light should be disconnected. Only battery-operated electric shavers, toothbrushes, or radios may be used. An AC-powered television may be used if it is operated by someone who is not in contact with the patient. The nurse should avoid simultaneous contact with the patient and any electrical equipment. The patient's bed must be kept dry at all times. Diathermy and electrocautery equipment should not be used because their waves may be sensed by and inhibit the demand pacemaker.

If an older model temporary pacemaker generator with exposed metal catheter tips or terminals is in use, these metal parts must be insulated. A rubber glove can be cut and taped over the exposed metal to provide insulation from external current sources.

The plastic cover supplied with the temporary generator must be kept in place over the dials to prevent inadvertant change in settings. The generator should be securely attached to the patient's arm or abdomen. The catheter should be securely taped to the patient's skin without direct tension on the catheter. Motion of the extremity nearest the catheter entry site should be minimized, especially if the femoral site has been used.

According to manufacturers of permanent pacemaker generators, there are very few electrical hazards associated with the permanent generators currently in use. These generators are shielded from external elec-

Teaching the Patient with a Pacemaker

1. KNOWLEDGE OF CONDITION

- Elicit the patient's previous knowledge of pacemakers and clarify any misconceptions.
- If appropriate, clarify the difference between heart block and heart attack. (A patient may confuse cardiac monitoring with pacing and become very anxious when the monitoring electrodes are removed.)
- Don't assume *anything* about the patient's understanding.
- The anatomy of the heart should be discussed in general terms when explaining the need for pacing and how the pacemaker takes the place of or complements spontaneous rhythm.
- The difference between temporary and permanent pacing should also be discussed.

2. PATIENT ACTIVITY

- Passive and active range of motion exercises should be started on the affected arm 48 hours after pacemaker implantation in the pectoralis major muscle to avoid "frozen shoulder."
- The patient should be instructed to repeat these exercises several times daily until the implantation site is completely free of discomfort through all ranges of arm motion.
- Explain that the pacemaker is relatively sturdy and that touching or bathing the implantation site will not damage it.
- The patient's activities of daily living and recreational activities should be discussed *before* permanent pacing to ascertain an appropriate site for implantation; for example, the right pectoralis muscle should not be used in the right-handed rifle hunter.
- Abdominal implantation may be preferable for the avid swimmer because of the strenuous arm activity.
- Activities that may result in high impact or stress at the implantation site should be avoided. This includes all contact sports.
- Instruct the patient to report any activity that may have damaged his pacemaker.
- The patient can return to work at the discretion of his physician.
- Discuss the type of work he will do and what his job entails. He may return to whatever degree of sexual activity he wants or tolerates.
- The patient should be aware that his pacemaker may set off the alarm on metal-detector devices in airports.

3. SIGNS OF PACEMAKER MALFUNCTION

- The symptoms of pacemaker malfunction are those associated with decreased perfusion of the brain, heart, or skeletal muscles.
- The patient should be instructed to report any dizzi-

ness, fainting, chest pain, shortness of breath, undue fatigue, or fluid retention.
- Fluid retention should be described in terms of sudden weight gain, "puffy ankles," "tightness of rings," and so forth.
- Patient should be instructed to take his pulse once daily upon awakening. He should report a pulse rate that is more than 5 beats per minute slower than that at which his pacemaker is set.
- Patient should be aware that his pulse may be somewhat irregular if he has a demand pacemaker and has some spontaneous beats as well as paced beats. It must be stressed that this does not signify pacemaker malfunction.

4. SIGNS OF INFECTION

- The patient should report any redness, swelling, drainage, or increase in soreness at the implantation site.

5. PULSE GENERATOR REPLACEMENT

- Instruct the patient regarding the expected life of his pacemaker battery.
- He should know that generator replacement requires hospitalization for about 3 days and that usually only the generator will need to be replaced.

6. MEDICATIONS

- The patient should be instructed regarding any medication he will be taking at home.
- He should know the name of the medication, as well as the dose, frequency of administration, side effects, and use of each medication.

7. SAFETY MEASURES

- The patient should inform any physician or dentist by whom he is seen of his pacemaker and of the medications that he is taking.
- He should carry a pacemaker identification card with him at all times. This card shows the brand and model of his pacemaker, the date of insertion, and the rate at which it is set.
- It is also advisable to wear a medical alert bracelet or necklace stating that he has a pacemaker.

8. FOLLOW-UP CARE

- The importance of physician or clinic follow-up visits should be stressed.
- The follow-up visit will include an interval history and physical examination and a 12-lead ECG.
- Many pacemaker clinics have specialized equipment available to measure the rate, amplitude, duration, and contours of the pacemaker artifact. This information is very helpful in predicting battery depletion. Some clinics have the capability for obtaining this information by telephone, reducing the necessity for travel to the clinic.

trical sources and are not affected by microwave ovens or small appliances. There have been rare reports of unipolar pacemakers being affected by large electromagnetic fields, such as radio transmitters. Defibrillator paddles should not be placed directly over or adjacent to the implanted generator.

PATIENT TEACHING

A planned and systematic approach to teaching the patient to live with his pacemaker is a vital part of nursing care. A helpful tool in patient teaching is a progress report accessible to the physician and other members of the team, along with written guidelines for the nurse who is instructing the patient. The patient's family should also be involved in the learning process.

Patient teaching relative to pacemakers begins at the time the decision for pacemaker insertion is made. The patient and his family should be told why the pacemaker is necessary. The insertion procedure should be explained, as well as the immediate postinsertion care that can be expected.

Many booklets and media presentations are available to aid the nurse in teaching the pacemaker patient. It is helpful to have written guidelines for the patient to review after discharge from the hospital.

The depth of teaching that is appropriate and the teaching tools used depend on such variables as the patient's age, intellect, attention span, vision, and interest in learning. An occasional patient will demonstrate difficulty in accepting the prospect of living with a pacemaker. His initial teaching should be confined to the positive aspects of life with a pacemaker. Knowledge of the function and care of the pacemaker are of no interest to him until he is able to accept it as part of his life. Many misconceptions can be negated by asking the patient what he knows or has heard previously about pacemakers and if he has any preconceived expectations relative to his pacemaker.

The teaching areas listed in the accompanying chart should be covered with the patient during the course of his hospitalization.

The nurse who cares for the patient with an artificial pacemaker must have thorough knowledge of the heart, the pacemaker, and the patient as a person. This knowledge must be applied continuously from the time the decision for pacemaker insertion is made until the patient is discharged from the hospital and sometimes beyond, to follow-up care. The nurse plays a vital role in assuring successful pacing and in reassuring the patient, whose well-being depends on successful pacing. Caring for the pacemaker patient is a challenging but most rewarding experience when the nurse is secure in her knowledge of the subject.

BIBLIOGRAPHY

Bognolo D et al: Atrial and atrioventricular sequential pacing rationale and clinical experience. J Fla Med Assoc 66:1028–1033, 1979

Dreifus L, Ohm O, Pennock R et al: Long-term monitoring of patients with implanted pacemakers. Heart Lung 11:417–421, 1982

Hyman AL: Permanent programmable pacemakers in the management of recurrent tachycardias. Pace 2:28–39, 1979

Kruse I, Arman K, Conradson TB, Ryden L: A comparison of the acute and long-term hemodynamic effects of ventricular inhibited and atrial synchronous ventricular inhibited pacing. Circulation 65:846–855, 1982

Lasche P: Permanent cardiac pacing technology and follow-up. Focus on Critical Care 10:28–36, 1983

Mansour KA et al: Further evaluation of the sutureless, screw-in electrode for cardiac pacing. J Thorac Cardiovasc Surg 77, No. 6:858–862, 1979

Parsonnet V et al: Transvenous insertion of double sets of permanent electrodes. JAMA 243, No. 1:62–64, 1980

Parsonnet V, Rodger T: The present status of programmable pacemakers. Prog Cardiovasc Dis 23:401–420, 1981

Satler L, Shepard R: New trends in permanent cardiac pacing. Ala J Med Sci 20:192–202, 1983

Sutton R, Citron P: Electrophysiological and hemodynamic basis for application of new pacemaker technology in sick sinus syndrome and atrioventricular block. Br Heart J 41, No. 5:600–612, 1979

Yashar JJ et al: Atrioventricular sequential pacemakers: Indications, complications, and long-term follow-up. Ann Thorac Surg 29, No. 1:91–98, 1980

Cardiopulmonary Resuscitation

Lane D. Craddock

DEFINITIONS

Because of the dual nature of resuscitation—that is, availability (ventilation) and transport (circulation) of oxygen—the more appropriate term is *cardiopulmonary resuscitation (CPR)*.

Cardiac arrest is the abrupt cessation of effective cardiac pumping activity resulting in cessation of circulation. There are only two types of cardiac arrest: cardiac standstill (asystole) and ventricular fibrillation (plus other forms of ineffective ventricular contraction, such as ventricular flutter and rarely ventricular tachycardia). The condition referred to as "profound cardiovascular collapse" will not be specifically included because its recognition and definition are nebulous and management less specific. One form, referred to as *cardiogenic shock,* is included in Chapters 10 and 11.

Resuscitation, liberally interpreted, is the restoration of vital signs by mechanical, physiological, and pharmacological means.

The application of cardiopulmonary resuscitation is made possible by the concept of clinical versus biological death.

Clinical death is defined as the absence of the vital signs, and *biological death* refers to irreversible cellular changes. As determined both experimentally and clinically, the interval between clinical and biological death is approximately 4 minutes.

WHO SHOULD BE RESUSCITATED

It is easier to determine who should *not* be resuscitated than who should be resuscitated. People who should not be resuscitated include those with known terminal illness and those who have been clinically dead for longer than 5 minutes. Both represent situations in which resuscitation would likely prove impossible and survival would be meaningless.

All others should be regarded as candidates for resuscitation. *Remember* that resuscitation can always be abandoned, but it cannot be instituted after undue delay.

One additional point is that the term *the very elderly* is often used to differentiate likely degrees of vitality and therefore of survival probability. On the surface, this is perhaps reasonable, but age alone should rarely, if ever, determine treatment. Bear in mind that, regardless of chronologic age, a person who is alert and able to carry on any sort of thoughtful conversation is a candidate for resuscitation.

"DO NOT RESUSCITATE" (DNR)

There has been much debate about the application of costly technology to prolong life; this use of all available methods in support of a patient's viability is not only reasonable but inevitable because it represents the natural progression of medical care as a dedicated scientific effort. Society is addressing the issue from a very important aspect: cost. It is also asserting its personal rights in various ways (*e.g.,* instituting living wills and insisting on the "right to be informed"). These are pertinent issues and will be the subjects of much debate, and they will perhaps result in hard choices in the near future. Many hospitals throughout the United States have active bioethics groups who grapple with these problems. None of this, however, alters the application of major efforts in support of a critically ill patient, including CPR, because it clearly cannot. It has, however, stimulated a more structured approach to patients who are considered to be inappropriate candidates for CPR. The present approach in many hospitals is to designate such patients as DNR after full discourse with family or responsible persons and to record such information in clear terms on the hospital record. From the beginning, this should always include the nursing personnel because they frequently have much to offer about the patient's attitude and the family's feelings. To leave them out is usually a bad mistake.

This situation should not be thought of as an encroachment into our domain as decision makers, but as a growing appreciation of its complexities. The major decision must, as always, be our responsibility.

RECOGNITION

The recognition of cardiac arrest depends on the finding of signs of absence of circulation, such as (1) unconscious state (preceded, of course, by less profound states of mental obtundation), (2) pulselessness, (3) dilated pupils, and (4) minimal or absent respirations. Two things should be noted. First, the pupils require a certain amount of time to dilate, which has been estimated at approximately 45 seconds but may be longer than 1 minute. It is therefore occasionally a valuable sign for pinpointing the time of cardiac arrest. Second, inadequate respiratory excursions may be noted in the early seconds of cardiac arrest, and these should not cause delay in recognition of the other signs.

Pulselessness is best determined by palpation of either the carotid or femoral arteries. Palpation of the carotid is almost always immediately available, whereas palpation of the femoral is not. Brachial or radial pulse palpation is of lesser value. Pulselessness should not be determined by attempting to obtain a blood pressure.

An ideal situation should exist in coronary care units or well-equipped critical care units that include continuous monitoring, electronic warning signals, automatic conditioned response of a skilled team without the delay of feeling pulses, auscultating over the precordium, and the like.

THE RESUSCITATION TEAM

An organized approach to resuscitation is essential. Resuscitation should be approached by a team made up of trained personnel, including nurses, physicians, ECG technicians, inhalation therapy technicians, and individuals to transport special instruments (*e.g.,* defibrillators, pacemakers, and special tray sets).

The team should also include an administrative or secretarial member who can do the legwork, make all necessary phone calls, and perform other miscellaneous duties that are a minor but necessary part of every prolonged resuscitation attempt. A common method of organizing a resuscitation team is to designate specific individuals who will respond to all cardiac emergencies; this works quite well, but it is not the only method nor is it always feasible.

Following is an illustration of a successful method of resuscitation geared to an institution with trained resuscitative personnel. The team includes a nurse who serves as the primary member. The first nurse present becomes the initial captain of the team, who also institutes the resuscitation attempt as outlined.

A single call, preferably by the secretary, should immediately summon the entire team—ECG technicians, inhalation therapy technicians, available physicians including house staff and senior staff members in the area, nurses from the appropriate intensive care unit who will immediately transport the necessary equipment (defibrillator, monitor, and pacemaker instrument) to the site of the emergency, and the nursing supervisor.

The last but not least important member of the team is the switchboard operator, who must immediately alert the entire team in preference to all other duties. A single digit on the telephone dial should be used to alert the switchboard. The switchboard operator will often know where to find key physician members of the team and can summon them individually.

Hospitals with house officers who carry emergency electronic communication equipment are at an obvious advantage and should have the best resuscitation statistics. Many smaller institutions, however, may be just as successful using only nursing personnel and well-trained technicians. Minor variations in approaches may bring the same results.

Two additional factors are crucial to the team's success. The team must have a definite routine that is kept up-to-date by all members. Furthermore, nursing personnel and other key nonphysician members must be sanctioned to act spontaneously.

Because many episodes of cardiac arrest occur outside a hospital setting, there has been a sharp growth of well-trained teams in mobile units who can respond in minutes to emergency calls. The reported success rates vary greatly, with many factors operative, but on the whole they are more effective than many health care personnel predicted. In any case, they have made an impact, and as more spontaneous activities are allowed (*i.e.,* immediate defibrillation by first responders), further improvement in overall survival can be expected.

STEPS IN CPR

There are two settings in which health care personnel may encounter a person in need of CPR: (1) that of a patient whose ECG is being continuously monitored, as in the coronary care unit, and (2) that in an area where the patient is not under continuous monitoring, such as an ordinary hospital room or unit.

For the continuously monitored patient, the arrhythmia sets the alarm, and if it is ventricular fibrillation, the patient is immediately defibrillated (without prior attempts by other means), after which a physician is summoned for evaluation.

In the unmonitored patient, proceed immediately as described subsequently. (For a summary of the following steps see the chart titled "Steps in CPR," later in this section.)

1. Sharp Blow to the Precordium
A sharp blow to the precordium requires virtually no time and may institute a cardiac rhythm; if so, it may be the only required resuscitation. This is referred to as *thumpversion* and is especially effective in ventricular tachycardia.

2. Call for Help
To call for help simply relay the message "code zero" or "red alert," together with the location of the patient to a second individual who then places the emergency call to bring the team together.

3. Achievement of Adequate Airway
Artificial ventilation (mouth-to-mouth) is instituted immediately.

4. External Cardiac Compression
External cardiac compression is a simple technique that one performs by standing at either side of the patient, placing the heel of one hand over the lower half of the sternum and the heel of the other hand over the first. Vigorous compression is applied directly downward, and the sternum is depressed between $1\frac{1}{2}$ and 2 inches and released abruptly. This rhythm is maintained at the rate of 60 to 80 times per minute. To be effective this technique must be learned correctly and applied skillfully. All that is required to learn this technique is a little attention to instructors, two hands, and a lack of timidity.

If one person must apply both ventilation and massage, it is best to give two or three quick inflations by mouth-to-mouth or other readily available means of inflating the lungs, followed by 12 to 15 external cardiac compressions. This routine may be maintained until additional members of the team arrive.

The generally accepted theory underlying CPR maintains that the heart functions as a pump and the valves operate appropriately as one-way passages during external compression. More recent work, involving two-dimensional echocardiography during CPR in animals and humans, indicates that different mechanisms may necessitate some minor alterations in the standard CPR procedure. The new studies emphasize that the heart serves primarily as a conduit, not as a pump, and that the properties of veins as capacitors and arteries as conduits influence cerebral and coronary circulation during CPR. Venous beds may act as reservoirs, while some venous circuits function as barriers to retrograde flow owing to the presence of valves. Arteries show less tendency to collapse and therefore should receive more blood during artificial massage. The splanchnic venous bed, however, may form a large static pool that robs the total circulation during CPR. Some advocate abdominal compression to prevent this. Although present techniques should not be changed until more evidence shows these newer techniques to be superior, it is imperative to keep an open mind because even small improvements could prove salutary.

5. External Countershock

External countershock should be applied as soon as the instrument is available. This procedure should be done even if the specific rhythm diagnosis is unknown if there is a delay in determining this.

If *cardiac standstill* is present, the countershock will take only moments and will do no harm. If *ventricular fibrillation* is present, the earliest possible countershock delivered is the one most likely to be effective and should be done at a time when the rhythm may more likely be maintained.

Here it is imperative to stress that any adult is capable of doing this; thus, all personnel involved should be allowed training in defibrillation techniques and be expected to execute them without need of supervision.

A specific *diagnosis* now is required (the word *recognition* has been used up to now, not diagnosis). As mentioned earlier, this will be either cardiac standstill or ventricular fibrillation (discussed in items 9 and 10 of this section).

6. Intravenous Infusion

This item is devoted to a very important member of the team—the nurse who is first available after two members are applying ventilation and massage. This person will be in charge of the emergency cart and therefore responsible for preparing the drugs to be used and an intravenous infusion set (with several types of ventipuncture equipment). Moreover, she must handle whatever is necessary to see that an intravenous infusion is started, thus paving the way for drug therapy. The importance of this function underlies the continuously available venous cannula maintained in patients in critical care units.

At this point the need for an intravenous infusion is obvious and must be fulfilled by whatever route is feasible. The simplest of all is the insertion of a needle, cannula, or scalp needle into an *arm vein.* If this fails, the *femoral vein* is readily accessible, and a very large

cannula can easily be inserted into the largest blood vessel in the body (the *inferior vena cava*) by simple puncture. A cutdown on a branch of the *basilic system* just above the elbow crease on the medial aspect of either arm or on the *external jugular vein* will allow insertion of a large cannula into the *superior vena cava* or right atrium.

The *subclavian venipuncture* is perhaps ideal, being readily available and easily done. In addition, it may be used for rapid infusion or withdrawal and monitoring of central venous pressure (CVP) and O_2 saturation, and it is well tolerated for long periods of time. The *internal jugular route* is also excellent but is less desirable than the subclavian.

The *intracardiac route* should be reserved for situations in which urgency takes precedence over availability of the intravenous route. This should be a rare occurrence.

7. Endotracheal Intubation

Endotracheal intubation is required for the patient whose spontaneous cardiac rhythm and respiration have not resulted from the measures already outlined.

8. Pharmacologic Agents

Pharmacologic agents and appropriate preparations to be made ready immediately include the following:

a. *Sodium bicarbonate* in a 5% solution is given in 50 ml aliquots every 5 to 10 minutes and is the initial drug used. Tromethamine (THAM) can also serve as a buffer, but it has disadvantages and is used much less often than sodium bicarbonate.

It has been argued that giving sodium bicarbonate intravenously results in a rise in PCO_2 (by the reaction $HCO_3^- + H^+ \rightarrow H_2CO_3 \rightarrow H_2O + CO_2$) and an increase in osmolality. This is often the case, but there is little choice when significant acidosis is present, as is the situation in virtually all instances of cardiopulmonary arrest. Thus, consensus holds that alkalinization is important, even vital, and that increased osmolality is seldom sufficient to be a major factor.

b. *Epinephrine* (Adrenalin) in a 1:1000 aqueous solution.

c. *Isoproterenol* should be available in an intravenous preparation; 2 mg in 250 ml of appropriate vehicle solution is an adequate routine preparation.

d. *Calcium chloride* 10% solution.

e. *Lidocaine* (Xylocaine) should be prepared in an intravenous solution of varying concentration, but 1 mg/ml is an adequate solution for initial use. This drug is used most frequently by intravenous push in 50-mg doses.

f. A *vasopressor,* preferably a peripheral vasoconstrictor such as methoxamine (Vasoxyl) or phenylephrine (Neo-Synephrine, an alphamimetic) or nor-epinephrine (both alpha-and beta-stimulating) should be available in an intravenous infusion of appropriate concentration.

g. Magnesium ion is second only to potassium in intracellular concentration and is vital in energy metabolism (including membrane transport function). Studies have shown its administration to be effective in certain life-threatening arrhythmias, notably torsade de pointes. Its role in regulating intracellular concentrations of potassium, calcium, and phosphorous suggests its usefulness in cardiac arrest due to ventricular tachycardia and ventricular fibrillation. Also, this cation may be depleted in a manner parallel to potassium depletion, and thus its use may be especially beneficial in patients on diuretics or digitalis or both. It is, in my opinion, underutilized. In the absence of known hypermagnesemia or renal failure it is quite safe. It may be given in a 10% solution at a rate of 1 to 2 ml/minute in doses of 3 to 4 mEq and may be repeated, depending on response.

Intravenous Push. The critical emergency drugs given by intravenous push (sodium bicarbonate, epinephrine, calcium chloride, lidocaine) are all supplied in ready-to-use forms and should be readily available.

Other preparations such as procainamide (Pronestyl); quinidine; diuretics such as ethacrynic acid (Edecrin) and furosemide (Lasix); mannitol, dexamethasone (Decadron); and propranolol (Inderal) should be available, although they are not routinely prepared for immediate use. Metoprolol has become available for IV use and should be equivalent to propranolol in CPR.

The inotropic and chronotropic agent *glucagon* has gained use in some situations. Its effects are less predictable, and it should not be considered a routine drug. Its inotropic effect is substantial, but less than that of isoproterenol, and it has the advantage of a lesser chronotropic effect and generally induces less hyperexcitability.

The catecholamine *dopamine* has emerged as perhaps the inotropic agent of choice. Its central inotropic effect is comparable to that of isoproterenol, but is has the advantage of augmenting renal blood flow. It has largely replaced isoproterenol and norepinephrine for enhancing perfusion pressure (although isoproterenol is still more effective as a temporary medical "pacemaker").

Other drugs that have become useful in cardiopulmonary emergencies include bretylium and dobutamine; the class referred to as *calcium antagonists* (*e.g.,* verapamil) are not yet fully evaluated but are unlikely to be important except in very special situations (*e.g.,* recurrent arrhythmias associated with variant angina). Animal work suggests that calcium antagonists may prevent microvascular spasm, a potential factor in ischemia and necrosis. Their use in CPR for this purpose is uncertain, although it appears promising, with further work anticipated.

Disopyramide (Norpace) is not yet available for parenteral use and probably will have limited value.

Bretylium has proved of great value in persistent ventricular arrhythmias in CPR. Its actions are complex and include adrenergic influences that give it a modest inotropic effect (unlike other antiarrhythmics). Its major action is a striking antifibrillatory effect produced by prolongation of both the action potential duration and the effective refractory period. Occasionally, it causes defibrillation without use of countershock. This sharp rise in threshold for ventricular fibrillation and ventricular tachycardia makes it extremely effective when these rhythm disturbances are recurrent, and it is becoming the drug of choice in this circumstance. It is given by intravenous bolus, in a usual dose of 500 mg, and it can be repeated one or more times within 1 hour.

Dobutamine, a derivative of isoproterenol, has the advantage of possessing minimal chronotropic effect. When dopamine produces tachycardia, dobutamine may provide potent inotropy without the harmful effects of excess heart rate.

Experimental drugs useful in cardiac arrhythmias are proving effective; it is not anticipated, however, that any presently in trials will be especially useful in CPR.

9. Countering Cardiac Standstill
If cardiac standstill is present, epinephrine should be given routinely, usually 1 mg intravenously, and artificial ventilation and circulation should be continued; if unsuccessful, epinephrine should be repeated and the isoproterenol drip started. At this point, calcium chloride, 0.5 to 1.0 g, is given intravenously.

If there is no response, continued artificial ventilation and circulation, continued intravenous epinephrine injections, and insertion of a transvenous pacemaker are indicated (less often a percutaneous transthoracic pacemaker is used).

10. In Case of Ventricular Fibrillation
If ventricular fibrillation is present, epinephrine is given intravenously (it is important that the continuous artificial ventilation and circulation are maintained and that interruptions not exceed 5 seconds and external *countershock* is given at the maximum setting of the instrument with immediate resumption of artificial circulation and ventilation. If unsuccessful, the cycle should be repeated (see further on).

If ventricular fibrillation persists in spite of the preceding intervention or if reversion to ventricular fibrillation occurs each time it is applied, intravenous *antiarrhythmics* should be given without delay.

It is here that *bretylium* is probably the drug of choice (dosage as given previously) and should be administered before time is wasted going "down-the-line" of other more commonly used agents.

If bretylium is ineffective, *lidocaine* is given by push in 50- to 100-mg aliquots. *Procainamide,* if preferred, may also be given by intravenous push, and either drug may be given by intravenous drip. *Beta-blocking drugs* such as propranolol (Inderal) may be effective here. *Quinidine* is preferred by some, but its tendency to lower peripheral blood pressure and reduce myocardial contractility (resulting in a diminished cardiac output should a rhythm be resumed) constitute important disadvantages.

It should also be emphasized that regardless of the initial mechanism (whether it be an irritable or a depressive phenomenon), once cardiac arrest has gained foothold with some duration it must be assumed that the heart is depressed, making the routine use of depressive drugs unwarranted.

Because uneven tissue perfusion, particularly myocardial perfusion, may be a factor in perpetuating the ventricular fibrillation or standstill, a *vasopressor agent* of the peripheral constrictor type may be of value at this point. Digitalis and potassium chloride are rarely indicated in resuscitative attempts, their use being based on knowledge of special preexisting situations.

As already indicated, depressive cardiac mechanisms are often the cause of repetitive ventricular fibrillation, and, paradoxically, pacing the heart (pharmacologically with isoproterenol or electronically by transvenous pacing catheter) is the treatment of choice in some cases (after resumption of rhythm, of course).

Much has been written about defibrillation regarding energy level, type of paddles, and so forth. Some believe that instruments should provide greater energy bursts, especially for large patients. Conversely, others have demonstrated that lesser energy (*e.g.,* 200 joules) is as effective as maximum levels. In my experience, the most important single factor in delivering shocks is the constant and rather heavy-handed pressure applied by the operator at the instant the button is pushed. It should also be remembered that all instruments deliver less than the setting indicates. Lastly, there seems no justification for insisting on front-to-back paddles.

11. Pericardial Tap

If the preceding measures fail

a. Pericardial tap should be performed, preferably by the subxyphoid route; although an uncommon

factor in cardiac arrest, it may result in dramatic recovery.

b. Consider further underlying causes subject to treatment, such as pneumothorax (insertion of chest tubes); pulmonary embolism (assisted circulation, surgery); ventricular aneurysm or rupture of papillary muscle or interventricular septum (assisted circulation, surgery); subvalvular muscular aortic stenosis with extreme gradients (propranolol, reserpine, etc.).

12. Terminating Resuscitation

If these interventions fail, the decision to terminate resuscitative attempts is imminent, based on central nervous system (CNS) changes or the assumption of a nonviable myocardium.

POSTRESUSCITATIVE CARE

If there is resumption of spontaneous cardiac activity, the situation should be thoroughly evaluated as to the clinical state, underlying causes, and complicating factors in order to determine proper management. A routine as follows has been found successful: intravenous diuretic (*e.g.,* furosemide 80 to 240 mg), a steroid such as dexamethasone for its salutary effect on cerebral edema, and electrical and physiological monitoring in a critical care unit. A portable chest roentgenogram is routine, and arterial blood gases should be obtained as indicated. Continuous oxygen therapy is maintained; an intravenous infusion is of course essential. Routine measurements other than continuous ECG monitoring include frequent blood pressures (ideally done by intra-arterial cannula), hourly urine volumes, frequent bedside estimates of tissue perfusion, and CVP and O_2 saturation measurements.

If CNS damage is evident, hypothermia should be instituted immediately, additional mannitol or intravenous urea should be given, and dexamethasone for cerebral edema should be continued. Monitoring otherwise is continued as already outlined.

If oliguria or anuria is present, massive doses of furosemide should be given immediately. If there is no response to these, management like that used in acute renal insufficiency should be instituted.

The specific approach in the postresuscitative period will depend not only on the patient's condition at the time but also on the underlying disease process, the previous condition of the patient, and the events in the immediate postresuscitative period. More patients are being studied by catheter techniques acutely to evaluate them for emergency surgical procedures such as saphenous bypass grafts, percutaneous transluminal coronary angioplasty, and thrombolysis. The state of this art is changing rapidly, and it is frequently necessary to transfer the patient to a facility in which these procedures are available.

It has long been known that abnormalities of coagulation may result from, or be aggravated by, cardiac arrest, especially in ischemic heart disease. Antithrombin III activity, fibrinolytic activity, as well as fibrinogen, PT, and PTT should be evaluated.

COMPLICATIONS OF RESUSCITATION

Resuscitation has come a very long way; it has changed drastically with time and undoubtedly will continue to do so. It has proved its worth beyond doubt. There are of course complications, including (1) injuries to sternum, costal cartilages, ribs, esophagus, stomach, liver, pleura, and lung, any one of which can be serious; (2) the production, fortunately rare, of permanent CNS damage in a live patient, which renders the patient totally dependent; and (3) medicolegal considerations, which originally leaned against the attempt because of the frequency of undignified failures.

This last medicolegal consideration should probably be ignored for the most part, since we are dealing with an earnest and reasonable approach to the treatment of sudden death in reversible situations. Nonetheless, it does emphasize that resuscitation should always be applied by well-trained, responsible people. The aim of resuscitation is to reverse the reversible and not to inflict suffering in situations involving the irreversible. The alternative in both, of course, is death. Differentiation between reversible and irreversible requires good judgment, which, as someone has said, "is difficult to learn, impossible to teach."

Commonly Used Antiarrhythmic Agents

Phillip S. Wolf

PHARMACOLOGIC AGENTS

Features of those agents most commonly used for management of arrhythmias are listed in Table 9-3.

Digitalis Preparations

Digoxin
This agent is often the first selected for patients with supraventricular arrhythmias, such as paroxysmal atrial tachycardia, atrial fibrillation and atrial flutter. Digoxin has little effect on multifocal atrial tachycardia. Digitalization often produces reversion to a normal sinus rhythm or, in the case of atrial fibrillation or flutter, slowing of the ventricular rate to a more satisfactory level. Digoxin should not be used to treat sinus tachycardia except when the tachycardia is secondary to congestive heart failure. The reduction in heart rate in such instances results from improved cardiac output.

Table 9-4 lists the chief characteristics of three digitalis preparations. Because digoxin receives the widest use, it merits further discussion.

Seventy percent to 80% of an oral dose of digoxin is absorbed. Digoxin is also absorbed when given intra-

---

Steps in CPR

1. Deliver a sharp blow to the precordium if patient is unmonitored. If patient is being monitored and ventricular fibrillation has occurred, patient is defibrillated immediately without administering the thump.
2. Call for help—"cor zero" or "red alert." Give code and location to second person who then places emergency call.
3. Establish airway and institute artificial mouth-to-mouth ventilation.
4. Apply external cardiac compression.
5. Apply external countershock as soon as the instrument is available.
6. If cardiac standstill has occurred
   - Give epinephrine routinely—usually 1 mg intravenously.
   - Continue artificial ventilation and circulation.
   If *unsuccessful*
   - Repeat epinephrine.
   - Start isoproterenol drip.
   - Give calcium chloride, 0.5 to 1.0 g intravenously.
   If *no response*
   - Continue artificial ventilation and circulation.
   - Continue intravenous epinephrine injections.
   - Insert transvenous pacemaker.
7. If ventricular fibrillation is present
   - Administer epinephrine intravenously.
   - Maintain artificial ventilation and circulation (any interruption not to exceed 5 sec).
   - Give external countershock at maximum setting, followed by immediate resumption of artificial ventilation and circulation.
   - If unsuccessful, repeat the cycle and give intravenous antiarrhythmics without delay.
   - Consider using a vasopressor agent at this point.

TABLE 9-3
PHARMACOKINETICS OF MOST COMMONLY USED ANTIARRHYTHMIC DRUGS

Drug	Effect on ECG	Dose and Interval	Route	Adverse Effects	Therapeutic Plasma Level
Digoxin	Prolongs P–R (±) S–T depression	0.5 mg initially; 0.25 mg q 2–4 hr total 1.0–1.5 mg first 24 hr	IV or PO	Nausea; vomiting; abdominal pain; blurred or colored vision; weakness; psychosis; VPCs; heart block	0.8–1.8 ng/ml
Quinidine	Prolongs QRS, Q–T, and P–R (±)	100–600 mg q 4–6 hr	PO	GI symptoms; cinchonism; thrombocytopenia; hypotension; heart block; ventricular tachycardia	2.3–5.0 μg/ml
Procainamide (Pronestyl)	Prolongs QRS, Q–T, and P–R (±)	500 mg–1 g; then 2–5 g/day	PO	GI symptoms; psychosis; hypotension; rash; lupus-like syndrome	4–10 μg/ml
		250–500 mg q 3–6 hr	IM		
		100 mg q 5 min to 1 g total Maintenance: 2–4 mg/min	IV		
Disopyramide (Norpace)	Prolongs QRS, Q–T, and P–R	Loading: 200–300 mg Maintenance: 100–200 mg q 6 hr	PO	Anticholinergic effects; hypotension; heart failure; heart block; tachyarrhythmias	2–8 μg/ml
Propranolol (Inderal)	Prolongs P–R, no change QRS, shortens Q–T	10–80 mg q 6 hr 0.3–5 mg total (not > 1 mg/min)	PO IV	Hypotension; heart failure; heart block; asthma	Not established; 50–100 ng/ml needed for beta-blockade

TABLE 9-4
DIGITALIS PREPARATIONS

Agent	Onset of Action (Minutes)	Peak Effect (Hours)	Average Half-Life	Principal Excretory Path	Average Digitalizing Dose		Usual Daily Oral Maintenance Dose
					Oral	IV	
Ouabain	5–10	½–2	21 hr	Renal; some gastrointestinal	—	0.3–0.5 mg	—
Digoxin	15–30	1–2	33 hr	Renal	1.25–1.5	0.75–1.0 mg	0.25–0.5 mg
Digitoxin	25–120	4–12	4–6 days	Hepatic	0.7–1.2 mg	1.0 mg	0.1 mg

muscularly, but this route is painful and has few advantages. When given intravenously (preferable for many seriously ill patients), the usual starting dose is 0.5 mg, followed by 0.25 mg every 2 to 4 hours. Total dosage requirements vary widely, although most patients will respond to a total dose of 1.0 to 1.5 mg IV. As stated previously, some patients will not respond to customary doses of digoxin.

In order to minimize the risks of *digitalis toxicity,* a serious and sometimes lethal complication, one should consider the following options for the patient with a supraventricular tachycardia:

• Stop treatment if the heart rate has reached a satisfactory, although not ideal, level and further doses of digoxin produce no further slowing (an example

is atrial fibrillation with a ventricular rate of 100 to 120/min).
• Choose a second drug for control of heart rate such as propranolol or verapamil.
• Attempt electrical cardioversion.
• Use an agent such as quinidine, procainamide, or disopyramide, which may reestablish normal sinus rhythm.

Alternate forms of digitalis are useful in specific circumstances.

Ouabain
Given only intravenously, ouabain exerts an effect on atrial arrhythmias within minutes. Its chief benefits are for the two following types of patients: those in whom

speed of rhythm control is important and those in whom the status of digitalization is uncertain. In each group, small increments of ouabain (0.1 mg IV q ½ hr) may produce either a favorable response or evidence of toxicity, such as the development of ventricular premature beats. The latter indicates that safe levels of digitalization have been exceeded. The small, stepwise doses and the shorter half-life make this approach somewhat safer than the use of digoxin for this purpose.

Digitoxin

By virtue of its relatively slow excretion, digitoxin is especially useful in some patients with chronic atrial fibrillation or atrial flutter who continue to exhibit rapid ventricular rates. The vagotonic action of digitoxin on the AV node is more consistent than that of digoxin, leading to more dependable rate control.

Digitalis Toxicity

All digitalis glycosides should be used with great caution in patients with Wolff-Parkinson-White (WPW) syndrome who develop atrial fibrillation or flutter. Digitalis reduces the refractory period of the accessory pathway. This action leads to transmission of potentially very rapid atrial rates to the ventricle. Ventricular fibrillation may result.

Excessive doses of digitalis can be avoided if consideration is given to some principles of its metabolism. When renal function is normal, one third of the digoxin stored in the body is excreted daily. The renal clearance of digoxin directly relates to the creatinine clearance. When serum creatinine is elevated to 2 to 5 mg/dl, the maintenance dose of digoxin should be reduced by at least one half. More severe levels of renal failure require an even further reduction of dosage. Because creatinine levels rise only after considerable loss of renal function, a normal serum creatinine does not assure a normal clearance of digoxin.

It is prudent to reduce the maintenance dose of digoxin in the elderly patient. Creatinine clearance declines with age. A second factor that favors accumulation of digoxin in this age group is the age-related decrease in muscle mass. Skeletal muscle is the major body depository for digoxin. A decrease in muscle mass is reflected in increased glycoside concentration in the serum and in the heart. Features of digitalis toxicity are listed in the accompanying chart.

Other conditions that may lead to digitalis toxicity include hypokalemia, hypomagnesemia, hypothyroidism, pulmonary hypertension, and severe heart disease of any etiology. Concomitant therapy with quinidine or verapamil is also known to increase the serum digoxin level. Certain of these states, such as severe heart failure, are themselves associated with atrial arrhythmias. The utmost care is required in choosing the dose of digitalis for these patients.

Measurements of serum digoxin levels have assisted in many cases in arrhythmia management. The normal range is 0.8 to 1.8 ng/ml (Table 9-3). It cannot be stressed too strongly that the serum level is only a guide and not an absolute indicator of the adequacy of digitalization. The clinical status of the patient, in particular the adequacy of rate control, often provides more useful information about the status of digitalization than absolute serum levels. As a common clinical example, a patient with chronic atrial fibrillation may require larger than customary doses of digoxin for maintenance of a satisfactory ventricular rate. A serum level above the "therapeutic range" in this instance may be misleading as an indicator of toxicity.

Manifestations of Digitalis Toxicity	
Gastrointestinal	Anorexia
	Vomiting
	Abdominal pain
	Diarrhea
	Unexplained weight loss
Neurologic	Weakness
	Blurred or colored vision
	Psychosis
Cardiac (entirely manifest as arrhythmias)	Atrial tachycardia, commonly with AV block
	Junctional tachycardia
	Ventricular ectopic rhythm
	SA node depression
	AV block
	Bidirectional tachycardia

Quinidine

Quinidine is highly effective in the management of atrial and ventricular ectopic rhythms. These include supraventricular tachycardia, atrial fibrillation, atrial flutter, multifocal atrial tachycardia, ventricular premature contractions, and ventricular tachycardia. Quinidine has been found superior to placebo treatment in maintaining sinus rhythm after cardioversion from atrial fibrillation or flutter.

Quinidine has two modes of action. First, it is vagolytic and by this mechanism enhances conduction through the AV node. This action tends to speed the ventricular rate in atrial fibrillation or flutter; prior digitalization prevents this undesirable effect. Second, quinidine exerts a direct myocardial effect that prolongs AV conduction, His-Purkinje conduction times, and the duration of repolarization (the Q–T interval on the ECG).

Quinidine sulfate is well absorbed orally and reaches a peak serum level at about 1.5 hours. In contrast, quinidine gluconate absorbs more slowly, with a peak level occurring at about 4 hours. It would be expected that quinidine gluconate could be given less frequently (every 8 to 12 hours) than the sulfate compound (every 6 to 8 hours) because of the more prolonged absorption of the gluconate salt, which also results in lower peak levels. The effective dose in any given patient will vary quite widely as a result of patient variation, the disease state, the presence of other drugs, and differences in composition of other products. An initial total dose of 600 to 900 mg daily is usually given. The dose should be gradually increased as needed with attention directed to ECG signs of toxicity (prolonged QRS and QT intervals).

Blood levels offer a guideline for management and should be obtained after the first 6 to 8 doses. With current techniques, the therapeutic levels range from 2.3 to 5.0 μg/ml. An occasional patient may show signs of toxicity with "therapeutic" serum levels. In some of these patients, the Q–T interval may show considerable prolongation over the pretreatment ECG and warn of impending toxicity. Excessive serum levels are associated with a high frequency of toxicity. Conversely, some patients may be controlled at "subtherapeutic" blood levels. The dosage of the drug should not be raised further in this situation.

Quinidine should not be given intramuscularly because of erratic absorption and the tendency to produce pain at the injection site. The intravenous route is hazardous because quinidine produces vasodilatation and sometimes circulatory collapse. Intravenous quinidine, given by slow drip, should be reserved for patients with serious rhythm disorders that have not responded to other modes of therapy.

Quinidine Toxicity

About 30% of the patients on quinidine cannot tolerate the drug because of troublesome side effects. Diarrhea is the most common, is unrelated to plasma concentrations, and is often associated with nausea and vomiting. Cinchonism (headache and visual, auditory, and vestibular symptoms) occurs with increased plasma concentrations. Arrhythmias, especially ventricular ectopic rhythms, occur more frequently in patients with advanced cardiac failure. A very slow ventricular rate in patients with atrial fibrillation or flutter also predisposes to ventricular arrhythmias. Transient ventricular flutter or fibrillation may produce the entity known as "quinidine syncope."

Sudden death occurs in a small percentage of patients on maintenance quinidine. A retrospective look at patients with quinidine syncope reveals a prolonged Q–T interval in many cases. Other patients may show AV block. Finally, idiosyncratic reactions occur in some patients; these include fever, rash, thrombocytopenia, hemolytic anemia, and hepatic dysfunction.

As a rule, the maintenance dose of quinidine should be reduced to 70% in the presence of congestive failure and to 50% with renal failure. The blood level should be checked at the peak serum concentration (1.5 hour after oral use) and at the trough (1 hour before the next dose).

Procainamide (Pronestyl)

Procainamide is highly effective for atrial and ventricular ectopic rhythms whether given orally, intramuscularly, or intravenously. Like quinidine, procainamide has a mild vagolytic effect on the AV node, which in some patients will prove deleterious by increasing the ventricular rate. Procainamide has the potential for myocardial depression. It decreases conduction throughout the heart and can prolong the QRS and Q–T intervals. A reduced cardiac output and hypotension may occur after rapid intravenous use or when the oral dose accumulates as a result of renal failure.

A metabolite of procainamide, N-acetylprocainamide (NAPA), also has antiarrhythmic activity. NAPA has a longer serum half-life than procainamide. Renal failure produces a toxic level of NAPA that is not detected by the usual serum measurements. Patients with renal failure should therefore be treated with lower doses of procainamide and followed closely to detect QRS prolongation.

Procainamide is well absorbed orally, reaching a peak level at 1 hour. The usual dose ranges from 250 to 500 mg every 3 to 6 hours. Therapeutic plasma levels range between 4 to 10 μg/ml. Earlier investigations indicated that the serum level fell to subtherapeutic levels after 3 to 4 hours. Many patients, however, exhibit a continued response for longer periods. This effect probably results from the more prolonged antiarrhythmic action of NAPA.

Procainamide is given intravenously in initial doses of 100 mg by slow infusion and repeated every 5 minutes until either a therapeutic effect is obtained or toxicity (hypotension or widening of the QRS complex) is noted. The total intravenous dose should not exceed 1 g. The loading dose is followed by a maintenance infusion of 2 to 3 mg/minute. The dose should be reduced in patients with heart failure or hepatic or renal insufficiency.

Procainamide Toxicity

Commonly encountered side effects of procainamide include nausea, vomiting, and diarrhea with the oral route. Rash, fever, agranulocytosis, and frank psychosis are occasionally seen. Long-term use leads to a very high incidence (80%) of antinuclear antibodies (ANA). Thirty percent of patients develop a lupuslike syndrome characterized by high ANA titer, fever, pleuropericarditis, and arthritis. Cessation of the drug usually reverses these findings.

Lidocaine (Xylocaine)

This drug is of great value in the management of ventricular ectopic rhythms in the critically ill. Lidocaine has the advantages of rapid effectiveness and minimal effect on cardiac contractility.

An initial intravenous bolus of 50 to 100 mg will usually suppress ectopic activity for approximately 20 minutes. Recurrence of ventricular premature contractions (VPCs) calls for a repeat intravenous bolus followed by a sustained intravenous infusion of 1 to 4 mg/minute. The dosage is adjusted to control ventricular ectopic beats. Care is taken to avoid excessive doses, which produce agitation or seizures. As a rule, lidocaine is not helpful in the management of supraventricular arrhythmias.

Evidence indicates that the usual protocol of lidocaine use may not provide adequate plasma levels during the early hours of therapy. Some authorities have recommended giving multiple doses of lidocaine to a total of 225 mg over 16 minutes followed by a constant infusion of 2 to 4 mg/minute.

Because lidocaine is metabolized by the liver, the dose should be reduced when hepatic blood flow is decreased, as in congestive heart failure. AV block with a slow junctional or ventricular focus is also a contraindication to the use of lidocaine.

Bretylium

Intravenous bretylium tosylate has been approved for those life-threatening ventricular arrhythmias (recurrent ventricular tachycardia or fibrillation) occurring during myocardial infarction that fail to respond to lidocaine or procainamide. The recommended dose, 5 to 10 mg/kg, is delivered intravenously over 10 to 12 minutes and is followed by an intravenous infusion of 1 to 2 mg/minute. Hypotension, which may occur even when the patient is supine, and nausea and vomiting are the most common adverse effects.

Phenytoin (Dilantin)

This drug is usually ineffective for atrial arrhythmias. It is largely reserved for digitalis-toxic rhythms, in which it has moderate success. Such rhythms include atrial tachycardia, with or without block, and atrial fibrillation or flutter with a very slow ventricular rate and multiple VPCs. In this setting phenytoin may increase the ventricular rate to a more normal range and abolish the ventricular ectopic activity.

Phenytoin should be given slowly and intravenously undiluted from the vial. The rate of administration should not exceed 50 to 100 mg every 5 minutes. The drug should be given until the arrhythmia is controlled or a maximal dose of 1 g is given. Phenytoin is seldom used in maintenance by the oral route.

Beta-Adrenergic Blocking Agents

Propranolol (Inderal), currently the only beta-blocking agent authorized for treatment of arrhythmias in the United States, is useful for a variety of atrial and ventricular tachyarrhythmias. Propranolol increases the degree of block at the AV node and reduces the heart rate in patients with atrial fibrillation or flutter. In some, these rhythms may revert to a sinus rhythm. Propranolol may be useful alone or as an adjunct to digitalis or quinidine. Beta-blockade is especially helpful in some patients with chronic atrial fibrillation or flutter in whom digitalization is insufficient to control the ventricular rate. Propranolol is the agent of choice for rapid atrial arrhythmias due to hyperthyroidism.

The oral dose of propranolol varies over a wide range owing to differences in the rate of removal by the liver. The usual dose is between 80 and 320 mg/day given in three or four divided doses. On occasion, however, even low doses of propranolol (10 to 20 mg/day) increase the degree of block at the AV node and provide satisfactory control of the heart rate. The dose in each situation must be "titrated," beginning with small amounts of the drug and adjusting further doses according to the degree of response. Therapeutic serum level measurements have not been established. Beta-blockade is usually present at 50 to 100 ng/ml.

The intravenous use of propranolol requires great caution. Hypotension, acute pulmonary edema, and cardiovascular collapse may occur with intravenous doses as low as 1 mg. Doses of 0.3 to 0.5 mg IV should be used initially with close ECG and blood pressure monitoring. The dose should be repeated every 1 to 2 minutes and increased slowly as needed. The total intravenous dose should not exceed 7 to 10 mg in the first 2 to 3 hours.

Propranolol Toxicity

Side effects are common. Sinus bradycardia, usually well-tolerated, need *not* be regarded as a complication. Fatigue, depression, nausea, diarrhea, alopecia, impotence, increased peripheral vascular insufficiency, and hypoglycemia have been noted.

Propranolol depresses cardiac output in patients with preexisting congestive heart failure and therefore is contraindicated in such patients. An exception to this statement is the patient with heart failure due to atrial fibrillation or flutter with a very rapid ventricular response. Reduction of the ventricular rate in this instance may improve cardiac output and offset the depressant action of propranolol on the heart.

The drug should be used with great caution in patients with asthma, in whom it may induce irreversible and fatal bronchospasm. Finally, in the insulin-dependent diabetic patient, propranolol may mask the symptoms of hypoglycemia and therefore should be given with great care.

Disopyramide (Norpace)

Disopyramide is effective for both atrial and ventricular arrhythmias. By prolonging the refractory period of the accessory pathway, disopyramide may be especially effective in patients with WPW syndrome who develop supraventricular trahyarrhythmias.

Disopyramide is well absorbed by the oral route. Peak plasma levels occur in 2 hours; plasma half-life approximates 6 hours. Excretion occurs mainly by the renal route. Oral doses range from 100 to 300 mg every 6 hours. Effective plasma levels occur at about 2 to 8 μg/ml. The intravenous route has not been approved for general use.

Disopyramide Toxicity

Disopyramide causes a slight to moderate decrease in cardiac output. It may precipitate overt cardiac failure in patients with limited myocardial reserve. The drug should be avoided in patients with advanced heart block. The most frequent side effects of this drug are anticholinergic, namely, dry mouth, blurred vision, and, especially in males with prostatic enlargement, urinary retention.

Disopyramide, similar to quinidine and procainamide, can prolong the Q–T interval. Patients with marked prolongation of this interval appear especially susceptible to malignant ventricular rhythms and sudden death.

Verapamil

Given intravenously, verapamil has become the drug of choice in the treatment of paroxysmal supraventricular tachycardia (PSVT). The drug also has antianginal and antihypertensive properties. Verapamil has a potent depressant action on the AV node. It thereby slows conduction and prolongs the effective refractory period in the AV node. Verapamil interrupts the pathways used by reentrant atrial rhythms such as PSVT and, when given intravenously, causes reversion to normal sinus rhythm in the majority of cases. The agent is also useful in retarding the ventricular response in patients with atrial fibrillation or atrial flutter and is often used alone or in conjunction with digoxin for this purpose. Verapamil is less successful in restoring sinus rhythm in patients with atrial fibrillation or flutter.

The usual dose of verapamil is 5 to 10 mg IV given over 1 to 3 minutes. The dose may be repeated in 20 minutes if necessary. When administered orally, the dose ranges from 80 to 120 mg given 3 to 4 times daily.

Verapamil Toxicity

Adverse effects include hypotension (especially with IV use), bradycardia, gastrointestinal intolerance, headache, anxiety, and edema. In susceptible patients with SA or AV nodal disease, verapamil should be avoided. It should also not be given to patients on beta-blocking agents if such patients exhibit left ventricular dysfunction or significant bradyarrhythmias. Verapamil may safely be used in combination with digoxin, but because verapamil increases the serum level of digoxin by 50 to 70%, the maintenance dose of digoxin should be adjusted downward.

INVESTIGATIONAL AGENTS

The following drugs are being evaluated for clinical use and are used chiefly for the treatment of ventricular premature beats and ventricular tachyarrhythmias.

Tocainide

This drug is an analogue of lidocaine, but unlike lidocaine, it is effective orally. Tocainide is primarily useful in the therapy of ventricular arrhythmias. The dose ranges from 400 to 600 mg every 8 hours. Adverse effects involve the gastrointestinal tract (nausea, vomiting, abdominal pain, or constipation) and the central nervous system (dizziness, tremor, or paresthesias).

Mexilitene

Mexilitene is also structurally similar to lidocaine. It may be given intravenously or orally. The oral dose is 200 to 300 mg given 3 to 4 times daily. Effectiveness has been established for ventricular arrhythmias, whether given intravenously in the setting of acute myocardial infarction or administered orally for chronic symptomatic ventricular arrhythmias. Dose-related neurologic and gastrointestinal adverse effects are common, but hemodynamic reactions are minor.

Encainide

Encainide effectively suppresses ventricular ectopy in doses of 75 to 300 mg/day in divided doses given every 4 to 6 hours. Adverse effects include exacerbation of ventricular ectopy, especially the production of sustained ventricular tachycardia in approximately 15% of patients. Both neurological and gastrointestinal side effects have been reported.

Flecainide

This highly promising agent appears more potent than quinidine or disopyramide in the management of ventricular premature beats and complex ventricular rhythms. Therapeutic doses (100 to 200 mg twice a day) appear to be well tolerated by most patients. The drug exerts a modest negative effect on cardiac performance, probably of importance only in patients with markedly compromised ventricular function. The chief adverse effects include dizziness and blurred vision. The role of flecainide in the therapy of supraventricular arrhythmias has not yet been clarified.

Lorcainide

This is a potent drug that acts against supraventricular and ventricular arrhythmias. The oral dose is usually 100 mg given twice daily. As is true of other experimental antiarrhythmic agents, gastrointestinal and neurological symptoms are common side effects and tend to occur at the beginning of therapy. Sleep disturbances such as vivid dreams have also been recorded with lorcainide.

Propafenone

This drug is also under investigation for therapy of ventricular arrhythmias and has shown a high degree of effectiveness in clinical trials. Doses range from 150 to 300 mg every 8 hours. The chief adverse effects include nausea, bitter taste, hypotension, and, in susceptible patients with AV nodal disease, heart block.

Amiodarone

Initially introduced in the 1960s as an antianginal agent, amiodarone has shown great promise as an antiarrhythmic drug. A unique feature of amiodarone is that it has an extraordinarily long duration of action, with a half-life of 14 to 52 days. This characteristic makes less frequent dosing possible but increases the duration of toxic effects when they occur.

Amiodarone is useful for recurrent supraventricular and ventricular tachyarrhythmias not responsive to conventional agents. The oral dose ranges from 200 mg 5 days a week to 600 mg once a day. Adverse effects are seen commonly and are sometimes life-threatening. When looked for, corneal microdeposits are found in nearly all cases; impaired vision is occasionally present. Hyperthyroidism and hypothyroid-

ism have both been reported. Cutaneous problems include photosensitivity and skin pigmentation. Other problems include neurological toxicity and an increase in hepatic enzyme levels. The most dreaded complication is pulmonary fibrosis, which may reverse when the drug is discontinued but progress in some instances to respiratory impairment and death.

CARDIOVERSION

Direct current (DC) cardioversion has become the treatment of choice for many patients with supraventricular arrhythmias, including atrial fibrillation and atrial flutter, and ventricular tachycardia. Only a brief discussion of the technique follows. The reader is referred to Lown's classic review for more comprehensive information.[1]

1. It is helpful to begin the patient on quinidine, 0.2 g every 6 to 8 hours for 24 hours prior to conversion, which will produce reversion to sinus rhythm in up to 15% of such patients.
2. The patient is maintained in a fasting state for 8 hours before cardioversion.
3. An intravenous infusion is begun with the patient on a monitor and with all necessary resuscitation apparatus readily available.
4. Ideally, digitalis should be withheld for 24 hours prior to cardioversion, although cardioversion may be attempted in an emergency situation without this precaution.
5. Sedation is induced with the use of intravenous diazepam (Valium) in graduated doses of 5 to 10 mg.
6. Care should be taken to synchronize the electrical impulse with the apex of the R wave of the monitored lead.
7. Two paddles are then placed, one at the upper right sternal area and the other behind the left scapula or over the cardiac apex. A generous amount of electrode jelly is used to prevent skin burns and to decrease electrical resistance; firm pressure is exerted. One should avoid contact with the patient or the bed.
8. Initially, begin with 25 to 50 watt/second (J) and increase until either reversion is achieved or a single shock level of 400 watt/second is delivered.
9. Following the procedure, the patient should be observed closely for changes in rhythm, blood pressure, and respirations.

REFERENCES

1. Lown B: Electrical reversion of cardiac arrhythmias. Br Heart J 29:469, 1967

BIBLIOGRAPHY

Anderson JL, Harrison DC, Meffin PJ, Winkle RA: Antiarrhythmic drugs: Clinical pharmacology and therapeutic uses. Drugs 15:271, 1978

Bigger JT Jr (ed): Symposium on flecainide acetate. Am J Cardiol 53:1–122, 1984

Danahy DT, Aronow WS: Lidocaine-induced cardiac rate changes in atrial fibrillation and atrial flutter. Am Heart J 95:474, 1978

Gillis AM, Clusin WT, Mason JW: New horizons in antiarrhythmic therapy. J Cardiovasc Med 8:959–964, 1983

Harrison DC (ed): Symposium on perspectives on the treatment of ventricular arrhythmias. Am J Cardiol 52:1–59, 1983

Wolf PS: Arrhythmias in chronic pulmonary disease. Angiology 30:676, 1979

Zipes DP, Troup PJ: New antiarrhythmic agents. Am J Cardiol 41:1005, 1978

Percutaneous Transluminal Coronary Angioplasty

Sally V. Zouras
Daniel Liberthson
John B. Simpson

DEFINITION

In percutaneous transluminal coronary angioplasty (PTCA), a coaxial catheter system is introduced into the coronary arterial tree and advanced into an area of coronary artery stenosis. A balloon attached to the catheter is then inflated, increasing the luminal diameter and improving blood flow through the dilated segment.[1] PTCA is a relatively new nonsurgical technique being applied as an alternative to coronary artery bypass surgery in the treatment of obstructive coronary artery disease (CAD). When indicated and if successful, PTCA can alleviate myocardial ischemia and relieve angina pectoris.

HISTORY

"Atherosclerotic coronary artery disease is a progressive process that is responsible for more deaths in this country than any other single affliction."[2] The first major advance in the palliative treatment of CAD was the implantation of an aortocoronary saphenous vein bypass graft in 1967. Since that time, coronary artery bypass graft surgery (CABG) has been continually refined and has been the treatment of choice for many patients with CAD. However, the first percutaneous transluminal coronary angioplasty, performed by Gruentzig in 1977, marked another major innovation in the treatment of coronary artery disease.

The path to PTCA began in 1964, when Dotter and Judkins introduced the concept of mechanically dilating a stenosis in a blood vessel with a technique of inserting a series of progressively larger catheters to treat peripheral vascular disease. After experimenting with this technique, Dr. Andreas Gruentzig modified the procedure by placing on the tip of a catheter a polyvinyl balloon, which was passed into a narrowed vessel and then inflated. Because it produced a smoother luminal surface with less trauma than the Dotter/Judkins approach, this new method reduced the risk of complications such as vessel rupture, subintimal tearing, and embolism. At first, Gruentzig continued to apply his technique only to peripheral vascular lesions. Then, after successful dilatation of more than 500 peripheral lesions, he designed a smaller version of the dilatation catheter for use within the coronary artery tree. This new design was initially tested on dogs with experimentally induced coronary stenoses. After extensive canine experimentation, Gruentzig performed the first human PTCA in 1977.[3] Since then, considerable improvements in technique and equipment have made PTCA the treatment of choice for appropriate cases of CAD.

COMPARISONS BETWEEN PTCA AND CABG

As an alternative treatment in appropriate cases of coronary artery disease, angioplasty compares favorably to bypass surgery in terms of risk, success rate, the patient's physical capacity following the procedure, and cost.

Mortality rates associated with first-time angioplasty and CABG are quite similar. The National Heart, Lung and Blood Institute (NHLBI) PTCA registry (1983) estimates the in-hospital death rate for angioplasty to be 0.85% for single vessel disease and 1.9% for multivessel disease.[4] The CABG mortality rate is about 0.8%, with no variance from single to multivessel disease. However, if a second surgical operation becomes necessary to alleviate the symptoms of progressive disease, the mortality and complication rates for the bypass procedure are significantly greater than for second angioplasty.

Published primary success rates for PTCA range from 59% to 90%.[5] Such inconsistency is to be expected because many factors bear on the success and the risk of the procedure. One such factor—perhaps the most significant—is the experience of the physician in performing the procedure, and his related abilities to select appropriate patients and equipment.

PTCA is more complex than routine diagnostic cardiac catheterization, and requires greater skill and knowledge. Gruentzig maintains that after the physician has performed 100 procedures, the primary success rate rises above 80%. To shorten the learning period, he recommends that practitioners of angioplasty be trained in centers with physicians who are already well experienced in the procedure.[6] The physician lacking experience in the procedure should consider referring the patient or working with an experienced practitioner. Also, since angioplasty techniques and equipment evolve continually, even the experienced physician should participate in a continuing education program to maintain and enhance his skills.

Another major factor that affects the success rate of angioplasty is the attempt to dilate multiple vessels in one session. When dilatation of more than one vessel is considered, "if you have even a 10% probability of failure of adequate dilatation per lesion and you dilate three lesions in a single patient, the overall probability of an inadequate technical result rises perhaps to 20% or 25%."[7]

Staged bicycle ergometer studies have demonstrated superior physical capacity for angioplasty patients as opposed to CABG surgery patients both immediately following and 1 year after the respective procedures. With angioplasty patients for whom the procedure was a primary success, the working capacity 1 year post procedure reached 90% of the expected non-CAD capacity, adjusted for age, sex, and body length.[8] Working capacities for patients who underwent CABG were 80% 1 year later, regardless of whether they also underwent angioplasty.[9] The decrease in exercise tolerance in CABG patients as compared with exercise tolerance in PTCA patients is attributed to the trauma of the operation, which restricts the patient's capacity for physical activity. "This result indicates better physiological function for the [angioplasty] patient and may be linked to other non-medical issues favoring angioplasty."[10] These factors may include better psychological and emotional response to a less traumatic procedure that enables faster and fuller recovery of physical capability.

Other psychological advantages of PTCA over surgery may argue favorably for the procedure. The emotional stress of awaiting dilatation is less than that of awaiting surgery. However, this reduction in anxiety is partly offset by the risk of psychological crisis if the angioplasty fails and surgery—especially immediate surgery—is needed. The psychological impact of this discouraging situation is significant, but it occurs in a relatively low percentage of cases, as evidenced by the 80% success rate associated with PTCA procedures.[11]

If there are no complications with either procedure, PTCA requires a hospital stay of 2 to 3 days, whereas CABG requires a stay of 7 to 10 days. In 1982, the average cost for PTCA was $4646 ± $1338 per case (assuming an 80% primary PTCA success rate); for CABG, the average cost was $16,093 ± $9807.[12] Obviously, angioplasty costs much less than bypass surgery on a case-by-case basis. On an overall basis, with current indications for patient selection and with 17,000 cases of coronary artery disease diagnosed annually in the United States in patients who are candidates for the procedure, approximately $170,000,000 could be saved yearly if angioplasty were performed instead of bypass surgery. One could calculate an even greater saving by taking into account that 79% of angioplasty patients return to work, with an average delay of 3 weeks, whereas only 69% of bypass surgery patients return to work after an average delay of 11 weeks.[13] Furthermore, current indications for candidate selection may expand considerably in the future if the technique and applications of angioplasty continue to progress.

To summarize: The major advantages of angioplasty over bypass surgery include reduced mortality and morbidity, shorter convalescence, and lower cost to the patient. However, as discussed in the following sections, it is important to bear in mind that with all its advantages, PTCA is currently indicated in only 15% to 20% of diagnosed CAD cases.[14]

DIAGNOSTIC TESTS FOR PTCA AND CABG PATIENT SELECTION

Prior to deciding between PTCA and bypass surgery, one must document all objective evidence of coronary insufficiency. Noninvasive methods of evaluation that may be used before and after PTCA include standard treadmill stress testing and thallium stress and redistribution myocardial imaging. These tests allow the physician to discover the areas of ischemia in the myocardium when the patient is subjected to stress (*i.e.,* exercise). In treadmill stress testing, the patient is attached to a 12-lead electrocardiogram (ECG) machine and exercised on the treadmill, which allows the physician to observe changes in the ECG that reflect hypoperfusion associated with obstructive coronary disease. In a thallium study, a radioisotope of thallium is injected into the patient intravenously during bicycle or treadmill exercise. The isotope is absorbed by the myocardial muscle; then the heart is scanned with a gamma camera, which maps (i.e., creates images from) the distribution of gamma radiation from the isotope. Thus, an image of the heart muscle reflecting myocardial perfusion is obtained. An area that is hypoperfused or ischemic during exercise lacks radioisotope and consequently appears as a "cold spot" in the image. The nurse should be familiar with the results of the thallium stress test indicated on the examination report because an understanding of the patient's diagnosis and related symptoms, and thus of the reasons for interventional angioplastic therapy, promotes more informed patient care.

Coronary arteriography with cardiac catheterization, another method of documenting coronary insufficiency, is done if the previous tests indicate coronary disease. Although this procedure is more invasive than treadmill testing and thallium imaging, it is required to pinpoint the location of any stenoses and the degree of involvement of the artery or arteries. The technique should be carried out in a radiology laboratory that is properly equipped for cardiac diagnostic studies. With the patient under local anesthetic, a guide wire is inserted into the aorta and advanced to the origin of the coronary arteries. A catheter is then placed over the wire and advanced until it is engaged in either the right or the left coronary ostium. the guide wire is then removed, radiopaque contrast material injected through the catheter, and a series of x-ray films are obtained (Figs. 9-23 and 9-24). Then the catheter is withdrawn to the abdominal level of the aorta, the guide wire is reinserted into the catheter and repositioned, the catheter is removed completely, and a second catheter placed over the wire and advanced to engage the other coronary artery. A second series of x-ray films of that second artery are then obtained. This procedure yields a 35-mm movie of the coronary artery anatomy. The physician can then closely analyze areas of narrowing, gaining precise information with which to decide the mode of treatment. From 15% to 20% of patients scheduled for coronary arteriography have coronary conditions for which PTCA is indicated.[15]

INDICATIONS AND CONTRAINDICATIONS FOR PTCA

In choosing to treat with PTCA (as with CABG), the physician's sole purpose is to alleviate angina pectoris unrelieved by maximal medical treatment. At this time, the ideal candidate for the procedure is the patient who has had angina for no longer than 3 years, and preferably less than 1 year; who presents with a hemodynamically significant, discrete, proximal, single-vessel lesion; and who has good left ventricular function. However, advances in technology have resulted in improved equipment over the past 6 years, so the spectrum of candidacy for coronary angioplasty has widened accordingly. In fact, there are at present no absolute contraindications in selection of patients for PTCA, and each case should be evaluated on the basis of the indications presented by the patient's condition, the physician's experience, and the sophistication of the laboratory.

The preceding statement is illustrated by a set of guidelines presented at a 1983 conference on guide wires and coronary angioplasty,[16] maintaining that patients with multivessel disease may be candidates for PTCA on one or more vessels if at least one of the following indications is present:

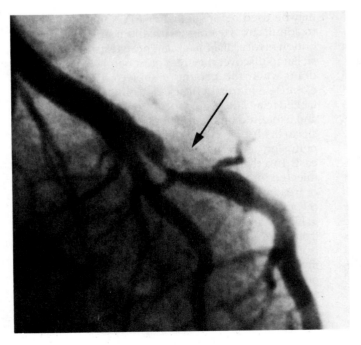

FIGURE 9-23
An eccentric stenosis in the left anterior descending (LAD) artery. The term "eccentric" defines a plaque involving only one side of the intraluminal wall. (Courtesy of John B Simpson, MD, Palo Alto, CA)

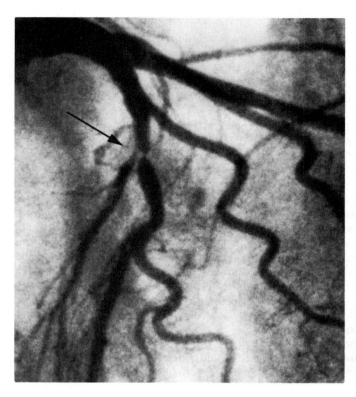

FIGURE 9-24
A coronary arteriogram of the circumflex artery (CX) illustrating a concentric stenosis. The term "concentric" defines a plaque involving the intraluminal wall circumferentially, giving a dumbell appearance. (Courtesy of John B Simpson, MD)

1. Two vessels, each with an ideally suited (proximally located and optimally shaped for the procedure) lesion for PTCA.
2. Severe stenosis in one vessel and a less than significant stenosis of another vessel not thought to be causing ischemia.
3. Severe stenosis in one vessel supplying viable myocardium and occlusion of a second vessel supplying noncontractile myocardium.
4. Severe stenosis in one vessel and significant stenosis in a branch of a second major vessel that would not be bypassed if coronary artery surgery were done.
5. Graft or native vessel stenosis in a patient with multivessel disease after CABG surgery.

Another example of the rapid expansion of the spectrum of candidacy for PTCA since its introduction is the change over time in the approach to treating the patient with a totally stenosed vessel. Early in PTCA practice, total occlusion disqualified a patient for the procedure because the stenosis could not be crossed with the guidewire and dilatation catheter without severe trauma. Currently, owing to refinement of equipment, technical advances, and greater experience, dilatation of totally obstructed vessels may be attempted in appropriate candidates.

In the evaluation of the diseased vessel or vessels,

location and condition of the lesion are more significant for PTCA than for CABG. Ideally, stenoses should be proximal, although this is not essential. With improved equipment, the distance of the lesion from the coronary ostium is now less significant. However, the position of the lesion is important; it may be in a location such that PTCA would compromise adjacent vessels, or it may be inaccessible to the balloon catheter owing to the patient's coronary anatomy tree. Furthermore, the shape of the lesion should be considered: Is it tapered, concentric, eccentric, discrete, or subtotal (Figs. 9-23 and 9-24). In vessels with very eccentric lesions, a segment of normal arterial wall may be dilated rather than the atherosclerotic plaque, compromising the success of the procedure. Moderately eccentric stenoses, however, do not seem to affect the results of angioplasty adversely. Lastly, the extent of calcification is a factor in the success of angioplasty because heavily calcified lesions may be too inflexible for dilatation.

To be considered for PTCA, a stenosis should close at least 50% of the vessel. In patients with mild stenoses, PTCA has favorable immediate and long-term results yet involves a significant risk of myocardial infarction and may accelerate the disease process in the dilated coronary lesion. The high risk of infarction may be due to the absence of the collateral circulation that normally develops over the years with moderate to severe obstructions. Thus, careful patient selection is essential when the physician is considering dilatation of mild stenosis. "This also applies to patients who undergo PTCA for a severe stenosis but have an additional mild lesion in another vessel, the 'preventative' dilatation of which in the same operating session is tempting. The possible complications and a recurrence rate of almost 30% with potential disease acceleration in the dilated lesion should caution against using PTCA in patients with mildly diseased vessels."[17]

All candidates for PTCA must be candidates for CABG because emergency surgery may be necessary if an intraoperative complication develops during angioplasty. The only exception to this rule is the group of patients who have severe underlying noncardiac diseases (*e.g.,* neoplasms, uremia, or lung disease) that make them unlikely candidates for coronary artery bypass surgery. These patients are particularly suited for PTCA because successful dilatation obviates the need for an operation that they would tolerate poorly.

Other candidates who might benefit from PTCA are those who have previously undergone CABG in who symptoms have recurred owing to stenosis and closure of grafts or progression of coronary disease in the native vessels. For these candidates, successful angioplasty makes second surgery, with its increased potential for complications, unnecessary. Aortocoronary graft stenosis usually results from thrombosis and/or fibrous intimal proliferative changes within the graft. The fibrous stenotic process may develop as a result of trauma (ischemia) to the saphenous vein graft during transplantation and because of the tendency of the vein graft to assume arterial characteristics (thicker walls) when placed in a higher-pressure arterial system. Studies show that within 1 month after surgery, 10% to 15% of vein grafts develop thrombosis and that the same percentage have significant stenosis, and that another 10% to 15% occlude within the first year.[18] However, it is thought that the proliferative disease in the graft wall generates fibrous stenosis that is much less dense than most fibrotic tissue in the native vessels, and so it responds very favorably to dilatation. In fact, whereas total occlusion of a native coronary vessel contraindicates PTCA, some totally occluded grafts have been recanalized with this technique. "Even partial improvement can be enough to relieve angina, and there is no apparent contraindication to repeated dilatations."[19]

In the past, if a patient had an acute myocardial infarction documented by significant S–T elevation, increased cardiac enzyme levels, and pain unrelieved by medication, surgery or pharmacological treatment with complete bedrest in a coronary care unit were the only alternatives for treatment. Now, if thrombosis and underlying stenosis are causing the infarction, strepto-

kinase and PTCA offer another alternative. When a blood clot has impeded flow to the distal myocardium and thus caused an ischemic episode, streptokinase, a thrombolytic drug, can be administered directly into the involved coronary artery with a cardiac catheter or intravenously at a higher dosage. Upon lysis of the thrombus, an underlying stenosis may be found to be causing the accumulation of blood cells. Immediate dilatation by PTCA of a subtotal stenosis often further enhances blood flow to the reperfused myocardium, reducing the risk of rethrombosis or critical narrowing caused by normal or spastic vasomotion superimposed on an organic stenosis.

PTCA may also be a first step in treating patients with multivessel disease who are presenting with an acute episode of unstable or preinfarction angina and are intended for elective bypass surgery. Dilatation of the most critical or involved stenosis minimizes the risk of infarction before the operation. As a first-stage treatment in such patients, PTCA immediately relieves pain and improves blood flow to the jeopardized myocardium.

Patients with left main artery disease are generally not considered candidates for angioplasty. The obvious drawback of PTCA in left main disease is the possibility of acute occlusion or spasm of the left main artery during the procedure, which would result in severe left ventricular dysfunction. The only exception to this rule is the patient who has had previous bypass surgery to the left anterior descending and/or circumflex arteries with patent grafts present. Only then might a physician consider dilating a left main artery stenosis. However, at present, most of these patients are still considered surgical candidates.

Table 9-5 summarizes the indications for PTCA and gives a list of those factors that would usually contraindicate the procedure for most patients.

PATIENT PREPARATION

Once the decision has been made to proceed with coronary angioplasty, the patient is usually admitted to the hospital the day before the procedure. It then becomes the nurse's responsibility to coordinate and carry out care for that patient. The nurse should monitor all preliminary lab tests, such as evaluations of cardiac enzymes, serum electrolytes, and prothrombin time (assessing coagulability), and should notify the physician of any abnormalities. The serum levels of potassium, creatinine, and blood urea nitrogen (BUN) are particularly important.

It is essential that potassium levels be within normal limits because low levels result in increased sensitivity and excitability of the myocardium. The cardiac muscle is also sensitive and becomes irritable when the

---

TABLE 9-5
INDICATIONS AND CONTRAINDICATIONS FOR PTCA

Indications	*Contraindications*
Discrete lesion	
Proximal lesion (ideally)	Less than 50% stenosis
Hemodynamically significant lesion (angina unrelieved by medical therapy)	
Single/multiple vessel disease	Diffuse multiple vessel disease
Favorably positioned lesion	Lesion located inaccessibly
Accessible coronary artery segment	Tortuous, inaccessible tree
Atherosclerosis of side branches	Nondilatable type of lesion (very calcified)
Evidence of collateral circulation	Evidence of preexisting dissection or thrombosis

Morphology to Be Considered for Candidacy
Vessel tortuosity
Number of vessels involved
Position of lesion
Atherosclerotic involvement of side branches
Evidence of preexisting dissection or thrombosis

---

flow of oxygen-rich blood decreases, as happens for a controlled period of time during placement and inflation of the dilatation balloon across the lesion. The irritability arising from hypokalemia or ischemia or both can give rise to ventricular arrythmias that pose a threat to the patient.

Elevation in the levels of serum creatinine or BUN or both may indicate problems in kidney function. Good kidney function is important because, during angioplasty, radiopaque contrast material (which allows fluoroscopic visualization of the coronary anatomy and of catheter placement) is introduced into the bloodstream. This contrast material is a hyperosmotic solution that the kidneys must filter from the blood and excrete. High levels of creatinine and BUN may reflect decreased renal filtration capability and vulnerability of the kidney to processing the extra load of radiopaque solution. Instances of acute renal failure have resulted from high doses of radiopaque contrast. However, because false high serum levels may result from hypovolemia, the nurse should take care to keep the patient adequately hydrated either by mouth with clear liquids or by means of intravenous solutions. If the efficacy of kidney function is in question, it can best be monitored by trends in creatinine and BUN levels in conjunction with measurement and documentation of urine output.

Once it is determined that the patient's physical condition permits angioplasty, the nurse must obtain from the patient an informed consent to the procedure. The physician will explain how the angioplasty is done, the reasons for the treatment, and the risks and potential benefits of PTCA and of the available alternative, surgery. The nurse should answer any questions that the patient may have left and should explain the course of post-PTCA care.

Prior to the procedure, the patient's medications may include aspirin, 325 mg three times a day; dipyridamole (Persantine), 75 mg three times a day; or sulfinpyrazone (Anturane), 200 mg three times a day for their antiplatelet effect. Also prescribed to reduce vasospastic events are nitroglycerin and calcium-blocking agents, such as nifedipine (Procardia), 10 mg three times a day, and diltiazem (Cardizem), 30 mg three times a day. Low molecular weight dextran (500 ml intravenously) may be given to combat platelet cohesiveness, and routine sedation is usually administered.

Surgical standby during PTCA is essential because of the possibility of complications requiring emergency revascularization. Therefore, the patient must be surgically prepped (shaved) as if for elective coronary artery bypass surgery. "Experience to date indicates that immediate coronary artery bypass surgery with an elapsed time from occlusion to restoration of flow of approximately 90–120 minutes will usually avert progression from ischemia to infarction."[20]

EQUIPMENT

Since the introduction of PTCA, there has been continual refinement of the equipment, resulting in lower rates of mortality and of emergency bypass surgery.

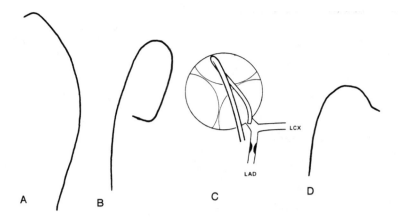

FIGURE 9-25
Judkins and Amplatz guiding catheters with preshaped tips suitable for selectively engaging the appropriate coronary ostia. (A) Judkins right coronary guiding catheter. (B) Judkins left coronary guiding catheter. (C) Judkins left shown engaged in the left coronary ostium, as seen from above the aortic valve. (D) Amplatz guiding catheter. (Reprinted with permission of Advanced Cardiovascular Systems [ACS] Inc, Mountain View, CA)

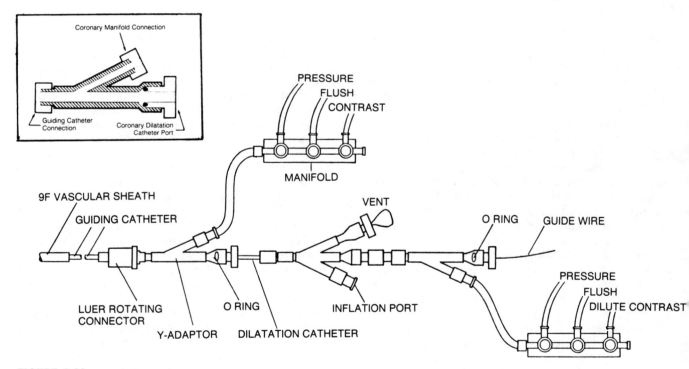

FIGURE 9-26
Advanced cardiovascular systems (ACS) balloon dilatation catheter and manifold system showing how angioplasty equipment is assembled, with a detail of the Y-adaptor. Equipment to the right of the vascular sheath is outside the patient's body. (Reprinted with permission of Advanced Cardiovascular Systems [ACS] Inc, Mountain View, CA)

Currently, the guiding catheter used to direct the dilatation catheter into the appropriate coronary artery ostium measures 8 to 8.8 Fr across the outer diameter. Like the Judkins[21] and Amplatz[22] coronary angiography catheters, the tips of the guiding catheters have curves that are preshaped for selective access to either the right or the left coronary artery (Fig. 9-25).

A Y-type (side arm) adaptor attached to the guiding catheter permits introduction of the dilatation catheter into the guiding catheter with minimal blood loss (Fig. 9-26). This Y-adaptor is connected to the guiding catheter with a Luer rotating connector, and its side arm is in turn attached to a three-port manifold. Each manifold port is connected to appropriate apparatus to enable the physician to measure coronary ostial pressure through a pressure monitoring line, to flush with saline solution, or to inject contrast medium through the guiding catheter while simultaneously positioning the dilatation catheter.

The catheter mechanism has evolved since Gruenzig's original system, which had a small, flexible guidewire preattached to the end of the dilatation catheter. In 1982, Simpson introduced a coaxial system, an improvement that has become predominant in current catheter designs. The main innovation is an independently movable guidewire within the balloon dilatation catheter.[23] This guidewire can be manipulated to select the correct vessel despite side branches and permits safe advancement of the dilatation catheter across the lesion (Fig. 9-27). Currently, the available guidewires measure between 0.009 and 0.018 inches in diameter and thus usually pose little threat of interference with the blood flow through a stenosis.

The dilatation catheter is 4 to 4.5 Fr across the outer diameter, narrow enough for easy passage through the guiding catheter. The dilatation catheter's interlumen allows passage of the teflon-coated wire and of contrast medium injected to visualize placement of the wire (Fig. 9-28) or to measure transstenotic intracoronary pressures when necessary.

The physician manually or mechanically inflates the balloon with contrast from a 10-ml syringe attached to the side inflation port on the dilatation catheter. This port communicates directly with the balloon via the catheter lumen (Fig. 9-26). A pressure gauge between the syringe and the lumen of the catheter indicates the amount of pressure exerted against the wall of the balloon as the physician applies force to the syringe plunger. Balloon pressure is usually measured in pounds per square inch (psi). The average dilatation is between 80 and 120 PSI and lasts from 15 to 60 seconds. Balloons have been strengthened over the years so that they now can apply and withstand greater pressure against calcified lesions.

In the Advanced Cardiovascular Systems (ACS) dilatation catheter, the balloon has, at its distal and proximal ends, radiopaque markers that can be imaged by the fluoroscope (Fig. 9-29). Thus, the physician always knows the balloon's exact position. The inflated balloon ranges from 2.0 to 4.0 mm in diameter and from 20 to 25 mm in length. The size (inflated diameter) of the balloon to be used for a particular PTCA is usually the same as the diameter of the coronary artery proximal and distal to the stenosis (*e.g.,* 3 mm-vessel, 3 mm-balloon). However, severe stenoses may require that a smaller balloon be used initially.

FIGURE 9-27
Advancing the guidewire (A) through the inner lumen of the dilatation catheter, (B) past the side branches, and (C) across the stenosis. (Reprinted with permission of Advanced Cardiovascular Systems [ACS] Inc, Mountain View, CA)

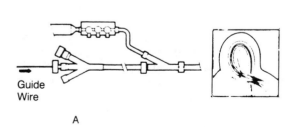

Guide Wire

A

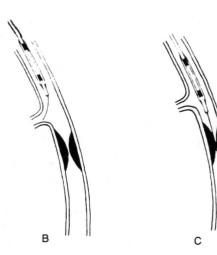

B   C

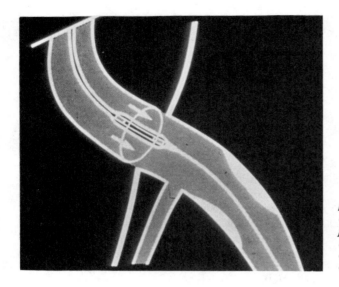

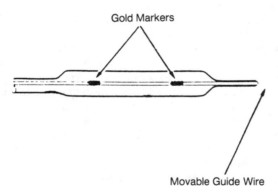

Gold Markers

Movable Guide Wire

One of the most frequent causes of failure of PTCA is inability to cross the lesion. "Severe stenoses of greater than 90% diameter narrowing pose the greatest problems for success in PTCA and are associated with the highest rate of complications."[24] Because a large percentage of candidates for angioplasty have high-grade stenoses, a new low profile steerable (LPS) catheter with smaller shaft and uninflated balloon diameters has been developed for use in the dilatation of lesions greater than 95%. This catheter increases the initial rate of success and decreases complications in stenoses that are hard to cross. For example, a coronary artery may measure 3.0 mm in diameter, but stenosis may narrow the artery too much (greater than 95%) to allow initial passage of the 3.0-mm balloon normally used for this vessel size. This lesion could be crossed

and dilated initially with a 2.0 or 2.5-mm LPS balloon so that it could then be recrossed and dilated further with a 3.0-mm balloon. This staged dilatation minimizes trauma to the vessel.

Many factors must be considered in selecting the most appropriate equipment for performing PTCA upon any one patient. In terms of the particular procedure, the outcome of PTCA is greatly affected by the following: (1) the size of the guiding catheter and of the dilatation catheter in relation to the size of the target artery, (2) the balloon type and size in relation to the severity and type of the lesion, and (3) other factors related to choice of equipment. In terms of making appropriate choices of equipment, there is no substitute for experience on the part of the physician.

TECHNIQUE

The entire PTCA procedure is carried out in a sterile fashion, with the use of local anesthesia and either the Judkins (percutaneous femoral) technique or, less often, the Sones (brachial cutdown) technique (Fig. 9-30).

With the Judkins technique, one cannulates the femoral vein and artery percutaneously by inserting a needle (usually 18-gauge) containing a removable obturator.[25] The obturator can then be removed to confirm by the presence of blood flow that the outer needle is within the lumen of the vessel. Once proper placement is established, a 0.035- or 0.038-inch guidewire is introduced through the needle into the artery to the level of the diaphragm. The needle is then removed, and a standard angiographic catheter is placed over the wire and advanced to the arch of the aorta. The procedure may also be approached by the Sones technique,

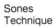
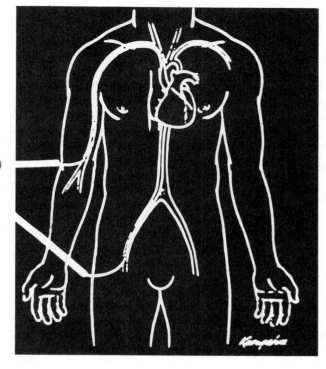

Sones
Technique

(brachial)

Judkins
Technique

(femoral)

FIGURE 9-30
Two approaches to left heart catheterization. The Sones
technique uses the brachial artery, and the Judkins technique
uses the femoral artery. With either method, the catheter is
passed retrograde through the ascending aorta to the left
ventricle. (Reprinted with permission of Advanced Cardiovas-
cular Systems [ACS] Inc, Mountain View, CA)

in which a brachial cutdown is used to isolate the brachial vein and artery.[26] A small arteriotomy is made, and the catheter is passed to the level of the arch in the aorta.

Regardless of the mode of access, repeat coronary arteriography is then carried out to determine whether the patient still meets the criteria for PTCA. A candidate's status can change quickly, and it is to reevaluate just prior to the procedure. Factors that might be grounds for cancelling PTCA are (1) progression of the disease, (2) coronary spasm, (3) large branch involvement, (4) previously unapparent additional stenotic lesions, and (5) total occlusion of the artery.

If PTCA is to proceed, the patient is anticoagulated with 10,000 units of heparin to prevent clots from forming on or in the catheter system during the procedure. Intracoronary nitroglycerin is usually administered at the start of the procedure as a prophylactic measure against vasospasm and to obtain maximal coronary vasodilation. Also, nitroglycerin is kept on the sterile field throughout the procedure and given intermittently as needed. A temporary pacing electrode is

positioned in the apex of the right ventricle and placed on standby in case emergency pacing is required.

The angiographic catheter is then removed and replaced by an 8 or 9 Fr introducer sheath. The sheath provides support at the puncture site in the groin and reduces potential arterial trauma if multiple catheter exchanges are necessary. The guiding catheter is then inserted through the sheath and positioned precisely in the appropriate coronary ostium. A manifold is attached to the side arm of the Y adaptor (Fig. 9-26). The manifold contains three entry ports to which are attached a saline flush, contrast medium, and a pressure-monitoring line. By manipulating the stopcocks to the appropriate ports, the operator can, in an entirely closed system, flush the catheter intermittently with saline, visualize positioning with contrast and fluoroscopy, or monitor intra-arterial pressure. The dilatation catheter is inserted through the guiding catheter port (Fig. 9-31). The dilatation catheter and guidewire are advanced to the tip of the guiding catheter while their position is checked by fluoroscopy (Fig. 9-32). The guidewire is then advanced and manipulated to nego-

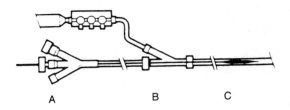

FIGURE 9-31
The coronary dilatation catheter passing through (A) *the coronary dilatation catheter port,* (B) *the side-arm adaptor (Y-connector), and* (C) *the guiding catheter. (Reprinted with permission of Advanced Cardiovascular Systems [ACS] Inc, Mountain View, CA)*

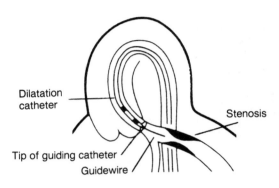

FIGURE 9-32
Advancing the coronary dilatation catheter to the tip of the guiding catheter while checking position by fluoroscopy. (Reprinted with permission of Advanced Cardiovascular Systems [ACS] Inc, Mountain View, CA)

tiate branch vessels. Proper advancement can be confirmed by injecting contrast through the guiding catheter and fluoroscopically visualizing the coronary tree.

Once the guidewire is safely across the stenosis, the dilatation catheter can be advanced slowly over the guidewire through the narrowing without the risk of dissecting beneath the atheroma or of entering the wrong vessel (Fig. 9-33). The advantage of the coaxial system is that "if symptomatic myocardial ischemia develops when the balloon dilation catheter is within the stenosis, the dilatation catheter can be withdrawn into the guiding catheter system as the guidewire is advanced, thus maintaining guidewire position across the stenosis."[27] Once the symptoms resolve, the balloon can be replaced across the lesion and the procedure continued. Also, the guidewire can be removed entirely while the balloon is still within the lesion and can then be replaced by an exchange wire that allows the present balloon to be removed and replaced by a balloon of smaller or larger diameter, without ever losing the position in the coronary artery.

Exact placement of the dilatation balloon within the stenosis is facilitated under fluoroscopy by the proxi-

mal and distal radiopaque markers on the balloon (Fig. 9-29) as well as by contrast injections for visualization (Fig. 9-28). Because the guidewires are so fine that they do not impede flow, the physician can measure transstenotic pressure gradients while the wire is in place across the lesion. Before starting dilatation, simultaneous transstenotic pressure gradient measurements are obtained from the tip of the guiding catheter proximal to the stenosis and from the tip of the dilatation catheter distal to the stenosis (Fig. 9-34). These measurements, made using the pressure-monitoring line attached to the three-port manifold, help confirm that the dilatation catheter and balloon are correctly positioned across the stenosis.

After the baseline gradient has been obtained, dilatation of the balloon begins. Initially, the balloon is fully inflated with 80 psi of pressure for 5 to 6 seconds and then deflated. At first it expands at both ends and not in the center, where it is pinched in by the stenosis (Figs. 9-35 and 9-36). The central indentation usually disappears as the stenosis is dilated. "After each inflation, arteriography through the guiding catheter assesses coronary blood flow around the deflated balloon. If the coronary blood flow is compromised, the guidewire may be advanced as the deflated balloon is removed from the stenosis."[28] Once reperfusion is established, the balloon is readvanced over the wire and inflations are continued until the desired results are obtained.

After dilatation is complete, as indicated by free contrast flow around the deflated balloon, the residual transstenotic gradient is determined via simultaneous measurement of ostial and distal coronary pressures. "If a significant residual gradient (greater than 15 mm Hg) persists, additional balloon inflations are performed until the gradient resolves or fails to improve with subsequent inflations to a maximal pressure of 90 psi."[29] Once it is decided that maximum dilatation has been obtained, the guiding catheter and the dilatation catheter are removed. Postdilatation arteriography is performed with a standard angiographic catheter to define more clearly the results of the PTCA. Successful dilatation can be defined as "a greater than 20% arteriographic improvement in the vessel lumen, a residual transstenotic gradient of less than 20 mm Hg, improved treadmill exercise response and resolution or marked alleviation of the anginal syndrome."[30]

Reasons for failure to complete a PTCA procedure include (1) inability to engage the guiding catheter adequately in order to advance the balloon catheter smoothly into the correct coronary artery, (2) coronary anatomy that does not allow passage of the catheter selectively into the stenotic vessel, (3) atherosclerotic plaque that is too fibrotic or too calcified to allow dilatation even with proper positioning of the wire and balloon within the lesion, (4) a stenosis too narrow to

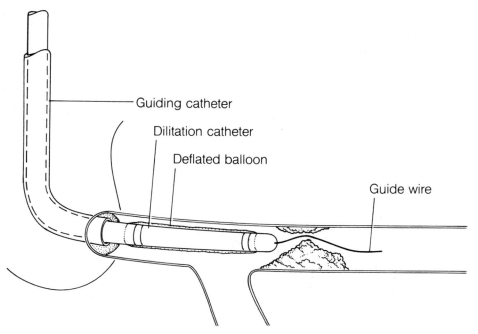

FIGURE 9-33
Cross-sectional view of the balloon dilatation catheter within the guiding catheter proximal to a stenosis. (Reprinted with permission of Advanced Cardiovascular Systems [ACS] Inc, Mountain View, CA)

allow the balloon to pass across, and (5) lack of experience or expertise or both on the part of the cardiologist.[31]

Arteriography after successful angioplasty demonstrates an immediate increase in the intraluminal diameter of the involved vessel (Fig. 9-37). A decrease in transstenotic gradient results from the increase in luminal diameter followed by increased blood flow through the dilated segment to the previously ischemic myocardium. Clinical improvement of the patient is demonstrated by improved or normalized myocardial perfusion deficits as shown by comparison of a post-PTCA thallium stress image to the pre-PTCA stress image. Postangioplasty treadmill test results compared with the preprocedure test results reveal increased exercise endurance and a decrease in exercise-induced chest pain.

NURSING RESPONSIBILITIES DURING PTCA

During the preparation for angioplasty and throughout the procedure, the nurses in the cardiac catheterization laboratory are responsible for understanding all aspects of equipment use and patient care. They should be experienced in advanced life support and knowledgeable about the proper administration of emergency medications and the correct application of emergency equipment, including the defibrillator, the ventilator, and the pacemaker. They should observe and communicate with the patient intermittently and report any changes in patient status to the physician. The nurse monitors the ECG and arterial pressure scopes constantly and is aware of changes in tracing that may accompany the administration of drugs, symptoms of ischemia, or chest pain. The nurse must recognize signs and symptoms of contrast sensitivity, such as urticaria, blushing, anxiety, nausea, and laryngospasm. The nurse should understand the proper assembly and use of all angioplasty equipment and should be able to "troubleshoot" any malfunction that might arise.

After the PTCA is complete, the nurse instructs the patient in the precautions necessary to prevent bleeding from the puncture site. These include the following:

- Six to 8 hours of bed rest
- Maintenance of the involved leg in a straight position (for Judkins technique)
- Avoidance of the upright position
- Avoidance of vigorous use of the abdominal muscles, as in coughing, sneezing, or moving the bowels

The patient is then transferred to a telemetry unit where he can be observed closely for possible complications requiring immediate action.

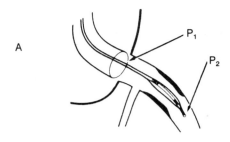

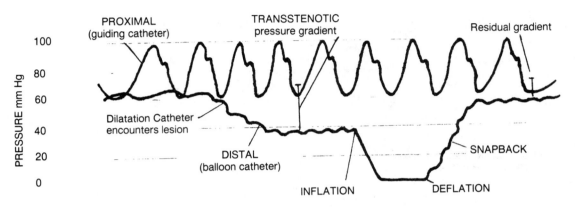

FIGURE 9-34

(A) *Positions at which transstenotic pressure gradients are recorded. P₁ represents the arterial pressure recorded at the guiding catheter ostium proximal to the stenosis, and P₂ represents coronary arterial pressure recorded at the balloon dilatation catheter ostium distal to the stenosis.* (B) *Recording of transstenotic pressure gradients. (Reprinted with permission of Advanced Cardiovascular Systems [ACS] Inc, Mountain View, CA)*

MECHANISMS OF ACTION

Understanding of the mechanisms of action of PTCA is currently based on postulations by various investigators. The process that leads to successful dilatation is complex and is not clearly defined; further research will be necessary before a consensus on an exhaustive definition can be reached. Studies of human cadavers, on which much current postulation is based, have indicated that PTCA initially traumatizes the dilated arterial segment. "Transluminal angioplasty produces endothelial desquamation and shearing of superficial plaque elements in all areas where the angioplasty balloon is inflated. Some plaque compression may occur."[32] Where the vessel is moderately stenosed, intimal healing and reendothelialization lead to a larger vessel lumen by 1 to 2 weeks after PTCA. With tightly stenosed vessels, in which there is considerable disparity in size between the stenosed lumen and the inflated balloon, splits occur in the atheromatous plaque and occasionally in the internal elastic membrane. This controlled trauma to the stenosis immedi-ately increases lumen size. The trauma to the dilatation site is visible fluoroscopically as a hazy arteriographic appearance and as filling defects that seem to arise when contrast fills in the splits in the plaque during postdilatation arteriography. "As fibrosis and healing occur, retraction and endothelialization of the separated intimal flaps further enlarge the lumen and smooth its inner contour in 2 to 3 weeks after the procedure."[33]

RESULTS

The latest report from the PTCA Registry Data Coordinating Center (National Heart, Lung, and Blood Institute, 1983) indicates a 61% primary success rate, a 6% rate of complications requiring emergency surgery, a 5% rate of myocardial infarction, and a 0.9% rate of mortality.[34] These data reflect clinical practice at over 100 sites and may be skewed by results reported by angiographers with inadequate experience or skills in

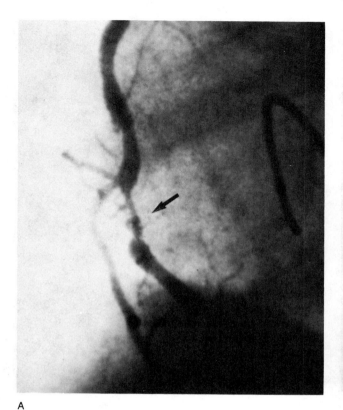
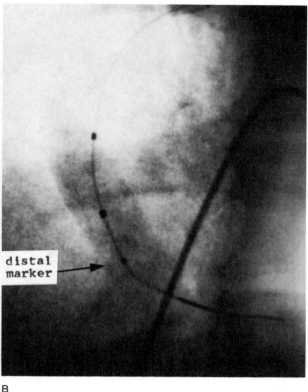

A   B

FIGURE 9-35
Thirty-five–spot frames showing (A) *stenosis involving the midright coronary artery (RCA), and* (B) *the first and second radiopaque markers revealing the position of the dilatation balloon across the stenosis, with the distal marker referring to the tip of the catheter beyond the narrowing. (Courtesy of John B Simpson, MD)*

PTCA. By contrast, it is instructive to examine these rates in 114 PTCA procedures performed during September, 1983, at Emory University Hospital by Gruentzig, a pioneer in and expert practitioner of angioplasty. Of 114 cases treated, 109 (96%) were successfully dilated and 5 (4%) were failures, and there were no myocardial infarctions or emergency bypass surgeries.[35] These rates reflect the current potential of coronary angioplasty in a specialized center with highly skilled practitioners.

COMPLICATIONS

Three basic factors increase the incidence of complications in patients undergoing angioplasty: (1) lack of experience and consequent lack of mastery of PTCA technique on the part of the physician; (2) the presence of unstable angina pectoris, which significantly increases nonfatal complications; and (3) severely stenotic lesions occluding more than 90% of the coronary artery. Prior coronary bypass surgery is the only

major factor that has been shown to influence significantly the rate of mortality in PTCA patients. A second CABG is technically more difficult and, when performed on PTCA patients as an emergency procedure, is associated with greater morbidity and mortality.[36] This result is anticipated because initial CABG causes damage such as scarring, adhesions, and accelerated aging of the heart and vessel tissue, which increase the risk of severe bleeding upon a second surgery.

Complications from angioplasty can occur during the procedure or even after it is completed. Thus, close observation and monitoring of the patient are imperative after successful PTCA. Major complications that can result in ischemia and possible severe left ventricular dysfunction necessitating emergency surgery include (1) angina unrelieved by maximal administration of nitrates and calcium channel blockers (see Table 9-7), (2) myocardial infarction, (3) coronary artery spasm, and (4) coronary artery dissection leading to occlusion.

Normally, angina is an anticipated complication during coronary angioplasty due to the temporary oc-

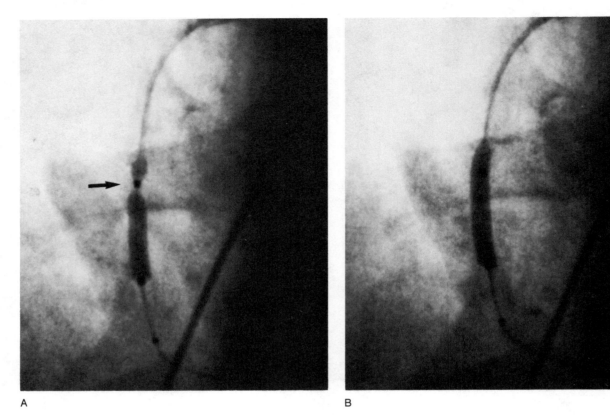

A   B

FIGURE 9-36
Thirty-five–spot frames showing (A) *inflation of the balloon revealing the position of the
stenosis by the "dumbbell" effect, and* (B) *absence of stenosis after dilatation. (Courtesy of
John B Simpson, MD)*

clusion of the involved vessel during dilatation. Such
incidence of angina is handled with intracoronary nitroglycerin or removal of the dilatation balloon as
needed. Evidence of persistent chest pain after PTCA,
reflected in changes in heart rate and blood pressure
and elevated S–T segments, indicates ischemia predisposing to an insult to the myocardium and requiring immediate intervention.

Coronary artery dissection or an intimal tear in the
inner lining of the artery can be visualized in the form
of intraluminal filling defects or extraluminal extrava-
sation of contrast material. Mild interruptions in the
intraluminal wall are an expected result of the splitting
and stretching of the intima upon inflation of the dilatation balloon at the lesion site. Therefore, in the absence of adverse effects early after PTCA, angiograph-
ically apparent dissection does not usually represent a
major complication. However, a dissection may sometimes cause a major luminal obstruction associated
with coronary artery occlusion, leading to a deterioration in blood flow with resultant severe ischemia or
myocardial infarction that requires emergency bypass
surgery.[37]

Coronary artery spasm also requires surgical inter-

vention when the vasoconstriction, occlusion, and ischemia cannot be reversed through the administration
of nitrates.

Other major complications of PTCA requiring medical intervention are (1) bradycardia, which requires
temporary pacing; (2) ventricular tachycardia or ventricular fibrillation, which require immediate defibrillation; and (3) a central nervous system event causing
transient or persistent neurologic deficit.

Peripheral vascular complications occurring primarily at the catheter site include (1) arterial thrombosis,
(2) excessive bleeding that causes a significant hematoma, (3) pseudoaneurysm, (4) femoral arteriovenous
fistula, and (5) arterial laceration. If any of these complications persists or compromises distal blood flow to
the involved extremity, surgical intervention may be
required.

Restenosis of a dilated lesion occurs in about 30% of
PTCA cases, with greater frequency in the first 5
months after angioplasty. According to the NHLBI
PTCA Registry (1983), the basic factors associated with
increased incidence of restenosis are (1) male sex, (2)
PTCA of a bypass graft, (3) severe pre-PTCA angina,
and (4) no history of a prior myocardial infarction.[38]

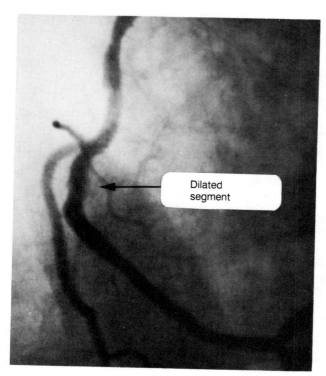

FIGURE 9-37
Repeat angiography after PTCA of a right coronary artery stenosis showing increased flow and increased diameter of the dilated segment. (Courtesy of John B Simpson, MD)

Because a great deal of variability exists in the data collected thus far, and many other factors have been proposed, further research will be necessary to define clearly the common characteristics of patients who restenose.

If a patient undergoes repeat angioplasty of a previously involved artery, the primary success rate increases to 98%, the complication rate decreases from 15% to 8%, and the possibility of emergency surgery decreases from 5% initially to 1%.[39] Thus, since the success rate increases and the rate of complication decreases, PTCA would be the indicated mode of therapy for recurrent stenosis in selected patients.

Table 9-6 is a summary of complications that may result from PTCA, including general signs of the complications and possible interventional actions.

NURSING ASSESSMENT AND INTERVENTIONS POST PTCA

Once the patient has returned to the coronary care or telemetry unit, the nurse plays an important role in observing and assessing his recovery. Postangioplasty care is designed to monitor the patient closely for signs and symptoms of myocardial ischemia. The most overt symptom of a possible complication—early recurrence of angina pectoris after PTCA—requires swift nursing action.

As soon as possible upon receiving the patient from the cardiac catheterization lab, the nurse should attach him to the ECG monitor, which allows a quick initial cardiac assessment and establishes a baseline to refer to if the patient's condition should change suddenly. While the patient is transferred from the gurney to the bed, the nurse should assess his status from head to toe, noting the overall skin color and temperature and carefully observing the level of consciousness. After the patient is transferred to the bed and attached to the monitor, the nurse should listen closely to the heart and breath sounds. The nurse should evaluate the peripheral circulation by noting peripheral skin color and temperature and the presence and quality of dorsalis pedis and/or posterior tibialis pulses in the limbs.

Because the Judkins technique is most often used in PTCA to access the vasculature, most patients will have an entry port in either the right or the left groin through which sheaths will have been placed percutaneously in a vein and artery to allow catheterization. (If the Sones technique was used, there will be an arterial catheter in the brachial area [Fig. 9-30]). The sheaths are not removed immediately after PTCA because the patient was anticoagulated at the start of the procedure to avoid complications of clot formation; consequently, the effects of the warfarin or heparin are not reversed but allowed to dissipate naturally, over 3 to 4 hours. The nurse should pay careful attention to the area distal to the puncture site, checking pulses frequently and reporting to the physician immediately any changes that may indicate clotting. Bleeding at the sheath site may result in a major hematoma that can require surgical evacuation or compromise distal blood flow to the lower extremity. To prevent excessive bleeding and to aid hemostasis, the physician may order a 5-pound sandbag placed over the puncture site.

The nurse should impress on the patient the importance of keeping the involved leg straight and the head of the bed angled up no more than 45°. To prevent clotting within the lumens of the introducing sheaths, an intravenous infusion is attached to the venous sheath, and a pressurized arterial flush is attached to the arterial line. This arrangement also ensures patency should an immediate return to the cardiac catheterization laboratory be necessary because of a complication. The physician chooses both the type of solution infused (via the venous sheath) and the rate of infusion, which depends on the patient's fluid volume state.

Initial post-PTCA laboratory blood tests should include (1) prothrombin time, to assess the patient's coagulability; (2) cardiac enzymes, with particular at-

TABLE 9-6
COMPLICATIONS OF PTCA

Complications	General Signs/Symptoms	Possible Interventions

Prolonged angina
Myocardial Infarction
 	
Coronary occlusion
Dissection/intimal tear
 	
Hypotension
Coronary branch injury
Coronary embolism
	Angina pectoris
	Arrhythmias: tachycardia,
	  bradycardia, V-tach/V-fib
	Marked hypotension
	Acute ECG changes (S–T
	  segment change)
	Nausea/vomiting
	Pallor
	Restlessness
	Cardiac/respiratory arrest
		CABG
		Redo PTCA
		Oxygen
		Medications:
		  vasodilators-(nitrates),
		  calcium-channel
		  blockers, analgesics,
		  anticoagulants,
		  vasopressors
		Complete bedrest
		Increase IV fluid volume
		  within patient tolerance

Marked change in heart
  rate: bradycardia,
  ventricular tachycardia,
  ventricular fibrillation
	HR below 60/minute
	HR above 250/minute
	No discernible cardiac
	  rhythm
	Pallor
	Loss of consciousness
	Hypotension
		Temporary pacemaker
		Defibrillation
		Medications:
		  antiarrhythmics,
		  vasopressors

Vascular: Excessive blood
  loss
	Hypotension
	Decreased urine output
	  (from hypovolemia)
	Decreased H & H
	  (hemoglobin/
	  hematocrit)
	Pallor
	Hematoma at puncture site
		Possible surgical repair
		Fluids
		Transfusion
		Oxygen
		
		Flat in bed or in
		  Trendelenburg's position

Allergic	Hypotension, urticaria,
	  nausea/vomiting, hives,
	  laryngospasm, erythema,
	  shortness of breath
		Medications:
		  antihistamines, steroids,
		  antiemetics
		Clear liquids/NPO
		Oxygen
		With anaphylaxis: fluids for
		  volume expansion,
		  epinephrine, vasopressors
		  for hypotension

Central nervous system
  events
	Changes in level of
	  consciousness
	Hemiparesis
	Hypoventilation/respiratory
	  depression
		Oxygen
		
		Discontinue/hold sedatives

Miscellaneous complications: Conduction defects, pulmonary embolism, pulmonary
  edema, coronary air embolism, respiratory arrest, febrile episode, nausea, minor bleeding

tention to CPK and CPK isoenzymes; and (3) serum electrolytes. Elevation of the cardiac enzymes can indicate that a silent myocardial infarction has occurred (*i.e.,* infarction unannounced by prolonged chest pain). If an abnormal cardiac enzyme laboratory value appears, the nurse should immediately notify the physician because the patient's postoperative care might need to be modified to prevent further injury.

The nurse plays a significant role in observing and assessing angina that recurs soon after PTCA. Any chest pain demands immediate and careful attention because it may indicate either the start of vasospasm or impending occlusion. The patient may describe angina as a burning, squeezing heaviness or as sharp midsternal pain. Other signs and symptoms of myocardial ischemia include (1) ischemic electrocardiographic changes (elevation of the S–T segments or T wave inversion), (2) arrhythmias, (3) hypotension, and (4) nausea. The nurse should immediately notify the physician of any such change in the patient's condition because it is impossible to tell merely by observation whether the change indicates a transient vasospastic episode, which can be resolved with vasodilation therapy, or an accute occlusion requiring emergency surgery.

If vasodilation therapy is indicated, it may be administered as described subsequently unless the patient is severely hypotensive; in that case, vasodilation is contraindicated. At the first sign of vasospasm, one must first give oxygen by mask or nasal cannula. For fast, temporary (and possibly permanent) relief, 0.4 mg of nitroglycerin, 5 mg of isosorbide, or 10 mg of nifedipine should be administered sublingually. The most effective method of vasodilation, an intravenous drip of nitroglycerin in dextrose and water (concentrations vary among institutions), should be set up while the aforementioned remedies are applied. This drip should be started and appropriately titrated to maintain a blood pressure adequate to ensure coronary artery perfusion and to alleviate chest pain.

In conjunction with the onset of the chest pain, a 12-lead electrocardiogram should be taken to record any acute changes. If the angina resolves and any acute ECG changes caused by medical therapy disappear, it is safe to assume that transient vasospastic episode occurred. However, if the angina continues and the ECG changes persist, redilatation or emergency bypass surgery should be considered.

If the postangioplasty course is uncomplicated, the sheaths are removed after 3 to 4 hours and a mild pressure dressing is applied to the site. The patient must continue complete bed rest for 6 to 8 hours after removal of the sheaths. A normal, low-sodium or low-cholesterol diet may be resumed, depending on the preference of the physician and the needs of the patient.

During the recovery period, the nurse can introduce the patient to the rehabilitation process, emphasizing ways to combat the advance of coronary artery disease. During this instruction, she should reinforce the importance of aerobic conditioning with regular, moderate exercise with reasonably paced increases. Also, she should explain that such abuses as frequent stress, excessive weight, and smoking promote CAD and that the patient has the power and responsibility to avoid these abuses by modifying his behavior.

As preventive therapy, the patient will, for 6 months after angioplasty, take medications that help prevent thrombus formation and maintain maximal dilatation at the angioplasty site. The patient is routinely sent home on aspirin; dipyridamole (Persantine), 75 mg given orally three times a day; or sulfinpyrazone (An-

turane), 200 mg given orally four times a day, for the antiplatelet effect, and a nitroglycerin patch (Nitro-Dur) or 5 mg of isosorbide (Isordil) for vasodilation. If it is suspected or has been documented during cardiac catheterization that the patient has experienced intermittent coronary artery spasm, he will be sent home on calcium-channel blockers, such as nifedipine (Procardia), 10 mg given three times a day for 2 weeks, or diltiazem (Cardizem), 30 mg given three times a day for 2 weeks. The nurse is ultimately responsible for explaining to the patient the indications for the specific medications ordered by the physician, including side effects and signs of overdose, and should answer any questions the patient may have regarding the follow-up care, making sure that all aspects are clearly understood.

Prior to the patient's discharge, an exercise treadmill stress test and a thallium rest-stress imaging study are done to test the efficacy of the PTCA. In comparison to the pre-PTCA tests, an increase in exercise capacity and a decrease in or disappearance of exercise-induced chest pain (without S–T segment changes) suggest improved blood flow and normalization of cardiac function to the previously hypoperfused muscle. Treadmill stress testing should be repeated at 1 month, 3 months, 6 months, and 1 year after angioplasty. Cardiac catheterization should be repeated 6 months after angioplasty unless it is indicated sooner, primarily by recurrent chest pain.

THE FUTURE OF CORONARY ANGIOPLASTY

If the rapid strides in improving PTCA technique and equipment continue in the future, the hope and the promise are that coronary angioplasty will replace bypass surgery in treating more and more patients with coronary artery disease. In France, current research includes inquiry into the value of laser therapy to treat CAD in conjunction with PTCA. By the late 1980s, we may witness another revolution in CAD treatment in which the laser and the balloon dilatation catheter together are applied to plaque-occluded arteries. By then, it may be standard treatment to use a microscopic laser beam to create an opening in a total occlusion, allowing insertion of an angioplastic catheter and inflation of its balloon.

Pharmacology has much to offer in treating angina pectoris due to CAD, and advances in this field have sometimes proved directly or indirectly helpful in bettering PTCA practice. For example, in the past, angina would have been treated with nitrates in the form of a nitropaste placed on the skin and absorbed over 3 to 4 hours for a continual vasodilation effect. This method was messy and inconvenient and at times led to inter-

TABLE 9-7
SUMMARY OF DRUGS MOST OFTEN ASSOCIATED WITH PTCA

Anticoagulants/Antiplatelets

Aspirin

Indications: Prophylaxis of coronary and cerebral arterial thrombus formation
Actions: Blocks platelet aggregation
Dosage: 100–200 mg qid
Adverse effects: Well tolerated. Nausea, vomiting, diarrhea, headache, and vertigo are seen occasionally.

Dextran (Rheomacrodex)

Indications/actions: Prevents venous thrombus/thromboembolism in high-risk patients
Dosage: 10–20 ml/kg of body weight (for shock). Total daily dose not to exceed 20 ml/kg
Adverse effects:

1. Hypersensitivity, nausea, vomiting, acute hypotension
2. Increased bleeding time due to interference with platelet function (may not appear until 6–9 hours after infusion)
3. Acute tubular failure when renal flow is decreased owing to increased viscosity and specific gravity

Dipyridamole (Persantine)

Indications

1. Angina pectoris
2. Prophylaxis in thromboembolic disease by decreasing platelet aggregation

Actions: Primarily affects the small resistance vessels of the coronary bed
Dosage: 25–75 mg tid
Adverse effects: Well tolerated. Nausea, vomiting, diarrhea, headache, and vertigo are seen occasionally.

Heparin

Indications: An anticoagulant used in prophylactic treatment of coronary occlusion with acute myocardial infarction and in
   prophylaxis of peripheral arterial embolism
Actions: Inhibits clotting of blood and formation of fibrin clots. Inactivates thrombin, preventing conversion of fibrinogen to
   fibrin. Also prevents formation of a stable fibrin clot by inhibiting the activation of fibrin stabilizing factor. Inhibits
   reactions that lead to clotting but does not alter normal components of blood. Prolongs clotting time but does not affect
   bleeding time. Does not lyse clots.
Dosage: Varies with indications. IV or IA: 10,000 units at start of PTCA
Adverse effects: Uncontrollable bleeding, hypersensitivity

Sulfinpyrazone (Anturane)

Indications: Prophylaxis in thromboembolic disease
Actions: Blocks platelet aggregation
Dosage: 100–200 mg qid
Adverse effects: GI irritation (lessened if taken in divided doses with meals), hypersensitivity (rash and fever), blood dyscrasias

Coronary Vasodilators

Isosorbide Dinitrate (Isordil, Sorbitrate)

Indications: Prophylaxis of angina
Actions: A nitrate that acts as a smooth muscle relaxant. Causes coronary vasodilation without increasing myocardial oxygen
   consumption. Secondary to general vasodilation, blood pressure decreases.
Dosage:

1. Sublingual: 2.5–10 mg q2–3 hours prn angina
2. Oral: 5–30 mg qid
3. Sustained-action oral: 40 mg q6–12 hours

Adverse effects:

1. Cutaneous vasodilation that can cause flushing
2. Headache, transient dizziness, and weakness
3. Excessive hypotension

Nitroglycerin

Indications: Control of blood pressure and angina pectoris
Actions: Potent vasodilator that affects primarily the venous system. Selectively dilates large coronary arteries increasing blood
   flow to ischemic subendocardium.
Dosage:

1. Sublingual: 0.3–0.4 mg prn chest pain
2. Topical (patch): 2.5–10 mg/day. Indicated for primary, secondary, or nocturnal angina owing to more sustained effect.
3. IV: 5 mcg/minute to start—titrate to patient response. (No fixed dose owing to variable response in different patients.)

TABLE 9-7
(Continued)

Nitroglycerin

Adverse effects:

1. Excessive and prolonged hypotension
2. Headache
3. Tachycardia, palpitations
4. Nausea, vomiting, apprehension
5. Retrosternal discomfort

Calcium-Channel Blockers

Nifedipine, Diltiazem
Indications:

1. Angina pectoris due to coronary artery spasm and chronic stable angina
2. Hypertension (investigational)
3. Arrhythmias

Actions: Inhibits calcium ion flux across the cell membrane of the cardiac muscle and vascular smooth muscle without changing serum calcium concentration. Decreases afterload through peripheral arterial dilatation and

1. Reduces systemic and pulmonary vascular resistance
2. Vasodilates coronary circulation
3. Decreases myocardial oxygen demands and increases myocardial oxygen supply

Dosage:

1. Nifedipine (Procardia): 10 mg tid
2. Diltiazem (Cardizem): 30 mg tid

Adverse effects:

1. Contraindicated in patients with sick sinus syndrome
2. Hypotension after IV use
3. GI distress
4. Headache, vertigo, flushing
5. Peripheral edema, occasional increase in angina, tachycardia

rupted dosage. Now nitrates are administered in the form of a disc (Nitro-Dur) that lasts 24 hours before it must be replaced. Similarly, calcium-blocking agents have evolved, improving the treatment of angina pectoris. Table 9-7 is a summary of drugs currently associated with PTCA. future progress in pharmacology may make available still more potent intracoronary vasodilators, which would help sustain patency and thus favorably influence the PTCA success rate.

Lastly, the future may bring a broad shift in emphasis to the early detection, prevention, and treatment of coronary artery disease. CAD is a process that develops over many years, mainly in persons ranging in age from 40 to 60 years. Currently, treatment is begun only when a patient has symptoms of ischemia. Gruentzig, the inventor of coronary angioplasty, believes that PTCA should be applied as early as possible, when a patient is still in the single vessel disease stage, and repeated at intervals throughout life.[40] He states that it is important to identify at an early stage patients who will likely develop single and double vessel disease in

30 to 50 years. Early on we should ask, could this patient be developing CAD? If the answer is *yes,* angioplasty should be considered preventive therapy that might avert the development of one of the leading causes of death in the United States. "Today's patient requiring bypass surgery for multivessel disease may give way to tomorrow's patient with serial angioplasties over several decades for single- or double-vessel disease in multiple vessels."[41]

REFERENCES

1. McCarty CL: Percutaneous transluminal coronary angioplasty: Therapeutic intervention in the cardiac catheterization Lab. Heart Lung 11, No. 6:499, 1982
2. Hall D, Gruentzig AR: Percutaneous transluminal coronary angioplasty: Current procedure and future direction. Am J Roentgenol 142:13, 1984
3. Gruentzig Dilaca Coronary Balloon Dilatation Catheter, p 1. USCI Cardiology & Radiology Products, Division of CR Bard, Inc. Box 566, Billerica, MA, 01821
4. Dorros G, Cowley MJ, Simpson J et al: Percutaneous translu-

minal coronary angioplasty: Report of complications from the National Heart, Lung, and Blood Institute PTCA Registry. Circulation 67, No. 4:726, 1983

5. McAuley BJ, Sheehan DJ, Simpson JB: Use of a low profile steerable dilatation catheter for percutaneous transluminal coronary angioplasty. Unpublished paper, 1984

6. Bailey K, Erman J, Marks D et al: Percutaneous transluminal coronary angioplasty: An alternative to coronary artery bypass surgery. Unpublished paper, 1983

7. Gruentzig AR, Collins JJ: Controversies in cardiology, proposed: Angioplasty should be utilized in double vessel and triple vessel coronary disease. Hosp Prac 17, No. 9: 152, 1982

8. Bailey K, Erman J, Marks D et al: Op cit

9. Gruentzig AR: Results from coronary angioplasty and implications for the future. Am Heart J 103:779–783, 1982

10. Baily K, Erman J, Marks D et al: Op cit

11. Hall D, Gruentzig AR: Op cit, p 16

12. Jang GC, Block PC, Cowley MJ et al: Comparative cost analysis of coronary angioplasty and coronary bypass surgery: Results from a national cooperative study (abstr), Circulation (suppl II) 66:II-124, 1982

13. Hall D, Gruentzig AR: Op cit, p 15

14. Ibid

15. Ibid

16. Simpson JB: Multivessel PTCA, 1983. Presented at the Conference on Guidewires in Coronary Angioplasty, Canada College, Redwood City, CA, August, 1983

17. Ischinger T, Gruentzig AR, Hollman J et al: Should coronary arteries with less than 60% diameter stenosis be treated by angioplasty? Circulation 68, No. 1:153, 1983

18. Ford WB, Wholey MH, Zikria EA et al: Percutaneous transluminal dilation of aorotocoronary saphenous vein bypass grafts. Chest 79, No. 5:529, 1981

19. Ibid, p 534

20. Williams DO, Gruentzig AR, Kent KM et al: Guidelines for the performance of percutaneous transluminal coronary angioplasty. Circulation 66, No. 4:694, 1982

21. Judkins MP: Percutaneous transfemoral selective coronary arteriography. Radiol Clin North Am 6:467–497, 1968

22. Amplatz K, Formanek G, Stanger P et al: Mechanics of selective coronary artery catheterization via femoral approach. Radiology 69:1040–1047, 1967

23. Simpson JB, Baim DS, Robert EW et al: A new catheter system for percutaneous transluminal coronary angioplasty. Am J Cardiol 49:1216–1222, 1982

24. McAuley BJ, Sheehan DJ, Simpson JB: Op cit

25. Judkins MP: Op cit

26. Sones FM, Shirey EK, Proudfoot WL et al: Cine coronary arteriography. Circulation 20:773, 1959

27. Simpson JB, Baims DS, Robert EW et al: Op cit

28. Ibid, p 1220

29. Ibid

30. Ibid

31. McCarty CL: Op cit, p 502

32. Block PC: Percutaneous transluminal coronary angioplasty. Am J Roentgenol 135, No. 5: 958–959, 1980

33. Ibid

34. Hall D, Gruentzig AR: Op cit, p 15

35. Ibid

36. Dorros G, Cowley MJ, Simpson J et al: Op cit, p 729

37. Ibid, p 724

38. Holmes P, Vlietstra R, Smith H et al: Restenosis following PTCA: A report from the NHLBI PTCA Registry. Circulation 68, No. 4, 1983. Quotation from abstract No. 379, Abstracts of the 56th Scientific Sessions, p III-95

39. Meier B, King SB III, Gruentzig AR et al: Repeat coronary angioplasty. Circulation 68, No. 4, 1983. Quotation from abstract No. 381, Abstracts of the 56th Scientific Sessions, p III-96

40. Gruentzig AR, Collins JJ: Op cit, p 147

41. Hall D, Gruentzig AR: Op cit, p 16

BIBLIOGRAPHY

The ACS Simpson-Robert Vascular Dilatation System for Percutaneous Transluminal Coronary Angioplasty. Advanced Cardiovascular Systems (ACS), Inc, 1500 Salado Drive, Suite 101, Mountain View, CA 94043

Amplatz K, Formanek G, Stanger P, Wilson W: Mechanics of Selective Coronary Artery Catheterization via Femoral Approach. Radiology 69:1040–1047, 1967

Bailey K, Erman J, Marks D, Smith J: Percutaneous transluminal coronary angioplasty: An alternative to coronary artery bypass surgery. Unpublished paper, 1983

Block PC: Percutaneous transluminal coronary angioplasty. Am J Roentgenol 135, No. 5:955–959, 1980

Cowley MJ, Vetrovec GW, Wolfgang TC: Efficacy of percutaneous transluminal coronary angioplasty: Technique, patient selection, salutary results, limitations and complications. Am Heart J 101, No. 3:272–280, 1981

Dorros G, Cowley MJ, Simpson JB et al: Percutaneous transluminal coronary angioplasty: Report of complications from the National Heart, Lung, and Blood Institute PTCA Registry. Circulation 67, No. 4:723–730, 1983

Ford WB, Wholey MH, Zikria EA, et al: Percutaneous transluminal dilation of aorotocoronary saphenous vein bypass grafts. Chest 79, No. 5:529–535, 1981

Ford WB, Wholey MH, Zikria EA et al: Percutaneous transluminal angioplasty in the management of occlusive disease involving the coronary arteries and saphenous vein bypass grafts. J Thoracic Cardiovasc Surg 79, No. 1:1–11, 1980

Galan K, Gruentzig AR: Significance of early chest pain after coronary angioplasty (abstr). Circulation (Part II) 68, No. 4:III-291, 1983

Gruentzig AR: Results from coronary angioplasty and implications for the future. Am Heart J 103:779–783, 1982

Gruentzig AR, Collins JJ: Controversies in cardiology, proposed: Angioplasty should be utilized in double-vessel and triple-vessel coronary disease. Hosp Pract 17, No. 9:143–155, 1982

Gruentzig Dilaca Coronary Balloon Dilatation Catheter. Pamphlet by USCI Cardiology and Radiology Products, Division of CR Bard, Inc, PO Box 566, Billerica, MA, 01821

Gunby P: Future seems promising for coronary angioplasty. JAMA 251, No. 3:302, 1984

Hall D, Gruentzig AR: Percutaneous transluminal coronary angioplasty: Current procedure and future direction. Am J Roentgenol 142, No. 1:13–16, 1984

Holmes D, Vlietstra R, Smith H, et al: Restenosis following PTCA: A report from the NHLBI PTCA Registry (abstr). Circulation (Part II) 68, No. 4:III-95, 1983

Ischinger T, Gruentzig A, Hollman J et al: Should coronary arteries with less than 60% diameter stenosis be treated by angioplasty? Circulation 68, No. 1:148–154, 1983

Jang GC, Block PC, Cowley MJ et al: Comparative cost analysis of coronary angioplasty and coronary bypass surgery: Results from a national cooperative study (abstr). Circulation (suppl II) 66:II-124, 1982

Judkins MP: Percutaneous transfemoral selective coronary arteriography. Radiol Clin North Am 6:467–497, 1968

McAuley BJ, Sheehan DJ, Simpson JB: Use of a low profile steerable dilatation catheter for percutaneous transluminal coronary angioplasty. Unpublished paper, 1984

McCarty CL: Percutaneous transluminal coronary angioplasty: Therapeutic intervention in the cardiac catheterization lab. Heart Lung 11, No. 6:499–504, 1982

Meier B, King SB III, Gruentzig AR et al: Repeat coronary angioplasty (abstr). Circulation 68, No. 4:III-96, 1983

Meyer J, Schmitz H, Erbel R et al: Treatment of unstable angina pectoris with percutaneous transluminal coronary angioplasty (PTCA). Cathet Cardiovasc Diag 7, No. 4:361–371, 1981

Meyer J, Merx W, Schmitz H et al: Percutaneous transluminal angioplasty immediately after intracoronary streptolysis of transmural infarction. Circulation 66, No. 5:905–913, 1982

Partridge SA: The nurse's role in percutaneous transluminal coronary angioplasty. Heart Lung 11, No. 6:505–511, 1982

Pluth J: Balloon angioplasty in multivessel coronary artery disease. Mayo Clin Proc 58:624–625, 1983

Simpson JB: Multivessel PTCA, 1983. Presented at the Conference on Guidewires in Coronary Angioplasty, Canada College, Redwood City, CA, August, 1983

Simpson JB, Baim DS, Robert EV, Harrison, DC: A new catheter system for percutaneous transluminal coronary angioplasty. Am J Cardiol 49:1216–1222, 1982

Sones FM, Shirey EK, Proudfit WL, Wescott RN: Cine coronary arteriography. Circulation 20:773, 1959

Williams DO, Gruentzig AR, Kent KM et al: Guidelines for the performance of percutaneous transluminal coronary angioplasty. Circulation 66, No. 4:693–694, 1982

Intra-Aortic Balloon Pump Counterpulsation

Julie A. Shinn

Prior to the advent of critical care units, cardiac patients frequently died as a result of arrhythmias following acute myocardial infarction. Critical care units, offering continuous ECG monitoring, effectively reduced mortality due to arrhythmias by early detection and treatment. Acute left ventricular power failure, resulting in cardiogenic shock, emerged as a major cause of death following myocardial infarction. Since the 1960s, research emphasis and clinical therapy have been directed toward minimizing or preventing myocardial infarct extension and acute left ventricular power failure. Mortality rates ranged from 80% to 100% in patients suffering from cardiogenic shock. Invasive hemodynamic monitoring, diuretic agents, and vasoactive and inotropic drugs offered little assistance in decreasing mortality. Similar problems were encountered as cardiac surgery became more sophisticated and more complex surgery was performed. Among its complications was the development of acute left ventricular power failure, resulting in an inability to wean patients from cardiopulmonary bypass.

Therapeutic goals were directed toward (1) increasing oxygen supply to the myocardium, (2) decreasing left ventricular work, and (3) improving cardiac output. Prior to intra-aortic balloon pumping (IABP), no one therapeutic agent was capable of meeting these three goals.

IABP counterpulsation was designed to increase coronary artery perfusion pressure and blood flow during the diastolic phase of the cardiac cycle by inflation of a balloon in the thoracic aorta. Deflation of the balloon, just prior to systolic ejection, was designed to decrease the impedance to ejection and thus left ventricular work. Inflation and deflation counterpulsated each heart beat. With improved blood flow and effective reduction in left ventricular work, the hoped for results were improved myocardial pump function and increased cardiac output.

IABP was first introduced clinically by Kantrowitz and associates in 1967. This therapeutic approach was instituted for treatment of two patients with left ventricular power failure following acute myocardial infarction. Since that time, IABP has become a standard treatment for medical and surgical patients with acute left ventricular power failure that is unresponsive to pharmacologic and volume therapy.

DESCRIPTION

The intra-aortic balloon catheter is constructed of a biocompatible polyurethane material. Polyurethane is also used to make the balloon that is mounted on the end of the catheter. Filling of the balloon is achieved with pressurized gas that enters through small perforations in the catheter. There are several configurations of balloons available, one model having two chambers and the others having single chambers (Fig. 9-38). Inflation patterns differ in that some inflate from one end to the other, whereas some inflate from the center. Types of balloons used are determined by physician preference and the type of equipment used to drive the balloon pump catheter. It is felt that configuration of the balloon may affect performance characteristics. However, it is not the purpose of this text to advocate any one particular model.

Proper position of the balloon is in the thoracic aorta just distal to the left subclavian artery and proximal to the renal arteries (Fig. 9-39). Insertion of the catheter is achieved through a dacron graft that has been anastomosed to either a femoral or iliac artery. The catheter is advanced until proper position has been achieved. End-to-side anastomosis of the graft to the artery allows for proper securing of the catheter without obliteration of blood flow to the extremity. Suture is used around the graft to secure the catheter in position so that it will not slip out of the artery. Saphenous vein

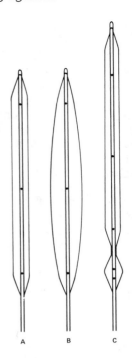

FIGURE 9-38
Balloon configurations include (A) *cylindrical shape,* (B) *fusiform shape, and* (C) *dual chamber.*

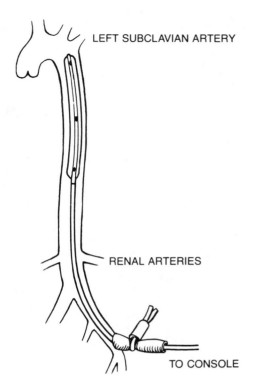

LEFT SUBCLAVIAN ARTERY

RENAL ARTERIES

TO CONSOLE

FIGURE 9-39
Proper position of the balloon catheter illustrating exit site through a dacron graft.

may also be used for the graft. In some selected patients with healthy vascular tissue, a purse string suture may be run through the adventicial layer of the artery to secure the catheter. In this situation, a graft is not necessary. One type of catheter allows for percutaneous insertion using a Seldinger technique. Currently, the majority of physicians use a temporary graft for insertion. Other approaches have been described. The most common alternative used is direct insertion into the thoracic aorta. Because this requires a throacotomy incision, it is essentially restricted to use in cardiac surgery patients.

Once in place, the catheter is attached to a machine console that has three basic components: (1) a monitoring system, (2) an electronic trigger mechanism, and (3) a drive system that moves gas in and out of the balloon. Monitoring systems have the capability of displaying the patient's ECG, an arterial waveform showing the effect of balloon inflation/deflation, and a balloon waveform that illustrates the inflation and deflation of the balloon itself. The standard trigger mechanism for the balloon pump is the R wave that is sensed from the patient's ECG. This trigger will cause the balloon to inflate with each cardiac cycle. Adjustment of exact timing is controlled on the console of the machine. Precise timing will be discussed later. The drive system is the actual mechanism that drives gas into and out of the balloon by alternating pressure

and vacuum. Each machine must have pressurized tanks of either helium or carbon dioxide to drive the balloon.

Prior to discussing the actual timing of balloon inflation and deflation, we will examine the physiologic principles of IABP.

PHYSIOLOGIC PRINCIPLES

In the failing heart, greater work is required to maintain cardiac output. With this added work requirement, oxygen demand increases. This may occur at a time when the myocardium is already ischemic and coronary artery perfusion is unable to meet the oxygen demands. As a result, left ventricular performance diminishes even further, resulting in decreased cardiac output. A vicious cycle ensues that is difficult to interrupt (Fig. 9-40). Without interruption of the cycle, cardiogenic shock may be imminent. This cycle can be broken with IABP by increasing aortic root pressure during diastole through inflation of the balloon. With increased aortic root pressure, the perfusion pressure of the coronary arteries will be increased.

Effective therapy for the patient in left ventricular power failure also involves decreasing myocardial ox-

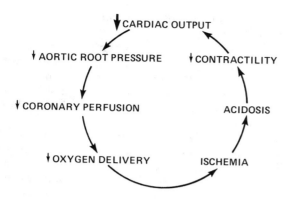

FIGURE 9-40
Cycle leading to cardiogenic shock.

ygen demand. Four major determinants of myocardial oxygen demand are (1) afterload, (2) preload, (3) contractility, and (4) heart rate. IABP can have an effect on all these factors. It will directly decrease afterload and will indirectly affect the other three determinants as cardiac function improves.

Afterload. This is the amount of wall tension that must be generated by the ventricle to raise intraventricular pressure, allowing the ventricle to overcome impedance to ejection. When adequate intraventricular pressure is reached, the semilunar valve is forced open and ejection occurs. This occurs in either ventricle. Because IABP assists the left heart, only the left ventricle will be discussed. Impedance to ejection is a result of the aortic valve, aortic end-diastolic pressure, and vascular resistance. With greater impedance, afterload increases, and thus more oxygen is demanded by the ventricle for energy. The aortic valve is a factor that does not change unless stenosis, which increases afterload, is present. Greater aortic end-diastolic pressures require higher afterload to overcome this impedance to ejection. Vascular resistance will increase impedance when vessels become vasoconstricted. Vasodilation or lower vascular resistance will decrease impedance to ejection, and thus afterload decreases.

Deflation of the balloon in the aorta, just prior to ventricular systole, lowers aortic end-diastolic pressure, which decreases impedance. The greatest amount of oxygen required during the cardiac cycle is for the development of afterload. With decreased impedance, the workload of the ventricle also decreases. In this way, IABP can effectively decrease the oxygen demand of the heart.

Preload. This is the volume or pressure in the ventricle at end-diastole. Volume in a chamber creates pressure. A person in acute left ventricular power failure has increased volume in the ventricle at end-diastole

owing to the heart's inability to pump effectively. This excessive increase in preload also increases the workload of the heart. Clinically, preload of the right heart is measured by central venous pressure or right atrial pressure, and preload of the left heart is measured with the pulmonary capillary wedge pressure or left atrial pressure. These pressures increase when the ventricles are in failure.

IABP helps decrease excessive preload in the left ventricle by decreasing impedance to ejection. With decreased impedance, there is a more effective forward flow of blood. Preload is decreased, with more efficient emptying of the left ventricle during systole.

Contractility. This refers to the velocity of contraction during systole. With greater velocity, the workload of the heart is increased. Although contractility requires oxygen, good contractility is a benefit to cardiac function because it ensures good, efficient pumping, which serves to increase cardiac output. In failure, contractility is depressed. The biochemical status of the myocardium directly affects contractility. Contractility is depressed when calcium levels are low, when catecholamine levels are low, and when ischemia is present with resultant acidosis.

IABP can increase oxygen supply, thereby decreasing ischemia and acidosis. In this way, IABP contributes to improve contractility and better cardiac function (Fig. 9-40).

Heart Rate. This is a major determinant of oxygen demand because the rate determines the number of times per minute the high pressures must be generated during systole. Normally, myocardial perfusion takes place during diastole. Coronary artery perfusion pressure is determined by the gradient between aortic diastolic pressure and myocardial wall tension. It can be expressed by the following equation:

coronary perfusion pressure
    = aortic diastolic pressure
                         − myocardial wall tension

Tension in the muscle retards blood flow, which is why approximately 80% of coronary artery perfusion occurs during diastole. With faster heart rates, diastolic time becomes shortened, with very little change occurring in systolic time. A rapid heart rate not only increases oxygen demand but also decreases the time available for delivery of oxygen. In acute ventricular power failure, a person may not be able to maintain cardiac output by increasing the volume of blood pumped with each beat (stroke volume) because contractility is likely to be depressed. Cardiac output is a function of both stroke volume and heart rate.

cardiac output = stroke volume × heart rate

Direct Physiologic Effects of Intra-Aortic Balloon Pump (IABP)

Inflation: 1. ↑ aortic diastolic pressure
2. ↑ aortic root pressure
3. ↑ coronary perfusion pressure
4. ↑ oxygen supply

Deflation: 1. ↓ aortic end-diastolic pressure
2. ↓ impedance to ejection
3. ↓ afterload
4. ↓ oxygen demand

If stroke volume cannot be increased, heart rate must increase to maintain cardiac output. This is very costly in terms of oxygen demand.

By improving contractility, IABP helps improve myocardial pumping and the ability to increase stroke volume. Decreasing afterload also increases pumping efficiency. With improved myocardial function, heart rate will decrease. IABP will also increase coronary artery perfusion pressure by increasing aortic diastolic pressure during inflation of the balloon, resulting in improved blood flow and oxygen delivery to the myocardium.

Physiologic effects of IABP are summarized in the chart that follows. Proper inflation of the balloon will increase oxygen supply, and proper deflation of the balloon will decrease oxygen demand. Timing of inflation and deflation is crucial and must coincide with the cardiac cycle.

TIMING

Systole and diastole are the two major components of the cardiac cycle.

The first step to proper timing of the balloon pump is the identification of the beginning of systole and diastole on the arterial waveform. Every patient must have an arterial catheter in place to monitor timing. The cycle of the left heart will be used to describe the events of the cardiac cycle. Systole begins when left ventricular pressure exceeds left atrial pressure, forcing the mitral valve closed.

There are two phases to systole: (1) isovolumic contraction and (2) ejection. Once the mitral valve is closed, isovolumic contraction begins and continues until enough pressure is generated to overcome impedance to ejection. When ventricular pressure exceeds aortic pressure, the aortic valve is forced open, initiating ejection, or phase two. Ejection continues until pressure in the left ventricle falls below pressure in the aorta. At this point, the aortic valve closes and diastole begins.

Closing of the valve creates an artifact on the arterial waveform that is called the dicrotic notch. The dicrotic notch is used as a timing reference to determine when balloon inflation should occur. Inflation should not occur before the notch because systole has not been completed.

After aortic valve closure, two phases of diastole begin: (1) isovolumic relaxation and (2) ventricular filling. Following aortic valve closure, there is a period of time in which neither the aortic nor mitral valve is open. The mitral valve remains closed because left ventricular pressure is still higher than left atrial pressure. This phase is isovolumic relaxation. When left ventricular pressure falls below left atrial pressure, the mitral valve is forced open by the higher pressure in the left atrium. This begins the filling phase of diastole. Balloon inflation should continue throughout diastole. Deflation should be timed to occur at end-diastole, just prior to the next sharp systolic upstroke on the arterial waveform.

Figure 9-41 illustrates the cardiac cycle with left atrial, left ventricular, and aortic pressure superimposed on one another. Note the systolic upstroke seen on the aortic tracing and the appearance of the dicrotic notch.

Figure 9-42 illustrates a radial artery waveform with the beginning of systole and diastole marked. One can estimate the amount of time balloon inflation should last by knowing the patient's heart rate. Systole is roughly one third of the cardiac cycle, and diastole is approximately two thirds. Each R to R interval on the ECG represents one cardiac cycle. Heart rate per minute is actually the number of cardiac cycles per minute. With each minute equaling 60,000 msec, 60,000 msec

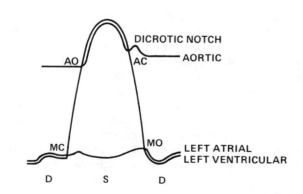

FIGURE 9-41
Cardiac cycle of the left heart with aortic, left ventricular, and left atrial pressure waveforms. (AO) aortic valve opening; (AC) aortic valve closure; (D) diastole; (MO) mitral valve opening; (MC) mitral valve closure; (S) systole.

Calculation of Inflation and Deflation Time for a Heart Rate of 60

msec in one R to R interval

$$= \frac{60,000 \text{ msec/min}}{\text{patient's heart rate (60 beats/min)}}$$

one R to R interval = 1000 msec
systole ($\frac{1}{3}$) ~ 400 msec
diastole ($\frac{2}{3}$) ~ 600 msec

---

divided by heart rate equals the total milliseconds in each cardiac cycle, or R to R interval. Approximately one third of the R to R interval will be systole, or the number of milliseconds the balloon is deflated, and two thirds will be diastole, or the balloon inflation interval. It is wise to add extra time to the deflation period until fine adjustment of the waveform can be made.

The accompanying chart outlines the steps taken to determine inflation and deflation time for a patient with a heart rate of 60. This method can be used as a guide for initial establishment of balloon pumping.

CONTRAINDICATIONS

Now that the principles of IABP have been outlined, it will be clear why IABP is advantageous in a variety of patients. Few contraindications are associated with its use.

A competent aortic valve is necessary if the patient is to benefit from IABP. With *aortic insufficiency,* balloon inflation would only increase aortic regurgitation and offer little, if any, augmentation of coronary artery perfusion pressure.

Severe peripheral vascular occlusive disease is also a contraindication to use of IABP. Occlusive disease would make insertion of the catheter quite difficult and possibly interrupt plaque formation along the vessel wall. In patients who absolutely require IABP, insertion can be achieved by way of the thoracic aorta, thus bypassing diseased peripheral vessels.

Any previous aortofemoral or aortoiliac *bypass graft* would also contraindicate femoral artery insertion.

The presence of an *aortic aneurysm* is also a contraindication to the use of IABP. A pulsating balloon against an aneurysm may predispose the patient to dislodgement of aneurysmal debris with resultant emboli. A more serious complication would be rupture of the aneurysm. The chart that follows lists the contraindications to IABP.

Contraindications to IABP

- Aortic valve incompetence
- Severe peripheral vascular occlusive disease
- Previous aortofemoral or aortoiliac bypass grafts
- Aortic aneurysm

INDICATIONS

Two major applications of IABP currently employed are for treatment of cardiogenic shock following myocardial infarction and for acute left ventricular power failure following cardiac surgery. In additon, other applications have been made for other types of patients with cardiac pathophysiology (see accompanying chart). Successful support of the septic shock patient and the cardiovascular patient undergoing general surgery has also been reported.

Cardiogenic Shock

Treatment of cardiogenic shock is complicated, and the mortality remains high. Approximately 15% of patients with myocardial infarction will develop cardiogenic shock. The presence of cardiogenic shock is confirmed by the following accepted criteria:

- Low cardiac output syndrome
- Cardiac index of 2.0 liters/minute/M² or less
- Systolic blood pressure < 80 mm Hg or < 100 mm Hg in a formerly hypertensive patient
- Urine output < 20 ml/hour

Patients will first be given a short period of treatment with various inotropic drugs, vasopressors, and volume. A lack of or minimal response in arterial pressure, urine output, and mental status following this

Indications for IABP

- Cardiogenic shock following acute infarction
- Left ventricular power failure in the postoperative cardiac surgery patient
- Severe unstable angina
- Postinfarction angina
- Postinfarction ventricular septal defect or mitral regurgitation
- Refractory ventricular tachyarrhythmias
- Septic shock
- General surgery for the patient with cardiovascular disease

therapy will indicate a need for assisted circulation with IABP. Once hypotension is present, the self-perpetuating process of injury will be in effect. Control of further injury and improvement in survival require early reversal of the shock state.

Most research centers agree that patients who hemodynamically exhibit left ventricular end-diastolic pressures or pulmonary capillary wedge pressures of >18 mm Hg with cardiac indexes of <2.0 to 2.2 liter/minute/m^2 carry high mortality and should be considered for IABP if they are unresponsive to a short period of pharmacologic therapy.

Response Patterns

Once IABP is instituted, improvement should be seen in 1 to 2 hours. At this time, steady improvement should be seen in cardiac output, peripheral perfusion, urine output, mental status, and pulmonary congestion. With improved cardiac function, one should also see a decrease in CVP and pulmonary capillary wedge pressure. Average peak effect should be achieved within 24 hours.

There are three general responses to IABP therapy. One group of patients will achieve hemodynamic stabilization and survive with the support of medical therapy and IABP. The second group of patients will continue to deteriorate with the support of IABP and will die from irreversible cardiogenic shock. The third group of patients will become dependent on IABP for circulatory support. Attempted withdrawal of IABP in this group results in hemodynamic deterioration. Some or the patients in this group may achieve some benefit from cardiac surgical intervention. There are centers that advocate early resection of infarcted tissue or coronary artery bypass grafting for this group of patients. Surgery on patients in cardiogenic shock will carry extremely high risk. Many of the nonoperated patients will die from complicatons of their illness.

Postoperative Left Ventricular Power Failure

Successful reduction in mortality has been achieved by utilizing IABP for patients with acute left ventricular power failure or cardiogenic shock following cardiac surgery. There are two major conditions that might lead to postoperative pump failure: (1) severe preoperative left ventricular dysfunction and (2) intraoperative myocardial infarction.

IABP can be used to wean patients from cardiopulmonary bypass and to provide postoperative circulatory assistance until left ventricular recovery occurs. In these situations, early recognition of failure is evidenced by the heart's inability to support circulation following cardiopulmonary bypass.

Early recognition and treatment is crucial if left ventricular power failure is to be reversed. Later development and recognition of failure following cardiac surgery results in much higher mortality, even with the assistance of IABP.

High-Risk Cardiac Surgery Patients

IABP has also been used in the high-risk cardiac surgery patient for safer induction of anesthesia. Patients who develop signs of acute cardiac ischemia unresponsive to pharmacologic therapy may benefit from IABP during *anesthesia induction* and for support prior to *cardiopulmonary bypass.*

IABP may also be employed during *cardiac catheterization* for this same group of high-risk patients. In this situation, cardiac catheterization studies are generally followed by emergency cardiac surgery. In this category are patients with unstable angina, postinfarction angina and postinfarction ventricular septal defects, or mitral regurgitation with resultant cardiac failure. IABP has been successfully used to abolish or markedly decrease the incidence of angina attacks in patients in whom previous medical therapy has failed. The use of IABP for patients with cardiac failure following ventricular septal rupture or mitral valve incompetence will aid in the promotion of forward blood flow. This will decrease shunting through the septal defect and decrease the amount of mitral regurgitation.

Postoperative Complications

Complications in the postoperative period, related to ventricular performance, might also indicate the use of IABP. Limited use of IABP in the pulmonary artery for right ventricular afterload reduction has been reported following right ventricular infarction resulting in severe failure following cardiac surgery. A small number of patients with refractory ventricular tachyarrhythmias may benefit from the physiological effects of IABP. This group is composed of patients with myocardial ischemia, infarction, or ventricular aneurysms. IABP is instituted when pharmacologic management fails to suppress irritable foci. In these situations, IABP is used as support until blood blow can be restored by surgical revascularization or by resection of irritable foci, the ventricular aneurysm, or the area of infarction.

Septic Shock

A newer application of IABP is for the support of patients in septic shock. Patients in septic shock have very low systemic vascular resistance owing to vasodilatation caused by the endotoxin. To review, mean arterial blood pressure is a function of cardiac output and systemic vascular resistance. In order to maintain adequate perfusion pressure to vital organs, the patient in septic shock must maintain a very high cardiac output. IABP has been used when traditional vasopressor support fails to maintain adequate mean arterial pressure. Prolonged, inadequate perfusion pressure will result in possible renal failure or myocardial infarction. IABP is advocated by some clinicians to assist blood pressure maintenance and increase coronary perfusion when traditional support fails.

General Surgery for High-Risk Patient

Another newer application of IABP is for the high-risk cardiovascular patient undergoing a general surgical operation. Any patient with ischemic heart disease will be at higher risk for general anesthesia and the surgical procedure. IABP is used to ensure adequate coronary artery perfusion pressure during the procedure.

NURSING PROCESS

Patients requiring IABP are managed much like any other critically ill patient in cardiogenic shock or acute left ventricular power failure. Nursing assessment and management of these conditions are discussed elsewhere in Chapters 10 and 11. There are additional nursing skills and assessment considerations specific to IABP therapy that must be included in the care of these patients.

Assessing the Cardiovascular System

Monitoring the cardiovascular system is extremely important in the determination of the effectiveness of balloon pump therapy. The basis for this assessment should include vital signs, cardiac output, heart rhythm and regularity, urine output, color, perfusion, and mentation.

Vital Signs

Three important vital signs with respect to IABP are heart rate, mean arterial blood pressure (MAP), and pulmonary capillary wedge pressure.

Because timing of the balloon pump is based on *heart rate,* any variation of heart rate may significantly affect the performance of the balloon pump. Any variation in heart rate of 10 or more beats necessitates an evaluation and possible readjustment of inflation and deflation timing. Large variations in heart rate may also indicate a change in the patient's overall clinical status.

MAP should improve with effective IABP. An acute change in MAP may require a quick evaluation of timing and then a further assessment of other vital signs. In such cases, patients tolerate very little change in

volume status, and an acute drop in MAP may also indicate volume depletion.

The *pulmonary capillary wedge pressure* is an important parameter for monitoring volume status. It will provide an early indication of volume depletion or volume overload.

Blood pressure readings require special consideration. Because the balloon inflates during diastole, peak-diastolic pressure may be higher than peak-systolic pressure. It is important to remember that monitoring equipment cannot distinguish systole from diastole but only peak pressures from low-point pressures. For this reason, a monitor digital display of systolic pressure may actually represent peak-diastolic pressure. It is advisable to record blood pressure as systolic, peak-diastolic, and end-diastolic; that is, 100/110/60. These pressures can be read from a strip recording of the arterial waveform.

To determine the effect of the balloon pump, one can record pressures (systolic, diastolic, and MAP) with the pump either on or off.

Heart Rhythm and Regularity

Heart rhythm and regularity are also important considerations. Early recognition and treatment of *arrhythmias* are crucial not only for patient safety but also for effective IABP. Irregular arrhythmias may inhibit efficient IABP because timing is set by the patient's regular R to R interval on the ECG. A safety feature of all balloon pump consoles is automatic deflation of the balloon for premature QRS complexes. Any patient who develops a bigeminal rhythm will then lose 50% of the balloon assistance. If the arrhythmia persists, another alternative might be use of the systolic peak on the arterial waveform as the trigger mechanism for balloon inflation.

Other Observations

Urine output, color, perfusion, and *mentation* all are important assessment parameters for determining the adequacy of cardiac output. Any deterioration in these signs might also indicate a fall in cardiac output. If the patient is responding to IABP, these signs should also show improvement. Cardiac output measurement with a pulmonary artery catheter is indicated when deterioration is evident or when a major change in volume or pharmacologic therapy has been instituted. Monitoring the patient's ability to maintain cardiac output is also important during weaning procedures from IABP.

Special attention should be given to the *left radial pulse.* A decrease or absence of the left radial pulse may indicate that the balloon has advanced up the aorta and may be partially or totally obstructing the left subclavian artery.

The presence of the balloon catheter in the femoral or iliac artery predisposes the patient to impaired circulation of the involved extremity. The extremity with the catheter in place will also be relatively immobile. Any flexion of the hip may kink the catheter and impair balloon pumping. Extremities should be checked hourly for pulses, color, and sensation. Any deterioration in the affected extremity should be reported to the physician. Severe vascular insufficiency will necessitate the removal of the catheter. Patients should be encouraged to flex their feet frequently every hour to avoid venous stasis. If they are unable to do this, the nurse can do it for them.

Some physicians advocate the use of heparin therapy to prevent possible thrombus formation around the catheter and vascular insufficiency. Each physician will determine whether the risks of anticoagulation outweigh the benefits for the individual patient. If anticoagulation is used, it is advisable to perform a guaiac test periodically on nasogastric drainage and stools for the presence of blood. Observation of *urine* for hematuria, *skin* for petechiae, and any *incisions* for oozing of blood should also be part of patient assessment. If any of these are noted, the physician should be alerted. Heparin therapy may require adjustment or possible reversal with protamine sulfate.

Assessing the Pulmonary System

The majority of patients on IABP will require intubation and ventilatory assistance. Many will have suffered respiratory insufficiency as the result of the fluid overload associated with cardiac failure. Any intubated patient has an increased risk of *respiratory tract infection*. This risk increases greatly in the debilitated patient. Invasive hemodynamic monitoring catheters and the balloon catheter will also restrict the patient's mobility, requiring modification in turning. This may increase the risk of *atelectasis*. Turning is appropriate as long as the extremity with the balloon catheter is kept straight. It may be helpful to use a soft restraint around the ankle of the affected extremity to remind the patient to avoid flexion of the hip. For the same reason, the head of the bed cannot be elevated more than 30°. In addition, elevation may cause the catheter to advance up the aorta.

Some patients might require horizontal lifting for placement of a chest x-ray film when portable roentgenograms are taken. Daily chest roentgenograms are needed to follow pulmonary status and to inspect intravenous catheter placement. The position of the balloon catheter can also be determined in this manner.

Assessing the Renal System

Patients in cardiogenic shock are at risk for the development of acute renal failure. Urine output and quality should be monitored closely. Serum levels of blood urea nitrogen and creatine should be included in daily laboratory studies to monitor renal function. It is advisable to study creatine clearance in addition to serum creatine. Creatine clearance will indicate renal dysfunction and possible failure much earlier than serum creatine. Serum creatine does not rise until significant renal function is lost. Also, any acute, dramatic drop in urine output might be an indication that the catheter has slipped down the aorta and is obstructing the renal arteries. A portable roentgenogram can confirm this suspicion. Predisposition to urinary tract infection is also present in patients with indwelling Foley catheters. Good catheter hygiene and maintenance of an acidic urine will help prevent infection.

Assessing Psychosocial Problems

Balloon insertion is usually an unplanned, emergent procedure for patients with deteriorating conditions. Abundant monitoring is frightening for both the patient and family. Every effort should be made to explain surroundings and procedures to patients. The goal is to make them feel more secure in their environment and to alleviate anxiety.

Family members need to be prepared for the first visit after balloon insertion. Good preparation helps them deal with the stress of the situation and be more supportive of the patient. Honest communication with the family is very important. This helps them interpret the situation realistically and view changes in the patient's condition with appropriate significance. Families will also be carrying the responsibility of making decisions regarding the patient's care. It is often helpful to provide contact with another nonmedical personnel member, such as a social worker or clergyman. These people can provide additional support to the family. Sometimes it is easier to express feelings of hopelessness or fear of the patient's death when dealing with a person who is not directly involved in the patient's care.

Critically ill patients often suffer from sleep deprivation and disorientation. Immobility and unfamiliar noises and machinery also increase stress and anxiety in the patient. Frequent orientation by staff and family visits can help alleviate some of this stress. Good care planning can help organize procedures such as suctioning, turning, and dressing changes so that patients receive longer periods of uninterrupted rest.

Assessing Other Parameters

Nutrition should be an early consideration to promote healing and strength. Hyperalimentation can be instituted to provide nutrients and essential vitamins. Tube feedings might also be considered in patients who are able to tolerate them.

Infection is a major problem in the debilitated patient. Thus, it is extremely important to maintain sterile technique, particularly in relation to the dressing over the balloon catheter exit site. Many patients will have a dacron graft lying beneath subcutaneous tissue. The presence of the graft increases the risk of wound infection. Once bacteria lodge in the graft, infection is relatively impossible to treat. Intravenous antibiotics have little effect because the graft has no blood supply. Once the wound is infected, the graft must be removed for successful treatment. For that reason, dressings should be changed with sterile gloves and ideally, a sterile mask. Dressings should be kept clean and dry. In some institutions, sterile, occlusive dressings are used for this type of wound care.

WAVEFORM ASSESSMENT

An important nursing function in the care of patients on IABP is the analysis of the arterial pressure waveform and the effectiveness of IABP. Nurses must be able to recognize and correct problems in balloon-pump timing.

Step 1. The first step in timing assessment is the ability to recognize the beginnings of systole and diastole on the arterial waveform (Fig. 9-42). Systole begins at point *A* on Figure 9-42, where the sharp upstroke begins. Point *B* marks the dicrotic notch, which represents aortic valve closure. It is at this point that diastole begins and the balloon should be inflated. Balloon deflation occurs just prior to point *A*, at end diastole.

The chart that follows lists five criteria that can be used to measure the effectiveness of IABP on the arterial pressure waveform. To effectively evaluate the waveform, one must view the patient's unassisted pressure tracing alongisde the assisted pressure tracing. This can be accomplished through adjustment of

FIGURE 9-42
Arterial waveform with A *representing the point of balloon deflation prior to the systolic upstroke and* B *representing balloon inflation at the dicrotic notch.*

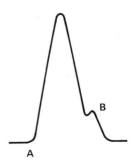

the machine so that the balloon inflates and deflates on every other beat (*i.e.,* a 1:2 assist ratio). Most patients will tolerate this well for a brief period of time. Many machine consoles are capable of freezing the waveform on the console monitor so that it would only be necessary to assist 1:2 for one screen. The machine can then return to 1:1 assistance while the nurse assesses the tracing. Another alternative would be to obtain a strip recording of the 1:2 assistance for analysis. These two approaches might be necessary if the patient's MAP drops significantly on 1:2 assistance.

Criteria for Assessment of Effective IABP on the Arterial Pressure Waveform

- Inflation occurs at the dicrotic notch.
- Inflation slope is parallel to the systolic upstroke.
- Diastolic augmentation peak is greater than or equal to the preceding systolic peak.
- An end-diastolic dip in pressure is created with balloon deflation.
- The following systolic peak (assisted systole) is lower than the preceding systole (unassisted systole).

Step 2. Using the first criterion, one should identify the patient's dicrotic notch. Comparison is then made with the assisted tracing to see that inflation occurs at the point of the dicrotic notch. Inflation before the dicrotic notch will abruptly shorten the patient's systole and increase ventricular volume as ejection is interrupted. Late inflation, past the dicrotic notch, will not raise coronary artery perfusion pressure as effectively. The peak diastolic pressure may not be as high as it would be with proper timing. Also, the duration of assistance during diastole will be unnecessarily shortened.

Step 3. Next, the slopes of systolic upstroke and diastolic augmentation should be compared. The diastolic slope should be sharp and parallel the systolic upstroke. A diastolic slope that reaches its peak slowly indicates that the increase in aortic root pressure rises slowly and is not as effective in immediately increasing coronary perfusion pressure. The greater the peak in diastolic pressure, the greater the increase in aortic root pressure. For this reason, balloon assistance should be adjusted until the highest peak possible is achieved. The method of doing this will vary with different brands of consoles. The nurse should be familiar with the particular console used by the institution.

Step 4. Deflation should occur just prior to systole, causing an acute drop in aortic end-diastolic pressure.

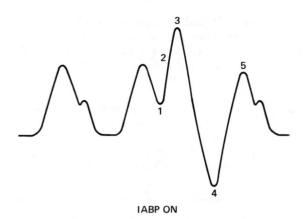

IABP ON

FIGURE 9-43

Inspection of the arterial waveform with intra-aortic balloon assistance should include observation of (1) inflation point; (2) slopes; (3) diastolic peak pressure; (4) end-diastolic dip; (5) next systolic peak.

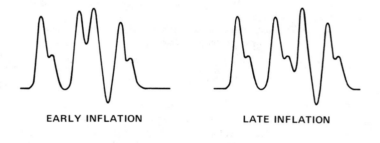

EARLY INFLATION   LATE INFLATION

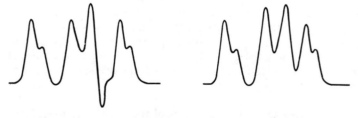

EARLY DEFLATION   LATE DEFLATION

FIGURE 9-44

Illustration of possible errors occurring with timing.

This quick deflation displaces between 20 to 40 ml of volume, depending on the size of the balloon. This displacement of volume causes a drop in pressure because the volume was contributing to pressure. The result is an end-diastolic dip in pressure that reduces the impedance to the next systolic ejection. The end-diastolic pressure without the balloon assistance should be compared with the end-diastolic pressure with the dip created by balloon deflation. Optimally, a pressure difference of at least 10 mm Hg should be obtained. Better afterload reduction is achieved with the lowest possible end-diastolic dip.

The point of deflation is also crucial. Deflation that is too early will allow pressure to rise to normal end-diastolic levels preceding systole. In this situation, there will be no decrease in afterload. Early deflation may actually have a "sink-like" effect on the aortic root, impairing coronary perfusion because blood is distracted to the area of the pressure drop. Late deflation will encroach upon the next systole and actually increase afterload owing to greater impedance to ejection.

Step 5. Finally, if afterload has been reduced, the next systolic pressure peak should be lower than the unassisted systolic pressure peak. This implies that the ventricle did not have to generate as great a pressure to overcome impedance to ejection. This may not always be seen because the systolic pressure peak also represents the compliance of the vasculature. If the vasculature is noncompliant owing to atherosclerotic disease, the systolic peak may not change very much. Figure 9-43 illustrates the five points that must be assessed on the waveform. Figure 9-44 demonstrates possible errors in timing.

Balloon Fit. The fit of the balloon to any particular patient's aorta will determine how well each of these criteria is met. Ideally, approximately 80% to 90% of the aorta should be occluded with balloon inflation. Any occlusion greater than this may damage aortic tissue. Occasionally, the larger balloon cannot be threaded through the femoral or iliac arteries, so a smaller balloon must be used. In this situation, the effect of inflation and deflation will not be as dramatic on the waveform. In a patient who is hypotensive or hypovolemic, the balloon will not have as pronounced an effect on the waveform because there is less volume displacement as the balloon inflates or deflates.

TROUBLESHOOTING

Conduction Problems

Some console units require a separate set of ECG leads for input into the trigger mechanism. Some units can be jacked into the primary monitor, requiring only one set of ECG leads. The nurse should be familiar with the capabilities of the particular console. Maintenance of good conduction through the skin is important.

Any ECG artifact will interfere with the console's ability to recognize the trigger, or R wave, and will result in ineffective assistance. Any interference will cause an automatic deflation of the balloon. If the amplitude of the R wave is too low to trigger effectively, one can correct this by changing lead placement. Any pacemaker artifact may also be interpreted as a trigger. This is generally not a problem with ventricular pacemakers. Atrial pacing artifact occurs just before atrial contraction during diastole. Because it is not desirable for balloon deflation to occur before end-diastole, adjustments must be made. Inflation time can be delayed until the dicrotic notch is seen on the arterial waveform. This delay time will be longer than the normal delay set before inflation occurs.

A cardiac arrest due to ventricular fibrillation or asystole will not provide a trigger for IABP. In this situation, the machine can be turned off. It should not be left off for more than 5 minutes because this will likely result in platelet aggregation around the balloon. It should be inflated periodically to avoid this problem. Some consoles are capable of pumping at a preset rate regardless of the patient's ECG pattern. Cardioversion or defibrillation can be performed while the machine remains on. The machines are insulated so that this electric current will not damage the internal mechanisms. Tachycardias may also impair pumping ability. Often, switching the machine to a 1:2 assist will increase its ability to follow the rapid rate with increased effectiveness.

Balloon Problems

A small amount of gas will normally diffuse out of the balloon. This necessitates that the balloon be evacuated and filled periodically. Normally, this is required approximately every 3 to 4 hours. Some consoles do this automatically whereas others require manual refilling by the nurse. Loss of balloon volume will be evident when the diastolic pressure peak and end-diastolic dip begin to decrease. Any increase in frequency required for refilling might suggest a leak in catheter connection. Normal diffusion of gas should be only 1 to 2 ml/hour. Rarely, a balloon may develop a leak. Initally, a loss in balloon effectiveness will be noted. With refilling, a greater loss of volume will be observed. Eventually, blood will back up into the catheter. The physician should be notified immediately because the faulty balloon will have to be removed to avoid the possibility of gas embolus. Because carbon dioxide is highly soluble in blood, a small leak is rarely a serious problem. Helium does not have this characteristic, and a leak—even a small one—is therefore more serious. In this situation, it is important to keep the balloon moving slightly while decreasing its volume. The frequency of inflation should be decreased to the absolute minimum.

Vacuum Problems

Each machine will have an alarm system that will alert the nurse to any loss of vacuum. The vacuum will be responsible for deflation of the balloon. Any decrease in vacuum will interfere with the balloon's ability to deflate. However, a loss of pressure from the compressor pump will interfere with effective inflation. Any fault in the drive system (the vacuum or compressor) requires that the console be changed. The malfunctioning console should then be inspected by a biomedical engineer or the service representative from the particular company.

WEANING

Indications

Weaning patients from a balloon catheter generally can begin 12 to 24 hours after insertion. Some patients will require longer periods of support. Weaning can begin when a patient shows evidence of *hemodynamic stability.* A patient should not require excessive vasopressor support to maintain hemodynamic stability. Ideally, vasopressor support should be minimal when weaning begins. After the balloon is removed, it is much easier to increase vasopressor support than to reinsert a balloon catheter for hemodynamic support. Each physician will determine his own criteria for hemodynamic stability. General guidelines might include a cardiac index >2 liters per minute, a pulmonary wedge pressure <20 mm Hg, and a systolic blood pressure >100 mm Hg.

The patient should also exhibit signs of *adequate cardiac function,* demonstrated by good peripheral pulses, adequate urine output, absence of pulmonary edema, and improved mentation. *Good coronary artery perfusion* will be evidenced by an absence of life-threatening arrhythmias and no evidence of ischemia or injury on the ECG.

Complications may also require abrupt cessation of IABP. This may or may not result in a reinsertion of another balloon catheter. Severe vascular insufficiency evidenced by a loss of pulses in the distal extremity, pain, and pallor is definitely an indication to remove the balloon catheter from that particular insertion site. Any balloon that develops a leak also requires removal for obvious reasons. The physician may choose to reinsert the balloon catheter in another extremity or to replace the faulty balloon if the patient is hemodynamically unstable. Depending on the philosophy of the institution and physician, a deteriorating, irreversible situation might also be an indication for weaning or discontinuing balloon pump support. The accompanying chart lists major indications for weaning the patient from IABP.

Approaches

Weaning may be achieved by any combination of the approaches listed in the chart that follows. The first likely step would be to decrease the assist ratio from 1:1 to 1:2 and so on until the minimum assist ratio is achieved on any particular console. A patient might be assisted at the first decrease for up to 4 to 6 hours. The minimal amount of time should be 30 minutes. During this time, the patient must be assessed for any change in hemodynamic status. An increasing heart rate with decreasing blood pressure indicates a deterioration in hemodynamic status. Cardiac output should also be assessed at this time. A decrease in cardiac output or any evidence listed previously indicates that the patient is not tolerating the weaning. Weaning should be temporarily discontinued. Therapy may be adjusted for the patient prior to another weaning attempt. If the first decrease in assist ration is tolerated, the assist ration is decreased to minimum, with 1 to 4 hours allowed for each new assist ratio. Again, the patient must be continually assessed for any indications of intolerance to the process.

Indications for Weaning From IABP

- Hemodynamic stability
  - Cardiac index >2 liters/minute
  - Pulmonary capillary wedge pressure <20 mm Hg
  - Systolic blood pressure >100 mm Hg
- Minimal requirements for vasopressor support
- Evidence of adequate cardiac function
  - Good peripheral pulses
  - Adequate urine output
  - Absence of pulmonary edema
  - Improved mentation
- Evidence of good coronary perfusion
  - Absence of life-threatening arrhythmias
  - Absence of ischemia on the ECG
- Severe vascular insufficiency
- Balloon leakage
- Deteriorating, irreversible condition

Approaches to Weaning from IABP

- Gradually decrease assist ration
- Decrease diastolic augmentation
- Decrease balloon volume

Another approach, which might be utilized in conjunction with decreasing assist ratio, is the decrease of the diastolic augmentation. This will result in decreased aortic root pressure, which should be tolerated by the patient who is ready for weaning. At this time, and also during decreasing assist ratio, the patient's ECG should be monitored for any S–T segment changes. In addition, a return of angina is an indication that this procedure is not being tolerated.

The preceding steps may be all that are required to assess the patient's ability to maintain hemodynamic stability without IABP. Some physicians might also choose to decrease balloon volume so that the balloon merely quivers at the lowest assist ratio. It is important to maintain movement of the balloon to avoid platelet aggregation around the balloon. By maintaining a quiverlike state, the balloon never completely inflates. At this point, IABP has essentially been discontinued because the patient receives no hemodynamic benefit from balloon inflation.

Removal of the Balloon Catheter

Removal is a surgical procedure; therefore, the patient will most often return to the operating room after weaning is complete. Prior to removal, the patient is heparinized. After the balloon catheter has been removed, a Fogarty catheter is passed proximally to the aortic bifurcation and distally to the popliteal artery. The purpose of this procedure is to remove any clot formation that may be present and to prevent thromboembolic complications. The graft is then removed, and the arteriotomy is closed with either a dacron or saphenous vein patch. The patch secures hemostasis and decreases the potential for late femoral artery or iliac artery stenosis. Upon return to the intensive care unit, the patient will require frequent assessment of perfusion to the distal extremity.

COMPLICATIONS

Insertion of the catheter in a patient with severe atherosclerotic vascular disease might result in arterial perforation or occlusion. Iatrogenic dissection of the aorta is rare but has been reported. Vascular insufficiency is the most common complication of IABP. Vascular insufficiency may be permanent, or it may possibly be relieved by aortofemoral or ileofemoral bypass grafting. Neuropathy in the catheterized extremity is another reported complication.

Decreased circulating platelets in the first 24 hours of IABP and a minimal decrease in red blood cell count have been reported; however, they are not thought to be significant problems. There is a low incidence of balloon leakage and rupture. These complications might result from balloon inflation against a calcific, atherosclerotic plaque in the aorta. This disruption in the balloon surface may be as small as a pinhole or may be a large tear. The associated danger is gas embolism. There is some safety advantage in using carbon dioxide when leaks are small; however, either carbon dioxide or helium would be dangerous if a patient received a large bolus of gas through a large tear.

Finally, a complication of any catheter insertion is the possibility of infection at the insertion site. This can be a considerable problem in the unstable, critically ill patient because of the necessity of catheter removal. However, the advantages of IABP clearly outweigh the risks associated with its use for appropriately selected patients.

BIBLIOGRAPHY

Bolooki H: Clinical Application of Intra-Aortic Balloon Pump. Mount Kisco, Futura, 1977

DeWood MA et al: Intra-aortic balloon counterpulsation with and without reperfusion for myocardial infarction shock. Circulation 61, No. 6:1105–1112, 1980

Kerber RE et al: Effect of intra-aortic balloon counterpulsation on the motion and perfusion of acutely ischemic myocardium: An experimental echocardiographic study. Circulation 54, No. 5:853–859, 1976

Miller DC et al: Pulmonary artery balloon counterpulsation for acute right ventricular power failure. J Thorac Cardiovasc Surg (Nov) 80:760–763, 1980

O'Rourke MF, Sammel N, Chang VP: Arterial counterpulsation in severe refractory heart failure complicating acute myocardial infarction. Br Heart J 41:308–316, 1979

Reed EA: Intra-aortic balloon pump. AORN J 23, No. 6:995–1001, 1976

Stewart S, Biddle T, DeWeese J: Support of the myocardium with intra-aortic balloon counterpulsation following cardiopulmonary bypass. J Thorac Cardiovasc Surg 72, No. 1:109–114, 1976

Swank M et al: Effect of intra-aortic balloon pumping on nutrient coronary flow in normal and ischemic myocardium. J Thorac Cardiovasc Surg 76, No. 4:538–544, 1978

Whitman G: Intra-aortic balloon pumping and cardiac mechanics: A programmed lesson. Heart Lung 7, No. 6:1034–1050, 1978

Autotransfusion

Rae Nadine Smith

PURPOSE

Autotransfusion is the collection, filtration, and reinfusion of the patient's own blood. The purpose of autotransfusion is to avoid or decrease the requirements of homologous or bank blood and its potential complications. Autotransfusion is cost-effective and saves bank blood for use when no other alternative is available. Although reported by Blundell in 1818 and performed successfully in 1914, autotransfusion has gained widespread use and acceptance only since the technological advances made in the 1970s. It is now a well-accepted procedure that in many instances is lifesaving.

ORIENTATION AND FOCUS

The patient's own blood (autologous) may be reinfused as whole blood or as washed, packed red blood cells (RBC's), depending on the needs of the patient, the type of autotransfusion equipment utilized, and the preference of the physician. Autotransfusion methods may be classified into four types: emergency, preoperative, intraoperative, and postoperative. Regardless of the technique that is used, the advantages and contraindications remain the same.

Advantages

There are many advantages associated with reinfusing the patient's own blood, otherwise known as autotransfused, or autologous, blood (Table 9-8). These advantages are discussed subsequently.

Safety

Elimination of Disease Transmission. The risks of donor-related diseases such as AIDS (acquired immune deficiency syndrome), hepatitis, malaria, syphilis, cytomegalovirus, and Epstein-Barr virus are avoided.

Elimination of Transfusion Reaction. Autologous blood is type-specific and cross-match compatible. This eliminates the hemolytic, febrile, allergic, or graft-versus-host reactions sometimes associated with homologous (bank) blood. In addition, there is no risk of isoimmunization to erythrocyte, leukocyte, platelet, or protein antigens.

Bank blood is associated with a 5% risk of serious transfusion reaction, including deaths secondary to posttransfusion hepatitis and hemolytic reactions. It is estimated that 8% to 10% of bank blood recipients develop posttransfusion hepatitis, with a significant incidence of cirrhosis.

Absence of Anticoagulants. Whereas all bank blood contains anticoagulants, intraoperative (washed) blood and postoperative shed mediastinal autologous blood contain no anticoagulants.

TABLE 9-8
ADVANTAGES OF AUTOTRANSFUSION

Safety
Availability and Compatability of Blood
Superior Blood Quality
Reduction of Religious Objections
Conservation of Bank Blood
Cost-Effectiveness

Availability of Blood

Because type-matching and cross-matching are not required on autotransfused blood, the blood is often available immediately for initial stabilization of the patient.

Inexpensive systems are available that are simple and fast to set-up, eliminating the need for special operators or technicians.

Superior Blood Quality

Platelets in autologous blood remain viable with nearly normal platelet count and function, whereas platelets in stored blood become nonviable within 24 hours.

2,3 diphosphoglycerate (DPG), which is essential to adequate tissue oxygenation, is within normal levels in autologous blood. Bank blood shows a decreased amount of 2,3-DPG stored in the red blood cells, with blood stored more than 10 days containing no 2,3-DPG. This results in a shift to the left in the oxyhemoglobin dissociation curve that lead to impairment of oxygen transfer at the tissue level.

Autotransfused RBC's have a near-normal survival time. Also, clotting factors V (labile factor) VIII (antihemophilic factor), and IX (Christmas factor) remain near normal in autologous blood but not in bank blood. In addition, autologous blood has normal PTT, potassium, and ammonia levels and is near body temperature.

Reduction of Religious Objections

Religious groups whose beliefs forbid transfusion, such as Jehovah's Witnesses, often permit autotransfusion.

Cost-Effectiveness

Autotransfusion eliminates the need for type- and cross-matching and reduces the need for bank blood.

ASSESSMENT

Patients who are candidates for transfusion should be evaluated for autotransfusion.

Contraindications

Autotransfusion is contraindicated in patients with malignant neoplasms, intrathoracic infections or infestations, and coagulopathies. The use of a substance such as an antibiotic not suitable for IV use at the injury site and excessive hemolysis, such as found in injuries more than 6 hours old, are also contraindications to autotransfusion.

Contamination of the blood with abdominal contents, such as feces, urine, or bile, is a relative contraindication. If bank blood is available, its use is recom-

TABLE 9-9
CONTRAINDICATIONS TO AUTOTRANSFUSION

Malignant Neoplasm
Infections and Infestations
Blood Contamination
Coagulopathies
Excessive Hemolysis

mended. Cell washing reduces but does not eliminate enteric contamination. When contamination of the blood is suspected, autologous blood is used only if failure to transfuse would be life-threatening (Table 9-9).

Risks

Although autotransfusion has proved safe and effective, there are certain risks associated with the procedure. These include hemolysis, air and particulate emboli, coagulation, and thrombocytopenia.

Knowledgeable selection of equipment used according to the manufacturer's instructions makes risks negligible. No major complications have been reported with the use of autotransfusion equipment currently on the market, although complications were reported with early systems.

Indications

Emergency Autotransfusion. Although most commonly used for hemothorax, emergency autotransfusion can also be used in primary injuries of the lungs, liver, chest wall, heart, pulmonary vessels, spleen, kidneys, inferior vena cava, and iliac, portal, and subclavian veins.

Preoperative Autotransfusion. This is used primarily for patients with rare blood types, for procedures with which massive blood loss is anticipated, and for patients in whom isoimmunization may present a future complication.

Preoperative phlebotomy with hemodilution is used primarily with open heart surgery.

Intraoperative Autotransfusion. This is used most often during thoracic and cardiovascular surgery. Its use has also been reported with gastric liver resection, orthopedic surgery (hip resection), gynecological surgery (for ruptured ectopic pregnancy), and neurosurgical (spinal fusion) procedures. A cell washer-processor is routinely used to reduce anticoagulated whole blood to washed packed RBCs for reinfusion.

Postoperative Autotransfusion. This is utilized to collect shed mediastinal blood after cardiac surgery.

PLANNING AND INTERVENTION

Autotransfusion systems are available for whole blood autotransfusion and washed or processed (component) autotransfusion. The type of system selected depends primarily on the type of patient being managed. Whole blood systems are most frequently used in emergency and trauma facilities and in the postoperative management of cardiovascular patients. These are simple systems requiring minimal in-servicing. A system that involves a cell washer-processor is most commonly selected for the operating room. The cell washer-processor requires a specially trained operator.

It is recommended that autologous blood be collected and reinfused within a 4-hour period. Aseptic technique is used with all autotransfusion procedures. A 20- to 40-micron depth or screen microaggregate filter is used for reinfusion so that microaggregate debris (consisting of degenerating platelets, white cells, red cells, fibrin and fat particles) can be eliminated. Adult respiratory distress syndrome has been reported less frequently with filtered autotransfusion blood than with bank blood.

Regional anticoagulants are used during intraoperative autotransfusion and usually during emergency autotransfusion. Regional anticoagulants such as CPD (citrate-phosphate-dextrose), ACD (acid-phosphate-dextrose), and sometimes heparin are added only to the autotransfusion collection system. CPD is the anticoagulant used in bank blood and the one most frequently used in autotransfusion. It consists of a buffered citrate solution, phosphate, and dextrose. The citrate prevents the blood from coagulating by chelating calcium, thus preventing calcium catalysis of the coagulation cascade. Dextrose and phosphate provide metabolic support of the blood.

Heparin is often used in conjunction with intraoperative autotransfusion. Heparin interferes with the formation of thromboplastin and thrombin, preventing clotting.

Laboratory evaluations done before and after autotransfusion include urinalysis, chest radiograph, CBC, CO_2 content, and serum levels of NA^+, K^+, Cl^-, Cr, Glucose, and BUN. Additional studies on selected patients include calcium levels, blood cultures, arterial blood gases, and intravenous pyelograms.

Emergency Autotransfusion

Emergency autotransfusion is for the immediate collection of whole blood that is filtered and reinfused. Hemothorax is the most common indication. Because the source of bleeding is not always apparent in an emergency situation, a regional anticoagulant, most commonly CPD, is added to the collection device before and during blood collection. Although a 7 : 1 ratio of blood to CPD is usually used, variations in ratio are reported. If the blood is known to be mediastinal in origin and therefore defibrinogenated, regional anticoagulants such as CPD and ACD are sometimes omitted.

Blood Collection

Blood is usually collected through chest tubes into a sterile, disposable liner with a gross particulate filter (170-micron) that has been primed with CPD (Fig. 9-45). A vacuum of 10 to 30 mm Hg is maintained so that hemolysis can be reduced. Should there be a loss of vacuum during blood collection, the chest tube must be immediately clamped. Failure to do so may result in pneumothorax. Prior to discontinuing auto-

transfusion vacuum, one must establish an underwater seal.

During aspiration of blood, the quantity of added anticoagulant is controlled to provide approximately 100 ml of anticoagulant for every 700 ml of blood. This 1 : 7 ratio is the same "CPD:Blood ratio" used in bank blood.

Blood Reinfusion

Reinfusion is initiated when all blood is evacuated from the site, when immediate transfusion is clinically indicated, or when the autotransfusion collection liner is full.

A microaggregrate (microemboli) filter and recipient set are attached to the disposable autotransfusion collection container, usually a flexible, sterile liner. All air should be removed from the blood container prior to initiation of reinfusion so that risk of air emboli is reduced.

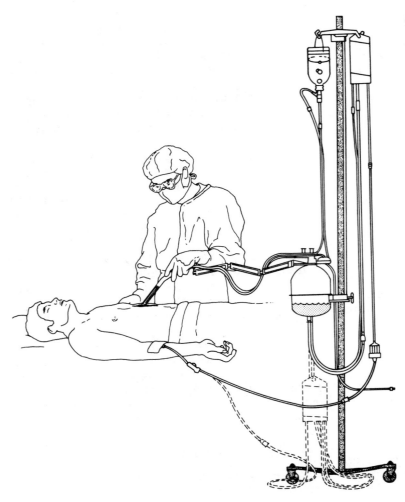

FIGURE 9-45
Whole-blood intraoperative autotransfusion system. (Courtesy of Thoratec Medical Products)

One may use blood pumps or pressure administration cuffs to expedite rapid blood infusion.

Although whole blood is most commonly used in an emergency situation, one may use a cell washer-processor in selected patients to salvage the patient's erythrocytes for reinfusion and discard contaminants and debris in the plasma.

Preoperative Autotransfusion

Preoperative autotransfusion is the collection of whole blood up to 35 days prior to surgery.

Phlebotomy

CPD or CPD with adenine (35 days) is routinely used as the regional anticoagulant. Four to 8 units may be drawn at a blood bank, usually for patients with rare blood types scheduled for surgery with anticipated high blood loss. The blood is reinfused as necessary, either intra- or postoperatively.

Phlebotomy with Hemodilution

Used primarily with open heart surgery, 1 or 2 units of blood are withdrawn immediately following induction of anesthesia and prior to heparinization. One replaces the blood with equivalent amounts of crystalloids or colloids, such as Ringer's lactate, 5% serum albumin, or 5% dextran to produce normovolemic anemia. All blood removed is reinfused into the patient intraoperatively.

Intraoperative Autotransfusion

Intraoperative autotransfusion usually consists of the collection of anticoagulated blood during surgery, cell processing, and the reinfusion of washed, packed red blood cells in the operating room. In selected patients, whole blood autotransfusion is used (Fig. 9-46).

Blood Collection

Systemic anticoagulation of the patient is used as medically indicated. Regional anticoagulation of the aspirated blood with CPD, ACD, or heparin is routinely performed. To keep the operative field dry, one uses a standard suction wand in conjunction with the autotransfusion suction wand. For reduction of hemolysis secondary to air-blood interface, only pooled blood is aspirated into the autotransfusion system. Both systemic and regional anticoagulants are removed from the blood prior to reinfusion by cell washing-processing.

A cell washer-processor is a centrifuge device that separates the plasma from the red blood cells. The red blood cells are washed and resuspended in normal

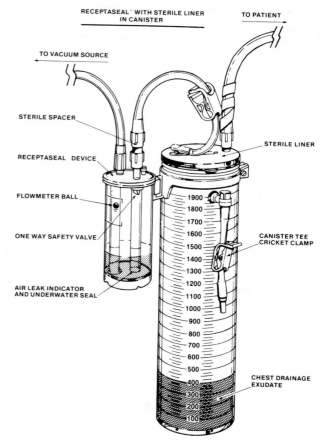

FIGURE 9-46
Autotransfusion set-up. This figure illustrates an autotransfusion system set-up with a thoracic drainage system for postoperative autotransfusion. For emergency autotransfusion, the pleural drainage system may be added after hemothorax evacuation. (Courtesy of Sorenson Research, Division of Abbott Laboratories)

saline by continuous centrifugation. The discarded plasma contains debris and activated clotting factors.

Advantages of washed-processed blood include increased hemoglobin and hematocrit levels secondary to volume reduction, elimination of anticoagulants, and reduction of microemboli. Enteric contamination is reduced by cell washing, but not eliminated.

Blood parameters that remain relatively unchanged by cell washing include mean corpuscular volume and 2,3-DPG levels. There may be a slight drop in white blood cells.

Disadvantages of washed-processed blood include cost, complexity, and time delay as well as loss of clotting factors, white blood cells, plasmaproteins, and platelets. Blood leaving the operating room for processing should be labeled.

TABLE 9-10
AUTOTRANSFUSION TROUBLESHOOTING GUIDELINES

Complication	Cause	Intervention
Coagulation	Insufficient anticoagulant added	Add regional anticoagulant such as CPD at a ratio of 7:1 blood to CPD Shake collection device periodically to mix blood and CPD Check reversal of anticoagulant
	Mediastinal blood not defibrinogenated	Strip chest tubes PRN
Hemolysis	Blood trauma secondary to turbulence or roller pumps	Avoid skimming operative field Avoid using equipment containing roller pumps Maintain vacuum below 30 mm Hg when collecting blood from chest tubes, below 60 mm Hg when aspirating from a surgical site
Coagulapathies	Decreased levels of platelets and fibrinogen Platelets trapped in filters Increased levels of fibrin split products	Patients autotransfused with more than 4000 ml of blood may require transfusion of fresh frozen plasma or platelet concentrate
Particulate and air emboli	Microaggregate debris	Use 20 to 40-micron microaggregate filter during reinfusion
	Air emboli	Avoid roller pump and pressure infusion systems Remove air from blood liners prior to reinfusion
	Nonparenteral medication at site	Avoid use of blood containing non-IV medications
Sepsis	Breakdown of aseptic technique	Broad-spectrum antibiotics as indicated Maintain good aseptic technique Reinfuse within 4 hours
	Contaminated blood	Avoid use of blood from infected areas and/or with known contaminants, such as stool and urine
Citrate toxicity (rare and unpredictable)	Chelating effect of citrate in the CPD on calcium	Monitor for hypotension, dysrrhythmias, and myocardial contractility When more than 2000 ml of CPD anticoagulated blood is given over a 20-minute period, calcium chloride may be given prophylactically
	Hyperkalemia, hypocalcemia, acidosis, hypothermia, myocardial dysfunction, and liver or renal dysfunction are predisposing factors	Stop CPD infusion, correct acidosis Monitor toxicity with frequent blood gases and serum calcium levels

Blood Reinfusion

The processed blood is reinfused according to the standard protocol for the infusion of packed red blood cells.

Postoperative Autotransfusion

Postoperative autotransfusion is the collection of shed mediastinal blood from chest tubes placed during open heart surgery. Anticoagulation is not required because mediastinal blood is defibrinogenated by its contact with serosol surfaces and the beating action of the heart.

Blood Collection

The blood is collected in a sterile system with a gross filter, usually 170 microns. An underwater seal chest drainage system may be incorporated, usually set at 20 cm of H_2O (15 mm Hg) (Fig. 9-45). Chest tubes are stripped as necessary. Excessive stripping may result in clot formation.

Blood Reinfusion

Prior to initiation of reinfusion, all air is removed from the blood collection system. Blood is reinfused through a microaggregate filter within a 4-hour period. Although mediastinal blood is usually defibrinogenated, some clotting may occur. The presence of clots in the gross filter in the sterile liner is not a contraindication to reinfusion of the shed mediastinal blood. Reinfusion may be expedited by placement of the blood liner in a pressure administration cuff. See Table 9-10 for troubleshooting guidelines.

EVALUATION

Hemolysis remains the primary effect of autotransfusion on blood. Elimination of roller pumps from autotransfusion systems has reduced but not eliminated this effect. Reduction of the air-blood interface by maintenance of a vacuum no greater than 30 mm Hg on chest tubes and 60 mm Hg during the surgical aspiration of pooled blood limits damage to RBCs. Hemolysis causes a reduction in hematocrit, an increase in serum and urine hemoglobin, and accumulation of erythrocyte debris. Significant renal failure secondary to hemoglobinuria has not been reported. Hemolysis tends to continue for a period of time following autotransfusion.

Defibrinogenated blood aspirated from the mediastinum, such as during hemothorax drainage or postoperatively, is devoid of fibrinogen with prolonged prothrombin (activity 30% to 50% of normal) and par-

tial thromboplastin time and increased levels of fibrin split products. Values usually return to normal by the second postoperative day.

There have been no reports of coagulopathies directly related to the use of autotransfusion systems currently available commerically.

Although it is often difficult for one to assess the exact amount of blood that the patient is losing, precise measurement is usually not essential because autologous blood is usually reinfused.

Record the duration of collection and reinfusion and the approximate volume. Note the type and amount of anticoagulant used. Record the amount of vacuum used and any complications encountered, such as clots.

CONCLUSION

Autotransfusion is a safe, effective method for reducing the risks associated with homologous (bank) blood transfusion in selected patients. It is lifesaving for patients who are bleeding rapidly and for those who have blood types that are unavailable in bank blood. Autologous blood is compatible and often immediately available, and its use allows conservation of bank blood for use when required. Whole blood autotransfusion is less expensive than most bank blood.

BIBLIOGRAPHY

Boudreaux JP et al: Emergency autotransfusion: Partial cleansing of bacteria-laden blood by cell washing. J Trauma 23, No. 1:31–35, 1983

Cowley RA, Dunham CM (eds): Shock Trauma/Critical Care Manual, pp 39–41. Baltimore, University Park Press, 1982

Davidson SJ: Current use of autotransfusion in the emergency patient. ER Reports 2, No. 17:73–78, 1981

DeCrosta T: Autotransfusion: Risks and rewards in emergency care. Nursing Life, pp 52–55, November/December, 1983

Engman S, Hauer JM: Autotransfusion Units. Guideline Report. AHA Hospital Technology Series 2, No. 19, 1983

Glover J, Groadie TA: Intraoperative autotransfusion. Massive transfusion in surgery and trauma, pp 151–170. New York, Alan R Liss, Inc, 1982

Gruendeman BJ, Meeker MH: Alexander's Care of the Patient in Surgery, 7th ed, pp 201–205. St Louis, Mosby, Co, 1983

Hauer JM: Current uses of autotransfusion in surgery. NITA 6:261–264, 1983

Johnson RG et al: The efficacy of postoperative autotransfusion in patients undergoing cardiac operations. Ann Thorac Surg 36, No. 2:173–179, 1983

Rosen et al: Emergency Medicine Concepts and Clinical Practice, pp 153–154, 164–165. St Louis, CV Mosby, 1984

Smith RN: Autotransfusion: Procedures, 301–307, 364–365. Springhouse, Intermed Communications, Inc, 1983

Thurer RL, Hauer JM: Autotransfusion and Blood Conservation. Chicago, Year Book Medical Publishers, Inc, 1982

10
Heart Failure

H. L. Brammell
Julie J. Benz

The heart, a complex structure composed of fibrous tissue, cardiac muscle, and electrical conducting tissue, has a single function: to pump blood. In order to do its job well, a good heart pump requires good functioning muscle, a good valve system, and an efficient pumping rhythm. An abnormality of sufficient severity of any component of the pump can affect its pumping efficiency and may cause the pump to fail.

RESERVE MECHANISMS OF THE HEART: RESPONSES OF THE HEART TO STRESS

When the heart is stressed, several reserve mechanisms can be called upon to maintain good pumping function—that is, to provide a cardiac output sufficient to meet the demands of the body. These mechanisms are increased heart rate, dilatation, hypertrophy, and increased stroke volume.

Increased Heart Rate

The first response is an increase in *heart rate*. This adjustment is rapid and has been experienced by everyone during periods of exercise or anxiety. Increasing the heart rate is an excellent way of quickly increasing the cardiac output and meeting the demands of the body for blood. Its utility and effectiveness, however, are functions of age, the functional state of

Supported by a Research and Training Center Grant (16-P-56815) from the Rehabilitation Services Administration, Department of Health, Education and Welfare, Washington, D.C.

the myocardium, and the amount of obstructive coronary artery disease, if any.

The maximum heart rate that can be achieved is related to age (Table 10-1). For example, heart rate in a 20-year-old person will plateau at approximately 200 beats per minute at maximum effort, whereas at 65 years of age, maximum heart rate is about 150 beats per minute. After 25 years of age, maximum heart rate capability drops approximately 6 beats for each 5 years. There is, of course, considerable spread around these mean maximum heart rates for each age—some persons will exceed the average value, whereas others will fail to achieve it. As heart rate increases, the time for diastolic ventricular filling decreases, and at high heart rates the time available for ventricular filling may be so small that filling is inadequate and cardiac output starts to fall.

In addition to advancing age, the functional state of the heart muscle (how capable it is of maintaining repeated rapid contractions) and the state of the coronary circulation are important determinants of the effectiveness of heart rate as a response to stress. In persons with coronary artery disease and significant obstruction to one or more coronary arteries, a substantial increase in heart rate can be a potentially dangerous event. Coronary artery blood flow to the left ventricle takes place primarily in diastole. With increasing heart rates, decreased diastolic filling time, and increased demands of the heart for oxygen (heart rate being one of the major determinants of myocardial oxygen demand), coronary blood flow may become critical, and angina pectoris, congestive failure, or occasionally myocardial infarction may be produced. Furthermore, if the heart muscle contracts poorly and

TABLE 10-1
MAXIMUM HEART RATE ACCORDING TO AGE

Age (Years)	Maximum Heart Rate (BPM)
20	200
22	198
24	196
26	194
28	192
30	190
32	189
34	187
36	186
38	184
40	182
45	179
50	175
55	171
60	160
65+	150

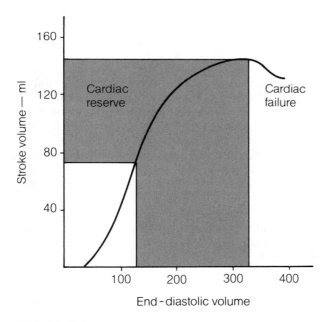

FIGURE 10-1
The Starling curve. (From Langley LL: Review of Physiology, 3rd ed. New York, McGraw-Hill, 1971.)

cannot sustain strong contractions at moderate or rapid rates, heart failure may follow.

Heart rate, then, is an immediate response to stress that is effective in maintaining or increasing cardiac output but whose value depends on the patient's age, functional state of the myocardium, and amount of obstructive disease in the coronary arteries.

Dilatation

The second reserve mechanism of the heart is *dilatation*. With dilatation, the muscle cell stretches. The relationship between the cardiac output (the amount of blood the heart pumps in each unit of time) and the length of the heart muscle cell at the end of diastole is expressed in the well-known *Starling relationship,* which states that as the end-diastolic fiber length increases, so does the cardiac output (Fig. 10-1).

Like heart rate, however, the usefulness of dilatation is self-limiting. There is a point beyond which the stretching of the muscle cell leads not to an increase in cardiac output but to a decrease. This is partly explained by the *Laplace relationship,* which states that the tension in the wall of a chamber such as the left ventricle is directly related to the pressure in that chamber and its radius. Put another way, as the radius of the chamber increases (dilatation), so does the wall tension, as long as the pressure in the chamber rises or does not fall.

Because wall tension is directly related to the demand of the myocardium for oxygen, it is not difficult to see that eventually the radius will dilate to such a degree that the demand of the heart for oxygen cannot be met. In this instance, dilatation has advanced to the point where it is no longer providing an increase in cardiac output, and the pump has started to fail.

Hypertrophy

The third reserve mechanism of the heart is the ability of the individual cardiac muscle cells to *hypertrophy.* The process of hypertrophy requires time and is not an acute adjustment to stress. However, if the stress is applied long enough, such as with systemic or pulmonary hypertension or significant stenosis of the aortic or pulmonary valve (pressure loads), the muscle of the chamber pumping against the resistance may hypertrophy to such a degree that it effectively outgrows its blood supply and becomes ischemic. When this happens, hypertrophy ceases to be a useful compensatory mechanism, and the heart's pumping ability decreases. A similar situation may occur with the imposition of a volume load on the pumping ventricle, as occurs with mitral or aortic regurgitation.

Stroke Volume

The fourth reserve mechanism of the heart is to increase its *stroke volume,* the amount of blood that it ejects into the circulation with each systole. It can do this either by increasing the percentage of the end-diastolic volume ejected with each beat (increase the ejection fraction through an increase in contractility) or by increasing the amount of blood presented to the heart (increased venous return). This is commonly accomplished by the reflexive increase of sympathetic nervous system activity, which increases venous tone. Venous pressure is then raised, and thus venous return to the heart is increased.

Venous return is also increased by elevated body temperature, which shortens the time required for blood to circulate completely through the body; by recumbency, in which case the volume of blood that is held in the legs as a result of gravity is largely returned to the central circulation and presented to the heart; or by taking a deep breath, which increases intrathoracic negativity, thereby "sucking" more blood into the chest. Also, any increase in intravascular volume will increase venous return. By an increase in either ejection fraction (contractility) or venous return (volume), stroke volume and cardiac output will increase. As with other mechanisms of response to stress, increased venous return ("preload" to the physiologist) and increased contractility may not function to increase cardiac output. For example, the myocardium may be so fatigued (depressed contractility) that it cannot respond to further attempts to improve its force of contraction. Similarly, an increase in venous return may cause increased dilatation and decrease, rather than improve, cardiac output.

This simplistic review of cardiovascular responses to stress is designed to promote a basic understanding of the topic and to indicate how the responses can be overwhelmed. In addition, it will assist in generating an appreciation for approaching clinical situations, both diagnostic and therapeutic, from a physiological cause-and-effect point of view.

PATHOPHYSIOLOGY OF HEART FAILURE

When the normal cardiac reserves for responding to stress are inadequate to meet the metabolic demands of the body, the heart fails to do its job as a pump, and heart failure results. Also, as stated earlier, dysfunction of any of the components of the pump may ultimately result in failure. Heart failure was very simply and appropriately defined in 1933 by Lewis as "a condition in which the heart fails to discharge its contents adequately." This definition is as good today as it was in the 1930s.

Causes of Failure

Arrhythmias
Disorders of the cardiac *rhythm* can produce or contribute to failure in several ways. *Bradycardia* allows for increased diastolic filling and myocardial fiber stretch with an associated increase in stroke volume

(Starling relationship). Cardiac output is therefore preserved. This is well tolerated in healthy persons; resting bradycardia is, in fact, a result of high levels of aerobic physical conditioning. However, in the diseased heart contractility is decreased, the useful limits of the Starling relationship are exceeded, and cardiac output may be diminished.

With *tachycardia,* diastolic filling time is decreased, myocardial oxygen demand is increased, and the diseased myocardium or the heart with significant coronary artery disease may tolerate the burden poorly and fail or develop ischemia, injury, or infarction. Furthermore, frequent premature contractions may decrease the cardiac output, a circumstance that may be poorly tolerated in a patient with marginal pump function.

Valve Malfunction
Valve malfunction can lead to pump failure either by *pressure load* (obstruction to outflow of the pumping chamber, such as valvular aortic stenosis or pulmonary stenosis), or by *volume load* (the valve may be regurgitant as with mitral and aortic insufficiency, which present an increased volume of blood to the left ventricle.

Valve abnormalities that impose either a pressure load or a volume load on one or more chambers usually are slowly progressive conditions that cause the heart to use its long-term defense mechanisms of dilatation and hypertrophy. Both these mechanisms can be overcome, with resultant pump failure.

Less commonly, an acute volume load is imposed on the heart, causing a rapid onset of pump failure. Bacterial endocarditis of the aortic or mitral valves, rupture of a portion of the mitral valve apparatus (papillary muscle or chordae tendineae), or rupture of the interventricular septum is the usual cause. In these cases, initial therapy is designed to support the heart during the period of acute insult so that the long-term compensatory mechanisms can be used. However, if this is not successful, emergency replacement of the abnormal valve or closure of the septal defect is indicated.

Heart Muscle Abnormalities
Abnormalities of the *muscle* causing ventricular failure include myocardial infarction, ventricular aneurysm, extensive myocardial fibrosis (usually from atherosclerotic coronary heart disease or prolonged hypertension), endocardial fibrosis, primary myocardial disease (cardiomyopathy), or excessive hypertrophy due to pulmonary hypertension, aortic stenosis, or systemic hypertension.

Myocardial Rupture. In acute myocardial infarction, *myocardial rupture* presents as a dramatic and often catastrophic onset of pump failure and is associated with a high mortality. Rupture usually occurs during the first 8 days following infarction, during the period of greatest softening of the damaged myocardium. Fortunately, myocardial rupture is a relatively rare complication of infarction. Rupture of a papillary muscle, of the interventricular septum, or of the free wall of the left ventricle may occur.

We will first examine the mechanisms of *rupture of a papillary muscle.* There are two papillary muscles in the left ventricle that are thumblike projections of muscle to which the restraining "guidewires" of the mitral valve, the chordae tendineae, are attached. The papillary muscle may be involved in the infarction process and very occasionally may rupture. When it does, there is a sudden loss of restraint of one of the leaflets of the mitral valve, and free mitral regurgitation occurs with each contraction of the left ventricle. This sudden profound pressure and volume load on the left atrium is reflected through the pulmonary veins to the pulmonary vascular bed, and the acute onset of symptoms of pulmonary vascular congestion is noted. This is usually manifested as severe dyspnea and frank pulmonary edema. At the bedside, a loud murmur lasting throughout systole is present. Very often, nothing can be done to save the patient, although occasionally emergency mitral valve replacement can be successfully accomplished.

Sudden heart failure is seen occasionally in acute myocardial infarction as a result of *rupture of the interventricular septum.* Like rupture of the papillary muscle, septal rupture is uncommon, but when it does appear is also usually noted in the first week after damage. Septal rupture is clinically characterized by chest pain, dyspnea, shock, and a rapid onset of evidence of pump failure. There is a loud murmur that lasts throughout systole at the lower left sternal border and is often accompanied by a thrill that one can feel by placing the hand over the precordium at the left sternal border. As with all myocardial ruptures, the prognosis of septal rupture is poor. However, it is occasionally possible to repair these ventricular septal defects by emergency surgery involving cardiopulmonary bypass.

Ruptures of a papillary muscle and the interventricular septum are virtually indistinguishable at the bedside, with both presenting as sudden onset of left ventricular failure, a new murmur, and occasionally a palpable thrill. The location of the infarction is not helpful, and the clinical course in each is rapidly downhill. Emergency cardiac catheterization is the only way to differentiate the two clearly.

Mechanical failure of the heart seen in acute myocardial infarction is another relatively rare event and is due to *rupture of the free wall of the left ventricle* and the spilling of blood into the pericardial cavity. This results in acute compression of the heart or tamponade

and the inability of both chambers to fill adequately. There is then very sudden pumping failure with associated shock and death.

Rupture of the free wall may be preceded by or associated with a return of chest pain as the blood dissects through the necrotic myocardial wall. Sudden vascular collapse as occurs with ventricular fibrillation, but with an unchanged rhythm on the electrocardiogram (electromechanical dissociation), suggests rupture of the ventricular free wall. As with rupture of the papillary muscle and interventricular septum, rupture of the free wall of the left ventricle carries with it an extremely poor prognosis.

Responses to Failure

When the heart's normal reserves are overwhelmed and failure occurs, certain physiological responses to the decrease in cardiac output are important. All these responses represent the body's attempt to maintain a normal perfusion of vital organs.

The primary acute adjustment to heart failure is an increase in sympathetic nervous system influence on the arteries, veins, and heart. This results in increased heart rate, increased venous return to the heart, and increased force of contraction; in addition, sympathetic tone helps maintain a normal blood pressure. The price extracted for this adjustment is an increase in myocardial oxygen demand and oxygen consumption, a request that may inadequately be met in the patient with significant coronary artery obstructive disease or poor pump contractility.

As a result of the autonomic nervous changes and other factors, the blood flow to the essential organs, specifically the brain and heart, is maintained at the expense of less essential organs such as the skin, gut, and kidneys. With severe congestive heart failure, there is sufficient decrease in blood flow to the skeletal muscles to cause a *metabolic acidosis* that must be considered when a treatment program is planned.

When the kidneys sense a decreased volume of blood presented for filtration, they respond by retaining sodium and water and thereby try to do their part in increasing the central blood volume and venous return. With an increase in circulating blood volume and venous return to the heart, there is an increase in end-diastolic fiber length (dilatation) and, within limits, an increase in stroke volume and cardiac output. However, with a failing heart, an increased circulatory volume may be too great a burden for the ventricle, and failure may be worsened.

In some patients with prolonged failure, remaining heart cells with hypertrophy, increasing pumping efficiency, and the clinical findings of heart failure may improve or disappear.

Assessment of Failure

Left Ventricular Failure

It is useful to think of the clinical features of heart failure as coming from failure of either the left ventricle, the right ventricle, or both. When the *left ventricle* fails, its inability to discharge its contents adequately results in dilatation, increased end-diastolic volume, and increased intraventricular pressure at the end of diastole. This results in the inability of the left atrium to empty its contents into the left ventricle adequately, and pressure in the left atrium rises. This pressure rise is reflected into the pulmonary veins, which bring blood from the lungs to the left atrium. The increased pressure in the pulmonary vessels results in pulmonary vascular congestion, which is the cause of the most specific symptoms of left ventricular failure.

Pulmonary Vascular Congestion. The symptoms of pulmonary vascular congestion are dyspnea, orthopnea, paroxysmal nocturnal dyspnea, cough, and acute pulmonary edema.

Dyspnea, characterized by rapid, shallow breathing and a sensation of difficulty in obtaining adequate air, is distressing to the patient. Occasionally, a patient may complain of insomnia, restlessness, or weakness, which is caused by the dyspnea.

Orthopnea, the inability to lie flat because of dyspnea, is another common complaint of left ventricular failure related to pulmonary vascular congestion. It is important to determine whether the orthopnea is truly related to heart disease or whether elevating the head to sleep is merely the patient's custom. For example, if the patient states that he sleeps on three pillows, one might hasten to conclude that he is suffering from orthopnea. If, however, when the patient is asked why he sleeps on three pillows, he replies that he does this because he likes to sleep at this evelation and has done so since before he had symptomatic heart disease, the condition does not qualify as orthopnea.

Paroxysmal nocturnal dyspnea (PND) is a well-known complaint characterized by the patient's awakening in the middle of the night because of intense shortness of breath. Nocturnal dyspnea is thought to be caused by a shift of fluid from the tissues into the intravascular compartment as a result of recumbency. During the day, the pressure in the veins is high, especially in the dependent portions of the body, owing to gravity, increased fluid volume, and increased sympathetic tone. With this increase in hydrostatic pressure, some fluid escapes into the tissue space. With recumbency, the pressure in the dependent capillaries is decreased, and fluid is resorbed into the circulation. This increased volume represents an additional amount of blood that is presented to the heart to pump each minute (increased preload) and places an additional burden on an already congested pulmonary vascular bed, with acute onset of dyspnea the resultant symptom. Keep in mind that PND occurs not only at night but also at any time during acute hospitalizations that require bedrest.

An *irritating cough* is one symptom of pulmonary vascular congestion that is often overlooked but that may be a dominant symptom. It may be productive but is usually dry and hacking in character. This symptom is related to congestion of bronchial mucosa and an associated increase in mucus production.

Acute pulmonary edema is the most florid clinical picture associated with pulmonary vascular congestion. It occurs when the pulmonary capillary pressure exceeds the pressure that tends to keep fluid within the vascular channels (approximately 30 mm Hg). At these pressures, there is transduction of fluid into the alveoli, which in turn diminishes the area available for the normal transport of oxygen into and carbon dioxide out of the blood within the pulmonary capillary bed. Acute pulmonary edema is characterized by intense dyspnea, cough, orthopnea, profound anxiety, cyanosis, sweating, noisy respirations, and very often chest pain and a pink, frothy sputum from the mouth. It constitutes a genuine medical emergency and must be managed vigorously and promptly.

Decreased Cardiac Output. In addition to the symptoms that result from pulmonary vascular congestion, left ventricular failure is also associated with nonspecific symptoms that are related to decreased cardiac output. The patient may complain of weakness, fatigability, apathy, lethargy, difficulty in concentrating, memory deficit, or diminished exercise tolerance. These symptoms may be present in chronic low output states and may dominate the patient's complaints. Unfortunately, these symptoms are nonspecific and are often ascribed to depression, neurosis, or functional complaints. Therefore, these potentially important indicators of deteriorating pump function are often not recognized for their true value, and the patient is either inappropriately reassured or placed on a tranquilizer or mood-elevating preparation. Remember, the presence of the nonspecific symptoms of low cardiac output demands a careful evaluation of the heart as well as the psyche—an examination that will yield the information that will dictate proper management.

Heart Sounds and Rales. Physical signs associated with left ventricular failure that are easily recognized at the bedside include third and fourth heart sounds and rales in the lungs.

The fourth heart sound, or *atrial gallop,* is associated with and follows atrial contraction and is best heard with the bell of the stethoscope very lightly applied at the cardiac apex. The left lateral position may be required to elicit the sound. It is heard just before the first heart sound and is not always a definitive sign of congestive failure but may represent decreased compliance (increased stiffness) of the myocardium. It therefore may be an early, premonitory indication of impending failure. A fourth heart sound is common in patients with acute myocardial infarction and likely does not have prognostic significance, but it may represent incipient failure.

The third sound, or *ventricular gallop,* is an important sign of left ventricular failure and in adults is almost never present in the absence of significant heart disease. Most physicians would agree that treatment of congestive failure is indicated upon the appearance of this sign.

The third sound is heard in early diastole following the second heart sound and is associated with the period of rapid passive ventricular filling. It is also best heard with the bell of the stethoscope applied lightly at the apex, with the patient in the left lateral position, and at the end of expiration.

The fine *moist rales* most commonly heard at the bases of the lungs posteriorly are often recognized as evidence of left ventricular failure, as indeed they may be. Before these rales are ascribed to pump failure, the patient must be instructed to cough deeply in order to open any basilar alveoli that may be compressed as a result of recumbency, inactivity, and compression from the diaphragm beneath. Rales that fail to clear after cough (posttussic) need to be evaluated; those that clear following cough are probably clinically unimportant. It is, however, important to note that the patient may have good evidence of left ventricular failure on the basis of a history of symptoms suggesting pulmonary vascular congestion or the finding of a third heart sound at the apex and yet have quite clear lung fields. It is not appropriate to wait for the appearance of rales in the lungs before instituting therapy for left ventricular failure.

Arrhythmias. Because an increase in heart rate is the heart's initial response to stress, sinus tachycardia might be expected and is often found in the examination of a patient with pump failure. Other rhythms associated with pump failure include atrial premature contractions, paroxysmal atrial tachycardia, and ventricular premature beats. Whenever a rhythm abnormality is detected, one must attempt to define the underlying pathophysiological mechanism; therapy can then be properly planned and instituted.

Other Signs. Other signs of left ventricular failure that may be noted in addition to a third heart sound, rales in the lungs, and supraventricular rhythms include wheezing breath sounds, pulsus alternans (an alternating greater and lesser volume of the arterial pulse), a square-wave response to a standard Valsalva maneuver (see further on), weight gain, and Cheyne-Stokes respirations. Indeed, patients may awaken at night during respiratory height of a Cheyne-Stokes cycle, a situation that may falsely be interpreted as PND but that may have the same pathophysiological significance. Weight gain resulting from retention of salt and water by the kidneys is a useful sign that the patient may follow at home. Daily weight should be recorded in the morning after voiding and before breakfast.

Radiographic Findings. Radiographic examination of the chest often helps one diagnose heart failure. Careful evaluation of the chest roentgenogram may demonstrate changes in the blood vessels of the lungs that result from an increase in pulmonary venous pressure. Radiographic findings may be present in the absence of rales, and careful examination of the chest film is necessary if left ventricular failure is suspected.

Right Ventricular Failure

Failure of the *right ventricle* alone is often the result of severe underlying lung disease and such conditions as severe pulmonary hypertension (primary or secondary), stenosis of the pulmonary valve, and a massive pulmonary embolus. The right ventricle tolerates a volume load well, and pure right ventricular failure is usually due to resistance to outflow (pressure load). More commonly, however, right ventricular failure is the result of failure of the left ventricle. In this situation, symptoms and signs of both left and right ventricular failure are present, and the symptoms of left ventricular failure may improve as the right ventricle fails through relief of left ventricular preload and decrease in pulmonary vascular congestion.

Low Cardiac Output. In contrast to left ventricular failure, in which specific symptoms can usually be related to a single underlying mechanism—pulmonary vascular congestion—the symptoms of right heart failure are not so specific, and many are related to a low cardiac output. Fatigability, weakness, lethargy, or difficulty in concentrating may be prominent. Heaviness of the limbs (especially the legs), an increase in abdominal girth, inability to wear previously comfortable shoes, and weight gain reflect the ascites and edema associated with right ventricular failure.

In addition, symptoms of the underlying pulmonary disease usually dominate complaints if failure is due to a primary pulmonary problem, usually chronic bronchitis or emphysema. Occasionally bronchiectasis or restrictive lung disease may be the primary pulmonary problem, but chronic bronchitis and emphysema are by far the most common pulmonary causes of right ventricular failure.

Jugular Vein Distention. When the right ventricle decompensates, there is dilatation of the chamber, an increase in right ventricular end-diastolic volume and pressure, resistance to filling of the ventricle, and a subsequent rise in right atrial pressure. This increasing pressure is in turn reflected upstream in the venae cavae and can be recognized by an increase in the jugular venous pressure. One can best evaluate this by looking at the veins in the neck and noting the height of the column of blood. With the patient lying in bed and the head of the bed elevated between 30° and 60°, the column of blood in the external jugular veins will be, in the normal person, only a few millimeters above the upper border of the clavicle, if it is seen at all (Fig. 10-2).

When an observation of venous pressure is recorded, the height of the column of blood above the sternal angle and the elevation of the head of the bed should be included. This will then provide a useful basis for comparison of future observations.

Edema. Edema is often considered a reliable sign of heart failure, and, indeed, it is often present when the right ventricle has failed. However, it is the least reliable sign of right ventricular dysfunction. Many people, particularly the elderly, spend much of their time sitting in a chair with the legs dependent. As a result of this body position, the decreased turgor of subcutaneous tissue associated with old age, and perhaps primary venous disease such as varicosities, ankle edema may be produced that reflects these factors rather than right ventricular failure.

When edema does appear related to failure of the right ventricle, it is dependent in location. If the patient is up and about, it will be noted primarily in the ankles and will ascend the legs as failure worsens. When the patient is put to bed, the dependent portion of the body becomes the sacral area, and edema should be looked for there. In addition, other signs of right ventricular failure should be present before the diagnosis is made. Dependent edema alone is inadequate documentation of the status of the right ventricle. With congestion of the liver, this organ may enlarge and become tender, ascites may be present, and jaundice may be noted.

Other Signs. As with left ventricular failure, sinus tachycardia and the other rhythms associated with pump failure may be present. In addition, right ventricular third and fourth heart sounds are not uncommon. They are best heard at the lower left sternal border, with the bell of the stethoscope applied lightly to the chest, and can be recognized by an increase in intensity with inspiration. Finally, signs of any underlying cause of right ventricular failure may be present, such as hyperresonance with percussion, low immobile diaphragms, decreased breath sounds, increased anteroposterior chest diameter, and use of the accessory muscles of respiration in patients with severe pulmonary emphysema.

Valsalva Maneuver in Diagnosis

The Valsalva maneuver has been used in the diagnosis of heart failure and has a long and interesting history. It is discussed here for its general clinical interest rather than as an important diagnostic maneuver in suspected heart failure.

The Valsalva maneuver has also been implicated as causing an occasional fatality either through the production of a cardiac arrhythmia or through the dislodging of venous thrombi, producing massive pulmonary embolization.

One performs a standard Valsalva maneuver by blowing into a mercury manometer to a pressure of 40 torr and sustaining this effort for 10 seconds. Naturally, a patient does not do this on his own during the day but may closely simulate the maneuver during a prolonged effort of straining at stool. Intermittent positive pressure breathing may produce short periods of a similar type of strain, as may a cough or sneeze.

In the normal response to the Valsalva maneuver there are four phases.

Phase I occurs with the onset of strain, at which time there is an increase in intrathoracic pressure, which is

FIGURE 10-2
Estimation of jugular venous pressure as a noninvasive determination of central venous pressure. (A) Phlebostatic axis (4th intercostal space at the sternum, intersecting the mid anteroposterior line). (B) Internal jugular vein. (C) External jugular vein. (D) Vertical distance in centimeters from the meniscus to the phlebostatic axis equals the CVP in cm H$_2$O. (From Brunner LS, Suddarth DS: Textbook of Medical-Surgical Nursing, 5th ed. Philadelphia, JB Lippincott, 1984)

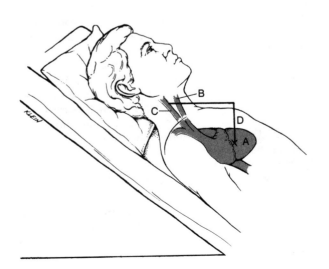

transmitted to the great vessels (aorta and pulmonary artery), and leads to a rise in arterial blood pressure.

During *phase II,* as a later result of the increased intrathoracic pressure and limitation of venous return to the heart, there is a decrease in right atrial filling and a decrease in left ventricular stroke volume, producing a fall in arterial blood pressure and pulse pressure (the difference between the systolic and diastolic pressures). This fall in pressure stimulates the receptors in the carotid sinus, aortic arch, and common carotid artery, which are sensitive to pressure and which in turn cause an increase in sympathetic activity, resulting in an increase in heart rate and peripheral vasoconstriction. At the bedside, phase II is characterized by an increase in heart rate and a fall in blood pressure.

With *phase III,* or release of the strain, there is an increased venous return to the right heart and an increase in blood volume in the pulmonary vascular bed. This is ultimately transmitted to the left side of the heart, with an associated increase in the left ventricular stroke volume as the left ventricle once again fills. Because it takes a few seconds for the pulmonary vascular bed to fill with blood before it reaches the left heart, there may be a continuous fall in cardiac output and blood pressure for 2 to 3 seconds immediately upon the release of the strain.

Phase IV is called the *overshoot* and is characterized by bradycardia and a rise in blood pressure over the resting observed values. This occurs because the increased left ventricular stroke volume is ejected into a constricted peripheral vascular bed. This constricted bed causes an increase in peripheral resistance, and the pressure therefore rises. The pressure-sensitive receptors in the carotid body sense the higher pressure, and parasympathetic activity through the vagus nerve is stimulated, causing a reflex slowing of the heart. The overshoot period is then characterized by blood pressure that is greater than the initial resting values and by bradycardia.

In *heart failure,* the response to the Valsalva maneuver is quite different. As the strain begins, there is a rise in intrathoracic pressure. This rise in pressure is transmitted and is noted as an increase in the peripheral arterial pressure. However, as the strain continues, there is no decrease in pressure and no increase in the heart rate. Upon release of the maneuver, the blood pressure returns to the baseline values, and there is no overshoot.

This kind of response, in which there is only a rise in arterial pressure without any heart rate changes and no overshoot response, has been called *the square-wave response* and is due to the fact that the failing myocardium, with its already maximized preload, will not change total stroke volume enough to decrease cardiac output further and stimulate the pressor receptors. The same kind of response is seen in patients with a signifi-

cant atrial septal defect because the preload to the right ventricle remains high owing to the shunt from the left to the right atrium.

A pilot study designed to serially evaluate the Valsalva maneuver in 51 postinfarction patients showed it to be an insensitive indicator of an impending acute event.*

Intervention in Heart Failure

Heart failure may be present in varying degress of severity. In acute myocardial infarction, heart failure has been simply and usefully classified by Killip into four classes: I, no failure; II, mild to moderate failure; III, acute pulmonary edema; and IV, cardiogenic shock (Table 10-2).

Early, moderate (Killip class II) failure and chronic failure are often characterized by a third heart sound, increased heart rate (usually sinus rhythm), and possibly fine posttussic crackling rales at the lung bases. In addition, evidence of pulmonary vascular congestion (often without pulmonary edema) is often evident on the chest roentgenogram, and arrhythmias may be present: atrial premature contractions, atrial fibrillation, atrial flutter, paroxysmal atrial tachycardia, and junctional rhythms. The patient may be reasonably comfortable at rest or may have symptoms of low cardiac output or pulmonary vascular congestion. Symptoms are increased with activity.

Acute pulmonary edema (Killip class III) is a life-threatening situation characterized by transudation of fluid from the pulmonary capillary bed into the alveolar spaces, with associated extreme dyspnea and anxiety. Immediate care is required if the patient's life is to be saved.

Cardiogenic shock (Killip class IV) is the most ominous pump failure syndrome and is associated with the highest mortality, even with aggressive care. Cardiogenic shock is recognized clinically by

- A systolic blood pressure less than 80 torr (often it cannot be measured)
- A feeble pulse that is often rapid

---

* HL Brammell: Unpublished observations.

TABLE 10-2
KILLIP CLASSIFICATION OF HEART FAILURE

Class	Status
I	No failure
II	Mild to moderate failure
III	Acute pulmonary edema
IV	Cardiogenic shock

- Pale, cool, and sweaty skin that is frequently cyanotic
- Restlessness, confusion, and apathy
- Possible coma, although not usual
- Decreased or absent urine output

These manifestations of shock are a reflection of the profound inadequacy of the heart as a pump and usually reflect a large amount of muscle damage (40% or more of the left ventricular mass).

Some patients with significant, long-standing arterial hypertension will have manifestations of cardiogenic shock at relatively normal pressures. These people require a higher pressure to perfuse vital organs and maintain viability. Knowledge of the preceding blood pressure history is of great importance in recognizing these people. Not all clinical circumstances of cardiogenic shock are associated with an inadequate cardiac output, however. Depending on modifying circumstances, such as fever, the cardiac output may occasionally be normal or even increased.

The failure to decrease coronary care unit mortality below 10% to 15% is largely due to only modest improvement in the management and mortality of severe pump failure syndromes, especially cardiogenic shock.

Plan

The physiological responses to heart failure form a rational basis for treatment. The goals of the management of congestive heart failure are to reduce the work of the heart, to increase cardiac output and myocardial contractility, and to decrease retention of salt and water (Table 10-3).

Bed Rest. Because the heart cannot be put to complete rest to heal in the same fashion as a broken bone, the best that can be done is to put the entire patient to rest; thereby, through inactivity, the overall pumping demand on the heart is decreased. *Bed rest* is therefore an important part of the treatment of congestive heart failure, especially in acute and refractory stages.

In addition to decreasing the overall work demands made on the heart, bed rest assists in lowering the work load by decreasing the intravascular volume through a recumbency-induced diuresis. Studies of prolonged bed rest have demonstrated that within 48 to 72 hours of inactivity there is a decrease of plasma volume of 300 ml or more. Although this is not a great volume in terms of the overall intravascular fluid compartment, it does assist in decreasing the volume load that is presented to the failing heart. It therefore assists in decreasing dilatation of the heart chambers and establishing a compensated state. This effect results from stimulation of atrial stretch receptors that sense the increased volume of blood returning to the right side of the heart, which would be sequestered in the lower extremities if the patient were upright. These receptors then "turn off" the production of antidiuretic hormone, and a diuresis follows. By decreasing intravascular volume and therefore the amount of blood presented to the heart to pump (preload), compensation of the heart may be enhanced.

Diuretics. In addition to bed rest, *salt* and *water restriction* and *diuretics,* either oral or parenteral, will decrease preload and the work of the heart.

All diuretics, regardless of the route of administration, may cause significant changes in the serum electrolytes, especially potassium and chloride. Therefore, regular determination of serum electrolytes is important in patient follow-up. This is particularly true when the patient is also receiving digitalis because low potassium produced by diuretics predisposes to digitalis toxicity, a life-threatening but avoidable complication. Because of this possibility, potassium supplements are customarily ordered when potassium-depleting diuretics are given, especially when digitalis is given as well.

The choice of route of administration of the diuretic is largely a function of the gravity of the clinical situation. Mild to moderate left ventricular failure (manifested by sinus tachycardia, posttussic rales, and a third heart sound) can usually be managed with oral preparations. However, acute pulmonary edema, a life-threatening situation, demands more drastic approaches, and the parenteral route should be chosen.

Other modifiers of preload and afterload are valuable approaches to the management of acute and chronic failure states. Both pharmacologic and mechanical methods are useful.

Morphine. *Morphine* is the single most useful drug in the treatment of pulmonary edema. It achieves its primary physiological usefulness through a peripheral vasodilating effect, forming a peripheral pool of blood (bloodless phlebotomy) that decreases both venous return and the work of the heart. In addition, morphine allays the great anxiety associated with severe dyspnea and quiets the patient, thereby decreasing the respiratory pump mechanism for increasing venous return. Morphine also decreases arterial blood pressure and

---

TABLE 10-3
GOALS FOR MANAGEMENT OF HEART FAILURE

Reduce work of the heart
Increase cardiac output and myocardial contractility
Decrease retention of salt and water

resistance, lessening the work of the heart (decreased afterload).

Reduction of Circulating Blood Volume. An even more dramatic method of decreasing preload and the work of the heart is *phlebotomy,* a procedure that is often useful in the patient with acute pulmonary edema because it immediately removes a volume of blood from the central circulation, decreases venous return and filling pressure, and provides rather prompt reversal of some basic hemodynamic problems.

Phlebotomy may be bloodless (*rotating tourniquets*), or whole blood may be directly removed from the circulation. Tourniquets are less effective than direct removal of blood.

Although phlebotomy is often helpful in managing acute pulmonary edema, it may be dangerous in the patient who does not have an increased intravascular volume. This situation most commonly occurs in patients with acute myocardial infarction in whom there is extensive muscle damage and rapid onset of pulmonary edema before the kidneys can compensate for a diminished cardiac output by sodium and water retention.

Patients with normal blood volume and pulmonary edema usually demonstrate a normal-sized heart on chest roentgenogram. Removing a unit of blood from the circulation either by use of tourniquets or by venesection may cause a significant drop in blood pressure in these patients. However, patients who have more chronic congestive heart failure with an increased intravascular volume and dilatation of the heart in association with pulmonary edema are often excellent candidates for rotating tourniquets or venesection.

Nitrates. The use of *nitrates,* both acutely and chronically, has been advocated in the management of heart failure. By causing peripheral vasodilatation, the heart is "unloaded" (decreased afterload), with a subsequent increase in cardiac output, decrease in pulmonary artery wedge pressure (a measurement that reflects the degree of pulmonary vascular congestion and the severity of left ventricular failure), and decrease in myocardial oxygen consumption. This form of therapy has been found useful in mild to moderate failure and acute pulmonary edema failure associated with myocardial infarction, chronic refractory left ventricular failure, and failure associated with severe mitral regurgitation. At present, parenteral vasodilator therapy (intravenous nitroglycerin or sodium nitroprusside) requires accurate hemodynamic monitoring of arterial and pulmonary wedge pressure (arterial cannula and Swan-Ganz catheter) and use of an infusion pump to carefully titrate the dose delivered.

Nitroprusside must be used with care. Long-acting nitrate therapy is usually given with isosorbide dinitrate (sublingual or oral, with the former being preferred) or nitroglycerin ointment. Some patients who have received maximal benefit from other forms of therapy for left ventricular failure have been substantially improved by vasodilator treatment.

Digitalis. Although modification of the work of the heart by decreasing preload and afterload is indicated in heart failure and at times permits avoidance of drugs that increase the force of myocardial contraction, inotropic agents remain important therapeutic tools.

Digitalis is the primary drug for increasing contractility. This inotropic drug has a multiplicity of uses in cardiology and is also potentially one of the most dangerous, a fact recognized in 1785 by William Withering, discoverer of the pharmacologic value and toxicity of digitalis (foxglove): "Foxglove when given in very large and quickly repeated doses occasions sickness, vomiting, purging, confused vision, objects appearing green or yellow, increased secretion of urine with frequent motions to part with it and sometimes inability to retain it; slow pulse even as low as 35 in a minute, cold sweats, convulsions, syncope and death." In the failing heart, digitalis slows the ventricular rate and increases the force of contraction, increasing cardiac efficiency. As cardiac output increases, a greater volume of fluid is presented to the kidneys for filtration and excretion, and intravascular volume decreases.

In early failure with acute myocardial infarction, digitalis may increase the potential amount of damaged myocardium by causing increased contractility and therefore increased myocardial oxygen demand. Treatment of failure in this circumstance is probably best if preload or afterload is decreased through the use of diuretics or nitrates. Of course, if either agent causes a significant drop in central aortic pressure, coronary artery perfusion may fall and the area of damage increase. The key lessons here are that any medication has potentially ominous side effects, that a management regimen must be selected with care and with a full understanding of potential adverse effects, and that close patient monitoring is mandatory.

Other Measures. Cardiogenic shock unfortunately is not a completely understood situation at this time. Accordingly, the management of cardiogenic shock is generally unsatisfactory. At the very least, treatment requires administration of bicarbonate to correct the metabolic acidosis, oxygen, and agents to elevate the blood pressure. The most commonly used pressor agents at this time are dopamine, norepinephrine, and dobutamine. Depending on the pulmonary artery wedge pressure (left ventricular filling pressure), the administration of small amounts of fluid may be indicated. Mechanical life-support devices such as intra-aortic balloon counter-pulsation, direct ventricular assistors, or left heart bypass are occasionally used. The intra-aortic balloon assist device has been the most successful to date and has established a place in cardiac care.

The general outlook for patients with cardiogenic shock is poor for both the short and the long term. Heart failure, with its accompanying symptoms of low cardiac output or pulmonary vascular congestion or both, is one of the major sources of disability in cardiovascular disease. Its recognition and pathophysiologically based management are of paramount importance if a patient's functional capacity and vocational and community viability are to be optimized and maintained.

BIBLIOGRAPHY

Cohen S: New concepts in understanding congestive heart failure—Part I: How the clinical features arise. Am J Nurs 81:119–142, 1981

Cohen S: New concepts in understanding congestive heart failure—Part II: How the therapeutic approaches work. Am J Nurs February, 1981, pp 357–380

Little RC, Little WC: Cardiac preload, afterload and heart failure. Arch Int Med 142:819–822, 1982

Miller D, Borer J: Cardiomyopathies: A pathophysiologic approach to therapeutic management. Arch Int Med 143:2157–2162, 1983

Sclant RC, Sonnebleck E: Pathophysiology of heart failure. In Hurst JW (ed): The Heart, Arteries and Veins, Vol 1, pp 382–407. New York, McGraw-Hill, 1982

Withering W: An Account of the Foxglove and its Medical Uses, with Practical Remarks on Dropsy and Other Diseases. London, CGJ and J Robinson, 1785

11
Acute Myocardial Infarction

Julie J. Benz

Although the mortality associated with problems of the heart and vessels has decreased by 25% since the 1970s, cardiovascular disease remains the most serious threat to life and health in the United States. For men, the chance of developing heart disease before 60 years of age is one in three; the risk for women is one in ten. It has been estimated that 20% of Americans have one or more cardiovascular diseases. Each year, 1,250,000 people have myocardial infarctions, which result in approximately 650,000 deaths. Sixty-four percent of all cardiovascular deaths are related to arteriosclerosis, and strokes account for 17% of the annual mortality rates.

As overwhelming as the mortality and morbidity statistics appear, much progress has been made in diagnosis, management, and therapy to combat cardiovascular disease successfully. The mortality rate is declining by 2% per year. Since the Framingham study of risk factors in 1951 and the development of coronary care units in the same decade, the critical care nurse has played a major role in reducing the mortality associated with heart disease.

Sophisticated prehospital care and continuous cardiac monitoring have dramatically decreased the number of deaths due to dysrhythmias. Following an acute myocardial infarction, the most frequent cause of death is now left ventricular heart failure.

The role of the critical care nurse has evolved rapidly. To combat cardiovascular disease, the nurse must have finite assessment skills, intervene quickly, and reevaluate the results of the interventions. Complete discharge planning and "cardiac rehabilitation" programs have enabled patients to return home, maximiz-ing their health status. The role of the nurse, in both acute and nonacute settings, cannot be minimized.

PATHOPHYSIOLOGY

Myocardial infarction (MI) is a "segmental" disease of the myocardium. Therefore, physiological considerations of global heart disease will not always apply. Rather than an epidemic loss of myocardial function, the myocardial infarction creates a partial loss, based on location and severity of tissue necrosis.

An MI is the result of coronary artery disease with concomitant tissue damage and necrosis. The coronary artery damage may be traced to thrombosis, atherosclerosis, or spasm. The cardiac tissue dependant upon blood flow from the diseased artery will become ischemic and necrotic, resulting in an infarct.

Atherosclerosis

For many years, the etiology of "coronary thrombosis," or clot occlusion, of a coronary artery was believed to cause an MI. The thrombosis found on postmortem examination usually resulted in blood flow that was compromised to the extent of a full myocardial wall thickness, or "transmural" infarct, and tissue death.

As dissection study continued, it became clear that the final event may have been thrombotic but that the narrowing of the coronary artery had begun by the development of plaque, known as atherosclerosis. The term "atherosclerosis" comes from the Greek word "athere," which means "porridge" or "gruel." This term seems to describe the gross appearance of the plaque substance.

Atherosclerosis is actually an insidious process, beginning long before symptoms occur. In atherosclerosis, the intima (inner lining) of the artery undergoes focal changes. Muscular arteries, such as the coronaries, carotid, aortic, iliac, femoral, and popliteal arteries, are most susceptible.

Spots develop on the artery's intimal wall. These minor elevations cause a proliferation of intimal cells, and eventually a "cap" of cells is formed. The center of this small cap consists of necrotic intimal cells and cholesterols. As the cap becomes larger, it is known as plaque. Plaque develops best in plasma that is rich in low-density lipoproteins (cholesterol). The inflammatory process causes these cholesterols to gravitate towards disruptions in the otherwise smooth intimal lining. Although the origin of intimal injury resulting in intimal spotting is unclear, cigarettes and hypertension are known to aggravate intimal injury.

As the plaque increases in size, platelet adhesion begins. This process can continue to the point of slowing arterial blood flow from a rushing state to merely a trickle by reducing arterial diameter.

Much attention has been given to coronary artery spasm. A blood vessel, narrowed by atherosclerosis, can be occluded if spasm occurs. It is believed that many partial wall thickness infarcts, or nontransmural infarcts, are the result of coronary spasm. This process is not fully understood and will likely be the focus of research in the 1990s.

As arterial blood flow is decreased, the myocardial tissue's need for oxygen and nutrients continues. The same work of pumping blood must be accomplished with less available energy and oxygen. The tissue that depends on the blood supply becomes ischemic as it functions with less oxygenated blood. Anaerobic metabolism can provide only 6% of the total energy needed. Glucose uptake by the cells is markedly increased as glycogen and ATP stores are depleted. Potassium rapidly moves out of the myocardial cells during ischemia. An acidotic cellular bath develops, further compromising cellular metabolism.

Myocardial Infarction

If the reduced blood flow is reestablished to normal levels, the ischemic event will terminate. This transient myocardial ischemia is known as "angina." If the ischemia were to continue while myocardial oxygen requirements persevered, the tissue would become necrotic because the energy demands would exceed the oxygenated blood's energy supply. This is a myocardial infarction.

Necrotic myocardial tissue cannot be revived. Surrounding the dead tissue is a zone of ischemic tissue that has suffered less, remaining viable on severely compromised blood flow. It is a major therapeutic goal to prevent the ischemic concentric rings of tissue from becoming necrotic. If the ischemic rings cannot be saved, the resulting damage is referred to as an "extension" of the acute MI.

Transmural Infarction

As mentioned before, infarct size and location have enormous impact on prognosis and survival. Transmural infarcts include necrosis of all layers of the myocardium. Because the heart functions as a squeezing pump, systolic efforts to empty the ventricle can be markedly reduced by a segment of the myocardial wall that is dead and nonfunctional. If the area of the transmural infarct is small, the necrotic tissue may be "dyskinetic." As this muscular wall squeezes during systole or relaxes with diastolic filling, dyskinetic tissue does not remain in synchronous motion with the healthy myocardial wall. If the transmural infarct area is larger, the dead tissue may become "akinetic," lacking any motion and therefore interfering with efficient pumping.

During the process of necrosis, the transmural infarct area may weaken. As the rest of the chamber goes through isotonic contraction, the necrotic area may bulge with an aneurysm or even rupture under the efforts to create an adequate systolic contraction.

Subendocardial Infarction

Not all infarcts affect the full wall thickness. Subendocardial infarcts are common and involve necrosis of the inner layers of the myocardium. The subendocardial tissue is most vulnerable to ischemia; the outer wall, the epicardium, is the least vulnerable. Because myocardial muscle layers are "wrapped" for efficient squeezing (layers criss-cross over each other), a subendocardial infarct will have less impact on wall motion than a transmural infarct will.

CORONARY CIRCULATION

Infarct location can affect prognosis. Because the process of an MI begins with coronary artery disease leading to decreased blood flow, it is imperative that one understand the functional anatomy of the major coronary arteries.

There are two major coronary arteries, the left and the right. The left main coronary artery has two branches. The left anterior descending, or LAD (also called the "widow maker"), passes down the anterior wall towards the apex of the myocardium. It supplies blood flow to two thirds of the intraventricular septum, most of the apex, and the anterior left ventricle. The left circumflex (Circ) flows from the left coronary

TABLE 11-1
THE CORONARY ARTERY BLOOD SUPPLY

Left main coronary artery
   Left anterior descending supplies
      Anterior two thirds of ventricular septum
      Anterior left ventricle
      Entire apex
   Left circumflex supplies
      Posterior ventricular septum
      Left atrium
      Entire posterior wall
Right coronary artery supplies
   Posterosuperior ventricular septum
   Part of the left atrium
   Right atrium
   Sinoatrial node
   Atrioventricular node
   Right ventricle
   Posterior left ventricle
   Diaphragmatic left ventricle

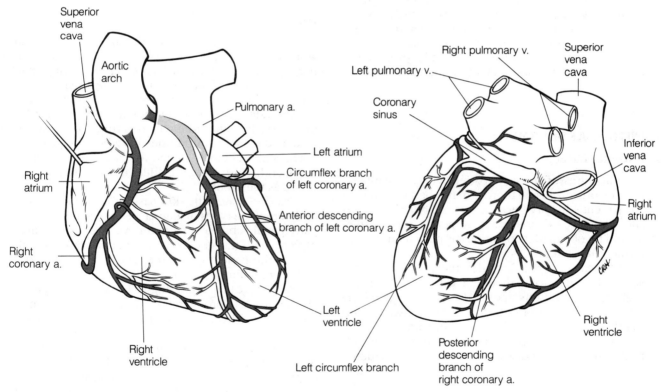

FIGURE 11-1
Coronary circulation.

towards the left lateral wall of the left ventricle. The circumflex supplies blood flow to the left atrium, the entire posterior wall, and the posterior one third of the intraventricular septum (Table 11-1 and Fig. 11-1).

The right coronary artery (RCA) comes off the aorta on the right side of the pulmonary artery and travels along the right lateral wall to the posterior heart. The RCA supplies the right atrium, right ventricle, sinoatrial node, atrioventricular node, posterosuperior intraventricular septum, part of the left atrium, and the posterior and diaphragmatic surface of the left ventricle. Thus, the coronary arteries manage to distribute blood flow to the very active heart tissue.

Forty-eight percent of the population has dominant flow through the RCA; 18% have dominant flow through the LCA; and 34% have an even balance of blood flow. People with left dominant flow are more likely to succumb to a coronary occlusion. Although infarcts can occur on any wall of the myocardium, the term myocardial infarction commonly refers to a left ventricular infarct. The impact of a left ventricular infarct is dramatically symptomatic, and our common diagnostic tools can recognize and locate left ventricular damage. As diagnostic skills expand, more attention may be given to infarcts of the other chambers.

Collateral Circulation

Collateral circulation has received much attention. During ischemic attacks, homocoronary anastomosis occurs. The blood flow is unable to pass through the occluded vessel. As pressure builds on the proximal side of the occlusion, flow is redirected and new vessels develop. This collateral circulation allows the vascular pressure to be relatively equal and provides alternate coronary circulation routes, minimizing ischemia potential.

INITIAL ASSESSMENT

Patient History

The nursing assessment of a patient with a probable MI must be organized and thorough. It is best to start with the patient's history because this establishes rapport and provides valuable data. A generalized history should be obtained, with emphasis placed on the cardiovascular system.

Historical data that includes the presence or absence of "risk factors" should be gathered. The Framingham Massachusetts study of the late 1940s and early 1950s identified five risk factors of heart disease. During this prospective study of a large, random population, several factors were noted to increase a person's propensity for heart disease. The major factors identified were elevated blood cholesterol, cigarette smoking, obesity, hypertension, and sedentary life style (Table 11-2).

Other factors that may potentiate the development of coronary artery disease include the following:

- Familial history of heart disease
- Type "A" personality (intense ambition, competitive outlook and fast pace)
- Diabetes mellitus or abnormal glucose tolerance test
- Excessive sucrose or saturated fat consumption
- Use of oral contraceptives
- Menopause

The patient's description of the acute event is important. Often the precipitating events involve cold weather, exercise, heavy meals, stress, emotional events, or Valsalva actions such as a bowel movement. Some people develop symptoms at rest, but usually there is an activity involved that increases the metabolic requirements of the body.

Angina

Typically, the pain is precordial. Angina (from a Latin word meaning "squeezing") often presents as a crushing, squeezing, constricting, choking, or burning pain. The sensation is sharp, stabbing, or sore, aching, and dull. The pain may radiate behind the sternum to the left chest, left arm, neck, jaw, or left shoulder. Visceral pain from the myocardium is sometimes poorly localized, and over 100 conditions have been improperly diagnosed as angina. Commonly, gastric distress, peptic ulcer disease, and gallbladder disease are misdiagnosed as the problem.

Advanced diagnostic skill has enabled practitioners to differentiate types of angina. "Stable angina" is the paroxysmal substernal pain, relieved by rest or nitroglycerin. This transient bout of ischemia presents similarly to the patient each time. The pain can be controlled with nitroglycerin.

More severe than stable angina is "unstable angina," also known as "preinfarction angina" or "crescendo angina." Unstable angina is characterized by more severe or more frequent attacks, occurring with less provocation or at rest. Usually, two nitroglycerin tablets are insufficient to relieve pain. About 16% to 20% of patients with unstable angina will have MI. During an unstable anginal attack, the electrocardiogram will reveal significant S–T segment depression.

The last category of angina is known as "Prinzmetal's," or "variant," angina. Typically, the pain occurs without precipitating factors because it is due to coronary artery spasm. The ECG will show S–T segment elevation (usually seen only with an MI) rather than the ischemic S–T depression seen in typical angina.

The pain of an acute MI is similar to anginal pain, but

TABLE 11-2
FRAMINGHAM'S RISK FACTORS

Hypercholesterolemia	>275 mg/dl
Cigarette smoking	>20/day
Obesity	>120% of ideal weight
Hypertension	>160/90
Sedentary life style	

more severe. While anginal pain may last minutes and be relieved with nitroglycerin, MI pain can last hours and is best relieved with narcotics such as morphine. As many as 25% of patients with acute MI will experience little or no pain.

As the nurse assesses the patient, it is likely that symptoms of a severe autonomic response will be apparent. Patients with cardiac pain (anginal or MI) often are very still. Pallor and diaphoresis often occur. Cyanosis may be present, but the skin will often look gray or washed out. Vomiting and bradycardia may be present. Syncope is not rare. Some patients will complain of the feeling of "impending doom," and most are very frightened.

It is of value to be able to differentiate between symptoms of right-sided and left-sided heart disease. Right-sided failure (congestive heart failure) presents with edema, distended jugular veins, peripheral venous congestion, an enlarged liver, cyanosis, and rales. Left-sided heart failure presents with a "shock" picture of gray skin, mottled lower extremities, dyspnea, orthopnea, low blood pressure, and low urine output. Further diagnostic studies are often needed to establish a conclusive etiology.

Diagnostic Studies

Critical care nurses will need to anticipate diagnostic studies required to verify the medical diagnosis. Continuous cardiac monitoring for dysrhythmias and response to treatment will begin on admission. A 12-lead ECG may confirm the presence of heart disease.

Electrocardiographic Findings
On the 12-lead ECG, ischemic but functional myocardial tissue will produce changes in the T wave, causing inversion as the electrical current is directed away from the ischemic tissue. More seriously, ischemic tissue will alter the S – T segment, causing S – T depression.

With an infarct, the dead myocardium does not conduct electricity and fails to repolarize normally. This results in S – T segment elevation. As the necrosis develops, with healing of the ischemic rings around the necrotic area, Q waves develop. The necrotic area is an electrically inactive scar, but the ischemic zone will reflect T wave changes as ischemia recurs. Initially, with a myocardial infarction, the S – T elevation is accompanied by tall T waves. Hours to days later, the T waves invert. As the myocardial infarction ages, Q waves remain and the S – T segments return to normal.

The 12-lead ECG also identifies the location of the ischemic or infarcted tissue. By the presence of the specific lead changes, as well as reciprocal changes occurring on the other walls, infarct area and size are determined (Table 11-3 and Figs. 11-2 to 11-4).

Subendocardial infarcts of partial wall thickness are documented by persistent S – T depression and/or T wave inversion with Q waves. The presence or absence of permanent Q waves will not always indicate MI. For example, right ventricular hypertrophy causes Q waves in V_5 and V_6. Because Q waves are not always abnormal, further diagnostic studies are needed.

Cardiac Enzymes
Traditionally, serial studies of cardiac enzymes are obtained through blood samples drawn every 8 hours for 1 to 2 days. When tissue injury occurs, large proteins escape from inside the cardiac muscle cell and enter the circulation. The enzymes that should be observed are creatine kinase (CK), lactic dehydrogenase (LDH), and serum glutamic oxaloacetic transaminase (SGOT). False-positive results occur in as many as 15% of patients. Isolated enzymes are now available to assist in determining the cardiac origin of CK and LDH. (See discussion of serum enzyme studies in Chap. 8.)

Other Diagnostic Procedures
If the physician desires durther diagnostic data, exercise stress testing can be used to determine functional capacity of the heart under stress in a controlled environment. The blood pressure, heart rate, rhythm, and ischemic ECG changes are monitored during a graded treadmill workout.

Vectorcardiography is a noninvasive measure of electrical axis for speed and direction of conduction and disturbances such as left ventricular and right ventricular hypertrophy and heart blocks. Thallium scintiphotography allows for myocardial imaging after an injection of thallium 201. A "cold spot" occurs in the image corresponding to the area of ischemia.

Invasive diagnostic tests are not without risk, but they provide valuable and accurate data. Coronary angiography (heart catheterization) allows for the direct visualization of the major coronary arteries and direct measurement of left ventricular function. Under the fluoroscope, a catheter is passed through the femoral artery to the aortic arch. The vessel to be studied can be located and a dye injection selectively administered. Coronary artery lesions are visualized, and permanent visual recordings are made.

Pressure readings of all cardiac chambers can be made during a heart catheterization. Radiopaque dye allows the left ventricle to be studied in peak systole and peak diastole. The still films of the functioning ventricle can be compared with the cardiac cycle (determined by ECG) to determine left ventricular end-diastolic volume, stroke volume, and ejection fraction. A comparison of these three values is helpful in determining the degree of compromise in an infarcted left ventricle. (See Chap. 8 for a full discussion of cardiovascular diagnostic techniques.)

TABLE 11-3
SPECIFIC ECG CHANGES FOR ACUTE TRANSMURAL MYOCARDIAL INFARCTIONS

Infarct Area	ECG Changes
Anterior	S–T segment elevation in leads V_3–V_4; reciprocal changes (S–T depression) in leads II, III, aVF (Fig. 11-2)
Inferior	S–T segment elevation in leads II, III, aVF; reciprocal changes (S–T depression) in V_1–V_6, I, aVL (Fig. 11-4)
Lateral	S–T segment elevation in I, aVL, V_5–V_6 (Fig. 11-3)
Posterior	Reciprocal changes in II, III, aVF; predominant R waves in V_1–V_2
Right ventricle	Mimic inferior wall changes

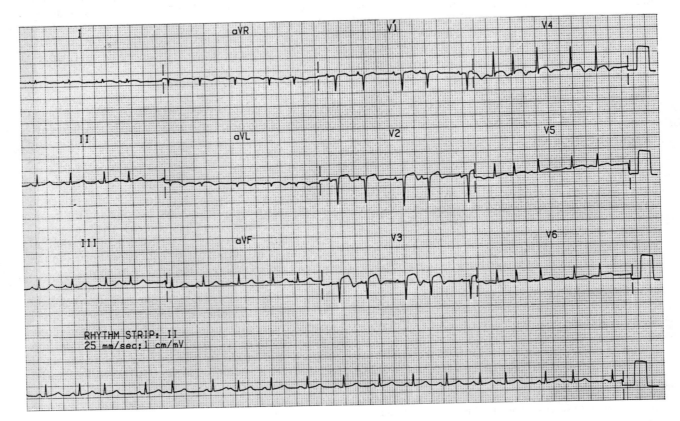

FIGURE 11-2
Acute anterolateral infarct. Note the S–T segment elevation in V_2 to V_6, I, and aVL. There are no reciprocal changes. The rhythm is a sinus tachycardia with premature atrial contractions (PACs).

ONGOING ASSESSMENT AND INTERVENTIONS

After the history and diagnostic studies determine the presence of an acute MI, an ongoing assessment becomes crucial to the goal of minimizing tissue necrosis.

Pain Assessment and Management

Chest pain can be assessed for location, duration, and the patient's description. It is helpful to have the patient evaluate his pain on a scale of 1 to 10, with 10 being the worst. This helps quantitate a subjective experience. Duration and onset factors should be identi-

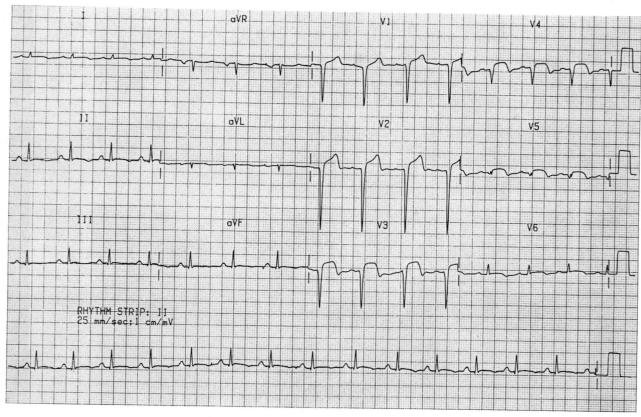

FIGURE 11-3
Acute lateral infarct, with an old inferior infarct that extended into an acute anterior lateral infarct later in the day. Note the elevated S–T segments and T wave inversion in V₃ to V₆, I, and II. The rhythm is a normal sinus rhythm. The old inferior infarct presents as residual Q waves in leads II, III, and aVF.

fied. A rhythm strip can be placed in the patient's record. Although ischemic changes are best noted by 12-lead ECG, dysrhythmias may occur during chest pain.

The definitive treatment of ischemic chest pain is administration of an agent in the nitrate group. Nitroglycerin (tablets or continuous infusion) acts on the vascular bed. A relative hypovolemia occurs with a lessened venous return as the result of peripheral pooling of blood. Nitrates act more on veins than on arteries but selectively dilate the coronary arteries. They cause a significant decrease in the left ventricular filling pressure and a slight increase in cardiac index and stroke volume. Nitroglycerin eases the myocardial work load by decreasing preload. Nitroglycerin tablets can be repeated every 5 minutes until relief is obtained, but long-acting nitrate administration is best accomplished intravenously.

The pain accompanying an MI is best treated with narcotics. Morphine given in small increments of 1 to 2 mg by intravenous push is the traditional choice. Morphine, a potent vasodilator, decreases preload and

provides an analgesic effect. Some patients benefit from the euphoric side effect of morphine, finding that it relaxes and calms them.

Either method of pain relief can result in hypotension. Again, the patient's pain relief should be assessed on a scale of 1 to 10. The blood pressure should be checked frequently (every 5 to 10 minutes) until the pain has subsided.

The presence of hypotension (<100 mm Hg systolic) can indicate impending shock or an adverse response to therapy. Modified Trendelenburg position, with the feet slightly elevated, may help. Some patients with acute MI cannot tolerate having their bed flat so positions should be changed carefully. Hypotension seen only during chest pain indicates a compromised mechanical pump during ischemia.

Hypertension causes the myocardium to work harder. Convalescing hearts need to have their workload limited. A blood pressure of less than 150 mm Hg systolic is ideal.

After relief of chest pain, the most important therapeutic goal is to maximize the cardiac output while

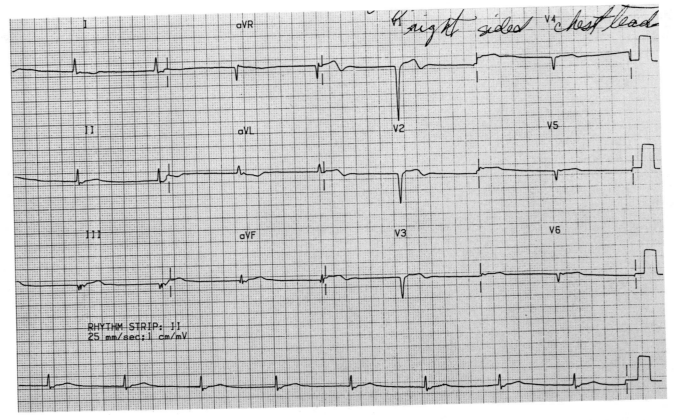

FIGURE 11-4
Acute inferior infarct. The S–T segments are elevated in II, III, and aVF. Reciprocal change of S–T segment depression is seen in I and aVL. The unusual precordial lead configuration (leads V_1 to V_6) occurred because the tracing was done across the right chest, since a transthoracic pacemaker wire was on the left chest. The rhythm is complete heart block, at a rate of less than 50 bpm, which was not tolerated by this patient. The patient was stabilized with a temporary pacemaker, and this heart block resolved as the acute infarct evolved.

limiting the cardiac workload. This requires a delicate balance of pharmacologic interventions and continuous assessment of the hemodynamic state.

Arrhythmia Assessment and Management

The pulse should be assessed ideally by an apical auscultation and simultaneous radial palpation. Apical/radial pulse assessment will document whether extrasystoles perfuse to the radial artery. It is important to remember that extrasystoles on a rhythm strip may be electrical events without a mechanical response, resulting in a decreased cardiac output.

Dysrhythmias must be treated and minimized in the presence of an acute myocardial infarction. Ischemic myocardium has a lower fibrillatory threshold, and few ventricular dysrhythmias are considered benign after an infarct. The management of dysrhythmias is considered in Chapter 9, in the discussion of commonly used antiarrhythmic agents.

Some rhythm disturbances have special implications during an acute MI. Heart block, when accompanying an inferior infarct, tends to be transient, whereas heart block in the setting of an anterior wall infarct is often permanent. Bradycardia is common among inferior infarct patients, probably owing to vagal nerve ischemia, and is generally considered to be more benign than bradycardia seen with anterior infarcts. The temporary support of slow or heart block rhythms with a pacemaker may be necessary.

Minimizing the cardiac work load can be accomplished in various ways. Beta-adrenergic blockade (*e.g.,* propranolol) will decrease heart rate and contractility. This is indicated if a third heart sound develops (heard at the end of rapid ventricular filling) and a gallop rhythm exists, indicating the presence of heart failure. Because propranolol will decrease rate and contractility, the patient should have an adequate heart rate (≥ 55 bpm) and blood pressure (≥ 95 mm Hg systolic) and no heart block prior to the onset of therapy.

Calcium antagonists are often used to decrease afterload (the pressures the ventricle must push against to pump blood) and decrease contractility. Calcium antagonists also act directly on the coronary arteries, producing vasodilatation. Nifedapine is the most effective calcium antagonist. Verapamil and diltiazem provide less direct arterial dilatation but have strong antiarrhythmic qualities, slowing transmission through the sinus and atrioventricular nodes. Verapamil and diltiazem are effective in terminating supraventricular tachycardias.

The use of low-flow oxygen assists in maximizing the oxygen saturation of arterial blood and is very beneficial to the recovering myocardium.

Myocardial work can be limited only through the reduction of energy expenditures by the entire body. Small meals that are easily digestable should be encouraged. Bedrest with a gradual increase in the activities of daily living can help keep the metabolic rate lowered. It is important to keep the environment calm and to reduce stressors during the early stages of recovery. Often, minor tranquilizers are given. Stool softeners are used to prevent Valsalva action during bowel movements.

Accurately recorded intake and output records along with daily weights help the fluid balance assessment. An intravenous line must be maintained so that emergency drugs can be given if needed.

Anticoagulation Drug Therapy

The use of anticoagulation agents has been controversial. Heparin therapy at one time was standard during the acute phase of a myocardial infarction. Recent studies show that patients who have large anterior MIs with large dyskinetic areas are most at risk for systemic arterial embloli and may benefit from systemic anticoagulation. Minidose heparin (5000 units given subcutaneously every 8 hours) will effectively prevent venous emboli for patients with heart failure, obesity, edema, or established vascular disease.

An exciting therapy involving intracoronary streptokinase has been developed. With intracoronary streptokinase, thrombus dissolution can occur. Eighty percent of patients with transmural infarcts have acute thrombosis. Streptokinase, administered in the early stage (first 4 hours) of infarction can dissolve this thrombus. Many times, the atherosclerotic lesions are flattened with a balloon dilatation at the site of the lesion by a procedure known as angioplasty. This acute recanalization of the diseased coronary arteries can promptly relieve ischemic pain and reduce infarct size. (See discussion of percutaneous transluminal coronary angioplasty in Chap. 9.)

The nursing care provided to patients after streptokinase or angioplasty is similar to the care given to patients following heart catheterization. Systemic anticoagulation with heparin can be expected to continue for 48 to 72 hours. Although these patients require close observation, their recovery is often dramatic because the ischemic process is arrested.

Cardiogenic Shock: Assessment and Management

The previously outlined therapy and assessments allow one to manage the patient with an uncomplicated infarction quite well. Many patients who experience infarcts will have more dramatic symptoms of heart failure and present in a shock state. When the patient's blood pressure falls below 95 mm Hg systolic or climbs above 150 mm Hg systolic, rales develop, and urine output decreases, a more aggressive approach is needed.

In order to monitor fluctuations in hemodynamic status adequately, one must use a thermodilution cardiac output catheter (*e.g.,* Swan-Ganz). Because most myocardial infarctions involve the left ventricle, measurement of the central venous pressure (CVP) will not reflect changes in left ventricular filling pressures. The pulmonary capillary wedge pressure (PCWP) will indicate an indirect measurement of left ventricular filling pressures. If the pulmonary artery diastolic pressure (PAD) is within 1 to 3 mm Hg of the PCWP, this value can be used as well. Optimal filling pressure is below 18 mm Hg, as long as satisfactory systemic flow is maintained.

Using the thermodilution technique, one can determine cardiac output and index. A cardiac index (CI) $\left(\dfrac{\text{cardiac output}}{\text{body surface area}} \right)$ of 2.2 liters/minute will provide adequate systemic flow. One can further assess the clinical status by comparing the cardiac index with the PCWP (Table 11-4).

If the clinical picture is one of volume depletion, the patient's PCWP will be less than 18 mm Hg, while the CI will be less than 2.2 liters/minute/m^2. Tachycardia, low urine output, and elevated serum sodium and hematocrit may be present. Careful volume replacement with crystalloid intravenous fluids is indicated. Nitrates and narcotics must be used with care because further systemic lowering of the blood pressure may occur. Although a vasopressor (dopamine or dobutamine) may elevate the systemic pressure, vasopressors are least effective in the setting of volume depletion. Pulmonary congestion will present as a PCWP over 18 mm Hg and a high CI, over 2.2 liter/minute/m^2. This

TABLE 11-4
HEMODYNAMIC ASSESSMENT OF THE MYOCARDIAL INFARCTION

Pulmonary Capillary Wedge Pressure (mm Hg)	Cardiac Index (L/minute/m²)	Clinical State	Anticipated Therapy
<18	>2.2	Normal	Reduced metabolic needs
<18	<2.2	Volume depletion	Volume expansion with crystalloids
>18	>2.2	Pulmonary congestion	Diuretics Nitrates
>18	<2.2	Cardiogenic shock	Vasopressors Inotropic agents Afterload reducers Intra-aortic balloon pump

volume overload state presents with tachycardia, rales, dyspnea, orthopnea, possible hypoxemia, and diaphoresis. The blood pressure may be elevated in the early stages. Diuretics such as furosemide will effectively reduce intravascular volume. Careful monitoring of serum potassium is needed because diuretic therapy will deplete potassium. Potassium replacement should maintain a serum level of 3.5 mEq/liter for the convalescing myocardium.

Diuresis is also obtained through the use of low-dose dopamine (2 mcg/kg/minute). Dopamine will enhance the systemic blood pressure and increase the renal blood flow, allowing for increased urine formation through normal physiologic mechanisms. It is important to maintain low dose levels because higher dopamine doses have catecholamine-like effects and will decrease renal blood flow.

Digitalis has been used extensively in the management of congestive failure. Digitalis will decrease heart size and therefore decrease myocardial oxygen consumption (MVO_2). MVO_2 is determined by evaluation of heart rate, contractility, and preload/afterload. Digitalis has a negative chronatropic effect (slows heart rate), a positive inotropic effect (increases contractility), and a negative dromotropic effect (slows electrical impulses). Response to digitalis is delayed in the presence of ischemic myocardium. Although a popular therapy, digitalis can increase infarct size by stimulating MVO_2 if failure is not present.

Cardiogenic shock will present with a PCWP greater than 18 mm Hg and a CI less than 2.2 liters/minute/m². The patient will be fatigued and restless and eventually experience drowsiness and stupor. In addition, hypotension of ≤ 80 mm Hg systolic and oliguria or anuria may ensue. The skin appears gray, mottled, and cool, and diaphoresis is often present. Hypoxemia and acidosis are common.

Shock is accompanied by an intense neurohumoral response. Usually, 40% or more of the left ventricle must be infarcted to cause cardiogenic shock. In an attempt to improve the weakened left ventricle's pumping action, norepinephrine and epinephrine are released. Plasma glucose, free fatty acids, and glucagon are increased as potential energy sources. The MVO_2 increases and lactate acids form as a result of anaerobic metabolism. The catecholamine response causes increased capillary permeability, resulting in interstitial edema and intravascular volume depletion. All the physiological responses to shock increase the MVO_2 while decreasing the myocardial pumping action.

In cardiogenic shock, vasopressors are needed to maintain systemic blood pressures. Dopamine may be used, but often dobutamine is preferred. Dobutamine in small doses of 2 to 5 mcg/kg/minute will improve cardiac contractility and decrease afterload and systemic vascular resistance, and it has less of a tachycardic side effect than dopamine. There is also less renal artery vasodilatation with dobutamine.

The severe hypotension of cardiogenic shock is often managed with norepinephrine (Levophed). At dosages of 2 to 6 mcg/kg/minute, norepinephrine will increase the blood pressure by arterial constriction, which results in an increased peripheral vascular resistance. Although this increases MVO_2, norepinephrine causes direct coronary artery dilatation.

Often, vasodilators are added to the therapy to reduce the afterload. Nitroprusside is an effective vasodilator that reduces systemic vascular resistance and therefore enhances stroke volume. The systemic vascular vasodilatation can markedly reduce venous return, and it is important to keep the diastolic blood pressure ≥ 60 mm Hg. Having a short half-life of only minutes, nitroprusside can be titrated to the desired effect. Long-term nitroprusside therapy (over 72 hours) may cause thiocyanate or cyanide toxicity, and follow-up therapy is often accomplished with intravenous nitroglycerin or long-acting nitrates applied topically (Nitrobid).

The maximum support that can be offered to the

failing left ventricle is the intra-aortic balloon pump. Occupying 40 cc of space in the proximal aorta, the inflated balloon will, during diastole, displace arterial blood into the coronary arteries and systemic circulation. Coronary artery perfusion is enhanced, and the MVO_2 is lowered. Lactate production is decreased as systemic circulation is augumented. This treatment is as complex as it is successful. It is discussed in depth in Chapter 9.

As in all myocardial infarctions, the goal of minimizing further tissue necrosis is also a goal in cardiogenic shock. The challenge to improve myocardial oxygen consumption while decreasing the work of the ventricle and maintaining systemic circulation is enormous. Modern pharmacologic therapies and treatment modalities require constant bedside assessment and intervention. The role of the critical care nurse in dealing with cardiogenic shock is vital, challenging, and dynamic.

COMPLICATIONS OF ACUTE MYOCARDIAL INFARCTION

Special clinical conditions may develop during the convalescence of the patient with an acute infarct. These events, although not entirely predictable, can be managed at the time of occurrence.

Pericarditis

Pericarditis occurs at the 48- 72-hour postinfarct period with chest pain that may be confused with ischemic pain. This precordial pain intensifies with deep breathing, and often a friction rub can be heard. Some friction rubs are transient, and therefore the absence of such a rub is not conclusive. Anti-inflammatory agents such as aspirin, indomethacin, and corticosteriods, given in usual dosages, can bring dramatic relief.

Ischemic Chest Pain

Recurrent chest pain that is ischemic in nature should be treated aggressively. There may be ischemic ECG changes (S – T segment depression) and enzyme elevations. Angiography and possible revascularization (coronary artery bypass grafting) should be considered while nitrates are administered. Further progressive loss of myocardial tissue can be minimized and the extension of the infarct aborted with careful hemodynamic assessment for decreasing the MVO_2.

Dysrhythmias

Dysrhythmias often accompany acute infarcts. Often the arrhythmia is caused by a failing left ventricle rather than a direct consequence of conduction system ischemia.

Supraventricular rhythms may be the result of high left atrial pressures caused by left ventricular failure. Although most rhythm disturbances are manageable with drugs or cardioversion, adequate response to therapy may be delayed until the ventricle heals. Synchronized cardioversion may convert atrial fibrillation, atrial flutter, and nonparoxysmal atrial tachycardias. Paroxysmal atrial tachycardia will respond to verapamil (5 to 10 mg IV infusion over 10 minutes). Digitalis can be effective but does not work promptly in the ischemic heart. Propranolol is often used if heart failure is not severe.

Many ventricular dysrhythmias will respond to lidocaine therapy. After a bolus loading dose of 50 to 100 mg intravenous push, a continuous infusion of 1 to 4 mg/minute is begun. Lidocaine will decrease the automaticity of the Purkinje fibers and prevent a reentry circuit of tachydysrhythmias by depressing the action potential duration.

Some ventricular dysrhythmias will not respond to lidocaine. The ischemic myocardium may suffer left ventricular failure, hypoxia, hypokalemia, or acidosis, all contributing to a less than predictable response. Bretylium, given with a loading dose of 5 mg/kg and followed by a maintenance infusion of 1 to 2 mg/minute is effective therapy for recurrent ventricular tachycardia/fibrillation. Bretylium produces a slow initial response (often 20 to 25 minutes after the loading bolus), so supportive resuscitative measures should be maintained during this time. Orthostatic hypotension may become a problem during continuous infusion.

Other ventricular antiarrhythmic agents may be employed. Procainamide, quinidine, propranolol, and phenytoin are sometimes effective. Overdrive pacing may be indicated. The therapeutic goal of dysrhythmia control is to maintain cardiac output while reducing cardiac work load. This can be assessed by monitoring hemodynamics, blood pressure, urine output, general appearance, and level of consciousness.

Inferior infarctions or occlusion of the right coronary artery will result in conduction disturbances at the atrioventricular node for about 10% of the population. Because the inferior wall is small in area and AV node infarcts are rare, these conduction disburbances are transient. Usually Mobitz I (Wenckebach) block will appear and may progress to atrioventricular dissociation. If the ventricular rate is too bradycardiac to maintain a sufficient blood pressure, transvenous pacing is indicated.

When the lesion is high in the left anterior descending artery, resulting in an anterior infarct, the development of heart block has serious consequences. The conduction system may be critically damaged at the level of the bundle branches. Multifascicular block occurs, involving two of the three bundles. Mobitz II block (intermittent, nonconducted P waves) may occur, and the cardiac output will fall dramatically.

Care Plan: Acute Myocardial Infarction

NURSING DIAGNOSIS	PATIENT OUTCOMES	INTERVENTIONS
Alteration in comfort: chest pain due to angina, MI	Relief from chest pain Hemodynamic stability	1. Assess history: onset location, duration description, severity of pain (using the scale of 1 to 10), radiation, precipitating events 2. Check BP, apical/radial pulse, respirations; q 5–10 minutes 3. Check skin color, temperature 4. Document rhythm strip 5. Initiate or maintain IV line and oxygen (2–4 L/minute) 6. Administer pain medication (nitrates or narcotics) as ordered 7. Assess relief of pain (using the scale of 1–10) 8. Instruct the patient to notify staff of further pain 9. Minimize MVO_2; encourage bedrest; provide quiet environment, easily digestable meals, stool softeners 10. Obtain 12-lead ECG as ordered
Reduced cardiac output: electrical factors affecting rate, rhythm, or conduction	Maintenance of cardiac rhythm with adequate systemic perfusion	1. Conduct continuous cardiac monitoring in MCL_1 or lead II 2. Document rhythm strip during every shift and as changes in rhythm occur 3. Assess BP, apical/radial pulse for exrasystoles, perfusion of extrasystoles 4. Administer antiarrhthymics as ordered 5. Obtain 12-lead ECG as ordered
Reduced cardiac output: mechanical factors relating to preload, afterload, left ventricular failure	Maintenance of hemodynamic stability	1. Assess BP, dyspnea, level of consciousness, hypoxemia, tachypnea, orthopnea, rales, S_3 ventricular gallop, jugular vein distention, urine output, daily weight, peripheral edema, skin color, and temperature 2. Maintain IV line, I & O, oxygen, and bedrest 3. Assess hemodynamic parameters: PCWP, Co, and CI 4. Give medication as ordered: diuretics, crystalloid fluids, nitrates, vasopressors, inotropic agents, afterload reducers 5. Assess blood gases 6. Monitor cardiac rhythm 7. Assess electrolyte balance, especially serum potassium 8. Minimize hypoxemia, acidosis, dysrhythmias, pain 9. Assess anxiety level of patient and family; instruct and inform at the appropriate level 10. If needed, prepare for intra-aortic balloon pumping

Knowledge deficit: related to illness and impact on patient's future	Demonstration of compliance with ADL limitations Articulation of pertinent questions	1. Initiate nurse–patient relationship that encourages questioning and utilize both formal and informal styles 2. Include family in care and teaching 3. Begin cardiac rehabilitation education: risk factors, pathophysiology, when to seek medical attention, medications, progressive ADL, diet, sexual activity, returning to work, stress reduction 4. Evaluate patient's understanding; document teaching and patient's response on the record
Anxiety: stress due to fear or illness/death and critical care environment	Recognition and expression of concerns and fears Utilitzation of effective coping mechanisms Demonstration of reduction in fear and anxiety	1. Explain environment, all procedures, expectations and equipment 2. Allow patient to express himself freely 3. Maximize patient's control of ADL 4. Include family in patient's care 5. Assess for normal grieving process: anger, denial, depression, acceptance 6. Sedate as needed if ordered by physician 7. Maximize effective coping styles 8. Spend quiet time with patient so that he may explore feelings and fears if he is ready 9. Document patient's emotional response to critical illness
Potential for alteration in comfort: chest pain due to pericarditis	Relief from pain	1. Assess pain: onset, location, duration, description, severity (using scale of 1–10), radiation, precipitating factors 2. Determine whether pain increases with deep breathing, presence of friction rub 3. Assess rhythm, BP, and heart rate during pain 4. Administer anti-inflammatory agents as ordered 5. Explain pathology to patient 6. Assess pain relief (using scale of 1–10)
Potential for alteration in cardiac output: profound shock and heart failure due to acute structural changes (septal rupture, papillary muscle rupture, or cardiac muscle rupture	Maintenance of hemodynamic stability No signs of acute structural changes	1. Assess for sudden onset hypotension, systolic murmur, and pulmonary edema 2. Assess hemodynamic parameters: PCWP, CO, CI 3. Prepare for IABP support and possible surgery 4. Administer afterload reducers and vasopressors as ordered 5. Minimize MVO_2: bedrest, supplemental oxygen, NPO, quiet environment 6. Monitor cardiac rhythm 7. Provide emotional support and appropriate explanations to patient and family

Mortality is high for clients with anterior infarcts with heart block; 70% to 80% will succumb. Pacemakers are indicated for all anterior infarcts with heart block. Some patients will not respond to pacing if the tissue damage to the left ventricle is extensive.

Patients with inferior wall infarcts should be suspected of also having suffered right ventricular infarcts. This will present as acute congestive failure with hypotension, jugular vein distention, dyspnea, rales, and an elevated CVP. Management of right ventricular infarcts is similar to that of any other infarct with a moderate amount of failure.

The most catastrophic complications of an infarct are intraventricular septal rupture, papillary muscle dysfunction or rupture, and cardiac rupture. These clinical situations develop rapidly and result in almost immediate physiologic deterioration.

Septal Rutpure

Intraventricular septal rupture presents as a new, loud, systolic murmur, progressive dyspnea, tachycardia, and pulmonary congestion. Oxygen samples taken from the right atrium, right ventricle, and pulmonary artery will show higher pO_2 in the right ventricle than in the right atrium because the oxygenated left ventricular blood is shunted to the right ventricle. This testing can be accomplished during pulmonary artery catheterization. Urgent cardiac catheterization and surgical correction is needed. The patient can be supported with afterload reducers (nitroprusside) and diuretics until emergency surgery is possible. Some fibrosis of the tissue is needed for suturing and it is often impossible to maintain the patient medically until this occurs.

Papillary Muscle Rupture

Papillary muscle rupture carries a 95% fatality rate. Clinical presentation of sudden onset valvular failure is similar to that of septal rupture, except that progressive oxygen testing will show equal pO_2 levels in the right atrium, right ventricle, and pulmonary artery. Pulmonary artery pressures will be very high and the wave form will reflect a large V wave. Emergency surgery is required within hours of the onset of symptoms.

Cardiac Rupture

Cardiac rupture presents with sudden neck vein distention, hypotension, and electromechanical dissociation. This event occurs so suddenly and with such severity that life-saving efforts are futile.

NURSING DIAGNOSIS AND OUTCOME EVALUATION

After assessment data are gathered, the nurse must design a plan of care that provides for the patient's current needs and anticipates potential problems. The plan of care should be designed in a manner that permits evaluation of the care given by observation of patient outcomes and interventions and by quality assurance assessments of patient records.

The following is a sample standardized plan of care for the patient with an acute myocardial infarction. This plan would need to be individualized prior to implementation for a specific patient.

SUMMARY

Critical care nursing began as complex care and assessments were made by nurses specially trained to care for cardiac patients. Although the role of the critical care nurse has evolved enormously, the challenge of caring for patients with acute myocardial infarction remains. The nurse can no longer "watch" patients but must rapidly assess complex physiologic processes and anticipate sophisticated interventions. The declining mortality rate speaks to our success in meeting the challenge of the patient with an acute MI.

BIBLIOGRAPHY

Conn RD: Acute myocardial infarction. In Bone RC (ed): Critical Care: A Comprehensive Approach, pp 316–334. American College of Chest Physicians, 1984

Goldberger E: Textbook of Clinical Cardiology, St Louis, CV Mosby, 1982

Guzzetta CE, Dossey BM: Nursing diagnosis: Framework, process and problems. Heart Lung 12, No. 3:281–291, 1983

Huang S, Dasher L, Larson C, McMullough C: Coronary Care Nursing. Philadelphia, WB Saunders, 1983

Hurst JW: The Heart, Arteries and Veins, 5th ed. New York, McGraw-Hill, 1982

Rushmer RF: Cardiovascular Dynamics. Philadelphia, WB Saunders, 1976

Shoemaker W, Thompson WL, Holbrook P: Textbook of Critical Care. Philadelphia, WB Saunders, 1984

12
Disseminated Intravascular Coagulation Syndrome (DIC)

Judith Ives

Disseminated intravascular coagulation syndrome has the distinction of being the oldest universally accepted hypercoagulable clinical state known. In most "clotting circles," the syndrome has been dubbed "DIC" and will be referred to as such throughout this chapter.

The veins, venules, capillaries, arterioles, and arteries constitute an intricate network of conduits for the transportation of blood to and from the body tissue. The patency of the conduits and the containment of blood within the vasculature depend on the maintenance of the integrity of the transporting conduits. States of physiologic disequilibrium that increase permeability or weakening of the vessel walls may lead to leaking of the blood outside the vasculature, resulting in hemorrhage. If the response of the hemostatic system to this threat to vascular integrity is too great, thrombus formation that occludes the vasculature may result, inhibiting the transportation of blood.

It is clear that a delicate balance must be maintained in the vasculature to ensure the patency of the vasculature and liquid state of the blood, tending towards neither thrombosis nor hemorrhage. This delicate balance is provided by the interrelationship of the hemostatic and fibrinolytic systems working in concert. To understand the pathogenesis and the diagnostic and therapeutic modalities of DIC, one must first be familiar with the physiology of these two systems.

HEMOSTATIC SYSTEM

The components of the hemostatic system are the blood vessels, platelets, and blood clotting factors of the intrinsic and extrinsic systems. These interdependent components are responsible for maintaining hemostatic homeostasis.

In the course of normal wear and tear, the endothelial lining of blood vessels is subject to numerous insults that require local repair to prevent leakage of the blood. Damage to the endothelium or sloughing of the endothelium exposes the underlying collagen. This exposed collagen attracts and activates platelets to adhere to the exposed collagen; that begins the formation of platelet plugging.

With the attraction of platelets to the exposed collagen of a blood vessel, an initial barrier of platelets is formed. These platelets release small amounts of adenosine diphosphate (ADP), which causes additional platelets to be attracted and to stick to each other. Lastly, there is a release of platelet factor 3 from the platelet membrane, which interacts with various blood coagulation proteins, resulting in thrombin generation, fibrinogen to fibrin conversion, and ultimately the platelet plug. Thus, the exposed collagen initiates the formation of a platelet plug to prevent leakage of the blood and to maintain vascular integrity.

The last component of the hemostatic system consists of the blood coagulation proteins, commonly referred to as the coagulation factors of the intrinsic and extrinsic pathways to coagulation.

Intrinsic Pathway

In the normal state, the blood coagulation factors circulate in the blood in an inactive state and are designated by Roman numerals. Following an initiating stimulus, changes in the coagulation factors start immediately. The changes that occur bear the relationship of enzyme (organic catalyst) to substrate (specific substance upon which an enzyme acts). The initiation of change causes molecular alteration in one coagulation factor. The unaltered coagulation factor, known as a proenzyme, is converted to an altered state—an active enzyme. The product of this enzymatic reaction (the enzyme) activates the next coagulation factor (substrate). Thus, one molecule of enzyme acts on a specific substrate, which is also a proenzyme coagulation factor. The activated factor is designated by a lower case "a" (*e.g.,* XIIa).

This is only one event in what is to become an entire series of enzyme-substrate reactions. A chain reaction evolves whereby activation of a single proenzyme molecule may lead to activation of the entire clotting mechanism, resulting in thrombin generation, fibrinogen to fibrin conversion, and, finally, the fibrin clot.

As mentioned previously, disruption of the endothelial membrane lining blood vessels attracts platelets, which in turn releases platelet factor 3. This platelet factor initiates the activation of the intrinsic pathway by activating Factor XII, and it is a necessary component for complex reactions at Factor V and Factor VIII levels. The exposed collagen, phospholipids from injured erythrocytes and granulocytes, antigen-antibody complexes, and endotoxins are thought to be other activators of Factor XII.

These activators convert inactive Factor XII (Hageman factor) to the active enzymatic form of XIIa. The enzyme XIIa acts upon the next clotting proenzyme, inactive factor XI, converting it to the active enzyme XIa. Active XIa is responsible for the activation of Factor IX and requires calcium ions. The activation of the next factor, Factor X, requires Factor VIII and platelet factor 3. The conversion of prothrombin (Factor II) to thrombin requires Factor V, platelet factor 3, and calcium ions. Thrombin acts on fibrinogen, converting it to fibrin. This initial soluble fibrin clot is stabilized by Factor XIII in the presence of calcium.

A self-perpetuating effect in the intrinsic pathway

FIGURE 12-1
Sequence of coagulation.

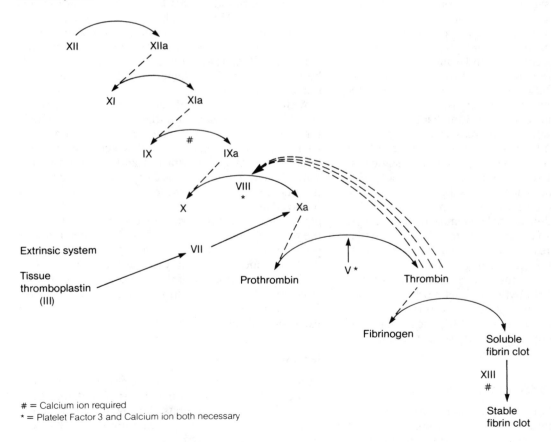

Intrinsic system

Extrinsic system

Tissue thromboplastin (III)

\# = Calcium ion required
* = Platelet Factor 3 and Calcium ion both necessary

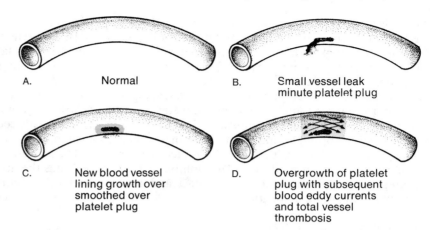

A.   Normal

B.   Small vessel leak
minute platelet plug

C.   New blood vessel
lining growth over
smoothed over
platelet plug

D.   Overgrowth of platelet
plug with subsequent
blood eddy currents
and total vessel
thrombosis

FIGURE 12-2
Sequence of thrombus formation in blood vessels.

occurs as the result of the ongoing cycle of activation of Factor X through the effect of thrombin on Factor VIII. Thrombin enhances the activity of Factor VIII so that it interacts more rapidly with Factor IXa and thus catalyzes the activation of Factor X. Also, thrombin attacks platelets, resulting in the release of platelet factor 3, which activates Factor XII.

Extrinsic Pathway

The triggering event initiating the extrinsic pathway is injury to tissues and blood vessels, resulting in the release of Factor III, tissue thromboplastin, into the circulation. As in the intrinsic pathway, a chain of events occurs that leads to clot formation. Tissue thromboplastin catalyzed by Factor VII activates Factor X. In the presence of calcium ions, Factor V, and platelet factor 3, active Factor X catalyzes the conversion of prothrombin to thrombin and fibrinogen to fibrin clot.

The result of the interaction of the blood vessels, platelets, and blood coagulation factors is the formation of Factor Xa, which converts prothrombin to thrombin and results in fibrin formation. Thus, it can be seen that at Factor Xa, the intrinsic and extrinsic pathways merge into a final common pathway to clot formation. Figure 12-1 depicts diagrammatically the sequence of clot formation. Notice that the activation of Factor VIII by thrombin creates the activation of Factor X, resulting in the self-perpetuating effect.

Unchecked activation of the blood clotting factors would cause clots to form on top of the platelet plug, releasing thrombin in the process of clotting, further attracting platelets to the clot site and causing additional clots to form at the local site of vessel leak. The result of this activation would be total vessel occlusion (Fig. 12-2) if there were no mechanisms operating to maintain the blood in a fluid state and prevent uncontrolled clotting.

COAGULATION INHIBITORS

Within humans, there is a well-controlled balance between clotting and lysis. Through the action of physiological coagulation inhibitors, the blood is maintained in its fluid state and vessels remain patent. These inhibitors work by limiting reactions that promote clotting and by breaking down any clots that do form, preventing total occlusion of the vessels. Coagulation inhibitors include the reticuloendothelial system, antithrombin III, adequate blood flow, mast cells, and the fibrinolytic system.

Reticuloendothelial System

The reticuloendothelial system inhibits coagulation by clearing activated factors from the blood, and the maintenance of an adequate blood flow acts to dilute activated clotting factors. The liberation of antithrombin III in response to thrombin inactivates the circulating thrombin, as well as neutralizes activated Factors XII, XI, IX, and X. This retards the conversion of fibrinogen to fibrin, thus stopping sequential activation of clotting factors. Mast cells located in most body tissues produce heparin with anticoagulant activity that is low compared with that of commercial heparin. Lastly, the system antagonist, the fibrinolytic system, interferes with thrombin at its site of action on fibrinogen. Similar to the coagulation mechanisms, the fibrinolytic system also involves a chain reaction whereby activation of a series of proenzymes produces lytic enzymes capable of dissolving clots.

Fibrinolytic System

Circulating in the blood is the proenzyme plasminogen, waiting for activation. It is believed that the endothelial cells that constitute the endothelial lining of blood vessels release plasminogen activator, converting plasminogen to plasmin. In addition, activated Factor XII, thrombin, kallikrein, and substances in the tissues are thought to be involved in the conversion of plasminogen to plasmin. Plasmin is the dissolving or lytic enzyme that acts to lyse fibrin and attacks Factor V, Factor VIII, Factor IX, and fibrinogen. Plasminogen activator levels are found to be transiently elevated in response to exercise, stress, anoxia, and pyrogens.

The lysis of fibrinogen and fibrin results in the liberation of degradation products. These products, known as fibrin degradation products (FDP), inhibit platelet aggregation, exhibit an antithrombin effect, and interfere with formation of the fibrin clot.

Fibrinolytic System Inhibitors
Similar to the coagulation system inhibitors, there are inhibitors of the fibrinolytic system. The reticuloendothelial system clears the fibrin degradation products from the circulation. Antiplasmin, a protein circulating in the blood, binds with plasmin and renders it inactive. The level of circulating antiplasmin far outweighs plasmin concentration and rapidly neutralizes plasmin. Figure 12-3 depicts fibrinolytic activation.

It is evident that the systems of hemostasis and fibrinolysis in conjunction with their system inhibitors function within a narrow margin to ensure the liquidity of the blood and patency of the vasculature. An upset in these systems may result in clinical evidence of thrombosis, hemorrhage, or the catastrophic event of disseminated intravascular coagulation.

DISSEMINATED INTRAVASCULAR COAGULATION SYNDROME (DIC)

Pathophysiology

DIC, a syndrome of transient coagulation, causes transformation of fibrinogen to fibrin clot and is often associated with acute hemorrhage. Paradoxically, DIC is a bleeding disorder resulting from an increased tendency to clot. The syndrome is triggered by a host of diverse states of physiological disequilibrium resulting in systemic activation of coagulation and fibrinolysis. States of physiological disequilibrium that act as precipitating factors in DIC include crush syndrome, hemorrhagic shock, abruptio placentae, septic abortion, leukemia, carcinoma, incompatible blood transfusion, and endotoxic shock.

Regardless of the precipitating event in DIC, the triggering stimulus initiates systemic coagulation activity, resulting in diffuse intravascular fibrin formation and deposition of fibrin in the microcirculation. The ultimate result is the accumulation of clot in the body's capillaries, the length of which exceeds 100,000 miles in the average adult. The amount of blood clot seques-

tration in the capillaries due to DIC is enormous. Because of the rapidity of intravascular thrombin formation, clotting factors are effectively used up in the capillary clotting process at a rate exceeding factor replenishment. Circulating thrombin persists in the extravascular space waiting for its substrate, fibrinogen, to arrive. The availability of the inhibitor, antithrombin III, is greatly reduced by the excessive thrombin formation.

The activation of the coagulation mechanisms also activates the fibrinolytic system. Recall that activated Factor XII, thrombin, endothelial cells, and tissue substances stimulate the release of plasminogen activators. The breakdown of fibrin and fibrinogen results in fibrin degradation products that interfere with platelet function and the formation of the fibrin clot. Thus, the patient has a simultaneous, self-perpetuating combination of thrombotic and bleeding activity occurring in response to the precipitating event.

Almost uniformly, there is arterial hypotension, often associated with activation of the kallikrein and complement systems. Kallikrein perpetuates the activation of XII to XIIa, further enhancing clotting activity. In addition, kallikrein releases kinins that increase vascular permeability and vasodilation, increasing hypotension. The activation of the complement system results in an increased vascular permeability and lysis of erythrocytes, granulocytes, and platelets. This activ-

FIGURE 12-3
Sequential fibrinolytic activation.

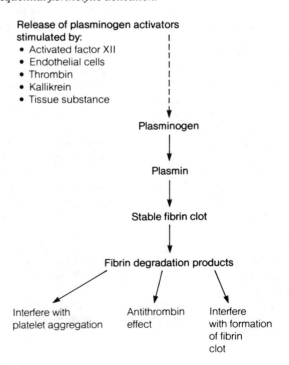

ity produces phospholipids, which provide fuel for accelerating clotting activity by activating Factor XII.

As the result of the activation of the kallikrein and complement systems, there are arteriole vasoconstriction and capillary dilatation. Blood is then shunted to the venous side, bypassing dilated capillaries owing to the opening of arteriovenous shunts. The dilated capillaries now contain stagnant blood, which accumulates metabolic by-products that render the blood acidotic. We now have three concomitant procoagulating effects in the capillary blood: acidosis, blood stagnation, and the presence of coagulation-promoting substances. Figure 12-4 depicts the effect of AV shunting.

The DIC patient bleeds not only because of increased clotting that results in consumption of clotting factors but also because of increased fibrinolysis and diminished antithrombin III. As mentioned earlier, the thrombin concentration is regulated by antithrombin III, and in DIC antithrombin III cannot keep up with the excessive generation of thrombin. This circulating thrombin continues to activate the conversion of plasminogen to plasmin, which compounds the bleeding diathesis. Figure 12-5 depicts the self-perpetuating cycle of thrombosis and bleeding in DIC.

Diagnosis

"All that glitters is not gold." Likewise, all that bleeds is not DIC. All too often, every bleeding crisis is diag- nosed as DIC. There are numerous bleeding situations that mimic DIC; unfortunately, routine laboratory data do not differentiate these syndromes readily. Because treatment of the different bleeding disorders varies, correct diagnosis is essential if the person's life is to be prolonged. Incorrect diagnosis and subsequent improper treatment will hasten death. Therefore, the interpretation of laboratory tests must be correlated with the clinical presentation of the patient. Table 12-1 represents tests that are abnormal in DIC.

Management

The backbone of therapy in the management of DIC is elimination of the cause. If one's basement is flooded by a broken pipe, the problem will not be solved by mopping alone: The water supply to the broken pipe must be turned off. In DIC, the factor that activates the clotting factors must be "turned off." If the initiating state of physiological disequilibrium is septic shock, volume must be restored and antibiotic therapy initiated to eliminate the precipitating event.

Attention should also be directed at correction of hypovolemia, hypotension, hypoxia, and acidosis, all of which have procoagulant effects. Correction of these imbalances must be the focus of the treatment of DIC bleeders. Additionally, correction of hemostatic deficiencies that compromise the clotting mechanisms is necessary.

Heparin Therapy

If the underlying cause of DIC cannot be eliminated, one can control it by stopping the cycle of thrombosis-hemorrhage with heparin administration. Heparin helps prevent further thrombus formation, but it does not alter clots that have already formed. Heparin also slows coagulation and permits restoration of coagulation proteins. It does this by combining with antithrombin III, and in the presence of thrombin, forms a reversible combination in which thrombin is inactivated. Also, this combination of heparin and antithrombin III neutralizes activated Factors XII, XI, IX, and X, thus blocking the progression of the sequential activation of the coagulation factors. Furthermore, heparin inhibits platelet aggregation that is mediated by thrombin by neutralizing effects on thrombin. The administration of heparin therefore inhibits thrombin generation, thrombin–fibrinogen interactions, and platelet aggregation.

The dose of heparin required to treat DIC must agree with the clinical status of the patient and his individual needs. There are advocates for both the subcutaneous and the intravenous routes of administration. Those who advocate intravenous administration favor continuous infusion of doses ranging up to 20,000 to 30,000 units in 24 hours. Proponents of sub-

FIGURE 12-4
Arteriole-capillary-venule relationship in normal circulation as opposed to the DIC patient. The diagram shows the effect of AV shunting in DIC.

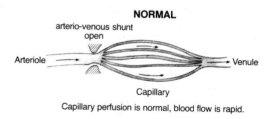

NORMAL

Capillary perfusion is normal, blood flow is rapid.

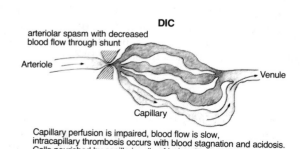

DIC

Capillary perfusion is impaired, blood flow is slow, intracapillary thrombosis occurs with blood stagnation and acidosis. Cells nourished by capillaries die of ischemia due to blood clotting.

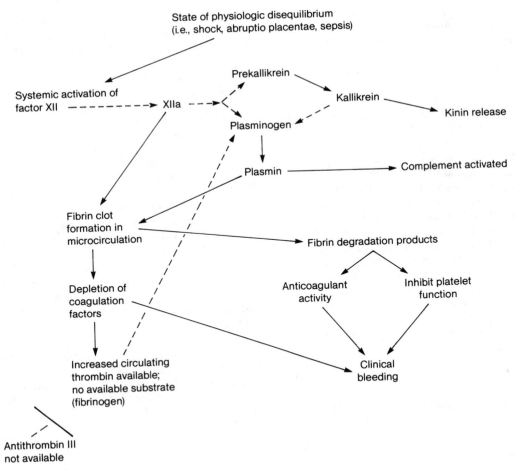

FIGURE 12-5
Self-perpetuating cycle of thrombosis and bleeding in DIC.

TABLE 12-1
LABORATORY FINDINGS IN ACUTE DISSEMINATED INTRAVASCULAR COAGULATION (DIC)

Test	Values
Prothrombin time (PT)	Prolonged
Partial thromboplastin time (PTT)	Prolonged
Platelet count	Decreased
Fibrinogen level	Decreased
Antithrombin III level	Decreased
Thrombin time	Prolonged
Fibrin degradation products	Elevated
Plasminogen levels	Decreased
Plasmin levels	Present

cutaneous heparin favor low doses that range from 2500 to 5000 units every 4 to 8 hours. One must conduct sequential coagulation studies to regulate the heparin dose and to determine the patient response to the heparin. Heparin should be continued until the primary precipitating cause has been removed and the clinical and the laboratory data suggest that the patient is on the way to recovery.

Depleted Factor Replacement
Continued bleeding despite treatment of the underlying cause and heparin administration may indicate depletion of the coagulation factors. Some advocate administration of depleted factors only *after* heparin therapy is initiated so that the infused fibrinogen present in whole blood or fresh frozen plasma does not add "fuel to the fire" of circulating thrombin waiting for its substrate. Others do not support this rationale and advocate the administration of depleted factors as the patient's condition dictates.

Antithrombin III Concentrate
Clinicians are awaiting the results of the use of investigational antithrombin III concentrate in DIC patients. Thus far, the studies have been favorable, and perhaps

in the future there will be antithrombin III concentrate available to replenish the depleted stores in the patient with DIC.

NURSING PROCESS

All critically ill patients are at risk for developing DIC because many are in the state of physiological dysequilibrium characterized by hypovolemia, hypotension, hypoxia, and acidosis, all of which have procoagulant effects. The increased awareness of DIC as a potentially catastrophic complication in the critically ill has resulted in earlier recognition and intervention. The critical care nurse who is armed with a knowledge of physiological norms and who uses a systematic approach to assessment may be the first person to identify the early signs of coagulation dysfunction.

As the backbone of management in DIC is the removal of the precipitating cause, the backbone of critical care nursing is the decision-making process inherent in the nursing process. The assessment phase of the nursing process provides the foundation on which decisions are based for the identification of defined clinical problems and nursing diagnoses or potential problems to be addressed both in planning interventions and in evaluating patient response to interventions.

A focused assessment format is often utilized with critically ill patients concentrating on the current state of physiological dysequilibrium that necessitated admission to the critical care unit. The amount of psychosocial data gathered depends on the condition of the patient at the time of data collection. Initially, a rapid "A-B-C" approach to assessment is utilized on admission, followed by a head-to-toe system assessment correlated with the admitting diagnosis, history and physical, laboratory data, and other clinical data. Analysis of these data identifies the clinical problems and nursing diagnoses to be addressed in the planning of care and provides the baseline for evaluating response to interventions and decision-making.

Nursing Diagnoses

Patients with DIC present a challenge to any critical care nurse because they exhibit a varied constellation of problems and have the potential for developing more. The critical care nurse will be confronted with a patient bleeding from the nose, gums, and injection sites; a patient covered with purpura, petechiae, and ecchymosis; a patient immobilized by a variety of drainage tubes, IV lines, and hemodynamic monitoring equipment and attached to a mechanical ventilator; a patient frightened by the loss of his life fluid — blood — and at risk for renewed bleeding if on heparin; a family feeling frightened by their loved one's appearance and the blood loss and lacking understanding of this catastrophic event.

Based on the preceding scenario, the following nursing diagnoses may be derived:

• Impaired verbal communication related to inability to speak secondary to intubation
• Alteration in mucous membranes related to hemorrhagic gingivitis and oral intubation
• Impaired physical mobility related to mechanical monitoring and life support systems preventing full range of motion
• Impairment of skin integrity related to immobility
• Alteration in family processes related to ill family member
• Fear related to critical illness

Nursing Care Plan

In the critical care unit, the nursing care plan incorporates clinical problems and nursing diagnoses. Clinical problems are those problems for which the physician orders the interventions, whereas nursing diagnoses represent problems that nurses are responsible for diagnosing, prescribing and treating.

Clinical problems are included in the care plan because the nurse in the critical care unit is responsible for assessing and monitoring the patient.

Based on the pathophysiology of DIC, some clinical problems addressed in the nursing care plan are as follows:

• Cardiac output decrease related to hemorrhage
• Alteration in tissue perfusion related to intravascular thrombosis
• Alteration in respiratory function related to increased pulmonary capillary permeability
• Cardiac output decrease related to dysrhythmias secondary to acidosis and electrolyte imbalance
• Sepsis related to stagnation of blood

These clinical problems and diagnoses are only a few that will be addressed in the nursing care plan. Not only the nurse's assessment skill but also her ingenuity in planning care and interventions to meet the DIC patient's needs will be challenged.

Nursing Intervention

Recognition of the signs of coagulation dysfunction depends on knowing what to look for, based on a knowledge of physiological norms. Remember: All that bleeds is not DIC. The nurse must be suspicious of the subtle signs of bleeding that may be heralding the onset of this medical catastrophe. Clues to the onset of DIC (*e.g.,* the appearance of petechiae, ecchymosis, or prolonged bleeding from injection or venipuncture sites) may be so subtle that they are overlooked until the patient manifests overt signs of bleeding. Thus, an integral part of the nursing care plan is continual monitoring of the patient for signs of increased bleeding, with the sites and amount of bleeding noted. Because bleeding may occur in any system, a systems approach is necessary.

1. *Assess for bloody drainage.* Not only does persistent oozing from injection sites, venipuncture, or arterial puncture sites require close monitoring, but also surgical sites, mucous membranes, drain sites, and chest tube sites need to be carefully checked for bleeding and the amounts carefully noted. Monitoring the drainage from the genitourinary and gastrointestinal tracts as well as the tracheal aspirates includes checking the urine, stool, emesis, nasogastric drainage, and sputum for the presence of blood.
2. *Observe for signs of thrombosis.* The formation of thrombus may also be evidenced, and if it does occur, the symptoms exhibited are also associated with the system involved. Often arterial and venous thrombi occur at the sites of intravascular cannulization; thus, the distal and proximal pulses should be ascertained frequently, with the quality of the pulse and capillary filling noted.

   Frequent assessment of the patient's neurologic status — level of consciousness, orientation, pupillary reaction, and movement and strength of extremities — will indicate manifestations of intracranial bleeding or thrombosis. The use of any painful stimulus should be tempered with caution because it could initiate a new bleeding site.

   The kidneys are most often affected by thrombosis; decreased urinary output is the warning sign. Remember, there are other etiologic factors of decreased urinary output such as dehydration, hypovolemia, or hypotension that must also be addressed in the assessment.
3. *Check for petechiae, ecchymosis, or cyanosis.* Many of the signs of bleeding are manifested in the integumentary system, and the patient should be inspected for petechiae, purpura, ecchymosis, and peripheral and central cyanosis.

   Petechiae are pinpoint-size, flat lesions caused by hemorrhage into the skin, and purpura are larger skin hemorrhages. These signs may be obscured in the ethnic person of color; however, the nurse who is an alert observer and knows where to look will not miss them.

   Petechiae appear as reddish-purple pin points on the buccal mucosa and also in the conjunctiva. They may be observed on the volar surface of the forearms in moderately dark-skinned individuals. *Ecchymosis* can also be observed on the buccal mucosa, and neither it nor petechiae will blanch when momentary pressure is applied.

   Evidence of *cyanosis* may be observed in the sclera, conjunctiva, buccal mucosa, tongue, lips, nailbeds, palms, and soles. In order to recognize early changes, the nurse must be familiar with the patient's color before the onset of cyanosis and should adapt her assessment to the dark-skinned person so that these signs of bleeding will not be missed.
4. *Provide meticulous care to avoid infection.* Infection predisposes the patient to bleeding. All IV, hemodynamic monitoring, and incisional sites as well as open bleeding areas require meticulous care to prevent infection.
5. *Assess for fluid volume.* DIC patients usually lose large quantities of blood and receive frequent transfusions and other fluids to maintain the intravascular and extracellular fluid volume at a level that provides optimal blood pressure, cardiac output, and urinary flow. It is important for the nurse to be alert for signs of fluid overload because these patients already have fragile capillaries.
6. *Assess for respiratory and cardiovascular problems.* Assessment of the respiratory and cardiovascular systems must be made at frequent intervals. It is important to detect as soon as possible the presence of basilar rales, cyanosis or pallor, hypoxia or hyperventilation, tachycardias, dysrhythmias, gallop rhythm, and increases in central venous pressure and pulmonary artery wedge pressure.
7. *Provide gentle care to avoid trauma.* Another nursing goal is to protect the patient from trauma or stresses that may predispose him to further bleeding. All nursing procedures and interventions should be carried out with extra *gentleness*. Particular, gentle care is necessary for the patient's skin, as an inadvertent scratch or removal of a scab on an old bleeding site may initiate another episode of bleeding. Skin care should be such as not to disturb scabs. Fingernails and toenails should be trimmed to prevent scratches. Electric razors should be used to shave male patients. Mouth care should be performed with cotton swabs and diluted mouthwash to avoid injury to the mucous membrane.

   Medication should be given intravenously, but if a medication must be given by injection, the smallest gauge needle possible for the solution being injected should be used. The same is true of venipuncture and arterial puncture procedures. Following injections or punctures, pressure must be applied to the site for a minimum of 15 minutes and frequent inspections made for evidence of continued bleeding.

8. *Attend to IV therapy lines and heparin infusion.* If the patient has an arterial line, it may be tempting to draw blood samples for coagulation tests from this heparinized line, but it must be remembered that any heparin picked up from the line can distort the values. If hospital protocol permits the aspiration of blood from central venous lines, laboratory work may be drawn from these lines without picking up heparin. When invading a catheter for blood, one must observe strict aseptic technique.

Because the administration of heparin is of prime importance in the care of the DIC patient, the continuous infusion rate must be carefully monitored. The use of a self-regulating IV infusion apparatus, such as an IVAC, assists in controlling the rate of fluid infused. Machines are prone to dysfunction and depend on the operator to ensure the proper rate of infusion.

9. *Provide psychosocial support.* In the assessment and planning of nursing care for the patient with DIC, the critical care nurse's knowledge, skill, resourcefulness, creativity, and decisiveness will be challenged. Any illness requiring hospitalization stresses a person, and when an illness requires placement in an intensive care unit, he is exposed to additional stress. The nurse's assessment must include the patient's psychosocial status and nursing interventions directed at preventing or alle-viating stresses resulting from unmet psychosocial needs that may stimulate the fibrinolytic system.

Just as the patient with DIC requires extra gentleness, so does the patient's family. The nurse should direct interventions at allaying their anxieties by explaining simply what is happening to their loved one and providing emotional support by encouraging the family to verbalize their fears without judging them.

BIBLIOGRAPHY

Berk JL, et al (eds): Handbook of Critical Care. Boston, Little, Brown, 1976

Bick RL: Disseminated Intravascular Coagulation and Related Syndromes. Boca Raton, CRC Press, 1983

Carpenito LJ: Nursing Diagnosis Application to Clinical Practice. Philadelphia, JB Lippincott, 1983

Katcher BS, et al (eds): Applied Therapeutics: The Clinical Use of Drugs, 3rd ed. San Francisco, Applied Therapeutics, 1983

Kline DL, Reddy KNN (eds): Fibrinolysis. Boca Raton, CRC Press, 1980

McKay DG: Disseminated Intravascular Coagulation: An Intermediary Mechanism of Disease. New York, Harper & Row, 1965

Minna JD, et al: Disseminated Intravascular Coagulation in Man. Springfield, Charles C Thomas, 1974

Murano G, Bick RL (eds): Basic Concepts of Hemostasis and Thrombosis. Boca Raton, CRC Press, 1980

Nilsson IM, et al: Physiology of Fibrinolysis. In Kline DL, Reddy KN (eds): Fibrinolysis. Boca Raton, CRC Press, 1980

Platt WR: Color Atlas and Textbook of Hematology. Philadelphia, JB Lippincott, 1979

Unit Two

Respiratory System

13
Normal Structure and Function of the Respiratory System

Barbara Brockway-Fuller

Oxygen is required for the complete catabolism of chemicals that occurs in the production of cellular energy. Although some energy can be stored, cells differ in the amount of energy they can store. Neurons, for example, are thought to have less capacity to store energy than skeletal muscle cells. Also, the amount of energy stored can fuel cell activities for only a short time. Neuronal energy storage and the duration of cell life it will support are partially reflected by the limited time available in which cardiopulmonary resuscitation can be started.

Catabolic energy-producing reactions produce carbon dioxide. High levels of this waste product can seriously impair cell function. Thus, there is a critical need for providing oxygen to body cells and at the same time removing carbon dioxide from the body. Strictly defined, *respiration* is the exchange and transport of oxygen and carbon dioxide between cells (of the body) and the external environment (atmosphere).

Accomplishing this in vertebrates (including humans) involves both the respiratory and the cardiovascular systems: the former to provide exchange of these gases between atmosphere and blood, the latter to transport these gases to and from the cells of the body. At times it is difficult to establish priorities between these two systems; it is better to consider them as being equally critical to the dynamic stability of the human body.

In this chapter, we will examine four general phases or areas of respiration in the following order:

1. Pulmonary ventilation — actual flow of air in and out between the atmosphere and the alveoli of the lung

2. Exchange of oxygen and carbon dioxide between the alveoli and the blood
3. Transport of oxygen and carbon dioxide in the blood and body fluids to and from the cells
4. Regulation of ventilation by control mechanisms of the body with regard to rate, rhythm, and depth

VENTILATION

Mechanics of Respiration

The downward and upward movement of the diaphragm, which lengthens and shortens the chest cavity, combined with the elevation and depression of the ribs, which increases and decreases the anteroposterior diameter of the cavity, causes the expansion and contraction of the lungs. It is estimated that about 70% of the expansion and contraction of the lungs is accomplished by the change in anteroposterior measurement and about 30% is achieved by the change in length due to movement of the diaphragm.

Respiratory Pressures

The lungs — two air-filled spongy structures — are attached to the body only at their hila. Thus the outer surfaces have no attachment. However, the membrane lining the interpleural space constantly absorbs fluid or gas that enters this area, thereby creating a partial vacuum. This phenomenon holds the visceral pleura of the lungs tightly against the parietal pleura of the chest wall.

As the volume of the chest cavity is increased by the

muscles of inspiration, the lungs also enlarge; as it is decreased during expiration, the lungs in turn become smaller. The two pleurae slide over each other with each inspiration and expiration, lubricated by the few millimeters of tissue fluid-containing proteins in the intrapleural space.

With each normal inspiration, the pressure within the alveolar sacs, the intra-alveolar pressure, becomes slightly negative (-3 torr) with regard to the atmosphere. This slightly negative pressure sucks air into the alveolar sacs through the respiratory passage.

During normal expiration and resultant compression of the lungs, the intra-alveolar pressure builds to about $+3$ torr and forces air out of the respiratory passages. During maximum respiratory efforts, the intra-alveolar pressure can vary from -80 torr during inspiration to $+100$ torr during expiration.

The lungs continually tend to collapse. Two factors are responsible for this phenomenon. First, there are many elastic fibers contained within the lung tissue itself that are constantly attempting to shorten. The second and more important factor contributing to this tendency to collapse is the high surface tension of the fluid lining the alveoli. If surface tension is high, the moist interior surfaces of an alveolus are difficult to separate from one another. This increases the energy required to open and fill the alveolus with air during inspiration. If it is low, the alveoli walls more easily separate, making alveolar filling during inspiration less effortful. A lipoprotein substance called *surfactant,* which is constantly secreted by the epithelial alveolar lining, decreases the surface tension of the fluids of the respiratory passages 7- to 14-fold. The lack of the ability to secrete surfactant in the newborn is called *hyaline membrane disease* or *respiratory distress syndrome.*

No single factor or phenomenon is responsible for the body's ability to maintain inflated functional lungs; rather, it is the combination of all these factors.

Gravity and Respiratory Pressure

In an erect adult, the force of gravity increases the intrapleural pressure (and thus the intra-alveolar pressure) at the bases of the lungs. Consequently, more air exchange occurs in the upper regions of the lungs than at the bases. Similarly, in any other body position, gravitational forces increase the effort required to ventilate dependent portions of the lungs. This causes a shift in ventilation wherein ventilation of these portions is decreased and ventilation of other less dependent areas is increased.

Compliance and Respiratory "Work"

As can be seen from the preceding discussion, both the lungs and the thorax itself have elastic characteristics and thus exhibit expansibility. This expansibility is called *compliance* and is expressed as the volume increase in the lung for each unit increase in intra-alveolar pressure. Normal total pulmonary compliance, that is, both lungs and thorax, is 0.13 liter per centimeter of water pressure. In other words, every time alveolar pressure is increased by an amount necessary to raise a column of water 1 cm in height, the lungs expand 130 ml in volume.

Conditions or situations that destroy lung tissue, cause it to become fibrotic, produce pulmonary edema, block alveoli, or in any way impede lung expansion and expansibility of the thoracic cage reduce pulmonary compliance and decrease the efficiency of meeting the need for oxygen to carry on the necessary functional activities of the total organism.

It is extremely important to emphasize that when the lungs are expanded and contracted through the action of the respiratory muscles, energy is required for the muscular activity involved.

In addition to this work, energy is also required to overcome two other factors that tend to prevent expansion of the lungs: (1) nonelastic tissue resistance, and (2) airway resistance, meaning that energy is required to rearrange the large molecules of viscous tissues of the lung itself so that they slip past one another during respiratory movements. In the presence of tissue edema, the lungs lose many of their elastic qualities, and increased viscosity of the tissues and fluids increases the nonelastic resistance. Thus the work of breathing is increased, and the energy expended to accomplish the task is also greatly increased.

Under normal conditions, the airway resistance is low, and the amount of energy required to move air along the passages is only slight. When the airway becomes obstructed, such as in chronic obstructive lung disease, asthma, or diphtheria, airway resistance is greatly increased, and the energy required simply to move air in and out is greatly increased.

Ventilatory Function Tests

Ventilatory function tests can be subdivided into tests to measure static values and capacities and tests to measure dynamic values and capacities. These measurements will be influenced by exercise and disease. Age, sex, body size, and posture, when measured, are other variables that are taken into consideration when the test results are interpreted. Static values for women are usually 25% less than those for men.

Static Measurements

There are eight static measurements: four volumes and four capacities.

- *Tidal volume* (V_T) is the volume of air moved in and out with each normal respiration and measures about 500 ml in normal young males.

- *Inspiratory reserve volume (IRV)* represents forced inspiration over and beyond V_T, amounting to about 3000 ml.
- *Expiratory reserve volume (ERV)* is the volume of a forced expiration following the normal tidal expiration and amounts to about 1100 ml.
- *Residual volume (RV)* is the volume of air remaining following forced expiration. This volume can be measured only by indirect spirometry, whereas the others can be measured directly.

When one studies the actual moment-to-moment events of the pulmonary cycle, it is sometimes more convenient to consider some volumes in combination with others. These various combinations are known as the four pulmonary capacities:

- *Inspiratory capacity (IC)* is equal to the V_T plus the IRV. This is about 3500 ml and is the amount of air that, when starting from normal expiratory level, can be forcibly inspired.
- *Functional residual capacity (FRC)* is the sum of the ERV and the RV. It is the amount of air remaining in the lungs at the end of normal expiration, about 2300 ml.
- *Vital capacity (VC)* is the sum of the IRV, V_T, and ERV. Stated another way, it is the maximal amount of air that can be forcibly expired following a forced maximal inspiration. This volume is about 4600 ml in a normal male.
- *Total lung capacity (TLC)* is equal to the volume to which the lungs can be expanded with greatest inspiratory effort. The volume of the capacity is about 5800 ml.

These static volumes and capacities provide information about compliance. In persons with reduced compliance (restrictive) disorders, these measurements will be reduced. Increases in TLC, FRC, and RV may occur in persons with obstructive disorders that have resulted in chronic hyperinflation of the lungs. In contrast, the dynamic measurements provide data about airway resistance and the energy expended in breathing (respiratory work).

Dynamic Measurements

There are eight such dynamic measures, discussed subsequently:

- Respiratory rate or frequency (f)
- Minute volume, or minute ventilation (V_E)
- Dead space (V_D)
- Alveolar ventilation
- Lung resistance
- Forced expiratory volume (FEV)
- Forced vital capacity (FVC)
- Maximal midexpiratory flow (MMEF)

Respiratory rate or frequency (f) is the number of breaths per minute. At rest, f equals about 15.

Minute volume, sometimes called minute ventilation (V_E), is the volume of air inhaled and exhaled per minute. As such, it is calculated by multiplying V_T by f. At rest V_E equals approximately 7500 ml/minute.

Dead space (V_D) is the part of the V_T that does not participate in alveolar gas exchange. V_D (measured in ml) comprises the air contained in the airways (anatomical dead space) plus the volume of alveolar air that is not involved in gas exchange (physiological dead space, *e.g.,* air in an unperfused alveolus due to pulmonary embolism or, more commonly, air in underperfused alveoli).

Adult anatomical dead space is usually equal to the body weight in pounds (*e.g.,* 140 ml in a 140-lb person). In the healthy person, V_D is composed only of anatomical dead space. Physiological dead space occurs in certain disease states.

One obtains V_D by subtracting the partial pressure of arterial carbon dioxide ($PaCO_2$) from the partial pressure of the carbon dioxide of alveolar air ($PACO_2$). The normal value of V_D in healthy adults is typically less than 40% of the V_T. This value of the V_D/V_T ratio is used to follow the effectiveness of mechanical ventilation.

Alveolar ventilation is the complement of V_D expressed as the *volume of tidal air that is involved in alveolar gas exchange*. This volume is represented as volume per minute by the symbol V_A. As such, V_A indicates effective ventilation. It is more relevant to the blood gas values than either V_D or V_T because these last two measures include physiological dead space. One calculates V_A by subtracting V_D from V_T and multiplying the result by the respiratory rate/minute:

$$V_A = (V_T - V_D) \times f$$

About 2300 ml of air (FRC) remains in the lung at the end of expiration. Each new breath introduces about 350 ml of air into the alveoli. The ratio of new alveoli air to total volume of air remaining in the lungs is $\dfrac{350 \text{ ml}}{2300 \text{ ml}}$. Thus, new air is only about one seventh of the total volume contained within the lungs. The normal V_A is 5250 ml/minute (350 ml/breath $\times$ 15 breaths/min = 5250 ml/min).

A normal breath (V_T) can replace 7500 ml of air per minute (500 ml/breath $\times$ 15 breaths/min = 7500 ml/min), requiring a time of .008 second per ml $\left(\dfrac{1 \text{ min}}{7500 \text{ ml}} \times \dfrac{60 \text{ sec}}{1 \text{ min}} = .008 \text{ sec/ml}\right)$. Thus, the FRC of the lungs can be completely replaced in 18.4 seconds (2300 ml $\times$ .008 sec/ml = 18.4 sec), if there is uniform air diffusion. This slow turnover rate prevents rapid fluctuations of gas concentrations in the alveoli with each breath.

In order for these three volumes to be moved into and out of the lungs, work must occur to overcome the resistance of the abdomen, thorax, and lung tissue.

This work is the amount of energy expended to operate the chest bellows. The energy required for ventilation is proportional to the nature of *lung resistance* encountered. There are two kinds of such resistance: (1) elastic, which is measured by compliance indices, and (2) nonelastic, which is best reflected by measures of airway diameters — patency.

Compliance may refer to distensibility of lung or thorax. Relevant data are collected by simultaneous measurement of intraesophageal balloon pressure (as a reflection of intrapleural pressure) and of lung volume (with a manometer attached to an oval or nasal breathing tube). The subject then inflates the lungs to varying degrees and the two measurements attained at each point are plotted on a graph. The slope of this pressure-volume curve reflects compliance. The equation is as follows:

$$\text{compliance} = \frac{\text{change in lung volume (liters)}}{\text{change in balloonic measure (cm/H}_2\text{O)}}$$

Elasticity in the alveolar walls and the presence of normal amounts of surfactant contribute to normal compliance. Fibrosis, atelectasis, or fluid in the alveoli (pneumonia) or around them (edema) will decrease compliance. With decreased compliance, a greater pressure is associated with a given volume than would be normally seen. With increased compliance, the reverse would occur.

Common measures of airway diameters are the forced expiratory volume (FEV), the forced vital capacity (FVC), and the maximal midexpiratory flow (MMEF). FEV is the volume of air exhaled in a given time period — usually during the first second of the FVC (FEV_1). FVC measures the amount of air in a forceful maximal expiration. Normally it is approximately the same as the VC. MMEF is the volume of air that is exhaled during the midpoint record of the FVC. This also may be termed $FVC_{50} - FVC_{25}$.

The FEV is expressed in terms of the FVC or the VC. Normally, the FEV_1 is about 80% of a VC. In obstructive disorders such as chronic bronchitis or emphysema, this FEV_1 is a smaller percentage of the VC (or FVC).

As stated before, the work of breathing is proportional to the compliance and airway resistance (diameters). A normal person at rest expends less than 6% of his total bodily oxygen consumption upon the work of breathing. This percentage increases as the airway diameters (FEV, MMEF) or compliance decreases.

VENTILATION-PERFUSION

Maximal efficiency in the exchange of gases between blood and alveolus results when ventilation and perfusion correspond equally. In other words, if an acinus (group of alveoli — the basic unit of respiration) is less ventilated, it needs less perfusion; if it is more ventilated, perfusion must be increased. Ventilation would be, in effect, wasted on an unperfused unit. Similarly, perfusion would be wasted on an unventilated unit. Two reflexes operate normally to facilitate such matching of ventilation and perfusion.

One reflex adjusts perfusion to ventilation. Here, a low concentration of alveolar oxygen (PAO_2) causes a lowered PaO_2, which, in turn, triggers vasoconstriction of nearby pulmonary arterioles. This effectively shunts blood away from an un(der)ventilated area. The other reflex adjusts ventilation to perfusion. If perfusion through an area is impeded (*e.g.,* an embolus plugging the vessel), it will result in a local decrease in $PaCO_2$. This will cause a decrease in $PACO_2$, which, in turn, will cause a constriction of the bronchioles and smaller bronchi in the underperfused area. Thus, the underperfused area is not ventilated as much as before. These reflexes keep the ventilation (V = 4 liters/minute) to perfusion (Q = 5 liters/minute) ratio at 4:5. Thus, the V/Q ratio is 0.8 under normal circumstances. V/Q mismatch occurs in many respiratory disorders. If ventilation is in excess of perfusion, the disorder is termed a *dead space–producing* one (with a V/Q > 0.8). When perfusion exceeds ventilation, the disorder is a *shunt-producing* one (with a V/Q < 0.8).

Exchange of Gases Through the Pulmonary Membrane

The pulmonary membrane in humans is composed of all the surfaces in the respiratory wall that are thin enough to permit the exchange of gases between the lungs and the blood. The total area of this membrane in the average normal adult male is about 60 m², or about the size of a moderate-sized classroom. It is 0.2 to 0.4 μ thick, or less than the thickness of the average red blood cell. These two outstanding features combine to allow large quantities of gases to diffuse across the pulmonary membrane in a very short period of time.

Partial Pressure

The air that is taken into the respiratory passages is a mixture of primarily nitrogen and oxygen (99.5%) and a small amount of carbon dioxide and water vapor (0.5%). The molecules of the various gases behave as in solution and exhibit Brownian movement. Thus, a mixture of gases such as air has all molecular species evenly distributed throughout the given volume. Because of this constant molecular bombardment, the volume of gases exerts pressure against the walls of the container. This pressure can be defined as the force with which a gas or mixture of gases attempts to move from the confines of the present environment. Therefore, each of the components of a mixture such as air will account for part of the total pressure of the entire mixture. Consequently, if we take 100 volumes of air and place them in a container under 1 atmosphere of pressure (760 torr), by analysis we would find that nitrogen constitutes 79 of the 100 volumes and oxygen accounts for 21 volumes, or 79% and 21% concentration, respectively.

Both these gases are contained at 760 torr pressure in this container. If we now take the same volume of nitrogen and move it to a container of the same volume and allow it to expand until it completely fills all of the volume (100%), we will observe that the pressure in the second container drops from 760 to 600 torr. If we do the same thing with the 21 volumes of oxygen and allow them to expand to 100% of the volume, we observe that the pressure in the third container drops from 760 to 160 torr. We conclude then that in the original container the *part* of the total pressure due to nitrogen was 600 torr and the *part* due to oxygen was 160 torr. This pressure of nitrogen is called the *partial pressure* of nitrogen (PN_2) and that of oxygen the *partial pressure* of oxygen (PO_2).

The partial pressure of a gas in a given volume is the force it exerts against the walls of the container. If the walls of the container are permeable, like the pulmonary membrane, the penetrating or diffusing power of a gas is directly proportional to its partial pressure.

It is extremely important to point out that atmospheric air differs from alveolar air in partial pressures of the components. The comparative concentrations of each are shown in Table 13-1.

The difference between atmospheric air and alveolar air is in the increased concentration of carbon dioxide and water in alveolar air. There are two reasons for these differences. First, the air is humidified as it is inspired by the moisture of the epithelial lining of the respiratory tract. At normal body temperature, water vapor has a partial pressure of 47 torr and mixes with and dilutes the other gases, decreasing their partial pressures.

Second, molecules in a given volume of gas behave like molecules in a solution and diffuse from an area of high concentration to one of lower concentration.

Factors Affecting Diffusion

The factors that govern the rate of diffusion of the gases through the pulmonary membrane are as follows.

- The greater the pressure difference across the membrane, the faster the rate of diffusion.
- The larger the area of the pulmonary membrane, the larger the quantity of gas that can diffuse across the membrane in a given period of time. The thinner the membrane, the more rapid the diffusion of gases through it to the compartment on the opposite side.
- The diffusion coefficient is directly proportional to the solubility of the gas in the fluid of the pulmonary membrane and inversely proportional to molecular size. Therefore, small molecules that are highly soluble diffuse more rapidly than do large molecular gases that are less soluble.

The diffusion coefficients are as follows:

- Oxygen   1
- Carbon dioxide   20.3
- Nitrogen   0.53

The coefficients indicate that CO_2 is the most soluble and N_2 the least soluble of these three gases. They are very similar to one another with regard to molecular size but have quite different solubilities in the fluids of the pulmonary membrane. These differences account for the difference in the rate of diffusion of the gases through the pulmonary membrane.

Transport of Oxygen and Carbon Dioxide Through the Tissues

As oxygen diffuses from the lungs to the blood, a small portion of it becomes dissolved in the plasma and cell fluids, but more than 60 times as much combines immediately with hemoglobin and is carried to the tissues. Here the oxygen is used by the cells, and carbon dioxide is formed.

As the carbon dioxide diffuses into the interstitial fluids, about 5% is dissolved in the blood, and the remainder diffuses into the red blood cells where one of two things occurs:

- Carbon dioxide combines with water to form carbonic acid and then reacts with the acid base buffer and is transported as the bicarbonate ion.
- A small portion of the carbon dioxide combines with hemoglobin at a different bonding site than oxygen and is transported as carbaminohemoglobin.

TABLE 13-1
COMPARISON OF GASES IN ATMOSPHERIC AND ALVEOLAR AIR

Gas	Atmospheric Air (%)	Alveolar Air (%)
N_2	78.62	74.90
O_2	20.84	13.60
CO_2	0.04	5.30
H_2	0.50	6.20
	100.00	100.00

TABLE 13-2
RELATIVE PARTIAL PRESSURES

Gas	Atmospheric Air	Alveolar Air	Venous Blood	Arterial Blood
PO_2	159	104	40	100
PCO_2	0.15	40	45	40
PN_2	597	569	569	569

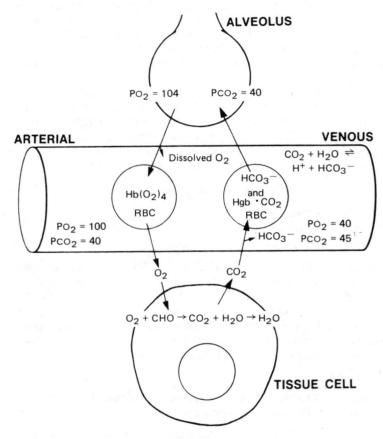

FIGURE 13-1
*Gaseous diffusion through pulmonary membrane
in respiration.*

Nitrogen diffuses from the alveolus into the blood. Because there is no carrier mechanism and under standard conditions nitrogen has only slight solubility in tissue fluid, it quickly establishes an equilibrium state on either side of the membrane and thus is essentially inert.

The relative partial pressure (torr) in the various compartments is summarized in Table 13-2.

It can readily be seen that concentration gradients are established that then foster the diffusion of these gases in the direction that is physiologically advantageous.

Figure 13-1 summarizes the events of gaseous diffusion through pulmonary membrane and transport to and from the tissues.

Oxyhemoglobin Dissociation Curve
The influence of PaO_2 (the arterial level of oxygen) on the attachment of oxyen to hemoglobin is not a straight-line function. In other words, the relationship

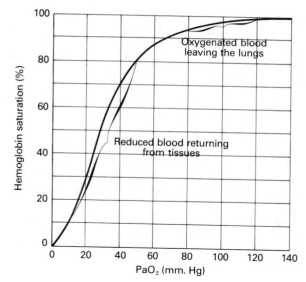

FIGURE 13-2
Oxyhemoglobin dissociation curve. (From Guyton AC:
Textbook of Medical Physiology. Philadelphia, WB Saunders,
1976)

is not directly proportioned on a 1:1 basis. The relationships involved are shown in Figure 13-2. The upper right-hand corner illustrates conditions in arterial blood when the normal PaO_2 is at about 100 torr. Then, as the blood circulates through the capillaries, losing oxygen to the interstitial fluid, the curve falls until the PO_2 of venous fluid (40 torr) is reached. At a PO_2 of 40, hemoglobin molecules are still about 70% to 75% saturated (combined) with oxygen. This provides a reserve supply of oxygen that can be provided to the tissues in cases of emergency or strenuous exercise. Thus, only about 25% to 30% of the arterial oxygen supply is used to meet tissue needs.

Owing to the relationships represented by this curve, oxygen can be applied to the tissues even if the PaO_2 is under 100 (hypoxemia or high-altitude living). Indeed, hemoglobin is approximately 95% saturated at a PaO_2 of 80.

Several factors influence the affinity of hemoglobin for oxygen. Clinically important are the *p*H, PCO_2, and temperature. These factors exert a Bohr effect on the oxyhemoglobin dissociation curve: They shift it to the right or left. A shift to the right is caused by acidity, hypercarbia, and elevation in temperature and means a decrease in the affinity of hemoglobin for oxygen. This means that less oxygen can be picked up in the lungs but that oxygen is more readily given up to the tissues in the capillaries. A shift to the left, as produced by alkalinity and a fall in PCO_2 and temperature, will increase the affinity of hemoglobin for oxygen. Thus,

more oxygen can be picked up in the lungs, but oxygen is less readily released in the capillaries. This could cause tissue hypoxia even in the face of adequate PaO_2. Respiratory alkalosis (*e.g.,* as caused by mechanical hyperventilation) has the greatest clinical potential for producing such a condition.

REGULATION OF RESPIRATION

Brain Stem Centers

Unlike the heart, the lungs have no spontaneous rhythm. Ventilations depend on rhythmic operation of brain stem centers and intact pathways from there to the respiratory muscles. There are two centers in the medulla: (1) a center that stimulates inspiration by diaphragmatic contraction (by way of phrenic nerves), and (2) another center that innervates both inspiratory and expiratory intercostal and accessory muscles.

The pons also contains two centers included in respiration. One is called the *pneumotaxic* center. The other, the *apneustic* center, produces sustained inspiration when stimulated. Voluntary control and involuntary control are further established by descending fibers from other brain centers. (These facilitate the alterations in respiration seen, for example, during swallowing, coughing, yawning, and willed action.)

In breathing at rest, the following sequence is thought to occur. The neurons innervating the inspiratory muscles fire bursts of impulses to these muscles. These neurons also stimulate the pneumotaxic center. This center, in turn, fires inhibitory impulses back to these inspiratory neurons. This causes a halt in inspiration. Expiration is thought to follow passively. After this, the inspiratory neurons are again stimulated to fire automatically. During exercise or other occasions when more vigorous ventilation occurs, the expiratory neurons of the medulla are postulated to participate in this sequence. A more comprehensive picture of the breathing process awaits further data.

External Regulations

The rate and depth of ventilations are potentially influenced by four factors: concentrations of (1) hydrogen ions, (2) carbon dioxide, (3) oxygen, and (4) exercise.

Carbon Dioxide. The most powerful stimulus for the respiratory center is the carbon dioxide content of the blood and tissue fluids of the body. When the carbon dioxide level rises above normal, both inspiratory and expiratory neurons are stimulated, and thus both rate and depth of respiration are increased. Approximately one half of the effect of carbon dioxide on respiration is due to its direct effect on the respiratory neurons themselves. The other half is due to the indirect effect of carbon dioxide in the cerebrospinal fluid. As carbon dioxide diffuses into the cerebrospinal fluid, it combines with water to form carbonic acid, which then dissociates to hydrogen and bicarbonate ions. The increased hydrogen ion concentration directly stimulates the neurons of the respiratory center as the fluid bathes the sides of the brain stem.

The respiratory system's response to carbon dioxide concentrations is extremely important because it is the main pathway for regulating carbon dioxide levels in body fluids. Should carbon dioxide accumulate in the tissues and fluids of the body, all chemical reactions of the body are essentially inhibited. If the carbon dioxide level drops too low, alkalosis develops, which is also incompatible with life.

Hydrogen Ion Concentration. As implied in the previous section, hydrogen ion concentration is the second most powerful influence on alveolar ventilation. In the equation showing carbon dioxide combining with water in body fluids, it is noted that the reactions are reversible. Therefore, if there is an accumulation of hydrogen ion concentration (a low *p*H tending toward acidemia), the center neurons respond, increasing the rate of respiration, which drives the reaction to the left and lowers the hydrogen ion concentration. If the hydrogen ion concentration is low (high *p*H tending toward alkalemia), alveolar ventilation is depressed, and the reaction is driven to the right. This response of the respiratory system in conjunction with the kidneys to a large extent controls the acid-base balance of the body.

Oxygen. Although normally hemoglobin is almost completely saturated with oxygen, the body does have chemoreceptors located in the carotid bodies in the neck and in the aortic arch that monitor blood oxygen levels. These receptors are sensitive to oxygen diffusion, and the respiratory center is stimulated by the vagus and glossopharyngeal nerves.

The chemoreceptor mechanism is not as powerful a respiratory stimulus as either carbon dioxide or hydrogen ion concentration, but it is important in some persons with chronic obstructive pulmonary disease (COPD). These persons eventually become physiologically acclimated to their chronically high $PaCO_2$. Their hydrogen ion mechanisms no longer operate to stimulate ventilation. Instead, they rely on the PaO_2 mechanism. Thus, administration of oxygen to such a COPD patient can actually depress ventilation and even cause respiratory arrest if it raises PaO_2 levels high enough.

There is also a mechanism for preventing lung over-inflation. It is called the *Hering-Breuer reflex*. Scattered throughout the lung tissue (between acini) are stretch receptors. When they are stimulated by lung inflation, they cause sensory impulses to travel up fibers in the vagus. These impulses reflexively cause inhibition of the inspiratory center, which halts further inhalation and consequent stretch.

Exercise. The rate and depth of respiration are directly proportional to the amount of work done during exercise. It is not the chemical factors that appear to cause increased rate and depth of respiration during exercise, except secondarily. The primary cause of increased respiration during exercise is the simultaneous stimulation (by the cerebral cortex) of the muscle exercised and of the sensory pathway from the cord that stimulates the respiratory center.

The Respiratory System and *p*H Homeostasis

Erythrocytes contain the enzyme carbonic anhydrase, which catalyzes the formation of carbonic acid from carbon dioxide and water ($CO_2 + H_2O \rightarrow H_2CO_3$). Carbonic acid readily dissociates to form a hydrogen ion (H^+) and a bicarbonate radical (HCO_3^-). It may be remembered that acidity represents the concentration of unattached or free hydrogen ions. Thus, the more carbon dioxide in the blood, the more free hydrogen ions or acidity that may be produced. The less carbon dioxide, the less acid (or more boric) the blood.

The hydrogen ions produced in this way are normally buffered, thereby maintaining homeostasis of extracellular fluid (ECF) *p*H. However, if there is more carbon dioxide–produced acid than the buffers can handle, acidosis will result. This is called *respiratory acidosis*. It occurs whenever there is a situation that produces alveolar hypoventilation and consequent decrease in the elimination of carbon dioxide from the bloodstream (*e.g.,* depression of the respiratory centers in the brain by certain drugs). Conversely, hyperventilation reduces the amount of carbon dioxide in the bloodstream. Less carbon dioxide means fewer hydrogen ions. This results in respiratory alkalosis.

In addition to its potential for causing *p*H imbalances, the respiratory system plays a role in compensating for metabolically caused acidosis or alkalosis. Respiratory compensation for metabolically caused acidosis is hyperventilation. This maneuver decreases the plasma carbon dioxide, thereby decreasing the plasma hydrogen ion concentration. Fewer hydrogen ions mean less acidosis. For metabolic alkalosis, respiratory compensation involves decreased ventilation. This increases plasma carbon dioxide (or free hydrogen ions), thereby reducing the alkalosis. Such compensation can occur immediately when blood and time buffers are inadequate to handle the *p*H imbalance. In 48 to 72 hours, the renal compensatory mechanism also comes into play in order to restore *p*H homeostasis.

SLEEP APNEA

Two different types of sleep apnea have been discovered. Although they are not usually fatal, they do disrupt sleep and can lead to severe sleep loss and its attendant sequelae—most notably a sense of fatigue and daytime sleepiness. If not recognized, they can obfuscate the clinical picture of the critical care patient.

The first type is termed *obstructive sleep apnea*. It occurs in some persons because, during certain stages of sleep when skeletal muscles are most relaxed, the muscles of the oropharynx and tongue of these patients relax to such an extent that they obstruct the upper airway. Ventilatory chest and diaphragm movements continue, but gas exchange can be so severely inhibited as to cause a decrease in PaO_2. The decreased PaO_2 usually arouses the person, and the arousal decreases the relaxation of tongue and oropharynx, thereby relieving the obstruction. A person may have several to a hundred such apneic episodes per night.

The second type is called *central sleep apnea*. In this condition, something periodically goes awry in one or more of the respiratory centers in the brain stem, causing a cessation in outgoing nerve impulses to the respiratory muscles. Intercostal and diaphragmatic movements cease, gas exchange is impaired, and the PaO_2 rapidly falls. After a few missed breathing cycles, the decreased PaO_2 is usually sufficient to arouse the patient. The fall in PaO_2 or rise in PaO_2 stimulates the respiratory centers to resume their rhythmic activities, and breathing begins again.

BIBLIOGRAPHY

Ganong WF: Review of Medical Physiology, 11th ed. Los Altos, Lang, 1983

Price SA, Wilson LM: Pathophysiology: Clinical Concepts of Disease Processes. New York, McGraw-Hill, 1978

Stephens G: Pathophysiology for Health Practitioners. New York, Macmillan, 1980

14
Assessment: Respiratory System

Joseph O. Broughton

Assessment of the Chest

Nurses contribute significantly to the care of patients with respiratory problems by taking an illness-specific history and performing a chest physical examination. This assessment allows the nurse an opportunity to establish a baseline of information and provides a framework for detection of some of the rapid changes in the patient's condition. Because the nurse is with the patient more frequently than the physician is, it makes sense that it will often be the nurse who detects the patient's changing condition rather than the physician, who visits the patient only once or twice a day, and who, even with the information provided by daily chest roentgenograms, is less likely to be alert to changes in the status of the patient.

PATIENT HISTORY

The patient history should start with information about the present illness. Often when the patient is very ill, a relative or friend provides more information.

If dyspnea is present, one should ask whether it occurs only with exertion or only when the patient is lying flat (therefore requiring the patient to sit up, as is seen more commonly in heart failure) and whether it awakens him at night (paroxysmal nocturnal dyspnea). The last two circumstances of paroxysmal nocturnal dyspnea and orthopnea often signify heart failure but can be seen in severe dyspnea of any cause. How long the shortness of breath has been present and when it became worse also are important details.

Often the dyspnea seen with lung disease is associated with an anterior chest discomfort that must be distinguished from angina.

One should ask how much sputum is produced in 24 hours, giving the patient a frame of reference (*e.g.,* a tablespoonful or one half cup). The color of the sputum provides important information about infection. Yellow, green, or brown sputum usually signifies bacterial infection, but clear or white sputum usually indicates absence of bacterial infection. The color usually comes from white blood cells in the sputum. However, yellow color can occur if there are many eosinophils in the sputum, thereby signifying allergy rather than infection. An increase in either the color or the amount of sputum often means infection. Sometimes in infections, the patient is unable to cough up the sputum; a decrease in sputum production associated with worsening hypoxemia and a silent chest may signify bronchiolitis. Usually, though, cough without sputum production means that bacterial infection is not present. One must try to determine whether mucus production comes from the nose or sinuses as postnasal drainage or whether the mucous originates in the chest.

It is important for one to ask whether there has been blood in the sputum; sometimes the patient is afraid to mention it. The amount of blood should be evaluated —from streaks or specks, to blood-colored mucus, to pure blood (bright red or dark). One should also determine whether the blood is associated with sputum production, as it often is in bronchitis and pneumonia, or whether it occurs alone, as is often the case in a pulmonary embolus.

If chest pain is present, one should determine whether there is more than one type of pain. For each type of chest pain, one should determine duration, related factors (*e.g.,* exertion — which usually is seen with cardiac pain — position, or eating habits), whether pain is worsened by breathing or movement (*e.g.,* in pleurisy), and what it is relieved by (*e.g.,* rest, nitroglycerin, antacids, or belching).

Especially in elderly people, it is important to determine whether regurgitation and aspiration of gastric contents, often occurring at night, cause symptoms of cough, wheeze, or dyspnea.

EXAMINATION OF THE CHEST

Sometimes a chest examination by the nurse is the quickest and most reliable assessment of the situation.

EXAMPLE

A 69-year-old hypertensive man fainted in the shower and fell, breaking five ribs on the left side. When he recovered consciousness, it was clear that he had had a cerebrovascular accident (CVA), with left-side hemiparesis. He did well until the third day of hospitalization, when he developed respiratory distress. The working diagnosis was congestive heart failure, but the nurse was able to convince those in attendance that the breath sounds and thoracic movement on the left side — which everyone agreed were depressed due to rib fractures — were more depressed than they had been previously. A chest roentgenogram showing atelectasis of the entire left lung confirmed the nurse's observations. The roentgenogram showed the lung returned to normal the next day after tracheostomy, vigorous bronchial hygiene, and tracheal suction.

This is just one of many examples in which the nurse's ability to do a competent chest physical examination results in improved patient care.

Physical diagnosis of the chest includes four procedures:

• Inspection, or looking at the patient (Fig. 14-1)
• Palpation, or feeling the patient
• Percussion, or thumping on the patient
• Auscultation, or listening to the patient's chest with a stethoscope

INSPECTION

Inspection of the patient involves checking for the presence or absence of several factors.

Cyanosis is one of the factors in which we are most interested. Cyanosis is notoriously hard to detect when the patient is anemic, and the patient who is polycythemic may have cyanosis in his extremities even when he has a normal oxygen tension.

We generally differentiate between *peripheral* and *central* cyanosis: peripheral cyanosis occurs in the ex-

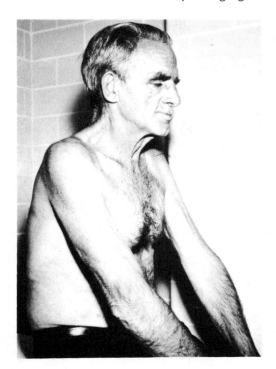

FIGURE 14-1
Frequently observe the patient's overall aspect.

FIGURE 14-2
Feel the patient's extremities and assess their temperature.

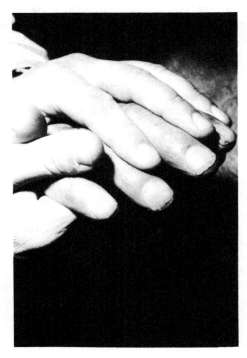

tremities or on the tip of the nose or ears, even with normal oxygen tensions, when there is diminished blood flow to these areas, particularly if they are cold or dependent (Fig. 14-2). Central cyanosis, as noted on the tongue or lips (Fig. 14-3), has a much greater significance; it means the patient actually has a low oxygen tension.

Labored breathing is an obvious sign to check; we are particularly interested in knowing whether the patient is using the accessory muscles of respiration. Sometimes, the number of words a patient can say before having to gasp for another breath is a good measure of the amount of labored breathing. *An increase in the anteroposterior (AP) diameter of the chest* (i.e., an increase in the size of the chest from front to back) also is checked. This often is due to overexpansion of the lungs from obstructive pulmonary disease, but an increase in AP diameter also may be present in a patient who has kyphosis (forward curvature of the spine).

Chest deformities and scars are important in helping us determine the reason for respiratory distress. For instance, a scar may be our first indication that the patient has had part of his lung removed. A chest deformity such as kyphoscoliosis may indicate why the patient has respiratory distress.

The patient's posture also must be noted because patients with obstructive pulmonary disease often sit and prop themselves up on outstretched arms or lean forward with their elbows on a desk in an effort to elevate their clavicles, thereby gaining a slightly greater ability to expand their chests.

The position of the trachea also is an important factor to observe (Fig. 14-4). Is the trachea in the midline as it should be or deviated to one side or the other? A pleural effusion or a tension pneumothorax usually deviates the trachea away from the diseased side. With atelectasis, however, the trachea often is pulled toward the diseased side.

The respiratory rate is an important parameter to follow; it should be counted over at least a 15-second period rather than merely estimated. Often the respiratory rate is recorded as 20 breaths/minute, which frequently means that the rate was estimated instead of counted.

The depth of respiration is often as meaningful as the respiratory rate. For instance, if a patient were breathing 40 times/minute, one might think he had severe respiratory problems, but if he were breathing quite deeply 40 times/minute, it might mean that he had Kussmaul respirations due to diabetic acidosis or other acidosis. However, if the respirations were shallow at a rate of 40 times/minute, it might mean that he had severe respiratory distress from obstructive lung disease, restrictive lung disease, or other pulmonary problems.

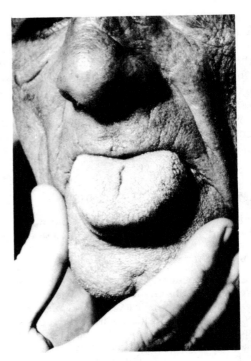

FIGURE 14-3
Examine the tongue and lips for cyanosis.

FIGURE 14-4
Note the position of the trachea.

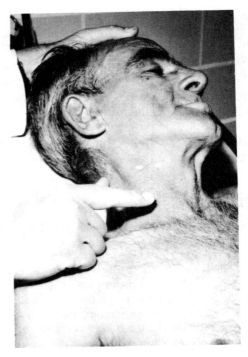

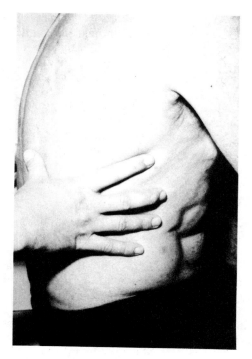

FIGURE 14-5
Note the general chest expansion.

FIGURE 14-6
In palpation, place the heel of your hand flat against the patient's chest.

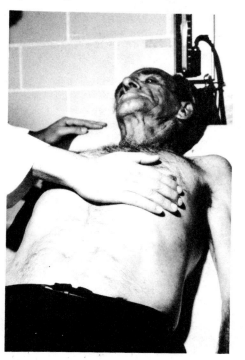

The duration of inspiration versus the duration of expiration is important in determining whether or not there is airway obstruction. In patients with any of the obstructive lung diseases, expiration is prolonged, more than $1\frac{1}{2}$ times as long as inspiration.

General chest expansion is an integral part of examining a patient. Normally we expect about a 3-inch expansion from maximal expiration to maximal inspiration (Fig. 14-5). Ankylosing spondylitis, or Marie-Strümpell arthritis, is one condition in which general chest expansion is limited. We compare the expansion of the upper chest with that of the lower chest and use of the diaphragm to determine if the patient with obstructive pulmonary disease is concentrating on expanding his lower chest and using his diaphragm properly. We look at the expansion of one side of the chest versus the other side, realizing that atelectasis, especially that caused by a mucus plug, may cause unilateral diminished chest expansion.

A pulmonary embolus, pneumonia, pleural effusion, pneumothorax, or any other cause of chest pain, such as fractured ribs, may lead to diminished chest expansion. An endotracheal or nasotracheal tube inserted too far, so that it extends beyond the trachea into one of the main stem bronchi (usually the right), is a serious and frequent cause of diminished expansion of one side of the chest. When the tube slips into the right main stem bronchus, the left lung is not expanded, and the patient usually develops hypoxemia and atelectasis on the left side. Fortunately, the nurse who is aware of this potential problem usually recognizes it.

If present, *intercostal retractions* (*i.e.,* sucking in of the muscles and skin between the ribs during inspiration) usually mean that the patient is making a larger effort at inspiration than normal. Usually this signifies that the lungs are less compliant (stiffer) than usual.

The effectiveness and frequency of a patient's cough are important to note, as are sputum characteristics such as amount, color, and consistency.

PALPATION

Palpation of the chest is done with the heel of the hand flat against the patient's chest (Fig. 14-6). Often we are determining whether tactile fremitus is present. We do this by having the patient speak, particularly asking him to say "ninety-nine." Normally, when a patient follows these instructions, a vibration is felt on the outside of his chest by the examiner's hand. This is similar to the vibration one feels when putting a hand on the chest of a cat when the cat is purring. In normal patients, tactile fremitus is present. It may be diminished or absent when there is something that comes between the patient's lung and the hand on the chest

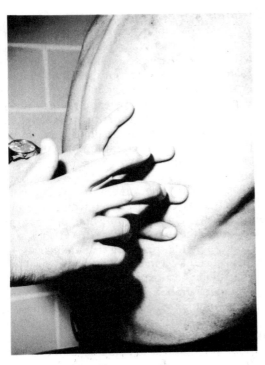

FIGURE 14-7
In percussion, press a finger flat against the patient's chest or back and strike this finger over the knuckle with the end of a finger from the opposite hand.

wall. For instance, when there is a pleural effusion, thickened pleura, or pneumothorax, either it is impossible to feel this vibration or the vibration is diminished. When the patient has atelectasis due to an occluded airway, the vibration also cannot be felt. Tactile fremitus is slightly increased in conditions of consolidation, but detection of this slight increase may be difficult. Just by palpating over the patient's chest with quiet breathing, one may sometimes feel palpable rhonchi that are due to mucus moving in large airways.

PERCUSSION

In percussing a patient's chest (Fig. 14-7), one must use a finger that is pressed flat against the chest; this finger is struck over the knuckle by the end of a finger from the opposite hand. Normally, the chest has a resonant or hollow percussion note. In diseases in which there is increased air in the chest or lungs, such as pneumothorax and emphysema, there may be hyperresonant (even more drumlike) percussion notes. Hyperresonant percussion notes, however, are sometimes hard to detect. More important is a dull or flat percussion note such as is heard when one percusses over a part of the body that contains no air. A dull or flat percussion note is heard when the lung underneath the examining hand has atelectasis, pneumonia,

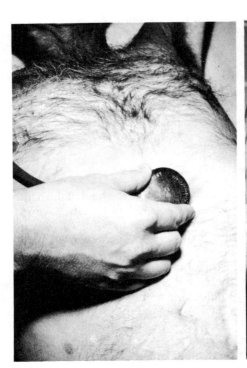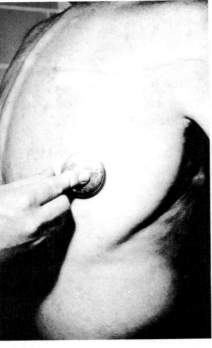

FIGURE 14-8
In auscultation, press the stethoscope firmly against the chest wall (left) *or the back* (right).

TABLE 14-1
CHECKLIST OF ABNORMAL RESPIRATORY FINDINGS

Bronchitis
Increased respiratory rate (occasional)
Use of accessory muscles (occasional)
Intercostal retraction (occasional)
Prolonged expiratory phase (frequent)
Increased AP diameter of the chest (frequent)
Decreased motion of the diaphragm (frequent)
Decreased intensity of breath sounds
Fine, medium, and coarse rales (rhonchi)
Wheezes (frequent)
Coarse rales (rhonchi) and wheezes clear after cough
    (frequent)

Pneumothorax
Increased respiratory rate
Trachea deviated to side of pneumothorax
Cyanosis (occasional)
Decreased movement of chest on side of pneumothorax
    (splinting)
Hyperresonance (unreliable sign)
Decreased breath sounds
Decreased tactile fremitus and decreased vocal fremitus
    (the most reliable signs)

Emphysema
Increased respiratory rate (frequent)
Use of accessory muscles (neck)
Intercoastal retractions
Propped up on outstretched arms
Prolonged expiratory phase
Increased AP diameter
Decreased chest expansion
Decreased motion of diaphragm
Hyperresonance to percussion
Decreased intensity (loudness) of breath sounds
Little or no increase in loudness of breath sounds with
    deep breath
Fine rales at bases (frequent)
Wheeze (occasional)

Pneumonia
Increased respiratory rate
Cyanosis (occasional)
Decreased expansion (splinting) (frequent)
Increased fremitus (tactile and vocal)
Palpable rhonchi—usually are removed by coughing or
    suctioning (occasional)
Dullness to percussion
Bronchial breathing, whispered pectoriloquy, and E to A
    changes (usual if consolidation is extensive)
Fine or medium rales
Coarse rales (rhonchi)—usually clear with cough or
    suctioning (occasional)
Pleural friction rub (occasional)

Atelectasis
Increased respiratory rate
Increased pulse
Cyanosis (frequent)
Trachea deviated to side of atelectasis
Decreased chest expansion on side of atelectasis
    (splinting)
Decreased fremitus (tactile and vocal)
Dull or flat percussion note
Decreased breath sounds
Rales (occasional)

Pleural effusion
Increase in respiratory rate (occasional)
Trachea deviated away from side of effusion
Decreased fremitus (tactile and vocal)
Decreased breath sounds
Above effusion
    Bronchial breathing ⎫
    E to A changes   ⎬ due to compressed lungs
    Whispered pectoriloquy ⎭ with open airway
Friction rub—after fluid is removed and visceral pleura
    rubs against parietal pleura

Large mass lesion (tumor)
Dullness over tumor
Fine rales (frequent)
Decreased breath sounds if airway is occluded
Bronchial breathing, E to A changes, and whispered
    pectoriloquy if airway is open
Pleural friction rub (occasional)

Subcutaneous emphysema
Crackling sounds similar to rales that come from air
    outside the chest in the soft tissue

Pulmonary edema (congestive heart failure)
Increased respiratory rate
Cyanosis (frequent)
Use of accessory muscles (usual)
Apprehension
Sitting upright (frequent)
Increased fremitus (due to interstitial edema)
Dull percussion note (due to interstitial edema)
Bronchovesicular sounds (due to interstitial edema,
    often obscured later by rales)
Fine rales → medium rales later
Coarse rales (rhonchi) (occasional)
Wheezing (occasional)

Pulmonary interstitial fibrosis
Increased respiratory rate (frequent)
Intercostal retractions
Cyanosis (late)
High-pitched, fine, and medium rales
Bronchovesicular breathing (occasional)

pleural effusion, thickened pleura, or a mass lesion. A dull or flat percussion note also is heard when one is percussing over the heart.

AUSCULTATION

In auscultation, one generally uses the diaphragm of the stethoscope and presses this firmly against the chest wall (Fig. 14-8). It is important for one to listen to the intensity or loudness of breath sounds and to realize that normally there is a fourfold increase in loudness of breath sounds when a patient takes a maximum deep breath as opposed to quiet breathing. The intensity of the breath sounds may be diminished owing to decreased airflow through the airways or to increased insulation between the lungs and the stethoscope. In airway obstruction, such as chronic obstructive pulmonary disease or atelectasis, the breath sound intensity is diminished. With shallow breathing, there is diminished air movement through the airways, and the breath sounds also are not as loud. With restricted movement of the thorax or diaphragm, there may be diminished breath sounds in the area of restricted movement. In pleural thickening, pleural effusion, pneumothorax, and obesity there is an abnormal substance (fibrous tissue, fluid, air, or fat) between the stethoscope and the underlying lung; this substance insulates the breath sounds from the stethoscope, making the breath sounds seem less loud.

Generally, there are three types of sounds that are heard in the normal chest:

- Vesicular breath sounds, which are heard in the periphery of the normal lung
- Bronchial breath sounds, which are heard over the trachea
- Bronchovesicular breath sounds, which are heard in most areas of the lung near the major airways

Bronchial breath sounds are high-pitched, seem to be close to the ear, are loud, and include a pause between inspiration and expiration. *Vesicular breath sounds* are of lower pitch, having a rustling quality, and include no noticeable pause between inspiration and expiration. *Bronchovesicular breath sounds* represent a sound halfway between the other two types of breath sounds.

Bronchial breathing, in addition to being heard over the trachea of the normal person, is also heard in any situation in which there is consolidation—for instance, pneumonia. Bronchial breathing is also heard above a pleural effusion in which the normal lung is compressed. Wherever there is bronchial breathing, there also may be two other associated changes: (1) "E to A" changes, and (2) whispered pectoriloquy.

An *E to A change* merely means that when one listens with a stethoscope and the patient says "E," what one hears is actually an A sound rather than an E sound. This occurs when there is consolidation.

Whispered pectoriloquy is the presence of a loud volume as heard through the stethoscope when the patient whispers. For bronchial breathing and these two associated changes to be present, there must be either (1) an open airway and compressed alveoli, or (2) alveoli in which the air has been replaced by fluid.

Extra sounds that are heard with auscultation include rales, rhonchi, wheezes, and rubs.

Rales are divided into three categories: fine, medium, and coarse. Fine rales are also called *crepitant rales* and are produced in the small airways in patients with diseases such as pneumonia and heart failure. Medium rales are sounds produced in the medium airways and occur later in pneumonia, heart failure, and pulmonary edema. Coarse rales, also called *rhonchi,* are continuous, bubbling, gurgling, or rattling sounds, often musical and usually coming from the large airways.

Extra sounds such as wheezing mean there is airway narrowing. This may be caused by asthma, foreign bodies, mucus in the airways, stenosis, and so forth. If the wheeze is heard only in expiration, it is called a *wheeze;* if the wheezing sound occurs in both inspiration and expiration, it is usually due to retained secretions and is best called a *rhonchus.*

A *friction rub* is heard when there is pleural disease such as a pulmonary embolus, peripheral pneumonia, or pleurisy and is often difficult to distinguish from a rhonchus. If the abnormal noise clears when the patient coughs, it usually means that is was a rhonchus rather than a friction rub.

Certainly, critical care nurses and respiratory nurse therapists and, it is hoped, unit nurses and inhalation therapy technicians should learn to participate in chest physical diagnosis so that they can detect changes in the patient's condition as soon as they occur, rather than waiting for the physician's visit once or twice a day or depending on a daily chest film. See Table 14-1 for a checklist of abnormal respiratory findings in a number of common pulmonary disorders.

Respiratory Diagnostic Procedure: Blood Gases

Blood gases are obtained in a variety of clinical situations, but they are obtained for two major reasons:

- To determine whether the patient is well oxygenated
- To determine the acid-base status of the patient, concentrating on either the respiratory component, the metabolic (nonrespiratory) component, or, most often, both respiratory and metabolic components.

In the following discussion, the term *nonrespiratory* will be used interchangeably with the term *metabolic*.

ARTERIAL VERSUS VENOUS BLOOD MEASUREMENTS

Most often blood gases are measured on arterial blood rather than on venous blood for two reasons:

- Studying arterial blood is a good way to sample a mixture of blood that has come from various parts of the body.
- Arterial blood gives the added information on how well the lungs are oxygenating the blood.

Blood obtained from a vein in an extremity gives information mostly about that extremity and can be quite misleading if the metabolism in the extremity differs from the metabolism of the body as a whole, as it often does. This difference is accentuated if the extremity is cold or underperfused as in a patient in shock, if the patient has done local exercise with the extremity such as opening and closing his fist, if there is local infection in the extremity, and so forth.

Sometimes blood is sampled through a central venous (CVP catheter) in hopes of getting mixed venous blood, but even in the superior vena cava or right atrium, where a CVP catheter ends, there is usually incomplete mixing of venous blood from various parts of the body. For complete mixing of the blood, one would have to obtain a blood sample from the pulmonary artery through a Swan-Ganz catheter, for example; even then one would not get information about how well the lungs are oxygenating the blood.

The second reason for selecting arterial blood is that it gives the added information of how well the lungs are oxygenating the blood. Oxygen measurements of mixed venous blood indicate whether the tissues are being oxygenated but cannot separate the contribu-

tion of the heart from that of the lungs. In other words, if the mixed venous blood oxygen is low, it means that either heart or lungs or both are at fault, and this may indicate either (1) that the lungs have not oxygenated the arterial blood well and that when the tissues extract their usual amount of oxygen from arterial blood, the resulting venous blood has a low oxygen concentration, or (2) that the heart is not circulating the blood well so that it is taking blood a long time to circulate through the tissues. The tissues, therefore, must extract more than the usual amount of oxygen from each cardiac cycle because the blood is flowing slowly. This produces a low venous oxygen concentration.

If it is known that the arterial oxygen concentration is normal (indicating that the lungs are doing their job), but the mixed venous oxygen concentration is low, then one can infer that the heart and circulation are failing.

One advantage of using mixed venous blood instead of arterial blood is that if the oxygen concentration in mixed venous blood is normal, one can infer that the tissues are receiving enough oxygen—usually this means that both ventilation and circulation are adequate. Thus, when the mixed venous oxygen saturation is monitored and is found to be normal, it ensures both normal oxygenation of blood by the lungs and normal or near normal cardiac function. If the oxygen saturation is low, one should measure arterial O_2 saturation and cardiac output. However, as long as the mixed venous oxygen saturation is normal, one can infer that both the arterial oxygen saturation and the cardiac output are normal. Therefore, these two determinants of the mixed venous oxygen saturation would not have to be measured as frequently as long as the mixed venous oxygen saturation remains normal. The development of a pulmonary artery flotation (Swan-Ganz) catheter that allows continuous monitoring of oxygen saturation with an oximeter built into its tip so that one can constantly monitor oxygen saturation in the pulmonary artery and display it as a constant digital read-out makes the aforementioned procedure a reality that should see more use in the future. Even if the exact mixed venous oxygen saturation measured by this catheter is not completely accurate, certainly the trends recorded are just as useful. Alternatively, one

---

TABLE 14-2
CAUSES OF LOW MIXED VENOUS OXYGEN SATURATION

- Low arterial saturation due to abnormal lungs, but normal cardiac function.
- Normal oxygen saturation and decreased cardiac function (slower blood flow) allowing more tissue extraction of oxygen (increased arteriovenous oxygen difference).
- Combination of the two.

Procedure for Drawing Blood for Arterial Blood Gas Analysis

A. Equipment
1. 5- or 10-ml glass syringe or plastic syringe with vented plunger
2. 10-ml bottle of heparin, 1000 units/ml (reusable)
3. No. 21 or No. 22 needle or even No. 25 disposable needle (short level)
4. Cork
5. Alcohol swab
6. Container of ice (emesis basin or cardboard milkshake cup or plastic bag)
7. Request slip on which to write patient's clinical status, etc., including
   a. Name, date, time
   b. Whether receiving O_2, and if so how much and by what route
   c. Whether in shock
   d. Recent bicarbonate Rx, etc.
   e. If on continuous ventilation: tidal volume, respiratory frequency, inspired oxygen concentration (FIO_2), amount of PEEP or CPAP, and amount of dead space

B. Technique
1. Call the lab to notify them that you plan to draw a blood gas sample so that they can be calibrating equipment for 15 to 30 minutes.
2. Patients should be in steady state for at least 15 minutes (no recent change in inspired O_2, etc.).
3. Brachial artery is generally preferred, although radial may be used. Femoral artery sometimes must be used in hypotensive patients but should be avoided if possible.
4. Elbow is hyperextended and arm is externally rotated.
   a. Very important to have elbow *completely straight*—usually a folded towel or pillow under the elbow accomplishes this.
   b. For radial artery puncture, wrist is hyperextended after supporting lower arm on towels.
5. 1 ml of heparin is aspirated into the syringe, barrel of the syringe is wet with heparin, and then excess heparin is discarded through the needle, with care taken so that the hub of the needle is left full of heparin and there are no bubbles.
6. Brachial or radial artery is located by palpation with index and long fingers, and point of maximum impulse is found.
7. Needle is inserted into the area of maximal pulsation. This is easiest with the syringe and needle approximately perpendicular to the skin; however, if the needle is inserted at a more acute angle (such as used for venipunctures), there may be better hemostasis after the needle is removed.
8. Often the needle goes completely through both sides of the artery and only when the needle is slowly withdrawn does the blood gush up into the syringe.
9. The only certain indication that arterial blood is obtained is pumping of the blood up into the syringe under its own power.
   a. If one has to aspirate blood by pulling on the plunger of syringe—as is sometimes required with a tighter fitting plastic syringe—it is impossible to be positive that blood is arterial.
   b. *The blood gas results do not allow one to determine whether blood is arterial or venous.*
   c. If one suspects that blood may be venous, then another sample of obviously venous blood should be drawn and the two samples compared. If the two samples are similar, the first sample also was venous, but if the PO_2 and O_2

---

can draw blood from the pulmonary artery through a regular Swan-Ganz catheter and measure the PO_2 or oxygen saturation or both on a blood gas analyzer or oximeter or both and use the information in the same way.

Finally, there is another rare cause of arterial hypoxemia that is due to a combination of heart and lung failure. Low mixed venous oxygen saturation resulting from decreased cardiac function can occasionally lead to a low arterial oxygen saturation if the lungs cannot raise the oxygen saturation to normal as the markedly desaturated blood traverses the lungs. This is seen only if there is significant shunting of blood in the lungs away from ventilated alveoli. In this case, a decrease in cardiac output in a patient with a large pulmonary shunt can lead to a reduction in arterial PO_2 with-

out any change in the severity of the patient's lung disease. This cause of arterial hypoxemia—low cardiac output and large pulmonary shunt—is uncommon but important to remember (Table 14-2).

Noninvasive Measurement of PO_2 and PCO_2

Although transcutaneous PO_2 and PCO_2 measurements might become quite valuable in the future, at present, in the adult critical care patient, they are not accurate enough to be useful. Ear and finger oximetry are more accurate and frequently can be substituted for arterial blood gas measurements in the circumstance when one is most interested in the PO_2 and oxygen saturation and for use in titrating the oxygen up to a

saturation on the second (obviously venous) sample are significantly lower than the first sample, the first sample is probably arterial.

10. After 5 to 10 ml of blood are obtained, the needle is withdrawn and the assistant puts constant pressure on site of arterial puncture for at least 5 minutes.
    a. If the patient is anticoagulated or hypertensive or has a bleeding disorder, a longer period of pressure—10 minutes—is required.
    b. Even if an attempt is unsuccessful, pressure must be applied.
11. Any air bubbles should be squirted out of the syringe and needle immediately because these can change the blood gas values. The needle is then stuck into a cork, and the syringe is shaken to ensure that the blood mixes with the heparin.
12. Corked syringe and needle are labeled and immediately placed into ice or ice water, then taken to the laboratory.
13. Minimal analyses required are
    a. pH
    b. PCO_2 (by direct electrode or Astrup tonometer technique)
    c. PO_2
    d. Hgb
    Base excess and actual bicarbonate should be calculated (standard bicarbonate may be substituted for actual bicarbonate). Other calculated values such as buffer base should not be reported because they tend to be confusing.
14. *Other*
    a. If O_2 saturation is also measured, this provides a cross-check for accuracy of the PO_2 (use PO_2 and pH to calculate O_2 saturation on blood gas slide rule and see whether this calculated O_2 saturation agrees with the measured O_2 saturation plus carboxyhemoglobin (calculated O_2 saturation = measured O_2 saturation + carboxyhemoglobin).
    b. If CO_2 content is also measured, this provides a cross-check for accuracy of PCO_2. (Use PCO_2 and pH to calculate CO_2 content on blood gas slide rule and see whether this calculated CO_2 content agrees with the measured CO_2 content.)
15. Another way to ensure accuracy is to run the tests in duplicate on two different blood gas analyzers. If there is a discrepancy in the two determinations, the test must be run a third time.
16. If PO_2 and O_2 saturation do not seem to agree with the clinical situation, the patient's O_2 saturation should be measured with a finger or ear oximeter to resolve the discrepancy.
17. Results should be reported back to the unit on the same request slip that includes the patient's status, as listed in step A-7, so that results of blood gases can be related to clinical condition. (If all information is not on the same slip, it becomes impossible to interpret data hours, days, or weeks later. For instance, PO_2 has little meaning unless FIO_2 is known.
18. The technician performing analysis should report any suspicion that results are not reliable. For instance
    a. If syringe comes to her with air bubbles in it
    b. If she introduces air into the sample inadvertently
    c. If calculated O_2 saturation and measured O_2 saturation do not agree
    d. If calculated CO_2 content and measured CO_2 content do not agree
    e. If equipment does not appear to be functioning correctly

specified saturation. Occasionally, ear oximetry or finger oximetry measurements require confirmation with blood gas determinations. Measurement of end-tidal PCO_2 of the patient's expired gas is a satisfactory way of estimating the patient's arterial PCO_2.

The new technology in oximeters that demonstrates the patient's arterial waveform and allows accurate measurements even in the presence of high bilirubin levels and skin pigment is impressive. We can expect to see more use of noninvasive means of estimating oxygenation and PCO_2 in the future.

OXYGEN

There are three ways to measure oxygen in blood:
- Oxygen content, which is the number of milliliters of oxygen carried by 100 ml of blood

- The PO_2, or pressure exerted by oxygen dissolved in the plasma
- The oxygen saturation of hemoglobin, which is a measure of the percentage of oxygen that hemoglobin is carrying related to the total amount the hemoglobin could carry, or

$$O_2 \text{ sat} = \frac{\text{amount of oxygen that hemoglobin is carrying}}{\text{maximal amount of oxygen that hemoglobin can carry}} \times 100$$

The first of these methods is the easiest to understand but the most difficult to measure, so it is not used routinely. The last two methods, which are used routinely, are more understandable when compared with the first method in Table 14-3.

TABLE 14-3
HOW OXYGEN IS CARRIED IN BLOOD

Dissolved in plasma	0.3 ml/100 ml blood	Reflected by PO_2 90 torr
Combined with Hgb	19.4 ml/100 ml blood	Reflected by O_2 sat Hgb 97%
Total in whole blood	19.7 ml/100 ml blood	

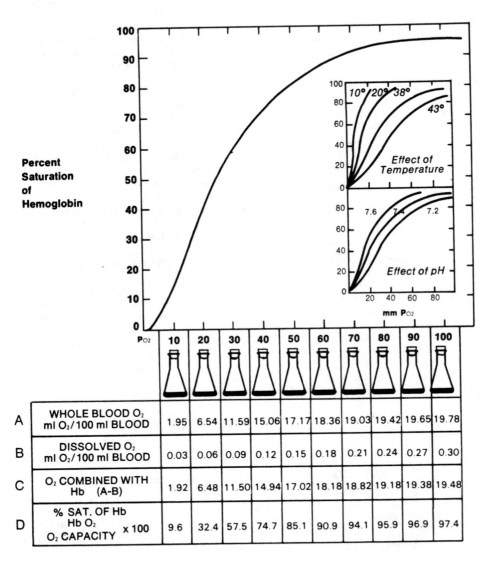

		10	20	30	40	50	60	70	80	90	100
A	WHOLE BLOOD O_2 ml O_2/100 ml BLOOD	1.95	6.54	11.59	15.06	17.17	18.36	19.03	19.42	19.65	19.78
B	DISSOLVED O_2 ml O_2/100 ml BLOOD	0.03	0.06	0.09	0.12	0.15	0.18	0.21	0.24	0.27	0.30
C	O_2 COMBINED WITH Hb (A-B)	1.92	6.48	11.50	14.94	17.02	18.18	18.82	19.18	19.38	19.48
D	% SAT. OF Hb $\frac{Hb\,O_2}{O_2\,CAPACITY}$ × 100	9.6	32.4	57.5	74.7	85.1	90.9	94.1	95.9	96.9	97.4

FIGURE 14-9
HbO_2 dissociation curves. The large graph shows a single dissociation curve, applicable when the pH of the blood is 7.40 and temperature 38° C. The blood O_2 tension and saturation of patients with CO_2 retention, acidosis, alkalosis, fever, or hypothermia will not fit this curve because the curve shifts to the right when temperature, pH, or PCO_2 is changed. Effects on the HbO_2 dissociation curve of change in temperature and in pH are shown in the smaller graphs. (Comroe JH: Physiology of Respiration, 2nd ed. Copyright © 1974 by Year Book Medical Publishers, Inc., Chicago. Used by permission.)

The table reminds us that the majority of oxygen carried by the blood is carried by hemoglobin and that a very small amount is dissolved in plasma. The percentage saturation of hemoglobin with oxygen, then, gives a close estimate of the total amount of oxygen carried in blood.

The PO_2 measurement, however, tells only of the pressure exerted by the small amount of oxygen that is dissolved in plasma.

PO_2 is widely used and is valuable because PO_2 (pressure of oxygen dissolved in plasma) and oxygen saturation of hemoglobin (which is closely related to the total oxygen content of whole blood) are related to each other in a definite fashion, and the relationship has been charted—the *oxyhemoglobin dissociation curve* (Fig. 14-9).

When the PO_2 in plasma is high, hemoglobin carries much oxygen. When the PO_2 is low, hemoglobin carries less oxygen. Once this relationship is known, PO_2 is just as valuable as a measurement of total O_2 content or the percentage of oxygen that hemoglobin is carrying.

Oxygen Content

Oxygen content refers to the total amount of oxygen that is present in blood in any form. Oxygen is carried in blood in only two ways: (1) dissolved in the plasma, and (2) combined with hemoglobin. By far the larger amount of oxygen is carried in combination with hemoglobin, and a very small amount is dissolved in plasma (Table 14-1). Oxygen is not very soluble in plasma or water, so only a very small amount can dissolve in plasma. Oxygen content and oxygen saturation of hemoglobin are indicators of the *amount* of oxygen in blood and in the red blood cells, respectively.

FIGURE 14-10
Effects of barometric pressure.

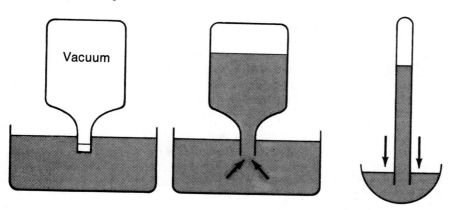

TABLE 14-4
COMPARISON OF PO_2 AT SEA LEVEL WITH PO_2 AT DENVER

At Sea Level		At Denver		Remarks
760		630	torr	Average barometric pressure
−47		−47	torr	Water vapor pressure at body temperature (subtracted because in the body this pressure is exerted by water vapor)
713		583	torr	Corrected barometric pressure (in body or completely humidified air at body temperature)
×21%		×21%		Percent of oxygen in the atmosphere
150	torr	123	torr	PO_2 in air that is completely humidified
−40		−36		PCO_2—pressure exerted by CO_2 in alveolus
110	torr	87	torr	PO_2 in alveolus
−5	torr	−5	torr	Gradient for diffusion of O_2 from alveolus into capillary
105	torr	82	torr	PO_2 in capillary blood in lungs
−10	torr	−10	torr	Due to venous shunting
95	torr	72	torr	PO_2 in arterial blood

PO$_2$ Measurement

The oxygen that is combined with hemoglobin exerts no pressure, but the oxygen that is dissolved in plasma exerts a pressure or tension. The pressure or tension of oxygen dissolved in plasma can be readily measured and is known as PO$_2$. The hemoglobin oxygen dissociation curve (Fig. 14-9) defines the relationship between the pressure exerted by dissolved oxygen and the amount of oxygen carried by hemoglobin. It should be made quite clear, though, *that PO$_2$ is a measure of the pressure or tension exerted by dissolved oxygen and that PO$_2$ is not a measure of the amount of oxygen in blood.*

Partial Pressure and Barometric Pressure.

An explanation of PO$_2$ must start with an explanation of barometric pressure. Barometric pressure may be thought of as the weight of the atmosphere or the pressure exerted by the atmosphere. At sea level, barometric pressure is 760 torr. We are not conscious of the weight or pressure exerted on us by the atmosphere, partly because the atmosphere is made up of gases. If we dive into water, we are much more aware of the weight or pressure exerted on us by the water, and this pressure increases as we dive deeper because there is progressively more water above us. Just as in water, the deeper we are in the atmosphere, the higher the barometric pressure. Thus, at the top of Pike's Peak (elevation 14,110 feet above sea level) we are near the top of the atmosphere and the barometric pressure is lower—425 torr. Denver and the other cities of Colorado as well as the cities of Wyoming are between these two extremes. The average barometric pressure in Denver is 625 torr. (Of course, as weather fronts approach, the barometric pressure may fluctuate slightly even though the elevation is constant.) With high-pressure weather fronts, the barometric pressure may increase by 5 to 10 torr, and with low-pressure fronts the barometric pressure may fall by 5 to 10 torr. In blood gas laboratories a barometer is necessary for determining the barometric pressure each day.

If one takes a bottle in which a vacuum has been created and inverts this bottle in a pan of water, when the cork is removed from the bottle the water in the pan will rise in the bottle (Fig. 14-10). The force that makes the water rise in the bottle is the difference between the barometric pressure exerted on the pan and the absence of barometric pressure in the vacuum bottle.

If we substitute a long tube for the bottle, create a vacuum in the tube, and invert the tube in a container of mercury instead of a pan of water, we have a barometer. Because the vacuum in the tube remains constant, the only factor influencing how high mercury rises in the tube is the barometric pressure (or weight of the atmosphere) pressing down on the mercury in the container.

Table 14-4 is a simplified explanation of why the arterial PO$_2$ in Denver is about 72 torr and at sea level about 95 torr.

It should be pointed out that the percentage of oxygen in the atmosphere is 21% (actually 20.93%) everywhere in the atmosphere and that changes in PO$_2$ with altitude are due to changes in barometric pressure with altitude and not to changes in percentage of oxygen present.

Hemoglobin Saturation

Each gram of hemoglobin in 100 ml of blood can carry a maximum of 1.34 ml of oxygen. As stated earlier in this chapter, the percentage of saturation of hemoglobin is defined as the amount of oxygen that hemoglobin *is* carrying compared with the amount of oxygen that hemoglobin *can* carry, expressed as a percentage:

$$\text{Percent O}_2 \text{ saturation of Hgb} = \frac{\text{Amount O}_2 \text{ Hgb is carrying}}{\text{Amount O}_2 \text{ Hgb can carry}} \times 100$$

Because the amount of oxygen that hemoglobin can carry is a constant 1.34 ml/g hemoglobin,

$$1.34 \text{ ml} \times \text{g Hgb} \times \% \text{ saturation Hgb} = \text{No. of ml O}_2 \text{ that Hgb is carrying}$$

(It should be noted that there are rare abnormal types of hemoglobin that cannot carry 1.34 ml oxygen/g. There also are rare situations in which normal hemoglobin has been poisoned so that it cannot carry 1.34 ml oxygen/g—*e.g.*, with sulfhemoglobin or methemoglobin).

In 100 ml of blood

$$\begin{cases} 1 \text{ g Hgb can carry } 1.34 \text{ ml O}_2 \\ 15 \text{ g Hgb can carry } 15 \times 1.34 \text{ ml O}_2 \end{cases}$$

In Denver, the normal oxygen saturation of hemoglobin in arterial blood is 93% (*i.e.*, hemoglobin *is* carrying 93% of the total amount of oxygen it *can* carry), then 93% of 20.1 ml equals 18.7 ml of oxygen carried by hemoglobin in Denver. At sea level, arterial oxygen saturation of hemoglobin is 97%, so hemoglobin is carrying 97% of 20.1 ml or 19.4 ml of oxygen.

The major factor that determines how much oxygen hemoglobin *is* carrying is the PO$_2$ that the hemoglobin is exposed to. At high PO$_2$ hemoglobin carries more oxygen; at low PO$_2$ hemoglobin carries less oxygen. The exact relationship between the amount of oxygen that hemoglobin is carrying and the PO$_2$ is shown by the oxyhemoglobin dissociation curve in Figure 14-9.

Oxyhemoglobin Dissociation Curve

The relationship between PO_2 and oxygen saturation of hemoglobin is not a linear one, so that for a given rise or fall in PO_2 there is not always the same amount of rise or fall in oxygen saturation of hemoglobin. Instead, for very low PO_2, a rise in PO_2 is associated with a more rapid rise in oxygen saturation, and for PO_2 in the normal range or higher, a rise in PO_2 is associated with a very small rise in oxygen saturation.

This relationship is much easier to understand if one looks at the oxygen dissociation curve for hemoglobin (Fig. 14-9). In simple terms, the dissociation curve indicates that in environments in which the PO_2 is high, such as the capillaries of the lungs, hemoglobin combines with and carries a high percentage of the total oxygen it could carry; in environments in which the PO_2 is low, such as the capillaries in the tissues, hemoglobin carries a lower percentage of the total oxygen it could carry, having given up the difference in oxygen for use by the tissues.

Shifts in the Curve. The dissociation curve presented applies only to normal conditions. In the presence of *acidosis* or fever, the entire dissociation curve is shifted to the right, so that for a given oxygen saturation the PO_2 is greater than usual and more oxygen is available for the tissues. In the presence of *alkalosis,* hemoglobin has a greater affinity for oxygen, and for a given oxygen saturation the PO_2 is lower than usual.

Certain abnormal types of hemoglobin may shift the dissociation curve to the right or the left, and the presence of certain compounds such as 2,3 diphosphoglycerate (2,3 DPG) may also shift the dissociation curve. Normal or high amounts of 2,3 DPG shift the curve to the right, thereby making more oxygen available to the tissues for a given oxygen saturation of hemoglobin because 2,3 DPG decreases the affinity of hemoglobin for oxygen. Conversely, blood with low amounts of 2,3 DPG, such as transfused blood from a blood bank, has a left-shifted oxyhemoglobin dissociation curve, which makes less oxygen available to the tissues because this hemoglobin has a greater than normal affinity for oxygen. The measurement of P_{50} (partial pressure of oxygen when hemoglobin is exactly 50% saturated) allows one to detect the shifted oxyhemoglobin dissociation curve, so that P_{50} is greater than 27 when the curve is shifted to the right and less than 27 when it is shifted to the left.

A − a Oxygen Gradient, a/A Ratio, and Fraction of Inspired Oxygen (FIO_2). One should always relate the oxygen content of blood to the FIO_2. For instance, an oxygen saturation of hemoglobin of 96% is normal if the patient is breathing room air, which has an FIO_2 of 21, but is quite abnormal if the FIO_2 is −40. It is useful to calculate the A − a oxygen gradient and a/A

ratio for every blood gas. However, much the same information can be obtained if one compares the arterial PO_2 or oxygen saturation with the FIO_2 that the patient was receiving and also looks at the PCO_2 to see the amount of ventilation required to produce the PO_2. The capital "A" is used to designate the alveolus, and the lowercase "a" is used to designate the artery.

A − a oxygen gradient is the difference between PO_2 in alveolar air and PO_2 in arterial blood. PO_2 is always higher in the alveolus. One calculates the alveolar PO_2 by making several assumptions, and although the result may not be precise, it is accurate enough to be quite useful clinically. One can estimate the alveolar PO_2 at the bedside by

- Subtracting the water vapor pressure from barometric pressure
- Multiplying the barometric pressure by the patient's FIO_2
- Subtracting from this $1\frac{1}{4}$ times the patient's arterial PCO_2.

These calculations give the alveolar PO_2. When the arterial PO_2 is subtracted from the alveolar PO_2, the A − a oxygen gradient has been calculated. Frequently, a computer is used to calculate a/A ratios and A − a gradients.

The A − a oxygen gradient is most useful for patients breathing room air because normal values are well established. An example of the usefulness of the A − a oxygen gradient would be in a patient suspected of having a pulmonary embolus, where arterial hypoxemia is often used as a screening test for pulmonary emboli. However, hyperventilation (which is common in patients with pulmonary emboli) can raise the arterial PO_2 into the normal range. The A − a oxygen gradient would remain abnormal and would suggest pulmonary embolus even if the PO_2 were normal. For example, a patient at sea level breathing room air with a PO_2 of 85 and PCO_2 of 20 would still have a widened A − a gradient of 40 (normal value is less than 20), suggesting pulmonary embolus. The normal range for A − a oxygen gradient increases with age. In young people, the A − a oxygen gradient may normally be as high as 15 torr, whereas in elderly people it may be normally as high as 27 torr. Often a range of less than 20 is used to encompass all age groups.

The a/A ratio is the percentage of alveolar PO_2 that arterial PO_2 represents. In the preceding example and in Figure 14-11, the a/A ratio would be as follows:

$$\frac{\text{Patient's measured arterial } PO_2}{\text{Patient's calculated alveolar } PO_2}$$

$$\frac{90}{100} = 0.9$$

The normal a/A ratio is greater than 0.75.

A − a Oxygen Gradient: Difference between PO₂ in alveolus and PO₂ in arterial blood.

PaO_2	minus	PaO_2	=	A − a Oxygen Gradient

$$\left(\begin{array}{c}\text{Barometric}\\\text{pressure}\end{array}\right) - \left(\begin{array}{c}\text{Water vapor}\\\text{pressure}\end{array}\right) \times \left(\begin{array}{c}\text{Patient's}\\F_IO_2\end{array}\right) - (1\tfrac{1}{4}) \times \left(\begin{array}{c}\text{Patient's}\\\text{Arterial}\\PCO_2\end{array}\right) - \begin{array}{c}\text{Patient's}\\\text{Arterial}\\PO_2\end{array} = \begin{array}{c}\text{A − a Oxygen}\\\text{Gradient}\end{array}$$

Example: In a patient at sea level, breathing room air (F_IO_2) with PO₂ of 90 and PCO₂ of 40, this is how the A − oxygen gradient is easily calculated:

$(760 - 47) \times (.21) - (1\tfrac{1}{4}) \times (40)$	− 90	=	
$(713 \times .21) - 50$	− 90	=	
$150 - 50$	− 90	=	
100	− 90	=	10

FIGURE 14-11
A−a oxygen gradient: difference between PO₂ in alveolus and PO₂ in arterial blood.

TABLE 14-5
DETERMINANTS OF a/A RATIOS AND A − a OXYGEN GRADIENTS

Right-to-left shunts
Diffusion abnormalities
Ventilation/perfusion mismatching

Abnormal A − a oxygen gradients and a/A ratios are seen in patients with right-to-left shunting, ventilation/perfusion mismatching, and diffusion abnormalities (Table 14-5). In patients who are receiving oxygen, the a/A ratio is more useful than the A − a gradient because the A − a gradient increases as the patient's FIO_2 increases. The a/A ratio does not vary as the FIO_2 is changed. In patients on ventilators, one can change the FIO_2 and still look at the a/A ratio to determine whether oxygen transfer is improving or worsening.

As previously mentioned, the normal values for oxygen in arterial blood in Denver or any other place above sea level are lower than those at sea level be-cause there is progressively lower PO₂ in the ambient air as one ascends (Table 14-6).

In mixed venous blood the normal values for oxygen may be slightly lower in Denver than at sea level, but not sufficiently lower to warrant memorization of a second set of values.

Oxygen Transport

The amount of oxygen that is transported to the tissues is more important than the PO₂. The PO₂ is a measure of intensity or pressure due to oxygen, and oxygen content is a measure of amount of oxygen.

O₂ transport to the tissues
= arterial O₂ content × cardiac output

The oxygen transported to the tissues depends on (1) the amount of oxygen in arterial blood (arterial oxygen content), and (2) the ability of the heart to pump this blood containing oxygen around to the tissues.

The arterial oxygen content depends in turn on (1) how well the lungs are able to get oxygen from air into

TABLE 14-6
OXYGEN VALUES IN DENVER VS SEA LEVEL

Denver	Sea Level
Arterial Blood O_2	
Oxygen content . . . . .18.9 ml O_2/100 ml of blood	19.7 ml O_2/100 ml of blood
PO_2 . . . . .70 torr (range 65–75)	>80 torr
O_2 saturation of Hgb . . . . . . .93% (range 92%–94%)	≥95%
Mixed Venous Blood O_2	
Oxygen content . . . . .14–16 ml O_2/100 ml of blood	14–16 ml O_2/100 ml of blood
PO_2 . . . . .35–49 torr	35–49 torr
O_2 saturation of Hgb 65–80%	65–80%
Ratios and gradients	
a/A ratio . . . .>.75	>.75
A − a oxygen gradient . . . . .<20	<20

the blood, and (2) a normal amount of functioning hemoglobin to carry the oxygen.

In summary, oxygenation of the tissue depends on the following:

1. Arterial O_2 content, which depends on
   a. Lungs' ability to get O_2 into blood
   b. Ability of hemoglobin to hold enough O_2
2. Cardiac output (circulation)

Tissue Hypoxia

There are varied pulmonary and nonpulmonary causes for tissue hypoxia, which results from insufficient oxygenation. Four pulmonary reasons can be listed to explain why arterial blood may not be carrying the normal amount of oxygen.

1. Alveolar hypoventilation. Associated with high PCO_2.
2. Diffusion defect (at alveolar-capillary level). Associated with low or normal PCO_2.
3. Right-to-left shunt (in lung or heart). Associated with low or normal PCO_2.
4. Mismatching of ventilation and blood flow in the lungs. (Blood goes by alveoli that are poorly ventilated. This blood, as it passes through the lungs, picks up little oxygen. This poorly oxygenated blood then returns to the heart and is pumped out into the arteries to the body, thus causing arterial blood to have less than the normal amount of oxygen.) Associated with low or normal PCO_2.

The nonpulmonary causes of tissue hypoxia are (1) reduced blood flow to the tissues (reduced cardiac output); (2) anemia—not enough hemoglobin to carry oxygen; (3) nonfunctioning hemoglobin—enough hemoglobin but hemoglobin that exists cannot carry oxygen because it has been "poisoned"; and

(4) right-to-left cardiac shunts — most frequently seen in cyanotic congenital heart disease.

1. *Reduced blood flow* to the tissues (reduced cardiac output) might be caused by
   a. Myocardial infarction
   b. Abnormal cardiac rhythm
   c. Reduced cardiac function (other causes): congestive heart failure, valvular heart lesion, etc.
   d. Hypovolemia (intimately related to anemia)
2. *Anemia:* 1 g Hgb carries 1.34 ml O_2, and normally there are 15 g Hgb to carry 15 × 1.34 ml O_2 or 20.1 ml O_2. If there is anemia so that only 7.5 g Hgb are present, 7.5 × 1.34 ml O_2 = 10 ml O_2 are all that can be carried; if anemia is milder (between 7.5 and 15 g Hgb), more O_2 can be carried; if anemia is more severe (less than 7.5 g Hgb), even less O_2 can be carried. Usually the body compensates for anemia by having the heart circulate faster the lesser amount of hemoglobin that is present.
3. *Nonfunctioning hemoglobin:* A few rare conditions exist in which there might be a normal amount of hemoglobin, but even this normal amount cannot function because it has been poisoned. Some examples of this are
   a. Carbon monoxide poisoning
   b. Methemoglobinemia
   c. Sulfhemoglobinemia
   In each of these situations, something (*e.g.,* carbon monoxide) has combined with hemoglobin, making it hard for oxygen to combine with and be carried by this hemoglobin.
4. In *right-to-left cardiac shunts,* oxygen gets through the lungs normally into the bloodstream, there is enough functioning hemoglobin to carry the oxygen, and the heart is strong enough to circu-

late the oxygenated blood. However, some venous blood that never passes through the lungs to get oxygenated is *shunted* into the systemic arterial system, and the combination of oxygenated blood plus venous unoxygenated blood is carried through the arteries to the tissues, supplying them with less oxygen than they need.

Compensatory Mechanisms

The patient who is hypoxemic compensates for hypoxia in the following ways:

- Tachypnea (rapid breathing)
- Tachycardia (rapid heartbeat)
- Erythrocytosis (high hemoglobin and hematocrit)

The tachypnea and tachycardia represent extra energy expenditure by the patient. Erythrocytosis simply means increased production of red blood cells by the hypoxic patient's bone marrow in an attempt to get more oxygen to the tissues. If the fault is lack of enough red blood cells, this can be remedied. However, if the fault is in getting enough oxygen through the lungs, increasing the number of red blood cells helps little or not at all. The hypoxemic patient tries all these means of compensating for hypoxemia, and often all of them together are inadequate.

Hypoxia often leads to pulmonary hypertension (high blood pressure in the arteries of the lungs), and this can lead to strain or failure of the right side of the heart.

Oxygen Therapy

If oxygen is administered to the patient to treat his hypoxemia, tachypnea and tachycardia do not occur, there is no erythrocytosis, and pulmonary hypertension may go away. Complete compensation is possible with oxygen treatment, but sometimes patient compensation is not complete.

It can be seen that supplemental oxygen is rational treatment for the patient with hypoxemia, but long-term continuous oxygen is usually reserved for the patient who, when completely stable, has a PO_2 below 50 torr (oxygen saturation below 85%) and who also has one or more of the following:

- Right heart failure that is difficult to manage with digitalis and diuretics
- Significant secondary erythrocytosis
- A progressive downhill course with weight loss, progressive muscle wasting, or decreased mental function

Often such a patient responds to nocturnal oxygen (oxygen for 8 hours at night). If the patient is living at a high altitude, a move to a lower altitude may make supplemental oxygen unnecessary.

Possible CO_2 Retention. Oxygen treatment may lead to CO_2 retention if the oxygen is not carefully controlled.

There are two major reflex stimuli to breathing:

- CO_2 retention (hypercapnic stimulus to breathe)
- Low PO_2 (hypoxic stimulus to breathe)

Small elevations of PCO_2 are a major stimulus to breathing. Increasing the PCO_2 by 4 torr can cause a 100% increase in ventilation. Large elevations in PCO_2 reduce the amount of ventilation by reducing all brain functions including function of the respiratory center.

In patients with large elevation of PCO_2, hypoxemia may be the most important stimulus to breathing. If a patient who no longer has a hypercapnic stimulus to breathing is treated with oxygen, thereby eliminating the hypoxic stimulus to breathe, he may breathe even less, significantly worsening his condition. It has become apparent that administration of a controlled amount of oxygen (just enough to raise the PaO_2 to approximately 60 torr) allows the patient to benefit from the oxygen and usually does not reduce ventilation.

It should be clear that oxygen therapy, although often given in a haphazard fashion, requires just as much understanding and precision in dosage as any other form of drug therapy.

BLOOD GAS ANALYSIS

Normal Values

Normal values for blood gases are given in Table 14-7. Following this the main emphasis will concern acid-base interpretation (Table 14-8).

Note that in Table 14-7 only two measurements, PO_2 and PCO_2, are actually measurements of gases. However, all should be determined in blood gas analyses. It is imperative that a measure of the nonrespiratory (metabolic) component be included, and actual HCO_3^- and base excess are the most useful. Many other terms may be given on a blood gas report, but one need be concerned only with those listed in Table 14-7.

Older persons have values for PO_2 and oxygen saturation near the lower part of the normal range, and younger people tend to have high normal values.

Normal values for mixed venous blood are more variable than for arterial blood, but representative normals are given in Table 14-7. Because there is not much difference in normal values of HCO_3^- and base excess between arterial and mixed venous blood and because venous blood is not often used, one does not need to remember a different set of values for venous blood.

TABLE 14-7
NORMAL BLOOD GAS VALUES

	Arterial Blood	Mixed Venous Blood
pH	7.40 (7.35–7.45)	7.38 (7.33–7.43)
PO_2	80–100 torr	35–49 torr
O_2 sat	95% or greater	65%–80%
PCO_2	35–45 torr	41–51 torr
HCO_3	22–26 mEq/liter	24–28 mEq/liter
Base excess (BE)	−2–+2	0–+4

TABLE 14-8
DEFINITIONS

Acid: A substance that can donate hydrogen ions, H^+.
Example:

$$H_2CO_3 \longrightarrow H^+ + HCO_3^-$$
(acid)

Base: A substance that can accept hydrogen ions, H^+. All bases
are alkaline substances. Example:

$$HCO_3^- + H^+ \longrightarrow H_2CO_3$$
(base)

TABLE 14-9
ACID-BASE TERMS

pH measurements = Only way to tell if body is too acid or too
   alkaline
Acidemia = Acid condition of the blood—$pH < 7.35$
Alkalemia = Alkaline condition of the blood—$pH > 7.45$
Acidosis = Process causing acidemia
Alkalosis = Process causing alkalemia

TABLE 14-10
PCO₂, THE RESPIRATORY PARAMETER

PCO_2 = pressure (tension) of dissolved CO_2 gas in blood;
   influenced only by respiratory causes

$$\text{Food} \xrightarrow[\text{by body}]{\text{converted}} H_2O + CO_2 + \text{energy}$$

$$CO_2 + H_2O \rightleftharpoons H_2CO_3 \rightleftharpoons HCO_3^- + H^+$$

Normal PCO_2 = normal ventilation
High PCO_2 = hypoventilation
Low PCO_2 = hyperventilation

An acid is any substance that can donate a hydrogen
ion, H^+, which can be thought of as the most important
part of an acid.

Many substances may include H in their chemical
structure, but some cannot donate the H because it is
too tightly bound. Only those substances that can give
up their H^+ are acids.

Bases are substances that can accept or combine
with H^+. The terms *base* and *alkali* are used interchangeably. (Table 14-9). Each of the acid-base terms
in Table 14-9 will now be discussed in more detail.

The pH measurement is the only way to determine
whether the body is too acid or too alkaline. Low pH
numbers (below 7.35) indicate an acid state, and high
pH numbers (above 7.45) indicate an alkaline state.

If the numbers are lower than 7.35 there is acidemia,
and if they are higher than 7.45 alkalemia is present.
Acid*emia* refers to a condition in which the *blood* is
too acid. Acid*osis* refers to the *process* in the patient
that causes the acidemia, and the adjective for the process is acid*otic*. Alkal*osis* refers to the *process* in the
patient that causes the alkal*emia*, and the adjective for
this process is alkal*otic*.

This much time has been spent in defining the terms
because later it will be seen that in a patient there may
be more than one process occurring at the same time.
For instance, if both an acidosis and an alkalosis are
occurring at once, the pH will indicate which is the
stronger of the two processes. The pH will be below
7.35 if the acidosis is the stronger, above 7.45 if the
alkalosis is the stronger, and between 7.35 and 7.45 if
the acidosis and alkalosis are of nearly equal strength.
The pH value of blood represents an average of the
acidoses and alkaloses that may be occurring.

Respiratory Parameter: PCO₂

The PCO_2 refers to the pressure or tension exerted by
dissolved CO_2 gas in the blood (Table 14-10). The
PCO_2 is influenced *only* by respiratory causes. Although this is an oversimplification, remember that
PCO_2 *is influenced only by the lungs.*

Where does the CO_2 come from? It is present only in
very tiny amounts in the air we breathe. It comes directly from foods we eat. As a result of metabolism for
the production of energy, foods are converted by the
body tissues to water and CO_2 gas. When the pressure
of CO_2 in the cells exceeds 40 torr (the normal arterial
value), the CO_2 spills over from the cells into the
plasma. In plasma, CO_2 may combine with H_2O to
form H_2CO_3 (carbonic acid), but there is actually 800
times as much CO_2 in the form of dissolved gas in
plasma as is converted to H_2CO_3.

CO_2 gas should be considered an acid substance
because when it combines with water, an acid is
formed—carbonic acid, H_2CO_3.

H_2CO_3 dissociates into hydrogen ion, H^+, and bicarbonate, HCO_3^-. Much of the H^+ forms a loose association with the plasma proteins (*i.e.,* it is buffered), thus
reducing the free H^+.

The body has to get rid of the waste product, CO_2,
and can do so in two ways:

• The less important way is conversion of the CO_2 gas to carbonic acid, H_2CO_3, which dissociates to H^+ and HCO_3^-. The H^+ can be excreted by the kidneys, mainly in the form of NH_4^+.
• A much more important way is expulsion of the CO_2 by lungs.

Getting rid of CO_2 gas, then, is one of the main functions of the lungs, and a very important relationship exists between the amount of ventilation and the amount of PCO_2 in blood. If the PCO_2 in blood (*i.e.,* the dissolved CO_2 gas in blood) is too high, it means that the lungs are not providing enough ventilation. This is called *hypoventilation.* One can thus detect hypoventilation by finding high levels of PCO_2 in the blood. If the PCO_2 is too low, there is excessive ventilation by the lungs, or *hyperventilation,* and if the PCO_2 is normal, there is exactly the right amount of ventilation.

PCO_2 is much more important than PO_2 in the determination of whether there is normal ventilation, hyperventilation, or hypoventilation because there are other factors (*e.g.,* shunting and diffusion abnormalities) that lower the PO_2 without reducing ventilation.

As seen in Table 14-11, there are only two abnormal conditions associated with abnormalities in PCO_2: respiratory acidosis (high PCO_2) and respiratory alkalosis (low PCO_2).

Respiratory Acidosis

The term *respiratory acidosis* means elevated PCO_2 due to hypoventilation. The causes of respiratory acidosis (high PCO_2) are as follows:

• Obstructive pulmonary disease (mainly chronic bronchitis, emphysema, and occasionally asthma)

• Oversedation, head trauma, anesthesia, and other causes of reduced function of the respiratory center
• Neuromuscular disorders such as myasthenia gravis and the Guillain-Barré syndrome
• Hypoventilation with a mechanical ventilator
• Other rarer causes of hypoventilation (*e.g.,* the pickwickian syndrome) (Table 14-12).

It should be noted that *respiratory* acidosis may occur even with normal lungs if the respiratory center is depressed.

Respiratory Alkalosis

The term *respiratory alkalosis* means low PCO_2 due to hyperventilation. The causes are hypoxia, congestive heart failure, anxiety, pulmonary emboli, pulmonary fibrosis, pregnancy, hyperventilation with mechanical ventilator, gram-negative septicemia, hepatic insufficiency, brain injury, salicylates, fever, asthma, and severe anemia (Table 14-13). In gram-negative septicemia, the hyperventilation may precede other evidence of septicemia. In patients with congestive heart failure, pneumonia, asthma, pulmonary emboli, and pulmonary fibrosis, the hyperventilation (respiratory alkalosis) continues even if the hypoxia is corrected; thus, hypoxia is not the only cause in these conditions.

Nonrespiratory (Metabolic) Parameters: HCO_3^- and Base Excess

The term *base excess* refers principally to bicarbonate but also to the other bases in blood (mainly plasma proteins and hemoglobin). Bicarbonate and base excess are influenced *only* by nonrespiratory causes, not

---

TABLE 14-11
RESPIRATORY ABNORMALITIES

Parameter	Condition	Mechanism
↑ PCO_2	Respiratory acidosis	Decreased elimination by lungs of CO_2 gas (hypoventilation)
↓ PCO_2	Respiratory alkalosis	Increased elimination by lungs of CO_2 gas (hyperventilation)

TABLE 14-12
CAUSES OF RESPIRATORY ACIDOSIS (↑ PCO_2)

Obstructive lung disease
Oversedation and other causes of reduced function of the respiratory center (even with normal lungs)
Neuromuscular disorders
Hypoventilation with mechanical ventilator
Other causes of hypoventilation

TABLE 14-13
CAUSES OF RESPIRATORY ALKALOSIS ($\downarrow$ PCO$_2$)

Hypoxia
Nervousness and anxiety
Pulmonary embolus, fibrosis, etc.
Pregnancy
Hyperventilation with mechanical ventilator
Brain injury
Salicylates
Fever
Gram-negative septicemia
Hepatic insufficiency
Congestive heart failure
Asthma
Severe anemia

TABLE 14-14
METABOLIC ABNORMALITIES

Parameter	Condition	Mechanism
$\uparrow$ HCO$_3^-$ or $\uparrow$ BE	Nonrespiratory (metabolic) alkalosis	1. Nonvolatile acid is lost or 2. HCO$_3^-$ is gained
$\downarrow$ HCO$_3^-$ or $\downarrow$ BE	Nonrespiratory (metabolic) acidosis	1. Nonvolatile acid is added (using up HCO$_3^-$) or 2. HCO$_3^-$ is lost

by respiratory causes. Again, this is a simplification, but a very important fact to remember—*bicarbonate and base excess are influenced only by nonrespiratory processes.*

For our purposes we can define a *metabolic process* as anything other than respiratory causes that affects the patient's acid-base status. Examples of common metabolic (nonrespiratory) processes are diabetic acidosis and uremia.

When a nonrespiratory process leads to the accumulation of acids in the body or losses of bicarbonate, bicarbonate values drop below the normal range, and base excess values become negative. However, when a nonrespiratory process causes loss of acid or accumulation of excess bicarbonate, bicarbonate values rise above normal, and base excess values become positive. Base excess may be thought of as representing an excess of bicarbonate or other base. Bicarbonate, then, is base or, in other words, an alkaline substance.

As seen in Table 14-14, there are only two abnormal conditions associated with abnormalities in HCO$_3^-$ or base excess: metabolic alkalosis and metabolic acidosis. (Nonvolatile acid is any acid other than PCO$_2$—H$_2$CO$_3$.)

Metabolic Alkalosis

The *causes* of metabolic alkalosis (increased HCO$_3^-$ and base excess) are (1) loss of acid-containing fluid from the upper gastrointestinal tract as by nasogastric

suction or vomiting (this loss of acid from the stomach leaves the body with a relative excess of alkali); (2) rapid correction of chronic hypercapnia (it will take the body several days to correct its compensation for hypercapnia—accumulation of excess HCO$_3^-$—after the hypercapnia is suddenly relieved); (3) diuretic therapy with mercurial diuretics, ethacrynic acid, furosemide, and thiazide diuretics; (4) Cushing's disease; (5) treatment with corticosteroids (*i.e.,* prednisone or cortisone); (6) hyperaldosteronism; (7) severe potassium depletion; (8) excessive ingestion of licorice; (9) Bartter's syndrome; (10) alkali administration; and (11) nonparathyroid hypercalcemia.

A rare cause of nonrespiratory alkalosis, which unfortunately is not reflected by an elevated bicarbonate in the blood, is the intravenous infusion of phenytoin (Dilantin), which has a very alkaline *p*H. Infusion of this alkaline substance causes a short-lived alkalemia not associated with elevated HCO$_3^-$. Any condition that is associated with a reduction in blood volume (*e.g.,* the preceding examples 1 and 3) is said to cause a contraction alkalosis because of a contraction of blood or plasma volume.

Hypokalemia and Hypochloremia. The first three causes of alkalosis listed—fluid losses from the stomach, rapid correction of chronic hypercapnia, and diuretic therapy—will all show correction of the alkalosis in response to administration of sodium chloride.

TABLE 14-15
CAUSES OF METABOLIC (NONRESPIRATORY)
ALKALOSIS ($\uparrow HCO_3^-$)

Fluid losses from upper GI tract—vomiting or nasogastric tube causing loss of acid
Rapid correction of chronic hypercapnia
Diuretic therapy—mercurial, ethacrynic acid (Edecrin), furosemide (Lasix), thiazides
Cushing's disease
Therapy with corticosteroids (prednisone, cortisone, etc.)
Hyperaldosteronism
Severe potassium depletion
Excessive ingestion of licorice
Bartter's syndrome
Alkali administration
Nonparathyroid hypercalcemia

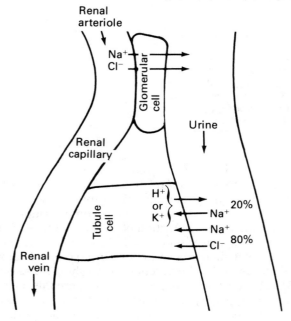

FIGURE 14-12
Process by which low Cl⁻ and low K⁺ can cause metabolic alkalosis.

Treatment with potassium chloride may be more reasonable if the potassium is low or if one is trying to prevent accumulation of salt and water. Treatment with two other diuretics, spironolactone (Aldactone) and triamterene (Dyrenium), does not cause metabolic alkalosis. With causes 4 through 9 in Table 14-15, the metabolic alkalosis cannot be corrected by administration of sodium chloride. With the last two causes listed, the response of sodium chloride is variable.

The following is an explanation of the relationship between hypokalemia (low K⁺), hypochloremia (low

Cl⁻), and metabolic alkalosis. Normally in the kidney, sodium (Na⁺) and chloride (Cl⁻) pass from the blood into the urine at the glomerulus. Further along in the tubules of the kidney this Na⁺, which is in the urine, must be reabsorbed from the urine into the kidney tubule cells and then into the blood.

Because Na⁺ has a positive charge (+), when it is reabsorbed into the cells it must either

• Be reabsorbed with something that has a negative charge (−), such as Cl⁻, or

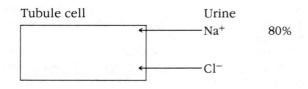

• Enter the tubule cell in exchange for something else that has a positive charge, such as K⁺ or H⁺ (which passes from the tubule cell to the urine)

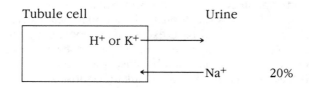

Normally, 80% of the Na⁺ is reabsorbed while accompanied by Cl⁻, and 20% is exchanged for K⁺ or H⁺ (Fig. 14-12).

When there is hypochloremia ($\downarrow$ Cl⁻), the amount of Na⁺ that is reabsorbed in the company of Cl⁻ is reduced, and more Na⁺ must be exchanged for K⁺ or H⁺. When Na⁺ is exchanged for K⁺ and H⁺, the loss of

---

TABLE 14-16
CAUSES OF METABOLIC (NONRESPIRATORY) ACIDOSIS
($\downarrow HCO_3^-$ AND $\downarrow$ BE)

With Increase in Unspecified Anions	Without Increase in Unspecified Anions
Diabetic ketoacidosis	Diarrhea
Starvation ketoacidosis	Drainage of pancreatic juice
Alcoholic ketoacidosis	Ureterosigmoidostomy
Poisonings	Obstructed ileal loop
Salicylate	Therapy with acetazolamide
Ethylene glycol	(Diamox)
Methyl alcohol	Therapy with ammonium
Paraldehyde (rarely)	chloride (NH_4Cl)
Lactic acidosis	Renal tubular acidosis
Renal failure	Intravenous hyperalimentation
	(rarely)
	Dilutional acidosis

H^+ represents a loss of acid, leaving the patient alkalotic—therefore a hypochloremic alkalosis.

When Na^+ is exchanged for K^+ or H^+, only a small amount of K^+ is available, and when this is used up the patient becomes hypokalemic, and H^+ is lost. The loss of H^+ is a loss of acid, leaving the patient with an alkalosis—hypokalemic alkalosis.

Metabolic Acidosis

Substances that have a negative charge are attracted to an anode and are called *anions*. The anions that are normally measured (specified) are HCO_3^- and CL^-. The anions that are not regularly measured but are normally present in blood are called *unspecified* or *unmeasured* anions. They are phosphates, sulfates, creatinates, and proteinates.

The causes of nonrespiratory (metabolic) acidosis (low HCO_3^- and low base excess) can be divided into those causes in which there is an increase in the unspecified anions and those causes in which bicarbonate has been lost and there is no such increase in unspecified anions (Table 14-16).

The normal value for unspecified anions is 12 ± 3.

An increase in unspecified anions may be due to accumulation of phosphates, sulfates, and creatinates, as seen in renal failure or the accumulation of an unusual negatively charged substance such as lactic acid, ketoacids, or the like. Often the unspecified anions are referred to as the *anion gap*. If one subtracts the sum of HCO_3^- and Cl^- concentration from Na^+ concentration and finds a difference greater than 15, there is said to be an increase in unspecified anions (increased anion gap). Conditions causing this are diabetic ketoacidosis, alcoholic ketoacidosis, poisonings (salicylate, ethylene glycol, methyl alcohol, paraldehyde), lactic acidosis, and renal failure. In these cases there is accumulation of or ingestion of an unusual acid.

Conditions that cause a metabolic acidosis *without an increase in unmeasured anions* are associated with a high serum chloride. These conditions are diarrhea, drainage of pancreatic juice, ureterosigmoidostomy, obstructed ileal loop, treatment with acetazolamide (Diamox), renal tubular acidosis, treatment with ammonium chloride or arginine monohydrochloride, and intravenous hyperalimentation. In most of these latter conditions, there is a deficit of bicarbonate, leaving relatively too much acid.

In all the conditions in the left-hand column in Table 14-16, there is an accumulation of an abnormal acid substance in blood, which then reacts with and uses up some of the usual amount of bicarbonate, leaving the patient with reduced levels of bicarbonate and base excess.

One of the most important causes of metabolic acidosis is *lactic acidosis*. Whenever body tissues do not have enough oxygen, they lose their ability to metabolize lactic acid, which then accumulates in the blood. This lactic acid then combines with some of the normal amount of bicarbonate, using up the bicarbonate.

In a cardiac arrest, we customarily administer bicarbonate, about 1 ampule (44.6 mEq) every 5 minutes, to resupply the bicarbonate that is used up by combining with lactic acid. Other conditions besides cardiac arrest that may be associated with lactic acidosis are shock, severe heart failure, and severe hypoxemia. Tissue hypoxia, seen in all these conditions, leads to the lactate production.

If a patient has a metabolic acidosis with an anion gap of greater than 15, the nurse can consult the left-hand column of Table 14-16 and ask the laboratory technician to measure whichever unspecified anion she guesses might be elevated; for example, if the patient is an uncontrolled diabetic, ketoacids should be measured; if the patient is in shock, lactic acid should be measured.

CO_2 Content

PCO_2 is a respiratory parameter, a gas, and an acid, and it is regulated by the lungs. HCO_3^- and base excess are both nonrespiratory parameters occurring in solution and are bases (alkaline substances), and they are regulated mainly by the kidneys (not by the lungs). To summarize:

- PCO_2—respiratory parameter
  Gas
  Acid
  Regulated by the lungs
- HCO_3^- or base excess—nonrespiratory parameter
  Solution
  Base
  Regulated mainly by the kidneys

TABLE 14-17
CO_2 CONTENT

HCO_3^-	24 mEq/liter
Dissolved CO_2 gas	1.2 mEq/liter = 40 torr PCO_2
CO_2 content	25.2 mEq/liter

TABLE 14-18
CAUSES OF ALKALEMIA AND ACIDEMIA

Types		Primary Abnormality
Alkalemia (high *p*H)	Nonrespiratory (metabolic)	↑ HCO_3^-
	Respiratory	↓ PCO_2
Acidemia (low *p*H)	Nonrespiratory (metabolic)	↓ HCO_3^-
	Respiratory	↑ PCO_2

Where does the CO_2 content fit in this scheme? Determination of electrolytes consists of Na^+, K^+, Cl^-, and CO_2. In this case CO_2 is an abbreviation for CO_2 content, which is composed mainly of bicarbonate; if the term *CO_2 content* were used, it would improve understanding. Note that in conversation CO_2 is sometimes used to mean CO_2 content (mainly bicarbonate) and sometimes to mean CO_2 gas. This double use of the term CO_2 is one of the main difficulties in understanding acid-base problems. One should use the terms *CO_2 content* and *CO_2 gas* to avoid confusion. Better yet, some hospitals are reporting HCO_3^- in place of CO_2 content when electrolytes are ordered.

Table 14-17 shows that CO_2 content is mainly bicarbonate (HCO_3^-) and, to a lesser extent, dissolved CO_2 gas. The normal value of CO_2 content, 25.2 mEq/liter, consists of 24 mEq/liter of HCO_3^- and 1.2 mEq/liter of dissolved CO_2 gas. The 1.2 mEq/liter of dissolved CO_2 gas is expressed in different terminology: PCO_2 of 40 torr equals 1.2 mEq/liter. For changing torr to mEq/liter, the conversion factor is 0.03, so 40 torr × 0.03 = 1.2 mEq/liter.

HCO_3^-/CO_2 Ratio. In Table 14-17, the ratio of HCO_3^- to PCO_2 is 24 : 1.2 or 20 : 1. The body always tries to keep this ratio of HCO_3^- to PCO_2 stable at 20 : 1. That is, the ratio of alkali (HCO_3^-) to acid (PCO_2) is normally 20 : 1. As long as the ratio remains 20 : 1, the *p*H remains normal. If bicarbonate (HCO_3^-) or base excess increases, there is alkalosis, causing the *p*H to rise. *If HCO_3^- or base excess falls, there is acidosis, and the*

*p*H *falls. If the pH change is due mainly to change in bicarbonate (or base excess), it is said to be due to nonrespiratory (metabolic) causes.*

Just the opposite happens with PCO_2, which, remember, is an acid substance. If the PCO_2 rises, there is an acidosis, causing the *p*H to fall. If the PCO_2 falls, there is an alkalosis, and the *p*H rises. *If the pH change is due mainly to changes in PCO_2, it is said to be due to respiratory causes.*

As seen in Table 14-18, acid-base abnormalities can be separated into just four categories for easier understanding. First they are divided by *p*H into either alkalemia or acidemia. Next they are subdivided into either nonrespiratory (metabolic) or respiratory causes. This is the procedure one uses in interpreting acid-base abnormalities.

*p*H Factor

***p*H and Alkalemia.** If *p*H is high, there is an alkalemia. There may be two types of alkalemia:

- *Nonrespiratory,* in which the primary abnormality is due to an increase in bicarbonate. An example of this is overingestion of bicarbonate or baking soda.
- *Respiratory,* in which the primary abnormality is hyperventilation with loss of CO_2 gas. CO_2 gas is an acid substance; when it is lost (owing to hyperventilation), an alkalosis occurs. An example is a hyperventilation attack in a nervous person.

***p*H and Acidemia.** If the *p*H is low, there is an acidemia, of which there are just two types:

- *Nonrespiratory,* in which the primary abnormality is loss of HCO_3^- usually due to reaction with excessive metabolic acids. An example is diabetic acidosis in which ketoacids accumulate; these acids then react with the normal amount of HCO_3^-, using up HCO_3^- and leaving HCO_3^- and base excess levels low.
- *Respiratory,* in which there is an accumulation of CO_2 gas (high PCO_2), an acid substance. An example is a patient with acute respiratory failure who *hypo*ventilates because his airways are obstructed by mucus. In respiratory acidosis there is an accumulation of volatile acid—CO_2 gas—but in nonrespiratory acidosis the acids that accumulate are not gases.

***p*H and Combined Acidosis/Alkalosis.** There may be more than one primary acid-base disturbance occurring at the same time. Occasionally two disturbances will be of equal magnitude, and if one is an acidosis and the other an alkalosis, they will balance each other and the *p*H will remain normal. On another occasion there may be several acidoses, for instance, occurring at the same time, all adding their effects to make the *p*H more acidemic than one alone would.

pH Compensation and Correction. There are two ways in which an abnormal *p*H may be returned toward normal: (1) compensation and (2) correction (Table 14-19).

In *compensation,* the system not primarily affected is responsible for returning the *p*H toward normal. For example, if there is respiratory acidosis (high PCO_2) the kidneys *compensate* by retaining bicarbonate to return the ratio of HCO_3^- to PCO_2 to 20 : 1; when the ratio is 20 : 1, the *p*H is normal.

Compensation is complete only in chronic respiratory alkalosis. In the other acid-base disorders the *p*H is returned nearly but not completely to normal because the compensation is not complete.

In *correction,* the system primarily affected is repaired, returning the *p*H toward normal. For example, if there is respiratory acidosis (high PCO_2) vigorous bronchial hygiene and bronchodilators may improve ventilation and lower PCO_2, returning the *p*H toward normal.

In most cases, physicians, nurses, and paramedical persons are more interested in correcting the abnormality than in helping the body compensate. In both compensation and correction the *p*H is returned toward normal. The body tries hard to maintain a normal *p*H because the various enzyme systems in all organs function correctly only when the *p*H is normal. According to newer terminology, *acute* respiratory

TABLE 14-19
COMPENSATION VERSUS CORRECTION OF ACID-BASE ABNORMALITIES

In both:	Abnormal *p*H is returned toward normal.
Compensation:	Abnormal *p*H is returned toward normal *by altering the component not primarily affected;* that is, if PCO_2 is high, HCO_3^- is retained to compensate.
Correction:	Abnormal *p*H is returned toward normal *by altering the component primarily affected;* that is, if PCO_2 is high, PCO_2 is lowered, correcting the abnormality.

TABLE 14-20
COMPENSATION FOR ACIDOSIS AND ALKALOSIS

Parameter	Normal	Abnormal (Uncompensated)	Compensated
Respiratory Acidosis			
HCO_3^- mEq/liter	24	24	36
PCO_2 mEq/liter	1.2	1.8	1.8
PCO_2 torr	40	60	60
ratio	20 : 1	13 : 1	20 : 1
*p*H	7.40	7.23	7.40
Respiratory Alkalosis			
BE	0	+2.5	−5
HCO_3^- mEq/liter	24	24	18
PCO_2 mEq/liter	1.2	0.9	0.9
PCO_2 torr	40	30	30
ratio	20 : 1	27 : 1	20 : 1
*p*H	7.40	7.52	7.40
Metabolic Acidosis			
BE	0	−17	−10
HCO_3^- mEq/liter	24	12	12
PCO_2 mEq/liter	1.2	1.2	0.6
PCO_2 torr	40	40	20
ratio	20 : 1	10 : 1	20 : 1
*p*H	7.40	7.11	7.40
Metabolic Alkalosis			
BE	0	+13	+9
HCO_3^- mEq/liter	24	36	36
PCO_2 mEq/liter	1.2	1.2	1.8
PCO_2 torr	40	40	60
ratio	20 : 1	30 : 1	20 : 1
*p*H	7.40	7.57	7.40

acidosis means *uncompensated; chronic* respiratory acidosis means *compensated.*

Compensatory Mechanisms

Next we will discuss how the body compensates for the various acid-base abnormalities. Remember, the body compensates for abnormalities by trying to return the ratio of HCO_3^- to PCO_2 to 20:1, for if this ratio is 20:1, the pH is normal. If the primary process is respiratory, the compensating system is metabolic and vice versa. When the lungs compensate for a nonrespiratory abnormality, compensation occurs in hours, but the kidneys take 2 to 4 days to compensate for a respiratory abnormality.

Remember, the PCO_2 in torr must be converted to mEq/liter by multiplying it by 0.03 before trying it in the 20:1 ratio mentioned above; for example, PCO_2 of 40 torr $\times$ 0.03 = 1.2 mEq/liter.

In four examples in Table 14-20, the first column lists normal values for the parameters listed in the second column. The uncompensated state is listed in the third column, and the last column demonstrates how compensation takes place. The primary abnormality is enclosed in a box.

In *primary respiratory acidosis,* characterized by elevated levels of PCO_2 (an acid), the system at fault is the respiratory system, and compensation occurs through metabolic process. To compensate, the kidneys excrete more acid and less HCO_3^-, thus allowing levels of HCO_3^- to rise, returning the ratio of HCO_3^- to PCO_2 toward 20:1, and therefore returning pH toward normal.

If the PCO_2 is high (respiratory acidosis) but the pH is normal, it means that the kidneys have had time to retain HCO_3^- to compensate for the elevated PCO_2 and that the process is not acute (has been present at least a few days to give the kidneys time to compensate). Usually the body does not fully compensate for respiratory acidosis.

In *primary respiratory alkalosis,* characterized by low PCO_2, compensation occurs through metabolic means. The kidneys compensate by excreting HCO_3^-, thus returning the ratio of HCO_3^- to PCO_2 back toward 20:1; this compensation by the kidneys takes 2 to 3 days.

Of the four acid-base abnormalities, it is only in compensation for respiratory alkalosis that the body is able to return the ratio to 20:1 and return pH entirely to normal.

In *primary metabolic acidosis,* the major abnormality is low HCO_3^- or base excess. In most cases excess acids, such as ketoacids in diabetic ketoacidosis, have reacted with the normal amounts of HCO_3^- using up some of the HCO_3^- and leaving a low level of HCO_3^-. The body compensates by hyperventilating, thus low-ering the PCO_2 so that the ratio of HCO_3^- to PCO_2 returns toward 20:1. Because the compensating system is the lungs, compensation can occur in hours. However, if the metabolic acidosis is severe, the lungs may not be able to blow off enough CO_2 gas to compensate fully. Actually, in metabolic acidosis the body never compensates fully (never gets the ratio back to 20:1 or the pH back to 7.40).

In *metabolic alkalosis (i.e.,* presence of excess HCO_3^-), the body compensates with the respiratory system by hypoventilating so that PCO_2 rises and the ratio of HCO_3^- to PCO_2 is returned toward the normal of 20:1, therefore returning the pH to normal. The body is usually unable to compensate completely for metabolic alkalosis.

In this instance, respiratory compensation is by hypoventilation, and this occurs over one or several hours. Hypoventilation allows PCO_2 to rise only to a maximum of 50 to 60 torr before other stimuli of ventilation such as hypoxia take over to prevent further hypoventilation.

In compensating for one abnormality, high HCO_3^-, the body creates another abnormality, high PCO_2, but in doing so brings the ratio of HCO_3^- to PCO_2 to 20:1, allowing the pH to return to normal in spite of two abnormalities. These two abnormalities balance each other.

Treatment

It is important to realize that in each of these situations the body's compensation is only an effort to return the pH toward normal, and the primary abnormality is not corrected. The physician's definitive treatment is aimed at correcting the primary abnormality.

Metabolic (nonrespiratory) alkalosis (excess HCO_3^-) is treated by getting rid of excess HCO_3^- rather than just allowing PCO_2 to rise and normalize the ratio. Excess HCO_3^- can be corrected by giving the patient acetazolamide (Diamox) to make his kidneys excrete more HCO_3^-, or more commonly by giving KCl to allow the kidneys to excrete K^+ and Cl^- rather than acids. Sometimes ammonium chloride (NH_4Cl), arginine monohydrochloride, or even hydrochloric acid (HCl) is given to react with the excessive HCO_3^-, thereby correcting the metabolic alkalosis.

Respiratory alkalosis (low PCO_2) is treated by having the patient stop hyperventilating.

Metabolic (nonrespiratory) acidosis, in which excess acids have used up HCO_3^- or HCO_3^- has been lost, is treated by supplying HCO_3^- in the form of sodium bicarbonate ($NaHCO_3^-$) orally or intravenously while also treating the cause of acid accumulation or HCO_3^- loss. Multiplying the body weight (in kg) by the deficiency of HCO_3^- (in mEq/liter) by 0.3 gives a rough guide to the amount of $NaHCO_3^-$ (in mEq) that should be administered. Thus a 60-kg patient with an HCO_3^- of 4 would be given 360 mEq $NaHCO_3^-$, or

$$24 - 4 = 20 \times .3 \times 60 = 360$$

Administration of large doses of $NaHCO_3^-$ can give the patient a large osmotic load, which may be more detrimental than the acidemia; thus, metabolic acidosis is not usually treated with $NaHCO_3^-$ unless the pH is below 7.25.

Respiratory acidosis (high PCO_2) is treated by increasing ventilation, enabling the lungs to expel CO_2. Although *overtreatment* may occur, *overcompensation* by the body usually does not occur. In fact, complete compensation seldom occurs, so that instead of the ratio returning to 20:1, it returns to nearly 20:1, and pH, instead of returning to 7.40, returns almost to this point. (See Fig. 14-12 and the accompanying explanation.)

pH As a Determinant

It is the fact that the pH usually does not return completely to 7.40 that allows us in some cases to decide just from blood gas values which is the primary process and which is the compensating process. We first look at the pH to see which side of 7.40 it is on. Even though it is in normal range, pH is usually either above or below 7.40. If the pH is above 7.40, the primary process is probably alkalosis, and if below 7.40, the primary process is probably acidosis. For example

pH	7.42	
PCO_2	52 torr	...... Respiratory acidosis
HCO_3^-	33 mEq/liter	. Metabolic alkalosis

Which is the primary process, respiratory acidosis or metabolic alkalosis? If one consults Figure 14-13, he finds that these numbers can be interpreted in either of two ways, for they fit into two 95% confidence bands — that is, those for chronic (fully compensated) metabolic alkalosis and chronic (fully compensated) respiratory acidosis. However, following our rule, we see that the pH, although normal, is tending toward alkalemia. Therefore, the primary process is probably alkalemia. Thus, this is a metabolic alkalosis with nearly complete compensation. Often it is clinically obvious which is the primary abnormality, but sometimes this is not the case.

It must be pointed out that there may be more than one *primary* acid-base abnormality; thus, if there is both a respiratory and a nonrespiratory acid-base abnormality, instead of one compensating for the other, both may be acidoses or both alkaloses, in which case the pH deviates more from normal than if either of the abnormalities was present alone.

EXAMPLES

1. Here is an example of blood gases to interpret:

pH	7.24
PCO_2	38 torr
HCO_3^-	15.5 mEq/liter
B.E.	-11

Coronary care nurses deciphering an arrhythmia are taught to first find the P wave; in trying to interpret an acid-base abnormality, one must look first at the pH to

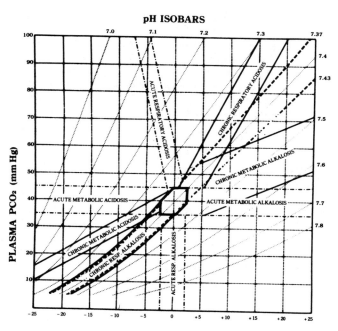

pH ISOBARS

FIGURE 14-13
Ninety-five percent confidence limits of respiratory or metabolic compensation.

Definitions for Acid-Base Disturbances

1. H^+: Hydrogen ion.
2. $[H^+]$: Hydrogen ion concentration.
3. pH: The negative log of the hydrogen ion concentration, or simply a way of representing the free H^+ in a solution. The pH of a solution is inversely proportional to the concentration of H^+ in the solution.
4. Acid: A substance that can donate hydrogen ions, H^+.

   $$\text{Example: } \underset{\text{(acid)}}{H_2CO_3} \rightarrow H^+ + HCO_3^-$$

5. Base: A substance that can accept hydrogen ions, H^+.

   All bases are alkaline substances.

   $$\text{Examples: } OH^- + H^+ \rightarrow H_2O$$
   $$\underset{\text{(bases)}}{HCO_3^- + H^+} \rightarrow H_2CO_3$$

6. Acidemia: Arterial pH below 7.35.
7. Alkalemia: Arterial pH greater than 7.45.
8. PCO_2: The tension exerted by carbon dioxide gas. The P in PCO_2 stands for pressure or tension exerted by CO_2 gas. CO_2 written without the preceding P does not refer to CO_2 gas but usually refers to total CO_2 content. (Usually CO_2 gas is dissolved in a solution.) Any deviation from the normal carbon dioxide tension (PCO_2) reflects a respiratory acid-base disturbance, either primary or compensatory. CO_2 combines reversibly with water to form carbonic acid, H_2CO_3.

   $$CO_2 + H_2O \leftrightarrows H_2CO_3$$

   In blood, there is 800 times as much CO_2 in the form of a gas, dissolved CO_2, as there is in the form of an acid, H_2CO_3. PCO_2 should be thought of as an acid. PCO_2 is inversely related to ventilation; thus, it tells a great deal about the lungs' function.

9. Base excess: Expresses directly, in mEq/liter, the amount of strong base (or acid) added per liter of blood with normal arbitrarily fixed at 0 (range of normal -2 to $+2$). Positive values express excess of base (or deficit of acid) and negative values express deficit of base (or excess of acid). Base excess reflects mainly the concentration of bicarbonate and is affected only by metabolic processes. Positive values reflect metabolic alkalosis, and negative values reflect metabolic acidosis.

10. Standard bicarbonate: The actual bicarbonate concentration measured at 37°C on blood that has been equilibrated to a high oxygen tension to saturate the hemoglobin completely and to a PCO_2 of 40 torr, thereby correcting any respiratory abnormalities that might have existed in the patient when the blood was drawn. Any abnormality remaining in standard bicarbonate, then, is due to metabolic causes.

11. Actual bicarbonate: The actual amount of bicarbonate, HCO_3^-, expressed in mEq/liter of plasma as it existed in the patient. (If the patient had a PCO_2 of 40 torr, completely saturated hemoglobin, and a temperature of 37°C, actual bicarbonate and standard bicarbonate are identical.)

12. Total CO_2 content (sometimes abbreviated as "CO_2"): The amount of CO_2 gas extractable from plasma in the presence of a strong acid. Total CO_2 content consists of bicarbonate (HCO_3^-), carbonic acid (H_2CO_3), and dissolved carbon dioxide gas (PCO_2).

    $$HCO_3^- + \text{dissolved } CO_2 \text{ gas and } H_2CO_3 = \text{total } CO_2 \text{ content}$$

    Because there is 800 times as much dissolved CO_2 gas at equilibrium as H_2CO_3, and because CO_2 gas and H_2CO_3 are interchangeable anyway, dissolved CO_2 gas is used instead of H_2CO_3.

    $$HCO_3^- + \text{dissolved } CO_2 \text{ gas} = \text{total } CO_2 \text{ content}$$
    $$HCO_3^- + PCO_2 = \text{total } CO_2 \text{ content}$$

    (Capital "P" stands for the pressure or tension exerted by the dissolved gas.)

    To convert PCO_2 from torr to mEq/liter, one multiplies it by 0.03

    $$HCO_3^- + (0.03 \times PCO_2) = \text{total } CO_2 \text{ content}$$
    Example: 24 mEq/liter + (0.03 × 40 torr)
    $$= \text{total } CO_2 \text{ content}$$
    24 mEq/liter + 1.2 mEq/liter
    $$= 25.2 \text{ mEq/liter}$$

    In normal plasma, more than 95% of the total CO_2 content is contributed by HCO_3^-, with the other 5% being contributed by dissolved CO_2 gas and H_2CO_3. Dissolved CO_2 gas (which is regulated by the lungs) therefore contributes little to the total CO_2 content. Total CO_2 content gives little information about the lungs.

---

determine whether there is an alkalemia or an acidemia. Here we have an acidemia because the pH is low.

Next look at the PCO_2 to see whether there is a respiratory abnormality. Here there is no abnormality; the PCO_2 is normal.

Next, look at either HCO_3^- or base excess to determine whether there is a metabolic abnormality. The HCO_3^- and the base excess are low, indicating a metabolic acidosis. We have an acidemia caused by a metabolic acidosis.

Consulting Figure 14-13, one sees that the example falls in the area labeled acute (uncompensated) metabolic acidosis.

2. Next is a tougher example:

pH	7.20
PCO_2	55 torr
HCO_3^-	20.5 mEq/liter
B.E.	-8

First, look at the pH to see whether there is an alkale-

13. Buffer: A substance that minimizes any change in *p*H when either acid or base is added to a solution containing the buffer.

APPROXIMATE CONTRIBUTION OF INDIVIDUAL BUFFERS TO TOTAL BUFFERING IN WHOLE BLOOD

Individual Buffers	% *Buffering in Whole Blood*	
Hemoglobin and oxyhemoglobin	35	
Organic phosphate	3	Total nonbicarbonate — 47%
Inorganic phosphate	2	
Plasma proteins	7	
Plasma bicarbonate	35	Total bicarbonate — 53%
RBC bicarbonate	18	

---

14. Metabolic acidosis: An abnormal physiological process characterized by the primary gain of strong acid or primary loss of bicarbonate from the extracellular fluid.
15. Metabolic alkalosis: An abnormal physiological process characterized by primary gain of strong base (or loss of strong acid) or the primary gain of bicarbonate by the extracellular fluid.
16. Respiratory acidosis: An abnormal physiological process in which there is a primary reduction in the rate of alveolar ventilation relative to the rate of CO_2 production.
17. Respiratory alkalosis: An abnormal physiological process in which there is a primary increase in the rate of alveolar ventilation relative to the rate of CO_2 production.
18. Henderson-Hasselbalch equation:
    (lowercase "p" stands for negative logarithm of a number)

$$pH = pK + \log \frac{HCO_3^-}{\left[\begin{array}{c} \text{dissolved } CO_2 \text{ gas} \\ \text{and } H_2CO_3 \end{array}\right]}$$

Although the equation is usually written simply as follows:

$$pH = pK + \log \frac{[HCO_3^-]}{[H_2CO_3]}$$

It is understood that most of the H_2CO_3 is in the form of dissolved CO_2 gas. In clinical practice we measure the pressure exerted by the dissolved CO_2 gas, so the equation could be rewritten as follows (capital "P" stands for pressure or tension exerted by dissolved gas):

$$pH = pK + \log \frac{[HCO_3^-]}{[PCO_2 \text{ in torr}]}$$

To convert PCO_2 from torr to mEq/liter, one multiplies by 0.03.

$$pH = pK + \log \frac{[HCO_3^-]}{[0.03 \times PCO_2]}$$

(pK is a constant 6.10)

Example: $7.40 = 6.10 + \log \dfrac{[24 \text{ mEq/liter}]}{[0.03 \times 40]}$

$$7.40 = 6.10 + \log \frac{24 \text{ mEq/liter}}{1.2 \text{ mEq/liter}}$$

$7.40 = 6.10 + \log 20$ (log of 20 is 1.30)
$7.40 = 6.10 + 1.30$
$7.40 = 7.40$

19. P_{50}: The partial pressure of oxygen (PO_2) when hemoglobin is exactly 50% saturated. This measurement is used to detect a shift in the oxyhemoglobin dissociation curve (*i.e.,* if the P_{50} is greater than 27, the curve is shifted to the right, and if the P_{50} is less than 27, the curve is shifted to the left).
20. Acute respiratory acidosis: Uncompensated respiratory acidosis.
21. Chronic respiratory acidosis: Compensated respiratory acidosis.
22. Acute metabolic acidosis: Uncompensated respiratory acidosis.
23. Chronic metabolic acidosis: Compensated metabolic acidosis.
24. Fully compensated: Compensated to the greatest extent that the body can in 95% of the cases.
25. Completely compensated: Compensated to the extent that the *p*H is within the normal range.

---

mia or an acidemia. Here the *p*H is low, indicating an acidemia.

Does the PCO_2 indicate a respiratory abnormality? Yes, PCO_2 is high, indicating respiratory acidosis.

Does the HCO_3^- or B.E. indicate a nonrespiratory abnormality? Yes, HCO_3^- and base excess are low, indicating nonrespiratory (metabolic) acidosis.

Therefore, this is an acidemia caused by combined respiratory and metabolic acidoses.

Consulting Figure 14-13, one sees that this example falls in the area between acute metabolic acidosis and acute respiratory acidosis, indicating that both are occurring.

THE NOMOGRAM

The foregoing is all that is necessary to solve most acid-base problems. Some experts feel that the use of "confidence limits" is a big help or even a necessity in solving acid-base problems. This concept will be briefly discussed subsequently and may help explain some of the intricacies of acid-base problems. The use of a nomogram will also be presented.

Some of the statements made in the preceding sections are true most of the time but not all of the time. For instance, according to the equation $CO_2 + H_2O \rightleftarrows HCO_3^- + H^+$ elevations of PCO_2 will raise the HCO_3^- solely because of the chemical reaction. Several days later, the HCO_3^- is elevated further because the kidneys excrete less HCO_3^- in an effort to compensate.

Ninety-five percent confidence limits have been compiled so that if, for example, the primary problem is chronic respiratory acidosis (fully compensated respiratory acidosis), one can look up the level of HCO_3^- that would be expected in 95% of the cases of chronic respiratory acidosis.

In Figure 14-12, base excess values are plotted on the horizontal axis and PCO_2 values are plotted on the vertical axis; pH isobars are the sweeping lines of small dots. Cohen, the author who produced this figure, prefers the narrow range of 7.37 to 7.43 for the normal pH range instead of 7.35 to 7.45. Cohen plotted 95% confidence bands for the acute and chronic (uncompensated and compensated) forms of each of the four basic acid-base disturbances. If one knows any two of the three parameters (pH, PCO_2, B.E.), one can calculate the third and also name the process and determine whether it is acute or chronic (fully compensated) or somewhere in between. Without using the 95% confidence limits or consulting the nomogram, one may occasionally miss the less obvious part of a combined acid-base problem.

COMPUTER INTERPRETATION

Based on the information shown in Figure 14-13, a computer program for acid-base interpretation has been developed. Computer interpretation of acid-base disorders, when combined with calculation of A − a gradients as well as a/A ratios and particularly when severely abnormal values are "flagged," is an extremely useful tool in alerting all members of the health care team that immediate action must be taken. The interpretive statements, combined with the printing of severely abnormal values in bold print, clearly indicate to the nurse or therapist that the physician must be called immediately to initiate corrective action. In some institutions, computer-generated reports have given the nurse and therapist the impetus and authority to notify the physician and to see that corrective action is taken.

BIBLIOGRAPHY

Broughton JO, Kennedy TC: Interpretation of arterial blood gases by computer. Chest 85:148–149, 1984

Divertie MB, McMichan JC: Continuous monitoring of mixed venous oxygen saturation. Chest 85:423–428, 1984

Masoro EJ, Siegel PD: Acid-Base Regulation: Its Physiology, Pathophysiology and the Interpretation of Blood Gas Analysis, 2nd ed. Philadelphia, WB Saunders, 1977

Schwartz AB, Lyons H (eds): Acid-Base and Electrolyte Balance. New York, Grune & Stratton, 1977

Wiedermann HP, Matthay MA, Matthay RA: Cardiovascular-pulmonary monitoring in the intensive care unit—Part I. Chest 85:537–549, 1984

15
Management Modalities: Respiratory System

Bronchial Hygiene
Patricia K. Brannin

Bronchial hygiene consists of any one or a combination of the following measures: inhaled bronchodilator therapy, aerosol therapy, deep-breathing maneuvers, coughing, and postural drainage. The therapeutic goals of bronchial hygiene are removal of secretions, improved ventilation, and oxygenation. Specific bronchial hygiene depends on existing pulmonary dysfunction.

The need for and the effectiveness of various modalities of bronchial hygiene must be assessed frequently. The evaluation process should be based on physical assessment, chest radiograph, measurement of arterial blood gases, and additional sources of information as indicated.

The following discussion is not intended as a specific instructional guide for bronchial hygiene. Techniques of delivery of bronchial hygiene are paramount in the prevention and treatment of pulmonary complications (i.e., retained pulmonary secretions in a chronic bronchitic who subsequently develops pneumonia). The nurse should integrate her knowledge of normal airway anatomy and lung function as she develops her techniques for the delivery of bronchial hygiene. She should concentrate on the primary phases of lung function that most techniques of bronchial hygiene should aim to improve, namely, ventilation and diffusion (Fig. 15-1).

Intermittent Positive Pressure Breathing (IPPB)

IPPB treatments are used for improved administration and deposition of aerosols. Successful IPPB treatments will be determined by the patient's position, ventilatory pattern, and ability to cooperate and follow instructions.

An adequate ventilatory pattern during an IPPB treatment consists of a deep inspiration aimed at increasing normal tidal volume two to three times. The patient is then instructed to hold his breath briefly to provide greater depth and deposition of aerosolized medication, water, or saline. Exhalation should take twice as long as inspiration, resulting in complete exhalation.

Possible contraindications to IPPB therapy include pneumothorax, active pulmonary tuberculosis in which infection or hemoptysis is hazardous, and hemoptysis. Caution should be taken in the use of IPPB treatment immediately following lung resection because of potential bronchial leakage.

The use and value of IPPB therapy have become controversial issues. Since the 1960s, this treatment modality has generated significant income for respiratory therapy departments at considerable expense to patients and third-party payers. At first, this form of therapy was considered acceptable and advised by many. What was the rationale for IPPB? Some of the reasons include the following: IPPB decreased the work and oxygen cost of breathing; IPPB was said to improve arterial blood gases (i.e., to elevate PaO_2 and to decrease $PaCO_2$); and IPPB provided a means for inhalation of therapeutic aerosols. In response to the

283

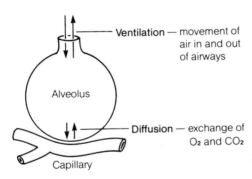

FIGURE 15-1
Lung functions: ventilation and diffusion.

last, the resultant decreased work and oxygen costs of breathing occur while the patient is using IPPB (*i.e.,* 10- 15-minute treatment). Changes in arterial blood gases last approximately 15 minutes after the treatment. There are a variety of devices available that— *when* used correctly—allow effective delivery of aerosols (Fig. 15-2). Which device will be most effective for the individual patient? Why (*i.e.,* cost, ease of use, availability, compliance, maintenance, effectiveness)? Does he use the device correctly?

IPPB may be the most effective mode of bronchodilator delivery for the patient with severe hand deformity (*e.g.,* rheumatoid arthritis or an abnormality secondary to trauma) and for the patient with neuromuscular disease causing such weakness that he is unable to generate adequate tidal volume, thus resulting in inadequate depth and deposition of an aerosolized bronchodilator.

In one multicenter trial, IPPB therapy was compared with compressor nebulizer therapy in 985 ambulatory patients with chronic obstructive pulmonary disease (Annals Internal Medicine, 1983). The reader is encouraged to review this reference to appreciate the controversy over IPPB and the findings of this important research.

If IPPB is indicated, the nurse must be aware of the importance of positioning the patient in the most effective position (one that is not contraindicated by any underlying condition, such as unstable vertebral fractures) to facilitate maximal ventilation. The nurse should remain with the patient to guide him through the treatment.

How can the nurse evaluate for an effective aerosolized bronchodilator treatment—*regardless of the mode of delivery?* Assessment includes the following before and after the treatment: bedside spirometry (tidal volume), breath sounds, pulse, and respiratory rate. The last two commonly increase during bronchodilator therapy and may remain elevated up to $1\frac{1}{2}$ hours after treatment. Measurement of arterial blood gases may be indicated but does not take the place of the

other assessments. Objective evaluation is certainly crucial, but what about the value of *subjective* information? How does the patient feel? Is his breathing better than before the treatment? Can he feel movement of air or medication in the lower part of his lungs? How long does the effectiveness of the treatments last? What, if any, side effects (*e.g.,* jitteriness, palpitations, inability to concentrate, increased heart rate) is he experiencing and how long do these symptoms last?

Inhaled Moisture

The primary purposes of inhaled moisture are hydration of normal mucociliary clearance mechanisms and liquefaction of secretions. Adequate systemic hydration is essential to obtaining optimal results of inhaled moisture.

The most important aspect of inhaled moisture therapy is active deep breathing by the patient followed by brief breath-holding to allow deposition of aerosolized particles and slow, complete exhalation. One must also remember the importance of helping the patient assume the most effective position (be cognizant of any factors such as unstable vertebral fractures that might be contraindications) to maximize ventilation and, thus, depth of deposition of aerosolized particles.

Potential hazards include bronchospasm in patients with hyperreactive airways and infection from contaminated equipment. The ultimate success of inhaled moisture therapy will depend on clearance of secretions with forceful, rigorous coughing.

Effective Cough

An effective cough is a necessary prerequisite to clearance of secretions. Various techniques are available to assist the patient in achieving an effective cough, such as a maximal exhalation followed by a maximal inspiration followed by a forceful cough. Gentle pressure to the trachea above the manubrial notch may be used to stimulate cough production in the comatose or uncooperative patient.

Chest Physiotherapy

Inadequate clearance of secretions dictates the need for chest physiotherapy. This technique involves use of gravity to aid flow of secretions to a point at which they can be expectorated with forceful coughing maneuvers or suctioned with a catheter. The effectiveness of positioning may be augmented by chest percussion. (Figure 15-3 demonstrates the positions for postural drainage.)

Modification or contraindication of chest physiotherapy may be necessary with the following: in-

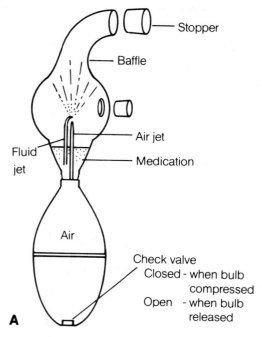

A

Hand-powered nebulizer

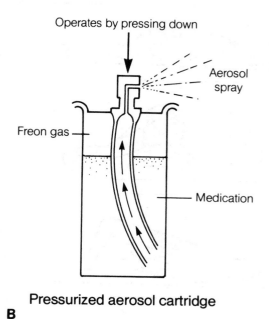

B

Pressurized aerosol cartridge

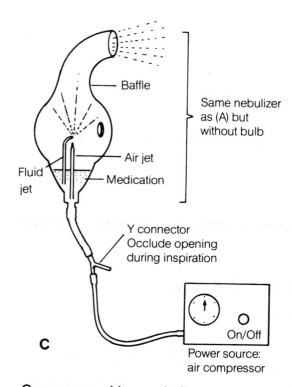

C

Compressor-driven nebulizer

D

IPPB

FIGURE 15-2
Common devices for inhaled bronchodilator delivery.

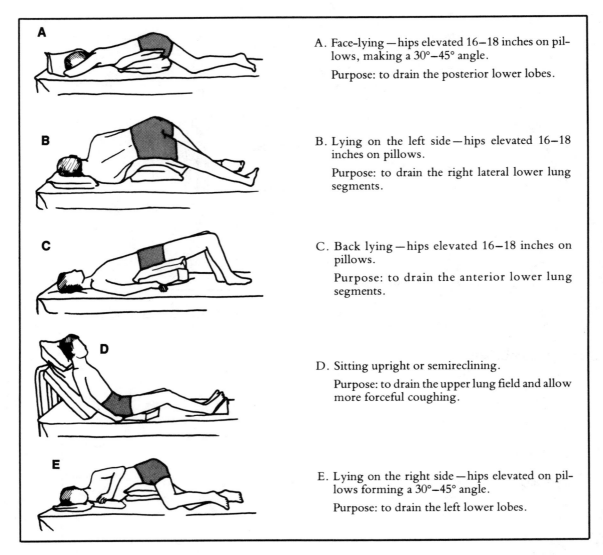

A. Face-lying—hips elevated 16–18 inches on pillows, making a 30°–45° angle.

Purpose: to drain the posterior lower lobes.

B. Lying on the left side—hips elevated 16–18 inches on pillows.

Purpose: to drain the right lateral lower lung segments.

C. Back lying—hips elevated 16–18 inches on pillows.

Purpose: to drain the anterior lower lung segments.

D. Sitting upright or semireclining.

Purpose: to drain the upper lung field and allow more forceful coughing.

E. Lying on the right side—hips elevated on pillows forming a 30°–45° angle.

Purpose: to drain the left lower lobes.

FIGURE 15-3
Positions used in lung drainage.

creased intracranial pressure, intravascular bleeds, cervical cord trauma, unstable fractures, chest and abdominal trauma, hiatal hernia, obesity, osteoporosis, and orthopedic appliances.

BIBLIOGRAPHY

Blodgett D: Manual of Respiratory Care Procedures. Philadelphia, JB Lippincott, 1980

Stevens P et al.: Intermittent positive pressure breathing therapy of chronic obstructive pulmonary disease—a clinical trial. Ann. Intern Med 99:612–620, 1983

Shapiro BA, Harrison RA, Trout CA: Clinical Application of Respiratory Care. Chicago, Year Book Medical Publishers, 1979

Artificial Airway

Patricia K. Brannin

Rigorous bronchial hygiene and carefully monitored oxygen therapy may eliminate the need for an artificial airway or ventilatory support. When these measures fail to provide adequate oxygenation and removal of carbon dioxide, an artificial airway or ventilatory support becomes mandatory. Artificial airways have a threefold purpose:

1. Establishment of an airway
2. Protection of the airway, with the cuff inflated
3. Provision of continuous ventilatory assistance

Knowledgeable, aggressive nursing care is required for maintenance of the patency of the airway as well as maximization of therapeutic effects and minimization of damage to the patient's natural airway.

The selection of the appropriate artificial airway is most important. Any artificial airway will increase airway resistance; therefore, it is essential that the largest tube possible be used for intubation. The cuff on the endotracheal or tracheostomy tube must be of low compliance (soft) so that barotrauma to the trachea, vocal cords, and subglottic area is minimized. The competency of the cuff must be established prior to intubation. Approximately 10 cc of air are injected into the cuff prior to use.

Placing the Tube. An artificial airway must be placed in the proper location and remain there. In order to ascertain tube placement properly, one must inflate the cuff. Anterior and lateral auscultation of the chest bilaterally aids in evaluation of tube position. It must be remembered that breath sounds can be transmitted to the nonventilated or inadequately ventilated lung field. The final analysis of tube placement must depend on roentgenography. Because of normal airway anatomy, endotracheal tubes have a tendency to enter the right main stem bronchus. Chest radiographs should be ordered immediately after tube placement. Evaluation of tube placement should be ongoing because endotracheal and tracheostomy tubes may become dislodged during routine care.

Proper securement of an endotracheal or tracheostomy tube must ensure airway patency, proper alignment, and stability of the tube, and it should minimize pressure at the insertion site. The tube should be immobilized so that it will not ride, slip, and twist unnecessarily and injure tissue with which it comes in contact (Fig. 15-4).

It should be noted that an endotracheal tube is a round tube that is inserted through an elliptic opening, the vocal cords. Therefore, a pathway is established for continual flow of oropharyngeal secretions and flora, which become potential pathogens to the lower respiratory tract. Use of minimal air leak technique reduces the flow of secretions and flora.

Inflating the Cuff. Appropriate inflation of a cuff on an artificial airway is based on the following rationale:

• It protects the airway in the presence of copious secretions

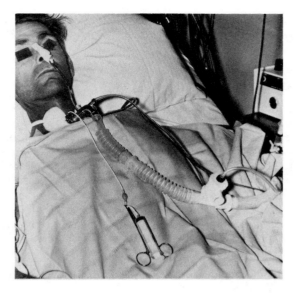

FIGURE 15-4
Proper alignment for securing endotracheal tubing.

• It establishes a seal necessary for ventilatory support

An inflated cuff requires only that amount of air necessary to achieve a minimal air leak. A minimal air leak may be achieved and ascertained by the application of positive pressure (ventilator or self-inflating bag) to the patient's airway, during which time air is injected into the cuff until no leak is heard over the trachea or felt over the mouth or nose. Once this is achieved, $\frac{1}{2}$ to 1 cc of air is removed, resulting in a minimal air leak. This method of cuff inflation minimizes airway trauma due to excessive cuff pressures.

Deflating the Cuff. *It has been proved that periodic deflation of a cuff of an endotracheal or tracheostomy tube is of no value in minimizing tracheal damage.*

Intelligent rationale for cuff deflation is based on the following:

• The presence and amount of upper airway secretions
• Continuous ventilatory support
• The patient's ability to protect his airway

The purpose of cuff deflation is to remove pooled secretions that have accumulated above the cuff, which may seed the upper airway with potentially pathogenic bacterial growth. The frequency of cuff deflation is dictated by individual patient needs.

Cuff deflation should be performed while positive pressure is applied during inspiration. This establishes retrograde flow of secretions into the oropharynx, where rapid removal of these secretions is achieved by suctioning. The minimal air leak is then quickly reestablished to provide adequate ventilation and protection of the airway.

SUCTIONING

The presence of an artificial tube prevents the patient from coughing, which functions as the normal clearing mechanism. It also increases production of secretions due to the presence of a foreign object. Suctioning therefore becomes paramount to removal of secretions and maintenance of patency. The need for suctioning is determined by visual observation of secretions and, more importantly, by chest auscultation for determination of the presence of secretions or mucus plugs in major airways. The author recommends the following suctioning procedure:

1. Hyperoxygenate the patient with 100% oxygen using a bag or the ventilator (this can be done while the nurse is preparing for suctioning).
2. Assemble the following equipment:
   a. Atraumatic sterile catheter
   b. Glove
   c. Sterile irrigation container
   d. Sterile normal saline
   e. Syringe containing sterile normal saline for tracheal irrigation when indicated
3. Once the first two steps have been completed, quickly but gently insert a sterile catheter as far as possible into the artificial airway without application of suction. Then withdraw it 1 to 2 cm and apply intermittent suction while rotating and removing the catheter. The aspiration should not exceed 8 to 10 seconds. Prolonged aspiration can lead to severe hypoxemia, changes in pulmonary pressure and volume, and ultimately cardiac arrest.
4. Reestablish ventilatory assistance, allowing the patient to receive 3 to 5 breaths before the procedure is repeated.

It should be noted that patients not on ventilators also need to be hyperoxygenated. The patient should be instructed to take deep breaths while connected to a 100% oxygen source. Patients incapable of taking a deep breath should be assisted by a positive pressure device.

If secretions are tenacious, 3 to 5 ml of sterile normal saline may be injected into the artificial airway. Secretions should be monitored for amount, consistency, odor, and color, and the observations should be recorded. Changes in any of these characteristics may necessitate changes in therapy. Laboratory analysis of secretions must be performed, based on patient assessment and response to existing therapy.

HUMIDIFICATION

An artificial airway excludes normal physiological airway humidification. Therefore, artificial humidification is essential to maintenance of airway patency and clearance of secretions. Determination of adequate airway humidification is based on the consistency and amount of secretions as well as condensation visible in the oxygen tubing leading to the patient. The humidification devices attached to oxygen therapy equipment often become media for bacterial growth. Appropriate care should therefore be taken in the maintenance of all oxygen therapy equipment. Policies should be established to monitor, by culture, the presence of organisms.

VENTILATORS

When ventilatory support is required, the nurse must be aware of the degree of hypoxemia present, the percentage of oxygen required, and the underlying cause and subsequent management of acute respiratory failure (ARF).

Ventilatory assistance does not negate the need for continued monitoring of the patient for signs of ARF but actually increases the need for rigorous assessment and aggressive pulmonary care. Ventilatory assistance in a sense buys time for the patient, and the amount we buy for a given patient is a direct reflection of the adequacy of management. Detailed information on ventilatory support is found in another section of this chapter.

BIBLIOGRAPHY

Borg N, Nikas D, Stark J, Williams SM (eds): Core Curriculum for Critical Care Nursing, 2nd ed. Philadelphia, WB Saunders, 1981

McPherson SP: Respiratory Therapy Equipment, 2nd ed. St. Louis, CV Mosby, 1981

Traver G (ed): Respiratory Nursing—The Science and the Art. New York, John Wiley & Sons, 1982

Wiedemann HP, Matthay MA, Matthay RA: Cardiovascular pulmonary monitoring in the intensive care unit (Parts 1 and 2). Chest 85:537–668, 1984

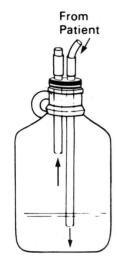

FIGURE 15-5
One-bottle system underwater seal drainage.

Chest Tubes

Patricia K. Brannin

CHEST TUBE MANAGEMENT

To understand the objectives for chest tube placement and drainage, one needs to review anatomy and physiology of the pleural space. The visceral and parietal pleurae provide a membranous covering of the lungs and lining of the thoracic cavity. A *potential* space filled with approximately 4 ml of pleural fluid is created by the visceral and parietal pleurae. There is normally negative (less than atmospheric) pressure in the pleural space, which ranges from -5 to 3 cm of water during expiration. The development of negative pressure during inspiration allows air to enter the lungs. As the extrapulmonary and atmospheric pressures equalize, active inspiration ceases, and passive exhalation occurs. When the integrity of the pleural space is disrupted, the air or fluid that accumulates prevents the development of negative pressure necessary for normal ventilation.

UNDERWATER SEAL DRAINAGE

Chest drains and underwater seal drainage are used to restore the physiological integrity of the pleural space. A chest tube (drain) inserted into the pleural space will remove air or fluid. The underwater seal drainage to which the chest tube is connected prevents backflow into the pleural space (Fig. 15-5).

A glass rod under water in a bottle establishes negative pressure in the water seal system. The depth of the rod in the water determines the degree of negative pressure. A basic law of physics states that gases and fluids move from areas of greater pressure to areas of lesser pressure. Therefore, the air or fluid disrupting the normal pressures in the pleural space will drain into the chest bottle in an attempt to equalize the more negative pressure of the underwater seal drainage system. The air vent in the chest bottle allows the drained air to escape, preventing pressure buildup in the bottle.

Larger amounts of blood or fluid draining from the pleural space necessitate modification of the underwater seal system. A second bottle may be added to accommodate large amounts of fluid (Fig. 15-6).

Suction may be added to the system if the air leak into the pleural space accumulates faster than the sys-

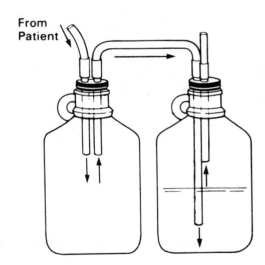

FIGURE 15-6
Two-bottle system underwater seal drainage.

tem can remove it (Fig. 15-7). A single self-contained underwater seal drainage unit that has the capacity to function as a two- or three-bottle system with suction has been developed.

The system must remain patent. Malfunction of the chest tube or underwater seal drainage system may result in inadequate removal of air or fluid from the pleural space. Occlusion of the system at any point may result in the development of a tension pneumothorax. The life-threatening seriousness of a tension pneumothorax has led to the consensus that clamping of chest tubes for more than a few seconds is a dangerous practice.

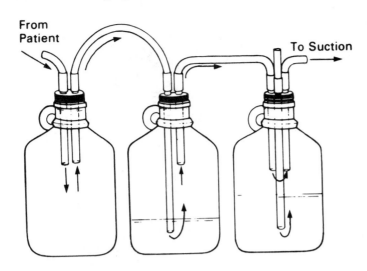

From Patient

To Suction

FIGURE 15-7
Underwater seal drainage with suctioning.

In addition to underwater seal drainage, there are a variety of disposable chest drainage units used to reexpand the involved lung or to provide a means for drainage, observation, and measurement. Become familiar with the equipment. Check the chest tube site for evidence of infection. Check all connecting points to be certain they are secure. Is there any drainage? If so, describe and note the amount. Does fluid in tubing fluctuate with patient's breathing? Why would this occur?

What physical findings were noted before placement of the chest tube? How will you know whether a pneumothorax is resolving? What might you expect to see? What might you expect to hear during chest auscultation?

Pharmacologic Agents

Patricia K. Brannin

The distinguishing feature of a group of diseases affecting the lower respiratory tract is spasm of the bronchial smooth muscle. Flow of air through the airways can fluctuate significantly within short periods of time secondary to an increased responsiveness to various stimuli (*e.g.,* noxious fumes and gases, air pollutants, animal dander, extreme cold, and exercise). Bronchospasm is an important component of reversible obstructive airway disease (asthma) and chronic bronchitis. In addition, bronchospasm is frequently associated with viral infections.

A basic understanding of pulmonary drugs and their sites of action (Table 15-1) and of specific pharmacologic agents with knowledge of action, dosage, and side effects (Table 15-2) is crucial for the delivery of safe pharmacologic support and meticulous assessment for drug effectiveness and side effects. Because a full discussion of the multiple pharmacologic agents is beyond the scope of this book, the reader should consult a current pharmacology text for added information.

BRONCHODILATORS

The choice of specific bronchodilator therapy depends on the physician's bias, drug availability, cost, the patient's tolerance, and the patient's compliance. Table 15-2 illustrates pulmonary drugs commonly used at this time, action, dosage and side effects. Therefore, only major points for emphasis will be discussed.

Theophylline, a member of the xanthine family, is the most useful bronchodilator for moderate to severe bronchospasm, and it increases diaphragmatic contractibility. It is a safe and effective drug that one can monitor relatively easily by obtaining serum theophylline levels that usually are between 10 and 20 mcg/ml. The incidence of drug toxicity increases at levels greater than 20 mcg/ml. Many physicians consider theophylline to be the "first-line" bronchodilator of choice, and this will be the first bronchodilator the patient receives. If after therapeutic levels have been achieved, the patient continues to be symptomatic, a second bronchodilator—an adrenergic agent—may be added.

The adrenergic bronchodilators are those drugs that mimic the sympathetic nervous system (sympathomi-

TABLE 15-1
SITES OF ACTION OF PULMONARY DRUGS

1. Receptors of Smooth Muscle — Airways

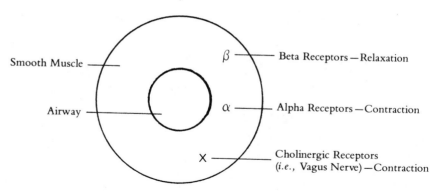

2. Cellular Metabolism

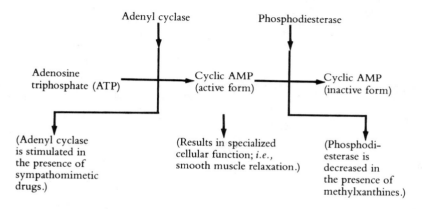

Cyclic AMP is one of the intermediaries of cellular metabolism in the sequence of energy production. It is present in almost all cell membranes and is influenced by a variety of agents, such as hormones and drugs.

3. Mast Cells

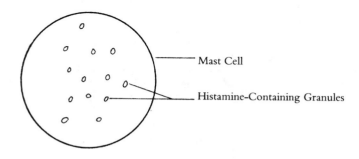

Mast cells with histamine-containing granules are abundant in allergic asthmatics.

TABLE 15-2
ACTION, DOSAGE, AND SIDE EFFECTS OF PULMONARY DRUGS

Pulmonary Drugs	Action	Dosage	Side Effects
1. *Bronchodilators* Methylxanthines	↓ phosphodiesterase with ↑ cyclic AMP (active form)	IV: loading—5 mg/kg; maintenance—0.9 mg/kg PO: aminophylline—1200 mg/24 hr; oxtriphylline (Choledyl)—1600 mg/24 hr NB: Dosages adjusted to maintain serum theophylline levels 10 μg–20 μg/ml	Nausea Vomiting Nervousness Arrhythmias Seizures

Theophylline—Dosage increased by 50% for smokers who can tolerate the drug if effect is less than optimal
Dosage decreased by 50% for patients with liver failure, heart failure, hypoxemia and in shock

Pulmonary Drugs	Action	Dosage	Side Effects
Sympathomimetics	Beta (β) stimulants		Relatively few side effects with recommended dosages
Isoetharine (Bronkosol)	Stimulates adenyl cyclase with ↑ cyclic AMP (active form)	Delivered via nebulizer—either hand-powered or IPPB 0.5 ml with sterile water or normal saline (1:3 conc.) q4hr	Tachycardia Palpitations Nausea Headache Changes in blood pressure Nervousness
Terbutaline (Brethine)	Stimulates adenyl cyclase with ↑ cyclic AMP (active form)	5 mg PO q8hr; 0.25 mg SC not to exceed 0.5 mg q4hr	↑ Heart rate Nervousness Tremor Palpitations Dizziness (Usually transient effects and do not require treatment)
Metaproterenol (Alupent, Metaprel)	Stimulates adenyl cyclase with ↑ cyclic AMP (active form)	Metered dose device: 0.65 mg/metered dose; 20 mg PO t.i.d.	Tachycardia Hypertension Palpitations Nervousness Tremor Nausea and vomiting
Albuterol (Salbutamol, Proventyl)	Same as for metaproterenol	Metered dose device: 1–2 inhalations q4–6hr Oral: 2–4 mg q6–8hr	Mainly fine finger tremors
Epinephrine	Same as for metaproterenol	0.2–0.5 mg of 1:1000 solution SC q2hr as necessary. Severe attacks: doses may be repeated every 20 minutes for maximum of three doses	Anxiety Tremors Palpitations Tachycardia Hirsutism (Contraindicated in hypertension, hyperthyroidism, ischemic heart disease, and cerebrovascular insufficiency)
2. *Steroids*	Stimulate adenylate cyclase with ↑ cyclic 3', 5'-AMP; may facilitate use of β-stimulants; anti-inflammatory action		
Prednisone		Variable; *e.g.,* 40–60 mg PO initially and decreasing according to PFT and eosinophil counts (in patients with ↑ Eos 2° to allergin-mediated responses)	Formation of glucose from body protein → ↑ blood sugar Depletion of bone calcium—osteoporosis Increase in fat production

TABLE 15-2
(Continued)

Pulmonary Drugs	Action	Dosage	Side Effects
			Impairment of immunologic response Reduction of inflammatory response Increase in gastric acidity Elevation of blood pressure Acne
Methylprednisolone (Solu-Medrol)		Variable; *e.g.,* 100 mg IV and repeat with one fourth original dose q6hr	Same as for prednisone
Beclomethasone (Vanceril)	Virtually same as for other steroids except it is an inhaled preparation with a high topical effect on the airways and low systemic activity	Inhalation device; 2 inhalations (100 μg) q.i.d.	Oral candidiasis Mild oropharyngeal symptoms—discomfort and dryness of throat
3. *Cromolyn sodium* (Aarane, Intal)	Prophylactic bronchospasmolytic in allergic asthma; *not* useful in acute bronchospasm; probably strengthens mast cell membrane, preventing release of histamine and therefore decreases bronchospasm in the allergic asthmatic	1 capsule via inhaler device q.i.d.	Maculopapular rash Urticaria Cough and/or bronchospasm
4. *Anticholinergics* Atropine sulfate	Parasympathetic antagonist	5 mg of solution	Tachycardia Dry mouth

metic) and are relatively short-acting because they are readily metabolized. The choice of a specific agent depends on the preferred route of administration (*i.e.,* oral versus inhaled), the rapidity of onset, the length of action, and prevalence as well as type of side effects. These drugs include metaproterenol, isoetharine, isoproterenol, albuterol, and terbutaline. Multiple trials may be needed to evaluate the maximal effectiveness of a timed-release preparation such as Slo-Phyllin or Theolair versus Bronkodyl. When possible, patients should participate in drug selection and schedule. This improves compliance with drug therapy and ultimately quality of life.

ANTICHOLINERGIC DRUGS

Atropine sulfate is an agent that has been used for many years preoperatively for drying oral secretions, and many physicians believe that such an agent would be contraindicated in patients with lung disease who have excessive secretion production. The parasympathetic action of atropine is effective in blocking neurotransmission by acetylcholine to smooth muscle. This agent may exert significant bronchodilator effect fol-

lowing inhalation while avoiding the drying effect of large systemic doses.

ASTHMA PROPHYLACTIC DRUGS

Cromolyn sodium may be used in asthmatic patients whose symptoms are not controlled adequately by bronchodilators. A trial of 1 month will be preceded and followed by pulmonary function testing to document response. If an appropriate response cannot be demonstrated, the drug is discontinued. The desired effects of cromolyn are to reduce severity of asthma attacks and to enhance effects of concomitantly administered bronchodilator and steroid therapy. As a result of the latter, one can anticipate a reduction of bronchodilator and steroid dosage.

ANTI-INFLAMMATORY CORTICOSTEROID

The reader should refer to Table 15-2 for a discussion of pulmonary drugs. Steroids apparently stimulate adenyl cyclase with a resultant increase of cyclic 3′,5′-

AMP. They may facilitate the action of β-stimulants. They also are anti-inflammatory agents. One must keep in mind that steroid side effects can occur with as little as 10 mg of prednisone per day. The inhaled form of corticosteroid, beclomethasone dipropionate (Beclovent or Vanceril inhaler), may be employed either for those patients who require 20 mg or less daily to control asthmatic symptoms or for those who require high-dose steroids. Beclomethasone supplementation may enable the physician to decrease the oral steroid dosage in the latter group. Regardless of whether the patient is transferred totally to inhaled steroids or to a combination of both oral and inhaled steroids, caution

must be exercised. Decrement of oral dosage should be very small (*e.g.*, 2 to 3 mg). Pulmonary functions should be monitored carefully. Stressful situations such as exacerbation of severe asthma, trauma, or surgery may indeed warrant a short course of systemic steroids in full therapeutic dosage.

OXYGEN

Oxygen is one of the most commonly used forms of medical therapy. Factors that determine tissue oxygenation include (1) alveolar oxygen concentration,

TABLE 15-3
ANTIBIOTIC THERAPY IN PULMONARY DISEASE*

Pulmonary Complication	Antibiotic	Dosage
Pneumococcal pneumonia with or without COPD	Penicillin	600,000 U procaine penicillin IM q12hr (a blood level of 0.02 mg/ml 12 hours after start of drug is adequate to kill organism) or IV prep: aqueous penicillin G 300,000–600,000 U IV q3–4hr
	Penicillin V	250 mg orally q6hr
	Cefazolin	500 mg IM or IV q8hr
	Cephalexin	500 mg orally q6hr
Staphylococcus pneumonia (production of enzymes that destroy lung tissue)	Antistaphylococcal agents: Nafcillin Methicillin Cloxacillin Penicillin	1–2 g IV q4–6hr
Klebsiella pneumonia (gram-negative): a very severe pneumonia with high mortality; seen more commonly in chronic/debilitated states	Cephalosporin (Cefazolin)	1 gm IM or IV q4–6hr
	Gentamicin	Dosage will be related to renal function (*i.e.*, creatinine clearance); commonly, 3–6 mg/kg/24 hr. Aim to achieve a trough blood level not less than 1.5 mg/ml and a peak level not over 10 mg/ml
Pseudomonas pneumonia (gram-negative)	Tobramycin	3–5 mg/kg/24 hr, producing blood levels of 2.5 mg/ml in presence of normal renal function
	Gentamicin	3–5 mg/kg/24 hr (see *Klebsiella* pneumonia, above)
Hemophilus influenza	Ampicillin	2.0–6.0 g/24 hr, increasing to 8–12 g/24 hr for serious infections
	Chloramphenicol	3.0–4.0 g/24 hr PO (50–100 mg/kg/24 hr)

* A complete discussion of antibiotic therapy related to pulmonary disease and/or complications is beyond the scope of this chapter.

(2) diffusion of gases (oxygen) at the alveocapillary membrane, (3) ventilation-perfusion ($\dot{V}/\dot{Q}$) relationships within the lung, (4) the amount and carrying capacity of hemoglobin, and (5) cardiac output.

Therapeutic oxygen is potentially harmful. The dosage of oxygen must be prescribed precisely in terms of percent concentration in the inspired air (*i.e.*, FIO_2 0.5) or in liters per minute. According to the 1982 report of Good and Waite,[1] a PaO_2 less than 50 mm Hg is the degree of hypoxemia that indicates a need for supplemental O_2. The goal of this therapy will be to raise the PaO_2 to approximately 60 mm Hg with a subsequent reduction of hypoxic vasoconstriction of the pulmonary vascular bed and pulmonary artery pressure and, it is hoped improvement in right ventricular function and tissue delivery of oxygen.

A detailed discussion of the devices employed commonly for oxygen delivery can be found in Table 15-16. The critical care nurse must become knowledgeable in the techniques and rationale for the various oxygen delivery devices, even though respiratory therapists may be responsible for oxygen therapy. If they have responsibilities in addition to ICU, they may not have adequate staff to provide constant ICU coverage. The nurse should develop the habit of checking this equipment and assessing the patient. What are the blood gases? Is the patient demonstrating signs and symptoms of hypoxemia—tachycardia, tachypnea, diaphoresis, and confusion or behavioral change?

ANTIBIOTIC THERAPY

Troleandomycin (TAO) is an antibiotic that may be initiated on a trial basis for those severe, chronic corticosteroid-dependent asthmatics who have been refractory to therapy, requiring high doses of corticosteroids in an attempt to control the disease. A major concern with sustained high steroid dosage is the potential for developing severe side effects, such as steroid-induced diabetes mellitus, gastric ulcers, bleeding disorders, and osteoporosis. The goal of combined TAO and steroid therapy in this instance is to reduce steroid dosage so that associated complications are avoided, minimized, or better controlled. In 1980, Zeiger and colleagues[2] reported that daily doses of TAO at 250 mg per day or less resulted in clinical improvement (documented by spirometry) within a 2-week introduction of the drug. Use of TAO is attended by the risk of hepatic toxicity. Liver function (*i.e.*, SGPT, SGOT, alkaline phosphatase, and bilirubin) should be monitored at regular intervals. Because TAO is not a commonly used pharmacologic agent for asthmatics at this time, it has been omitted from Table 15-2.

Current antibiotic therapy commonly employed for the treatment of pneumococcal, staphylococcal, and *Klebsiella* pneumonia and of *Hemophilus influenzae* is summarized in Table 15-3. The reader is encouraged to review the subject in a current pharmacologic text. Pneumonia with or without preexisting lung disease can be a serious complication. Side effects from potent antibiotic therapy can significantly complicate the situation with such problems as renal and hepatic complications and ototoxicity.

REFERENCES

1. Good JA, Waite D: Respiratory therapy including cardiopulmonary resuscitation. In Mitchell RS, Petty TL (eds): Synopsis of Clinical Pulmonary Disease, 3rd ed, p 90. St. Louis, CV Mosby, 1982
2. Zeiger RS, Schatz M, Sperling N, et al: Efficacy of troleandomycin in outpatients with severe, corticosteroid-dependent asthma. J Allergy Clin Immunol 66:438–446, 1980

BIBLIOGRAPHY

American Medical Association: AMA Drug Evaluations, 5th ed, p 589. Chicago, 1983.
Good JA, Waite D: Respiratory therapy including cardiopulmonary resuscitation. In Mitchell RS, Petty TL (eds): Synopsis of Clinical Pulmonary Disease, 3rd ed, p 90. St. Louis, CV Mosby, 1982
Zeiger RS, Schatz M, Sperling N, et al: Efficacy of troleandomycin in outpatients with severe, corticosteroid-dependent asthma. J Allergy Clin Immunol 66:438–446, 1980

Ventilatory Support

Eileen Brent-Hemman

Once a patient has been intubated and resuscitated successfully, the commitment to mechanical ventilation has been made. This commitment poses a high financial and psychological burden on the patient and family. Because mortality is reduced very little, every effort and consideration must be given to prevent mechanical ventilation.

Two approaches that may eliminate the need for mechanical ventilation are as follows:

• Identification of high-risk patients
• Institution of appropriate measures to forestall or prevent respiratory failure

Patients are predisposed to developing respiratory failure when any of the systems involved in respiration are compromised or overwhelmed (Table 15-4). The

TABLE 15-4
BODY SYSTEMS AND POSSIBLE EVENTS LEADING TO RESPIRATORY FAILURE

Systems	Events
1. Nervous system: Brain stem Spinal cord and nerves	Head trauma Poliomyelitis Cervical (C1–C6) fractures Overdose
2. Muscular system: Primary—diaphragm Secondary— respiratory	Myasthenia gravis Guillain-Barré
3. Skeletal system: Thorax	Flail chest Kyphoscoliosis
4. Respiratory system: Airways	Obstruction Laryngeal edema Bronchitis Asthma
Alveoli	Emphysema Pneumonia Fibrosis
Pulmonary circulation	Pulmonary embolus
5. Cardiovascular system	Congestive heart failure Fluid overload Cardiac surgery Myocardial infarction
6. Gastrointestinal system	Aspiration
7. Hematological system	DIC
8. Genitourinary system	Renal failure

degree of risk for developing respiratory failure depends on the patient's ability to move air, secretions, and blood. Inability to do the latter is reflected clinically as pulmonary edema due to poor cardiac output.

ASSESSMENT

Respiratory failure is defined as an inability to maintain an adequate pH, $PaCO_2$, and PaO_2. *Adequate* means a pH greater than 7.25, a $PaCO_2$ less than 50 torr, and a PaO_2 greater than 50 torr with the patient on oxygen. As the arterial blood gases deteriorate and the patient fatigues, mechanical ventilatory support is indicated.

Many times, it is the nurse who initially recognizes the onset of respiratory failure. Simple bedside monitoring can alert the nurse to signs of patient decompensation. Two simple, noninvasive, and inexpensive indicators that can be used are respiratory rate and vital capacity.

Normal *respiratory rate* is 16 to 20 breaths per minute. If the rate increases to 25 breaths per minute, the patient's status must be evaluated and appropriate measures instituted—namely, suctioning, postural drainage, and cupping. (See previous section.) Once the rate reaches 40 or more per minute, the "work of breathing" to maintain less than acceptable blood gas values is high. Eventually, exhaustion occurs, and ventilatory assistance is required. This process may occur over hours or minutes, depending on the patient's respiratory reserve (Table 15-5).

Vital capacity, the second parameter, is a measure of ventilation. Using a simple bedside spirometer, the patient is asked to take a deep breath and exhale through the spirometer until he has completely emptied his lungs. If the vital capacity is less than 10 to 20 ml/kg, respiratory reserve is minimal. Serial monitoring of this parameter is more meaningful than a one-spot check. A good clinical example is a patient with a cervical spine injury. Serial monitoring of vital capacity may show the progression of ascending edema and

TABLE 15-5
INDICATIONS FOR MECHANICAL VENTILATION

Parameters	Values	Action
Respiratory rate	<10 breaths/minute (diminished drive to breathe)	Evaluate patient and eliminate cause
	16–20 breaths/min	Normal
	28–40 breaths/min	Evaluate patient and institute appropriate measures
	>40 breaths/min	Consider elective intubation/ventilation
Vital capacity	<10–20 ml/kg (poor ventilatory reserve)	Watch for signs of respiratory failure
		Prepare to initiate ventilatory support
Inspiratory pressures	<20 cm water or decreasing trend	
Arterial Blood Gases		
pH	<7.25	Evaluate in combination with $PaCO_2$, if it is rising
$PaCO_2$	>50 torr	Evaluate in combination with pH, if it is decreasing
PaO_2	<50 torr while on oxygen	Evaluate in combination with the pH and $PaCO_2$
A – a gradient	≥300 mm hg	
Shunt	≥25%–30%	
Chest auscultation	Diminished or no breath sounds	Deliver 100% oxygen
		Prepare ventilatory support
Heart rate and rhythm	Pulse over 120, arrhythmias	Monitor for arrhythmias
Activity	Extreme fatigue	Evaluate with above and take appropriate measures
Mental status	Confusion, delirium, somnolence	Monitor for hypoxic seizure activity
Physical observation	Use of accessory muscles, fatiguing, extreme dyspnea	Prepare for ventilatory support

dictate elective rather than crisis intubation and resuscitation.

In summary, identification of high-risk patients, serial monitoring and evaluation of progressive respiratory status, and institution of appropriate measures may forestall or negate the need for mechanical ventilation.

MECHANICAL VENTILATORS

Generally, today's ventilators can be divided into two categories — *volume* cycled and *pressure* cycled. Realistically, the type selected will depend on the models present in the hospital and the familiarity of the physicians with one type over the other. Regardless of which type or model is used, the ventilator's function and limitations must be intimately known. A mechanical device used to sustain life is only as good as its design and the patient team using it.

Ambu Bag

Before discussing the two aforementioned types of ventilators, a brief note about a simple, man-powered model is necessary. Frequently overlooked is the nurse's first important line of defense for acute respiratory failure (ARF) — the ambu bag. This respiratory bag provides a satisfactory method of artificial resuscitation. Connected to an oxygen source with a reservoir bag or cuff, it can deliver close to 100% oxygen. Knowledge of the bag, along with skill in using it, is vital. The function of this simple ventilator can be compared with that of the more sophisticated models. With the ambu bag,

- The *force* of squeezing the bag determines *tidal volume* (V_T) delivered to the patient
- The *number* of hand squeezes per minute determines the *rate*
- Both the *force* and *rate* at which the nurse squeezes the bag determine the *peak flow*

When the bag is used, one must carefully observe the patient's chest to determine whether the bag is performing properly and whether any gastric distention is developing. In addition, the ease or resistance encountered can roughly indicate lung compliance. If a patient becomes progressively harder to "bag," an increase in secretions, hemothorax, pneumothorax, or worsening bronchospasms must be considered.

The following criteria are suggested for selection of an ambu bag:

- The ability of the ambu bag to deliver 100% oxygen in acute situations. (In nonacute maintenance situations, less oxygen concentration is acceptable.)
- If used with a face mask, the need for the mask to be transparent to enable visualization of vomitus or blood, which is a potential for aspiration.
- A valve system that functions without jamming in acute situations.
- The cleaning and recycling endurance of the bag.

Volume Ventilators

The volume ventilator is the most frequently used type in critical care settings. The basic principle of this ventilator is that once a *designated volume* of air is delivered to the patient, inspiration is terminated. A piston or bellows pushes a predetermined volume (V_T) into the patient's lungs at a set rate. Oxygen concentrations can vary from 21% to 100%. The advantage of a volume ventilator is that despite a change in patient lung compliance, a consistent V_T will be delivered.

Some examples of volume ventilators are the MA-I, MA-II, Ohio, Monaghan, Emerson, Bourns-Bear-I, Searle, and the Engstrom.

Pressure Ventilators

In contrast to the volume ventilator, the pressure-cycled ventilator works under the basic principle that once a *preset pressure* is reached, inspiration is terminated. At this pressure point, the inspiratory valve closes and exhalation occurs passively. Ultimately this

TABLE 15-6
METHODS OF DELIVERING HIGH-FREQUENCY VENTILATION

Methods	Features
High-frequency positive pressure ventilation (HFPPV)	Positive pressure ventilator Rates 60–100/minute Uses a small cannula IE ratios 1:6–1:2
High-frequency oscillation (HFO)	Rates 600–900/minute Primarily used with neonates
High-frequency jet ventilation (HFJV)	Uses pressure jets Rates 60–300/minute Primarily used with adults

means that if a patient's lung compliance or resistance to flow changes, the *volume* of air delivered will *vary*.

Clinically, as a patient's lungs become stiffer (less compliant), the volume of air delivered to the patient will drop—sometimes drastically. Consequently, to ensure adequate minute ventilation and to detect any changes in lung compliance and resistance, one must frequently monitor inspiratory pressure, rate, and *exhaled* V_T. In a patient whose pulmonary status is unstable, the use of a pressure ventilator is not recommended. However, in a very stable patient with compliant lungs, pressure ventilators are adequate and can also be used as a weaning tool in selected patients.

Examples of pressure ventilators are the Bird Mark-I and the Bennett PR-I and PR-II.

Experimental Ventilators

Because of the complications associated with positive pressure ventilation, other methods that may be more physiologically compatible are being investigated. The technique of high-frequency ventilation (HFV) is one such method. At present, it is still considered experimental. The exact mechanism by which HFV sustains life remains unclear, but it accomplishes oxygenation by the diffusion of oxygen and carbon dioxide from high to low gradients of concentration. This diffusion movement is increased when the kinetic energy of the gas molecules is increased. (A patient experiencing high-frequency ventilation is somewhat analogous to a panting dog: The dog moves small volumes of air at a very fast rate.)

Basically, three different methods of delivering HFV can be identified (Table 15-6). Because the range of machines that deliver HFV is so varied, the resulting clinical research data are difficult to interpret. When used clinically, HFV has been found to maintain adequate oxygenation in patients with normal lungs. In patients with diseased lungs, adequate oxygenation is maintained, but PEEP requirements are not reduced.

In some cases, the elimination of carbon dioxide has been a problem. Patients with bronchopleural fistulas have also been ventilated adequately without production of an air leak through their chest tube. Animal studies indicate that HFV can be used without a balloon cuff as long as PEEP is not required.

Because HFV is more compatible physiologically, it does result in more efficient cardiac performance and oxygen transport than other traditional methods. Patients tend to require less analgesia and sedation because of a reduced tendency to fight the ventilator. The major concern is the design of a totally acceptable ventilator for delivery of HFV.

Ventilator Controls

Most ventilators have dials that are similar in function regardless of terminology. Understanding each dial's function will enable the nurse to manipulate the function of the ventilator to meet the changing needs of the patient.

Fraction of Inspired Oxygen (FIO_2). Most models enable direct dial-in oxygen percentage, FIO_2. However, the nurse must not assume that because 100% is dialed-in, the patient is receiving 100%. When a patient requires 50% or more of FIO_2 concentrations, the ventilator needs to be checked daily for accuracy with an oxygen analyzer. The newer models of volume ventilators, such as the MA-II and Bear, have oxygen analyzers in circuit with constant digital readouts of oxygen concentrations. However, the older models, such as the MA-I and Monaghan, have no oxygen analyzers in circuit. Indeed, as long as 50 psi (pounds per square inch) of compressed air is connected, the ventilator will function.

Respiratory Rate. The number of breaths per minute delivered to the patient can be directly dialed-in. In some models, the numbers are marked, whereas in models such as the Monaghan, the rate is timed for a full minute with a watch, and the dial set accordingly. Again, the nurse must not assume that just because the ventilator is set at a specified number of breaths per minute that this is what is being delivered. Double-check the functioning of the ventilator with a watch that has a second hand. The possibility of mechanical failure is always present.

In the pressure ventilator, the inspiratory time flow-rate control determines the duration of inspiration by regulating the velocity of gas flow. The higher the flow rate, the faster peak airway pressure is reached and the shorter the inspiration. The lower the flow rate, the longer the inspiration. A high flow rate produces turbulence, shallow inspirations, and uneven distribution of volume.

Tidal Volume. In the volume ventilator, a dial or crank is turned to the number of cc's (cubic centimeters) of air to be delivered with each breath. Again, in the pressure ventilator, manipulation of the inspiratory time flow-rate control determines the magnitude of inspiration. A low flow rate increases V_T and produces better alveolar ventilation than a high flow rate. Use of a Wright respirometer to measure exhaled air checks that the V_T dialed-in is being delivered (Figs. 15-8 and 15-9).

Peak Flow. This is the velocity of air flow per unit of time and is expressed as liters per minute. In the volume ventilator, this is a separate knob. In the pressure ventilator, this is manipulated, again, with the inspiratory time flow-rate control.

Installation of a demand valve in the newer volume ventilators enables a patient to receive the flow of air as he demands. The older models dump the air at the set rate (peak flow) dialed-in. The demand valve, besides decreasing airway turbulence, enhances patient comfort.

Pressure Limit. On the volume-cycled ventilators, this knob limits the highest pressure allowed in the ventilator circuit. Once the high pressure limit is reached, inspiration is terminated. Thus, if the pressure limit is being constantly reached, the designated V_T is not being delivered to the patient. The cause of this can be coughing, accumulation of secretions, kinked ventilator tubing, pneumothorax, decreasing compliance, or simply a pressure limit set too low.

Positive End Expiratory Pressure (PEEP). The PEEP knob adjusts the pressure that is maintained in the lungs at the end of expiration. If an intermittent mandatory ventilation (IMV) model is used, this knob may be labeled continuous positive airway pressure (CPAP). CPAP indicates that spontaneous breathing through the ventilator circuit is occurring (non-IMV breaths) and that at the end of these breaths, positive airway pressure is being maintained. PEEP can be visualized on the respiratory pressure gauge. Instead of dropping to zero at the end of expiration, the pressure needle drops to PEEP level (see Fig. 17-2).

In the newer ventilators, PEEP is built-in. The process by which one obtains PEEP on these ventilators is by keeping the exhalation valve inflated throughout the expiratory phase with a pressure equal to the amount of desired PEEP.

Several other devices can be used to apply PEEP externally on a ventilator or t-piece. They range from spring-loaded diaphragms and plastic cylinder ball valves to a container of water. These devices are applied on the exhalation port of the ventilator circuit. If water is used, for each 1 cm of exhalation tubing extending into the water, 1 cm of PEEP will be generated.

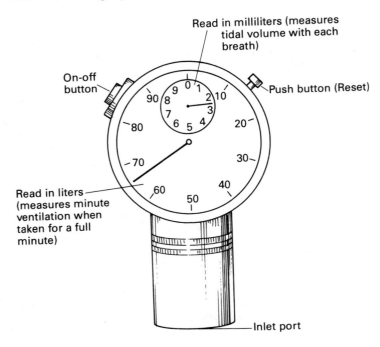

Read in milliliters (measures
tidal volume with each
breath)

On-off
button

Push button (Reset)

Read in liters
(measures minute
ventilation when
taken for a full
minute)

Inlet port

FIGURE 15-8
Wright respirometer — newer model.

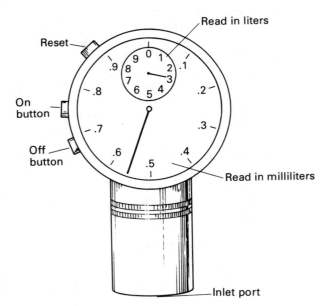

Read in liters

Reset

On
button

Off
button

Read in milliliters

Inlet port

FIGURE 15-9
Wright respirometer — older model.

Sensitivity. This controls the amount of patient effort as expressed by negative inspiratory pull needed to initiate an inspiration. Increasing the sensitivity decreases the amount of work the patient must do to initiate a ventilatory breath. Likewise, decreasing sensitivity increases the amount of negative pressure that the patient needs to initiate inspiration and increases the work of breathing. In some models, sensitivity may be totally dialed-out so that the ventilator is controlling the patient.

Sigh. To understand the function of this knob, a little history of initial attempts at mechanical ventilation must be reviewed. Because normal breathing consists of V_Ts at 5 ml/kg of body weight, patients were initially ventilated at these volumes. However, subsequent studies on dogs showed that atelectasis developed. In an attempt to mimic normal breathing, rather than V_T, a sigh mode was incorporated. A sigh mode delivers a bigger breath to patients at a designated volume and rate per hour. Presently, mechanical ventilation is performed at twice normal V_T; thus, with this practice, the need for sighs has been negated except in special cases such as refractive atelectasis.

Ventilatory Modes

Several different modes of ventilatory control can be found on ventilators. These modes can be separate dials, or they can be incorporated in the function of another knob such as sensitivity. Some of these modes are *assist, control, assist-control,* and *IMV*.

In the *assist mode,* only the breaths triggered by the patient at the designed V_T are delivered to the patient. In this mode, the patient *must* have a drive to breathe. If the patient is unable to trigger a breath, air will not be delivered.

In the *control mode,* the ventilator controls the patient. Breaths delivered to the patient will be at the rate and volume dialed-in on the ventilator, regardless of the patient's attempts to initiate an inspiration. If the patient is not unconscious or paralyzed, this mode can provoke high anxiety and discomfort.

The *assist-control mode* incorporates the preceding two modes. A basic rate can be set. If the patient wishes to breathe faster, he can trigger the ventilator (providing the sensitivity allows). If the patient's drive to breathe is negated, the ventilator will "kick-in" at the preset rate. This ensures that the patient will never stop breathing while on the ventilator. In the assist-control mode, all breaths—whether triggered by the patient or delivered at a set rate—are of the same tidal volume.

The *IMV mode* allows intermittent mandatory ventilation. As in the control mode, the rate and V_T are preset. If the patient wishes to breathe above this rate, he may. However, unlike the assist-control mode, any breaths he takes above the set rate are spontaneous breaths taken through the ventilator circuit. The V_T of these breaths may vary drastically from the V_T set on the ventilator because it is determined by the patient's ability to generate negative pressure in his chest. V_Ts may vary from 0 to 1 liter.

To understand IMV, one must review the basic functioning of the ventilator. Instantaneously, as the ventilator delivers a preset volume to the patient, a burst of air inflates a balloon in the exhalation port, forcing the air in only one direction—into the patient. When inspiration is terminated, the balloon deflates and air rushes into the area of least resistance—out the exhalation port. This occurs with every ventilator cycle in assist, control, and assist-control modes.

However, when the IMV mode is used, the balloon is inflated *only* during the *mandatory cycles.* The rate and V_T are dialed-in for only the IMV breaths. As the patient triggers above this rate, the balloon is not inflated. These are non-IMV breaths. Because the balloon is not inflated during these breaths, the ventilator bellows "dump" and air is delivered to the area of least resistance. If the patient generates negative pressure in his chest, some or all of the V_T dumped may be

FIGURE 15-10
Wright respirometer in-line circuit.

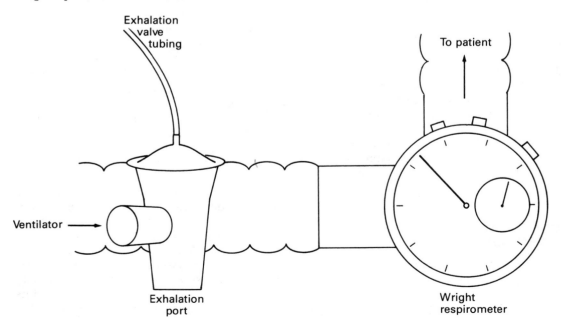

delivered to the patient. If the patient is unable to generate adequate negative pressure, all of the V_T dumped rushes out the exhalation port with none reaching the patient.

Because of this, accurate monitoring of *inspired* V_T must be done. On the newer ventilators, this is accomplished by a continuous digital readout of inspired V_T with alarms set accordingly. On the older models, such as the Monaghan, there are no such monitoring systems. The nurse or respiratory therapist *is the alarm system*. In these ventilators, Wright respirometers must be placed in line of the ventilator circuit between the patient and the exhalation port (Fig. 15-10). A total minute ventilation (MV) is calculated. From this, one subtracts the IMV MV to obtain the patient's MV.

$$\begin{array}{r} \text{Total MV} \\ -\ \text{IMV} \\ \hline = \text{Patient's MV} \end{array}$$

For example: the total MV, as measured in-line on the Wright respirometer, is 10 liters, and the ventilator is set for an IMV rate of 8 and V_T of 800. The following calculations produce the amount of patient's contribution to ventilation:

$$\begin{array}{lll} \text{Total MV} & 10 & \text{liters} \\ -\ \text{IMV MV} & \underline{6.4} & \text{liters} \quad (V_T \times \text{rate}) \\ \text{Patient's MV} & 3.6 & \text{liters} \end{array}$$

If the patient fatigues and drops his contribution to <3.6 liters, an arterial blood gas must be obtained to evaluate the $PaCO_2$. When the IMV rate is set very low and the patient fatigues, MV is reduced drastically. Because of this, the $PaCO_2$ elevates rapidly and the patient may have an arrest—on a mechanical ventilator. Use of IMV as a weaning tool will be discussed in the next section.

When selecting a patient for IMV, compliance and respiratory reserve must be evaluated. When compliance and reserve are both low and IMV is instituted, the work of breathing increases dramatically.

In the IMV mode, the mandatory breaths are delivered at a set rate regardless of whether the patient is in inspiration or expiration. Some ventilators have the IMV mode synchronized (SIMV) so that the mandatory breaths are delivered in synchrony with patient triggering. See Table 15-7 for clues to troubleshooting problems with the ventilator.

PHYSIOLOGICAL EFFECTS OF MECHANICAL VENTILATION

To understand the effects of mechanical ventilation, a review of normal respirations and their physiological effects is necessary.

With a normal respiration, *inspiration* is an *active* process. The intercostal muscles contract, pulling the rib cage upward and outward, and the diaphragm contracts downward, creating a *negative* pressure in the pleural cavity. When this subatmospheric pressure is generated, air moves into the lungs and ventilation occurs. In *expiration,* the thoracic cavity and lung tissue recoil, pushing air out of the lung and creating a *positive* pressure. This process is usually *passive.*

Hemodynamically, during inspiration, the fall in extrathoracic pressure decreases pressure in the great veins and atrium and acts as a suction pump. Venous return to the atrium is increased, resulting in increased ventricular output. During expiration, because of the positive pressures generated in the chest, venous return and cardiac output decrease.

In mechanical ventilation, the relationship between pressures in inspiration and expiration is *reversed.* The ventilator delivers air by virtually pumping it into the patient; thus, pressures during inspiration are positive. When a patient is placed on mechanical ventilation, hypotension may develop owing to the hemodynamic effects of the positive intrathoracic pressure. As PEEP is instituted, cardiac output may be affected even more because PEEP continues to keep positive pressure in the chest at all times. In addition, large V_Ts, greater than 10 to 12 ml/kg, which generate pressures greater than 40 cm H_2O, may not only influence the cardiac output but also increase the risk of pneumothorax.

The movement of air through the airways creates friction and turbulence. The more flow, the more friction. If the airway is narrowed, the friction increases even more. Thus, when inspiration is spontaneously generated, more negative pressure must be generated for a given flow of air to occur. During mechanical ventilation, more positive pressure is needed to deliver air through the narrowed airway.

Compliance. The lungs hold a volume of air. As more air is added, the lungs expand. Compare this with stretch or degree of elasticity. The resistance to stretch or lack of elasticity is compliance. Because volume determines stretch, compliance is equal to changes in volume divided by changes in pressure.

$$\text{compliance} = \frac{\text{volume (ml)}}{\text{pressure (cm } H_2O)} = \text{ml/cm}$$

Normal lung compliance is 200 ml/cm H_2O. Once the rib cage is added, this compliance drops to 100 ml/cm H_2O. As a lung becomes stiffer, as in adult respiratory distress syndrome (ARDS), increasing pressures are required to deliver the same volume. Therefore, compliance decreases. In contrast, where there is destruction of lung tissue, as in emphysema, elasticity is lost and the lung is more compliant. In terms of its compliance, the lung is frequently compared with a

TABLE 15-7
TROUBLESHOOTING THE VENTILATOR

Problem	Possible Causes	Action
Volume or pressure alarm on	*Patient-Related*	
	Patient disconnected from ventilator	Reconnect stat
	Loss of delivered tidal volume	Occlude endotracheal tube adaptor—if alarm goes off, there is a patient problem; if not, there is a ventilator problem
		Auscultate neck for possible leak around ET cuff
		Review chest film for endotracheal tube placement—may be too high
		Check for loss of tidal volume through chest tube
	Decrease in patient-initiated breaths	Evaluate patient for cause: check respiratory rate, ABGs, last sedation
	Increase in compliance	Good news! May be due to clearing of secretions or relief of bronchospasms
	Ventilator-related	
	Leaks	Check all tubing for loss of connection, starting at patient and moving towards the ventilator
		Tighten cascade humidifier
		Determine whether ventilator settings have changed
		Check for interference with spirometer dipstick
		Calibrate spirometer or pressure alarm
		If all else fails, replace exhalation valve

(*Note:* If problem is not corrected stat, bag-breathe patient until respirator problem is corrected)

Problem	Possible Causes	Action
	Decrease pressure to ventilator on pressure-driven ventilator (*e.g.,* Monaghan or Bird)	Have engineering dept. check pressure line; must deliver 50 psi
High-pressure or peak-pressure alarm	*Patient-Related*	
	Decreased compliance	
	Increased dynamic pressures	Suction patient
		Administer inhaled beta-agonists
		If sudden, evaluate for pneumothorax
		Alleviate coughing with sedation or lidocaine
		Try to change patient's position
		Evaluate chest film for endotracheal tube placement in right main stem bronchus
		Sedate if patient is bucking the ventilator or biting the ET tube
	Increased static pressures	Evaluate ABGs for hypoxia, fluids for overload, chest film for atelectasis
		Auscultate breath sounds
	Ventilator-Related	
	Tubing kinked	Check tubing
	Tubing filled with water	Empty water into a receptacle; do not drain back into the humidifier

(*Note:* Water in tubing will increase PEEP levels)

Problem	Possible Causes	Action
	Patient-ventilator asynchrony	Recheck sensitivity and peak flow settings
Abnormal ABGs	*Patient-Related*	
Hypoxia	Secretions	Suction
	Increase in disease pathology	Evaluate patient and chest film
	Positive fluid balance	Evaluate intake and output
Hypocapnia	Hypoxia	Evaluate ABGs and patient
	Increased lung compliance	Good news; evaluate for weaning potential
Hypercapnia	Sedation	Increase respiratory rate or tidal volume settings on ventilator
	Fatigue	
	Ventilator-Related	
Hypoxia	FIO$_2$ drift	Check ventilator with oxygen analyzer
		Possible blender piping failure
		Check oxygen source for failure
		Check oxygen reservoir for leaks
Hypocapnia	Settings not set correctly	Decrease respiratory rate, tidal volume, or minute ventilation settings. Consider dead space if assist control is used
Hypercapnia	Settings not set correctly	Increase respiratory rate, tidal volume, or minute ventilation settings.
Heater alarm	Addition of cool water to humidifier	Wait
	Altered setting	Reset
	Faulty temperature gauge	Replace gauge
	Thermostat failure	Replace heater

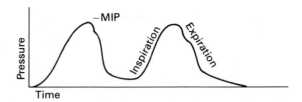

FIGURE 15-11
Graph depicting maximum inspiratory pressure. (MIP) *maximum inspiratory pressure.*

TABLE 15-8
FACTORS INFLUENCING MIP (MAXIMUM INSPIRATORY PRESSURE)

Flow resistance	Peak flow
	Size of airways
	Airway obstructions
	External obstructions (*i.e.,* kinked ventilator tubing or water in the tubing)
Lung resistance	Chest size
	Volume of air
	Elasticity of lung
Chest wall resistance	Chest wall deformities
	Position of patient
	External compression of chest wall or diaphragm (*i.e.,* distended abdomen)

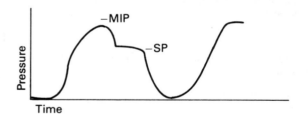

FIGURE 15-12
Graph depicting static pressure. (MIP) *maximum inspiratory pressure;* (SP) *static pressure.*

balloon. Initially it is hard to inflate, until it is stretched. After repeated inflations the elasticity is lost, and the balloon becomes very easy to blow up.

As the volume of gas is delivered to a patient on a mechanical ventilator, the respirator pressure gauge will slowly rise from zero to maximum inspiratory pressure (MIP). The rise in pressure is caused by resistance to flow or resistance to lung and chest wall inflation. A graph of pressure over time, depicting inspiration, would look like that shown in Figure 15-11.

Dynamic pressures and MIP can give an indication of flow properties of the airways (Table 15-8).

Static Pressure. Another measurement used to obtain compliance is static pressure (SP). SP is obtained by kinking the exhalation valve line when the patient is in maximum inspiration. This holds the volume of delivered air in the patient's chest by preventing exhalation. The pressure recorded at this moment is SP and reflects the force necessary to deliver the preset volume of air to the patient and hold the airways open. Graphically, it would appear as in Figure 15-12. Thus, dividing the V_T by the SP yields compliance.

Nursing Application. Clinically, compliance and airway dynamics can be applied in various situations. For example, an asthmatic patient being mechanically ventilated has a basic disease process affecting airway resistance with normal lung elasticity. In this situation, dynamic pressure would be high in contrast to SP, which would be near normal. When nebulized bronchodilators are administered, airway resistance decreases, and the respirator pressure gauge will reflect this by showing a lower dynamic pressure. In this way, the effectiveness of bronchodilators can be evaluated objectively.

In contrast, a patient with ARDS may have airway resistance near normal while compliance is very low, indicating a stiffness of the lung tissue. As the patient improves, compliance improves.

BIBLIOGRAPHY

Abu-Dbai J, Flatau E, Lev A, et al: The use of conventional ventilators for high-frequency positive pressure ventilation. Crit Care Med May, 1983, pp 356–358

Chin R, Pesce R: Practical aspects in management of respiratory failure in chronic obstructive pulmonary diseases. Crit Care Q Sept, 1983, pp 1–17

Davidson S: Nursing diagnosis: Its application in the acute care setting. Top Clin Nurs Jan, 1984, pp 50–56

Fletcher PR, Epstein MA, Epstein RA: A new ventilation for physiologic studies during high-frequency ventilation. Respiratory physiologic studies during high-frequency ventilation. Respir Physiol 1982, pp 21–37

Forman M: Nursing care planning. Am J Nurs June, 1979, pp 1086–1087

Froese A: High frequency ventilation. Am Rev Respir Dis Jan–Mar, 1981, pp 249–250

Hess D: Bedside monitoring of the patient on a ventilator. Crit Care Q Sept, 1983, pp 23–31

Kirby R: High-frequency positive pressure ventilation (HFPPV): What role in ventilatory insufficiency? Anesthesiology 1980, pp 109–110

Landis K, Smith S: The mechanically ventilated patient: A comprehensive nursing care plan. Crit Care Q 1980, pp 43–52

Malina JR, Nordstrom SG, Sjostrand UH, Wattwil LM: Clinical evaluation of high-frequency positive-pressure ventilation (HFPPV) in patients scheduled for open chest surgery. Anesthesia May, 1981, pp 324–330

Otto CW, Quan SF, Conahan TJ, et al: Hemodynamic effects of high-frequency jet ventilation. Anesth Analg Mar, 1983, pp 298–304

Smith RB, Klain M, Babinski M: Limits of high frequency percutaneous transtracheal jet ventilation using a fluidic logic controlled ventilator: Can Anaesth Soc J July, 1980, pp 351–356

Thompson WK, Marchak BE, Froese AB, Bryan AC: High-frequency oscillation compared with standard ventilation in pulmonary injury model. J Appl Physiol Mar, 1982, pp 543–548

Wattwil LM, Sjostrand UH, Borg UR: Comparative studies of IPPV and HFPPV with PEEP in critical care patients I: A clinical evaluation. Crit Care Med Jan, 1983, pp 30–37

Wattwil LM, Sjostrand UH, Borg UR, Eriksson IA: Comparative studies of IPPV and HFPPV with PEEP in critical care patients II: Studies on intrapulmonary gas distribution. Crit Care Med Jan, 1983, pp 38–43

Management of the Patient Requiring Ventilatory Support

Eileen Brent-Hemman

In most hospitals, the philosophy of respiratory care and ventilatory management depends on the philosophy of the pulmonary or anesthesia physicians who direct respiratory care. It is important that each team member be well acquainted with the basic guidelines of their philosophy.

ASPECTS OF THE MECHANICAL VENTILATOR

Humidification and Temperature

Mechanical ventilation bypasses the upper airway, thus negating the body's protective mechanism for humidification and warming. These two processes must be added—a humidifier with a temperature control. All air delivered by the ventilator passes through the water in the humidifier, being warmed and saturated. Because of this, no insensible water loss occurs. In most instances, the temperature of the air will be near body temperature. In some rare instances (severe hypothermia), the air temperature may be increased. Caution is advised because prolonged, high, inhaled temperatures can cause tracheal burns. Contrary to a dangerous myth, a dry humidifier does *not* decrease pulmonary edema! It only contributes to drying the airway, with resultant mucus plugging and an inability to suction-out secretions.

As the air is passed through the ventilator to the patient, large droplets are rained-out in the corrugated hose. This moisture is considered contaminated and must be drained into a receptacle and not back into the sterile humidifier. If the water is allowed to build up, resistance is developed in circuit and positive end expiratory pressure (PEEP) is generated. In addition, if left unchecked, the water may be aspirated by the patient. Attention to this is a primary nursing responsibility.

Initial Settings

Before placing a patient on a ventilator, attach it to a test lung to adjust the settings to the standard guidelines.

Standard Setting

- Fraction of inspired oxygen (FIO_2)   100%
- Tidal volume (V_T)   10–15 ml/kg body weight
- Respiratory rate (RR)   10–15 breaths/minute
- Inspiratory flow   40–60 liters/second
- Sensitivity   −2 cm H_2O
- Sigh rate (optional)   1–2/min, V_T 20 ml/kg
- Positive end expiratory pressure (PEEP)   0–5 cm

Settings for the patient will be determined by the goals of the therapy, and changes of the settings will be determined by the patient's response as reflected in arterial blood gases.

Fraction of Inspired Oxygen (FIO_2)

Initially the patient without a previous blood gas analysis is usually placed on 100% oxygen. When the PaO_2 on 100% has been established, calculation by the alveolar air equation can be used to determine an FIO_2 concentration for a *target* PaO_2 (see accompanying chart).

Respiratory Rate and Tidal Volume

RR times the V_T determines minute ventilation (MV). In turn, MV determines alveolar ventilation. These two parameters are adjusted according to the $PaCO_2$. Increasing MV decreases $PaCO_2$; conversely, decreasing MV increases $PaCO_2$. There are special cases, however, in which hypoventilation or hyperventilation may be desired. For example, in a head injury, the neurosurgeon may wish a respiratory alkalosis to occur to promote cerebral vasoconstriction. In this case, the V_T and RR are increased to achieve the desired alkalotic *p*H by $PaCO_2$ manipulation. In contrast, chronic obstructive pulmonary disease (COPD) patients

Calculating Alveolar Air

PAO_2 = partial pressure of O_2 in alveolus
PaO_2 = partial pressure of O_2 in arteries
PIO_2 = partial pressure of inspired O_2
$PACO_2$ = partial pressure of CO_2 in alveolus
$PaCO_2$ = partial pressure of CO_2 in arteries
($PACO_2$ = the patient's $PaCO_2$)
R = respiratory quotient = 1 on O_2 = 0.8
on room air and reflects $\dfrac{CO_2 \text{ production}}{O_2 \text{ consumption}}$

Pb = barometric pressure
PH_2O = water pressure

Alveolar Air Equation: $PAO_2 = PIO_2 - \dfrac{PACO_2}{R}$

STEP 1: $PIO_2 = FIO_2 (Pb - PH_2O)$

STEP 2: Substituting the following given values,

aPb of 647 torr
PH_2O of 47 torr

and a patient on 100% O_2 with a $PaCO_2$ of 40 torr, the equation would read:

$$PAO_2 = 1.00(647 - 47) - \frac{40}{1}$$

$$= 1.00(600) - 40$$
$$= 600 - 40$$
$$= 560 \text{ torr}$$

STEP 3: Blood gases are drawn on 100% FIO_2 with the following results:

$pH = 7.40$
$PaO_2 = 300$ torr
$PaCO_2 = 40$ torr

STEP 4: To calculate *target* PaO_2, set PaO_2 and PAO_2 in ratio form.
Because normal PaO_2 in Denver is 65 to 75 torr, target PaO_2 would be 75 torr.

(Equation) $\dfrac{PAO_2}{PaO_2}$ = $\dfrac{560}{300}$ = $\dfrac{x}{75}$
(Blood gas)

x = the PAO_2 to give a target PaO_2 of 75 torr

$$(560)\,75 = 300x$$
$$\frac{(560)\,75}{300} = x$$
$$140 = x$$

From these calculations, to have a PaO_2 of 75 torr, a PAO_2 of 140 is needed.

STEP 5: Now to find the FIO_2 that gives a PAO_2 of 140, substitute the values into the alveolar air equation. (Assume everything else stays constant.)

$$140 = x\,(647 - 47) - \frac{40}{1}$$

$$x = \text{target } FIO_2$$
$$140 = x\,(600) - 40$$
$$180 = 600x$$
$$.30 = x$$

STEP 6: Therefore, for a target PaO_2 of 75 torr, the FIO_2 on the ventilator can be reduced to 30%.

---

whose baseline arterial blood gases consist of elevated carbon dioxide need to be mechanically hypoventilated at their baseline, $PaCO_2$. These patients usually have a large acid load, and lowering their carbon dioxide levels rapidly may result in seizures. Patients with restrictive diseases need careful monitoring of their blood gases because they may need lower V_T and higher RR.

Peak Flow

If MV is high, peak flow may need to be increased to provide time for exhalation before a new inhalation is triggered. However, remember that increasing peak flow increases turbulence, which is reflected in increasing airway pressures.

Positive End Expiratory Pressure (PEEP)

Positive end expiratory pressure is primarily instituted for refractive hypoxemia. Currently, PEEP is also being used to control postoperative bleeding in patients who have undergone coronary artery surgery. PEEP is thought to exert a tamponade effect on the area of bleeding.

In patients who require greater than 50% oxygen concentrations for prolonged periods of time, the risk of oxygen toxicity increases. Because oxygen toxicity is time-dose related, PEEP is instituted to decrease the need for high FIO_2 concentrations. It is important to weigh the risk of PEEP against the risk of oxygen concentrations. The physiological effects of PEEP on cardiac output and tissue oxygenation must be monitored through the use of mixed venous and arterial blood gases. Mixed venous blood gases are drawn from the distal port of the Swan-Ganz catheter, slowly over 2 to 3 minutes. Mixed venous oxygen is a reflection of tissue oxygenation. Tissue oxygenation is determined by the following:

• The amount of oxygen that passes through the lungs and into the arteries (PaO_2)
• The number of oxygen carriers present (hemoglobin)

• The ability of the heart to circulate the oxygenated blood to tissues (cardiac output)

In the patient who does not have adequate circulating blood volume, institution of PEEP decreases blood return to the heart, decreases cardiac output, and decreases oxygen to the tissues. With an increase in PEEP, arterial oxygenation may improve, but if mixed venous oxygenation worsens, PEEP is not therapeutic. If hypotension or decreased cardiac output results from PEEP application, restoring circulating volume usually corrects the hypotension.

PEEP is usually increased in increments of 5 cm of water pressure. Mixed venous and arterial blood gases are drawn beforehand for baseline values and repeated 20 minutes after the setting is adjusted.

PEEP holds the alveoli open by maintaining a pressure greater than atmospheric pressure in the alveoli at the end of expiration. This end expiratory pressure increases functional residual capacity (FRC) by reinflating collapsed alveoli, keeping the alveoli open, and decreasing the pressure needed to ventilate them. In addition, there is some evidence that keeping the alveoli open may enhance surfactant regeneration. If a patient requires high levels of PEEP for a prolonged period of time, decreasing PEEP must be done slowly over a period of time. Within 4 hours after PEEP is decreased, airways may start to collapse again owing to hypoxia.

Hemodynamic measurements (PCWP, PAD, PAS) are taken at end-expiration. If PEEP is utilized, the patient is taken off the ventilator so that consistent readings can be obtained. PEEP can inflate hemodynamic values, depending on the lung zone into which the catheter has floated. For example, if the catheter has floated into the apical area, where vascular pressures are usually lower than airway pressures, PEEP is easily transmitted. If the catheter floats into the lung bases, where vascular pressures are usually greater than airway pressures, PEEP is not so readily transmitted unless higher levels are used.

Sensitivity

One can set sensitivity in some machines by turning the knob (increasing sensitivity) to the point that the ventilator "chatters." Chatter comes from the sound of the ventilator constantly dumping. The dial is then slowly decreased to the point at which the chattering stops. At this point, the ventilator can be triggered when a −2 cm is generated.

Some physicians prefer to have the patient trigger the ventilator. Keeping the patient in control of the ventilator enables him to adjust his own MV as needed. This will also be of benefit to the patient when he is weaned from the ventilator. In contrast, some physi-

cians prefer to paralyze, anesthetize, dial-out the sensitivity, or increase MV so the patient does not initiate respiration on the ventilator. They prefer to rest the patient while the ventilator does the work of breathing. In the latter case, psychological support must be provided if the patient is alert and awake.

Addition of PEEP may change the sensitivity on a ventilator. For example, if the machine is set so that generation of −2 cm initiates respiration, the patient triggers the ventilator by "sucking" the dial from zero to −2. If 10 cm of PEEP are added, the ventilator is still triggered at a −2 cm. However, now the patient must suck the needle from 10 to −2 (−12 cm pressure) to initiate a breath. This increases the patient's work of breathing. Because of this increased work, the patient may stop triggering the machine, decreasing his MV. To correct this, the sensitivity is increased so that inspiration is initiated at 8 cm of pressure. Thus, when the patient sucks the needle from 10 cm to 8 (−2 cm), the work of breathing is decreased to the initial level. If PEEP is decreased to levels less than 8 cm, sensitivity must also be decreased or oversensitivity occurs, resulting in a severe respiratory alkalosis from mechanical hyperventilation (Fig. 15-13).

Dead Space

Dead space is a term designating the addition of tubing between the patient and the exhalation valve. In essence, the patient is rebreathing his exhaled CO_2. Indication for additional dead space is a respiratory alkalosis not mechanically correctable through manipulation of RR and V_T. Clinically, for some physiological reason, the patient is hyperventilating. This type of high ventilatory output failure is often seen in adult respiratory distress syndrome (ARDS). Because it is desirable to correct this alkalosis by correcting the primary arterial blood gas abnormality (increased $PaCO_2$), dead space is sometimes added.

When adding dead space, an MV must be calculated before and after application. Some patients appear very sensitive to $PaCO_2$ levels. Indeed, if 5 inches of dead space are added, they may increase their MV so that the effect on the $PaCO_2$ values is negligible, and continued addition of vast inches of dead space may force the patient into agonal breathing.

There is no set formula for calculating inches of dead space for rises in $PaCO_2$. This is a trial-and-error process. Because 5 inches constitute a negligible amount, 10 inches are usually applied initially.

It must be stressed that *mechanical manipulation of $PaCO_2$ must be based on pH values*. In other words, if a patient is in metabolic acidosis and his $PaCO_2$ is low because of this, dead space is not indicated. Additional dead space at this time would force the patient into a more severe acidosis.

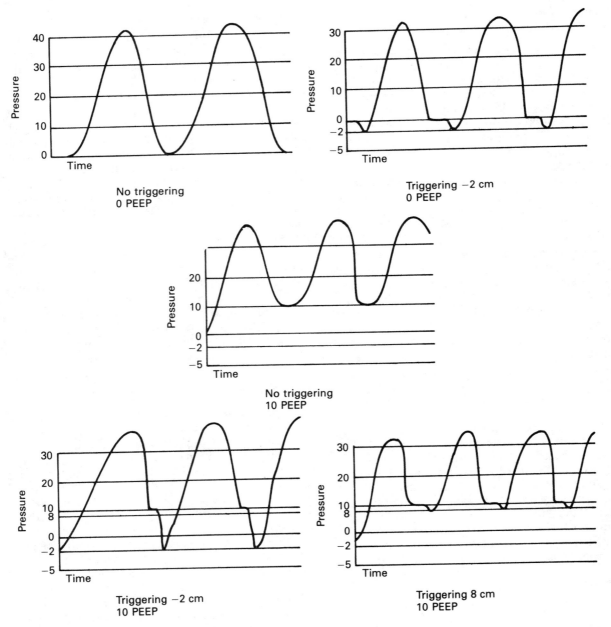

FIGURE 15-13
Respiratory wave forms with different settings of PEEP and triggering.

Lastly, because the partial pressures of CO_2 and O_2 largely determine the total pressure of inhaled gas on a ventilator, increasing the $PaCO_2$ may slightly lower the oxygen values.

Alarm Systems

Mechanical ventilators are used to support life. Alarm systems are necessary to warn the nurse of developing problems. Alarm systems can be categorized according to volume versus pressure and high versus low.

Low-pressure alarms warn of disconnection from the patient. High-pressure alarms warn of rising pressures. Low-volume alarms warn of leaks. Electrical failure alarms are a *must* for all ventilators.

NURSING CARE OF THE PATIENT REQUIRING VENTILATORY SUPPORT

The patient who needs ventilatory support also needs primary nursing care. Critical care units, mechanical ventilators, and intubation naturally evoke psychologi-

TABLE 15-9
NURSING CARE PLAN FOR THE MECHANICALLY VENTILATED PATIENT

Nursing Diagnosis	Goal	Nursing Interventions
Potential for ineffective breathing patterns related to ventilator failure	Identify and correct potential causes of ventilator failure	Every 2 hours, check ventilator and document findings. Respond to all alarms and diagnose etiology of problem stat. Keep manual resuscitator at bedside. Prevent tubing from kinking or disconnect.
Inadequate nutritional intake	Maintain nutritional status of patient	Develop a team plan based on routine nutritional assessment. Administer tube feedings, hyperalimentation, or phospholipids as ordered. Evaluate results and complications.
Potential for infection	Prevention of infection by use of basic infection control measures	Wash hands before and after suctioning. Evaluate color, consistency, and odor of sputum. Collect specimen for culture and sensitivity as indicated. Change ventilator tubing every 24 hours. Drain condensed water into a receptacle not back into the humidifier. Prevent aspiration of water into endotracheal tube.
Ineffective airway clearance	Maintain patency of endotracheal tube	Suction frequently with pre- and posthyperoxygenation. Instill and irrigate with normal saline if secretions are tenacious. Change tube as needed to maintain ventilation. Humidify airway to prevent plugging. Use a bite block or oral airway to prevent patient from biting endotracheal tube. Auscultate breath sounds frequently.
	Prevention of tracheal malacia or stenosis	Use low-pressure cuff tubes. Record cuff pressures every 2 hours. Maintain pressures in endotracheal tube cuff of $\leq$ 20 mm hg or use the minimal cuff leak technique. Tape tube securely in place without placing pressure on any facial area. Sedate or evaluate for weaning if patient is thrashing or restless. Restrain patient if needed to prevent self-extubation. Rotate tube from side to side every day; provide oral hygiene. Inspect daily the oral and nasal areas for signs of pressure or necrosis. Properly position and support ventilator tubing and use flexible connectors to keep the weight off patient's facial structures.
Alteration in comfort; potential pressure sores	Alleviation of physical stress through intervention by basic bedside nursing techniques	Administer sedatives or analgesics as needed. Turn the patient frequently and reposition. Be alert for pressure areas. Use flotation devices as necessary. Maintain comfortable environment. Allow patient to sit up in chair or walk outside if he can tolerate. Maintain cleanliness of patient and his environment. Be alert for signs of hypoxia and dyspnea. Evaluate patient for potential of stress ulcers.
Ineffective individual coping; sensory perception changes; powerlessness; impaired verbal communication	Lessening of stress	Reassure and support patient and family. Be visible. Provide call device for patient and answer as quickly as possible. Explain all procedures before doing them. Give patient an opportunity to make at least one decision per day. Provide media for conversation. Be present whenever patient is weaning. Treat patient in a humane manner. Be consistent and set limitations to manipulative behavior if it occurs. Provide the patient with privacy. Explain alarms to patient. Plan care around blocks of sleep time. Minimize noise. Provide stimulation and orientation of patient through use of familiar objects (*e.g.,* clock, newspapers)

cal stress. Communications are frustrating and anxiety-producing because the intubated patient will not be able to speak. Each patient must be told that the tube prevents him from talking and that there is nothing wrong with his voice. Perhaps he can write or use sign language to indicate his messages, and the nurse can be more aware of nonverbal communications and body language. A suggested plan of care is outlined in Table 15-9.

Airway Care

Airway care must consist of adequate humidification, suctioning, and monitoring.

Humidification and warming (discussed earlier) are accomplished by mechanical additions to the ventilator to prevent airway obstruction from dry secretions and mucus plugs.

Suctioning is done hourly *and* whenever necessary. Aseptic technique is used to reduce airway contamination, and the patient must be oxygenated with 100% oxygen both before and after suctioning.

Routine auscultation of the chest enables monitoring of results from therapy and alerts the nurse to any problems such as increasing fluid overload, secretions, bronchospasms, or slippage of the tube into the right main stem bronchus. If bronchospasms are present, administration of bronchodilators needs to be considered. When secretions become a problem, vigorous suctioning and "bagging" after postural drainage, percussion, and vibration must be instituted. The reader is referred to previous sections in Chapter 14 for details.

Tube Care

All endotracheal tubes must be anchored securely to prevent tube movement (Fig. 15-4). If taping obscures skin areas, septum or lip necrosis may occur. Because oral hygiene is given everyday, it is an opportune time

FIGURE 15-14
Monitoring cuff pressures.

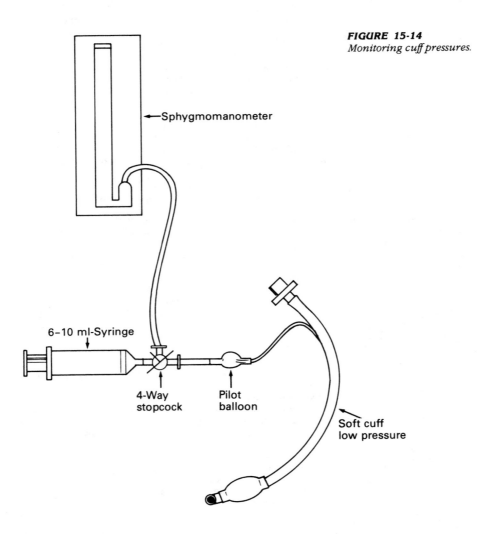

Sphygmomanometer

6–10 ml-Syringe

4-Way stopcock

Pilot balloon

Soft cuff low pressure

to inspect the skin, nose, and mouth for tissue breakdown. Placement of an oral bite block will prevent the patient from biting on the tube or displacing the tube with his tongue. The use of a swivel connector (connecting the tube to the ventilator circuit), along with anchoring a large loop of tubing to the bed, will facilitate patient movement without tube movement.

Tube Cuff Pressures

Tube cuff pressures are monitored every shift to prevent overdistention and excess pressure on the tracheal wall. When a patient is on the ventilator, the best pressure is the lowest possible pressure without having a leak of V_T. Physiologically, arterial circulation to the tracheal wall is obliterated by pressures near 30 torr. If a cuff leak is suspected by a discrepancy in actual versus measured V_T, auscultation at the neck for air turbulence can determine whether the seal is adequate. If the patient is not on a ventilator, the pressure is arbitrarily set at 20 torr. Figure 15-14 shows the procedure of cuff monitoring:

1. The pilot balloon tubing is attached to a syringe and mercury manometer by a four-way stopcock.
2. The stopcock is turned off to the patient.
3. Air pressure is added to the system by compressing the syringe until the mercury manometer reads 20 torr.
4. The stopcock is then turned on to the patient, manometer, and syringe. Pressure can be increased or decreased by manipulation of the syringe.
5. After the pressure is set, preferably at 20 or less, the stopcock is closed to the pilot balloon and the manometer.
6. The pressures are then recorded on the ventilator flowsheet.

Gastrointestinal (GI) Care

Owing to the increased physical and psychological stress, GI bleeds are a potential occurrence. Hourly antacids instilled by way of a nasogastric tube help neutralize gastric acidity. Also, cimetidine can be given prophylactically.

Nutritional Support

Nutritional support of ventilated patients should be instituted early. Current research verifies that there are many side effects of clinical starvation that can lead to pulmonary complication and death (Table 15-10).

Respiratory Muscles

Respiratory muscles, like all other body muscles, need energy to work. Once energy needs are not met, muscle fatigue occurs. Muscle fatigue leads to discoordination of respiratory muscles and a decrease in tidal volume. Hypomagnesemia and hypophosphatemia have been implicated in muscle fatigue due to depleted levels of ATP.

With prolonged starvation the body cannibalizes the intercostal and diaphragmatic muscles for energy. In addition, the respiratory muscles of a patient on long-term ventilation atrophy from inactivity and passive movement by the ventilator. If clinical starvation is not corrected weaning may be impossible.

Starvation has also been linked to emphysematous changes. In starvation, protein synthesis is decreased, which in turn adversely affects lung tissue elasticity and surfactant production. The potential for pulmonary infection is increased because the normal bacterial clearance mechanisms and immunological competence are impaired.

Central Nervous System

Normally hypoxia or hypercapnia stimulates an increase in the rate and depth of breathing. Starvation for 20 days in a normal person weakens this response. When starvation is corrected, the response is normalized. This response can also be acquired as the result of long-term residence at high altitudes or can be inherited.

Nutritional Replacement

If the gastrointestinal tract is intact, nutrition can be provided via a feeding tube. The concentration is initially diluted, and the rate of administration is slow. The patient is observed for side effects such as diarrhea or hyperosmolar dehydration. Blood sugar determinations and urinalyses for sugar and acetone are done. If the patient tolerates the tube feedings, first the rate and then the concentration are increased.

If tube feedings cannot be tolerated, parenteral hyperalimentation is considered. If used, one must observe strict aseptic technique to minimize the risk of infection. Basic caloric requirements are usually increased by 25% for hospital activity and stress associated with treatment. Large glucose loads increase

TABLE 15-10
RESULTS OF CLINICAL STARVATION

Atrophy of respiratory muscles
Decreased protein
Decreased albumin
Decreased cell mediated immunity
Decreased surfactant production
Decreased replication of respiratory epithelium
Intracellular depletion of ATP
Impaired cellular oxygenation
Central respiratory depression

CO_2 production and may precipitate respiratory failure in a compromised patient. High amino acid infusion also increases oxygen consumption.

Psychological Care

The ventilated patient is subjected to extreme physical and emotional stress in the critical care environment. Sleep deprivation and sensory overstimulation occur daily in a repetitive cycle. Treatment may often seem dehumanizing. In many cases, the prognosis is poor and the possibility of death is ever present. Feelings of helplessness and lack of control may be overwhelming. The patient may attempt to gain some element of environmental control through complaining or constant demanding. If the patient's coping mechanisms are incapable of dealing with stress, he may totally withdraw, exhibiting apathy and lack of emotional involvement.

If a patient has been struggling for years to breathe, assisted ventilation may precipitate a psychological dependence. It seems logical that if for the first time in years a patient is receiving enough oxygen to meet his metabolic needs and does not have to struggle for air, he would be reluctant to give up this feeling of normalcy. In this situation, weaning may become even more stressful for staff and patient. In fact, the patient may never wean because the staff is reluctant to "torture" the patient during the weaning process.

This is a stressful time for the family of a patient in the critical care unit. They must deal with a strange environment, a critically ill loved one, and the financial strain imposed by the illness. As soon as possible, the family should be familiarized with the physical surroundings, informed of visiting hours, and given progress reports on the condition of the patient. If the patient is critical, visiting hours can be made flexible until the patient stabilizes. Each member of the health care team should be aware of the established guidelines for family involvement in patient care.

Once the initial crisis is over, a nursing care plan for a coordinated approach to the patient should be developed. Inherent in the plan is the opportunity for the patient to gain some control over his environment and the activities of daily living. A plan must include ways to minimize the work of breathing, periods of rest, and ways to decrease traffic and noise (see Table 15-9).

COMPLICATIONS OF MECHANICAL VENTILATION

The patient on a mechanical ventilator requires observant, skillful, and *repetitive* nursing care. Complications that may occur with this therapy can be minimized—*prevention* is the key.

Airway Complications

Aspiration can occur before, during, or after intubation. One can minimize the risk of aspiration after intubation by securing the tube, maintaining an inflated cuff, and continuing adequate tube or oral suctioning. If resuscitation was prolonged and gastric distention occurred, the airway must be secured before one passes a nasogastric tube for stomach decompression. Once aspiration does occur, the potential for the development of ARDS increases.

Most ventilator patients need to be restrained on both hands because self-extubation with aspiration is an ever present complication. In addition, self-extubation with an inflated cuff can result in vocal cord damage.

The procedure of intubation itself is a high risk. Examples of intubation complications include the following:

• Prolonged and complicated intubation → increased hypoxia and tracheal trauma
• Mainstem intubation (usually right) → unequal ventilation, increasing the mortality rate
• Intubation of pyriform sinus (rare) → pharyngeal abscess

Mechanical Complications

Ventilator malfunctioning is a potentially serious problem at all times. Hourly checks of the ventilator by the nurse can minimize or spot potentials for existing problems. At this time, alarms must be checked for proper functioning and be noted.

If the tube is placed nasotracheally, a severe sinus infection can develop. Alternatively, because of the position of the tube in the pharynx, the orifice to the inner ear may become occluded, resulting in a severe otitis media. Whenever a patient complains of ear or sinus pain or develops a fever of unknown etiology, the sinuses and ears must be checked for possible sources of infection.

Some degree of tracheal damage results from prolonged intubation. Tracheal stenosis and malacia can be minimized if cuff pressures are minimized. Arterial circulation is occluded around cuff pressures of 30 torr. A decreased incidence of both stenosis and malacia has been reported when cuff pressures are kept near 20 torr. If laryngeal edema is present, life-threatening postextubation stridor can occur.

Pseudomonas pneumonia frequently develops in cases of prolonged intubation and is always a potential possibility from contaminated equipment.

The last frequently encountered problem involves alveolar ventilation. Alveolar hypoventilation is significantly associated with COPD and hypotension, whereas alveolar hyperventilation is associated with prolonged time on the ventilator. Hypoventilation increases the mortality of ventilation. Hyperventilation may or may not increase mortality, but it does produce a high alkalotic *p*H that can result in seizures and a significant drop in cardiac output. With a right mainstem intubation, the right lung is overventilated and develops significant atelectasis. The incidence of pneumothorax increases (Table 15-11).

WEANING FROM MECHANICAL VENTILATION

From the time the patient is placed on mechanical ventilation, the goal of weaning is present. The process to achieve this goal includes

• Correction of the cause of respiratory failure
• Maintenance of muscle strength
• Proper nutrition
• Psychological preparation

Each of these phases is as important as the other for a successful discontinuance of ventilatory support.

Each patient is evaluated daily for the possibility of weaning. Generally, patients are categorized as

• Short-term ventilation recipients experiencing uncomplicated extubation

---

TABLE 15-11
COMPLICATIONS OF MECHANICAL VENTILATION

Airway
  Aspiration
  Decreased clearance of secretions
  Predisposition to infection
Endotracheal Tube
  Tube kinked
  Tube plugged
  Rupture of pyriform sinus
  Tracheal stenosis
  Tracheal malacia
  Right main stem intubation
  Cuff failure
  Sinusitis
  Otitis media
  Laryngeal edema
Mechanical
  Ventilator malfunction
  Hypoventilation
  Hyperventilation
  Tension pneumothorax
Physiological
  Water and NaCl retension
  Left ventricular dysfunction → hypotension
  Stress ulcers
  Paralytic ileus
  Gastric distention

• Long-term ventilation recipients requiring prolonged weaning time

The former usually require only a short trial of 20 minutes before extubation; the latter require a tedious 3 to 4 weeks of weaning associated with numerous problems.

The criteria listed in Table 15-12 are suggested for assessing the patient's potential to be weaned. All criteria must be evaluated within the context of the patient's disease process and his capabilities.

Short-Term Weaning

Before any weaning is initiated, proper preparation of the patient is necessary. All patient resources must be mobilized. Patients ventilated for 24 to 48 hours meet the criteria for short-term weaning, provided that the initial cause necessitating ventilation is corrected. Standard steps in weaning are as follows:

TABLE 15-12
CRITERIA FOR POTENTIAL WEANING FROM VENTILATOR

RR	15–20 breaths/min
MV*	6–12 liters
V_T	5 ml/kg of body weight
VC	10 ml/kg of body weight
MVV†	12–20 liters
Inspiratory pressure‡	20 cm H_2O
Compliance	>20 ml/cm H_2O pressure
FIO_2 requirements	<50%
No PEEP	
Adequate ABG values§	
Physiologically stable§	

* Minute Ventilation. If MV is higher than 20 liters, the work of breathing is high. The patient may well wean, but after a couple of hours may fatigue and need to be reintubated. When MV is less than 6 liters, hypoventilation will occur. The etiology for hypoventilation needs to be investigated because often the cause will be sedation.

† Maximum Voluntary Ventilation (MVV) is obtained by having the patient breathe as hard and as fast as he can for 15 seconds. Multiply this by 4 and the answer is total MVV for one minute. MVV is an objective measurement of the patient's ventilatory reserve. If the patient's work of breathing postextubation is increased and ventilatory reserve is low, reintubation may be needed.

‡ Inspiratory Pressure. Inspiratory pressure gives an indication of inspiratory muscle strength. A pressure less than −20 ml/cm H_2O pressure indicates muscle weakness. The work of breathing will be very costly and fatigue will result.

§ Vital Signs and Blood Gases. When the decision has been made to have the patient try spontaneous breathing, baseline vital signs and arterial blood gases are obtained. It is preferable that the patient be well rested and that he receive an inhaled bronchodilator prior to weaning. Blood pressure, pulse, and respiratory rates are monitored frequently during the weaning, and at the end of 20 to 30 minutes arterial blood gases are drawn along with measurements of V_T, MV, and RR. These results will indicate the appropriateness of extubation.

TABLE 15-13
CRITERIA TO EVALUATE DURING WEANING

Category	Criteria	Termination Criteria
Physiological data	Pulse	Increase > 20 beats/minute
	Blood pressure	Systolic drop of 20 mm Hg
	Respiratory rate	Systolic rise of 30 mm Hg
		>25, <8/minute
Psychological/ subjective observations	Dyspnea	
	Panic	
	Pain	
	Fatigue	
Objective observations	Arrythmias	PVCs > 4/minute
	Accessory muscle use	Increased
	Intercostal retractions	Increased
	Flaring of nostrils	Increased
	Breathing pattern	Eratic

1. Start weaning in the morning, not at night when the patient is tired.
2. Explain the procedure to the patient.
3. Suction.
4. Obtain spontaneous parameters.
5. Administer bronchodilators if ordered.
6. Suction.
7. Rest the patient for 15 to 20 minutes.
8. Elevate the head of the bed.
9. Stay with the patient; support, reassure, and evaluate the patient's response to weaning.

T-Piece

If weaning by T-piece is selected, the following procedure is recommended. Collect all physiological data (Table 15-13). Connect the T-piece set at the desired FIO_2 to the patient. Usually, a period of 30 minutes on a T-piece is sufficient to evaluate the potential for extubation. Continue to collect physiological data every 5 to 10 minutes or as needed. At the end of 30 minutes, collect arterial blood gases and evaluate the patient for signs of fatigue. If the criteria for weaning (Table 15-12) are met at this time, extubation is warranted. Extubation should not be done unless someone qualified to reintubate is present. Postextubation stridor is sudden and can be fatal. Use of inhaled racemic epinephrine can be tried to constrict capillaries topically and to decrease edema.

Intermittent Mandatory Ventilation (IMV)

Short-term weaning by intermittent mandatory ventilation (IMV) is as effective as T-piece weaning. IMV may involve more time because each incremental rate decrease must be followed by a blood gas determination. The steps outlined for T-piece weaning apply to IMV.

The IMV rate is usually decreased by increments of two until a rate of two or zero is reached. At this point, the patient can be evaluated by the weaning criteria to determine the potential for extubation.

Weaning by any method should be terminated if any of the termination criteria are seen. Collection of arterial blood gases and vital capacity before termination can provide data on which to base further weaning plans.

Nursing Care Study

A 69-year-old man weighing 67 kg was admitted to the recovery room after coronary artery bypass. Initially he was placed on

IMV	10
FIO_2	100%
PEEP	5 cm
V_T	800 cc

Subsequent arterial blood gases revealed

pH	7.38
PaO_2	520
$PaCO_2$	38

The oxygen was reduced to 60%, then 40%, and arterial blood gases documented a normal oxygen level. The patient continued hemodynamically stable throughout the evening and was treated only with renal dose dopamine and two units of 5% albumin. At 11:00 P.M.

TABLE 15-14
ADJUNCTS TO WEANING

Fenestrated trach	Provides for communication during weaning periods
Kistner button	Provides for communication during weaning periods
	Less resistance to breathing and coughing up secretions than the fenestrated trach
Large ET tubes	Small diameter endotracheal tubes increase resistance to breathing, thereby increasing the work of breathing
Postural drainage and percussion	Aids in removal of secretions
Exercise	Provides increased stimulation to breathing
	Increases and changes environmental stimuli
Nutrition	Provides energy for breathing
	Maintains protein balance
	Aids in resistance to infection
IPPB	Provides periods of hyperinflation and rest during weaning periods
	May maintain patient when weaned
Ear oximetry	Provides noninvasive monitoring of oxygen saturation

TABLE 15-15
BASIC OXYGEN DELIVERY SYSTEMS

Method	Rate of Flow (Liters/Minute)	Oxygen Delivered (%)	Features
Cannula	2 3 4 5 6	23%–28% 28%–30% 32%–36% 40% max 44%	Convenient Comfortable Nasal passages must be patent Can be used in mouth breathers Exact O_2% depends on pt's minute ventilation >6 liters/minute dries mucous membranes Allows talking, eating
Catheter	Same as cannula		Less comfortable May cause abdominal distention >6 liters/minute dries mucous membranes
Simple mask	5 6 8	40 45–50 55–60	Confining Does not allow eating, coughing Tight face seal necessary Must have >5 liters/minute to flush CO_2 from mask
Partial rebreather	6 8 10 12 15	35 40–50 60 60 60	Confining Tight seal is necessary Does not allow eating or coughing Bag may twist or kink

(Continued)

TABLE 15-15
(Continued)

Valve

Non-rebreather

6	55–60	Same as partial	
8	60–80	Never let bag totally deflate	
10	80–90	All rubber diaphragms must be in	
12	90	place and not stick	
15	90		

Venturi mask

Jet adapter

*Color**			
Blue: 4	24	Delivers exact O_2 concentration despite pt's minute ventilation
Yellow: 4–6	28	Confining
White: 6–8	31	Must fit tight
Green: 8–10	35	Doesn't allow for coughing or eating
Pink: 8–12	40	If humidity is added, use compressed air so as to not alter O_2 concentration
Orange: 12	50	

T-tube

O_2% is dialed in on humidifier — Allows humidity for ET or trach tube
Flow should be high enough to cover pt's minute ventilation — Empty condensation in tubing — Mist should be visible on exhalation end

* Colors refer to Inspiron venturi ports, which are designed to deliver a factory-established percentage of O_2 when set at the specified rate of liter flow.

he awoke, made no effort to initiate ventilations, and drifted back to sleep immediately.

At 6:00 A.M. the patient was easily arousable, physiologically stable, and initiating an occasional breath. The IMV rate was decreased by increments of two until a rate of two was reached. Spontaneous parameters at this time revealed

V_T	400 cc
VC	1000 cc
V_E	4.8 liters
Respiratory rate	12/minute
MIF	−50 cm H_2O

Arterial blood gases continued to be normal. The patient was alert and communicated to the staff his desire to have the tube removed. After evaluation of the patient's clinical status and all available data, extubation was carried out. Postextubation blood gases were normal. The patient was awake and continued to present a good clinical picture. This patient demonstrates a short-term, easy, and safe wean from the ventilator.

Long-Term Weaning

Once a patient is ventilated for more than 48 hours, discontinuing ventilation is more difficult. The same principles that apply to short-term ventilation apply to long-term ventilation (see Table 15-12). The process is more prolonged, often taking weeks, and the criteria applied may have to be adjusted to chronic disease process.

When the decision is made to begin weaning, a team approach is necessary. The team should include the physician, nursing staff, respiratory therapist, physical therapist, nutritional therapist, and psychologist. A patient care plan is formulated to include daily exercise, walking, and wheelchair trips outside the critical care unit. The weaning process is reviewed at this time, short-term goals are formulated, and misgivings that may hinder the weaning process are expressed. Any manipulative behavior on the part of the patient is addressed at this time, and a systematic approach to the problem is defined. A designated primary nurse should coordinate and evaluate the weaning process daily.

Once the plan of care is formulated, the primary nurse discusses the plan with the patient and family. If the patient wishes to set personal goals, they should be incorporated. At this time, the patient may be informed of the consequences of not being able to wean from the ventilator.

T-Piece

If the T-piece is chosen as the weaning tool, the following schedule is suggested:

1. Initially, wean only during the day.
2. Obtain serial ABGs and other noted physiologic parameters.
3. Start with 5-minute weaning periods per hour.
4. Gradually increase the 5-minute weans further into the day.
5. Stress patient, but do not overfatigue.
6. Increase weaning periods to 10 minutes per hour.
7. Increase wean periods by 5-minute increments until 30 minutes per hour is attained.
8. Increase rest periods to 1 hour when weaning periods of 30 minutes are achieved.
9. Decrease tidal volume on the respirator by 50 cc per day.
10. When 8-hour wean periods are attained, extend weaning into late night and early morning.
11. Continue 1-hour rests between wean periods.
12. Wean through the night — *slowly;* this is the crucial period.
13. Wean accomplished!

During this prolonged weaning process, a record is maintained by the primary nurse and the patient as to the total number of hours accomplished off the ventilator each day. An additional record with ABG values and spontaneous parameters is also maintained. These records ensure that the patient is actually increasing his time off the ventilator and provide positive feedback for the patient and staff.

Usually, this process is not as progressive and uncomplicated as described. Many delays and setbacks occur. Weekly nursing care sessions provide staff support, redefine goals, and address new nursing diagnoses.

Intermittent Mandatory Ventilation

The preparations for IMV are the same as those described previously. The IMV rate is decreased slowly. Theoretically, this provides the patient time to exercise the muscles of respiration, although there are no clinical data to support this theory. Skillful evaluation by the team for hypoventilation and hypercapnia due to fatigue is essential. Tidal volume also may be slowly decreased as the weaning progresses. Monitoring is done with serial arterial blood gases and with the patient's contributory minute ventilation (see Table 15-13).

Table 15-14 outlines some equipment and techniques that may prove useful in the weaning process.

OXYGEN DELIVERY SYSTEMS

Once successful extubation is accomplished, supplemental oxygen is necessary. Oxygen therapy corrects hypoxemia, decreases the work of breathing, and decreases myocardial work. Oxygen delivery systems are traditionally divided into high-flow and low-flow systems. However, the approach to oxygen therapy is usually dictated by the physician, the nursing staff, and the respiratory staff's skill and familiarity with the oxygen equipment. A summary of basic oxygen delivery systems is depicted in Table 15-15.

BIBLIOGRAPHY

Bordow R, Stool E, Moser K (ed): Manual of Clinical Problems in Pulmonary Medicine. Boston, Little, Brown & Co, 1980

Bassili HR, Deitel M: Nutritional support in long term intensive care with special reference to ventilator patients: A review. Can Anaesth Soc J Jan, 1981, pp 17–19

Hemmer M, Viquerat CE, Suter PM, Vallothon MB: Urinary antidiuretic hormone excretion during mechanical ventilation and weaning in man. Anesthesiology 1980, pp 395–400

Hunker FD, Bruton CW, Hunker EM et al: Metabolic and nutritional evaluation of patients supported with mechanical ventilation. Crit Care Med Nov, 1980, pp 297–300

Larca L, Greenbaum DM: Effectiveness of intensive nutritional regimes in patients who fail to wean from mechanical ventilation. Crit Care Med May, 1982, pp 297–300

Schacter EN, Tucker D, Beck G: Does IMV accelerate weaning? JAMA Sept, 1981, pp 1210–1214

Scoggin CH: Weaning respiratory patients from mechanical support. J Respir Dis 1980, pp 13–23

Shapiro B: Respiratory intensive care state of the art: Chicago, Respiratory Care Seminars, Inc, 1983

Shasby DM, Dauber IM, Phister S et al: Swan-Ganz catheter location and left atrial pressure determine the accuracy of the wedge pressure when positive end-expiratory pressure is used. Crit Care Med July, 1983, pp 502–507

Vincent J: Medical problems in the patient on a ventilator. Crit Care Q 1980, pp 33–41

16
Common Pulmonary Disorders

Patricia K. Brannin

Alarming statistics reveal that lung disease is not only the third leading cause of death but also the fastest rising cause of death in the United States. According to Henson's 1984 study,[1] the number of deaths from COPD between 1968 and 1978 showed a 60% increase, with a 10% increase per year since 1978. The specialty of critical care nursing continually challenges its practitioners to expand their scope to meet the needs of the patient with pulmonary disease. Increased accountability for nursing practice demands continual development of the knowledge base from which the critical care nurse operates. The purpose of this chapter is to enable nurses to enhance their knowledge of normal pulmonary function and apply it to abnormal situations when assessing, applying, and evaluating therapeutic modalities. Patient observation and recognition of the signs of pulmonary insufficiency—tachypnea, tachycardia, diaphoresis, and anxiety—are the keys to recognizing abnormal pulmonary function. The ability of the clinician to anticipate, recognize, and intervene to treat pulmonary disorders may modify or prevent common lung disorders.

ATELECTASIS

Atelectasis can be defined as a diminution of volume or collapse of lung units. Several etiologic factors may precipitate atelectasis.

Reabsorption atelectasis occurs when communications between the alveoli and trachea are obstructed, for example, by plugging of a bronchus with mucus. The alveolar gas is rapidly absorbed into the circula-

tion and owing to the obstruction cannot be replenished; thus alveolar collapse ensues.

Passive atelectasis occurs when air and/or fluid in the pleural space prevents normal alveolar filling.

Compression atelectasis occurs in the presence of a space-occupying lesion such as a pulmonary mass. Atelectasis may also occur in patches, which may be caused by mucus plugging or altered compliance in the atelectatic area.

Atelectasis results in a pathologic shunting of blood from the right side of the heart to the left, resulting in desaturation of blood entering the systemic circulation. The degree of shunt present depends on the severity of the atelectasis. In the normal lung, there is a small amount of unoxygenated blood entering the systemic circulation. Contributing to the normal shunt are those vessels whose venous outflow bypasses pulmonary capillaries. Shunting is increased by atelectasis because blood flow passes through the pulmonary capillaries that are in contact with nonventilated alveoli (Fig. 16-1).

Signs and symptoms vary with the severity of atelectasis and degree of shunt present. With severe shunts (*i.e.,* large areas of atelectasis) cyanosis may become evident. Arterial blood gases will reflect the degree of hypoxemia as well as the adequacy of alveolar ventilation. There is frequently roentgenographic evidence of atelectasis. In compression atelectasis, there is roentgenographic evidence of air or fluid collection in the pleural space, resulting in atelectasis. All the roentgen signs are based on diminished volume of the affected lobe or segment. Cyanosis may become evident as atelectasis increases. Large areas of atelectasis may

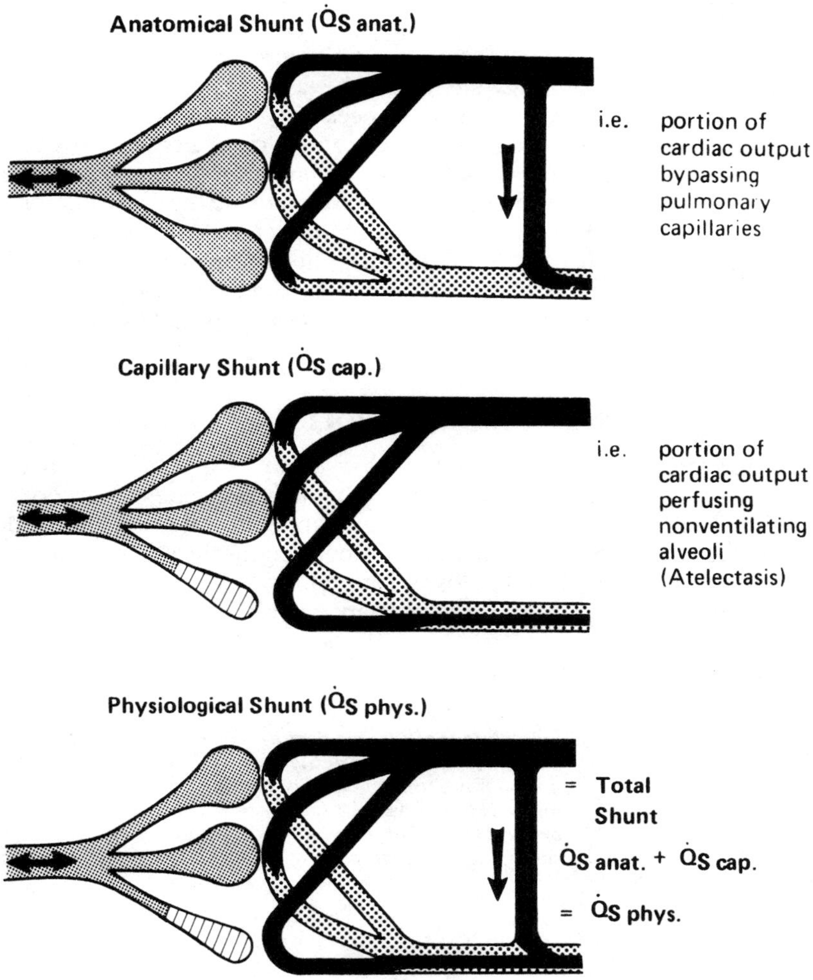

Anatomical Shunt ($\dot{Q}$S anat.)

i.e. portion of cardiac output bypassing pulmonary capillaries

Capillary Shunt ($\dot{Q}$S cap.)

i.e. portion of cardiac output perfusing nonventilating alveoli (Atelectasis)

Physiological Shunt ($\dot{Q}$S phys.)

= **Total Shunt**

$\dot{Q}$S anat. + $\dot{Q}$S cap.

= $\dot{Q}$S phys.

FIGURE 16-1
Subdivisions of the physiological shunt.
(Bendixen HH et al: Respiratory Care,
p. 13. St Louis, CV Mosby, 1965)

cause a shift of the mediastinal structures toward the affected side, which may be demonstrated roentgenographically. Auscultatory examination reveals decreased breath sounds over the atelectatic lung. There may be diminished chest expansion of the affected side. The patient may complain of shortness of breath (s.o.b.), dyspnea on exertion (d.o.e.), and weakness. He may have tachypnea, tachycardia, fever, anxiety, restlessness, and confusion.

Treatment is based on the etiology of the atelectasis. Meticulous bronchial hygiene (see discussion later in this chapter), mobilization of the patient when appropriate, and administration of oxygen in pharmacologic doses constitute the basic framework of therapy.

PNEUMONIA

Pneumonia is an inflammatory process in which alveolar gas is replaced by cellular material. The etiology may be due to viral, bacterial, fungal, protozoan, or rickettsial causes or to hypersensitivity, resulting in the primary presenting illness. Pneumonia may also result from aspiration.

The signs and symptoms will depend on the location and extent of involvement (*i.e.,* segmental or lobar) and etiology of the pneumonia. Subjective findings include dyspnea, tachypnea, pleuritic chest pain, fever, chills, hemoptysis, and cough productive of rusty or purulent sputum. Objective findings include fever, splinting of involved hemithorax, hypoxemia, percussion dullness, coarse inspiratory rales, and diminished breath sounds over the involved area.

Treatment of pneumonia depends on etiology (see Chapter 15, Table 15-3). Observation of the patient for tachycardia, tachypnea, diaphoresis, restlessness and confusion (signs of hypoxemia), increased sputum production, and increased splinting is essential in determination of progression or regression of the process. Careful attention must be directed toward improving ventilation through adequate pain medication followed by bronchial hygiene.

Complications of pneumonia include abscess formation, pleural effusion, empyema, bacteremia, and septicemia. Superinfection may occur as a complication of pharmacologic treatment.

BRONCHOSPASM

Bronchospasm implies a narrowing of the airways resulting in increased airway resistance, which can be caused by a variety of mechanisms: (1) inhalation of toxic or irritating substances, such as smoke, pollens, dust, and noxious gases; (2) bronchitis; (3) severe coughing episodes; (4) extreme cold; and (5) exercise. Although bronchospasm is usually associated with asthma, these mechanisms may precipitate bronchospasm in anyone.

Signs and symptoms vary with the degree of bronchospasm. The patient may complain of shortness of breath associated with wheezing respirations. Additional findings include tachycardia, tachypnea, retractions, restlessness, anxiety, inspiratory/expiratory wheezing, hypoxemia, hypercapnia, cyanosis, and coughing. One must be aware that a decrease in wheezing does not necessarily mean decreased bronchospasm, but rather progression of airway narrowing and markedly decreased ventilation.

Treatment is directed at removing the cause of bronchospasm and initiating bronchodilator therapy (see Chapter 15, Table 15-2). The patient must be observed for increasing bronchospasm and deteriorating pulmonary function manifested by a rising PCO_2.

PULMONARY EMBOLI

Pulmonary emboli may occur as a complication of many medical conditions that predispose to venous thrombosis, including postoperative states, prolonged bed rest, and trauma. Deep venous thrombosis, particularly in the lower extremities, is the main predisposing factor for pulmonary emboli.

Anatomical Deadspace (V_D anat.)

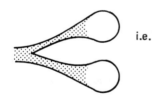

i.e. the portion of tidal volume not in alveoli

Alveolar Deadspace (V_D alv.)

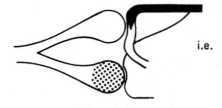

i.e. the portion of tidal volume in nonperfused alveoli

Physiological Deadspace (V_D phys.)

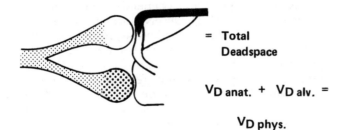

= Total Deadspace

V_D anat. + V_D alv. = V_D phys.

FIGURE 16-2
Subdivisions of physiological dead space. Only that part of the volume of ventilation that enters perfused alveoli is effective in blood-gas exchange and is labeled alveolar ventilation. The remainder is wasted, or dead space, ventilation. Total ventilation may be subdivided accordingly.

$$\begin{array}{c} \text{Total} \\ \text{ventilation} \\ (V) \\ - \\ \text{Alveolar} \\ \text{ventilation} \\ (V_A) \\ = \\ \text{Dead space} \\ \text{ventilation} \\ (V_D) \end{array}$$

This division applies equally to minute ventilation and to the individual tidal volumes. Dividing by the respiratory frequency we get

$$\begin{array}{c} \text{Tidal} \\ \text{volume} \\ (V_T) \\ - \\ \text{Alveolar} \\ \text{tidal} \\ \text{volume} \\ = \\ \text{Physiological} \\ \text{dead space} \\ (V_{D_{phys}}) \end{array}$$

(Berdixen HH et al: Respiratory Care, p 17. St Louis, CV Mosby, 1965)

Both pulmonary and hemodynamic changes occur as a result of occlusion of a pulmonary artery by an embolus. Alveoli are ventilated but not perfused, thereby producing areas of ineffective ventilation, that is, increased respiratory dead space (Fig. 16-2).

Pneumonconstriction resulting from a lack of carbon dioxide normally present in pulmonary arterial blood shifts ventilation from the underperfused alveoli. The decrease in pulmonary blood flow due to an embolus results in deficient nutrients for surfactant production, ultimately resulting in atelectasis. The severity of hemodynamic changes depends on the size of the embolus. Increased pulmonary vascular resistance occurs, which, if pulmonary blood flow remains constant, may result in right ventricular failure. Pulmonary embolus may resolve or infrequently may lead to death of tissue, that is, pulmonary infarction.

The symptom complex of a pulmonary embolus depends on its size. Dyspnea, one of the most frequent complaints, is often out of proportion to the physical findings. Tachypnea and tachycardia may be present in varying degrees. Mild fever may exist, although leukocytosis is rare. It should be noted that pleuritic chest pain and hemoptysis are associated with pulmonary infarction rather than with pulmonary embolus.

Massive pulmonary embolization results in a more dramatic clinical manifestation of acute illness. The patient develops pronounced tachypnea, usually with cyanosis, tachycardia, restlessness, confusion, and hypotension. The resulting shock state produces concomitant changes of decreased urinary output and cold clammy skin.

A suspected pulmonary embolus may be confirmed by radioactive lung scanning and pulmonary angiography. Treatment is anticoagulation and correction of predisposing causes of venous thrombosis. Anticoagulant therapy is administered by various ways in different institutions. The nurse must be aware that multiple drug interactions may occur with use of anticoagulant therapy.

HEMOTHORAX/PNEUMOTHORAX

A pneumothorax occurs when air enters the pleural space between the visceral and parietal pleurae. Blood in this location is called a *hemothorax*. There are two types of pneumothorax: spontaneous pneumothorax and tension pneumothorax.

A *spontaneous pneumothorax* may result from the rupture of a subpleural alveolar cyst or an emphysematous bleb. The signs and symptoms will vary with the size of the pneumothorax and may range from mild shortness of breath to chest pain and signs of increasing respiratory distress. Physical examination reveals decreased breath sounds and decreased respiratory

movement on the affected side. The diagnosis is confirmed by roentgenography.

Chest trauma, IPPB, positive and expiratory pressure (PEEP), cardiopulmonary resuscitation, thoracic and high abdominal surgery, and thoracentesis may precipitate an iatrogenic pneumothorax or hemothorax. A pneumothorax, regardless of etiology, becomes life-threatening as tension in the pleural space occurs.

When a *tension pneumothorax* develops, the tear in lung bronchus or chest wall acts as a one-way valve that allows air to enter the pleural space on inspiration, but not escape on expiration. If it is not immediately recognized and treated, massive atelectasis will result. In addition, the mediastinal structures are displaced toward the unaffected side, and tracheal deviation may be especially prominent. This mediastinal shift will result in a decreased venous return, decreased cardiac output, and ultimately death.

Clinically, the patient manifests severe respiratory distress. Agitation, cyanosis, and tachypnea are severe. Tachycardia and the initial increase in blood pressure are followed by hypotension as cardiac output decreases. The diagnosis is based on the clinical manifestations as well as the clinical setting. Any patient who is being ventilated and suddenly develops acute respiratory distress during ventilation evidenced by markedly increased inspiratory pressures is a prime candidate for a tension pneumothorax. Treatment must be immediate.

A 16- to 18-gauge needle inserted into the second, third, or fourth intercostal space at the midclavicular line on the affected side will relieve the pressure. Once this has been accomplished, a chest tube should be inserted and underwater seal drainage instituted to prevent any further development of tension.

PLEURAL EFFUSION

The pleural space is a potential space between the visceral and parietal pleura that line the lungs and interior chest wall. This space normally contains a small amount of fluid. Excess fluid may accumulate in neoplastic, thromboembolic, cardiovascular, and infectious disease processes. This is due to at least one of four basic mechanisms:

- Increased pressure in subpleural capillaries or lymphatics
- Decreased colloid osmotic pressure of the blood
- Increased intrapleural negative pressure
- Inflammatory or neoplastic involvement of the pleura

Subjective findings include shortness of breath and pleuritic chest pain, depending on the amount of fluid accumulation. Objective findings include tachypnea and hypoxemia if ventilation is impaired, dullness to percussion, and decreased breath sounds over the involved area.

Removal of the pleural effusion by thoracentesis or chest tubes is palliative treatment. Major treatment is that directed toward the underlying cause.

Empyema

Empyema is a collection of purulent material in the pleural space secondary to an inflammatory process of the mediastinum, lung, esophagus, or subdiaphragmatic space. The symptom complex may include shortness of breath and pleuritic chest pain. A major objective finding is continued fever during antibiotic administration. Other findings include those of pleural effusion. Treatment consists of rigorous antibiotic therapy and chest tube drainage (see discussion of chest tubes in Chap. 15). A serious complication of empyema is irreversible fibrotic changes that compromise pulmonary ventilation, due to trapping of the lung on the involved side.

FLAIL CHEST

Trauma to the thorax resulting in a flail chest is caused by the disruption of the normally semirigid structure of the chest cage from (1) fracture of three or more adjoining ribs in one or more places, (2) rib fracture(s) with costochondral separation, or (3) sternal fractures. Wherever fractures occur, that segment loses continuity with the remaining intact chest wall and subsequent paradoxical movement occurs.

During paradoxical ventilation, as the intact chest expands, the injured "flail" segment is depressed, thereby limiting the amount of negative intrathoracic pressure needed to move air into the lungs. During expiration the flail segment bulges outward, thus interfering with exhalation. The degree of ventilatory impairment that results from a flail chest is proportional to the extent of injury. The occurrence of concomitant hemothorax/pneumothorax further impairs ventilation.

During inspiration, the intrapleural pressures on the unaffected side are greater, thus displacing the mediastinum toward it. Conversely, during expiration the negative pressure on the unaffected side is less than on the affected side, and the mediastinum shifts toward the affected side. This phenomenon, known as *mediastinal flutter,* further impairs ventilation as well as cardiac output. Normally, venous return to the right heart is enhanced during inspiration. Reduced intrapleural negative pressure during inspiration impairs circulating dynamics, thus decreasing venous return to the heart, right atrial filling, and ultimately cardiac output.

Frequent patient assessment, including anterior and posterior visual inspection of chest movement, is essential to evaluation and intervention in the treatment of a patient with a flail chest.

Treatment is directed toward improvement of ventilation and oxygenation as well as stabilization of the chest wall. The increased ventilatory effort that is needed for adequate ventilation is difficult for the patient to maintain because of the pain caused by injury. A mechanically controlled volume ventilator, which will enhance chest wall stability and improve alveolar ventilation, is the treatment of choice. Ventilatory support is needed for approximately 14 to 21 days or until the chest is adequately stabilized.

A hemothorax or pneumothorax is treated by chest tubes, underwater seal drainage, and surgical intervention when repair of structural damage is necessary. Chest tubes with underwater seal drainage systems are usually maintained during the entire time the patient needs ventilatory assistance to manage not only the initial hemothorax/pneumothorax, but any that occur as a complication during positive pressure mechanical ventilation.

NONPULMONARY RESPIRATORY COMPLICATIONS

Patients who have surgery, notably high abdominal thoracic and low abdominal resection, are especially susceptible to respiratory embarrassment. The mechanism of pulmonary compromise is a restrictive entity in which there is a reduction of vital capacity, thus resulting in a limited ventilatory reserve. The major restrictive insult occurs sometime in the first 24 hours postoperatively. Patients without complications gradually resume their preoperative ventilatory status.

Postoperative pulmonary complications may be avoided or minimized by adequate preoperative cardiopulmonary evaluation by the critical care nurse. The nurse may thereby institute those measures that are directed toward monitoring pulmonary status and providing modalities aimed toward improving vital capacity.

Pharmacotherapy

Appropriate administration of narcotics and sedatives is a necessary adjunct to pulmonary care. The use of these drugs must be guided by the patient's clinical status. The aim of pharmacologic therapy is to minimize pain so that the patient will tolerate respiratory therapy and other therapeutic modalities. However, overzealous use of sedatives and narcotics may result in respiratory depression and acute respiratory failure.

The patient with a sedative or narcotic overdosage presents with respiratory insufficiency. The severity of the respiratory insufficiency depends on the specific drug(s), amount ingested, time of ingestion, and rate of metabolism of the drug(s).

Factors that may alter drug effects include multiple drug ingestion, hepatic or renal function abnormalities, and preexisting pulmonary disease such as COPD.

Care of patients with drug overdose is guided by this information as well as by the knowledge that patients with certain types of drug ingestion (*e.g.,* glutethimide) may show a fluctuation in level of consciousness. This presents a problem in the maintenance of an adequate airway. It must not be assumed that a patient who at one time appears alert and able to maintain his airway will continue to do so.

There are also drugs that in normal pharmacologic doses can cause neuromuscular blockage with resultant respiratory paralysis. These include kanamycin, gentamicin, streptomycin, neomycin, and polymyxin B.

Neuromuscular Involvement

Disease states or trauma involving the neuromuscular system may affect pulmonary function. The degree of dysfunction will depend on the extent of respiratory muscle involvement.

In certain neurologic diseases the gag and cough reflexes may be diminished, resulting in aspiration of food, fluid, or secretions. The aspirated contents can cause atelectasis and pneumonia, which, if not recognized, will lead to progressive respiratory failure. As impairment of respiratory muscles progresses, there is a resultant decrease in vital capacity.

Taking serial measurements of the vital capacity is an important method of assessing adequacy of pulmonary function. This assessment can be done quite readily by the nurse. Cardinal signs of respiratory embarrassment, pulmonary function measurements, and arterial blood gas analysis must be correlated with the clinical status of the patient.

Long-term management of a patient with a neuromuscular disorder includes maintenance of a patent airway, rigorous clearance of secretions, treatment of infections, maximal mobilization of the patient, and ventilatory assistance when indicated.

Restrictive Disorders

Several entities restrict chest wall expansion with resultant compromised pulmonary function. These include kyphoscoliosis, rheumatoid spondylitis, scleroderma, pectus excavatum, and use of orthopaedic appliances such as spica casts. These patients may, in a stable environment, have normal pulmonary function. A crisis such as trauma or a major medical illness such as drug overdose may precipitate severe respiratory impairment. In the management of these patients the nurse must use those measures that maximize ventilation and minimize pulmonary complications.

NonCardiac Pulmonary Edema

This type of pulmonary congestion occurs without cardiac malfunction. As opposed to cardiac pulmonary edema, the findings of heart failure are absent. Neck veins are not distended, there is no left ventricular gallop, and the pulmonary artery pressure is normal (*i.e.,* < 18 cm H_2O).

See Chapter 17 for a detailed discussion of possible pathophysiology, therapeutic modalities, and sequelae of noncardiac pulmonary edema.

ACUTE RESPIRATORY FAILURE (ARF)

ARF may be defined as respiratory dysfunction of such a degree that gas exchange is no longer adequate to maintain normal arterial blood gases. Quantitatively, ARF may be defined as a $PO_2 < 50$ torr with or without a $PCO_2 > 50$ torr (Fig. 16-3).

ARF may result from a variety of insults including pneumonia, atelectasis, and pneumothorax, Neuromuscular disease, drugs, toxins, and trauma may also lead to ARF.

The key to treatment of ARF is anticipation of its subsequent development in the face of a precipitating event. Management of the patient in the presence of ARF is twofold:

1. Establishment of adequate arterial oxygenation, thereby providing adequate tissue perfusion
2. Amelioration of the underlying cause(s) of ARF

CHRONIC OBSTRUCTIVE PULMONARY DISEASE (COPD)

The common pulmonary disorders discussed previously are potentially reversible causes of respiratory insufficiency, but several disease entities result in COPD. These include chronic bronchitis, bronchiectasis, emphysema, and asthma. Of major importance to the health care team is that fact that COPD is the most common cause of respiratory insufficiency.

Chronic Bronchitis

Chronic infection or irritation of the bronchi may result in bronchitis. The mucus-secreting glands of the tracheobronchial tree become thickened and encroach on the diameter of the airway lumen (Fig. 16-4). In addition, there is increased mucus produc-

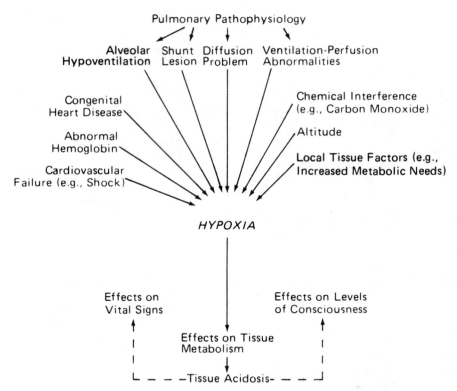

Pulmonary Pathophysiology

Alveolar   Shunt   Diffusion   Ventilation-Perfusion
Hypoventilation Lesion   Problem   Abnormalities

Congenital
Heart Disease

Abnormal
Hemoglobin

Cardiovascular
Failure (e.g., Shock)

Chemical Interference
(e.g., Carbon Monoxide)

Altitude

**Local Tissue Factors (e.g.,
Increased Metabolic Needs)**

HYPOXIA

Effects on
Vital Signs

Effects on Levels
of Consciousness

Effects on Tissue
Metabolism

— — —Tissue Acidosis— — —

FIGURE 16-3
*Hypoxia; mechanisms and effects.
(Brannin P: Oxygen therapy and
measures of bronchial hygiene. Nurs
Clin North Am 9, No. 1: 111, 1974)*

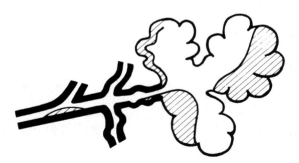

FIGURE 16-4
*Bronchitis. Inflammation and thickening produce narrowing
of airways. Lined areas indicate secretions.*

tion in peripheral airways. By far the most common cause is tobacco smoking.

The two most common bacterial organisms isolated from the secretions of the chronic bronchitic are *Hemophilus influenzae* and pneumococcus. Exacerbation of chronic bronchitis with resultant respiratory insufficiency most often is caused by an acute bacterial inflammation of the bronchial tree (Table 16-1). An essential prophylactic measure in preventing an acute inflammatory process is rigorous bronchial hygiene to promote clearance of secretions that provide an ideal medium for bacterial growth in the peripheral airways. In contrast to emphysema, chronic bronchitis may have a reversible component if the source of chronic infection or irritation is treated.

Bronchiectasis

The term *bronchiectasis* means an irreversible dilation of the bronchi that can be caused by repeated or prolonged episodes of pneumonitis, foreign body aspiration, or a mass (*i.e.,* neoplasm) encroaching on the bronchial lumen with resultant obstruction. The majority of cases are associated with severe chronic bronchitis. A hallmark of the diesase is the production of copious amounts of mucupurulent, often foul-smelling, sputum that settles out into three layers: cloudy mucus on top, clear saliva in the middle, and a cloudy purulent residue on the bottom. The diagnosis is made largely from the history and confirmed by bronchography. The primary treatment modality is *rigorous* bronchial hygiene several times daily. This therapy is essential because effective secretion clearance is altered in these patients as the result of abnormal widening of the airways.

Emphysema

Emphysema is an irreversible dilatation of the acinus accompanied by destructive changes of acinar walls, with resultant loss of lung elastic recoil. Experimental

studies have confirmed the key role of injury to the elastic fiber network in the structural changes of emphysema. Two possible sources of elastolytic activity are neutrophils and alveolar macrophages, both of which are increased in cigarette smokers. Cigarette smoking is a major factor in the development of emphysema. Does this factor play a role in an imbalance of an elastase/antielastase system? According to the 1978 report by Janoff,[2] elastase can be released from neutrophils because of components of smoke. What is the pathogenesis of emphysema? Extensive research has been reported and provides the potential for the development and testing of new hypotheses initially in the experimental animal and then in humans necessary to develop new approaches to the prevention of emphysema, a major cause of lung disease, disability, and death. The destructive process resulting in airway obstruction develops insidiously. In contrast to the chronic bronchitic, patients with emphysema usually have mild chronic hypoxemia because destruction of acinar walls is accompanied by destruction of corresponding vasculature. The ratio of ventilated to perfused lung tissue remains stable (Fig. 16-5).

The majority of patients with COPD will have a mixture of chronic bronchitis and emphysema rather than "pure" bronchitis or emphysema (Table 16-2).

Asthma

In comparison with emphysema and, to a lesser extent, chronic bronchitis, asthma is an acute reversible airways disease that occurs from a variety of causes (*e.g.,*

TABLE 16-1
MANIFESTATIONS OF SEVERE EXACERBATIONS OF CHRONIC BRONCHITIS

Constitutional signs	*Cardiovascular signs*
Temperature frequently subnormal	Diaphoresis
	Tachycardia
WBC varies—may be slightly ↑, normal, or ↓	Blood pressure varies: Normal, ↑, or ↓
	Vasoconstriction initially followed by vasodilation
CNS disturbances	*Neuromuscular signs*
Headache	Fine tremors
Confusion	Asterixis
Hallucinations	Flacidity
Depression	Convulsions
Drowsiness	
Somnolence	
Coma	
Papilledema	

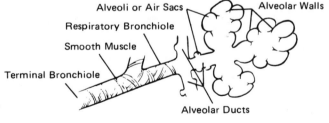

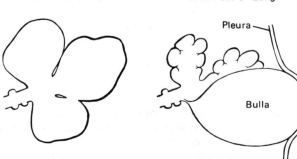

FIGURE 16-5
Emphysema. Airway showing normal primary lobule (top) *and emphysematous lobule* (bottom). *Introduction to Lung Diseases, 6th ed, p 71. New York, American Lung Association, 1975)*

TABLE 16-2
COPD: FEATURES THAT DISTINGUISH BRONCHITIS AND EMPHYSEMA

Features	Bronchitis	Emphysema
Primary location of pathology	Airways	Air sacs
Clinical Examination		
Subjective data	Frequent recurrent chest infections Sputum production Cough	Frequently only insidious dyspnea—initially with exercise only, then progressing
Objective data		
Appearance	"Blue bloaters"	"Pink puffers"
Chest examination	Noisy chest, *slight* overdistention	Quiet chest, marked over-distention
Sputum	Frequently copious and purulent	Usually scant and mucoid
Chronic cor pulmonale	Common—may occur relatively early	Infrequent until terminal stages
Laboratory Tests		
ABGs		
Chronic hypoxemia	Often significant	Usually mild
Chronic hypercapnia	Common	Uncommon
Spirometry		
FEV_1/FVC	Decreased	Decreased
FEV_1	Decreased	Decreased
Therapeutic Modalities		
Bronchial hygiene (measures to enhance secretion clearance)	Very important	Less important unless patient has respiratory infection

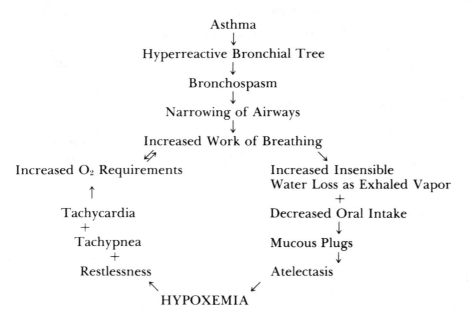

FIGURE 16-6
Sequence of events leading from asthma to hypoxemia.

allergens, infections, exercise) with resultant bronchospasm. Bronchospasm actually includes smooth muscle constriction, mucosal edema, and excessive mucus with plugging of the conducting airways in the advanced stages. Figure 16-6 illustrates a series of events that may become a vicious cycle resulting in life-threatening status asthmaticus unless bronchospasm is controlled.

Spontaneous remission of bronchospasm may occur; however, use of bronchodilating agents (see

Table 15-2) in addition to rigorous bronchial hygiene is the usual mode of treatment. The potential severity of an asthma attack is frequently minimized by these means.

Status Asthmaticus

Status asthmaticus is a medical emergency that is an attack of acute asthma that has not responded (refractory) to rigorous therapy with beta-adrenergic compounds or intravenous theophylline. The patient manifests a dramatic picture of acute anxiety, marked labored breathing, tachycardia, and diaphoresis. Deterioration of pulmonary function results in alveolar hypoventilation with subsequent hypoxemia, hypercapnia, and acidemia. A rising PCO_2 in a patient with an acute asthmatic attack is often the first objective indication of status asthmaticus.

Multiple therapeutic modalities must be instituted. All patients in status asthmaticus demonstrate hypoxemia and require oxygen therapy. Dehydration usually exists and requires correction. Pharmacologic agents consist of methylxanthines, sympathomimetic amines, and corticosteroids. If pulmonary function cannot be improved and respiratory failure ensues, the patient may require intubation and assisted ventilation.

For the purpose of teaching and learning, distinct pathophysiological differences among emphysema, chronic bronchitis, and asthma have been presented. There are times when the health care provider is uncertain whether the problem is asthma or chronic bronchitis. The asthmatic is often a nonsmoker; gives a history of a nonproductive cough that may be associated with chest tightness; states that symptoms are frequently triggered by allergens, cold air, exercise, or irritants; and tends to hyperventilate (defined by $PaCO_2$) and blow off CO_2 in acute attacks. The chronic bronchitic usually gives a history of smoking; coughs a minimum of 2 months per year for 2 or more years with excessive sputum production; may have right heart failure secondary to hypoxemia; and tends to hypoventilate and retain CO_2. There are certain signs and symptoms that may overlap. Some of these are chronic cough, shortness of breath, wheezing, airway obstruction, hyperinflation, and hypoxemia secondary to ventilation/perfusion ($\dot{V}/\dot{Q}$) mismatching and altered gas exchange.

The key to successful management of the asthmatic is *identification* of all possible factors that trigger bronchospasm and *prevention.* If a known cause of an asthma attack is exercise, the patient should be educated to take an inhaled bronchodilator treatment before starting. The adult patient should always have an inhaled bronchodilator with him (*i.e.,* metered dose device such as a metaproterenol inhaler or a dose of bronchodilator in a hand-powered nebulizer that is stored in a purse or pocket.

Sleep Apnea Syndrome

A disorder that is prevalent in patients with chronic obstructive lung disease is sleep apnea syndrome (SAS). This condition is more common in men than in women, although the incidence increases in women after the menopause, suggesting that female hormones are in some way protective. The patient's bed partner, when questioned directly, or the nurse in attendance for hospitalized patients will usually describe intermittent loud snoring followed by silence (apnea) lasting 10 to 100 seconds or longer.

Three classifications of apnea are (1) *obstructive*—associated with absence of airflow despite ventilatory efforts; (2) *central*—associated with absence of both airflow and ventilatory efforts; and (3) *mixed*—during which there is an initial period of central apnea followed by obstructive apnea. The site of obstruction in obstructive apnea is the oropharynx, which is apparently related to an abrupt loss of tone in the muscles surrounding the oropharynx just before the onset of inspiration. In 1985, Burrows and Colleagues suggested that a decreased ventilatory drive exists, for unknown reasons, in both central and obstructive apnea; ventilatory responsiveness to both hypoxemia and hypercarbia is depressed.[3]

In the obstructive type of sleep apnea due to laryngeal obstruction by the tongue or other neck structures, the patient often has struggling type respirations but no air flow, followed by loud snoring. However, in the central apneas, the reduced central nervous system drive to breathe is not associated with characteristic loud snoring. The obstructive apneas are more common.

Signs and symptoms of SAS include hypersomnolence, snoring, insomnia, abnormal motor activity during sleep, morning headache, personality and intellectual changes, altered relationships (*i.e.,* social, family, or job), bizarre behavior, sexual impotence, systemic hypertension, pulmonary hypertension and cor pulmonale, secondary erythrocytosis, cardiac arrhyth-

---

TABLE 16-3
SIGNS AND SYMPTOMS OF SLEEP APNEA

Daytime drowsiness
Headache on awakening
Intermittent loud snoring
Apnea spells of 10 to 100 seconds or longer
Difficulty concentrating
Personality changes
Reduced libido
Restless sleep
Cardiac rhythm disturbances
Pulmonary hypertension
Hypoxemia
Right ventricular failure

mias, and sudden nocturnal death (Table 16-3). Most cases of SAS occur in middle-aged men between 40 and 60 years of age. Suspicion of SAS is based on a middle-aged man who gives a history of sleep disturbance that may be accompanied by previously mentioned signs and symptoms. A definitive diagnosis is based on the results of polysomnography.

Conditions that can be predisposing to secondary sleep apnea include obesity, myxedema, acromegaly, anatomical upper airway obstruction (*i.e.,* nasal deformity with resultant obstruction), brain stem lesions, cervical spine injury, encephalitis, and myotonic dystrophy.

Treatment of SAS will be according to the type of apnea and the severity of symptoms. For example, a tracheostomy for obstrucive apnea may resolve all symptoms. Before this drastic measure is performed —unless the condition is life-threatening—a protriptyline trial is warranted. Protriptyline is a nonsedating tricyclic antidepressant that evidently improves pharyngeal muscle tone during inspiration. The usual dose is 10 to 30 mg taken at bedtime. When successful, this agent decreases somnolence, but according to the 1984 report of Perez-Padilla and Kryger,[4] these patients continue to have abnormal sleep patterns associated with many apneas and arousals. Other forms of treatment include medroxyprogesterone acetate (very useful in obesity-hypoventilation syndrome), continuous positive airway pressure (CPAP), and surgical enlargement of the pharyngeal airway by resection of excessive mucosa. By far the simplest treatment is nocturnal oxygen administration, which often prevents the nocturnal desaturation and many of the other symptoms.

REFERENCES

1. Henson PM: Deaths from lung disease on the increase. New Directions, National Jewish Hospital and Research Center/National Asthma Center, Summer, 1984, Vol. 14, No. 3
2. Janoff A, Blue ML: Possible mechanisms of emphysema in cigarette smokers. Release of elastase from human polymorphonuclear leukocytes by cigarette smoke condensate *in vitro.* Am. Rev. Respir. Dis. 117:17–325, 1978
3. Burrows B, Knudson RJ, Quan SF, Kettel LJ: Respiratory Disorders—A Pathophysiologic Approach, 2nd ed. Chicago, Year Book Medical Publishers, 1983
4. Perez-Padilla R, Kryger M: Upper airway obstruction. In Cherniack RM (ed): Current Therapy of Respiratory Disease 1984–85 pp 8–12. St Louis, CV Mosby, 1984

BIBLIOGRAPHY

Mitchell RS: Bronchiectasis. Mitchell RS, Petty TL (eds): In Synopsis of Clinical Pulmonary Disease, 3rd ed, p 177. St Louis, CV Mosby, 1982
Neff TA: Pulmonary thromboembolism and pulmonary hypertension. In Mitchell RS, Petty TL (eds): Synopsis of Clinical Pulmonary Disease, 3rd ed, p 115. St Louis, CV Mosby, 1982
Pierson DJ: Acute respiratory failure. In Sahn SA (ed): Pulmonary Emergencies, p 75. New York, Churchill-Livingstone, 1982
Scoggin CH, Petty TL: Clinical Strategies in Adult Asthma. Philadelphia, Lea & Febiger, 1981
Scoggin C: Noncardiac pulmonary edema. In Mitchell RS, Petty TL (eds): Synopsis of Clinical Pulmonary Disease, 3rd ed, p 268. St Louis, CV Mosby, 1982
Tobin MJ, Cohn MA, Sackner MA: Breathing abnormalities during sleep. Arch Intern Med 143:1221–1228, 1983

17
Adult Respiratory Distress Syndrome (ARDS)

Patricia K. Brannin

The adult respiratory distress syndrome (ARDS) is a pulmonary emergency that is a sudden and severe form of respiratory failure that usually occurs in previously healthy individuals who have been exposed to a variety of pulmonary or nonpulmonary insults. Some precipitating factors include near drowning, fat emboli, sepsis, pancreatitis, pulmonary emboli, aspiration, hemorrhage, and trauma of any kind. The precipitating event usually occurs 1 to 96 hours prior to the onset of ARDS. Table 17-1 provides an extensive list of disorders associated with ARDS.

ARDS was first described as a clinical syndrome in 1967. The prevalence of ARDS is estimated to be at least 150,000 cases per year. However, until there is an effective reporting mechanism based on a consistent definition, the true incidence of ARDS will remain unknown. The mortality rate depends on the etiology of the ARDS and is therefore variable. ARDS is a major cause of death among trauma and septic patients, with an overall mortality of approximately 50%. This distinct clinical syndrome of diverse etiology appears to manifest a common pathogenesis regardless of causative factors.

PATHOGENESIS

In spite of a wide spectrum of precipitating events associated with ARDS, the common pathogenesis is diffuse damage to the alveolocapillary membrane, postulated to be due to one of the two following primary categories of mechanisms:

1. Aspiration of certain chemicals or inhalation of nox-

ious gases into the airways is directly toxic to the alveolar epithelium, resulting in destruction and increased permeability of the alveolocapillary membrane.

2. Damage to the alveolocapillary membrane can be initiated in the pulmonary microvasculature.

Regardless of the mechanism of lung injury, the common denominator is increased permeability at the level of the alveolocapillary membrane with resultant leakage of fluid in a two-stage process. First, a disruption of the capillary endothelium occurs. Fluid leaks into the interstitial space. Second, a disruption of the alveolar epithelium occurs. Fluid leaks into the alveoli. Fluid in the interstitium and alveoli interferes significantly with gas transport; therefore, hypoxemia occurs. The role of suspected surfactant abnormalities in the development of ARDS remains speculative.

An increase in alveolocapillary membrane permeability leads to interstitial and alveolar edema and alveolar atelectasis. Thus, the amount of air remaining in the lungs at the end of a normal expiration, functional residual capacity (FRC), is decreased.

Mechanical properties of the lungs change. Lung distensibility (compliance) is decreased. The lungs become stiff. Therefore, greater than normal ventilator pressures will be needed to maintain adequate minute ventilation.

The ultimate outcome in the pathogenesis of ARDS is profound hypoxemia, which exists in spite of high inspired oxygen fractions (FIO_2). This cardinal feature may be secondary to extensive interstitial and alveolar edema, surfactant abnormalities, massive atelectasis, shunting, or ventilation-perfusion ($\dot{V}/\dot{Q}$) imbalance (Fig. 17-1).

TABLE 17-1
DISORDERS ASSOCIATED WITH ARDS

Shock of any etiology	Inhaled toxins:
	Oxygen
Infectious causes:	Smoke
Gram-negative sepsis	Corrosive chemicals
Viral pneumonia	
Bacterial pneumonia	Hematologic disorders:
Fungal pneumonia	Intravascular coagulation
Pneumocystic carinii	Massive blood transfusion
	? Postcardiopulmonary bypass
Trauma:	
Fat emboli	Metabolic disorders:
Lung contusion	Pancreatitis
Nonthoracic trauma	Uremia
Head injury	Paraquat ingestion
Liquid aspiration:	Miscellaneous:
Gastric juice	Lymphangitic carcinomatosis
Fresh and salt water	Increased intracranial pressure
Hydrocarbon fluids	Eclampsia
	Postcardioversion
Drug overdose:	Radiation pneumonitis
Heroin	
Methadone	
Barbiturates	

Hopewell PC: ARADS. Basics of RD 17(4), 1979

vere (*i.e.*, $PaO_2 < 50$ mm) as the process continues—in spite of increasing concentrations of supplemental oxygen. In contrast to refractory hypoxemia, the $PaCO_2$ is low. The latter finding reflects the significant compensatory increase of minute ventilation in an attempt to maintain PaO_2, which exists until the patient becomes fatigued.

Table 17-2 provides a summary of ARDS—clinical presentation through management process.

As previously stated, the physical examination is frequently not revealing. Therefore, one of the most powerful assessment tools is the constant awareness of the multiple causes of ARDS. Be suspicious! Train yourself to be an astute observer. Gather essential baseline data. Note changes and trends that can be early clues indicative of abnormal lung function—vital signs, sensorium, and arterial blood gases. A gradual increase in respiratory rate without apparent accompanying symptoms or signs may be the first clue. The clinical onset of ARDS may be insidious or sudden. Develop and learn to follow your index of suspicion. Prevention should be the major point of management.

ASSESSMENT

The clinical presentation and manifestations of ARDS will be a function of the acute pulmonary or nonpulmonary event that caused the syndrome. Unfortunately, in contrast to the magnitude of this medical emergency, the physical examination is usually not very revealing. Hallmarks of assessment are respiratory distress, profound hypoxemia, and diffuse bilateral alveolar infiltrates on the chest film. The last is secondary to increased alveolocapillary permeability with associated flux of fluid and protein into interstitium and alveoli.

Cardinal signs of respiratory distress and profound hypoxemia are changes in level of mental acuity, restlessness, tachycardia, and tachypnea. The respiratory rate frequently increases significantly with a high minute ventilation. Dyspnea with labored respirations and associated intercostal retractions is common. Cyanosis may or may not be present. One must remember that cyanosis is neither an early nor a reliable sign of hypoxemia.

Chest auscultation reveals few, if any, abnormalities. The bubbling rales of cardiogenic pulmonary edema are not present. Rhonchi secondary to secretions in large airways do not occur. Cardiac auscultation usually reveals normal heart sounds without gallops or murmurs unless myocardial disease is present or trauma has occurred.

Arterial blood gases document the severity of hypoxemia. The degree of hypoxemia becomes more se-

TABLE 17-2
ARDS: SUMMARY OF CLINICAL ASSESSMENT THROUGH INTERVENTION PROCESS

A. Precipitating pulmonary or nonpulmonary event
B. Clinical signs/assessment
  1. Tachypnea
  2. Tachycardia
  3. Labored respirations
  4. Use of accessory muscles
C. Laboratory findings
  1. Arterial blood gas analysis: $\downarrow\downarrow$ PaO_2 (*i.e.*, <50 mm with supplemental O_2)
                $\downarrow$ $PaCO_2$
  2. Chest radiograph: diffuse bilateral pulmonary infiltrates
  3. High minute ventilation (*i.e.*, >20 L/minute)
  4. Low left atrial pressure via pulmonary artery catheter
D. Intervention
  1. Establishment of definitive airway: endotracheal tube/tracheostomy
  2. Mechanical ventilation: volume ventilator with high pressure and flow capabilities
  3. PEEP
  4. Adequate arterial oxygenation
  5. Fluids
  6. Pharmacologic agents (*i.e.*, oxygen and diuretics; antibiotics for documented infection)
  7. Airway maintenance
  8. Prevention of infection
  9. Nutritional support
  10. Monitoring of *all* systems for response to therapy and potential complications
  11. Treatment of underlying condition
E. Prognosis: approximately 50% mortality
F. Sequelae on recovery: infrequent

Pathogenesis of ARDS

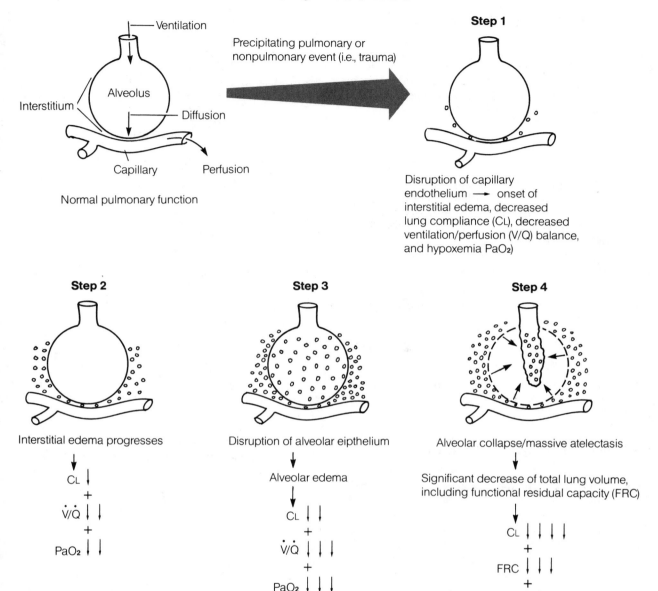

FIGURE 17-1
Pathogenesis of ards.

INTERVENTION

The primary goal of treatment is to reverse the immediate life-threatening problem: inadequate delivery of oxygen to the tissues secondary to the inability of the lungs to oxygenate, which is caused by severe $\dot{V}/\dot{Q}$ abnormalities and shunting. Oxygen delivery is determined by the amount of oxygen in the blood and the cardiac output. A second goal of treatment is to minimize pulmonary vascular pressures to prevent or inhibit the leakage of fluid at the alveolar capillary membrane.

Oxygen Therapy

Oxygen is a drug with essential therapeutic properties and potentially toxic side effects. According to the 1982 report by Albert, patients without underlying lung disease apparently tolerate 100% oxygen for 24 to 72 hours without physiologic abnormalities of clinical importance.[1] However, high fractions of inspired oxygen (*i.e.,* >0.5 torr) over a long period of time may cause increased permeability of endothelium and epithelium. The amount of oxygen prescribed for ARDS should be the lowest fraction of inspired oxygen (FIO_2) that produces an adequate oxygen content (*i.e.,* oxyhemoglobin content >90%). Intubation is almost always indicated to maintain constant high FIO_2.

Mechanical Ventilation

An important aspect of treatment of true ARDS is mechanical ventilation. (For a detailed discussion of general and specific principles of ventilatory management, refer to the ventilatory section of Chapter 15). A therapeutic goal of this treatment modality is to provide ventilatory support until the integrity of the alveolocapillary membrane is reestablished. Two additional goals are as follows:

- Maintenance of adequate ventilation and oxygenation during the critical period of severe hypoxemia.
- Reversal of the etiologic factors that initially caused the respiratory distress to occur.

To facilitate reversal or prevention of atelectasis, tidal volumes of 10 to 15 ml/kg of body weight are recommended.

Positive End Expiratory Pressure (PEEP)

Adequate ventilation and oxygenation are provided by volume ventilator with high pressure and flow capabilities to which PEEP may be added. PEEP is maintained in the alveoli throughout the entire respiratory cycle, thereby preventing or minimizing alveolar collapse at the end of expiration (Fig. 17-2). PEEP results in restored functional residual capacity (FRC) with improved airway resistance and compliance. The goal of continuous PEEP is improved oxygenation with subsequent decrease in inspired oxygen concentration needed to correct life-threatening hypoxemia.

The major complications of PEEP are barotrauma and decreased cardiac output. There are two types of barotrauma: pneumothorax and mediastinal, or subcutaneous, emphysema. According to the 1984 report of Albert, barotrauma occurs in up to 18% of patients treated with PEEP.[2] The relationship between the occurrence of barotrauma and the level of end expiratory pressure is unclear.

Decreased cardiac output secondary to PEEP results from decreased venous return or increased pulmonary vascular resistance. Careful monitoring of the patient's

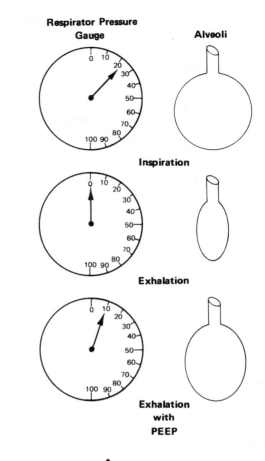

PEEP: Desired effect is: ↑ FRC (Functional Residual Capacity) ↓ F_IO_2 (Fraction of Inspired Oxygen)

FIGURE 17-2
With PEEP, the alveoli have more gas remaining after exhalation for O_2/CO_2 exchange to take place.

blood pressure, pulse, urine output, and sensorium is necessary. Infusion of dopamine or nitroprusside has been employed to return cardiac output to normal. Infusion of additional volume would also accomplish restoration of cardiac output but would ultimately increase lung water content.

The degree of PEEP for ARDS is highly controversial. Recall that the goal of PEEP is to correct life-threatening hypoxemia while using the safest therapeutic approach. Several pulmonologists [1-3] employ, for most patients, low levels of PEEP (*i.e.,* <15 cm H_2O). Owing to the potential cardiac effects of PEEP, additions and reductions in amount should be accomplished in 3- to 5-cm H_2O increments or decrements. Blood pressure should be noted before and after each change. Arterial blood gases will provide documentation for the effectiveness of PEEP (*i.e.,* improved oxygenation).

Hemoglobin

Most of the volume of oxygen is transported to the tissues in combination with hemoglobin. If anemia is present, O_2 content in the blood is reduced. As a result, the effects of mechanical ventilation, PEEP, and supplemental oxygen would be minimized. Serial hemoglobin measurements are necessary for calculation of O_2 content, which will determine the need for transfusing red blood cells.

Fluid Management

Recall the pathogenesis of increased alveolocapillary permeability, which results in interstitial and alveolar edema. Excessive administration of fluid in normal people can produce pulmonary edema and respiratory failure. The choice of colloid versus crystalloid fluid for replacement therapy remains controversial. In spite of advanced technology, an accurate *daily weight* (note trend) is frequently the most important indicator of fluid balance. The primary goal of fluid therapy is to maintain normal physiologic parameters (see Chapter 8, Hemodynamic Pressure Monitoring).

Pharmacologic Therapy

The use of corticosteroids is controversial. Previously, antibiotic therapy was initiated for prophylaxis, but experience demonstrated that this did not prevent dangerous gram-negative sepsis. Routine prophylactic antibiotic therapy is no longer acceptable.

Nutritional Management

The critically ill patient's demand for energy and protein increases while his supply all too often decreases—a classic dilemma in the critical care setting. Malnutrition is a relatively common problem in critically ill patients who are receiving ventilatory support. Nutritional management of ARDS is commonly overlooked during the early, as well as late, stages. Optimal nutrition during this pulmonary emergency may be difficult to achieve, but the establishment and maintenance of an adequate nutritional support program will be imperative for the successful management of every patient with this syndrome.

According to the 1984 report of Rochester and Esau,[5] one of the most outstanding effects of malnutrition on pulmonary function is to decrease the ability of patients to sustain appropriate levels of ventilation. This occurs secondary to the effects of nutritional deficit on both the central nervous system and the respiratory muscles. The diaphragm is the major muscle of respiration. According to Rochester and Esau, there are two ways in which the diaphragm is weakened secondary to malnutrition: (1) Actual muscle mass is reduced, and (2) marked reduction of the contractile strength of the remaining muscle fibers occurs.

A discussion of individual nutrients and minerals is beyond the scope of this chapter. However, it would be advantageous to discuss in brief proteins and the mineral phosphorus because both are essential to adequate nutritional balance.

Protein is stored as a nitrogen reservoir. Each molecule of protein is either part of the contractile force in muscle, part of the cellular content or membrane, or an enzyme. Protein depletion results in loss of essential function. Skeletal muscle undergoes the largest part of protein loss in starvation, with a resultant poor energy supply of less than 1 calorie per gram of muscle.

The mineral element, phosphorus, probably has more functions than any other. It is necessary for building bones and teeth, nucleic acids of all cells, phospholipids that regulate absorption and transportation of fats, enzymes involved in energy metabolism, buffer salts in the regulation of acid-base balance, and compounds involved in the sequential phases of muscle contraction. In other words, this mineral is involved in many metabolic pathways. The normal serum phosphate level is 2 to 5 mg/dl. Hypophosphatemia is said to occur with a serum level less than 1 mg/dl.

Assessment of nutritional status is crucial (Table 17-3). Body weight and body height are the most simple measurements. One must be aware that a major change in weight may be secondary to fluid shifts or to

TABLE 17-3
NUTRITIONAL ASSESSMENT

	Nutritional Depletion		
	Normal	Mild	Severe
Energy Reserves			
Weight change	Variable		
Protein Reserves			
Lymphocyte count	1800/mm³	1600	500
Cumulative nitrogen balance	0	−30 g	−300 g
Albumin	3 g/dl	2.5	1.5
Total protein	6 g/dl	5.5	4.0
Muscle strength Maximum volume ventilation	100% predicted	60	30

(From Bartlett RH: Assessment and management of nutrition in critical illness. In Bone RC (ed): Critical Care—A Comprehensive Approach, pp 60–81. Park Ridge, IL, American College of Chest Physicians, 1984

Protein intake		minus	Protein output	=	Balance
Grams of protein	Grams of protein		Urinary N₂ + 4 g		
$$\frac{\text{eaten}}{6.25}$$ +	$$\frac{\text{in TPN}}{6.25}$$ −		(stool and skin N₂)	=	Balance

Example of patient in negative nitrogen balance

$$\frac{60}{6.25}$$		−	8 + 4	=	
9.6		−	12	=	− 2.4

FIGURE 17-3
Nitrogen balance formula.

changes in body fat. Assessment of protein reserves includes lymphocyte count, cumulative nitrogen balance, albumin, total protein, and maximum voluntary ventilation (MVV) to test respiratory muscle strength.

Total parenteral nutrition (intravenous hyperalimentation) or enthusiastic tube feeding can correct the malnutrition and allow patients to avoid respiratory failure due to poor nutrition of inspiratory muscles. Certainly, malnourished patients with respiratory failure are difficult or impossible to wean from a ventilator until their malnutrition is corrected. In addition to calories and protein, phosphate must be supplied to allow the muscles to function properly (see Chap. 31).

Occasionally, a patient in respiratory failure who is receiving TPN has difficulty weaning from the ventilator because such a high percentage of total calories is being given as carbohydrates that the patient converts the excess carbohydrate to fat (lipogenesis), which produces a large amount of CO_2. Sometimes, this excessive CO_2 is more than the body can eliminate without the assistance of a ventilator.

Equipment that can accurately measure oxygen consumption and CO_2 production is available and useful in making sure that the patient is nourished correctly, especially when it is combined with nitrogen balance studies. Some new ventilators have a device for measuring CO_2 production that is sold as an accessory.

The nitrogen balance study is simple to do and is perhaps the best easy measure of adequate nutrition, particularly with regard to protein. One calculates the nitrogen in protein intake according to the formula in Figure 17-3. It is assumed that 4 g of protein are lost daily in the stool and skin. Positive nitrogen balance (more protein nitrogen in than out) means positive protein balance.

Airway Maintenance

A definitive airway—either an endotracheal or tracheostomy tube—is established not only as an airway but also as a means of protecting the airway (with the cuff intact), providing for continuous ventilatory support, and sustaining oxygen concentrations. Maintenance of the airway involves knowing *when* to suction; meticulous suctioning technique; adequate cuff pressures; prevention of pressure necrosis from endotracheal and oropharyngeal tubes; nasal and oral care to remove accumulated secretions, which, if aspirated into the lower respiratory tract, can cause secondary pulmonary infection; and constant monitoring of upper airway and tracheal secretions as well as the tracheostomy site for evidence of infections. This care is crucial. The new or inexperienced nurse should observe this process demonstrated and, in turn, demonstrate *both* assessment and technical skills before becoming responsible for this aspect of intensive therapy. One should remember that an artificial airway and ventilatory support buy time for the patient — *time* for the underlying conditions that precipitate ARDS to be treated and, it is hoped, *time* for ARDS to resolve. Maintenance of the airway and associated prevention of infection are paramount to recovery.

Surveillance for and Prevention of Infection

The importance of attention to upper and lower respiratory tract secretions and prevention of infection through meticulous suctioning techniques has been addressed. Nosocomial infections are hospital-acquired infections. In 1978, Dixon estimated that a staggering 2 million nosocomial infections occur annually in the United States.[6] The tremendous impact of such infections on economy (*i.e.,* extra hospital days) needs to be appreciated. In 1984, Bender and Bartlett reported that most common sites of infection are the urinary tract, surgical wound infections, lower respiratory tract, skin, and primary bacteremia.[7] The cause of infection may be exogenous (pathogen from any source other than the patient) or endogenous (patient's own microbial flora). Some of the important signs and symptoms of infection that the nurse should be alert to include pain, fever, redness, warmth or swelling associated with joints or wounds, and change in drainage or secretions (*i.e.,* amount, consistency, color, or odor).

Monitoring Respiratory Function

The patient in respiratory failure usually has monitoring of hemodynamic indices on a routine basis. The type of monitoring that is too commonly minimized — or completely overlooked — because of hemodynamic monitoring devices is that which is most simple. Astute observation by qualified personnel of *pulmonary function* (and the *total* patient) over time is vitally important. Physical diagnosis and radiological examination of the chest continue to be fundamental techniques that must be utilized. Technology should be considered a means of enhancing physical and radiographic findings rather than replacing them.

Physical examination of the intubated patient must include an attempt to elicit subjective information. If the patient is able to cooperate and write, paper and pen will provide a means for response to questions such as the following:

- How do you feel?
- How is your breathing?
- Are you getting enough air?
- Where are you?
- What are the date and time?
- Who is the president of the United States?

One must remember the deleterious effects of hypoxemia on central nervous system function. Asking questions of the patient in an attempt to determine mental acuity is an important part of assessment.

Objective assessment is next. What are the vital signs, and what do they mean at this time? Pulse rate is a nonspecific cardiopulmonary variable that, when elevated, can suggest hypoxemia, blood volume or flow deficits, fever, anxiety, cardiac impairment, and so forth. An increased respiratory rate is one of the earliest responses to either a decreased PaO_2 or an increased $PaCO_2$. When the rate exceeds 20 per minute with an upward trend, one must *be aware* of the likelihood of severe respiratory distress.

General assessment of ventilatory effectiveness can be gleaned by observation of chest movement. The nurse should stand at the foot of the bed with the patient's chest exposed, and observe the thorax for symmetry. Asymmetry can occur with right main stem bronchus intubation, pneumothorax, and atelectasis. Chest auscultation may or may not reveal unequal ventilation, depending on degree.

Assessment of breath sounds allows detection of ventilatory fluid and secretions, need for or adequacy of suctioning, and adequacy of tracheostomy or endotracheal tube cuff inflation. Wheezes, crackles, and dullness to percussion are usually considered late signs of respiratory failure. Again, the nurse must remember the importance of the physical examination as an essential conterpart of roentgenography and physiological studies in following the trend of ARDS, the underlying condition, and the course of treatment.

Chest roentgenography is an important way to document appropriate placement of an endotracheal tube and to determine the presence of pneumothorax following procedures such as thoracentesis and subclavian venous catheterization, following trauma, and secondary to PEEP. Chest radiography is also useful in following the course of ARDS and in detecting complications such as pneumonia and atelectasis. The nurse should develop a habit of reviewing and discussing chest films for her patient with the physician. Of what value could this process be to a nurse? For example, the current chest film reveals a right lower lobe pneumonia. Does the radiograph assist the nurse in determining optimal positioning of the patient for postural drainage and chest percussion of the right lower lobe? Will a repeat film in 24, 48, and 72 hours help her assess the success of care; does she need to be more rigorous? How does her physical examination of the patient correlate with the chest roentgenogram?

Cardiac arrhythmias are usually latent manifestations of pulmonary problems. It is important to monitor the patient with continuous cardiac monitoring or serial electrocardiograms or both. In addition to arrhythmia detection, how can the direct visibility of a cardiac monitor assist the nurse in the delivery of patient care? The nurse should glance at the monitor before, during, and after endotracheal suctioning. What

TABLE 17-4
BEDSIDE MEASUREMENTS OF RESPIRATORY FUNCTION

Physical Examination
  Subjective information (what patient says/writes)
  Objective information (what nurse observes)
    Daily weight
    Urine output/specific gravity
    Vital signs
    CNS: mental acuity, behavior
    Mouth: color of mucosa → ? central cyanosis
    Neck: ? prominent neck veins; ? supple
    Cardiopulmonary: heart sounds, breath sounds
    Abdomen: tenderness or distention?
    Extremities: ? cyanosis or clubbing

Pt/Ventilator
    Tidal volume (V_T)
    Minute ventilation ($\dot{V}_E$)
    Inspiratory pressure
    Compliance (C_L)

Laboratory
    CXR
    ECG
    ABG
    Hgb/Hct

happens to the heart rate? Why? What are the implications for nursing care?

Other equally important guides for monitoring bedside parameters of respiratory function in a patient with ARDS include ABGs, tidal volume, and minute ventilation. The nurse must learn to integrate each aspect of care with normal pulmonary anatomy and function, altered lung function (in this case, ARDS), and associated therapeutic modalities. A summary of bedside measurements of respiratory function has been developed as a guide for patient care and communication of patient information (*i.e.,* nursing report and patient record) (Table 17-4).

SEQUELAE ON RECOVERY

The significance of ARDS as an extreme pulmonary emergency with an average mortality of 50% could well indicate multiple sequelae upon recovery, yet the long-term prognosis appears to be good. Mild to moderate physiologic abnormalities that have been reported are restrictive/obstructive abnormalities (airflow limitation), moderate diffusion defects, and shift hypoxemia during exercise. The positive outcome for those who recover from ARDS is most likely a threefold function of the abilities of the health care team to protect the lung from further insult during the life support period, prevention of O_2 toxicity, and meticulous attention to sepsis reduction.

REFERENCES

1. Albert FK: Pulmonary edema. In Sahn SA (ed): Pulmonary Emergencies, p 180. New York, Churchill-Livingstone, 1982
2. Albert RK: Normal and increased-permeability edema. In Cherniack RM (ed): Current Therapy of Respiratory Disease 1984–85, pp 224–253. St Louis, CV Mosby, 1984
3. Hudson LO: Ventilatory management of patients with adult respiratory distress syndrome. Semin Respir Med 2:128–139, 1981
4. Petty TL: Adult respiratory distress syndrome (ARDS). Mitchell RS et al. (eds): In Synopsis of Clinical Pulmonary Disease, 3rd ed, pp 66–81. St Louis, CV Mosby, 1982
5. Rochester DF, Esau S: Malnutrition and the respiratory system. Chest 85:411–415, 1984
6. Dixon RE: Effect of infections on hospital care. Ann Intern Med 89:749–753, 1978
7. Bender BS, Barlett JG: Nosocomial infections. In Bone RC (ed): Critical Care — A Comprehensive Approach, pp 446–463. Park Ridge, Ill, 1984

BIBLIOGRAPHY

Bassili HR, Deitel M: Effects of nutritional support on weaning patients off mechanical ventilators. J Parenter Enter Nutr 5:161–163, 1981
Bone RC: Treatment of severe hypoxemia due to the adult respiratory distress syndrome. Arch Intern Med 140:85–89, 1980
Burrows B, Knudson R, Quan S, Kettel L: Respiratory Disorders, 2nd ed, pp 186–191. Chicago, Year Book Medical Publishers, 1983
Driver AG, Brun M: Iatrogenic malnutrition in patients receiving ventilatory support. JAMA 244:2195–2196, 1980
Larca L, Greenbaum DM: Effectiveness of intensive nutritional regimes in patients who fail to wean from mechanical ventilation. Crit. Care Med. 10:297–300, 1982
Sahn S: Pulmonary Emergencies, pp 169–172. New York, Churchill-Livingstone, 1982
Tisi G: Pulmonary Physiology in Clinical Medicine, pp 211–212. Baltimore, Williams & Wilkins, 1980

Unit Three

Renal System

18
Normal Structure and Function of the Renal System

Barbara Brockway-Fuller

NORMAL STRUCTURE OF THE KIDNEY

The regulation and concentration of solutes in the extracellular fluid of the body are the primary functions of the kidney. These are accomplished by removal of metabolic waste products and excess concentrations of constituents and by conservation of those substances that are present in normal or low quantities. Figure 18-1 is a schematic representation of the general macroscopic and microscopic structure of the kidney.

Urine, the end product of kidney function, is formed from the blood by the *nephron* and flows from the nephrons through *collecting tubules* to the *pelvis* of the kidney. From here it leaves the kidney itself by way of the *ureters* and flows into the *urinary bladder*. Each human kidney contains about 1 million nephrons, all of which function identically, and thus kidney function can be explained by describing the function of one nephron.

Figure 18-2 is a composite drawing of a functional nephron. Each nephron is made up of two major components: the *glomerulus,* in which water and solutes are filtered from the blood; and the *tubules,* which reabsorb essential materials from the filtrate and permit waste substances and unneeded materials to remain in the filtrate and flow into the renal pelvis as urine.

These two major divisions of the nephron are represented more schematically in Figure 18-3.

The *glomerulus* consists of a tuft of capillaries fed by the *afferent arteriole,* drained by the *efferent arteriole,* and surrounded by *Bowman's capsule.* Fluid that is filtered from the capillaries into this capsule then flows into the tubular system, which is divided into four sections: (1) the *proximal tubule,* (2) the *loop of Henle,* (3) the *distal tubule,* and (4) the *collecting tubule.*

Most of the water and electrolytes are reabsorbed into the blood in the *peritubular capillaries* and the *vasa recta,* and the end products of metabolism pass into the urine.

NORMAL RENAL PHYSIOLOGY

The Glomerulus and Filtration

The glomerular capillaries, nestled in Bowman's capsule, are composed of three layers: (1) an inner endothelium, (2) a glycoprotein-constituted basement membrane, and (3) an outer epithelial layer continuous from that lining Bowman's capsule.

Pore size determines permeability. Like other body capillaries, the glomerular capillaries are relatively impermeable to large plasma proteins and are quite permeable to water and smaller solutes such as electrolytes, amino acids, glucose, and nitrogenous waste. Unlike other capillaries in the body, the glomerular capillaries have an elevated hydrostatic (blood) pressure (70 torr versus 10 to 30 torr). This increased hydrostatic pressure in part forces (or squeezes) water and permeable solutes from the bloodstream into Bowman's capsule. This process is termed *glomerular filtration.* The material entering Bowman's capsule is called the *filtrate.*

The *hydrostatic pressure* of the glomerulus does not operate alone. Three other factors participate; (1) the

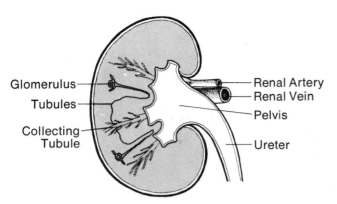

FIGURE 18-1
General characteristics of kidney structure. Note that the glomerulus is in the cortex of the kidney, whereas the proximal, distal, and collecting tubules are in the medulla.

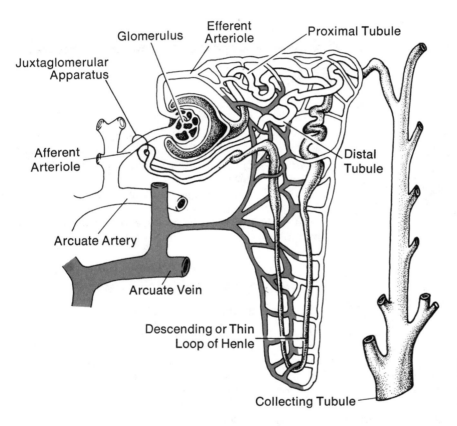

FIGURE 18-2
The nephron. (Guyton AC [ed]: Textbook of Medical Physiology, p 439. Philadelphia, WB Saunders, 1976)

hydrostatic pressure (HP) of the filtrate fluid (in Bowman's capsule), (2) the osmotic pressure (OP) of the blood, and (3) the osmotic pressure (OP) of the filtrate (in Bowman's capsule). Figure 18-4 illustrates the interaction of these factors. HP can be thought of as a "pushing" force, whereas OP can be viewed as a "pulling or attracting" force. Thus, the plasma HP (70 torr) cooperates with filtrate OP (close to zero) to move water and permeable solutes from plasma to Bowman's capsule, whereas the filtrate HP (20 torr) cooperates with the plasma OP to move water in the opposite direction (*i.e.,* from the capsule to blood-stream). Net effective forces can be equated as

from blood to capsule	versus	from capsule to blood
70 + 0		20 + 30

As can be noted, the left side of this equation has a greater force (70 torr) than the right side (50 torr). Thus, there is a pressure gradient of about 20 torr (70 − 50 = 20) that causes water and permeable solutes to filter out of the glomerulus into Bowman's capsule.

The *rate* at which the filtrate is formed is termed the *glomerular filtration rate (GFR).* In the typical healthy person, this amounts to the formation of

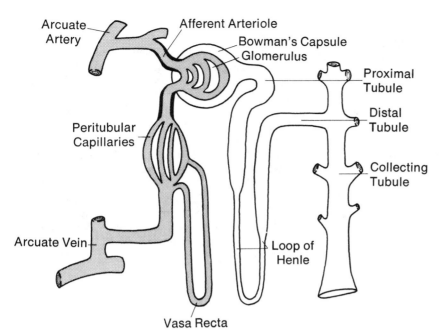

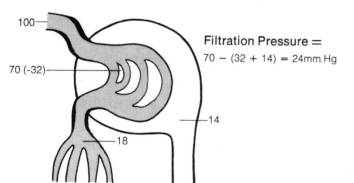

FIGURE 18-3
Schematic representation of the nephron. (Guyton AC: Function of the Human Body, Philadelphia, WB Saunders, 1969)

Filtration Pressure =
70 − (32 + 14) = 24mm.Hg

FIGURE 18-4
Normal fluid pressures at various points in the nephron. (Guyton AC: Function of the Human Body, p 197. Philadelphia, WB Saunders, 1969)

125 ml of filtrate per minute. Major factors that influence the GFR are the glomerular plasma HP and OP. Subnormal plasma OP, such as in hypoproteinemia, will increase the GFR. A fall in glomerular HP, such as that resulting from systemic hypotension or hypovolemia, would decrease the GFR. Other factors that will decrease the HP and thus the GFR are afferent arteriole constriction and renal artery stenosis.

Because of the influence of HP on the GFR, the kidneys were long thought to function in the normal homeostasis of systemic blood pressure. But we now know that the GFR is relatively stable over fluctuations of 20 to 30 torr in arterial blood pressure. The reason for this stability is that the afferent arterioles adjust their diameter in response to the pressure of blood coming to them. If the blood pressure decreases (*e.g.,* 10 torr), the smooth muscles of the afferent arterioles relax. This causes dilation of these arterioles, which, in turn, increases the perfusion of the glomeruli and maintains the GFR at its normal rate; conversely, with an increase in blood pressure, these vessels constrict. There is a limit, however, to this autoregulatory mechanism. If the systemic blood pressure falls greatly, such as in shock, the GFR will fall to near zero, thereby producing near anuria.

The Glomerular Filtrate

The glomerular filtrate is an ultrafiltrate of plasma containing only a small (0.03%) amount of protein. Roughly 23% of the cardiac output goes to the kidneys in a resting adult. From this, about 125 ml of filtrate are produced each minute. This totals 180 liters/day and is about 4½ times the total amount of fluid in the body. As this filtrate passes through the remainder of the nephrons, all but about 1.5 liters/day will be returned to the bloodstream by way of the peritubular capillaries (see Fig.18-3). The volume and content of the urine are the result of tubular reabsorption (accomplished by active transport, osmosis and diffusion, and tubular secretion). Reabsorption occurs in all parts of the nephron, whereas only tubule cells perform secretion.

Active transport involves the binding of a molecule to a carrier, which then moves the molecule from one side of the membrane to the other. The carrier acts somewhat like a pump. This process moves the transported molecule either into or out of a cell. In tubular cells, the carrier is located in the cell membrane nearest the peritubular capillaries, and it transports material out of the tubular cell into the peritubular fluid. This lowers the intracellular concentration of the type of molecule being transported. The decreased concentration enables more of those molecules to diffuse into the tubule cell. These molecules, in turn, exit the cell and enter the peritubular fluid by active transport. The movement of molecules increases the peritubular fluid concentration of the molecule, and this increase, in turn, stimulates the diffusion of the molecule into the peritubular capillaries. Thus, in the nephrons, active transport removes molecules from the filtrate (urine) back to the bloodstream.

Tubular secretion, thought also to be used as a carrier system, moves molecules from the bloodstream into the filtrate by a process similar to, but the reverse of, active transport. The carrier mechanism of both processes (active transport and secretion) requires energy (in the form of high energy adenosine triphosphate [ATP] bonds), the provision of which requires a healthy tubule cell. Thus, tests of secretion, for example, provide valuable data regarding tubular cell health. Similarly, a sign of diminished reabsorption of sodium (supernormal urinary sodium) provides evidence of damaged tubular cells in acute tubular necrosis.

The Proximal Tubule

Roughly 80% of the glomerular filtrate is returned to the bloodstream by reabsorption in the proximal tubule. Normally, all glucose and amino acids plus sodium, chloride, phosphate, bicarbonate, magnesium, calcium, other electrolytes, uric acid, water, and a little urea are reabsorbed here. Some urea, creatinine, hydrogen, and ammonia are secreted from the peritubular capillaries into the filtrate by these tubular cells. Some drugs (*e.g.,* para-aminohipuric acid [PAH] and penicillin) are also added to the filtrate by tubular secretion.

At plasma glucose levels of less than 200 mg/dl, all of the filtered glucose is returned back into the bloodstream by active transport. Amino acids, creatine, and some sodium, potassium, phosphate, sulfate, uric acid, and other organic molecules are also actively trans-

ported out of the filtrate (where they then diffuse back into the bloodstream).

The *active transport of sodium* is responsible for the osmotic reabsorption of water from the filtrate both here in the proximal and later in the distal tubule. As sodium ions are actively transported out of the cell and into the peritubular fluid, they make the osmotic pressure of this peritubular fluid higher than that of the cell or tubule fluid. Water is thus osmotically "pulled out" of the tubular fluid. Both water and sodium then diffuse into peritubular capillaries and are thus returned to the bloodstream.

The active transport of positively charged sodium ions also creates an electrochemical gradient that draws negatively charged ions—especially chloride—out of the tubular fluid and back into the bloodstream. This electrogenic sodium pump is inhibited by certain diuretics.

Loop of Henle

In the loop of Henle the filtrate (urine) becomes highly concentrated. This part of the nephron is composed of a thin-walled descending portion and a thick-walled ascending portion (see Fig. 18-3). Loops of Henle belonging to juxtamedullary nephrons dip into the medulla of the kidney, which contains a highly concentrated interstitial fluid. (The thin walls of the descending portion are quite permeable.) This permeability, together with the high concentration of the interstitial fluid at this point, causes water to osmose from the filtrate into the interstitial fluid. This makes the filtrate quite concentrated by the time it reaches the ascending limb of the Loop.

The thicker-walled ascending limb is relatively impermeable to water, but it contains ion carriers that actively transport chloride ions out of the filtrate. This creates an electrochemical gradient that "pulls" the positively charged sodium ions out of the filtrate also. This exit of electrolytes without water now makes the filtrate more dilute than before. Indeed, it may even become hypotonic to the blood at this point.

The Distal Tubule

In the distal tubule, sodium is again reabsorbed by active transport. Some ammonia diffuses into the filtrate. Also, hydrogen and potassium are added to the filtrate by means of tubular secretion.

The active transport of sodium uses a carrier system that is also involved in the tubular secretion of hydrogen and potassium ions (Fig. 18-5). In this relationship every time the carrier transports sodium out of the tubular fluid, it carries *either* a hydrogen *or* a potassium ion into the tubular fluid on its "return trip." Thus, for every sodium ion reabsorbed, a hydrogen *or* potas-

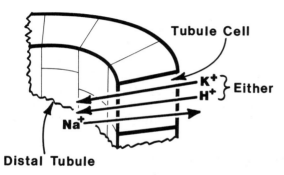

FIGURE 18-5
Cation exchange in the distal tubule.

sium must be secreted, and *vice versa*. The choice of cation to be secreted depends on the extracellular fluid (ECF) concentration of these ions (hydrogen and potassium).

Knowledge of this cation exchange system in the distal tubule helps us understand some of the relationships that these electrolytes have with one another. For example, we can understand why an aldosterone blocker may cause hyperkalemia or why there can be an initial fall in plasma potassium as severe acidosis is therapeutically corrected.*

Collecting Ducts

These structures, sometimes called collecting tubules, receive the contents of many nephrons (see Fig. 18-2). There is no further electrolyte reabsorption or secretion here, and in the normal well-hydrated person, there is no further water reabsorption either. Should the ECF become more concentrated (*e.g.,* dehydration), osmoreceptors in the hypothalamus respond by stimulating the hypothalamus to secrete antidiuretic hormone (ADH). ADH increases the permeability of the collecting tubule cells to water. This permits the (osmotic) reabsorption of water alone (without electrolytes), which in turn will decrease the concentration of the ECF. Negative feedback loops regulate ADH secretion. This means that as the concentration of the ECF returns to normal, the stimulus to ADH secretion disappears and ADH secretion is stopped.

* The aldosterone blocker reduces sodium reabsorption. Such reduced reabsorption of sodium also reduces the tubular secretion of either hydrogen or potassium. The hydrogen excess can be buffered, but the potassium simply rises to above-normal levels. In severe acidosis, the nephrons have been attempting to compensate by increasing their hydrogen-ion secretion rates. As acidosis is therapeutically corrected (*e.g.,* by sodium bicarbonate administration), one change is secretion of potassium ions (another concerns a shift of potassium into cells). As hydrogen ions no longer need to be secreted, potassium ions become the sole exchange for sodium ions, leading,it is thought, to a reduction in plasma potassium.

Juxtaglomerular Apparatus

The nephron is so arranged that the initial portion of the distal tubule lies at the juncture of the afferent and efferent arterioles, which is very near the glomerulus. Here, macula densa cells of the distal tubule lie in approximation to the juxtaglomerular cells of the wall of the afferent arteriole. Both these cell types plus some connective tissue cells constitute the juxtaglomerular apparatus. The juxtaglomerular cells of this apparatus are believed to secrete renin.

Renin causes plasma angiotensin (made in the liver) to be converted to angiotensin I, which in pulmonary capillaries is converted enzymatically into angiotensin II. This form of angiotensin acts to increase blood pressure and thus GFR by two mechanisms: (1) the constriction of peripheral arteries, and (2) the secretion of aldosterone by the adrenal cortex.

Aldosterone stimulates sodium reabsorption by the distal tubule cells. This causes increased water reabsorption, which then increases blood volume. This increase in volume can alleviate renal hypotension and restore the GFR to normal.

Stimulation of the juxtaglomerular apparatus may be varied. One hypothesis states that the macula densa cells are sensitive to the sodium concentration of distal tubule fluid. Sodium concentrations vary with the rate of glomerular filtration. The faster the filtration, the faster the fluid moves through the nephron. This decreases the time for sodium reabsorption, leading to high sodium concentrations in the distal tubule. With slower filtration and movement through the nephron, there is more reabsorption and, consequently, less sodium remaining in the fluid as it arrives at the macula densa. Decreased sodium concentration (acting as a "proxy variable" for the GFR) can then stimulate the secretion of renin by the juxtaglomerular apparatus. According to another school of thought, the juxtaglomerular cells themselves act as pressure receptors, sensitive to the HP of blood in the afferent arteriole. When these cells note a decrease in HP, they secrete renin. Both these modalities of stimulation may be correct. In addition, the juxtaglomerular apparatus seems to be stimulated by beta-adrenergics and possibly by the sympathetic stimulation as well (it appears to be enervated by sympathetic fibers).

Clearance

From the foregoing discussion a very important concept in renal function emerges—that of clearance. As the filtrate moves along the nephron, a large proportion of metabolic end products remain in it, unreabsorbed. These products are thus removed (cleared) from the blood and exit the body in the urine. Indeed, of each 125 ml of glomerular filtrate formed per minute, 60 ml leave urea behind in the fluid within the tubules. Stated another way, 60 ml of plasma are "cleared" of urea each minute in normally functioning kidneys. In the same way, 125 ml of plasma are cleared of creatinine, 12 ml of uric acid, 12 ml of potassium, 25 ml of sulfate, 25 ml of phosphate, and so forth each minute.

It is possible for one to calculate renal clearance by simultaneously sampling urine and plasma. By dividing the quantity of substance found in each milliliter of plasma into the quantity found in the urine, one can calculate the milliliters cleared per minute. This method is used as one means of testing kidney function.

Other methods of assessing renal function involve chemicals that are known to be either filtered only or both filtered and secreted. *Inulin,* for example, is only filtered and neither really absorbed nor secreted. Thus, the clearance of inulin provides a measure of glomerular filtration. *Mannitol* can be used similarly. PAH or iodopyracet (Diodrast) are drugs that are secreted in addition to being filtered. As such, their clearance provides an index of plasma flow through the kidneys. They also can be used together with a filtered-only drug in assessing tubular secretion and thus the health of tubular cells.

The sodium concentration in the urine can also serve as an index of tubular health in certain situations. For example, in acute renal failure, an increased clearance of sodium can indicate acute tubular necrosis. Accordingly, supernormal blood levels of filtered substances (creatinine and other nitrogenous wastes) indicate a fall in glomerular filtration and thus in nephron health.

Renal Regulatory Functions

In addition to excreting nitrogenous and other wastes, the kidneys can function in regulating (1) the osmotic pressure, (2) the volume, (3) the electrolyte concentration, and (4) the pH of the ECFs (blood and interstitial fluids) of the body. Let us look at specific mechanisms regarding these.

Osmotic Pressure. A rise in the ECF osmotic pressure stimulates osmoreceptors located in the hypothalamus. Such stimulation causes the hypothalamic supraoptic nuclei to secrete ADH. This hormone is thought to stimulate a sensation of thirst. It also increases the permeability of the collecting tubules to water. This increases water reabsorption, which makes the urine hypertonic and restores homeostasis of ECF osmotic pressure. Increased intake of water (due to thirst) can also serve to dilute the ECF. Conversely, a fall in ECF osmotic pressure serves to decrease the secretion of ADH, thereby enabling the kidneys to ex-

crete a more hypotonic (dilute) urine and thereby increase the ECF to normal.

Volume. Homeostasis of ECF volume is maintained by both the renin-angiotensin mechanism already discussed and the side effect of the ADH mechanism. Angiotensin also elevates blood pressure directly. Indeed, renin plays a pathologic role in one group of hypertensives.

Electrolyte Concentration. Decreased ECF *sodium* concentrations will directly stimulate aldosterone secretion from the adrenal cortex. Because decreased ECF sodium can also cause a decrease in tubular sodium, it may stimulate the juxtaglomerular secretion of renin, which will indirectly increase aldosterone levels. Aldosterone stimulates sodium reabsorption of the distal tubule cells. Thus, sodium homeostasis is restored. A rise in ECF sodium can cause the reverse.

A backup mechanism for *potassium regulation* is also found in renal function. If there are high levels of potassium in the face of normal sodium levels, the distal tubules and collecting ducts actively secrete (reverse of active reabsorption) potassium back into the urine. Similar specific reabsorption mechanisms appear to exist for divalent ions such as calcium, magnesium, and phosphates.

The regulation of the monovalent anions, chloride and bicarbonate, is secondary to sodium-ion regulation. As the positively charged cation, sodium, is reabsorbed, a negatively charged ion is electrochemically carried along. This maintains electroneutrality. Whether the negative ion is bicarbonate or chloride depends on the pH of the ECF, which is also regulated by buffers and respiratory and renal mechanisms.

pH Regulation. If buffers and the respiratory mechanism for pH homeostasis are insufficient, the kidneys then take part. Remember, the acidity of a solution is directly due to the number of unattached (free) hydrogen ions in it. In *renal compensation for alkalosis,* tubular reabsorption of hydrogen ions is increased and secretion is decreased. This increases the hydrogen-ion concentration of the ECF and thereby decreases the alkalosis.

Renal compensation for acidosis involves an increase in the hydrogen-ion secretion of the tubule cells, especially in the distal tubule cells. Now, bicarbonate and sodium ions are continually being filtered from the glomerulus. Also, as has been stated, hydrogen-ion secretion by distal tubule cells causes an increase in sodium reabsorption. Such sodium reabsorption can electrochemically increase bicarbonate reabsorption. Thus, as hydrogen ions are being eliminated from the ECF, sodium and bicarbonate ions are being added to it. Both will decrease the acidosis.

Now, the urine can only be acidified (by hydrogen-ion secretion) to a *p*H level of 4.0 to 4.5. If this mechanism operated alone, only a few hydrogen ions could be secreted before the critical shut-off level of 4.0 was reached because hydrogen would combine with urinary chloride to make hydrochloric acid. Not many of these strong hydrochloric acid molecules are needed to make the urine *p*H 4.0. This would then stop tubular hydrogen-ion secretion before sufficient compensation for acidosis could be obtained.

Fortunately this does not occur because ammonia (NH_3) is also secreted. The tubule cells deaminate certain amino acids and secrete the nitrogenous radicals from them in the form of ammonia (NH_3). This ammonia combines with hydrogen in the urine to form ammonium (NH_4^+), which in turn can combine with chloride to form ammonium chloride (NH_4Cl).

Because NH_4Cl is a neutral salt, the urine can hold many more secreted hydrogen ions than it otherwise could.

SUMMARY

The total blood flow into the nephrons of both kidneys is estimated to be about 1200 ml per minute. Of this total amount, about 650 ml is plasma. Approximately one fifth of the plasma filters through the glomerular membranes into the Bowman's capsules, forming 125 ml glomerular filtrate per minute. This filtrate is essentially plasma minus proteins. The *p*H of glomerular filtrate is equal to that of plasma, or 7.4.

As the glomerular filtrate passes through the proximal tubules, nearly 80% of the water and electrolytes, all of the glucose, proteins, and most of the amino acids are reabsorbed. The glomerular filtrate passes on through remaining tubules, where water and electrolytes are reabsorbed, depending on the need of body fluids and the effectiveness of the regulatory mechanism responsible for maintaining their normal levels.

The *p*H of the forming urine may rise or fall, depending on the relative amount of acidic and basic ions that are reabsorbed by the tubule walls. The osmotic pressure of the tubular fluid will depend on the amounts of electrolytes and water that are reabsorbed. Because of those factors, urine *p*H may vary from 4.5 to 8.2, and osmotic pressure may vary from one fourth that of plasma to approximately four times plasma pressure.

The amount of urine delivered to the renal pelvis is usually about $\frac{1}{125}$ the amount of glomerular filtrate produced or about 1 ml per minute. This 1 ml of urine will contain nearly one half the urea contained in the original 125 ml of glomerular filtrate, all of the creatinine, and large proportions of uric acid, phosphate, potassium, sulfates, nitrates, and phenols.

It should be pointed out that even though all glucose and proteins, nearly all amino acids, and large amounts of water and sodium in the original glomerular filtrate are reabsorbed, a very large proportion of the waste products are never reabsorbed and are found in the urine in highly concentrated form.

In addition to waste excretion, the kidneys function in the regulation of the osmotic pressure, volume, electrolyte concentrations, and *p*H of body fluids.

BIBLIOGRAPHY

Ganong WF: Review of Medical Physiology, 11th ed. Los Altos, Lange Medical Publications, 1983

Price SA, Wilson LM: Pathophysiology: Clinical Concepts of Disease Processes. New York, McGraw-Hill, 1978

Stephens G: Pathophysiology for Health Practitioners. New York, Macmillan, 1980

19
Assessment: Renal System

Donald E. Butkus

The nurse plays a vital role in the assessment and management of fluid and electrolyte disorders in the critically ill patient. Careful monitoring of the patient's symptoms and of his general appearance, weight, and vital signs as well as judicial interpretation of laboratory results may provide early clues to the diagnosis of disorders of water and volume imbalance as well as other complications of renal dysfunction. A thorough understanding both of the factors involved in the body's regulation of water and volume homeostasis and of the processes that alter those homeostatic mechanisms is therefore paramount in providing quality nursing care.

REGULATION OF BODY FLUIDS AND ELECTROLYTES

The human body has the rather remarkable capacity to regulate, within very narrow ranges, both the volume and composition of body fluids. Regulation of the volume of body fluids depends primarily on the intake of the cations sodium and potassium, which control the volume of the extracellular and intracellular spaces, respectively. Their balance in the body is normally governed by net intake in the diet minus their loss in sweat, feces, and urine. Elimination occurs primarily in the urine, except when increased sweating or diarrhea occur. Then the skin and intestinal tracts contribute significantly to these losses. During an excess or a reduced intake of either of these cations, homeostatic mechanisms including alterations of GFR, aldosterone production, natriuretic factor, catecholemines, and so forth may be called into play to maintain balance either by enhancing their excretion into, or by increasing their reabsorption from, the urine.

An example of this balancing activity is the reduction in extra cellular volume that occurs when sodium intake is restricted or when there are sodium losses, as with vomiting and diarrhea. This stimulates the renin-angiotensin system, which results in both peripheral vasoconstriction and increased aldosterone production. The aldosterone stimulates renal sodium conservation in exchange for potassium and hydrogen ions and prevents further loss of sodium in the urine. As volume depletion continues, renal blood flow decreases, with GFR initially remaining near normal. This produces an increased filtration fraction (GFR/RBF), due to renal efferent arteriolar constriction, which results in both a decrease in peritubular capillary hydrostatic pressure and an increase in oncotic pressure. This increases the net peritubular starting forces favoring reabsorption and results in an increased fraction of the filtered fluid being reabsorbed. Increased proximal sodium and fluid reabsorption and increased (aldosterone-stimulated) distal sodium reabsorption combine to remove most of the sodium from the urine and prevent further volume depletion. If volume depletion continued, renal blood flow would further decrease, GFR would fall, and the amount of sodium filtered would also decrease. Increased sympathetic tone and circulating catecholamines would further contribute to this sequence of events.

When excess sodium is taken in, the sequence is reversed, and the renin-angiotensin system and aldosterone production are shut off, allowing decreased renal sodium reabsorption. Other factors such as decreased catecholamines and increased renal prostaglandin production help maintain this homeostasis. When excess sodium is retained because of either primary aldosterone excess, the nephrotic syndrome, or congestive heart failure, the body may elaborate one or several "natriuretic factors" that stimulate renal sodium loss independent of the factors mentioned before.

The tonicity of body fluids, which maintain plasma osmolality within a narrow range, is controlled primarily by regulation of water intake and by excretion. For example, an increase in plasma osmolality of only 1% to 2% due to fluid loss or sodium addition will stimulate thirst and the release of the antidiuretic hormone vasopressin. This results in increased water intake and increased renal water reabsorption, which decrease the serum osmolality. This in turn decreases the stimulus to thirst and to vasopressin release. Excessive volume depletion (in the range of 7% to 10%), can also stimulate vasopressin release and result in fluid retention (at the expense of plasma tonicity) and produce hyponatremia and hypo-osmolality. The osmotic threshold for vasopressin release is set lower than the thirst threshold, so that during water restriction maximum urinary concentration is achieved before thirst is stimulated. This adapative mechanism allows a person to be deprived of water much longer than if the thirst threshold were set lower.

Urinary Concentration and Dilution

The kidney possesses a considerable capacity to reabsorb filtered water. In people with normal renal function, the final concentration of the urine depends on the state of hydration. A patient who is well hydrated will excrete a very dilute urine, whereas a patient who is dehydrated will excrete a very concentrated urine, as the kidneys attempt to either eliminate or conserve water, respectively.

The factor that governs the amount of water excreted and, therefore, the urine concentration is the amount of antidiuretic hormone (ADH) secreted by the pituitary gland and the ability of the kidneys to respond to ADH.

Urinary concentration may be measured by tests for specific gravity or osmolality (see later in this chapter).

Serum Sodium Concentration

The serum sodium concentration is generally maintained in a narrow range (135 to 145 mEq/liter) and depends on the body's state of fluid balance as governed by the release of ADH and water intake. Generally, it is relatively constant in a normal person who is not exposed to any physiological stress.

The measurement of the serum sodium by flame photometry is relatively accurate. However, in certain circumstances (*e.g.,* hyperproteinemia and hyperlipidemia), the "measured" serum sodium may be artificially low. This is because the sodium concentration is measured per volume of plasma or serum. For example, hyperlipidemia and hyperproteinemia, by occupying part of the volume of the sample, will result in an artificially lowered measured concentration of sodium, which is present primarily in plasma water. In this situation, measurement of the serum osmolality, which more accurately reflects tonicity in the water phase, will be normal and there will be a discrepancy between the measured serum osmolality and that calculated from the serum sodium. This condition of pseudohyponatremia is not clinically significant, except that it produces problems in interpreting the serum sodium concentration.

Regulation of Urinary Sodium Excretion (Volume Maintenance)

The normally functioning kidney has a considerable capability of adapting *urinary sodium excretion* to the person's needs. Normally the amount of sodium appearing in the urine in a 24-hour period will exactly equal sodium intake, minus a small amount that is excreted in the feces and in the sweat.

When excess sodium is ingested, adaptation begins within 24 hours to rid the body of excess sodium. When sodium intake is restricted, urinary sodium excretion decreases to match intake. This may take 2 to 3 days to occur in normal people or longer if chronic renal disease is present. During this time, a mild total body sodium deficit will occur. With extreme sodium restriction, the kidneys can reduce urinary sodium excretion to virtually zero to prevent further deficits in body sodium. Therefore, no absolute value for urinary sodium excretion is "normal"; instead, a range of normal exists, depending on the body's state of sodium balance.

Likewise, there is no normal value for *urinary sodium concentration* but rather a *range* of normal that depends on the amount of sodium excreted and on the amount of water that is simultaneously excreted. A low urinary sodium concentration might result from a low sodium intake, or it might reflect extreme dilution of the urinary sodium by a large amount of excreted water. In addition to being lowered as the result of decreased sodium intake, the urinary sodium concentration may be reduced by factors that reduce renal blood flow and result in excessive retention of sodium (and water) to maintain absolute or effective intravascular volume. This may be seen in hypotension and shock from any cause, in congestive heart failure, in decompensated cirrhosis, in the nephrotic syndrome, and in acute nephritis, all of which might be associated with both very low concentrations and absolute amounts of sodium in the urine. Administration of diuretics might artificially increase the urine sodium in these states and interfere with interpretations of urinary diagnostic indices (see further on).

ALTERED STATES OF FLUIDS AND ELECTROYLTES

Disorders of Water Balance

Primary disorders of water balance, *hyponatremia,* and *hypernatremia,* occur when water is retained or lost from the body in excess of sodium. Hyponatremia may be due to any of the following:

- A primary increase in thirst
- Decreased intravascular volume (with unbalanced fluid replacement with water without sodium salts)
- Inappropriate secretion of vasopressin
- Renal salt wasting

In contrast, hypernatremia may occur as the result of either of the following:

- Defective ADH release or renal responsiveness
- Water loss in excess of sodium as with excessive sweating or renal salt wasting.

Changes in body sodium concentration are reflected in parallel changes in serum osmolality, which is the primary stimulus for vasopressin release or suppression.

Hyponatremia

In a number of disease states, the serum sodium concentration may be reduced (hyponatremia) because of an inability of the kidneys to excrete free water. This is due to either a persistent release of ADH in response to a decrease in the total or effective intravascular volume or to some inappropriate stimulation of ADH release. (It is not due to volume or osmotic stimuli).* States of actual or effective intravascular volume depletion also contribute to the hyponatremia by decreasing distal delivery of fluid in the nephron and thereby limiting the amount of water that can be excreted.

Hyponatremia may be associated with (1) an increased total body sodium and edema, (2) a decreased total body sodium and hypovolemia, or (3) a normal or slightly increased total body sodium and increased blood volume, depending on the clinical disorder that gives rise to the hyponatremia (Table 19-1).

Volume Depletion. In patients with edema due to cirrhosis, congestive heart failure, or the nephrotic syndrome, hyponatremia occurs frequently and may be enhanced by the use of diuretics. In these conditions, although there is an overall increase in body sodium and water, ADH release is stimulated because the *effective* blood volume is decreased. As a result, the kidneys tend to reabsorb a greater percentage of filtered fluid in the proximal tubule. This causes further fluid retention and hyponatremia, especially if the patient has unlimited access to water, because the little fluid reaching the distal tubule is reabsorbed more completely owing to the high plasma ADH level.

CASE STUDY

A 46-year-old male alcoholic was admitted after a binge, with a 48-hour history of jaundice and increasing mental confusion. For 2 weeks he had noted increasing edema and increasing abdominal girth. During physical examination, he was moderately obtunded but arousable. Blood pressure was 98/68 mm Hg, pulse was 92/minute, and temperature was

---

* A significant decrease in blood volume can override the normal osmotic stimulus to ADH release.

TABLE 19-1
HYPONATREMIA

Accompanying Factors	Causes
Increased total body sodium and edema	Congestive heart failure
	Decompensated cirrhosis
	Nephrotic syndrome
Decreased total body sodium and hypovolemia	Diuretics
	Renal salt-wasting
	Adrenal insufficiency
	Hemorrhage
Normal total body sodium and hypervolemia	Syndrome of inappropriate ADH release, which may accompany CNS and pulmonary disease, tumors, porphyria, use of certain drugs, psychiatric disorders, myxedema

97°F. The patient had marked scleral icterus, tense abdominal ascites, and diffuse pitting edema below the waist. Initial laboratory studies revealed the following:

Serum:	Na	115 mEq/Liter
	Cl	75 mEq/Liter
	K	2.8 mEq/Liter
	CO_2	30 mEq/Liter
	BUN	10 mg/dl
	Creatinine	0.8 mg/dl
	Albumin	2.4 gm%
Urine:	Specific gravity	1.028; pH6.8
	U_{osm}890	mOsm/Liter
	U_{Na}	8 mEq/Liter
	U_K	33 mEq/Liter
	U_{Cl}	2 mEq/Liter

The serum bilirubin, SGOT, alkaline phosphatase, and LDH were all elevated, but the blood ammonium level was normal.

The patient had developed severe hyponatremia in the face of an increase in total body sodium and water, as reflected by the pronounced edema. Sodium retention is due to the combined effects of decreased renal perfusion secondary to (1) hypovolemia from hypoalbuminemia and ascites formation, (2) alcoholic peripheral vasodilatation, and (3) secondary hypoaldosteronism. The hyponatremia is due to the combined effects of volume-mediated vasopressin release, as reflected in the high urine specific gravity and osmolality, and to decreased distal nephron sodium and water delivery due to renal underperfusion.

The patient had acute alcoholic hepatitis and was treated with enteral hyperalimentation via a nasogastric tube. Initial treatment of his hyponatremia consisted of water restriction and a combination of a thiazide diuretic and aldactone, resulting in slow correction of his serum sodium.

It should be noted that in addition to his hyponatremia, the patient also had a hypokalemic metabolic alkalosis, probably resulting from the combined effects of volume and potassium depletion. His urinary sodium of 8 mEq per liter was considerably higher than his urine chloride concentration, probably owing to spilling of bicarbonate in the urine. Bicarbonaturia obligates urinary sodium excretion, even in the face of volume depletion. In this situation, the urinary chloride concentration is a better indication of volume depletion than is the urinary sodium concentration, as was noted in this patient.

Treatment with thiazide diuretics, furosemide, or ethacrynic acid can produce or seriously compound the hyponatremia because these drugs may further decrease the effective blood volume and because they decrease sodium transport in the ascending limb of Henle, which is necessary for the kidneys' ability to excrete free water and maximally dilute the urine.

Patients with volume depletion due to loss of sodium or blood may also develop hyponatremia when the volume depletion is great enough to stimulate ADH release. In this situation, body sodium and blood volume are reduced, and edema is not present. Diuretic administration, renal salt-wasting, adrenal insufficiency, and hemorrhage are examples of this type of condition. ADH release occurs and stimulates water reabsorption in an attempt to restore intravascular volume, irrespective of serum osmolality. If the patient ingests water without salt, or if hypotonic fluids are administered IV, hyponatremia will result.

Primary Excessive ADH Secretion. Hyponatremia may also occur in a number of conditions that are not associated with a decrease in either effective or absolute blood volume but in which either persistent release of ADH from the pituitary gland or ectopic production of ADH occurs. This unregulated production of ADH results in what is referred to as *the syndrome of inappropriate ADH release* (SIADH). This may occur with cerebral disease such as stroke, infection, and trauma; pulmonary diseases such as pneumonia, tuberculosis, and tumor; systemic disorders such as porphyria and systemic lupus erythematosus; certain drugs such as morphine, tranquilizers, and anesthetics, and with psychiatric disorders, such as schizophrenia.

When hyponatremia is due to the SIADH, blood volume is slightly increased owing to water retention, but edema does not occur. The BUN and serum uric acid concentration are generally low normal because of dilution, and the urine is abnormally concentrated in relation to the degree of plasma hypo-osmolality because of the persistent ADH effect.

The urine sodium concentration is frequently high despite the hyponatremia, probably because the mild volume expansion stimulates the kidneys to excrete sodium. The mechanism responsible for the persistent sodium excretion is unknown, but it may be the result of a humoral natriuretic factor (also called *third factor*) released in response to volume expansion or of altered peritubular physical factors (*i.e.,* oncotic pressure) that govern tubular sodium reabsorption. However, when sodium intake is decreased in these patients, urinary sodium may also decrease.

CASE STUDY

A 31-year-old woman with chronic schizophrenia was admitted with a history of syncope, incoherent speech, sluggishness, and combativeness. She had been on thorazine and artane for her psychiatric disorder.

Blood pressure was 130/70 mm Hg, pulse was 68/minute, temperature was 98°F, and respirations were 19/minute. Except for incoherence of speech and combativeness, findings on physical examination were normal. Specifically, there were no edema and no significant orthostatic drop in blood pressure or increase in pulse. Admission chemistries were as follows:

Serum:	Sodium	119 mEq/liter
	Potassium	3.4 mEq/liter
	CO_2	20 mEq/liter
	Chloride	87 mEq/liter
	BUN	4 mg/dl
	Creatinine	0.6 mg/dl

	Osmolality	253 mOsm/liter
Urine:	Osmolality	258 mOsm/liter
	Sodium	23 mEq/liter

The patient demonstrated euvolemic hyponatremia with decreased BUN and creatinine secondary to intravascular volume expansion. The urine osmolality and sodium were inappropriately high for her serum sodium (and osmolality). Urine osmolality would have been expected to be below 100 mOsm/liter in view of her euvolemic hyponatremia had this been due to simple water excess. The diagnosis of SIADH, due either to medication or to psychiatric disorder, was made. Water restriction and elimination of medications resulted in a return of electrolytes and mental status to normal in 48 hours. At that point, she was able to relate a history of two previous similar episodes when these medications had been prescribed in the past.

Hypernatremia

Hypernatremia results from primary water deficits in such situations as restricted intake, intestinal losses, and excessive insensible loss or from nephrogenic or pituitary diabetes insipidus. Hypernatremia due to primary water loss from either decreased intake, diarrhea, or increased sweating results in a concentrated urine, whereas hypernatremia due to either central or nephrogenic diabetes insipidus is associated with a dilute urine.

CASE STUDY

A 12-year-old girl was admitted with a 2-week history of diplopia and a 72-hour history of polydypsia and polyuria. There was no history of head trauma or seizures.

Findings on physical examination were normal except for oculomotor nerve paresis on the right and mild early papilledema. The following laboratory work was obtained:

Serum:	Na	155 mEq/liter
	Cl	114 mEq/liter
	K	4.0 mEq/liter
	CO_2	28 mEq/liter
	BUN	24 mg/dl
	Creatinine	0.8 mg/dl
	Glucose	95 mg/dl
	Osmolality	314 mOsm/liter
Urine:	Sodium	14 mEq/liter
	Osmolality	92 mOsm/liter

A radiological workup showed an extensive mass in the area of the third ventricle that proved to be a craniopharyngioma. Laboratory studies were consistent with a diagnosis of central diabetes insipidus: Urine osmolality was inappropriately low for the degree of hypernatremia and hypo-osmolality, both of which were corrected following exogenous pitressin administration.

Body fluid and electrolyte balance thus depend both on adequate access and intake of food and fluids and on intact hormonal and renal mechanisms to facilitate their excretion or conservation. Factors that interfere with intake or excretion of both solutes and water can therefore have significant effects on the volume and composition of body fluids and the well-being of the patient (Table 19-2).

NURSING ASSESSMENT: INTAKE, LOSSES, OUTPUT

An accurate history and physical examination will assist the nurse in estimating fluid and electrolyte problems that occur in the clinical setting. The variables to be assessed include the following:

- Intake
- Losses by any route
- Output

Assessment of Intake

An accurate history of intake of fluids as well as electrolytes and nonelectrolytes is important in assessing the clinical status of the patient. Either inadequate or excessive intake, in appropriate circumstances, can cause significant disturbances in the body's homeostasis of fluids and electrolytes.

Inadequate fluid intake in a conscious patient may result from anorexia, apathy, lethargy, difficulty in swallowing, or inaccessability to fluids and food (as might occur in debilitated or stroke patients). Because of physical limitations or socioeconomic restrictions or both, debilitated patients and the elderly may not have ready access to food and fluids, even though their hunger and thirst responses are appropriate. Infants, the elderly, and the incapacitated or feeble patient are especially vulnerable because they cannot make their needs known or do not have appropriate access to adequate intake without relying on others. In patients with psychiatric or central nervous system disorders, abnormalities of thirst may occur that either depress or increase the intake of fluids out of proportion to the body's needs and the kidney's regulatory abilities. Decreased intake leads to water depletion and hypernatremia (if sodium intake is normal). Increased intake may lead to water excess and hyponatremia if intake exceeds the excretory capacity of the kidneys. In patients who are unconscious or who are entirely dependent on nursing personnel for parenteral fluids and alimentation, it is mandatory that a record of intake and output be maintained so that the status of the patient can be assessed. For some patients, a daily record is sufficient, whereas for acutely ill patients hourly records may be crucial.

Excessive free water intake in a patient with relative or absolute hypovolemia from sodium depletion, diuretic administration, diarrheal losses, congestive heart failure, decompensated cirrhosis, and other conditions can lead to hyponatremia. In addition, increased thirst from CNS disease or decreased renal water excretion resulting from use of drugs that stimulate vasopressin release (*e.g.,* cyclophosphamide and valium) or that interfere with the action of vasopressin on the kidney (*e.g.,* chlorpropamide and nonsteroidal anti-inflammatory drugs) can cause hyponatremia

TABLE 19-2
FACTORS AFFECTING WATER BALANCE

	Water Excess	Water Deficiency
Intake		
Thirst	Decreased thirst threshold	Increased thirst threshold
	Increased osmolality	Decreased osmolality
	Potassium depletion	Lack of access
	Hypercalcemia	Psychiatric disorders
	Fever	
	Dry mucous membranes	
	Poor oral hygiene	
	Unmisted O_2 administration	
	Hypotension	
	Psychiatric disorders	
Parenteral fluids	Excessive D5W	Deficient replacement
		Osmotic loads
		Hyperalimentation
		Hyperglycemia
		Mannitol
		X-ray contrast agents
Output		
Sweating		High ambient temperature
		High altitude
		Fever
Renal Excretion	Inappropriate ADH release	Excess excretion
	Appropriate ADH release	Central
	Congestive failure	Nephrogenic
	Decompensated cirrhosis	Potassium depletion
	Volume depletion	Hypercalcemia
	Adrenal insufficiency	Lithium administration
	Renal salt-wasting	Declomicin
	Hemorrhage	Penthrane
	Diuretics	
	Burns	
	Hypothyroidism	
	Renal disease	
	Acute renal failure	
	Chronic renal failure	
	Nephrotic syndrome	
	Acute glomerulonephritis	
	Nonsteroidal anti-inflammatory agents	

even when intake appears appropriate. Excessive administration of IV fluids such as D5W without adequate saline can also result in hyponatremia, even when renal function and sodium conservation are normal.

Excessive sodium intake, either enteral or parenteral, can lead to hypernatremia when water intake is restricted if the patient has a decrease in effective circulatory volume is on drugs such as lithium or doxycycline, or has chronic renal disease, all of which interfere with the kidneys' ability to conserve water by responding appropriately to vasopressin.

Assessment of Losses

Losses of fluids and electrolytes can occur through the skin, respiratory tract, gastrointestinal tract, and kidney, from drainage from body cavities and fistulas, and from third-spacing into body compartments.

Sources of Excessive Losses

- *Fever.* A patient with a fever of 104°F (40°C) and a respiratory rate of 40 breaths per minute can lose as much as 2500 ml of fluid in a 24-hour period from the respiratory tract and from the skin.
- *Environment.* Hot, dry climates can increase evaporative sweat losses to 1500 ml/hour to maintain body evaporative heat loss. This can increase to between 2 and 2.5 liters/hour for short times in acclimatized individuals exercising in hot climates.
- *Hyperventilation.* Hyperventilation can increase respiratory water losses as the result of either disease or use of nonhumidified respirators.
- *Gastrointestinal Tract.* Vomiting, nasogastric suction, diarrhea, and enterocutaneous drainage or fistulas can increase gastrointestinal losses.
- *Third-Spacing.* Formation of pleural or peritoneal effusions and edema from liver, renal, or hepatic

disease or from the diffuse capillary leak syndrome can result in a loss of effective intravascular volume. Drainage of peritoneal or pleural fluid, when formation of these third spaces is still occurring, can result in further effective intravascular losses because of continued fluid shifts from the vascular compartment to the third space.

- *Burns.* Fluid loss into burned tissues can result in a significant decrease in effective intravascular volume. Because both evaporative and transulative losses through the burned skin can result in absolute losses of 1 to 2000 ml/day, the burned patient requires special attention to maintain fluid and electrolyte balance.

- *Renal Losses.* Inappropriate solute and fluid loss from the kidneys can occur because of renal salt-wasting, as seen in the diuretic phase of ATN, in some rare patients with true renal salt-wasting, and as the result of excessive diuretic administration. It also may occur as the result of solute diuresis from high-protein or high-saline enteral and parenteral alimentation and from administration of osmotic agents, such as mannitol and radiocontrast agents. Finally, there can be fluid loss during the generation phase of metabolic alkalosis, in which compensatory urinary bicarbonate excretion obligates renal sodium excretion, frequently in the face of volume depletion.

Assessment of Output

Output with Normal Renal Function

The *normal kidney* can maintain solute balance when urine volume is reduced to between 4 and 600 ml/day because the kidneys can increase the urine concentration from 1000 to 1200 mOsm/kg. In the average person producing 600 mOsm of metabolic solute from dietary intake and metabolic conversion, approximately 500 ml of urine is required to excrete this if solute urine concentrating ability is normal. If solute load is increased as a result of increased intake (*e.g.,* from high protein diets, hyperalimentation, or hypercatabolism), a greater urine volume will be required to excrete the metabolic solute load.

Because the urinary concentrating ability normally decreases progressively after 40 years of age, older people, who cannot maximally concentrate their urine, will require a greater urine volume to maintain homeostasis in the face of "normal" intakes. However, even if maximum urine concentrating ability is reduced to 600 mOsm/kg, only 1000 ml of urine would be required to excrete an "average" 600 mOsm solute load generated per day. Older people probably eat considerably less and thereby obligate a smaller urine volume to maintain homeostasis. The same sort of decreased urinary concentrating ability is noted in patients with chronic renal disease as their disease progresses. In addition to increased solute load from hyperalimentation, both glycosuria associated with poorly controlled diabetes and radiologic contrast agents can result in a solute diuresis and obligate a greater urine volume than normal.

Output With Impaired Renal Function

In *chronic renal disease,* the kidneys have the ability to adapt significantly to maintain water and electrolyte levels that are equivalent to normal levels until GFR decreases below 15 to 20 ml per minute. This is accomplished through increased solute and water excretion per nephron and is partially modulated by changes in systemic and local intrarenal hormone production, possibly by the so-called natriuretic factor.

At the extremes of intake (*i.e.,* sodium and water excess or restriction), the kidneys' ability to compensate may be restricted in chronic renal failure. This is especially true with abrupt decreases in sodium intake, with which the time required to adapt may be prolonged beyond the normal 2 to 3 days and a relative state of "salt-wasting" may occur. Some patients may actually have true sodium-wasting and require greater than normal sodium intakes to maintain sodium balance. However, this is rare, and most patients with chronic renal failure can adapt if sodium restriction is produced slowly. In addition, unless acidosis is present, as with hyporeninemic hypoaldosteronism or with more severe decreases in GFR, serum potassium levels and the ability to excrete potassium are also maintained. When the GFR decreases below 10 ml/minute, patients with end-stage renal disease may require restriction of sodium, potassium, and water intake to maintain balance. This usually requires major adjustments in the diet.

Output With Acute Renal Failure

Acute renal failure is quite different from chronic renal disease. Because patients with classic acute renal failure have oliguria or anuria (<500 ml/day or <100 ml/day, respectively), they demand much more attention to electrolyte and water balance than patients with comparable degrees of chronic renal failure. Sodium and water restriction, as well as protein and potassium restriction, become necessary because of the limited capacity of the kidney to excrete these substances. In addition, the hypercatabolic state, with generation of excess metabolic water and with shifts of solutes between intracellular and extracellular compartments as a result of acidosis, adds to the effects of uremia per se in most patients with acute renal failure. Attention to strict intake and output monitoring is mandatory in these patients if fluid overload and congestive heart failure are to be prevented. In the conservative management of these patients, replacement of fluids should be restricted to correction of measured losses (urine plus gastrointestinal products) and should be primarily in the form of D5W, unless measureable changes in serum electrolytes also occur. Insensible losses should not be corrected unless measurable sweating from fever occurs because the "metabolic" water generated will approach 5 to 600 ml/day and should not be replaced. A rough guide to appropriate restriction is a weight loss of 0.5 to 0.75 kg/day.

Nursing Intervention

The nurse's role in the evaluation, correction, and maintenance of fluid balance includes accurate recording of intake and output, weight, vital signs, and drug administration. The most sensitive indices of changes in body water content are serial weights and intake-output patterns. Although vital signs provide supporting data, they may not be abnormal until significant volume or water deficits occur. Assessment of fluid imbalance is based on observation and recognition of pertinent symptoms, and nursing action involves replacement or restriction of fluids. Knowing how the patient's medical condition and medications may affect fluid balance is important in predicting which patients are at risk and require closer supervision.

Intake and Output

An accurate intake and output record provides valuable data for evaluating and treating fluid and electrolyte imbalances. It is important that all nursing personnel, as well as the patient and his visitors, are involved and instructed. The severity of the circumstances will dictate how exact the record should be and what data will be included. For example, in a postsurgical patient who has no complications, fluid replacement may be projected on estimated and actual losses for a 24-hour period. All measureable intake and output are recorded and totaled at the end of every shift.

In the presence of excessive losses or deterioration of cardiac, hepatic, renal, or respiratory function, more detailed recording of every source of fluid intake and output is necessary, and calculations may be required every 1 to 4 hours.

Intake includes not only pure liquids such as water and juices but also those foods that are high in water content (*e.g.,* oranges, grapefruit, gelatin, and ice cream). Patients and their families frequently must be reminded that ice and water are the same and that ice therefore must be included in the measurements. It is useful to keep a list of equivalents for fruits, ice cubes, and other sources of water and electrolytes. Output should include intestinal and renal as well as respiratory and cutaneous losses if the patient's temperature or the ambient temperature is high. If enteric, thoracic,

abdominal, or ileostomy drainage is present, it should also be recorded.

In severe electrolyte and fluid imbalances, the time and type of fluid intake as well as the time and amount of each voiding should be recorded. These data are mandatory in the event that renal function decreases because of prerenal azotemia or acute renal failure, and they may aid immeasurably in the diagnosis of, and possible prevention of, acute renal failure.

Weight

Rapid daily gains and losses in weight are usually related to changes in fluid volume. Because of the difficulties in obtaining accurate figures for intake and output records, serial weights are often more reliable. In addition, *weight changes will usually pick up imbalances before symptoms are apparent.*

As with intake and output records, the weighing procedure should be consistent. The patient should be weighed on the same scale with the same attire, preferably in the morning before breakfast and after voiding. Variations in the procedure should be noted and made known to the physician.

A kilogram scale provides for greater accuracy because drug, fluid, and diet measurement are calculated with the metric system, and conversion from pounds to kilograms may lead to discrepancies.

Normally, a patient with a balanced nutritional intake will maintain his weight. A patient whose protein intake is limited or who is catabolic will lose about 2.2 kg/day (1 lb/day). A weight gain of more than 2.2 kg/day (1 lb/day) suggests fluid retention. *A generally accepted guide is that 473 ml (1 pt) of fluid is reflected in $\frac{1}{2}$ kg (1.1 lb) of weight gained.*

Assessment of Hypovolemia and Hypervolemia

One must be continuously on the alert to detect early changes in volume status of the patient. Seldom is the diagnosis made on the basis of one diagnostic parameter. The first clue to the nurse may be the patient's general appearance; after she observes this, she should seek and note more specific parameters.

Symptoms vary with the degree of imbalance, some being seen early in imbalance states and others not being evident until severe imbalances have occurred. Table 19-3 lists the physical assessment and symptoms of fluid imbalance and can be used as a guide for nursing assessment.

With volume depletion, the patient may complain of orthostatic light-headedness when he assumes the sitting or standing position (this can also occur from inactivity and autonomic dysfunction). Development of tachycardia on assuming the upright position and a decrease in blood pressure (orthostatic hypotension),

TABLE 19-3
PHYSICAL ASSESSMENT AND SYMPTOMS OF IMBALANCE

Assessed Factors	Hypovolemia	Hypervolemia
Skin and subcutaneous tissues	Dry; less elastic	Warm, moist, pitting edema over bony prominences; wrinkled skin from pressure of clothing
Face	Sunken eyes (late symptom)	Periorbital edema
Tongue	Dry, coated (early symptom); fissured (late symptom)	Moist
Saliva	Thick, scanty	Excessive, frothy
Thirst	Present	May not be significant
Temperature	May be elevated	May not be significant
Pulse	Rapid, weak, thready	Rapid
Respirations	Rapid, shallow	Rapid dyspnea, moist rales
Blood pressure	Low, orthostatic hypotension; small pulse pressure	Normal to high
Weight	Loss	Gain

as opposed to the normal rise, are frequent early findings. Later, the pulse may become rapid, weak, and thready. There may be early dryness of the skin, with loss of elasticity, sunken eyes, loss of axillary sweating, and dry, coated tongue. When severe volume depletion occurs, thirst, decreased urine volume, and weight loss may be noted. However, except for weight loss and orthostatic blood pressure and pulse changes, these findings are not usually present. Laboratory studies such as a high urine osmolality and low urinary sodium may facilitate the diagnosis.

Other guidelines such as a raised hematocrit, decreased central venous pressure (CVP), and decreased pulmonary wedge pressure may corroborate the diagnosis.

In fluid overload the patient, if alert, may complain of puffiness or stiffness in the hands and feet or state that rings feel tight. Later, periorbital edema or puffiness, followed by pitting edema of the dependent parts (feet and ankles if upright; sacral area and posterior thighs if supine) will occur, followed by dyspnea or ascites, depending on etiology (*i.e.,* cardiac decompensation and systemic fluid overload versus hepatic disease). Urine volume and urine sodium may be normal, increased, or decreased, depending on the etiology. In most diseases with fluid retention, except for SIADH, urine sodium will be reduced. The hematocrit will be decreased, reflecting hemodilution.

The pulse may be rapid, and respirations may be increased because of pulmonary congestion, and auscultation of the chest may reveal rales. A chest film may reveal pulmonary vascular congestion, increased aveolar lung markings, cardiac dilatation, or frank pulmonary congestion and pleural effusions.

All data should be evaluated in the light of other evidence. Trends are usually more significant than isolated values. For example, when the nurse notes a decrease in urine output, she should then do a systematic assessment in order to determine why this is happening and what nursing interventions are most appropriate. Any system of assessment will work when it is consistent and thorough.

Nursing Intervention in Hypovolemia and Hypervolemia

After reviewing the intake and output records for both the current and the previous day and making an assessment of the symptoms and parameters just discussed, the nurse can make a decision about whether to increase or decrease fluid intake. In the absence of symptoms of fluid retention, when intravenous fluids are behind schedule and intake is inadequate for the patient's condition, missed fluids should be given. The nurse should watch the patient's fluid status closely for the next few hours, especially his urine output, to evaluate whether or not the increase in fluid intake corrected the patient's fluid balance. If, however, urine output is zero or diminished in the presence of adequate fluid intake, no more fluids are given, and the physician is called immediately. If a patient presents any of the symptoms of fluid overload discussed earlier, all fluid intake is restricted, and the physician is notified immediately.

Fluid replacement, as stated previously, may be calculated for any given period of time, depending on the severity of the situation. For example, a 24-hour calculation of intake for a patient who is oliguric with normal insensible losses could be as follows:

Previous 24-hour urine output:	100 ml
Insensible loss replacement:	500 ml
Total 24-hour fluid allowance:	600 ml

TABLE 19-4
SIGNS AND SYMPTOMS RELATED TO HYPONATREMIA ACCORDING TO SERUM SODIUM CONCENTRATION

140–120 mEq/Liter	120–110 mEq/Liter	110–100 mEq/Liter	100–95 mEq/Liter
Generally none	Headache	Confusion	Delirium
	Apathy	Hostility	Convulsions
	Lethargy	Lethargy or violence	Coma
	Weakness	Nausea and vomiting	Hypothermia
	Disorientation	Areflexia	Cheyne-Stokes respiration
			Death

Although the physician will specify the total amount and kind of fluid replacement, the details of distribution are often decided by the nurse. Priority is given to requirements for administration of drugs, both intravenous and oral. Distribution of the remaining fluid is then made according to patient preference. The nurse guides the patient in his selection to help him avoid using up the entire day's allowance early in the day. Because sodium and potassium may be restricted in the patient with renal failure, fluids such as ginger ale, 7-Up, and Kool Aid, which are low in sodium and potassium, are given.

Assessment of Hyponatremia

Hyponatremia is important because it can produce a wide range of neurologic symptoms, including death. The severity of symptoms depends on the degree of hyponatremia and on the rate at which it has developed. Generally, symptoms do not occur until the serum sodium is below 120 mEq/liter. Table 19-4 depicts the symptoms to be expected in several ranges of hyponatremia. It is important to remember that for each level of sodium concentration, the severity of symptoms encountered will depend on how rapidly the sodium concentration was lowered.

Nursing Intervention in Hyponatremia

Treatment of hyponatremia depends on the level of serum sodium, the patient's symptoms, and the cause.

In most cases of mild hyponatremia associated with congestive heart failure or SIADH, fluid restriction to approximately 1000 ml/day is the only treatment necessary. In cases associated with true volume depletion, normal saline will usually correct the volume deficit and restore the sodium concentration to normal. For the most severe degrees of hyponatremia, with potentially life-threatening symptoms, hypertonic (3%) sodium chloride given intravenously may be necessary.

If fluid overload is also a problem, water restriction and intravenous furosemide or ethacrynic acid, both of which cause water loss in excess of sodium, may be the therapy of choice, sometimes with concomitant replacement with hypertonic saline. This type of therapy requires hourly urine collections and accurate measurements of electrolyte losses so that serious electrolyte disturbances are prevented.

For patients with chronic hyponatremia due to SIADH, demeclocycline, which blocks the renal ADH effect, may be the preferred treatment.

Assessment of Hypernatremia

Symptoms of hypernatremia are generally the same as those of hyperosmolality and result from CNS dehydration. Mental confusion, stupor, seizures, coma, and death may occur, in addition to other signs of dehydration such as fatigue, muscle weakness and cramps, and anorexia. The serum osmolality is generally above 350 mOsm/liter before significant symptoms are noted. This corresponds to a serum sodium of 165 to 170 mEq/liter.

Nursing Intervention in Hypernatremia

Treatment consists of administration of free water (without salt), vasopressin (Pitressin) in those cases due to pituitary diabetes insipidus, and elimination of conditions known to produce nephrogenic diabetes insipidus (hypercalcemia, hypokalemia, demeclocycline, and lithium administration).

SELECTED TESTS FOR ASSESSMENT AND MONITORING OF RENAL FUNCTION

The patient whose condition is serious enough to warrant observation in the critical care unit will frequently manifest abnormalities of renal function, as the result of either impaired ability to excrete nitrogenous waste products or an inability to handle water and electrolyte loads efficiently or both. It is therefore mandatory that certain aspects of renal function be monitored on an intermittent or a continuing basis in order that these complications can be detected early and appropriate therapy instituted.

In most circumstances, the parameters followed will include the urine output, the urine solute concentration (frequently in relation to the plasma solute concentration), and some parameter of the kidneys' ability to excrete nitrogenous waste products.

Creatinine and Creatinine Clearance

The most commonly used tests of renal function are the serum creatinine and the blood urea nitrogen (BUN), but the most accurate test readily available is the creatinine clearance. Creatinine is formed as a by-product of normal muscle metabolism and is excreted in the urine primarily as the result of glomerular filtration, with a small percentage secreted into the urine by the kidney tubules. It is therefore a useful indicator of the glomerular filtration rate. The amount of creatinine excreted in the urine of any given person is related to his muscle mass and will remain quite constant unless muscle-wasting occurs.

The actual creatinine clearance is calculated by the following formula:

$$\text{creatinine clearance} = \frac{\text{UV}}{\text{P}}$$

Where U is the urine creatinine concentration, V the urine volume, and P the plasma creatinine concentration. The most important technical aspect of this test is the *accuracy of the urine collection;* it is important to know the exact time it took to form the sample and the exact amount of creatinine present.

The expression UV tells how much creatinine appears in the urine during the period of collection, and this can be readily converted to milligrams per minute, which is the standard reference point. Dividing this value by the plasma creatinine concentration (which must be converted from mg/100 ml to mg/ml) tells the minimum number of milliliters of plasma that must have been filtered by the glomeruli in order to produce the measured amount of creatinine in the urine. The final result is expressed in milliliters per minute, and the normal range varies between 80 and 120, depending on the person's size and age. The results should be corrected to a standard body size of 1.73 m² (body surface area [BSA]), which can be derived from standard tables if the patient's height and weight are known, and averages 120 to 125 ml/minute/1.73 m² BSA.

If the kidneys are damaged by some disease process, the creatinine clearance will decrease and the serum creatinine concentration will rise. The urine creatinine excretion will initially decrease until the blood level rises to a point at which the amount of creatinine

appearing in the urine is again equal to the amount being produced by the body. For example, a normal person with a serum creatinine concentration of 1 mg/dl and a creatinine excretion of 1 mg/minute has a creatinine clearance of 100 ml/minute. If the person develops renal disease with 50% loss of renal function, his serum creatinine will rise to 2 mg/dl, and he will continue to excrete 1 mg of creatinine in his urine per minute when balance is restored. In many situations in which the patient has rapidly changing renal function and oliguria (*e.g.,* acute renal failure), the creatinine clearance becomes less reliable until the situation becomes more stable. It is therefore useful to follow the serum creatinine concentration as an indicator of the rate and direction of change until stability occurs. In patients with rhabdomyolysis, the serum creatinine will be elevated out of proportion to the deduction of GFR as the result of chemical conversion of muscle creatine to creatinine and is less reliable as an indicator of renal function.

Blood Urea Nitrogen

The BUN has also been used for many years as an indicator of kidney function, but, unlike the serum creatinine, its level tends to be influenced by a great many factors.

As mentioned in an earlier section, urea has a clearance less than that of creatinine, largely because some urea diffuses out of the tubule back into the bloodstream. This is particularly true at low urine flow rates, at which more sodium and water and, consequently, more urea are being reabsorbed. Therefore, in states of relative or absolute volume depletion, the BUN will tend to rise out of proportion to any change in renal function.

In addition, the amount of urea produced per day, unlike the quantity of creatinine, is quite variable, especially in seriously ill patients. Increased urea production can result from increased protein intake (tube feedings and some forms of hyperalimentation) or increased tissue breakdown, as with crush injuries, febrile illnesses, steriod or tetracycline administration, and reabsorption of blood from the intestine in a patient with intestinal hemorrhage. All these factors may cause an increase in urea production and an increase in BUN, even though renal function might be normal, and they would also contribute to the rate of rise in BUN in a person with renal failure.

The opposite is true for patients with decreased protein intake or liver disease (both of which reduce urea production) and for patients with large urine volumes secondary to excessive fluid intake.

The BUN is therefore less useful as a guide to changes in renal function than is the serum creatinine in most circumstances. The BUN is still of significant

TABLE 19-5
FACTS AFFECTING SERUM UREA: CREATININE RATIO

A. Decreased urea: creatinine (< 10 : 1)
   1. Liver disease
   2. Protein restriction
   3. Excessive fluid intake
B. Increased urea: creatinine (> 10 : 1)
   1. Volume depletion
   2. Decreased "effective" blood volume
   3. Catabolic states
   4. Excessive protein intake

value, however, especially when looked at in comparison with the serum creatinine concentration. Normally, these are present in a ratio of 10 : 1 (urea : creatinine). Discrepancies in this ratio might suggest a potentially correctable situation, as noted in Table 19-5).

Specific Gravity

The specific gravity of the urine is the time-honored test of the kidneys' ability to concentrate and dilute the urine. The specific gravity measures the buoyancy of a solution compared with water and depends on the number of particles in solution as well as their size and weight.

Two methods have been used to obtain this measurement in clinical practice, the *hydrometer* and the *refractometer* (or TS meter, as it is frequently called). The hydrometer has been in clinical use for many years and is the less preferred of the two methods because it requires a much larger volume of urine, its results are less reproducible, and it requires a greater amount of time.

The refractometer is highly reproducible and requires only a drop of urine for the measurement. In addition, this instrument can be used to measure the total solids of plasma (thus, the name TS meter), which are a good indicator of the plasma protein concentration and a useful indicator of the state of a patient's fluid balance, especially when serial determinations are made. The refractometer, because of its advantages, should replace the hydrometer for specific gravity determinations and should be used in the critical care unit.

The normal kidney has the capacity to dilute the urine to a specific gravity of 1.001 and to concentrate the urine to at least 1.022 (higher values are not unusual). Normally, a person's water balance will determine whether the urine is concentrated or dilute, with a dilute urine being an indicator of water excess, and a concentrated urine an indicator of water deficit. In many renal diseases, the ability of the kidneys to form a concentrated urine is lost, and the specific gravity becomes "fixed" at 1.010, a finding that might be seen in acute tubular necrosis, acute nephritis, or chronic renal disease.

Like many simple laboratory tests, the specific gravity determination has limited accuracy. The specific gravity is not always the most accurate indicator of the ability of the kidneys to concentrate the urine because this ability is a reflection of the concentration of particles in the urine. In addition to the concentration of particles, the size and weight of the particles in solution reflect, in part, the specific gravity. Therefore, a falsely high specific gravity determination will be found when high-molecular-weight substances such as protein, glucose, mannitol, and radiographic contrast material are present in the urine. A greater degree of accuracy can be obtained with urine osmolality determinations.

Osmolality

The *osmolality* of a solution is an expression of the total number (concentration) of particles in solution and is independent of the size, molecular weight, and electrical charge of the molecules. All substances in solution contribute to the osmolality to a certain degree. For example, a mol (gram molecular weight) of sodium chloride dissociates incompletely into NA^+ and Cl^- ions and produces 1.86 osmols when dissolved in a kilogram of solvent (such as plasma). A mole of nonionic solute (*e.g.,* glucose or urea) produces only 1 osmol when dissolved in a kilogram of solvent. The total concentration of particles in a solution is the osmolality and is reported in units of osmols per kilogram of solvent. In clinical situations, because we are dealing with much smaller concentrations, the osmolality is reported in milliosmols (thousandth of an osmol, abbreviated mOsm) per kilogram of solvent (plasma or serum).

In the laboratory, one generally determines osmolality by measuring the freezing point of the solution, which is directly related to the number of particles in solution. (More recent laboratory methods have taken advantage of another property of solutions, the vapor pressure, as an indicator of osmolality; one advantage is the much smaller sample required to perform the assay.)

The normal *serum osmolality* consists primarily of sodium and its accompanying anions, with urea and glucose contributing about 5 mOsm each. Therefore, knowing the serum sodium, urea, and glucose concentrations, we can calculate the osmolality of plasma by the formula

$$\text{osmolality} = 2\,\text{Na} + \frac{\text{BUN}}{2.6} + \frac{\text{glucose}}{18}$$

The calculated osmolality will normally be within 10 mOsm of the measured osmolality, which normally averages 290 ± 5 mOsm/kg. The plasma osmolality in normal people is quite constant from day to day.

Because water permeates freely between the blood, interstitial fluid, and tissues, change in the osmolality of one body compartment will produce a shift in body fluids. Therefore, the osmolality of the plasma is always the same as that of the other body compartments, except in the most rapidly changing conditions, where a slight lag may occur.

The *significance of the plasma osmolality* is that it is the main regulator of the release of ADH. When sufficient water is not being taken in, the osmolality will rise, stimulating the release of ADH, which signals the kidneys to conserve water and produce a more concentrated urine. When excessive amounts of water are ingested, the osmolality decreases, ADH release is inhibited, and the urine becomes more dilute. Under maximum ADH stimulation, the kidneys can concentrate the urine to approximately 1200 mOsm/kg, and with maximum ADH suppression (water load), the kidneys can dilute the urine to approximately 50 mOsm/kg.

Thus, there is no single normal urine osmolality, but a range in which predicted values might be expected, depending on the clinical setting. Also, when compared with the plasma osmolality, the urine osmolality depends less on the urine sodium concentration, and other substances, such as urea, play a more important role. In renal disease, one of the first renal functions to be lost is the ability to concentrate urine. As a reflection of this, the urine osmolality becomes fixed within +50 mOsm of the simultaneously determined serum osmolality. Therefore, the osmolality is a useful parameter of renal function.

The *serum and urine osmolalities* are useful in combination in a number of other circumstances. In the patient with diabetes insipidus, which results from neurologic disease or injury, the urine volume would be increased with a low urine osmolality (50 to 100 mOsm), and the serum osmolality would be increased (310 mOsm or greater) unless the fluid loss had been replaced. In contrast, the patient with carcinoma of the lung, porphyria, or central nervous system (CNS) disease might have an excess production of ADH or an ADH-like material and have the opposite picture, with a low serum osmolality and a disproportionately high urine osmolality (SIADH).

As already indicated, the serum osmolality may be increased or decreased in various states. A decrease in the serum osmolality can occur only when the serum sodium is decreased. An increase in the serum osmolality can occur whenever the serum sodium, urea, or glucose is elevated or when there are abnormal compounds present in the blood, including drugs, poisons, or metabolic waste products that are not usually measured, such as lactic acid. Symptoms due to increased osmolality usually occur when the osmolality is greater than 350 mOsm, and coma occurs when the osmolality is in approximately 400 mOsm or greater (see section on serum sodium concentration).

The usual close correlation between the measured and calculated osmolality has been mentioned. In certain circumstances, the measured serum osmolality might be significantly higher than the calculated osmolality when substances of an unusual nature are present in the blood. Many drugs and toxins such as aspirin and alcohol raise the serum osmolality. In a comatose patient, a discrepancy between the measured and calculated serum osmolalities might lead to the appropriate drug screen to provide the correct diagnosis. In patients with heart failure, hepatic disease, or shock, a discrepancy of 40 or more mOsm between the measured and calculated osmolalities, due to unknown metabolites, has been correlated with a mortality rate of 95% or greater.

Urinary Sodium Concentration. In the differentiation of the oliguria of acute renal failure from that due to prerenal causes, the urinary sodium excretion is frequently used as one indicator of intact renal function. As already noted, states of underperfusion of the kidney are associated with a decrease in urinary sodium concentration (usually <10 mEq/liter), whereas in acute renal failure, because of damage to the tubular transport mechanisms, urine sodium concentration is generally above 30 to 40 mEq/liter despite oliguria. When the urine pH is alkaline, however, urine sodium concentration will not accurately reflect sodium balance, and the chloride concentration becomes a better indicator of volume depletion.

Fractional Excretion of Sodium Test. Another test of renal function, used for the same purpose as the urine sodium concentration, is the fractional excretion of sodium (FE_{Na}). This test gives a more precise estimation of the amount of filtered sodium that remains in the urine and is more accurate in predicting tubular injury than the urinary sodium concentration. It is calculated by the formula

$$(U/P) \, Na \, / \, (U/P) \, Cr \times 100$$

in which U and P are the urinary and plasma concentrations of sodium and creatinine, respectively. (Although volume measurements are necessary to derive the absolute urinary excretion of both sodium and creatinine, these cancel out in deriving this formula.)

The test therefore requires the determination of both serum and urinary sodium and creatinine concentrations on simultaneously obtained samples. Values less than 1% indicate prerenal azotemia, or underperfusion. Values greater than 1% (and frequently greater than 3%) are indicative of acute renal failure.

This test appears to be a little more discriminating in detecting cases of acute renal failure than is measurement of urinary sodium concentration alone, especially in those patients who have borderline urinary sodium concentration values, and it is being used more frequently as a diagnostic tool.

The Anion Gap

In order to maintain chemical neutrality, the total concentration of cations and anions in the blood (as well as other body fluids) must be equivalent in terms of milliequivalents per liter. However, because there are a number of anions and cations present in blood that are not routinely measured, a "gap" exists between the total concentration of cations and anions and the concentration normally measured in plasma:

$$Na + K \text{ vs. } Cl + CHO_3$$

This gap is composed primarily of an excess of unmeasured anions, including plasma proteins, inorganic phosphates and sulfates, and organic acids. The unmeasured cations that exist in smaller concentration are primarily calcium and magnesium.

The anion gap is generally calculated by the following formula:

$$Na - (Cl + HCO_3)$$

and has a normal mean of approximately 12 mEq/liter (range: 8 to 16 mEq/liter). Potassium is generally, but not always, omitted from the formula because of its relatively low concentration and narrow range of fluctuation. Departures from this "normal" anion gap may have important diagnostic significance in acid-base disorders, especially metabolic acidoses, and may also assist in the diagnosis of other disorders.

The most common abnormality of the anion gap is an increase that is due most frequently to increased concentrations of lactate, ketone bodies, or inorganic phosphate and sulfate that are found in lactic acidosis, ketoacidosis, and uremia, respectively. Other forms of acidosis associated with ingestion of toxins such as ethylene glycol, methanol, paraldehyde, and salicylates may also produce significant increases in the anion gap. Increases in anion gap due to a decrease in unmeasured cations are rare but can be observed.

Decreases in the anion gap are less common but equally important and can occur because of increases in unmeasured cations or because of decreases in unmeasured anions, such as hypoalbuminemia. Causes are listed in Table 19-6.

Alterations of the anion gap may also be caused by laboratory error in measuring the electrolytes and must always be verified to avoid confusion and diagnostic error. Simultaneous occurrences of two dis-

TABLE 19-6
CAUSES OF AN ALTERED ANION GAP

Increased Anion Gap	Decreased Anion Gap
Laboratory error	Laboratory error
Increased unmeasured anions	Increased unmeasured cations
Endogenous metabolic acidosis	Normal cations
Lactic acidosis	Hypercalcemia
Ketoacidosis	Hyperkalemia
Uremic acidosis	Hypermagnesemia
Exogenous anion ingestion	Abnormal cations
Ethylene glycol	Increased globulins
Methanol	(myeloma, etc.)
Paraldehyde	TRIS buffer
Therapeutic agents	Lithium
Paraldehyde	Decreased unmeasured anions
Penicillin	Hypoalbuminemia
Carbenicillin	
Increased plasma proteins	
Hyperalbuminemia	
Decreased unmeasured cations	
Hypokalemia	
Hypocalcemia	
Hypomagnesemia	

orders having opposite effects on the anion gap could also obscure any potential diagnostic change.

Renal Biopsy

Renal biopsy is the ultimate diagnostic tool in renal medicine. It may provide an accurate histologic classification of the cause of renal dysfunction but, except in certain circumstances, cannot provide an etiologic diagnosis although it may be suggestive or confirmatory. Renal biopsy is performed to define the histologic counterpart of the clinical picture, provide for etiologic clues or diagnosis, assess prognosis, guide therapy, and provide assessment for insurability, employment, or disability.

The indications for renal biopsy depend on the clinical problem and opinions about the procedure vary considerably among physicians. Even when there is relative agreement among nephrologists as to when to perform a renal biopsy, there are generally few controlled studies to document how much a renal biopsy aids in therapy or prognosis above and beyond the other clinical parameters in a given clinical setting. The general indications for renal biopsy are given in Table 19-7. In each category, the timing of a renal biopsy will depend on the other clinical characteristics in each case. For instance, in the nephrotic syndrome in the pediatric age group, renal biopsy is generally not done unless the patient is steroid-resistant or has some other findings that suggest a primary renal disease or systemic disease other than lipoid nephrosis, the most

TABLE 19-7
INDICATIONS FOR RENAL BIOPSY

Clinical Condition	Biopsy Indicated	Expected Gain
Orthosatic proteinuria	No	—
Isolated hematuria and/or proteinuria	No*	—
Hematuria and/or proteinuria with ↓ GFR	Yes	D†,P‡,T$
Nephrotic syndrome	Yes	D,P,T
Systemic disease with renal abnormalities	Yes‖	D,P,T
Classic ARF	No	—
ARF with (1) azotemia > 3 wks	Yes	D,P
(2) moderate proteinuria	Yes	D,T
(3) anuria	Yes	D,T
(4) eosinophilia or eosinophiluria	Yes	D,T
Posttransplant ↓ in GFR	Yes	D,P,T

* Biopsy may be indicated for insurance, administrative reasons, and so forth.
† Diagnosis.
‡ Prognosis.
$ Therapy.
‖ Biopsy may or may not be indicated, depending on clinical picture.

common etiology of nephrotic syndrome in this age group. In adults with the nephrotic syndrome, renal biopsy is usually performed before therapy is started (although this is the subject of considerable debate at present). However, in certain patients (*e.g.,* an adult diabetic with the nephrotic syndrome and a benign urine sediment), renal biopsy is not universally performed. If clinical characteristics of other than diabetic nephropathy are present (*e.g.,* RBC casts), a biopsy may be indicated. Similar caviats may be employed in the other listed categories, depending on the circumstances. Thus, there are no general absolute indications for renal biopsy.

Contraindications for renal biopsy are relative. Serious bleeding disorders are the single generally accepted contraindication. Relative contraindications include excessive obesity, severe hypertension until blood pressure is controlled, uncooperative patients, renal malignancies, and inability to tolerate the procedure because of other serious medical conditions.

Procedure

Although renal biopsies are generally performed percutaneously with a biopsy needle, open renal biopsy under general anesthesia is still performed when percutaneous biopsy is impractical. Percutaneous renal biopsy is usually performed under either fluoroscopic or ultrasonographic control in the radiology department. The procedure generally requires about 30 minutes in the average patient when a regular routine is established.

Preparation for a renal biopsy should include the usual informed consent, prebiopsy clotting studies, some form of sedation (valium, 5 to 10 mg, is sufficient

in most patients), establishment of an intravenous access for treatment or prevention of complications, and preoperative blood typing in case replacement is necessary.

After biopsy, the patient's vital signs should be checked regularly every 15 minutes for the first 2 hours, hourly for 4 hours and then every 4 hours for the first 24 hours. The postoperative urine should be examined for blood. The major complication is bleeding, occurring either retroperitoneally or into the urinary tract. Although bleeding rarely is sufficient to require transfusion, it can be massive and, if occurring into the urinary tract, can result in clot formation and ureteral colic or obstruction. Intravenous fluids for maintenance of urinary flow can decrease the incidence of the latter two complications. Other complications include biopsy of other abdominal viscera (bowel, pancreas, liver, spleen, and vessels) and tears in the diaphragm or pleura.

Death occurs in less than 0.5% of cases. A late complication is infection in a perinephric hematoma, which can result in death if not adequately diagnosed and treated.

SUMMARY

The nurse plays a critical role in the assessment and management of patients with fluid and electrolyte disorders. Careful monitoring of patients' symptoms, general appearance, and changes in weight, blood pressure, and pulse may provide early clues to changes in volume status and to disorders of water balance. Knowledgeable application and interpretation of laboratory studies will facilitate the diagnosis and treatment of fluid and electrolyte disorders as well as other complications of renal dysfunction in the seriously ill patient.

The knowledgeable use and interpretation of the laboratory determinations described in the preceding paragraphs are of major importance in the assessment of the renal complications of the seriously ill patient. They are valuable in the prevention and the diagnosis of these complications. They are not cited to the exclusion of the usual parameters of close and accurate fluid and electrolyte balance, which are equally important in understanding the renal status of the patient.

BIBLIOGRAPHY

Duarte CG (ed): Renal Function Tests: Clinical Laboratory Procedures and Diagnosis. Boston, Little, Brown, 1980

Espinal CH: Non-invasive diagnosis of acute renal failure. In Lubek G (ed): Non-Invasive Diagnosis of Kidney Disease, pp 85–95. Basil, S Karger, 1983

Hostetter TH, Martinez-Maldonado M: Syndromes of ADH excess and deficiency. Miner Electrolyte Metab 5:159–194, 1981

Jamison RL, Oliver RE: Disorders of urinary concentration and dilution. Am J Med 72:308–322, 1982

Kokko JP: Renal concentrating and diluting mechanisms. Hosp Pract 14(2):110–116, 1979

Miller RT, Anderson RJ, Linas SL, et al: Urinary diagnostic indices in acute renal failure. Ann Intern Med 89:47–50, 1978

Oken DE: On the differential diagnosis of acute renal failure. Am J Med 71:916–920, 1981

Schrier RW, Bert T, Anderson RJ: Osmotic and non-osmotic control of vasopressin release. Am J Physiol 236:F321–332, 1979

Weitzman RE, Kleeman CR: The clinical physiology of water metabolism, part III: The water depletion (hyperosmolar) and water excess (hyposmolar) syndromes. West J Med 132(1):16–38, 1980

20
Management Modalities: Renal System

Christine M. Ceccarelli

HEMODIALYSIS

Principles of Operation

Dialysis refers to the diffusion of dissolved particles from one fluid compartment to another across a semipermeable membrane. *In hemodialysis,* the blood is one fluid compartment and the dialysate is the other.

The semipermeable membrane is a thin, porous cellophane. The pore size of the membrane permits diffusion of low-molecular-weight substances such as urea, creatinine, and uric acid. Water molecules are also very small and move freely through the membrane, but most plasma proteins, bacteria, and blood cells are too large to pass through the pores of the membrane. The difference in the concentration of the substances in the two compartments is called the *concentration gradient.*

The blood, which contains waste products such as urea and creatinine, flows into the blood compartment of the dialyzer, or artificial kidney, where it comes into contact with the dialysate, which contains no urea or creatinine. A maximum gradient is established so that these substances move from the blood to the dialysate. Repeated passages of the blood through the dialyzer at a rate of 200 to 300 ml/minute over 4 to 6 hours reduces the level of these waste products to a normal state. Hemodialysis is indicated in acute and chronic renal failure, drug and chemical intoxications, severe fluid and electrolyte imbalances, and hepatorenal syndrome.

The functions of the artificial kidney system are summarized as follows:

• Removes the by-products of protein metabolism such as urea, creatinine, and uric acid.

• Removes excess water by effecting a pressure differential between the blood and fluid compartments, usually consisting of positive pressure in the blood path and negative (suction) pressure in the dialysate compartment. This process is known as ultrafiltration.
• Maintains or restores the body buffer system.
• Maintains or restores the level of electrolytes in the body.

Major Components of the Artificial Kidney System

The Dialyzer, or Artificial Kidney. This apparatus supports the cellophane compartments. Dialyzers vary in size, physical structure, and type of membrane used to construct the blood compartment. All these factors determine the potential efficiency of the dialyzer, which refers to its ability to remove water (ultrafiltration) and waste products (clearance).

The three types of dialyzer designs currently available are the coil, parallel plate, and hollow fiber. These designs differ in structure of the dialyzing pathway and all come in different sizes, varying according to the needs of the patient. The coil dialyzer was the first design to become commercially available, but technological advances have made it almost extinct. Parallel plate and hollow fiber dialyzers are currently more popular owing to their lower blood volumes and increased predictability in ultrafiltration.

There are relative advantages and disadvantages to each dialyzer that must be considered when a selection is being made. Parallel plates should be used when

- Usual amounts of heparinization are contraindicated for patients with active or potential bleeding problems.
- Compliance of the blood compartment is desirable, as with a single vascular access for both blood inflow to, and blood outflow from, the dialyzer.

More efficient hollow-fiber dialyzers are generally used when

- A highly efficient, shorter dialysis is preferred, as in patients with drug intoxication and in some acutely ill patients in whom a longer dialysis is undesirable.
- Extracorporeal blood volume is the major concern (because this dialyzer design has the lowest priming volume).
- Chronic dialysis requires the most blood clearance in the shortest amount of time (to save time for both patients and staff).

Another consideration is dialyzer size. Smaller, low–blood volume dialyzers are preferable for children and some geriatric patients. Dialyzers with more surface area (and therefore more solute clearance) are used for large patients, for those who are very active and generate increased amounts of creatinine, and for those who require increased amounts of ultrafiltration. Most dialyzers are made of Cuprophane and other cellulosic membranes produced in Germany. Patients who exhibit adverse reactions to this membrane, however, can use dialyzers made of other materials, such as cellulose acetate.

The size and type of dialyzers depend on the aforementioned factors as well as the experience and philosophy of personnel in charge of the hemodialysis unit.

Dialysate, or Dialyzing Solution. The dialysate, or "bath," is a solution composed of water and the major electrolytes of normal serum. It is made in a clean system with filtered tap water and chemicals. It is not a sterile system, but because bacteria are too large to pass through the membrane, contamination from this source is not a major problem. Dialysate concentrates are usually provided by commercial manufacturers. A "standard" bath is generally used in chronic units, but variations may be made to meet specific patient needs.

Dialysate Delivery System. A single delivery unit provides dialysate for one patient; the multiple delivery system may supply as many as 20 patients units. In either system, an automatic proportioning device and metering and monitoring devices assure precise control of the water : concentrate ratio.

The single delivery unit is usually used in acute dialyses. It is a mobile unit, and dialysate requirements are easily tailored to meet individual patient needs.

Accessory Equipment. Hardware used in most dialysis systems includes a blood pump, infusion pumps for heparin delivery, and monitoring devices for detection of unsafe temperatures, dialysate concentration, pressure changes, air, and blood leaks. Disposable items used in addition to the artificial kidney include dialysis tubing for transport of blood between the dialyzer and patient, pressure transducers for protection of monitoring devices from blood exposure, and a normal saline bag and tubing for priming the system before use.

The Human Component. Expertise in the use of highly technical equipment is accomplished through theoretical and practical training in the clinical setting. The operation and monitoring of dialysis equipment will differ, however. Reference to the manufacturer's instruction manuals will give the nurse guidelines for the safe operation of equipment. Although the technical aspects of hemodialysis may at first seem overwhelming, they can be learned fairly rapidly.

The Nursing Process. A more critical aspect, one that takes long to achieve, consists of the understanding and knowledge that the nurse will use in caring for patients during dialysis. Because hemodialysis is a dynamic procedure, alterations in blood chemistries and fluid balance can occur. Therefore, the nursing process is in continued use throughout the treatment, with the nurse changing her plan of care according to changes in objective and subjective data. The nurse's observation skills, assessment of symptoms, and appropriate actions can make the difference between a smooth dialysis with minimal problems and one fraught with a series of crises for the patient and the nurse.

Predialysis Assessment

The degree and complexity of problems arising during hemodialysis will vary among patients and will depend on many factors. Important variables are the patient's diagnosis, stage of illness, age, other medical problems, fluid and electrolyte balance, and emotional state.

The essential first step in the hemodialysis procedure consists of a review of the patient's history, clinical records, consultation with other caregivers, laboratory reports, and, finally, the nurse's observations of the patient.

After reviewing the data and while consulting with the physician, the *dialysis nurse will establish objectives* for the dialysis treatment. The objectives will vary from one dialysis to the next in the acute renal failure patient, whose condition may change rapidly. For example, fluid removal may take precedence over correction of an electrolyte imbalance or vice versa. Bleeding problems — actual or potential — will determine the degree of anticoagulation with heparin.

The patient's emotional state should be included in this initial evaluation. Anxiety and apprehension, especially during a first dialysis, may contribute to change in blood pressure, restlessness, and gastrointestinal upsets. The security provided by the presence of a nurse during the first dialysis is probably more desirable than administration of a drug that might precipitate changes in vital signs.

A basic explanation of the procedure and its place in the total care plan for the patient may also allay some of the anxiety experienced by the patient and family. It is important that they understand that dialysis is being used to support normal body function rather than "cure" the kidney problem.

Risk Factors: Prevention, Assessment, and Nursing Intervention

Fluid Imbalances

Evaluation of fluid balance is desirable prior to dialysis so that corrective measures may be initiated early in the procedure. Parameters such as blood pressure, pulse, weight, intake and output, tissue turgor, and other symptoms will assist the nurse in estimating fluid overload or depletion.

The term *dry* or *ideal* weight is used to express the weight at which a patient's blood pressure is in a normal range for him and he is free of the symptoms of fluid imbalance. The figure is not an absolute one, but it provides a guideline for fluid removal or replacement. It requires frequent review and revision, especially in the newly dialyzed patient, in whom frequent changes in weight are occurring owing to fluid removal or accumulation and to tissue gains or losses.

Hypervolemia

The presence of some or all of the following may suggest fluid overload: blood pressure elevation, increased pulse and respiratory rate, increased central venous pressure, dyspnea, moist rales, cough, edema, excessive weight gain since last dialysis, and a history or record of excessive fluid intake in the absence of adequate losses.

A chest roentgenogram to assess heart size or pulmonary congestion may confirm the diagnosis of fluid overload but may not be essential in the presence of overt symptoms. Increase in abdominal girth will suggest accumulation of fluid in the abdominal cavity. If ascites is present, measurement of the abdominal girth will help one determine how to correct the problem.

An analysis of the causes of the fluid overload is essential to prevention of recurrences. Only after the causes are determined can a nursing diagnosis of "fluid volume excess related to . . ." be made accurately. Nursing interventions can then be planned appropriately. The intake and output record may provide a clue. For example, the patient may have been given excessive intravenous fluids in a "keep open" IV, or fluids used as a vehicle for intravenous medications may not have been calculated in the intake. The patient may not have adhered to his fluid restriction or may have had a decrease in his fluid losses. For example, gastric suction may have been discontinued. Often, after the institution of chronic dialysis, urinary output decreases. If the patient continues his normal fluid intake, he will become fluid-overloaded. In the chronic hemodialysis patient, fluid overload may be related to the intake of high-sodium foods. Moderate restriction is necessary for all patients so that extracellular fluid overload is prevented. Change in weight provides an indication of water load; an acceptable weight gain is 0.5 kg for each 24 hours between dialyses.

Treatment of fluid overload during dialysis is directed toward the removal of the excess water. Because this removal depends on shifting of fluid to the vascular space from other body compartments, one must take care to avoid too rapid volume depletion during dialysis. Excessive fluid removal may lead to hypotension, and little is gained if intravenous fluids are given to correct the problem. Thus, it is better to reduce the volume overload over a period of two or three dialyses, unless pulmonary congestion is life-threatening.

Ultrafiltration

Excessive water is removed from the vascular compartment by the process of ultrafiltration. This is accomplished by application of negative pressure to the effluent dialysate. This creates a "siphoning" effect on the dialysate, with water molecules being pulled across the membrane into the dialysate. As much as 4 to 5 kg (10 lb) of water may be removed in a 4- to 6-hour period. The amount of negative pressure that is applied is based on the ultrafiltration capability of the dialyzer, the amount of fluid that needs to be removed, and the individual patient's tolerance.

Symptoms of excessive ultrafiltration are similar to those of shock: hypotension, nausea, vomiting, diaphoresis, dizziness, and fainting.

Sequential Ultrafiltration (Diafiltration)

Aggressive ultrafiltration for the purpose of relieving or preventing hypertension, congestive heart failure, pulmonary edema, and other complications associated with fluid overload is often limited by the patient's tolerance of manipulations of intravascular volume.

Observation by several investigators suggests that there is a significant increase in patient tolerance to large, rapid fluid volume removal when the ultrafiltration process occurs in the absence of diffuse mass transfer. This has resulted in a mode of therapy designated *sequential ultrafiltration,* or *diafiltration,* in which the removal of body fluid is separated from the total dialysis procedure. This is accomplished by (1) initiation of dialysis without a dialysate flow, (2) maintenance of negative pressure in the dialysate compartment, and (3) return to the usual dialysis procedure following a predetermined amount of ultrafiltration time. It is thought that this technique is effective because plasma osmolality is kept constant without solute removal during ultrafiltration, thus enhancing fluid shifts from extravascular spaces.

High-Flux Membranes

Maximum ultrafiltration can also be achieved through the process of hemofiltration, in which highly permeable membranes are used to achieve convective fluid transfer. A dialysis bath is not used in this process, and a blood pump may or may not be utilized. Replacement fluid is required, usually in the form of Ringer's lactate and in an amount that depends on individual needs. This technique is especially valuable when hemodialysis is not available or practical and fluid removal is the patient's main requirement.

Hypovolemia

Assessment of hypovolemia also is based on the evaluation of trends in vital signs and symptoms. Clues to hypovolemia include falling blood pressure, increasing pulse and respiration rates, loss of skin turgor, dry mouth, a falling CVP, and a decreasing urine output. A history of excessive fluid loss through profuse perspiration, vomiting, diarrhea, and gastric suctioning with resulting weight loss will further substantiate the nursing diagnosis of fluid deficit.

Intervention is directed toward the replacement of previous losses and the prevention of further losses during dialysis.

It is usual practice to phlebotomize the patient at the onset of dialysis. The patient's blood is pumped through the dialyzer, displacing the priming normal saline solution. In the hypovolemic patient, the nurse can connect the venous return blood line immediately and infuse the normal saline into the patient. The 200 ml of solution might be sufficient to restore balance or at least prevent further hypotension. Ultrafiltration will be avoided in the hypovolemic patient, and he may even require additional fluids.

Normal saline is the solution used most frequently to replace depleted fluids during dialysis because small volumes usually produce the desired effect. Replacement in 50-ml increments is suggested, with frequent monitoring of blood pressure.

Blood-volume expanders such as albumin are some-times used in patients with a low serum protein. The treatment is expensive when the underlying cause of the hypoproteinemia is not corrected and repeated infusions become necessary.

Hypotension

Hypotension during dialysis may be caused by preexisting hypovolemia, excessive ultrafiltration, loss of blood into the dialyzer, and antihypertensive drug therapy. Hypotension at the beginning of dialysis may occur in patients with a small blood volume, such as children and small adults. Use of a small-volume dialyzer or initiation of dialysis at a slower blood flow rate may prevent or minimize problems. These nursing interventions should be included in the patient's care plan if effective and linked with the appropriate nursing diagnosis, such as "potential for decreased cardiac output related to blood removal during initiation of dialysis."

Hypotension later in dialysis is usually due to excessive or too rapid ultrafiltration. One may confirm this by weighing the patient and estimating fluid loss. Keeping the patient in a horizontal position and reducing the ultrafiltration rate may return the blood pressure to normal. If hypotension persists, saline or other plasma expanders may be administered. Intravenous fluids should be kept to a minimum and discontinued as soon as the patient is normotensive. Salty liquids or foods may be given, but their effect is slower than intravenous administration. If hypotension persists despite adequate fluid replacement, other medical causes for hypotension should be considered.

Clinicians have found that elevation of the sodium level of the dialysis bath also can help prevent hypotensive episodes and muscle cramps during and after the treatment. Dialysate sodium levels are often kept between 138 and 145 mEq/liter, depending on the patient's serum sodium. Personnel in some units are also experimenting with varying the dialysate sodium levels during the treatment, so as not to leave the patient with a high serum sodium at the end of dialysis (this can lead to increased thirst and excessive weight gains).

Nurse researchers are beginning to identify those types of patients at high risk for hypotensive episodes during dialysis, such as patients with impaired cardiovascular function. Interventions such as careful monitoring of vital signs and observation of specific symptoms can help limit the occurrence and severity of hypotensive episodes in these patients.

Blood loss due to technical problems such as membrane leaks and line separations also may lead to hypotension. The use of blood leak detectors and other monitoring devices has reduced the risk of excessive blood loss due to these causes, but they do occur. If separation of blood lines occurs, clamping the arterial blood line and stopping the blood pump immediately will minimize further blood loss.

The incidence of membrane leaks has decreased owing to improvements in dialyzer technology and the use of negative pressure dialyzers. In these systems, excessive pressure is not exerted in the blood compartment, so leaks are unusual unless the membrane is already damaged. If gross leaks do occur, dialysate may cross the membrane into the blood compartment. In this situation, the blood may be returned to the patient, but he should be observed for pyrogenic reactions. If the patient's hematocrit is low, the risk of blood loss may be greater than the possibility of dialysate contamination. Some units have standing policies to cover this contingency; however, decisions may be made according to individual circumstances.

The use of *antihypertensive drugs* in the dialysis patient may precipitate hypotension during dialysis. To avoid this, many units make it standard practice to omit antihypertensive drugs 4 to 6 hours before dialysis. Fluids and sodium restrictions are more desirable controls for hypertension. *Sedatives* and *tranquilizers* may also cause hypotension and should be avoided if possible.

Hypertension

The most frequent causes of hypertension during dialysis are fluid overload, disequilibrium syndrome, renin response to ultrafiltration, and anxiety.

Hypertension during dialysis is usually caused by sodium and water excesses. One can confirm this by comparing the patient's present weight to his ideal, or dry, weight. If fluid overload is the cause of hypertension, ultrafiltration will usually bring about a reduction in the blood pressure.

Some patients who may be normotensive before dialysis become hypertensive during dialysis. The rise may occur either gradually or abruptly. Although the cause is not well understood, it may be the result of renin production in response to ultrafiltration and an increase in renal ischemia. Careful monitoring of these patients is important because the vasoconstriction caused by the renin response is limited. Once a decrease in blood volume surpasses the ability to maintain blood pressure through vasoconstriction, hypotension can occur precipitously.

Hypertension is a common finding in dialysis disequilibrium syndrome (see following discussion) and will usually respond to correction of that condition. If the diastolic blood pressure is over 120 or the patient has symptoms, small doses of hydralazine (Apresoline) may be given intravenously. An initial dose of 10 mg may bring about a favorable response. Hydralazine is preferred to methyldopa (Aldomet) because its effect is more rapid. Blood pressure is monitored at frequent intervals following the administration of antihypertensive drugs.

Anxiety, fear, and apprehension, especially during the first dialysis, may cause transient and erratic hypertension. Sedatives may be necessary, but confidence in the staff and a smooth, problem-free dialysis will help reduce anxiety during subsequent treatments.

Dialysis Disequilibrium Syndrome

Dialysis disequilibrium syndrome is manifested by a group of symptoms suggestive of cerebral dysfunction. Symptoms range in severity from mild nausea, vomiting, headache, and hypertension to agitation, twitching, mental confusion, and convulsions. It is thought that rapid, efficient dialysis results in shifts in water, *p*H, and osmolality between cerebrospinal fluid and blood, which cause the symptoms.

Slow dialysis for short periods daily for two or three treatments may prevent disequilibrium syndrome in the acutely uremic patient. Phenytoin (Dilantin) is sometimes used prior to and during dialysis in the new patient to reduce the risk of central nervous system symptoms.

Restlessness, confusion, twitching, nausea, and vomiting may suggest early disequilibrium. Reduction of the blood flow rate and administration of sedatives may prevent more severe symptoms, but it may be necessary to discontinue dialysis if symptoms persist or worsen.

Electrolyte Imbalances

With the trend toward early and adequate dialysis, the severe extremes of electrolyte imbalances are not seen with the same frequency as before the widespread use of hemodialysis. Critical electrolyte changes and their management have been discussed in Chapter 19.

Maintenance and restoration of electrolyte balance in the dialysis patient are accomplished primarily with dialysis and to a lesser degree with dietary controls. Most of the dialysate electrolyte concentrations are standard for all patients, but the potassium concentration is determined according to the patient's individual serum level. Changes are often made in the calcium and sodium levels also, depending on the variety of dialysate concentrates available and sophistication of the machinery used.

Laboratory tests for evaluation of electrolyte status are performed before and after each dialysis in acute renal failure. The nurse's role includes knowing normal values, recognizing symptoms of imbalance, and evaluating probable causes. In many institutions, nursing intervention also includes taking the necessary corrective measures as defined by the policies of the critical care unit. For example, a patient complains of extreme muscle weakness. The nurse notes excessive amounts of gastric drainage during the previous 24-hour period. The situation suggests hypokalemia, and the nurse orders a stat serum K^+ level. If the result is low, the nurse increases the potassium level in the dialysate from the standard 2 mEq/liter to 3.5 mEq/liter. She also monitors the patient for possible cardiac arrhythmias during the procedure.

The electrolytes of main concern in dialysis, which are normally corrected during the procedure, are sodium, potassium, bicarbonate, calcium, phosphorus, and magnesium.

Serum Sodium. Serum sodium concentration normally varies between 135 and 145 mEq/liter and is a reflection of water volume.

A low serum sodium usually indicates water intake in excess of sodium and is characterized by an increase in body weight. A high serum sodium usually indicates water loss in excess of sodium and is reflected in weight loss. Serum sodium extremes do not, as a rule, become a problem unless the values fall below 120 or rise above 160 mEq/liter. The rate of change is probably more important than the absolute value (see Chap. 19).

Although serum sodium extremes are not usually seen in the adequately dialyzed patient, thirst may indicate sodium excess. The patient who is thirsty because of excessive sodium intake will drink excessive amounts of water, which can lead to hypertension and fluid overload. Evaluation of sodium intake should be made in the patient who retains excessive amounts of fluid between dialyses. Again, the recommended weight gain is approximately 2.2 kg (1 lb) for each day between dialysis. Shifts in sodium and water during hemodialysis may lead to muscle cramping. This can be alleviated by reducing the flow rate and ultrafiltration or supplementing the serum osmolality with an intravenous medication. Preparations frequently used to relieve muscle cramping include hypertonic saline, sodium bicarbonate, and 50% dextrose.

Potassium. Both hypokalemia and hyperkalemia occur in renal failure. Normal serum concentration is between 3.5 and 5 mEq/liter. Levels below 3 and above 7 mEq/liter may lead to generalized muscle weakness and cardiac arrhythmias (see Chap. 8).

Extremes in the serum potassium level are seen more frequently in the acutely ill patient and may result from either the disease or the therapy. Crushing injuries with extensive tissue destruction, blood transfusions, potassium-containing drugs, and acidosis all contribute to hyperkalemia. Vomiting, diarrhea, and gastric suction may lead to hypokalemia. Rapid correction of serum potassium in either direction should be avoided. Patients on digitalis are of special concern because a low serum potassium potentiates the effects of digitalis. Therefore, rapid lowering of the potassium level during dialysis can lead to hypokalemia, to increased effects of digitalis, and possibly to serious and sometimes fatal arrhythmias (see Chap. 8).

The potassium level in the bath is kept at 2 to 3.5 mEq/liter, whichever is more appropriate for the individual patient. Patients with overt or potential problems should be monitored for cardiac function during dialysis.

Bicarbonate. Bicarbonate protects the body from excessive acid loads. Normal concentration varies between 25 and 30 mEq/liter.

In uremia, the bicarbonate is depleted because it has been used to buffer the acidosis resulting from the inability of the kidneys to excrete acids. Acidosis in the uremic patient who has not been started on dialysis is corrected by administration of sodium bicarbonate.

During dialysis, acidosis is corrected by addition of either acetate or bicarbonate to the dialysate. Acetate diffuses into the blood, where it is metabolized to form bicarbonate. Although this has been the most common form of base buffer used in dialysis concentrates, it has been shown that some patients are either intolerant of the acetate itself or unable to utilize it effectively as a buffer. Acetate intolerance is exhibited by impairment of the cardiac contractile force that leads to a drop in blood pressure as well as nausea, vomiting, headache, and other neurologic symptoms.

Because dialysis of the critically ill patient can be further complicated by these symptoms, bicarbonate dialysis is often used. Depending on the type of dialysis machinery used, the production of bicarbonate bath usually requires special equipment, concentrates, and procedures.

Calcium. Normal serum calcium levels range between 8 and 10.3 mg/dl, although they will vary among laboratories. Disturbances in calcium metabolism that result in hypocalcemia occur in renal failure and are thought to involve impaired absorption of dietary calcium and resistance to the action of vitamin D.

The dialysate calcium is kept at 3 to 3.5 mEq/liter to prevent the loss of calcium from the blood to the dialysate. Dialysis, however, does not seem to correct the bone problems that occur in the chronic patient as a result of calcium-phosphorus imbalances (see Chap. 21). These must be controlled by a combination of dietary intervention and medications.

Phosphorus. In chronic renal failure, antacids are used to bind phosphorus in the intestinal tract and prevent its absorption. The lowered serum phosphorus reduces the risk of calcium-phosphorus imbalances and resulting bone problems.

Antacids are usually given during or after meals; however, because of the medication's unpleasant taste and consistency, patients often omit taking antacids. A high serum phosphorus indicates to the nurse that the patient is not tolerating the type of phosphate binder prescribed or that he is taking it at the wrong times. Nursing interventions should include appropriate patient teaching and consultation with the physician to find a more palatable antacid preparation for the patient.

Magnesium. The normal plasma level of magnesium is 1.5 to 1.7 mEq/liter. Magnesium accumulates in the serum, bone, and muscle in renal failure. It may be involved, along with calcium and phosphorus, in the bone problems accompanying chronic renal failure. Magnesium is generally maintained at an acceptable level with regular dialysis, but its intake should be limited so that symptoms of hypermagnesemia are avoided. Because it is difficult to reduce magnesium intake in the diet and provide palatable and nutritious meals, dietary limitations are problematic.

The regular use of magnesium-containing drugs should be avoided. This applies particularly to antacids that are taken regularly by patients on chronic dialysis. Acceptable nonmagnesium antacids include aluminum hydroxide gel (Amphojel), dihydroxyaluminum aninoacetate (Robalate), and basic aluminum carbonate gel (Basaljel).

Infection

The uremic patient has a lowered resistance to infection, which is thought to be due to a decreased immunologic response. Therefore, all possible foci of infection should be eliminated. Indwelling urinary catheters and intracaths should be removed as soon as possible, or their use should be avoided altogether. Strict aseptic technique is essential in catheterizations, venipunctures, wound dressings, and tracheal suctioning. Usual physiological responses to infection also may be altered in uremia. This effect is exhibited by a basal temperature that is lower than normal and by the absence of a usual temperature rise when infection is present.

Pulmonary infections are a leading cause of death in the acute uremic patient. Contributing factors include depression of the cough reflex and respiratory effort due to central nervous system disturbances, increased viscosity of pulmonary secretions due to dehydration and mouth breathing (especially in the unresponsive patient), and pulmonary congestion due to fluid overload. Fluid in the lungs not only acts as a medium for growing bacteria but also impedes respiratory excursion.

Nursing techniques that prevent or minimize pulmonary complications cannot be overlooked during the hemodialysis procedure. They include frequent turning, deep breathing and coughing, early ambulation, adequate humidification, hydration, tracheal aspiration, use of intermittent positive pressure machines, and oxygen therapy.

Oral hygiene is important because bleeding from the oral mucous membrane and the accumulation of dry secretions promote growth of bacteria in the mouth, which can lead to pneumonia.

Bleeding and Heparinization

Bleeding during dialysis may be due to an underlying medical condition such as an ulcer or gastritis or may be the result of excessive anticoagulation. Blood in the extracorporeal system, such as the dialyzer and blood lines, clots rapidly unless some method of anticoagulation is used. *Heparin* is the drug of choice because it is simple to administer, increases clotting time rapidly, is easily monitored, and may be reversed with protamine.

Specific heparinization procedures vary, but the primary goal in any method is to prevent clotting in the dialyzer with the least amount of heparin. Two methods are commonly used: intermittent and constant infusion. In both cases, an initial priming dose of heparin is given, followed by smaller doses either at intervals or at a constant rate by an infusion pump. the resulting effect is *systemic heparinization*, in which the clotting times of the patient and the dialyzer are essentially the same.

Absolute guidelines are difficult to provide because methods and dialyzer requirements vary. The normal clotting time of 6 to 10 minutes may be increased to the range of 30 to 60 minutes. The effect of heparin is usually monitored at the bedside by the activated clotting time (ACT) or whole blood partial thromboplastin time (WBPPT). These tests have replaced the use of the Lee White method because they can provide results in seconds, which gives the dialysis nurse the opportunity to make rapid adjustments in heparin administration.

Systemic heparinization usually presents no risk to the patient unless he has overt bleeding (*e.g.,* gastrointestinal bleeding, epistaxis, or hemoptysis), is 3 to 7 days postsurgery, or has uremic pericarditis. In these situations, *regional heparinization* may be employed. With this technique, the patient's clotting time is kept normal while that of the dialyzer is increased. This is accomplished by infusing heparin at a constant rate into the dialyzer and simultaneously neutralizing its effects with protamine sulfate before the blood returns to the patient.

Like systemic heparinization, regional heparinization has no associated standard heparin:protamine ratio. Frequent monitoring of the clotting times is the best way to achieve effective regional heparinization. Because of the rebound phenomenon that has been reported following regional heparinization and the use of activated coagulation-time methods, many dialysis units have switched to low-dose heparinization, even in the presence of overt bleeding. With this method, minimal heparin doses are used throughout dialysis. Although some clotting may take place in the dialyzer, the small blood loss is perferable to the risk of profound bleeding.

Bleeding problems occasionally occur because of accidental heparin overdose. This may be caused by infusion pump malfunction or carelessness in setting the delivery rate. Because of the hazards, the importance of careful, frequent monitoring of heparin delivery cannot be overemphasized.

Problems With Equipment

One of the major objectives of a dialysis unit is the prevention of complications resulting from the treatment itself. Hemodialysis involves the use of highly technical equipment. The efficiency of the dialysis, as well as the patient's comfort and safety, is compromised if both the patient and the equipment are not adequately monitored. Mechanical monitors provide a margin of safety but should not replace the observations and actions of the nurse.

Monitoring devices are designed to monitor many parameters, the most important of which are flow, concentration, and temperature of the dialysate, flow and leakage of blood, and air in the dialysis circuit. The design and operation of dialysis equipment and monitoring devices vary greatly; however, they have a common purpose.

Dialysate Flow. Inadequate dialysate flow will not harm the patient, but it will compromise dialysis efficiency. Flow is maintained at the rate recommended for each particular dialyzer, usually at 500 ml/minute. The nurse usually checks the flow at least every hour and makes adjustments as necessary.

Dialysate Concentrate. Sudden or rapid changes in dialysate concentration may result in red blood cell damage and cerebral disturbances. Mild symptoms include nausea, vomiting, and headache. In severe cases, convulsions, coma, and death may ensue. If a central delivery system is used to supply dialysis bath to several patients at the same time, the patients will develop similar symptoms simultaneously. If this occurs, dialysate concentrate imbalance should be thought of immediately. If a patient is accidently dialyzed against water or a hypotonic solution, hemolysis will occur and the first symptom may be sudden severe pain in the returning vein. Because of hemolysis, blood will immediately appear a clear cherry red in the dialysis return lines. When this occurs, dialysis is discontinued at once.

In a single delivery, proportioning system, monitoring devices are built into the system, and the concentrate is monitored continuously. If the concentrate exceeds the predetermined limits, dialysate automati-

cally bypasses the dialyzer until the problem is corrected. The problem may have been caused by an interruption in the water or concentrate delivery. Inflow lines should be checked for kinking, and the concentrate container should be inspected for quantity.

In a central delivery system, the electrolyte concentration also is checked continuously by a meter that measures the electrical conductivity of the solution. If the solution exceeds the limits, the transfer valve is automatically closed so that no solution in unsafe concentrations is delivered to the bedside. The solution is bypassed, and a system of visual and audible alarms alerts dialysis personnel to problems. This alarm condition should not be reset to function unless the problem has been corrected.

In a batch system, the bath may be checked in a number of ways. Tests for conductivity or chloride level of the solution are commonly used. Testing is done before dialysis commences and any time the bath is changed.

Temperature. Most dialysate delivery systems use a heating element to maintain dialysate temperature at optimal levels (98°F to 101°F, or 36.7°C to 38.3°C). Some systems include alarms; others require visual observation of the temperature gauge.

Cool temperatures may cause chilling and vessel spasm. Sometimes, chilling in the patient is the first indication of a drop in dialysate temperature. High temperatures (over 101°F, or 38.3°C) may produce fever and discomfort in the patient, whereas extremely high temperatures (110°F, or 43.3°C) will cause hemolysis. Corrections should be made as soon as the temperature reaches 101°F (38.3°C).

Blood Flow. Monitoring adequate blood flow rate throughout dialysis is essential to dialysis efficiency. Hemodialysis usually requires a blood flow rate of 200 to 300 ml/minute in adult patients; a somewhat lower rate is usually prescribed for children or very frail geriatric patients. Factors that influence blood flow rate are blood pressure, shunt and fistula function, and the extracorporeal circuit. A manometer, connected to the drip chamber is used to measure the pressure in the blood lines. Changes in blood line pressures are transmitted to the drip chamber and register on the manometer as high- or low-pressure alarms.

A high-pressure alarm indicates a problem in the venous blood line, vessel spasm, or a clotted vein. Vessel spasm is seen in new shunts or with chilling, and a heating pad over the shunt may help relax the vessel. If a clot is suspected, the vein is irrigated with a heparinized saline solution.

A low-pressure alarm reflects an obstruction to blood flow from the patient. Arterial spasm, clotting, displacement of a fistula needle, and a drop in blood pressure are possible causes. Correction is again directed to the cause.

Blood Leaks. A blood leak detector is invaluable when outflow dialysate is not visible, as in a single-pass delivery system. One type of blood leak detector is a color-sensitive photocell that picks up color variations in the outflow dialysate. Any foreign material, such as blood, will be detected and an alarm will be set off. Because false alarms are sometimes set off by air bubbles, the nurse will check the dialysate visually for a gross leak and with a hemostix for smaller leaks.

Dialysis is usually discontinued immediately with a gross leak. Whether or not the blood is returned to the patient is either a matter of unit policy or a determination based on individual circumstances. If the patient is severely anemic, the risk of losing the blood in the dialyzer may outweigh the risk of a reaction to dialysate-contaminated blood. Sometimes minor leaks, in which there is no visible blood in the dialysate and only a small hemostix reaction, seal over, and dialysis is continued.

Air Embolism. The risk of air embolism is one of the most serious patient safety problems in the hemodialysis unit. Air can enter the patient's circulation through defective blood tubing, faulty blood line connections, vented intravenous fluid containers, or accidental displacement of the arterial needle.

The use of air and foam detectors and nonvented plastic fluid containers has minimized air embolus risks, but the prevention of potential problems by strict attention to technical details and visual monitoring cannot be overemphasized.

Access to Circulation

Successful repeated hemodialysis depends on access to the patient's circulation. Methods commonly used are the external arteriovenous (AV) shunt, the internal arteriovenous fistula, bovine and Gortex grafts, and femoral and subclavian vein catheters.

Arteriovenous Shunt

The arteriovenous shunt consists of two soft plastic (Silastic) cannulas, one of which is inserted into an artery and the other into a vein. Between dialyses, the cannulas are joined by a hard, plastic (Teflon) connector, and blood flows freely between the two vessels. At the time of dialysis, the two cannulas are separated and attached to the blood tubing of the dialyzer.

Cannulation is a surgical procedure performed in the operating room under local anesthesia. The cannula is usually inserted in the forearm of the nondominant arm, although circumstances may dictate placement in other extremities.

Presurgical care should include avoidance of venipunctures, intravenous administrations, tourniquets, and blood-pressure cuffs in the affected limb. Nursing care is directed at maintenance of good function and prevention of clotting and infection beginning in the immediate postsurgical period.

General recommendations for promoting shunt life are as follows:

- *Limitation of activity in the postoperative period.* One can promote shunt functioning by elevating the affected extremity for 2 to 3 days to reduce swelling and discomfort and by avoiding weight-bearing in a leg shunt for at least 1 week.
- *Cleanliness.* The shunt site should be kept clean and dry. Good aseptic technique is essential in dressing changes and handling of the shunt. Daily dressing changes are not recommended unless infection with drainage is present or the dressing becomes wet. Cleansing at the time of dialysis is usually sufficient and should be done from the exit sites outward. Separate gauze and applicators are used for each exit to prevent cross-contamination. Picking at crusts should be avoided.
- *Proper alignment.* Misalignment may occur if the cannulas are twisted during either the hookup procedure or the reconnection at the end of dialysis. Distortions should be corrected immediately because tension at the exits may lead to small tears in the epithelium, which in turn contribute to clotting and infection. An outer dressing such as Kling, which conforms to the contours of the extremity, is recommended because it prevents the shunt and other dressings from slipping around with normal motions. One should take care, however, not to apply the dressing so tightly that circulation is compromised.
- *Gentleness.* Careful, gentle handling of shunt parts is important in extending shunt life. Therefore, jerking and pulling on the cannulas during dialysis procedures should be avoided.
- *Frequent observation.* Early detection and attention to symptoms may lead to the prevention of more serious problems. Clotting and infection are the two major complications.
- *Prevention of clotting.* A clue to good blood flow through the shunt is a sound or burst heard with a stethoscope. The sound has been likened to that of rushing water. Sometimes the bruit is so strong it can be palpated with the fingers. This is called a thrill. If the bruit is faint or absent, the dressing is removed so that the shunt can be observed. The color of the blood should be uniformly red, and the shunt should feel warm. If the shunt is clotted, the blood is quite dark and the red cells and serum may have already separated. Declotting may or

may not be successful, depending on the length of time that has elapsed between clotting and detection. The routine declotting procedure consists of evacuation of the clots by irrigation of each cannula with a weak heparinized saline solution. Aseptic technique is again emphasized. Once flow has been reestablished, the shunt is reconnected and observed closely. It has been the experience of dialysis personnel that once clotting occurs, it will recur unless the cause has been determined and corrective measures taken. A history of trauma, obstruction to flow caused by sleeping with a limb bent or legs crossed, hypotension, and infections is often found. The patient, however, may have an intrinsic clotting problem that may indicate the use of an anticoagulant such as sodium warfarin (Coumadin). This will necessitate the usual observations and precautions taken with anticoagulation therapy. The patient will also need a readjustment in heparin dosage during dialysis.

• *Prevention of Infection.* The shunt is routinely inspected at the time of dialysis. It is also inspected when the patient develops any unusual symptoms, such as pain or bleeding at exits, between dialysis. Any of the signs of inflammation, such as redness, swelling, tenderness, and drainage, are cause for concern and require prompt attention. Cultures are routinely done by the nurse if drainage is noted. Each exit site is cultured separately. Some physicians will treat the infection without cultures, assuming that most shunts are infected with *Staphylococcus aureus.* However, *Pseudomonas* and *Escherichia coli* are sometimes cultured out. Aside from the possibility of further shunt surgery, the most serious complication of a shunt infection is septicemia. To forestall this possibility, some physicians choose to remove an extremely infected shunt immediately. Whether or not this is done, the patient should be observed closely, especially during the hemodialysis procedure, when contamination of the bloodstream from an infected shunt is a strong possibility. The development of chills, fever, and hypotension in a patient with an infected shunt should be regarded as a serious sign. Blood cultures should be drawn immediately and the physician notified promptly.

Complications that occur rarely but that require immediate nursing intervention are accidental separation of the cannulas and displacement of the arterial cannula. The appearance of large amounts of bright red blood on the shunt dressing constitutes an emergency and should be investigated without hesitation.

If the arterial side of the shunt has become displaced, direct pressure should be applied to the site at which the shunt tip entered the vessel, usually on the suture line where the surgery was first performed. It is *not* correct to apply pressure where the shunt entered the skin because the tubing is generally tunneled subcutaneously before the exit site is formed. Medical help should then be sought immediately. If the cannulas have become separated, they should be clamped immediately and then reconnected. For this reason, it is essential that shunt clamps be attached to any person who has an arteriovenous shunt. Patients who are alert and able to learn about the care and function of their shunt should be instructed as soon as possible after shunt placement. The nursing diagnosis, "Knowledge deficit related to function and care of the arteriovenous shunt," is used until the patient has integrated this information.

Arteriovenous Fistula

The arteriovenous fistula technique was developed in response to the frequent complications encountered with the arteriovenous shunt.

In this procedure, the surgeon anastomoses an artery and a vein, creating a fistula or artificial opening between them. Arterial blood flowing into the venous system results in marked dilation of the veins, which are then easily punctured with dialysis fistula needles, usually 16 gauge in size. Two venipunctures are made at the time of dialysis, one for a blood source and one for a return.

The arterial needle is inserted toward the fistula to obtain the best blood flow, but the tip should not be placed closer than 2.5 to 4 cm from the fistula. A traumatic puncture might lead to damage and closure of the fistula. The venous needle is directed away from the fistula in the direction of normal venous flow. It may be placed in the vessel, in another vein in the same arm, or even in another extremity.

If both needles are inserted into the same vessel, the tips should be at least 8 to 10 cm apart to avoid mixing of the blood, which would result in inadequate dialysis. If it is necessary to place the needles close to each other, a tourniquet applied between the two needles may help prevent mixing.

Fistulated veins that have not matured well present a challenge to dialysis nurses whose goals are successful venipuncture and adequate blood flow rate. "Inadequate arterial flow from AV fistula due to vessel immaturity" is a common nursing diagnosis for these patients. Appropriate interventions include increased exercise of the fistulated arm, application of warm soaks to the arm during dialysis, and investigation of fistula revision if other measures fail.

Care of the arteriovenous fistula is less complicated than with the arteriovenous shunt. Normal showering or bathing with soap provides adequate skin cleansing. Traumatic venipunctures or repetition in the same site should be avoided because these lead to excessive bleeding, hematoma, and scar formation. Excessive manipulation and adjustment of the needles should also be avoided for the same reasons. Postdialysis care includes adequate pressure on the puncture sites after the needles are removed.

Most arteriovenous fistulas are developed and ready to use in 1 to 3 months following surgery. Patients are taught to exercise the arm after initial healing has occurred to assist in vessel maturation. The also are encouraged to become familiar with the quality of the "thrill" felt at the site of anastomosis so that they can report any deviation in its presence or strength.

Bovine and Gortex Grafts

Bovine and Gortex grafts were developed in response to a need for blood access in those patients with inadequate blood vessels of their own. A bovine graft is a segment of selected bovine carotid artery that is processed and sterilized for human use. A Gortex (polytetrafluorethylene) graft is a prosthetic material manufactured from an expanded, highly porous form of Teflon. Either type is anastomosed between an artery and a vein. After a suitable healing period, the vessel is used in the same manner as an arteriovenous fistula.

Gortex grafts have been shown to be extremely valuable for many patients whose own vessels are not adequate for fistula formation. Gortex segments are also used to patch areas of arteriovenous grafts or fistulas that have stenosed or developed areas of aneurysm. It is preferable to avoid venipuncture in new Gortex grafts while growth of the patient's tissue into the graft is occurring, usually 2 to 4 weeks. If tissue growth is allowed to progress satisfactorily, the graft has an endothelium and wall composition similar to the patient's own vessels.

The procedures for prevention of complications in grafts are the same as those employed for arteriovenous fistula; however, certain complications are seen more frequently with grafts than with fistulas, including thrombosis, infection, and aneurysm formation.

Femoral and Subclavian Vein Catheters

Catheters inserted into large veins, such as femoral and subclavian vessels, are used for hemodialysis when no other means of access to the circulation are available. They also are used temporarily for acute dialysis patients who are critically ill or chronic patients who are waiting for a more permanent access to mature. The advantages of large vein catheters are that they can be inserted at the bedside and do not produce permanent vessel alteration. Although usually thought of as a temporary means, subclavian catheters are being studied by some centers as a permanent means of access in patients in whom there is absolutely no other available vascular route of access and in whom peritoneal dialysis is contraindicated.

Use of femoral vein catheters (FVC; also called Shaldon catheters) involves insertion of one or two Teflon catheters into the femoral veins. If an arm vein can be used for blood return, only one catheter is used. It is possible to use only one catheter for both arterial inflow and venous outflow with a single-needle device, but this method is much less efficient. When an arm vein is not available, two femoral catheters are inserted, the lower one for the blood supply to the machine and the higher one for the return.

Subclavian vein catheters (SVC) are gaining wide acceptance as a temporary means of access because the location is more accessible and there are fewer complications than with femoral vein catheters. It is even possible to send patients home with a subclavian catheter in place, once careful instruction is given. Subclavian catheters are available with either a single lumen for use with a single-needle device or a double lumen; which provides avenues for both blood supply and blood return. A study by Raja and colleagues[1] showed that access-related hospitalizations and the number of catheter insertions were considerably fewer with the SVC than with the FVC. Insertion of the SVC is similar to that for any central line and must be performed by an experienced physician so that complications such as pneumothorax and pulmonary embolization are avoided. Proper placement of the SVC should always be verified by chest film before dialysis is initiated.

Whenever femoral or subclavian catheters are used, one must take care to avoid accidental slippage and dislodgement during hemodialysis. Femoral catheters are usually secured to the leg with tape, and subclavian catheters are sutured to the skin. The length of time for which catheters are left in place depends on catheter function and policy of the physician or institution or both. Subclavian catheters can generally be used for up to 3 to 4 weeks, but femoral catheters are usually removed within 24 to 48 hours after insertion to avoid infection. Catheters left in place between dialysis treatments are either filled with a concentrated heparin-saline solution after dialysis and plugged or irrigated periodically with a weak heparinized saline solution to prevent clotting. Cleansing and dressing of the insertion site are the same as with other central lines.

If the catheters are removed at the end of dialysis, pressure is applied to the puncture sites until complete clotting occurs. The site is checked for several hours thereafter so that any recurrent bleeding can be detected.

Limited experience has been described with use of the internal jugular vein for catheter insertion. Clinicians who use this vessel believe that they avoid problems associated with femoral and subclavian vein catheters. However, some problems with potential blood loss and extrusion of the catheter following suture breakage have been reported with this technique.

Whether wide use of this vessel for temporary access will develop remains to be seen.

Psychological Aspects

The psychological impact of acute renal failure is quite different from that of chronic renal failure. Even though the patient is dependent on a machine in both situations, the expectation in acute renal failure is that the patient may recover renal function. Thus, his concerns usually focus on the discomfort associated with insertion of the temporary vascular access and the dialysis treatment itself. Once these situations are dealt with, the patient and family must then cope with the uncertainty of how long renal failure will last and how long dialysis will be necessary.

Patients with chronic renal failure must deal with the fact that renal replacement therapy will be necessary for the rest of their lives. It is not uncommon for patients to deny a great deal of what is happening to them at first. This may continue over time and prevent some patients from accepting necessary aspects of their medical regimen. Other patients who feel considerably better after starting dialysis may enter a "honeymoon phase" and appear quite euphoric for a while. It is hoped that the normal grieving stages of depression will be followed by acceptance, with patients using their own coping mechanisms to deal with the chronicity of their treatment.

Issues of dependence versus independence also exist because the patient relies on equipment and personnel to maintain life. Education about their disease and involvement in the planning and implementation of care help most patients combat feelings of dependence and become motivated to keep themselves as well as possible.

PERITONEAL DIALYSIS

Peritoneal dialysis and hemodialysis accomplish the same function and operate on the same principle of diffusion. In peritoneal dialysis, however, the peritoneum is the semipermeable membrane, and osmosis is utilized to effect fluid removal rather than pressure differentials used in hemodialysis.

Intermittent peritoneal dialysis is an effective alternative method of treating acute renal failure when hemodialysis is not available or when access to the bloodstream is not possible. It is sometimes used as an initial treatment for renal failure while the patient is being evaluated for a hemodialysis program.

Peritoneal dialysis has some advantages over hemodialysis. First, the required technical equipment and supplies are less complicated and more available. Second, there is less need for highly skilled personnel. Third, the adverse effects associated with the more efficient hemodialysis are minimized, which may be important in patients who cannot tolerate rapid hemodynamic changes, such as those with severe cardiac disease.

There also are a few disadvantages associated with peritoneal dialysis. It requires more time to remove metabolic wastes adequately and to restore electrolyte and fluid balance than hemodialysis does. In addition, repeated treatments may lead to peritonitis, and long periods of immobility may result in such complications as pulmonary congestion and venous stasis. Because fluid is introduced into the peritoneal cavity, peritoneal dialysis is contraindicated in patients who have existing peritonitis, in those who have undergone recent or extensive abdominal surgery, and in those who have abdominal adhesions.

Materials Used In Peritoneal Dialysis

- Solutions. As in hemodialysis, peritoneal dialysis solutions contain "ideal" concentrations of electrolytes but lack urea, creatinine, and other substances that are to be removed. Unlike dialysate used in hemodialysis, solutions must be sterile. Dextrose concentrations of the solutions vary: A 1.5%, 2.5%, or 4.25% dextrose solution can be used. Use of 2.5% or 4.25% solutions is usually reserved for more fluid removal and occasionally for better solute clearance. Peritoneal dialysate usually contains no potassium, so potassium chloride may have to be added to the dialysate to prevent hypokalemia. One must monitor the patient's serum potassium closely to regulate the amount of potassium to be added.
- Peritoneal dialysis administration set.
- Peritoneal dialysis catheter set, which includes the catheter, a connecting tube for connecting the catheter to the administration set, and a metal stylet.
- Trocar set of the surgeon's choice.
- Ancillary drugs:
- Local anesthetic solution—2% lidocaine (Xylocaine)
- Aqueous heparin—1000 units/ml
- Potassium chloride
- Broad-spectrum antibiotics

Preliminary Steps

1. The bladder should be emptied just prior to the procedure to avoid accidental puncture with the trocar.
2. The patient may receive a preoperative medication to enhance relaxation during the procedure.
3. The dialyzing fluid is warmed to body temperature or slightly warmer.

4. Baseline vital signs, such as temperature, pulse, respirations, and weight, are recorded. An in-bed scale is ideal for frequent monitoring of the patient's weight so should be used if possible. Moving a lethargic or disoriented patient to a scale may create problems such as catheter displacement.

5. Specific orders regarding fluid removal, replacement, and drug administration should be written by the physician prior to the procedure.

Procedure

Under sterile conditions, a small midline incision is made just below the umbilicus. A trocar is inserted through the incision into the peritoneal cavity. The obturator is removed and the catheter secured.

The dialysis solution flows into the abdominal cavity by gravity as rapidly as possible (5 to 10 minutes). If it flows in too slowly, the catheter may need repositioning. When the solution is infused, the tubing is clamped, and the solution remains in the abdominal cavity for 30 to 45 minutes. Next, the solution bottles are placed on the floor, and the fluid is drained out of the peritoneal cavity by gravity. If the system is patent and the catheter well placed, the fluid will drain in a steady, forceful stream. Drainage should take no more than 20 minutes.

This cycle is repeated continuously for the prescribe number of hours, which varies from 12 to 36, depending on the purpose of the treatment, the patient's condition, and the proper functioning of the system.

Automated Peritoneal Dialysis Systems

Automated peritoneal dialysis systems are comparable to hemodialysis systems in that they mix water and dialysate in proper dilution and have built-in monitors and a system of automatic timing devices that cycle the infusion and removal of peritoneal fluid.

Automated peritoneal delivery systems are more appropriately used for chronic peritoneal dialysis in which a permanent, indwelling peritoneal catheter is used. Less sophisticated devices that minimize the necessity for manual bottle exchanges are more appropriate for the unit in which only an occasional peritoneal dialysis is performed.

Essential Features of Nursing Care

• *Maintenance of accurate intake and output records as well as accurate records of weights* obtained from the same scale for assessment of volume depletion or overload.
• *Frequent monitoring of blood pressure and pulse.* Orthostatic blood pressure changes and increased

pulse rate are valuable clues that help one evaluate the patient's volume status.
• *Early detection of signs and symptoms of peritonitis.* Low-grade fever, abdominal pain, and cloudy peritoneal fluid all are possible signs of infection.
• *Maintenance of the sterility of the peritoneal system.* Use of masks and sterile gloves while the abdominal dressing is being changed is mandatory.
• *Early detection and correction of technical difficulties* before they result in physiological problems. Slow outflow of the peritoneal fluid may indicate early problems with the patency of the peritoneal catheter.
• *Prevention of the complications of bedrest* and provision of an environment that will assist the patient in *accepting bedrest* for prolonged periods of time.
• *Prevention of constipation.* Difficult or infrequent defecation will decrease the clearance of waste products and cause the patient more discomfort and distention.

Complications of Peritoneal Dialysis: Nursing Assessment and Invervention

Technical Complications

Incomplete Recovery of Fluid. The fluid that is removed should equal or exceed the amount inserted. Commercially prepared dialysate contains approximately 1000 to 2000 ml of fluid. If after several exchanges the volume drained is less (by 500 ml or more) than the amount inserted, an evaluation must be made.

Signs of fluid retention include abdominal distention or complaint of fullness. The most accurate indication of the amount of unrecovered fluid is weight.

If the fluid drains slowly, the catheter tip may be buried in the omentum or be clogged with fibrin. Turning the patient from side to side, elevating the head of the bed, and gently massaging the abdomen may facilitate drainage.

If fibrin or blood exists in the outflow drainage, heparin will need to be added to the dialysate. The specific dose, which is ordered by the physician, will be in the range of 500 to 1000 units/liter. Nursing diagnoses for these patients may include "alteration in comfort . . ." or "alteration in fluid and electrolyte exchange . . ."

Leakage Around the Catheter. Superficial leakage may be controlled with extra sutures and a decrease in the amount of dialysate instilled into the peritoneum. A leaking catheter should be corrected because it acts as a pathway for bacteria to enter the peritoneum. "Potential for infection . . ." is an appropriate diagnosis in this situation. One must check the abdominal dressing frequently so that any leakage can be detected.

Blood-Tinged Peritoneal Fluid. This is expected in the initial outflow but should clear after a few passes. Gross bleeding at any time is an indication of a more serious problem and should be investigated immediately.

Physiological Complications

Peritonitis. This is a serious but manageable complication of peritoneal dialysis. Because peritonitis is a potential problem for any patient with a peritoneal catheter, it should be included on the patient's problem list and care plan. Early detection and initiation of treatment will lessen the patient's discomfort and prevent more serious complications.

Signs of peritonitis include low-grade fever, abdominal pain when fluid is being inserted, and cloudy peritoneal drainage fluid.

Treatment should begin as soon as a sample of peritoneal fluid is obtained. The specimen should be sent to the laboratory for culture and sensitivity. The patient should then start on a broad-spectrum antibiotic, which is usually added to the dialysate solution, although it also can be given intravenously. Depending on the severity of the infection, the patient's condition should improve dramatically within 8 hours of initiation of antibiotic therapy.

Catheter Infection. During the daily dressing change, the exit site should be examined closely for signs of infection, such as tenderness, redness, and drainage around the catheter. In the absence of peritonitis, a catheter infection is generally treated with an oral, broad-spectrum antibiotic.

Hypotension. This complication may occur if excessive fluid is removed. Vital signs are monitored frequently, especially if a hypertonic solution is used. Lying and sitting blood pressure readings are especially useful in evaluation of fluid status. A progressive drop in blood pressure and weight should alert the nurse to the potential problem of fluid deficit.

Hypertension and Fluid Overload. These problems may occur if all the fluid is not removed in each cycle. An increase in weight requires an assessment of the catheter and dialysate solutions. The exact amount in the bottles should be noted. Some manufacturers add 50 ml to a 1000-ml bottle. Over a period of hours, this can make a considerable difference.

The nurse should observe the patient for signs of respiratory distress, which may indicate pulmonary congestion. In the absence of other symptoms of fluid overload, hypertension may be the result of anxiety and apprehension. Reassurance of the patient and prompt correction of problems are preferable to the administration of sedatives and tranquilizers.

BUN and Creatinine. Close monitoring of the serum BUN and creatinine will assist in the evaluation of the effectiveness of the dialysis. Inadequate clearance of waste products needs prompt attention.

Hypokalemia. This is a common complication of peritoneal dialysis. Close monitoring of the serum potassium will indicate the need to add potassium chloride to the dialysate as well as the amount to be added.

Pain

Mild abdominal discomfort may be experienced by the patient at any time during the procedure and is probably related to the constant distention or chemical irritation of the peritoneum. If a mild analgesic does not provide relief, insertion of 5 ml of 2% lidocaine (Xylocaine) directly into the catheter may help.

The patient may be less uncomfortable if nourishment is given in small amounts, when the fluid is draining out rather than when the abdominal cavity is distended.

Severe pain may indicate more serious problems of infection or paralytic ileus. Infection is not likely in the first 24 hours. Aseptic technique and the use of prophylactic antibiotics minimize the risk of infection. Periodic cultures of the outflowing fluid will assist in the early detection of pathogenic organisms.

Complications from Immobility

Immobility may lead to hypostatic pneumonia, especially in the debilitated or elderly patient. Deep breathing, turning, and coughing should be encouraged during the procedure. Leg exercises and the use of elastic stockings may prevent the development of venous thrombi and emboli.

Psychological Aspects

Because peritoneal dialysis results in slower clearance of waste products than hemodialysis does, it is rarely associated with the disequilibrium seen with hemodialysis. However, because the treatment is longer, boredom is a frequent problem.

Nursing measures are directed toward making the patient as comfortable as possible. Diversions such as having visitors, reading, and watching TV should be encouraged. Educating the patient about peritoneal dialysis and involving him in his care may reduce some of the anxiety and discomfort.

Chronic Forms of Peritoneal Dialysis

Peritoneal dialysis has gained popularity as a chronic form of dialysis therapy, especially since *continuous ambulatory peritoneal dialysis (CAPD)* has become available. *Intermittent peritoneal dialysis (IPD)* has been used for chronic therapy for quite a few years, but it requires the patient to remain stationary for 10 to 14 hours three times per week. Because of this inconvenience to the patient and the increased staff time needed if this therapy is performed in-center, it is seldom used and is not available in many dialysis centers.

CAPD is easily taught to patients and does not limit ambulation between dialysate fluid exchanges. It utilizes the dialysis fluid that is continuously present in the peritoneal cavity, 24 hours per day, seven days per week. Dialysis fluid is drained by the patient and replaced with fresh solution three to five times per day. The number of solution exchanges needed per day depends on the patient's individual needs. Even though the patient is required to perform dialysis techniques every day, CAPD is attractive to many end-stage renal disease (ESRD) clients because they can accomplish it easily and independently.

Another variation of chronic peritoneal dialysis therapy is *continuous cyclic peritoneal dialysis (CCPD)*. Patients who choose this form of therapy perform IPD at night during sleep using a cycling machine and in the morning instill dialysis fluid, which remains in the abdomen during the whole day. This is most convenient for those who require the help of working family members to perform their exchanges.

As with acute peritoneal dialysis, peritonitis is the greatest potential problem with chronic forms of dialysis. The peritoneal catheters that are used are permanent and inserted in the operating room. They have one or two Teflon cuffs that the surgeon sutures to the abdominal wall or subcutaneous tissue or both to anchor the catheter and provide a permanent seal against invading bacteria. Patients are taught how to recognize any potential problem associated with the catheter or treatment and to seek help from the CAPD team when needed.

Patients who perform IPD, CAPD, or CCPD at home generally visit the dialysis unit every 4 to 8 weeks. At this time, a nursing assessment is done, techniques are reviewed, and required blood studies are drawn. All health team members, including the physician, nurse, dietitian, and social worker, work together with the patient and his family to ensure successful adaptation to his chosen mode of treatment.

REFERENCE

1. Raja, RM: Comparison of subclavian vein with femoral vein catheterization for hemodialysis. Am J Kidney Dis 2, No. 4:474–476, 1983

BIBLIOGRAPHY

Anderson, R et al: WBPTT and ACT clotting time methods for use in hemodialysis. AANNT J 9, No. 2:27–30, 1982

Burden, S et al: Meeting the immediate needs of the dialysis patient using the internal jugular catheter. AANNT J 11, No. 1:23–25, 1984

Ceccarelli, CM: Hemodialytic therapy for the patient with chronic renal failure. Nurs Clin North Am 16, No. 3:531–549, 1981

Coon, MH: Evaluation of hypotensive episodes during maintenance hemodialysis in patients with impaired cardiovascular function. AANA J 11 No. 5:45–51, 1984

Graife, U et al: Less dialysis—induced morbidity and vascular instability with bicarbonate in dialysate. Ann Intern Med 88:332–336, 1978

Gutch CF, Stoner MH (eds): Review of Hemodialysis for Nurses and Dialysis Personnel, 4th ed. St Louis, CV Mosby, 1983

Henderson, AE et al: Clinical use of the Amicon diafilter^R. Dial Transplant 12, No. 7:523–525, 1983

Lancaster, LE: The Patient with End-Stage Renal Disease. New York, John Wiley & Sons, 1979

Luckenbaugh, PR: An overview of nursing diagnosis and suggestions for use with chronic hemodialysis patients. Nephrol Nurse, 5(6):58–61, 1983

Norris, MK: Management of acute conditions in chronic renal failure. Dimens Crit Care Nurs 2, No. 6:328–337, 1983

Nursing '79 Skillbook Series: Monitoring Fluid and Electrolytes Precisely. Horsham, PA, Intermed Communications, 1978

Parisi, B et al: Nursing diagnosis: application for renal nurses. Dial Transplant 12, No. 5:362–370, 1983

Pflaum, SS: Investigation of intake-output as a means of assessing body fluid balance. Heart Lung 8, No. 3:495–498, 1979

Prowant, B et al: Continuous ambulatory peritoneal dialysis. Nephrol Nurse, Jan/Feb, 1980, pp 8–14

Reed, SB: Giving more than dialysis. Nursing '82 4:58–63, 1982

Roberts SL: Renal assessment: A nursing point of view. Heart Lung 8, No. 1:105–113, 1979

Rouby, JJ et al: Plasma volume changes induced by regular hemodialysis and controlled sequential ultrafiltration hemodialysis. Dial Transplant 8, No. 3:237–240, 1979

Sim, TW et al: Successful utilization of subclavian catheters for hemodialysis and apheresis access. AANNT J 10 (7):41–44, 1983

Stark, JL: BUN/creatinine: Your keys to kidney function. Nursing '80 10:33–38, 1980

Stark, JL: How to succeed against acute renal failure. Nursing '82 7:26–33, 1982

21
Acute Renal Failure

Donald E. Butkus

Acute renal failure refers to the sudden (hours to a few days) loss of renal function characterized by an increase in blood urea nitrogen (BUN) and serum creatinine. Although no exact criteria for BUN and creatinine can be set, an increase in BUN from 15 to 30 mg/dl and a rise in creatinine from 1 to 2 mg/dl suggest acute renal failure in patients with preexisting normal renal function. In patients with preexisting renal disease, larger variations may be required to suggest the diagnosis because small changes in renal function, not related to acute renal failure, may be magnified when nephron loss is already present. Early awareness of the diagnosis, however, is critical because of the persistent high mortality rate (60% to 65%) associated with acute renal failure despite the general availability of hemodialysis.

PATHOPHYSIOLOGY OF PRERENAL AZOTEMIA

The adverse effect of reduced renal perfusion on renal function, as a consequence of various shock states, has been recognized for over a hundred years. However, it was during and following World War II that most of the knowledge regarding the pathogenesis, physiology, and management of renal ischemia was obtained. Since about 1950, evidence has been accumulated to suggest that early diagnosis of renal failure in association with aggressive treatment of the shock state can reverse functional abnormalities and prevent acute tubular necrosis.

Because of the large amount of renal blood flow required to maintain normal renal function, changes in urinary composition occur early in the shock state when renal perfusion is decreased. Normally, the kidneys receive 20% to 25% of the cardiac output (approximately 1200 ml/minute). Almost 90% of the blood flow to the kidney is concerned with cortical distribution and, in turn, glomerular filtration. The kidney has an intrinsic ability to regulate blood flow (autoregulation) so that the glomerular filtration rate is kept constant over a blood pressure range of 80 to 180 torr. This is accomplished by variations in the tone of the preglomerular and postglomerular arterioles.

However, when renal blood flow is severely compromised as a result of either reduction in effective blood volume, fall in cardiac output, or decrease in blood pressure below 80 torr, characteristic changes occur in renal function. Thus, the capacity for complete autoregulation is exceeded. The glomerular filtration rate falls. The amount of tubular fluid is reduced, and the fluid travels through the tubule more slowly. This results in increased sodium and water reabsorption. Because of the reduced renal circulation, the solutes reabsorbed from the tubular fluid are removed more slowly than normal from the interstitium of the renal medulla. This results in increased medullary intonicity, which in turn further augments water reabsorption from the distal tubular fluid. Therefore, the urinary changes are typical in the shock state. The urinary volume is reduced to less than 400 ml per day (17 ml/hr), urinary specific gravity is increased, and urinary sodium concentration is low (usually less than 5 mEq/liter) (Fig. 21-1).

In addition, substances such as creatinine and urea, which are normally filtered but poorly reabsorbed from the renal tubule, are present in high concentra-

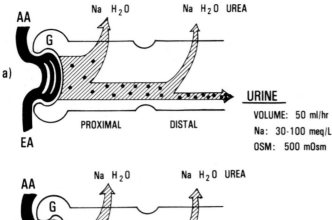

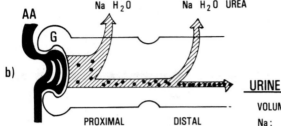

FIGURE 21-1
Normal perfusion of the kidney (a) *compared with underperfusion of the kidney* (b), *which results in decreased renal blood flow and glomerular filtration, with consequent increase in the fraction of filtrate reabsorbed in the proximal tubule and low urine flow with low sodium content and increased concentration.*

tion in the urine as a result of the increased water reabsorption. Because of the characteristic changes associated with renal underperfusion, measurement of urinary volume and specific gravity is a simple method of determining the effect of shock management on renal perfusion.

An increase in systemic blood pressure does not necessarily imply improvement in renal perfusion. This may be especially evident when drugs such as norepinephrine (Levophed) are used to correct the hypotension associated with states of volume depletion. These drugs may be associated with further reduction in renal blood flow as a consequence of constriction of renal arteries. This is manifested by a further fall in urinary volume and rise in specific gravity.

In turn, if the shock state is more appropriately and specifically treated by replacement of volume, improvement of cardiac output, correction of arrhythmias, or administration of isoproterenol (Isuprel), the improved renal perfusion will be manifested as an increased urinary volume and a fall in specific gravity of the urine.

PATHOPHYSIOLOGY OF ACUTE RENAL FAILURE

When renal underperfusion persists for a sufficient period of time (the exact duration of which is unpredictable and varies with the clinical circumstances), the kidneys may become damaged so that restoration of

renal perfusion no longer effects an improvement in glomerular filtration. In this situation, intrinsic renal failure (variously referred to as acute tubular necrosis, vasomotor nephropathy, and lower nephron nephrosis) occurs. This effect may be exaggerated by concomitant administration of nephrotoxic drugs or antibiotics such as the aminoglycosides. Alternatively, these agents and an increasing number of nephrotoxic substances may produce acute renal failure, even in the absence of systemic hypotension and renal ischemia, as a direct result of their toxic effects on the kidney. In both situations, the kidney may or may not reveal significant morphologic changes associated with the inciting insult. For example, in postischemic acute renal failure, the kidney may appear edematous and swollen but show only minor histologic changes on microscopic examination. In nephrotoxic acute renal failure, however, histologic changes, most commonly in the late proximal convoluted tubule and pars recta, may be seen more frequently in association with distal tubular dilatation and accumulation of cellular debris and intraluminal casts. Despite severe reduction in renal function, pathological changes may be minimal and may not reflect the nature of the underlying process unless detailed evaluation of the fine renal architecture is made by electron microscopy. Regardless of the extent of histologic damage, most patients recover complete renal function. Recovery time varies from a period of days to weeks, depending on the severity and etiology of the process.

The exact mechanism that reduces glomerular filtration in any given patient with acute renal failure may be difficult to ascertain owing to the complexity of clinical circumstances. The mechanisms that will be discussed subsequently represent those proposed for relatively pure circumstances of shock- and nephrotoxin-induced renal failure as defined by both human and laboratory animal studies. Even so, despite years of investigation, there is no overwhelming evidence that supports one potential mechanism over another, and it is likely that several operate together in any given clinical or experimental setting.

Renal blood flow has been found to be reduced to approximately one third of normal in acute tubular necrosis, whereas the glomerular filtration rate is almost completely suppressed. This is in contrast to other states in which a similar reduction in renal blood flow is accompanied by much better maintenance of glomerular filtration and renal function.

Numerous animal studies have suggested that intratubular obstruction from casts and cellular debris may be involved in the suppression of glomerular filtration. If this obstruction is relieved, renal function returns. Other studies have suggested that there is disruption of the tubule epithelium with excessive back flow of the filtrate out of the tubule lumen, thus explaining the lack of urine formation in the face of continuing, although reduced, renal blood flow (Fig. 21-2).

The mechanism responsible for the decreased superficial cortical blood flow in the kidney with acute tubular necrosis has not been defined. Earlier, discovery of converting enzyme in the kidney suggested that renin-angiotensin may play a role in this phenomenon. However, subsequent studies have clearly ruled out the renin-angiotensin system as the sole mediator of renal vasoconstriction and the decrease in glomerular

filtration rate. Rather, the abnormalities are mediated by excesses or deficiencies of numerous vasoactive substances, both vasoconstrictors and vasodilators, and by lack of intrinsic myogenic tone in the renal vasculature. It is likely that no single factor, but rather an imbalance of vasoconstrictors and vasodilators acting in unison on the glomerular vasculature, is at fault in the observed renal ischemia (Fig. 21-3). In certain cases, increases of angiotensin II or vasopressin or decreases in prostaglandins or bradykinin may be the overriding phenomenon that disrupts the maintenance of renal blood flow and GFR. Prostaglandin inhibitors, for example, may decrease renal blood flow and GFR in states of stress, such as volume depletion, and further induce acute renal failure. Prostaglandin inhibitors may also enhance renal failure caused by gentamicin and myoglobin, at least in the experimental setting. More studies are needed to define these etiologic associations.

Regardless of the mechanism, there are measurable physiologic changes that predictably occur. First, urine volume is generally reduced in most cases produced by ischemic and nephrotoxic etiologies. Exceptions do occur, however, especially with nephrotoxic acute renal failure caused by aminoglycosides, in which azotemia can occur without there ever having been an interruption of urine flow rate. The decreased GFR is accompanied by a rising serum creatinine and BUN and by characteristic urinary findings that differ from those seen in prerenal azotemia. First, urinary concentration, (osmolality or specific gravity) fall to levels similar to plasma concentration, and the urine concentration of urea and especially of creatinine are decreased, in contrast to findings made in the prerenal state of azotemia. Both reflect failure of distal tubules to concentrate the urine appropriately. The mechanism may be direct distal tubular toxicity or ischemia, or it may be disruption of the normal medullary solute concentration gradient necessary to produce a concentrated urine. Also, urinary sodium concentration no longer reflects systemic volume status and becomes disproportionately high (usually >30 mEq/liter), indicating an inability to modulate sodium concentration appropriate for the clinical circumstance. This is more accurately assessed by the fractional sodium excretion (or, alternatively, by the renal failure index), which is usually greater than 1% and often greater than 3%, probably also reflecting decreased tubular function in residual filtering nephrons.

Causes of Acute Renal Failure

The causes of acute renal failure are numerous but can be divided into two main groups: *ischemic* and *nephrotoxic*. In addition, acute interstitial nephritis due to drugs or infectious agents may produce secondary tubular damage and a clinical picture of acute renal

FIGURE 21-2
Potential mechanisms causing acute renal failure include decreased filtration pressure because of constriction in the renal arterioles (1 and 2); decreased glomerular capillary permeability (3); increased permeability of the proximal tubules with back-leak of filtrate (4); obstruction of urine flow by necrotic tubular cells (5); increased sodium delivery to the macula densa (6); which causes an increase in renin-angiotensin production and vasoconstriction at the glomerular level.

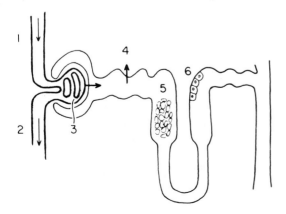

TABLE 21-1
CAUSES OF ACUTE RENAL FAILURE

Ischemic
    Hemorrhagic hypotension
    Severe volume depletion
    Surgical aortic cross-clamping
    Cardiac and biliary surgery
    Defective cardiac output, including open heart
        surgery
    Crush syndromes and other trauma
    Septic shock
    Pregnancy
    Pancreatitis
    Post–renal transplant

Nephrotoxic
    Antibiotics: aminoglycosides, penicillins,
        tetracycline, amphotericin
    Heavy metals: mercury, lead, *cis*-platinum, uranium,
        cadmium, bismuth, arsenic
    Hemoglobinuria
    Myoglobinuria
    Radiologic contrast agents
    Drugs: phenytoin, phenylbutazone, cimetidine
    Organic solvents: carbon tetrachloride
    Fungicides and pesticides
    Uric acid
    Ethylene glycol

Acute Interstitial Nephritis
    Drugs: methicillin, amoxicellen, thyazide diuretics,
        nonsteroidal anti-inflammatory agents
    Infection: septicemia, pyelonephritis, leptospirosis,
        hemorrhagic fevers

---

failure and is included in the differential diagnosis (Table 21-1).

Ischemic Acute Renal Failure

As indicated in Table 21-1, anything that reduces renal blood flow as a result of intravascular volume depletion can result in acute renal failure. In traumatic shock, both the duration and severity of hypotension play major roles in the development of acute renal failure. Over 40% of a large number of combat casualties in World War II developed acute renal failure. In contrast, the incidence of posttraumatic acute renal failure in Korea was 1 per 200 seriously injured, and in Vietnam was even lower, 1 per 600 seriously wounded. Similar findings have been noted in civilian trauma cases. The incidence and average duration of shock have been reduced because of prompter evacuation of patients to definitive treatment centers and more rapid institution of therapy with blood products and volume expanders. The Med-EVAC and MEDSTAR helicopter evacuation systems have contributed significantly to this. Not only has the incidence of acute renal failure decreased in posttraumatic shock, but also ARF is more likely to occur *after* hospitalization as a result of septic complications or nephrotoxic antibiotic administration than as a result of the shock itself.

Nephrotoxic Acute Renal Failure

A large number of diverse chemicals and drugs have been implicated in the production of acute renal failure (Table 21-1). In the hospitalized patient, the most common offending nephrotoxic agents are the antibiotics, especially the aminoglycosides. Examples of these agents are as follows, listed in decreasing order of the severity with which they produce dose-dependent damage to the proximal tubule: neomycin > tobramycin > kanamycin > gentamicin > amikacin > secomicin > netilmicin > streptomicin. Aminoglycoside nephrotoxicity accounts for up to 16% of all cases of acute renal failure, usually is nonoliguric, and frequently improves after cessation of the antibiotic therapy. However, because these agents accumulate preferentially in the renal cortex and are excreted slowly, they sometimes do not produce measurable toxicity until up to 1 week after cessation of administration. Routine monitoring of BUN and creatinine are therefore necessary when these agents are administered. Also, because these agents are primarily eliminated from the body by the kidneys, dosage must be adjusted in patients with preexistent renal function impairment. Peak and trough blood levels must be measured frequently so that drug dosage can be adjusted to the correct therapeutic range.

Acute Interstitial Nephritis (AIN)

Although acute interstitial nephritis is not traditionally listed as a cause of acute renal failure, it is now being included more frequently because of the overlapping clinical pictures and causative agents. Interstitial nephritis may be seen with gentamicin, for example, and may present with the same clinical picture as toxic nephropathy; the only differences are the histologic picture and the presence of more cellular elements in the urine. In this regard, AIN secondary to gentamicin may represent one end of a spectrum of toxicity. Many of the other agents in Table 21-1 produce AIN as an allergic type reaction with frequent eosinophils in the plasma and urine as well as in the kidney. Some of these agents may also produce significant proteinuria. Renal failure may be either oliguric or nonoliguric, although the latter is more common.

Infectious agents, especially those causing leptospirosis and the hemorrhagic fevers, may produce AIN with renal failure but should be recognized by their systemic clinical picture. Sepsis may also produce AIN and be difficult to recognize owing to the frequent accompaniment of shock and other ischemic causes of ARF in the same patient.

Urine Production in Acute Renal Failure

Nonoliguric ARF. Classically, patients have oliguria in association with acute tubular necrosis; however, this is not invariably so. A group of patients present with acute nonoliguria (partially reversible) renal failure. This state is especially common in patients receiving nephrotoxic antibiotics. If antibiotics are discontinued before renal function is markedly reduced, the patient frequently sustains moderate functional impairment for 7 to 10 days with gradual return to normal. In general, patients with nonoliguric acute renal failure have few symptoms, and the disease is much less serious than the oliguric form of acute tubular necrosis.

Oliguric ARF. The more classic or oliguric form of acute tubular necrosis begins with an acute precipitating event immediately followed by oliguria (urine volume less than 400 ml/day). The mean duration of oliguria is approximately 12 days, although it may last only 2 to 3 days or as long as 30 days. This is accompanied by a usual rise in BUN of 25 to 30 mg/100 ml/day and an increase in creatinine of 1.5 to 2 mg/100 ml/day. The most common complication in this period is overhydration with resulting cardiac failure, pulmonary edema, and death. In addition, the patient may develop acidosis, hyperkalemia, and symptoms of uremia.

Diuretic Stage. The oliguric phase is followed by gradual return of renal function as manifested by a stepwise increase in urine volume (the diuretic stage). The degree of diuresis is primarily determined by the state of hydration at the time the patient enters the diuretic stage. If the patient is markedly overloaded, urinary volume may eventually exceed 4 to 5 liters/day. This could result in marked sodium-wasting, with death resulting from electrolyte depletion in a few patients.

Because of the slow return of renal function during the diuretic phase, the degree of azotemia may increase during the early part of the diuretic period, and the patient will have complications that are similar to those noted in the oliguric phase. A period of several months is required for full recovery of renal function after the end of the diuretic period.

MANAGEMENT OF ACUTE RENAL FAILURE

Managing the Shock State

Primary management of renal function impairment is directed at the adequate and specific management of the shock state. The three most common causes for reduced renal perfusion are decreased cardiac output, altered peripheral vascular resistance, and hypovolemia.

Decreased Cardiac Output

Factors such as cardiac arrhythmias, acute myocardial infarction, and acute pericardial tamponade, all of which decrease cardiac output, may be associated with a reduction in renal blood flow. The reversibility of the renal failure thus depends on the ability to improve cardiac function. The specific management has been discussed in earlier chapters.

With the aforementioned conditions, cardiac output is usually acutely and severely compromised. However, when cardiac output is impaired to a lesser extent over a longer period of time, features of congestive heart failure occur. Again, there is reduced renal perfusion, although to a lesser extent. The major feature of this state, from the renal aspect, is avid sodium reabsorption, which results in increased extracellular fluid volume, elevation of central venous pressure, and edema.

Several mechanisms are responsible for the increased tubular reabsorption of sodium (Fig. 21-3). First, there is a greater reduction in renal blood flow than in glomerular filtration, bringing into play the mechanisms discussed earlier. Second, it has been suggested that blood flow to the superficial cortex is reduced, whereas blood flow to the inner cortical area is increased. It is also thought that the nephrons in the inner cortical region reabsorb a greater percentage of the filtered sodium than the nephrons in the outer cortex of the kidney.

Other factors include increased proximal and distal tubule sodium reabsorption. The mechanisms responsible for the increased proximal tubule sodium reabsorption are largely dependent on increased postglomerular oncotic pressure; however, aldosterone is largely responsible for the increased distal tubule sodium reabsorption. It can be seen that numerous mechanisms are responsible for the increased tubular reabsorption of sodium in congestive heart failure.

Therapy is largely directed at increasing urinary sodium excretion. At times this can be accomplished by improvement of cardiac output, which in turn increases renal perfusion. This is not always possible, however.

Diuretics are frequently used to increase sodium excretion. These agents directly inhibit sodium reabsorption in the renal tubule. The potency of a diuretic is primarily determined by the site in the renal tubule where sodium reabsorption is blocked.

The two most potent diuretics presently available are furosemide (Lasix) and ethacrynic acid (Edecrin). These agents block sodium reabsorption in the ascending limb of the loop of Henle and in the distal

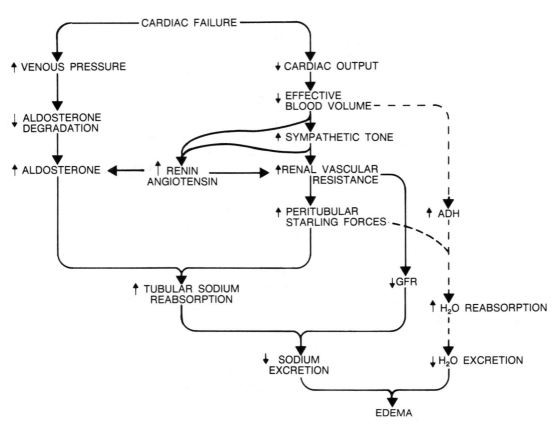

FIGURE 21-3
Factors affecting sodium reabsorption with decreased cardiac output.

tubule. It is still unclear whether they have an effect in the proximal tubule as well. The thiazide diuretics have their major site of action in the distal tubule and are therefore somewhat less potent than the above agents.

Another commonly used diuretic is spironolactone (Aldactone), which increases urinary sodium by blocking the renal tubular effect of aldosterone.

Spironolactone should be used with caution in patients with severe decreases in cardiac output and renal underperfusion because it decreases potassium excretion and can produce life-threatening hyperkalemia in such patients. The same is true of triamterene, another potassium-sparing diuretic.

Altered Peripheral Vascular Resistance
Renal perfusion is compromised in these states as a result of increased size of the intravascular compartment and redistribution of blood volume. This may be a consequence of gram-negative septicemia, certain drug overdoses, anaphylactic reactions, and electrolyte disturbances such as acidosis.

Management is primarily directed at treating the basic disturbance with appropriate specific therapy plus fluid, electrolyte, and colloid replacement. The controversy regarding the use of steroids and various pressor agents in gram-negative sepsis is beyond the scope of this discussion.

Hypovolemia and Hemorrhage
Restoration of extracellular fluid and blood volume is of major importance in the management of any shock state. Evidence for extracellular volume depletion is usually obtained from the history and physical examination.

Historically, the patient may give evidence of external sodium and water loss as a result of vomiting, diarrhea, excessive sweating, or surgical procedures. Blood volume also may be compromised as a result of fluid redistribution, as seen both with burns and with inflammatory processes in the abdomen, such as pancreatitis or peritonitis. The physical findings associated with extracellular volume depletion are sunken eyes, dry mouth, loss of skin turgor, and tachycardia. Postural hypotension may also be noted.

Therapy is directed at sodium and water replacement or blood when hemorrhage is the cause. Response to treatment can be judged by changes in urinary volume, specific gravity, central venous pressure, and the aforementioned physical findings.

Maintenance of Urinary Flow

At times, in spite of adequate treatment of the shock state, urinary volume remains low. This may be a result of either continuing functional impairment in the postshock period or parenchymal renal damage suffered as a consequence of the shock state. Besides recognizing the need to differentiate these two states from each other, a number of authors feel that prolonged oliguria, if allowed to persist, may eventually lead to acute tubular necrosis. Mannitol and furosemide have been used in this setting for both diagnosis and maintenance of urinary function.

Mannitol is the reduced form of the six-carbon sugar, mannose. It is distributed in the extra-cellular fluid and is essentially not metabolized. It is freely filtered at the glomerulus and not reabsorbed by the tubule. Because of its small molecular size (180), it exerts a significant osmotic effect and, in turn, increases urinary flow.

Mannitol is usually infused rather rapidly. The more rapid the infusion, the higher the blood level and, in turn, the filtered load. Urinary flow depends on the amount of mannitol filtered, and if the infusion is too slow, changes in urinary flow rate will be delayed and less apparent.

The usual test is 12.5 g given intravenously as a 25% solution over 3 to 5 minutes. If urine flow increases to greater than 40 ml/hour, the patient is felt to have reversible renal failure, and his urine volume is then maintained at 100 ml/hour with additional mannitol and fluid replacement as indicated.

More recently, *furosemide* and *ethacrynic acid* have largely replaced mannitol in the diagnosis of reversible renal failure. A number of patients who fail to develop a diuresis following infusion of mannitol will have an acceptable increase in urinary volume following administration of furosemide or ethacrynic acid.

After correction of volume depletion, furosemide in dosages of 200 to 1000 mg is given intravenously. The peak diuresis usually occurs within 2 hours of its administration. If furosemide is effective in increasing urinary volume, it is then repeated at 4- to 6-hour intervals to maintain the urinary flow rate as long as fluids are administered to maintain urine.

In patients failing to respond to furosemide, a diagnosis of acute tubular necrosis is seriously entertained. In patients who respond to furosemide and mannitol, it is important to realize that sodium and water depletion will occur if losses are not replaced. Usually urine volume is replaced by half-strength normal saline. In addition, potassium replacement is frequently required.

In 1981 Kopp and Thul[1] reported on the prevention and treatment of acute renal failure by IV bicarbonate loading. In their uncontrolled studies, bicarbonate loading in 41 patients with incipient ARF of various etiologies resulted in restoration of urine flow and 100% survival. In another group of 61 patients, the mortality rate due to ARF and sepsis was only 6.5%. Because these studies lacked matched controls, it cannot be stated that bicarbonate loading and urinary alkalization is definitely better than other methods of maintaining urine flow and preventing ARF. However, Ron and colleagues,[2] have shown a reduced incidence of myoglobinuric ARF by early alkalinization in crush injuries. These data, although suggestive, warrant confirmation in controlled studies.

Differential Diagnosis of Acute Renal Failure

Acute renal failure must be differentiated from prerenal azotemia, or decreased perfusion, and from obstruction. The latter can be distinguished by history and the appropriate use of ultrasonography and abdominal CT scanning. Very rarely will retrograde catheterization of the urinary tract be necessary to exclude this diagnosis in current practice.

Differentiation of acute renal failure from prerenal azotemia may be clinically difficult in many patients because both conditions are frequently accompanied by oliguria. However, a carefully collected urine sample may provide significant clues in making the distinction. The routine urine analysis may be of little diagnostic aid in and of itself because mild proteinuria may be present in both conditions in association with a few cellular elements and granular casts on microscopic examination. The latter are much more numerous in ARF than in prerenal azotemia and also tend to be pigmented; these are highly characteristic but not diagnostic.

Procurement of a urine specimen for diagnostic chemistries and indices as indicated in Table 21-2 is invaluable in establishing the diagnosis of ARF. This urine sample should preferably be obtained *before* a diagnostic challenge of diuretics because these agents may alter the urine chemical composition. As noted in Chapter 19, these urinary chemistry determinations distinguish between underperfusion of the kidney, in which most solutes except for sodium tend to be concentrated, and ARF, in which there tends to be a reduced solute concentration resulting from an inability of the injured tubules to alter the urine composition. Thus, in prerenal azotemia the urinary sodium is low, as are the renal failure index and Fe_{Na}, whereas the urine osmolality and concentration of nonreabsorbable solutes are high. In ARF, urine sodium is >30 mEq/liter, the renal failure index and Fe_{Na} are $>1\%$, and the urine osmolality is close to that of plasma, reflecting inability of the damaged kidney to reabsorb sodium and concentrate the urine.

Acute tubular necrosis must also be distinguished from all other intrinsic renal diseases that can rapidly reduce renal function (Table 21-3). Many of these can

TABLE 21-2
USE OF LABORATORY VALUES IN DIFFERENTIATING ACUTE TUBULAR NECROSIS FROM DECREASED RENAL PERFUSION

Test	Acute Tubular Necrosis	Reduced Renal Blood Flow
Urine		
Volume	<400 ml/24 hr	<400 ml/24 hr
Sodium	Between 40 and 10 mEq/liter	<5 mEq/liter
Specific gravity	1.010	Usually >1.020
Osmolality	250–350 mOsm/liter	Usually >400 mOsm/liter
Urea	200–300 mg/100 ml	Usually >600 mg/100 ml
Creatinine	<60 mg/100 ml	Usually >150 mg/100 ml
Fe_{Na}	>3.0%	<1.0%
Blood		
BUN:Cr	10:1	Usually >20:1
Responses to		
mannitol	None	None or flow increases to >40 ml/hr
Furosemide	None	Flow increases to >40 ml/hr

TABLE 21-3
DIFFERENTIAL DIAGNOSIS OF ACUTE RENAL FAILURE

1. Prerenal azotemia
   (a) Hypovolemia
   (b) Cardiovascular failure
       (1) Myocardial failure
       (2) Vascular pooling
   (c) Hepatorenal syndrome
2. Vascular obstruction
   (a) Arterial obstruction
       (1) Embolization
       (2) Thrombosis
       (3) Dissection
   (b) Venous obstruction
3. Intrinsic renal disease
   (a) Glomerulonephritis
   (b) Vasculitis
   (c) Microangiopathic disease
       (1) Hemolytic uremic syndrome
       (2) Thrombotic thrombocytopenic purpura
   (d) Malignant nephrosclerosis
4. Postrenal azotemia
   (a) Obstructive uropathy
   (b) Rupture of the bladder

be differentiated by their clinical picture, urine analyses, and so forth. In some circumstances, the diagnosis may be difficult, such as with rapidly progressive glomerulonephritis without significant urine sediment abnormalities. In this situation, urine chemistries look more like those seen in prerenal azotemia than those observed in acute tubular necrosis and should serve as a clue to the diagnosis because AIN patients are generally clinically volume-expanded rather than volume-contracted.

With regard to the etiology of acute renal failure, there are frequently subtle clues that will aid in the diagnosis, and these should be carefully sought (Table 21-4).

Managing the Postshock State

Because acute tubular necrosis continues to be associated with a high mortality, the major objective is prevention of this complication. The feasibility of pre-

TABLE 21-4
DIAGNOSTIC CLUES IN ACUTE RENAL FAILURE

Urine

Urate crystals	Tumor lysis, especially lymphoma (urate nephropathy)
Oxalate crystals	Ethylene glycol nephrotoxicity
	Methoxyflurane nephrotoxicity
Eosinophils	Allergic interstitial nephritis, especially methicillin
Positive benzidene without RBCs	Hemoglobinuria or myoglobinuria
Pigmented casts	Hemoglobinuria or myoglobinuria
Massive proteinuria	Acute interstitial nephritis, thiazide diuretics, hemorrhagic fevers (Korean, Scandinavian, etc.)
Anuria	Renal cortical necrosis, bilateral obstruction, hemolytic uremic syndrome, rapidly progressive glomerulonephritis

Plasma

Marked hyperkalemia	Rhabdomyolysis, tissue necrosis, hemolysis
Marked hypocalcemia	Rhabdomyolysis
Hypercalcemia	Hypercalcemic nephropathy
Hyperuricemia	Tumor lysis, rhabdomyolysis, toxin ingestion
Marked acidosis	Ethylene glycol, methyl alcohol
Eosinophilia	Allergic interstitial nephritis

venting development of acute tubular necrosis in patients with major traumatic injuries by rapid replacement of blood loss and correction of fluid and electrolyte disturbances has been clearly demonstrated.

Similarly, patients receiving potentially nephrotoxic agents should undergo serial determinations so that renal function can be evaluated during the course of the administration of these agents. One can most easily accomplish this by measuring serum creatinine levels on an every-other-day schedule. If the serum creatinine begins to rise, the drug should be discontinued. In the majority of patients, functional deterioration stabilizes, and the patient recovers without the development of severe impairment of renal function.

Drug Therapy

There is still considerable debate with regard to the effectiveness of *mannitol* and *furosemide* in the prevention of acute renal failure. In fact, some evidence has been accumulated that suggests that furosemide may actually increase the toxicity of certain nephrotoxic agents. However, most authors agree that a trial of furosemide up to 500 mg IV should be used. Often, this may correct oliguric to nonoliguric ARF, which is clinically easier to manage.

Volume Replacement

After development of acute tubular necrosis, the primary consideration is maintenance of fluid and electrolyte balance. During the oliguric phase, urinary volume is usually less than 300 ml/day. Insensible losses

average 800 to 1000 ml/day and are virtually free of electrolytes.

In general, fluid replacement should be approximately 500 ml/day. Additional water will be obtained from the water present in foods plus the water of oxidation from metabolism. Because of the utilization of body proteins and fats, the patient ideally should lose approximately 2.2 kg (1 lb) a day in order to maintain water balance. The *danger of fluid overload* with resulting congestive heart failure and pulmonary edema exists throughout the oliguric period. In contrast, during the diuretic phase of acute tubular necrosis there may be extensive *sodium-wasting* in association with the increased urinary volumes. It is thus necessary to keep accurate intake and output records as well as daily weights during both phases. This is especially important when there are other avenues of fluid and electrolyte losses such as vomiting, diarrhea, nasogastric suction, and drainages from fistulas. In general, losses occurring as a result of these problems should be replaced in full.

Nutritional Therapy

Besides replacing fluids and electrolytes, intake is directed at supplying the patient with calories in the form of carbohydrates and fats to decrease the rate of breakdown of body protein. Because 1 g of urea is formed from every 6 g of protein metabolized protein intake is usually restricted in order to prevent the BUN from rising at too fast a rate.

With the development of nutritional teams, there has been a growing tendency to provide more calories

TABLE 21-5
RECOMMENDED ANTIBIOTIC DOSAGE IN RENAL FAILURE

Antibiotic Group	Adjustment for Renal Failure				Dialysis Supplement
	Method	GFR (ml/minute)			
		>50	10–50	<10	
Aminoglycosides	I*	12–18	12	24	Yes
Amikacin					
Gentamicin					
Kanamicin					
Netilmicin					
Streptomicin					
Tobramicin					
Cephalosporins					Yes
All except Cefoperozone require reduction, but adjustments vary significantly between drugs.					
Cefaclor	D†	100	50–100	33	Yes
Cefadroxil	I	8	12–24	24–48	Yes
Cefamandole	I	6	6–8	8	Yes
Cefazolin	I	8	12	24–48	Yes
Cefoperazone	I	—	None‡	—	Yes
Ceforanide	I	12	24–48	48–72	Yes
Cefotaximine	I	6–8	8–12	12–24	Yes
Cefoxitin	I	8	8–12	24–48	Yes
Cefroxadine	D	65–100	15–65	10–15	?
Cefuroxime	I	8–12	24–48	48–72	Yes
Cefsulodin	D	50–100	15–50	10–15	Yes
Ceftizoxime	D	45–100	10–45	5–10	?
Cephalothin	I	6	6	8–12	Yes
Cephalexin	I	6	6–8	12	Yes
Cephapirin	I	6	6–8	12	Yes
Cephradine	D	100	50	25	Yes
Moxalactam	I	8	12	12–24	Yes
Clindamycin	D	—	None	—	Yes
Erythromycin	D	—	None	—	Yes
Lincomycin	I	6	12	24	Yes
Methenanime mandelate	D	100	Avoid§	Avoid	—
Nalidixic acid	D	100	Avoid	Avoid	—
Nitrofurantoin	D	100	Avoid	Avoid	—
Penicillins					
Amoxicillin	I	6	6–12	12–16	Yes
Ampicillin	I	6	6–12	12–16	Yes
Azlocillin	I	4–6	6–8	8	Yes
Carbenicillin	I	8–12	12–24	24–48	Yes
Cloxacillin	D	—	None	—	No‖
Cyclacillin	I	6	6–12	12–24	Yes
Dicloxacillin	I	—	None	—	No
Methicillin	I	4	4–8	8–12	No
Mezlocillin	I	4–6	6–8	8	Yes
Nafcillin	D	—	None	—	No
Oxacillin	D	—	None	—	No
Penicillin G	I	6–8	8–12	12–16	Yes
Piperacillin	I	4–6	6–8	8	Yes
Ticarcillin	I	8–12	12–24	24–48	Yes
Sulfonamides and trimethoprim					
Sulfamethoxazole	I	12	18	24	Yes
Sulfisoxazole	I	6	8–12	12–24	Yes
Trimethoprim	I	12	18	24	Yes

TABLE 21-5 (Continued)

Antibiotic Group	Method	Adjustment for Renal Failure GFR (ml/minute)			Dialysis Supplement
		>50	10–50	<10	
Tetracyclines					
Doxycycline	I	12	12–18	18–24	No
Minocycline	D	—	None	—	No
Vancomycin	I	24–72	72–240	240	No

* *I* refers to alteration in dosage interval in hours.
† *D* refers to percentage of alteration of usual dose.
‡ *None* means no dosage adjustment is necessary.
§ *Avoid* means drugs toxic in renal failure.
ǁ *No* means that hemodialysis does not significantly alter kinetics of the drug.
(Modified from Bennett WM et al: Drug prescribing in renal failure: Dosing guidelines for adults. Am J Kidney Dis 3:155–193, 1983)

and protein in the form of parenteral or enteral hyperalimentation in attempts to improve the overall condition of the patient and to hasten recovery of renal function. Diets containing 2000 to 3000 calories/day with 40 to 60 g of protein or essential amino acids have been used with increased frequency. These diets contain more than the 500 ml of fluid recommended earlier. Therefore, hyperalimentation requires more frequent dialysis, especially in the oliguric period, often in combination with hemofiltration. Controlled studies on the effects of hyperalimentation on survival are few, but in one study from England involving parenteral hyperalimentation with daily dialysis a mortality rate of only 30% was noted in patients with posttraumatic acute renal failure, a significant improvement over that reported in most similar patients.

Drug Precautions

Certain drugs should be avoided or dosage reduced in any patient with markedly impaired renal function. Because of the possibility of magnesium intoxication, *antacids* containing magnesium should be avoided. Because of the reduced renal function, *digitalis* excretion may be reduced. Dosage should be altered to avoid excessively high blood levels. In addition, certain *antibiotics* should be given in much smaller dosages than usually employed as indicated in Table 21-5. This table lists most commonly used antibiotics and gives general guidelines as to how dosage should be modified based on the level of GFR. Modifications may be made based on the dosage interval (I) or on alterations of the percentage of the normal dose (D) given at standard dosage intervals. In many cases, the modifications listed are only rough approximations and, when possible, serum levels should also be mea-

sured so that dosage can be more accurately determined. Table 21-5 also indicates which antibiotics may require supplemental doses because of their removal by hemodialysis.

Before administering a drug to a patient with renal failure, one should review the following questions:

- Does the drug depend on the kidney for secretion?
- Does an excess blood level affect the kidney?
- Does the drug add chemically to the pool of urea nitrogen?
- Does the effect of the drug alter electrolyte imbalance?
- Is the patient more susceptible to the drug because of kidney disease?

For additional information about the modification of drug dosages in uremia, see the article by Bennett and colleagues.

Acidosis

Metabolic acidosis of moderate severity is usually present in patients with renal failure. This results from the inability of the kidneys to excrete fixed acids (*e.g.,* H_2PO_4) produced from normal metabolic processes.

The acidosis can usually be easily controlled by giving the patient 30 to 60 mEq of sodium bicarbonate daily but does not require treatment unless the HCO_3^- falls below 12 to 15 mEq/liter.

Hyperkalemia

Hyperkalemia commonly occurs in patients with acute tubular necrosis. This is a consequence of both the reduced ability of the kidneys to excrete potassium and the release of intracellular potassium because of acidosis and tissue breakdown. The acidosis results in movement of the hydrogen ion into the cell, thus displacing potassium into the extracellular fluid. This maintains electrical neutrality but increases the hyperkalemic state.

An additional mechanism for producing hyperkalemia, often overlooked in acutely ill patients, is caloric restriction, especially glucose restriction. Transport of glucose and amino acids into cells is accompanied by potassium. In acutely ill, catabolic patients, when dietary intake is restricted or intravenous fluid therapy inadvertently disrupted, failure of transport of potassium intracellularly may contribute to hyperkalemia. Because this process requires insulin, insulin deficiency may have the same consequences, and diabetics may therefore be more prone to acute disturbances in potassium balance when renal failure occurs.

By interfering with catecholamine-induced translocation of potassium into cells, beta-blockers can also enhance hyperkalemia and should be avoided in patients with ARF.

Hyperkalemia is manifested clinically by cardiac and neuromuscular changes. Both cardiac conduction disturbances and acute flaccid quadriplegia are life-threatening complications. These hyperkalemic changes are rapidly reversed by administration of intravenous calcium gluconate, which has a direct antagonist effect on the action of potassium. Serum potassium can be reduced by intravenous administration of sodium bicarbonate for treatment of acidosis. In addition, administration of glucose and insulin is frequently used as an additional method of shifting extracellular potassium to intracellular pools.

Sodium polystyrine sulfomate resin (Kayexalate) given orally (25 g four times a day in 10 ml of 10% sorbitol) may reduce the body potassium burden more slowly and should be instituted when hyperkalemia begins to develop. In addition, when life-threatening hyperkalemia develops and emergency treatment with the aforementioned regimen fails or does not restore serum potassium to normal, emergency intervention, either hemodialysis or peritoneal dialysis, should be instituted. Although hemodialysis will reduce body burden of potassium to a greater degree than peritoneal dialysis, peritoneal dialysis generally can be instituted much more quickly. Because plasma potassium

TABLE 21-6
COMMON FLUID AND ELECTROLYTE IMBALANCES

Electrolyte Disturbance	Major Symptoms	Major Physical Findings	Etiology
Increased sodium and water	Dyspnea	Edema, anasarca, rales, increased jugular venous pressure	Congestive failure, renal disease, liver disease
Decreased sodium and water	Thirst Weakness	Tachycardia, postural hypotension, sunken eyes, dry mouth, decreased skin turgor	Excessive sweating, vomiting, diarrhea, Addison's disease, renal disease, diuretics without replacement
Decreased sodium and normal water	Headaches Psychological disorder	Hyperreflexia, pathologic reflexes, convulsions, coma	Water without sodium replacement in above states; excess ADH
Normal sodium and decreased water	Thirst	Often no findings or those found in decreased sodium and water	Lack of water intake, diabetes insipidus, excessive sweating, fever
Hyperkalemia	Weakness	Paralysis, ECG changes; spiked T waves	Renal disease, excess potassium replacement
Hypokalemia	Weakness	Paralysis, paralytic ileus, hypoventilation, ECG changes: T waves and prominent U waves	Diuretics, renal disease, diarrhea, vomiting, excess laxatives
Acidosis	Weakness	Kussmaul respiration	Renal disease, diabetic acidosis, certain intoxications
Hypermagnesemia	Weakness	Muscle weakness, hypoventilation, hypotension, flushing	Antacids with renal disease

equilibriates rapidly with peritoneal fluid, a prompt reduction of serum potassium can be effected and may be life-saving.

Hyperkalemia can usually be prevented by avoidance of potassium supplements, institution of chronic therapy for acidosis, and use of sodium polystyrene sulfonate resin (Kayexalate) when serum potassium is even slightly elevated.

Sodium and Water Diuresis

During the oliguric phase of acute tubular necrosis, sodium retention may occur. However, with the onset of the diuretic period, urinary volume and sodium excretion may markedly increase.

Urinary volume is largely determined by the state of hydration at the onset of the diuretic period. Because urinary sodium concentration is relatively fixed, sodium losses are largely determined by urinary volume. Therefore, if the patient is markedly overhydrated at the onset of the diuretic phase, sodium losses may be severe. Clinically, sodium depletion is characterized by either extracellular volume depletion, as manifested by tachycardia and postural hypotension, or water intoxication when sodium losses exceed water losses. This latter syndrome is characterized by markedly reduced serum sodium concentrations in association with personality changes, convulsions, coma, and death if allowed to progress untreated.

With acute water intoxication, treatment is directed at elevation of the serum sodium concentration. This can usually be accomplished by administration of hypertonic (3% to 5%) sodium chloride intravenously. Table 21-6 lists common fluid and electrolyte imbalances.

Uremic Syndrome

In addition to the aforementioned specific electrolyte disturbances, the patient may develop symptoms associated with any uremic state. Early findings are nausea, anorexia, and vomiting. Later, stupor, convulsions, and coma develop. In addition, bleeding abnormalities, uremic pneumonitis, pericarditis, pleuritis, and so forth may occur.

Dialysis is indicated prior to the development of clinical symptoms of uremia. With the availability of hemodialysis or peritoneal dialysis in most hospitals, there is little reason for the clinical features of uremia to occur in patients with acute tubular necrosis. Most patients having oliguria for more than 4 to 5 days will require dialysis sometime during the course of their acute tubular necrosis. There is little doubt that dialysis has improved survival in patients with acute tubular necrosis.

Continuous hemofiltration has been used to treat acute renal failure. With this method, the patient is connected to a low-volume ultrafiltration apparatus by an arteriovenous Scribner shunt. No extracorporeal pump or dialysate is required, and the procedure can be performed and monitored in the ICU. Ultrafiltrate must be measured and replaced with normal saline or a balanced salt solution. Further studies are required for assessment of how this treatment compares with standard hemodialysis, but from both the practical and physiologic standpoints, it is a potentially sound alternative.

Prognosis is largely determined by the primary event that led to the development of acute tubular necrosis. Among patients with acute tubular necrosis due to medical causes (*e.g.,* transfusion reactions, myoglobinuria, nephrotoxic agents, and simple volume depletion), the mortality rate is approximately 25%, whereas cases resulting from trauma and severe surgical complications are associated with a 60% to 70% mortality rate. Death usually results as a complication of poor wound healing and sepsis or the underlying disease.

In view of the continuing high mortality, every effort should be directed toward prevention of acute tubular necrosis early in the shock state by correction of the underlying disease.

CASE STUDY

An 85-year-old woman with calcific aortic stenosis was admitted with mild congestive heart failure. Admission examination revealed that the elderly woman, who appeared chronically ill, was mildly dyspneic but not edematous. Her weight was 53.3 kg, blood pressure was 120/60, pulse was 98 beats/minute, temperature 97.8° F, and respirations were 24/minute. BUN was 13.4 mg/dl, and serum creatinine was 0.4 mg/dl. The patient was maintained on her normal dose of digoxin (0.125 mg/day) and placed on a 2-g sodium diet and given hydrochlorthiazide, 50 mg two times a day.

The patient's cardiovascular symptoms gradually improved, but 1 week later she was slightly confused and complained of dizziness on sitting up. Her blood pressure was 150/60, pulse was 108 beats/minute, and weight was 37.7 kg. She did not recall voiding in the past 24 hours. A Foley catheter was passed, and 15 ml of dark yellow urine was recovered. The following laboratory values were obtained:

Serum	Na	149 mEq/liter
	Cl	112 mEq/liter
	CO$_2$	29 mEq/liter
	K	3.5 mEq/liter
	BUN	144 mg/dl
	Creatinine	2.1 mq/dl
	Osmolality	303 mOsm/liter
Urine	Na	11 mEq/dl
	K	33 mEq/dl
	Osm	482 mOsm/liter
	Creatinine	89 mg/dl

The hypernatremia suggested mild dehydration. BUN was alarmingly high, and the serum creatinine of 2.1 mg%, although seemingly low in relation to the BUN, was four times greater than the value recorded on admission, suggesting a loss of 75% of initial renal function. A diagnosis of acute renal failure secondary to volume depletion was entertained. However, when the patient's urine chemistries were returned, the low urinary sodium, the urinary osmolality (which was 1.6 × that of plasma), and the U/P creatinine ratio of 42/1 suggested intact renal function. The fractional excretion of sodium (U : P Na/U : P creatinine × 100) was calculated as follows:

$$11 : 149/88 : 2.1 \times 100 - .18\%$$

This was also consistent with volume depletion and prerenal azotemia.

This patient could have had either (1) acute renal failure resulting from excessive volume depletion or from emboli due to cardiac disease or (2) prerenal azotemia resulting from volume depletion, which was not appreciated because of failure to maintain daily weight or I and O records on the ward.

A challenge with 500 ml N/S IV over 1 hour produced a urine flow of 40 ml in the next hour. A slow infusion of N/S, 2 liters/day, was given over the next 4 days and followed by increasing urine volumes. The patient's weight increased to 41.1 kg, and the BUN and creatinine dropped to 22.4 and 0.9 mg/dl, respectively, without increased signs of cardiac decompensation. This dramatic response confirmed the laboratory-supported diagnosis of prerenal azotemia.

REFERENCES

1. Kopp KF, Thul GM: Prophylaxis and emergency treatment of acute renal failure. In Eliahou EH (ed): Proceedings of the Tel Aviv Satellite Symposium in the 8th Meeting of the International Society of Nephrology, pp 181–185, 1985
2. Ron D, Taitelman U, Michaelson M, Bar-Joseph G, Bursztein S, Better OS: Prevention of acute renal failure in acute rabdomyolysis. Archives of Internal Medicine 144:277–280, 1984
3. Bennett, WM et al: Drug prescribing in renal failure: Dosing guidelines for adults. Am J Kidney Dis 3:155–193, 1983

BIBLIOGRAPHY

Butkus DE: Persistant high mortality in acute renal failure: Are we asking the right questions? Arch Intern Med 143(2):209–212, 1983

Butkus DE: Post-traumatic acute renal failure in combat casualties—a historical review. Military Med 149(3):117–124, 1984

Butkus DE, Moore JA Jr: Acute renal failure. In Preuss HG (ed): Handbook of Clinical Nephrology—A Problem Oriented Approach. New York, John Wiley & Sons (in press)

Espinel CH, Gregory AW: Differential diagnosis of acute renal failure. Clin Nephrol 13:73–77, 1980

Schrier RW: Acute renal failure. Kidney Int 15:205–216, 1979

Schin B, Mackenzie CF, Cowley, RA: Changing patterns of post-traumatic acute renal failure. Am Sur 45:182–189, 1979

22
Endstage Renal Disease and Renal Transplantation

Karen Choate Robbins
Ann Marie Powers
Betty C. Irwin*

Transplantation research began in the early 1900s, although it was not until the early 1950s that transplantation became a realistic and therapeutic approach for chronic renal failure in humans.

Originally, kidneys were grafted into the thigh, with the femoral vessels used for vascularization. Experience with this procedure was limited to a very few patients. Because this site was obviously not practical for long-term graft survival, surgeons began grafting kidneys into the iliac fossa in the mid 1950s, the site still used today.

Since that time, many centers in the country are performing renal transplants as definitive therapy for *endstage renal disease* (ESRD)†. As more centers evolved, so too have a multitude of approaches and philosophies, with the major differences revolving around the immunosuppressive therapy.

This chapter does not encompass all possible management approaches but will, however, cover the major points of transplantation and care that are common to all centers and that are well-documented in the literature. It will provide the critical care nurse with sufficient information to provide competent care for the transplant recipient.‡

* The authors wish to acknowledge the help of Laurine S. Bow, B.S., in preparing the material on tissue typing.

† The recognized federal terminology for chronic renal failure is endstage renal disease (ESRD). As of July 1, 1973, patients with ESRD became eligible for Medicare coverage regardless of age. As a result, no one is denied replacement therapy due to lack of funds. This coverage extends for 3 years from the month of transplant procedure and includes the donor's medical expenses. Coverage for dialysis therapy is for the duration of treatment.

‡ If further information is desired please refer to *Standards of Clinical Practice. Section II: Transplantation*. Available from the Ameri-

ENDSTAGE RENAL DISEASE

Renal failure is rarely an "all or none" phenomenon but instead is a gradual loss of function involving either some or all of the nephrons, depending on the basic disease process.

When a patient has minimal renal damage, the body may compensate for certain lost functions, and the patient will have few symptoms. If the process is acute and reversible, the effects of long-term failure (*e.g.,* anemia, osteodystrophy) will not be seen. For many patients, however, the process is a long and exhausting one that affects all body systems.

It is not until irreversible damage to the majority of nephrons (approximately 2 million) occurs and the glomerular filtration rate decreases to 100 ml/minute that a patient is considered to have ESRD (see Chapters 18 and 21).

TRANSPLANT OR DIALYSIS: THE PATIENT'S CHOICE

Once a patient has reached ESRD, he has three options: no treatment and death, chronic dialysis (either peritoneal dialysis or hemodialysis), or transplantation (Fig. 22-1).

Although the option of no treatment and death is considered and occasionally chosen by the patient, the focus here will be on the treatment options of hemodialysis and transplant (two forms of *replacement therapy*). Intermittent peritoneal dialysis and continuous ambulatory peritoneal dialysis are two other forms of

can Nephrology Nurses Association. Box 56, North Woodbury Road, Pitman, New Jersey 08071.

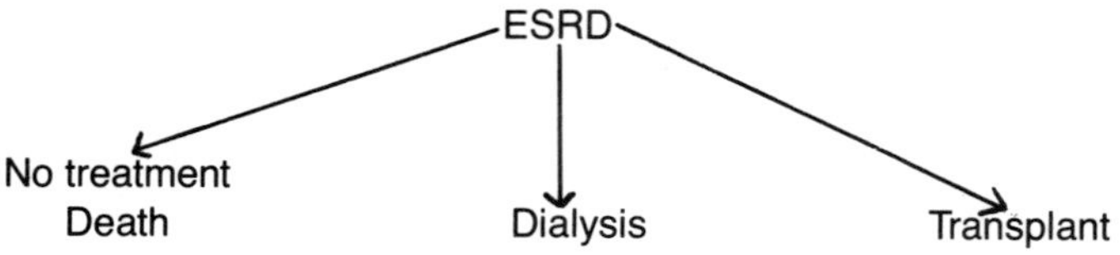

ESRD

No treatment
Death → Dialysis → Transplant

FIGURE 22-1
Options facing a person with endstage renal disease (ESRD).

TABLE 22-1
ALTERATIONS CREATED BY ENDSTAGE RENAL DISEASE MANAGED BY DIALYSIS AND WELL-FUNCTIONING TRANSPLANT

Function	Dialysis	Well-Functioning Transplant
Alteration in body fluids	Excess body fluids Renal filtration occurs only during dialysis Metabolic acidosis	Alteration in fluids resolved Acid-base balance maintained
Alteration in nutrition	Na, K, protein and fluid restrictions	Possible NA restriction for up to 1 year after transplant Possible alterations in diet for hyperglycemia
Alteration in hematologic system	Anemia, fatigue Shortened RBC survival Prolonged clotting time	Normal red blood cells and hematocrit Normal clotting time

Impaired physical mobility
  Bone disease
	Renal osteodystrophy:
	  Osteomalacia
	  Osteoporosis
	  Osteitis fibrosa cystica
		No further bone resorption
		
		Steroid-induced osteoporosis
		Possible tertiary hyperparathyroidism
		Avascular/aseptic necrosis

Decreased muscle strength	Decreased muscle mass due to dietary limits Decreased exercise tolerance	Myopathy that improves when steroid dosage decreases and patient's activity increases
Alteration in nervous system control	Peripheral, gastrointestinal, and genitourinary neuropathy Autonomic nervous system neuropathy	Neuropathy will not progress and may improve
Alteration of hepatic function	Increased risk of hepatitis from extracorporeal circulation in hemodialysis patient Increased risk of hepatitis B or non-A, non-B hepatitis from transfusions	Risk of hepatitis due to azathioprine or cyclosporine therapy Risk of hepatitis B or non-A, non-B hepatitis from transfusions Increased susceptibility to viral hepatitis
Alteration in cardiovascular system	Risk of vascular access infection, clotting, exsanguination, and frequent site changes Accelerated atherosclerosis Hypertriglyceridemia Ventricular hypertrophy, heart failure Uremic pericarditis Cardiac tamponade	No need for vascular access Effect on atherosclerotic process uncertain Increased cholesterol levels Ventricular size sometimes returns to normal
Alteration in gastrointestinal function	Increased gastric acid production Increased incidence of diverticulosis Constipation	Increased risk of ulceration Diverticulosis predisposes to perforation Increased incidence of ischemic colitis
Alteration in immune response	Increased susceptibility to infection from uremia	Increased susceptibility to infection from immunosuppressive drugs Increased incidence of malignancy (especially skin, lymph, and cervix)
Impaired gas exchange	Risk of pulmonary edema, congestive heart failure	Pulmonary infections secondary to immunosuppressive therapy
Alteration in self-concept; body image disturbances	Dependent on machine and solutions to support life Gradual, subtle physical changes (*e.g.*, change in skin color, muscle loss)	Dependent on medications to support renal function Rapid, abrupt early physical changes (*e.g.*, cushingoid appearance, hirsutism)

replacement therapy that will not be discussed in this chapter but that are covered in Chapter 20.

Hemodialysis and transplantation are presented here because they are the most prevalent therapeutic approaches. Although dialysis and transplant are separate options, each of these therapies is an integral part of the other. Transplantation cannot be done without the support of dialysis, and if the transplant fails, dialysis is resumed.

Both ESRD and replacement therapy change the patient's previous state of being. Therefore, the patient needs to consider the alterations created by the disease and the therapies and recognize that such alterations may persist post transplant. Table 22-1 outlines the alterations created by ESRD and the effects on them when managed by dialysis or a well-functioning transplant.

ALTERATIONS CREATED BY ENDSTAGE RENAL DISEASE

Alteration in Body Fluids

In ESRD, the glomerular filtration rate (GFR) and urinary output are grossly diminished, creating an excess of body fluids. Consequently, renal filtration occurs only during dialysis. With a well-functioning renal graft, however, renal filtration is constant.

Alteration in Nutrition

Diet is restricted in the majority of dialysis patients. These restrictions, which include protein, sodium, potassium, and fluid, are necessary because the equivalent of renal filtration occurs for only a limited number of hours per week.

When the diet is followed, it changes lifetime eating habits and poses severe limits on the patient's social activities. Gross abuse of the diet can result in malignant hypertension, congestive heart failure, pulmonary edema, hyperkalemia, or, potentially, cardiac arrest.

It may be necessary to restrict sodium following successful transplantation. If the recipient has diabetes mellitus or develops estrogenic diabetes mellitus, additional alterations in diet must be made. Rather than having fluids restricted, the patient is encouraged to drink at least 2 liters of fluid per day. Therefore, following successful transplant, the diet more closely approaches a normal one and is much more conducive to socialization.

Alteration in Hematologic System

Anemia is common to all patients with ESRD. Because the kidney is no longer able to produce adequate amounts of erythropoietic stimulating factor, red blood cell production is low. This, along with shorter red blood cell survival in the uremic patient, causes hematocrits one half that of normal. This anemia is thought to cause the fatigue that is one of the most frustrating problems for the ESRD patient.

If the diet has been severely limited in protein, iron and vitamin B_{12} intake will be diminished, thereby reducing the amount of iron that can be absorbed from the intestines. The use of iron and androgen therapy has been of benefit to many patients, although normal hematocrits are rarely seen in spite of such therapy. Increased blood losses in the hemodialysis patient further contribute to low hematocrits. Ruptures and clotting of the dialyzer, residual blood in the dialyzer following termination of the dialysis, and routine laboratory tests are sources of significant and chronic blood loss and contribute to this problem.[1]

The use of blood transfusions prior to transplantation has helped alleviate anemia-related problems. Several months after the transplant, anemia is seldom a problem, and the patient will have a near normal, if not normal hematocrit. Even though the kidney was denervated when transplanted, this does not affect the erythropoiesis of the graft. Although blood loss from laboratory tests is appreciable immediately following the transplant, it is markedly reduced following hospital discharge. The patient has a normal protein intake, an increased ability to absorb iron, and normal red blood cell survival time, all increasing the ability to maintain the hematocrit at a higher level.

Impaired Physical Mobility

Bone Disease

The kidneys play a major role in maintaining calcium-phosphorus balance in the body. They accomplish this function by excreting these elements and also by converting vitamin D to an active form. Loss of nephron (kidney) function, therefore, is accompanied by gross disturbances in calcium metabolism and the development of a complex set of comorbidity problems that are commonly referred to as *renal osteodystrophy.* Renal osteodystrophy refers to three bone disease processes that are caused by the malfunctioning kidneys as opposed to other etiologies: osteomalacia, osteoporosis, and osteofibrosa cystitis.

The ESRD patient may exhibit one or all three processes concurrently. The first process, *osteomalacia,* is defined as a softening of the bones. This process can cause bones to become flexible and brittle and can eventually result in spontaneous fractures. The second process is *osteoporosis,* which is defined as increased porosity of the bone and which occurs as bones continue to lose calcium.

Both osteomalacia and osteoporosis are caused by the lack of activated vitamin D to assist in maintaining calcium hemostasis. Activated vitamin D or D_3 acts by increasing renal calcium reabsorption and intestinal transport of calcium into the bloodstream as well as by assisting in calcium mobilization from the bone in conjunction with parathyroid hormone (PTH). Vitamin D is acquired from sunlight or dietary sources, but requires a functioning renal mass for complete activation.

In renal failure, dietary calcium is restricted, lessening the availability of this element to maintain serum calcium values. In addition, the continued serum phosphorus elevation is thought to shut off vitamin D conversion and to increase skeletal resistance to the effect of PTH. The long-term effect of this skeletal resistance is that the parathyroid gland enlarges to secrete enough PTH to increase serum calcium.

The enlargement of the parathyroid causes hyperplasia, or secondary hyperparathyroidism, and *osteitis fibrosa cystica,* the third bone disease process. Symptoms may include itching, metastatic soft tissue calcifications around joints and tendons, vascular calcifications of the large and small blood vessels, and diffuse or local skeletal pain. Continued gland enlargement can lead to tertiary or autonomic hyperparathyroidism diagnosed by hypercalcemia.

Medical management of these problems should be provided early in the course of renal failure through dietary restriction of phosphorus or administration of phosphate binders before initiation of dialysis or transplantation. Normal serum phosphorus is required before vitamin D or calcium supplements can be safely added to the management protocol; otherwise, calcium deposits can occur.

Once the patient is on dialysis, binders are given at mealtime. Calcium supplementation and vitamin D therapy can be initiated as needed. Even with adequate therapy, bone disease may continue, and a subtotal parathyroidectomy may be required to halt the progression of bone changes.

A successful renal transplant stops many of the osteodystrophic changes produced by ESRD because the kidney can again take an active role in calcium metabolism. Occasionally, the parathyroids continue to enlarge, causing *tertiary hyperparathyroidism.* In addition, the catabolic nature of the steroid medication contributes to the development of osteoporosis as well as of *aseptic necrosis of major joints.*

Decreased Muscular Strength

A *loss of muscle mass* is not uncommon in the ESRD patient. Limited dietary intake and inability to exert oneself due to the fatigue associated with anemia are probably the major contributing factors.

The transplant recipient will frequently experience *myopathies* due to steroid therapy. This loss in muscle mass can be recovered with exercise, particularly when the steroids are reduced. In an attempt to avoid severe myopathies, the transplant recipient is encouraged to walk, climb stairs, and exercise as much as possible.

Alteration in Nervous System Control

Although the mechanism is poorly understood, *neuropathies* may develop in the presence of severe or chronic uremia. The neuropathies cause muscle weakness, which sometimes requires the use of braces, walkers, or crutches for ambulation. Functions of the autonomic nervous system may be impaired to the extent that the gastrointestinal (GI) tract may be affected and blood pressure control is poor. Patients may actually have chronic hypotension from autonomic nervous system neuropathy.

Neuropathy should not increase in severity following transplantation, and, depending on the severity of the neuropathy, there may be partial or total reversal following successful transplantation.

Sexual Dysfunction

Impotence is prevalent among dialysis patients. Although women may be physically capable of engaging in sexual intercourse, libido is often markedly decreased, lowering their desire for sexual activity.

Most male patients are impotent, perhaps because of their disease or because of antihypertensive medications. The etiology of this complication is probably physiological as well as psychological. There are research data that suggest that certain trace elements (*e.g.,* zinc) may be implicated in sexual dysfunction. Marriages and other comparable relationships can be adversely affected, and the long-term effects can be devastating.

Some patients remain impotent following transplantation, although this is most frequently associated with antihypertensive medication and steroid therapy. The libido, which is decreased while the patient is on dialysis, seems to return to normal following transplant.

Women usually cease to have menstrual periods while on dialysis, but following transplant will once again ovulate and menstruate. Therefore, some means of contraception should be used for 2 years post transplant when renal function is stable and immunosuppression is at a minimum dosage. There is additional risk for the mother and fetus if pregnancy occurs with unstable renal function and higher doses of immunosuppressive medications.

Alteration in Hepatic Function

Problems associated with the dialysis treatments alone are considerable. Hepatitis is an ever present threat owing to the frequent extracorporeal circulation in the hemodialysis patient. If the transplant recipient receives blood transfusions prior to transplantation, he has the added risk of acquiring hepatitis from the transfusions. This risk was formerly limited to hepatitis B but is now also associated with non-A, non-B hepatitis. Even though blood donors may be screened for hepatitis B, screening for non-A, non-B hepatitis is not well defined, causing it to be an obscure but real threat to the integrity of hepatic function.

After the initial postoperative period, transplant recipients rarely receive transfusions. However, both azathioprine and cyclosporine are potentially hepatotoxic, as reflected by an elevation of liver function studies. When azathioprine is responsible for the alteration of function, the drug is withdrawn and replaced with cyclophosphamide, allowing for reversal of liver abnormalities. If it is necessary to decrease or stop cyclosporine, steroid therapy may be initiated or increased.

Alteration in Cardiovascular System

Vascular access must be maintained in the hemodialysis patient, and loss of sites can sometimes pose life-threatening problems.

Shunts, arteriovenous fistulas, and polytetrofluoroethylene (PTFE) grafts may be used in various combinations to gain permanent access to the circulation. Infections, clotting, high-output cardiac failure, and exsanguination are persistent threats with any type of access. With each access failure, the number of potential sites is reduced until finally all possible sites are exhausted. Access problems account for a significant number of hospital admissions of hemodialysis patients. For the peritoneal dialysis patient, the surgically placed peritoneal catheter is left in place, but the potential for peritonitis is always present.

The transplant patient need not maintain a vascular access site; in fact, the greatest problem of access is simply finding blood vessels from which to draw blood for laboratory studies to monitor renal function.

Perhaps the most dramatic complication of ESRD is the rate of accelerated *atherosclerosis.* The etiology is not understood, but the greatest cause of mortality in long-term dialysis patients is cardiovascular accidents.

Some of the most advanced atherosclerosis seen at postmortem examination has been in long-term dialysis patients. Because of protein restrictions, most calories are taken in the form of carbohydrates, which leads to an increased level of cholesterol. In addition, there is a hypertriglyceridemia thought to be due to increased synthesis by the liver and decreased clearing by the kidney of lipoprotein and lipase.

The effect of transplantation on atherosclerosis is uncertain but is under investigation. It is thought, however, that cholesterol levels increase after transplant. The return to a normal diet can decrease the dietary contributions to atherosclerotic changes.

Because the dialysis patient usually has little or no fluid output, an increased intake of sodium or fluid will cause *hypervolemia,* which, because the vascular system has difficulty accommodating this fluid excess, can lead to congestive heart failure. Some patients lose as much as 33 kg (15 lb) of fluid with a single dialysis treatment.

Hypervolemia can occur in the transplant recipient when decreased urinary output occurs as the result of rejection episodes or acute tubular necrosis and is managed by either diuretic therapy or dialysis support.

The specific mechanism causing *uremic pericarditis* is unclear. Depending on the severity and chronicity of pericarditis, a pericardial window or a pericardectomy is sometimes necessary to control this problem. If the patient has fluid overload, a pericardial rub may not be heard owing to the fluid contained in the pericardial sac. What seems to be an appropriate therapy — dialyzing to remove excess fluid — can actually increase the patient's pain because the fluid is removed and the friction is increased. At this point, a rub is very prominent. Conservative management of pericarditis varies greatly and may include anti-inflammatory agents.

A patient with uremic pericarditis may develop *cardiac tamponade.* The treatment for the ESRD patient is the same as for any other patient: an attempt to remove the blood from the pericardial sac before an arrest occurs. Cardiac tamponade is an ominous complication that is associated with high mortality.

Alteration in Gastrointestinal Function

Gastric acid production is increased in many ESRD patients. High levels of parathormone and decreased degradation of gastrin by the diseased kidneys both contribute to this.

Although these dysfunctions can be reversed by replacement of normal renal function, there is an increased risk of ulceration post transplant. This risk has been reported to be greatest during a period of compromised renal function, that is, during a rejection episode, when the patient is also receiving higher doses of immunosuppressants.[2] It has not been observed during periods of normal renal function and lower-dosage drug therapy.

The presence of diverticulosis before transplant has been shown to predispose the patient to *perforation* after transplant and should be treated by a colon resection prior to transplantation to reduce the risk of this serious problem.[3] *Constipation* is a problem for the dialysis patient that is contributed to by a limited fluid intake and the use of phosphorus binders. This can actually lead to development of an antacid bezoar causing impaction, possible perforation, and possible death.[4] GI complications are discussed in more detail later in the chapter.

Alteration in Immune System

It is known that both dialysis and transplant patients are more susceptible to *infections,* the former from uremia and the latter from medications that lower immunity.

There is a known increased incidence of *malignancy* among transplant patients, especially of the skin, lymph, and cervix, but the data for dialysis patients are obscure and controversial. The dialysis population is increasingly an elderly one, and comparison with the normal population should consider the age factor. In addition, patients with malignancies at the time of initiation of dialysis are increasing in number, so that the data have not been clearly segregated.

Impaired Gas Exchange

Hypovolemia as the result of ESRD can cause congestive heart failure, pulmonary congestion, and pulmonary edema. After transplantation, the risk of congestive heart failure and pulmonary edema diminishes because fluid balance can be maintained by the functioning kidney graft. However, after transplant there is greater risk of pulmonary infection as the result of immunosuppressant therapy (see discussion later in this chapter).

Alteration in Self-Concept and Body Image Disturbance

Patients with ESRD need dialysis to live and therefore are physiologically dependent on a machine or solutions. This dependence can alter the concept of one's self as an independent person. The average patient on hemodialysis spends approximately 12 hours/week attached to the machine, whereas a patient on continuous ambulatory peritoneal dialysis may spend several hours a day with solution exchanges.

Because of the life-sustaining value of dialysis as well as the time devoted to the procedure, patients have varying degrees of emotional dependence upon the treatment. Some patients keep their dependence in perspective by regarding dialysis as a necessary but not exclusive part of their lives and make an effort to keep the rest of their lives as fulfilling as possible. Others adapt to the dependency by having all their emotional energy revolve around the treatment and the personnel who provide care.

Conversely, the transplant recipient is no longer dependent on a machine, but on medication to support the function of the graft. Patients usually find dependence on the medication far more acceptable than dependence on a machine.

Changes in body image are more abrupt after transplantation because of the immunosuppressive drugs (see discussion later in this chapter and Table 22-2). The changes seen with chronic dialysis (*e.g.,* skin color changes associated with anemia and uremia as well as muscle wasting) are more gradual and sublet.

Summary

Endstage renal disease is chronic and complex and presents a multitude of problems for the patient, his family, and the health-care team, regardless of whether the decision is continued dialysis or transplantation. Many patients will choose transplantation. One of the next steps, then, is tissue typing to find a suitable donor.

FINDING A DONOR FOR RENAL TRANSPLANT

Just as red blood cells can be typed for both donor and recipient to prevent reaction between them, tissue can be typed, which may reduce the potential for reactions between donor and recipient when organs are transplanted. Antigens that denote a person's tissue type are coded by the major histocompatibility complex genes (MHC). These genes contain the genetic information to make antigens that are on the surface of all tissue cells. The antigens enable the body to differentiate self from nonself. Therefore, the greater the compatibility between donor and recipient, the better the chances for acceptance of an organ. This compatibility must also include ABO typing, although Rh factor compatibility is unnecessary.

The MHC establishes codes for four major allelic systems, A, B, C, and D loci, of which A and B code for the classic human leukocyte antigen (HLA) system. These antigens are found on the surface of lymphocytes and are used to determine a person's tissue type. Any peripheral blood sample can be used to determine tissue type. There are more than 60 known HLA antigens and thousands of combinations of antigen types. Each person has two A-locus and two B-locus antigens. These are inherited as a pair, or "haplotype," each of which consists of one A- and one B-locus antigen. Additionally, the D locus, which is part of the MHC, is inherited as part of the haplotype. The C locus is apparently insignificant in transplantation.

A test used to identify compatibility of the D locus of the MHC is the *mixed lymphocyte culture (MLC),* or *mixed lymphocyte response (MLR).* An MLC is a complex test that measures the reaction between donor and recipient when their lymphocytes are grown together in a culture. This test is not suitable for selection of cadaver kidney recipients because the test requires 5 to 7 days for cellular stimulation and division to occur.

Another test, called a *crossmatch,* is set up to screen the potential recipient for antibodies that he might have against the donor. This crossmatch takes 6 to 8 hours to complete and involves mixing serum from the potential recipient with donor lymphocytes. A positive crossmatch means that the recipient has antibodies against the donor. This response can be thought of as "in vitro" rejection. Thus, a "negative" crossmatch is necessary for recipient selection. Occasionally a crossmatch is negative when, in fact, the recipient has antibodies against the donor in insufficient titers to elicit a positive test. A number of other screening tests are being studied but are still research endeavors without clear-cut clinical application for predicting graft survival.

There has been an increasing trend to administer *blood transfusions* to potential recipients prior to transplantation. Although the mechanism of action of the transfusions on the immune system is still under study, improvement in graft survival in such patients has been observed by many centers.

One should note that the use of new terminology (*e.g.,* MHC) is reflective of new knowledge in immunology. MHC is broader than HLA and actually includes the HLA system as well as other antigen systems. Thus, an awareness of the complexity of the immune system should create an awareness of the complexity of organ transplantation. These mysteries of the immune system represent the thrust of transplantation investigation in the 1980s.

Living Related Donors

As the name indicates, a living related donor is a donor from within the family. The possibility of a compatible donor from within the family should be explored for every potential recipient.

If donor and recipient have inherited the same haplotypes, they are MHC identical, that is, they share the same A-, B-, and D-locus antigens, and this offers the greatest potential for a successful transplant. This match exists only among siblings. If only one haplotype is shared, they are compatible for only one half the MHC antigens. This "half-antigen match" is the most common match that can exist between parents and children or among siblings. A "no haplotype match" is considered a complete mismatch and is not a desirable situation in which to perform a transplant because no similarity exists between the tissues.

Once a potential living related donor is identified, he has a thorough medical evaluation so that it can be determined that he is free of underlying disease, that he has two kidneys, and that donation could in no obvious way jeopardize his well-being. Once this evaluation is successfully completed, a living related transplant may be performed.

A widely used technique of altering the immune responsiveness in living related donor situations is *donor specific transfusion* (DST). The technique involves transfusing blood from a potential living related donor to the recipient prior to transplanting the kidney. Depending on the transplant program's protocol, 50 to 100 ml of donor blood is administered to the recipient at 2-week intervals, two or three times. DST is thought to improve graft survival by two mechanisms: (1) by identifying recipients who would have reacted strongly to the antigens of the donor prior to actual transplantation, and (2) by inducing tolerance to the donor tissue, probably by stimulating the development of suppressor T cells. The risk in performing DST prior to transplantation is that the recipient will become sensitized (*i.e.,* develop antibodies) against the potential donor, thus eliminating that person as a donor. If sensitization does not occur and the transplant is performed, 1-year graft survival in a 1-haplotype-matched donor and recipient approaches 90%.[5]

Cadaver Donors

Approximately one fourth of the people who require a transplant have a suitable living donor, which means that three fourths of all potential recipients must wait for a suitable cadaver donor.* A potential cadaver kidney donor is a person who dies from a problem not involving the kidneys.

Some illnesses that exclude a person from becoming a donor are malignancy (except primary brain tumors), long-standing diabetes mellitus, chronic hypertension, hepatitis, tuberculosis, and sepsis. Patients with persistent hypotension resulting in oliguria or anuria are not acceptable donors.

Age is not necessarily a limiting factor: Donors have been younger than 1 year old and older than 60 years old. Many donors are trauma victims, whereas others die from cerebral aneurysms and surgery.

Criteria For Determining Death:
The Concept of Brain Death
Historically, death was acknowledged when irreversible cardiac or respiratory arrest occurred. In the mid 1960s, however, the concept of *brain death,* or *electrocerebral silence,* came into existence and is now medically accepted as an additional way in which death can be diagnosed. An increasing number of states have passed legislation that acknowledges brain death as a means of determining death. Brain death refers to the cessation of total brain activity at both

---

* Davis reported that there were 5358 renal transplants performed in 1982. Of these, 31% were from living related donors, and the remaining 69% were from cadaveric sources.[6]

cortical and lower levels even though heart and respiratory functions can be maintained mechanically.

The acknowledgement of brain death is important in obtaining kidneys from cadaver donors because the kidneys should be removed within 30 minutes after respiration and circulation cease. This time limit ensures viable organs for transplant.

As a result of technologic advances that sustain life, and because both physicians and the public want to be protected against premature diagnosis of death, various groups have tried to refine criteria that indicate death.

The Harvard Criteria for Determining Death
The most widely accepted criteria for defining death are referred to as the *Harvard criteria.*[7] All criteria must be met on two separate occasions, 24 hours apart, without any change in the findings, unless it is not possible to maintain respiratory and cardiac function.

The Harvard criteria include the following:

- Complete unresponsiveness: total unawareness of external stimuli (*i.e.,* irreversible coma).
- No spontaneous muscular movements, including respiration.
  - If the patient has been on a mechanical respirator, one can turn it off for 3 minutes to observe whether the patient breathes spontaneously. For this criterion to be valid, the patient must have a normal carbon dioxide tension and must breathe room air for at least 10 minutes before the test.
- Absent reflexes, spontaneous or elicited, except those that are spinal cord relfexes (*e.g.,* knee jerk).
- A flat electroencephalogram for at least 10 and preferably 20 minutes is a confirmatory rather than an essential criterion.
  - There are further procedural criteria for the way the test should be done.
  - Electroencephalographic data are not valid when there is hypothermia or central nervous system depression from drugs.

Alternate means of determining total and irreversible brain damage include intracranial blood flow studies performed by arteriography or isotope scan. It should be noted that the criteria for determining electrocerebral silence differs in patients under 14 years of age.

The issue of determining death is included in this chapter because of the increasing numbers of patients awaiting cadaver organs for transplant. The role of the transplant coordinator has evolved from this need for more organs. The tasks performed by the individual coordinator vary throughout the country and may include grief counseling for a potential donor's family as well as serving as a resource for the entire health care team. The coordinator should be a liaison between the transplant program and the critical care area. Cooperation between the critical care staff and the transplant program will help ensure the availability of organs for transplantation. So that no conflict of interest exists, the physician or physicians caring for the potential donor and pronouncing death cannot be involved in the removal or transplantation of organs.

Once kidneys are removed, they can be temporarily maintained for as long as 3 days by a preservation machine or a variety of preservation solutions. Recipient selection and preparation for transplantation are possible because of this time period. In addition, this time interval permits the transportation of kidneys so that a recipient has a greater chance to receive a well-matched graft. Increased sharing of kidneys among centers throughout the country ensures that kidneys will be transplanted even when there is no well-matched recipient locally.

The Nurse's Role
When a patient meets the criteria and becomes a potential donor, it is essential that the blood pressure be maintained as near normal as possible so that adequate perfusion of the organ can be provided.

At that time, there is also the need to support a family who may be troubled not only by the donor's impending death but also by ambivalence about the decision to donate organs. The chaplain or member of the clergy with whom the family has been associated can be an invaluable support for the family during this very stressful time. The clergy person can also be a positive influence in the decision to make an organ donation. Simmons has found that donation is often a positive experience for the donor's family and, in many instances, even helps in the grieving process.[8]

On the one hand, keeping an organ viable may be frustrating for the staff, particularly when the vigilant monitoring and regulation of blood pressure are viewed as taking care away from other patients who will survive. On the other hand, these efforts can be viewed as giving two people a chance at a longer and better life.

Visiting a transplant recipient, particularly one who has received a cadaver organ from a patient they cared for, has helped nurses realize that donation of an organ and the intervention needed to keep it viable are indeed worthwhile.

CARE OF THE TRANSPLANT RECIPIENT

The transplant recipient is usually cared for in a specially designated area throughout both acute and convalescent phases of recovery. This not only allows for highly proficient nursing care but also eliminates patient transfer, decreases fragmentation of care, and reduces exposure to infection for the newly immunosuppressed patient. In addition, the transplant recipient is usually not critically ill and therefore many times does not fit the criteria for admission to a critical care area. Nevertheless, there may be times when transplant patients will be cared for in a critical care area, especially during the acute postoperative phase or when complications occur.

Postoperative Phase of Care

Nursing Assessment

Immediately after surgery, the transplant recipient is cared for in a closely monitored area until his condition stabilizes. As the patient arrives in this recovery or intensive care area, the following assessment can be made:

1. Check the patient's level of consciousness and degree of pain.
2. Check the number of intravenous lines present, noting the site, type of solution, and flow rate.
3. Observe the abdominal dressing for drainage, noting whether a Hemovac or drain is present.
4. Check for the presence of Foley and ureteral catheters and observe the patency and urinary drainage of each.
5. Locate the vascular access site and determine its patency by placing either fingers or a stethoscope directly over the access site and feeling or listening for a characteristically loud pulsating noise called a *bruit.*
6. If the patient has been maintained on peritoneal dialysis, check the peritoneal dialysis catheter for closure and maintain sterility.
7. Check the blood pressure, apical pulse, respirations, temperature, and central venous pressure.
    Blood pressure should be taken on the extremity that does *not* have a functioning vascular access site because even momentary interference with arterial blood flow may lead to access malfunction.
8. If a nasogastric tube is present, attach it to an appropriate drainage system.
9. Obtain a baseline weight within 24 hours of surgery.
10. Measure abdominal girth at the iliac crest.
    This is baseline information used at a later time for assessment of complications (*e.g.,* ureteral leak, lymphocele, or bleeding).
11. In the case of a child, monitor more frequently than in an adult because of the dynamic nature of a child's fluid and cardiovascular status (*i.e.,* blood pressures, weights, and central venous pressures).

Answers to the following questions will provide additional baseline information.

- Are the patient's own kidneys present in addition to the graft, and, if so, how much urine do they produce daily?
    This information will help determine how much of the urine produced is from the transplanted kidney. If the chart does not provide answers, the patient and family can. In addition, flank scars usually indicate nephrectomy.
- When was the last dialysis treatment?
    The nurse should pay particular attention to the metabolic status if the patient has not been dialyzed within 24 hours of surgery.
- What are the preoperative results of laboratory tests (serum electrolytes, urea nitrogen, creatinine, liver function, calcium, phosphorus, complete blood count with differential and platelet counts, urine electrolytes, specific gravity, creatinine clearance)?
- How much and what kind of intravenous fluid has the patient received?
- Did the patient receive a loading dose of immunosuppressive drugs preoperatively?
- Is the patient to receive steroids, cyclosporine, azathioprine, antilymphocyte globulin, or other immunosuppressive therapy?
- Were any of these agents administered in the operating room, and, if so, what is the dosage schedule?
- Is the patient to receive antilymphocytic globulin or other immunosuppressive drugs?
    This drug information helps not only to clarify the regimen but also to estimate the degree of immunosuppression.
- What preoperative teaching has been done?
    Patients who have received some teaching tend to be less anxious and more cooperative because they know what to expect. A cadaver donor recipient who receives a graft shortly after being placed on the waiting list might be poorly informed because preoperative teaching was not done. In this case, additional explanation is needed. (See Chapter 4 for a more complete discussion of the effects of stress and anxiety on learning.)
- Which physician is to be called—how, where, and when—for on going medical care?
    Clarifying and recording this information may enhance communication and efficiency, especially in case of emergency.

Nursing Intervention

Many nursing responsibilities revolve around observing the function of the transplanted kidney, monitoring fluid and electrolyte balance, helping the patient avoid sources of infection, detecting early signs of complications, and supporting the patient and family through recovery phases.

Monitoring Renal Graft Function

The transplanted kidney may function immediately after revascularization and produce large amounts of urine (200 to 1000 ml/hour), small amounts of urine (<20 ml/hour), or no urine at all.

Ischemic Time. The amount of urine produced is related to the length of time the donor kidney was ischemic. The ischemic time tends to be shorter in the living related transplant situation than in the cadaver transplant situation. Therefore, the living related donor kidney has less ischemic damage and tends to produce more urine in the initial recovery phase.

However, the hourly production of large amounts of urine is called *post transplant diuresis* and is thought to be the result of a proximal tubular defect. The proximal tubule is responsible for 80% reabsorption of water, electrolytes, and glucose, and interference with its function allows more filtrate than normal to be excreted. This is a reversible state in which tubular reabsorptive functions are temporarily lost or greatly diminished because of an ischemic time period that begins with clamping the renal artery in the donor and concludes with the end of the venous revascularization of the recipient.

Preservation Time. The ischemic time is prolonged in the cadaver donor situation because it may take hours to find a suitable recipient after the donor has expired and the kidneys have been surgically removed. In this situation, the graft is placed on an organ preservation machine or in a preservation solution until a suitable recipient is found.

Acceptable time of preservation is under 50 hours. This preservation time, added to the extreme hypotensive period in cadaver donor patients, points out how long the ischemic period may be and why there is renal tissue damage and low output. Nevertheless, this damage is usually reversible.

The graft, in this situation, may produce either a small quantity or no urine at all for up to 4 weeks after the transplant operation. This output phase is referred to as *acute tubular necrosis.*

Laboratory Values. The quantity of urine does not have to correlate with the quality of graft function. Renal function is assessed by periodic serum urea nitrogen and creatinine levels and perhaps a beta$_2$-microglobulin test (β_2m). β_2m is a low-molecular-weight globulin that is readily filtered by the glomerular basement membrane and almost completely reabsorbed and metabolized by the proximal renal tubules.[9]

A renal scan is a radioisotope test used to determine renal perfusion, filtration, and excretion. It is frequently done in the first 24 hours for baseline data and periodically thereafter in the postoperative phase, depending on the patient's recovery and the presence of complications.

Drainage Problems. When a change in urinary output occurs, such as a large volume one hour to a diminished amount the next, mechanical factors that interfere with urinary drainage should be suspected. Clotted, kinked, or compressed tubing in the urinary drainage system may be the cause of the decreased output. When the catheter is occluded by a clot, the patient may complain of pain, feel an urgency to void, or have bloody leakage around the catheter. Milking is the preferred way to dislodge clots because irrigation, even under aseptic conditions, increases the risk of infection. However, gentle irrigation with strict aseptic technique may be necessary, regardless of inherent risks.

Urinary Leakage. Urinary leakage on the abdominal dressing and severe abdominal discomfort or distention may indicate retroperitoneal leakage from the ureteral anastomosis site.

Decreased urinary output or severe abdominal pain in the presence of good renal function and adequate pain medication should be reported because technical and surgical complications can result in loss of graft function.

Two major types of graft anastomoses are performed. In the first type, the donor kidney is anastomosed at the ureteropelvic junction to the recipient ureter. A Foley catheter is commonly used with this anastomosis. In the second type, which is more commonly used, the donor ureter is implanted into the recipient's bladder and a Foley or ureteral catheter may be used to provide drainage.

The urinary drainage from the ureteropelvic anastomosis tends to be bloody initially but turns pink in a few hours. The urinary drainage from the second type of anastomosis tends to be bloody for the first few days, and clotting is more problematic. The urine is bloody because the bladder is very vascular and tends to bleed after being sutured. With urine outflow, some clots are carried down the catheter while others occlude the lumen.

Maintaining Fluid and Electrolyte Balance

Maintaining fluid and electrolyte balance follows the same principles outlined in Chapter 19. Intake is provided intravenously while the patient is unable to take fluids by mouth.

Flow Rate. A standard maintenance solution of 600 to 1200 ml/24 hours for an adult is based on insensible water losses, whereas replacement solution is calculated for each patient according to such things as urine output, gastric and wound drainage, and central venous pressure (CVP) readings. When urinary output is high, as in posttransplant diuresis, replacement will be large, whereas in oliguric and anuric states replacement will be small. The solutions used most often include 0.9% normal saline, 5% dextrose in water, 0.45% saline, and 2.5% dextrose in water.

Infusion Site. The slow maintenance intravenous solution may be infused through a CVP line, but large amounts of fluid, such as 500 ml, should not be infused directly into the heart. Replacement intravenous solution is generally infused through a peripheral site on the extremity that does *not* have a vascular access site. It is important that one avoid placing intravenous lines in the extremity that has a vascular access site in order to preserve a patent and functional access for dialysis if it is needed. Dialysis may be required within the first few days if the renal graft does not function immediately.

Electrolyte Values. Serum electrolytes are drawn shortly after the patient arrives in the unit. The frequency of these tests usually depends on graft function. If the patient has a large volume of output, laboratory tests may be done every 4 to 6 hours for the first 24 to 36 hours. If the patient is anuric but otherwise stable, tests for electrolytes are done daily except for potassium, which may be ordered more frequently.

Excessive blood drawing should be kept to a minimum because the recipient is anemic in the initial recovery phase owing to ESRD.

The most frequent electrolyte disturbance in the acute postoperative phase is *hyperkalemia.* Most transplant recipients are dialyzed within 24 hours before surgery and therefore have a normal serum potassium in the operating room. If the graft functions and excretes a high volume of urine, it is also generally able to excrete the excessive serum potassium created by surgical tissue damage. If the patient is oliguric or anuric after surgery, serum potassium will increase to unacceptable levels and will need to be lowered initially by sodium polystyrene sulfonate (Kayexalate) enemas and then possibly by dialysis. Short-chain amino acid preparations (*e.g.,* Nephramine) also are used in some centers to control hyperkalemia.

Preventing Infection

Life-threatening infections are infrequent, but when present, they may compromise graft survival.

Immunosuppressive drugs are discontinued in the presence of a severe infection so that the patient can mobilize his immune response. Consequently, the graft may be sacrificed to save the patient. The immun-osuppressive drugs decrease the patient's defense system as they work to prolong graft survival.

The detrimental effect of immunosuppressive therapy is that patients are more susceptible to organisms, even those normally found in the environment. Because most infections are endogenous, strict isolation technique has been abandoned in the postoperative phase. It creates psychological problems for the patient, and compliance by all team members is difficult to enforce. Nevertheless, visitors, nurses, and other personnel who have upper respiratory or any other type of infection should not visit or give care to the patient. All personnel need to adhere to strict handwashing techniques. Everyone coming in contact with the patient should be aware of the need to protect these patients from infection.

General Preventive Measures. Following are several guidelines for preventing infection:

• Cleansing the catheter and perineal area around the urethral meatus with an antiseptic solution every 8 hours will decrease urinary tract infections.
• Changing intravenous tubing daily as well as when it is contaminated will also decrease the risk of sepsis.
• Changing wet dressings frequently will remove an excellent media for organism growth.
• Thorough handwashing before and after patient care is a simple and effective way to decrease organisms in the recipient's environment.

Avoiding Pulmonary Infections. Because pulmonary infections are high on the list of transplant recipient complications, enhancement of ventilation and promotion of drainage of secretions are paramount. Observation of the rate and character of respirations and auscultation of breath sounds will help determine how often the patient should turn, deep breathe, cough, walk, use incentive spirometer, or need postural drainage. Transplant patients can turn to the operative side; in fact, doing so promotes wound drainage and decreases the incidence of hematomas and lymphoceles.

COMPLICATIONS OF RENAL TRANSPLANTATION

Immunity and the Rejection Phenomenon

The most frequently occurring and poorly understood noninfectious complication is *graft rejection.* This process can be confusing because, like renal failure, graft rejection is rarely an "all or none" phenomenon.

Rejection can vary in degree from mild to severe reversible rejection (*i.e.,* rejection episode) to complete or irreversible rejection. Rejection episodes are reversible when treated with a variety of antirejection therapies discussed in the next section.

Antigen-Antibody Reaction

To begin to understand the rejection phenomenon, one needs to understand antigen-antibody reaction. There are two basic types of acquired immunity—humoral and cellular—and both are involved in the rejection process.*

Humoral Immunity. This type of immunity refers to the system responsible for antigen-antibody reactions. Antigens are large protein complexes that invade the body and elicit an antibody response. Antibodies are globulin molecules that are made in response to a specific antigen. Once formed, these antibodies are capable of attacking the antigen any time after the initial exposure.

Cellular Immunity. This type of immunity depends primarily on leukocyte activity. The lymphocytes, which constitute about 20% to 40% of the total number of leukocytes in a person who is not immunosuppressed, become specifically sensitized against a foreign agent. The lymphocytes involved in cellular immunity are thymus-dependent lymphocytes, also called T-lymphocytes. It is generally believed that monocytes or macrophages detect foreign antigens and "present" the antigen to a subset of T-lymphocytes called T-helper lymphocytes. These T-helper lymphocytes are activated by a chemical, a lymphokine, produced by macrophages called interleukin-1 (IL-1). These T-helper lymphocytes release a second chemical mediator, or lymphokine, known as interleukin-2 (IL-2), also referred to as T-cell growth factor. Interleukin-2 results in the maturation and proliferation of cytotoxic T-lymphocytes. Cytotoxic T-lymphocytes are the primary cells involved in tissue destruction due to cellular immune response.

The transplanted kidney is a foreign antigen implanted in a recipient. Eventually, the recipient's body will recognize the kidney as a foreign antigen and mobilize its defense system to try to rid itself of this foreign substance. This process is called *rejection*.

It is important to realize that all transplant recipients' defense immune systems eventually see the kidney as foreign and in some way respond to it. Exceptions to this are recipients who are nonresponders. Such persons either do not respond to any foreign antigen stimulation or respond poorly to stimulation. The nonresponders, however, are few in number; therefore, what becomes important is observing how strongly the immune defensive system responds.

---

* For an in-depth explanation of the immune system and antigen-antibody reaction, see John Stobo's article in the bibliography.

There are various ways by which a transplant recipient can become sensitized to donor cells prior to transplantation. Exposure to tissue antigens can occur as a result of blood transfusions, pregnancy, or previous transplant. This exposure could result in the formation of "preformed antibodies" or "sensitized lymphocytes."

Categories of Rejection

There are four basic categories of rejection:

• Hyperacute
• Accelerated
• Acute
• Chronic

Hyperacute Rejection. This type of rejection can occur within minutes to hours following transplantation. This may occur either because of a major blood group incompatibility or, more commonly, because preformed antibodies existed in titers too low to be detected in the tissue typing tests. There is no treatment for hyperacute rejection, and it always results in loss of the graft, which must be removed. With improved tissue typing methods, hyperacute rejection is very uncommon.

Accelerated Rejection. This type of rejection occurs within a few days to approximately 1 week following transplantation. It is due either to preformed antibodies against the donor antigens in the recipient's blood or to lymphocytes in the recipient, which are already sensitized to some of the donor antigens. Accelerated rejection, like hyperacute rejection, is infrequently seen because of improved techniques of tissue-typing and crossmatching. If it occurs, accelerated rejection must be aggressively treated with immunosuppressive medications. Even then, it may not respond to therapy and may result in loss of the transplanted kidney.

Acute Rejection. This occurs after the first postoperative week. It is the most frequently seen form of rejection and fortunately the type that responds best to therapy. One must *assess* for the following signs and symptoms because the patient may experience any, all, or none of the following during an acute rejection episode:

• Decrease in urine output
• Weight gain
• Edema
• A temperature of 100°F (37.8°C) or greater
• Tenderness over the graft site, with possible swelling of the kidney itself
• General malaise
• Increased blood pressure

Other findings indicating an acute rejection episode include

- Increased serum creatinine
- Decreased urine creatinine and creatinine clearance
- Possible decrease in urine sodium
- Increased BUN
- Increased serum β_2m
- Increased urine β_2m
- Decreased blood flow as demonstrated on renal scan

Chronic Rejection. This is a gradual deterioration of kidney function and is the result of repeated insults from acute rejection episodes. The symptoms are similar to those of acute rejection except that fever and graft enlargement may not occur.

Chronic rejection results in scarring of renal tissue and infarction of renal vessels from the vasculitis accompanying acute rejection. Therefore in chronic rejection the inflammatory signs are absent.

Laboratory findings are similar in both acute and chronic rejection, but chronic rejection also includes those changes consistent with chronic renal failure, including declining hematocrit, calcium-phosphorus imbalance, and so forth. The rate of deterioration in chronic rejection can vary, and the patient may have adequate renal function from a few months up to a year before replacement therapy is indicated.

There is no effective therapy known to treat this type of rejection. Unlike other forms of rejection, chronic rejection does not always require a transplant nephrectomy because the kidney does not always become necrotic and cause a life-threatening situation.

Immunosuppression Therapy

Drugs

As the term implies, immunosuppression is the use of drug therapy to suppress the immune response in order to permit acceptance of transplanted organs, most often with a type of tissue at least partially different from that of the recipient. The difficulty of this therapy is in providing enough suppression to prevent rejection without rendering the recipient grossly susceptible to opportunistic infections.

The drugs given to control the immune response are methylprednisolone (Solu-Medrol), prednisone, azathioprine (Imuran), cyclophosphamide (Cytoxan), antilymphocytic globulin and cyclosporine (Sandimmune). Major points about these drugs are summarized in Table 22-2.

Methylprednisolone is the parenteral steroid used in the initial postoperative period, and prednisone is the most commonly used oral steroid. *Prednisone* may be given in a variety of schedules and doses, and the philosophy varies from center to center, just as it does with the use of methylprednisolone in the treatment of rejection episodes.

Treatment of rejection episodes may include intravenous injections of methylprednisolone in boluses up to 1 g per dose. It is recommended that it be administered over 20 to 30 minutes. This is particularly important because several cardiac arrests have been reported following the administration of 1 g of methylprednisolone delivered by intravenous push.

Azathioprine, an antimetabolite, is the mainstay of immunosuppression. The patient's ability to tolerate 2 to 3 mg/kg consistently is important for long-term graft survival. Azathioprine cannot be increased to treat rejection because of its bone marrow suppression effects and its cumulative effects in the presence of little or no renal function.

Cyclophosphamide, an alkylating agent is used only in the presence of hepatotoxicity from whatever source. It has been shown to be inferior to azathioprine in prolonging graft survival but represents the most viable alternative to azathioprine therapy. The development of hemorrhagic cystitis increases the risk for later development of cancer of the bladder and also necessitates discontinuation of therapy.

Antilymphocyte (antithymocyte) globulin (serum) is used in a number of centers in an effort to prevent rejection by providing the patient with antibodies against lymphocytes or thymocytes, which are the cells responsible for rejection. These antibodies are produced by injection of human lymph or thymus cells into an animal (horse, rabbit, or goat), which then produces antibodies against these cells.

Cyclosporine, a fungal metabolite, is the most specific immunosuppressive agent currently available. During the controlled clinical trials conducted prior to its approval by the FDA, 1-year graft survival improved from 50% to 60% in most centers to 70% to 90% in patients treated with this very promising medication.[10] Cyclosporine acts by interfering with IL-2, a chemical mediator necessary for the proliferation and activation of helper and cytotoxic T-lymphocytes (see earlier discussion of cellular immunity). By acting in such a specific manner, it appears to spare other facets of a person's immune system, thus allowing for some protection from infectious organisms.

The usefulness of cyclosporine in renal transplantation is limited by its adverse effects, most notably nephrotoxicity. Other major known side effects include hepatotoxicity, marked hirsutism, tremors, hyperglycemia, and gum hypertrophy. Protocols for its use vary among institutions. Many centers use cyclosporine with low-dose steroids for a few months immediately after transplantation, then change the regimen to prednisone and azathioprine for long-term maintenance.

Radiation

Radiation therapy given locally to the graft is sometimes used as an adjunct to conventional immunosuppressive therapy during a rejection episode. This therapy has been used since the 1960s, and reports of its

TABLE 22-2
IMMUNOSUPPRESSIVE DRUGS USED IN RENAL TRANSPLANTATION

Drug	Adverse Reactions	Dosage	Comments
Methylprednisolone (Solu-Medrol) (IV) Prednisone (PO)	Increased susceptibility to infection	Initial: 0.5 to 3 mg/kg of body weight, tapered to an adequate oral maintenance dose	Methylprednisolone is given up to 1 week
	Masks symptoms of infection Peptic ulcer, GI bleeding		An antacid is given while patient is on steroids to reduce the risk of gastric irritation and ulceration; cimetidine may also be used to decrease ulcerogenic tendencies
	Increased appetite, weight gain	During rejection, methylprednisolone may be given in IV boluses up to 1 g/dose	Cardiac arrest can occur if IV bolus of 1 g is given rapidly
	Increased sodium and water retention, which exaggerate hypertension Delayed healing Negative nitrogen balance Adrenal gland suppression Behavior and personality changes Diabetogenic effect Muscle weakness Osteoporosis with long-term therapy Skin atrophy, striae Easy bruising Glaucoma, cataracts Hirsutism Acne Avascular/aseptic necrosis		Sodium restriction may be necessary when steroid dosage is high or when fluid retention increases
Azathioprine (Imuran) (IV or PO)	Bone marrow suppression: leukopenia, thrombocytopenia, anemia, pancytopenia Rash Alopecia Liver damage, jaundice Increased susceptibility to infection	Regulated to keep WBCs 5000 to 10,000. Drug usually stopped when WBCs are 3000 or less Initial 2 to 10 mg/kg of body weight Maintenance: 2 to 3 mg/kg of body weight During rejection: maximum of 3 mg/kg of body weight, dose not usually increased with rejection	Lower doses are given when 1. Renal function is poor 2. Given concurrently with allopurinol, which delays metabolism of azathioprine (allopurinol and azathioprine are synergistic) 3. WBC is low
Cyclophosphamide	Leukopenia, thrombocytopenia Increased susceptibility to infections Metabolites are direct irritants to bladder mucosa and may cause hemorrhagic cystitis	1 to 2 mg/kg (or $\frac{1}{2}$ to $\frac{2}{3}$ of Imuran dosage)	Given in place of azathioprine when it causes hepatotoxicity Administration should be suggested to patient upon his awakening to avoid accumulation of metabolites while he is sleeping Hematuria should be watched for Fluid intake should be encouraged to dilute metabolites
	Alopecia		

TABLE 22-2 *(Continued)*

Drug	Adverse Reactions	Dosage	Comments
Antilymphocyte globulin (ALG) Antithymocyte globulin (ATG) Antilymphocyte serum (ALS) Antithymocyte serum (ATS) (usually IV, IM, or deep SC)	Anaphylactic shock due to hypersensitivity to animal serum Fever (up to 105°F, or 40.6°C) and chills Increased susceptibility to infections due to decreased lymphocytes IM or deep SC injection site may be swollen, red, and painful, with abscess formation Difficulty walking if IM or SC injection given in thigh	Dosage may vary	Skin test for hypersensitivity to animal serum performed before initial dose Lymphocytes or platelets decrease sharply with drug administration; therefore, bloodwork for lymphocyte and platelet counts should be drawn before infusion is started Usually given only for short period of time to either prevent or treat rejection; not a long-term immunosuppressant
Cyclosporin A (Sandimmune) (IV, IM, or PO)	Nephrotoxicity Hepatotoxicity	Initial: 4 mg/kg/day (IV) Maintenance: protocols differ, generally patients require less than initially, some units plan to switch patients to conventional therapy after several months Dosage is altered by monitoring drug levels at least during initial period	Initially, nephrotoxicity and hepatotoxicity seem to be dose-related and respond to dose reduction Long-term nephrotoxicity is a major concern
	Hypertension Hirsutism Gum hyperplasia Malignancy		Incidence of malignancy (especially lymphoma) is increased when other immunosuppressants are used in conjunction with CyA (particularly Imuran and ATS or ATG)
	Nausea, vomiting, diarrhea Tremors Diabetogenic effects Anaphylactic reaction have been seen with IV administration		Risk of anaphylaxis is reduced if slow continuous infusion is given

efficacy have ranged from beneficial to ineffective. It continues to be used in some centers.

Thoracic Duct Drainage
Thoracic duct drainage (TDD) has been used since the 1960s by a diminishing number of centers. TDD involves cannulation of the left thoracic duct to remove lymph fluid. The purpose of lymph removal is to reduce the number of lymphocytes available that could become involved in the rejection process. The procedure is usually carried out for several weeks to 1 month prior to transplantation, depending on the amount of lymph fluid removed.

TDD requires hospitalization for the duration of drainage because the patient's physiological status must be carefully monitored. Replacement of fluids and protein is required, and thus close monitoring of the fluid and electrolyte balance is necessary; some patients may drain as much as 1 liter/hour.

Inclusion of TDD as part of the immunosuppressive protocol has been disappointing in that improved graft survival has not been consistently demonstrated. Furthermore, it is costly, increases risk to the patient, and prolongs the patient's hospital course.

Donor-Specific Transfusions
For a discussion of DST, refer to the earlier section on living related donors.

Total Lymphoid Irradiation (TLI)
Sublethal levels of fatal lymphoid irradiation have been used by a very few centers to improve the results of renal transplantation. This technique remains investigational and is now used even less frequently as improved drug therapy becomes available.

For the Future: Monoclonal Antibodies
Many experts in transplantation believe that monoclonal antibodies are the immunosuppressive agents of the future. These drugs are antibodies specifically made to recognize and bind to the surface markers expressed on the specific cell populations. By doing, so, they render those cells inactive. Because cloning techniques are employed in producing these antibodies, each molecule is identical with all other molecules in the solution. Impurities — antibodies aimed at other than the target cell population — are not in the solution. By identifying the specific cells in the immune system that cause graft rejection and by producing antibodies to inactivate just those cells, rejection, it is hoped, could be prevented and resistance to invading pathogens preserved. Some initial clinical trials with pan – T-cell monoclonal antibodies have been conducted. The use of monoclonal antibodies for immunosuppression remains an investigational technique but one that is very promising.

Infection

One of the greatest crises for the recipient is sepsis because it is still one of the greatest threats to recipient survival. The origin of sepsis may be the blood (septicemia); a single organ, such as the liver, lungs, or pancreas; or the entire body (*i.e.*, a disseminated infection).

The pathogens vary from the more commonly seen bacterial organisms to fungal, viral, or even protozoan organisms. The last three groups of organisms are referred to as *opportunistic pathogens*. These organisms, normally found in humans and in the environment, are generally considered harmless. However, the patient with a compromised immune system, such as a transplant recipient, is susceptible to infections from these organisms. The microorganisms "take advantage" of the decreased host defenses; thus the term *opportunistic*. Specific examples of these opportunistic infections include herpes simplex, herpes zoster, *Candida albicans, Aspergillus, Cryptococcus, Nocardia, Pneumocystis carinii,* and cytomegalovirus (CMV). The presence of any of these infections should be monitored closely because they can pose life-threatening crises.

Oral monilial infections are common, and precautions should be taken to prevent the development of or progression to monilial esophagitis, a serious infectious complication. Precautions should include daily observation of the mouth. Appearance of oral moniliasis should be treated with oral mystatin (Mycostatin).

If immunosuppressive therapy is reduced or discontinued in the presence of a life-threatening situation resulting from an opportunistic infection, the emphasis *must* be on the patient's life rather than on the graft. Therefore, rejection of the graft is permitted in an effort to save the patient's life. If the graft it totally rejected, the patient is supported with dialysis therapy, and once the infectious process is resolved, the patient can then be considered for retransplantation.

Another problem that contributes to loss of renal function is the antibiotic therapy necessary to control the infection. Amphotericin B, a drug used to treat fungal infections, is nephrotoxic in that it decreases renal perfusion. The use of mannitol in the amphotericin B solution can counteract the problem of decreased perfusion because it increases renal perfusion. Because many antibiotics and antifungal agents are nephrotoxic, treatment of infections can pose difficult management problems.

Cardiovascular Complications

Although cardiovascular accidents can occur in the acute postoperative period, more frequently they occur a year after transplant and are considered late complications of transplantation. Should the complications occur in the early postoperative period, graft survival and vascular problems are of concern. However, if they occur as late complications of transplantation, graft function has usually stabilized, and vascular complications are the major concern. Patients with a functioning graft may succumb to this type of complication. As stated earlier, it is unclear what the effects of transplantation are upon the atherosclerotic process and subsequent cardiovascular complications.

Since the early 1970s, higher risk patients, such as those with diabetes, vasculitis, systemic lupus erythematosus, and those 50 to 70 years old, have had transplants. In fact, patients with cardiac disease treated by coronary bypass surgery have later received renal transplants. Perhaps these higher risks have contributed to an increase in death from vascular complications. Because there is an increasing patient population 10 years or more post transplant, there is more opportunity to study the etiology of the long-term cardiovascular complications.

GI Complications

GI complications may pose serious and even life-threatening situations for the recipient.

Ischemic bowel disease has been observed in the early posttransplant period, but the appearance of this problem and its association with transplantation are uncertain.

Massive GI bleeding may occur as the result of steroid therapy, stress, and the decreased viability of tissues due to earlier protein restrictions.

GI complications most often will occur in the acute postoperative phase, at the point when graft survival is still of major concern. Again, forfeiture of the graft may be necessary to save the patient's life.

Other serious GI complications include acute pancreatitis, obstruction from bowel adhesions, and ulcerative colitis. If the patient has an intestinal perforation, then not only is the GI complication a threat, but so is infection.

Transplant recipients may have more than one complication occurring simultaneously. The following case studies point out how complex and interwoven complications become and how necessary it is to be thoughtful and thorough in assessing for clues.

CASE STUDY 1

A 42-year-old white male with ESRD secondary to radiation nephropathy underwent living-related transplantation with his paternal cousin as the donor. On tissue-typing, the patient and donor were found to be ABO-compatible and a 1-haplotype match. Stimulation was demonstrated in mixed lymphocyte culture. Donor-specific transfusions were given prior to transplantation. A crossmatch one day prior to surgery showed that the recipient demonstrated no preformed antibodies to his cousin's tissues. Surgery was performed without complication. Three days after surgery, the patient demonstrated evidence of an accelerated rejection episode: fever, greatly diminished urine output, graft tenderness, rising BUN and creatinine, and diminished perfusion as shown on renal scan. The rejection was treated with doses of methylprednisolone and antithymocyte globulin (ATGAM). Oral prednisone and azathioprine (Imuran) were continued. Because the rejection episode was not reversing despite this therapy, cyclosporine was added to the regimen. Renal function began to improve, as evidenced by increasing urine output and falling BUN and creatinine. The dose of prednisone was reduced and both Imuran and ATGAM were discontinued to avoid the complications of overimmunosuppression. The cyclosporine dosage was altered to maintain a therapeutic blood level (approximately 50 to 300 mg/ml) and to avoid toxicity. BUN stabilized at 40 to 45, and creatinine was maintained in a range of 2 to 2.3 mg/dl. The patient was discharged from the hospital $3\frac{1}{2}$ weeks after transplantation.

Three weeks after discharge, the patient was readmitted with a fasting glucose of 256 mg/dl. His 2-hour postprandial glucose level was 340. He was admitted for initiation of insulin therapy. He had developed insulin-dependent diabetes because of the steroids and cyclosporine. On further examination, it was determined that there was a strong family history of diabetes in the patient's grandfather's generation. After being stabilized on insulin and receiving instruction in self-care related to his diabetes, he was again discharged home.

The patient returned to work 3 weeks later. While out to dinner with a friend the following weekend, he suffered acute abdominal pain. He presented at a local emergency room, where an abdominal film revealed free air under the diaphragm. A perforated ulcer was feared. He was transferred to the transplant center, where more extensive evaluation showed a small duodenal ulcer that had perforated. The patient was prepared for emergency surgery. At surgery, a pinpoint-sized ulcer was located and oversewn. Minimal contamination of the peritoneum was noted. Multiple cultures were taken. The patient was started on triple antibiotic coverage with penicillin, clindamycin, and tobramycin. A nasogastric tube and Foley catheter were placed. Immunosuppression was continued with intravenous methylprednisolone and cyclosporine. Renal function, cyclosporine levels, and clinical evidence of infection were closely monitored. He recovered without complications. The preoperative immunosuppressive regimen of oral prednisone and cyclosporine was resumed. The patient was discharged after 3 weeks of hospitalization.

CASE STUDY 2

A 50-year-old man was the recipient of a cadaver transplant. The patient was known to have renin-dependent hypertension and was receiving propranolol four times per day. Throughout the immediate posttransplant period, the patient complained of "gas pains." Because of this chronic complaint, an evaluation was undertaken but with negative findings. Approximately 3 weeks post transplant, a duodenal ulcer perforated. Because of steroid therapy, the symptoms of perforation were masked to the extent that none of the classic signs of peritonitis were present. In addition, the myocardial effects of the beta blocker therapy prevented the patient's heart from responding to the sympathetic drive, and as a result his apical rate never varied from approximately 60, in spite of his perforation. About 8 hours following the perforation, the patient's blood pressure began to drop, and bowel sounds were no longer heard. The diagnosis of perforation was made. Thus, the combination of drugs markedly masked the otherwise classic symptoms the patient might have demonstrated.

CASE STUDY 3

A 14-year-old white girl developed endstage renal disease secondary to congenital anomalies of the urinary tract and recurrent episodes of obstruction and infection. Throughout her childhood, multiple surgical procedures had been performed to relieve the obstructions and prevent further destruction of renal parenchyma. Renal function continued to deteriorate, however, and she reached endstage disease by age 13. The patient began hemodialysis and then underwent bilateral nephrectomy in preparation for transplantation. Her mother was evaluated as a potential living related donor but was found to be unsuitable for numerous medical and psychological reasons. The patient underwent an uneventful surgical placement of the graft.

The kidney had an ischemic time of less than 24 hours and functioned immediately. Creatinine rapidly fell from over 10 to 2.1. Immunosuppression was begun preoperatively with intravenous cyclosporine and methylprednisolone. Once GI function had returned to normal postoperatively, intravenous immunosuppressants were discontinued and oral prednisone and cyclosporine instituted. One mild episode of rejection associated with low-grade fevers occurred, and the serum creatinine rose to a level of 3.5. This rejection episode was successfully reversed with intravenous methylprednisolone. The patient was discharged from the hospital 3 weeks postoperatively with a serum creatinine level of between 2 and 2.2.

The patient was seen 3 days later in renal clinic, where her creatinine was found to be elevated to 2.8. She had 2 + pitting edema in her lower extremities and had gained 3 kg (about 1½ lb). Another rejection was feared, and she was readmitted to the hospital. Sonogram demonstrated no obstruction. Renal scan was consistent with rejection. The patient was treated with intravenous and oral steroids over a 7-day period. Creatinine initially fell to 2.5 but then stabilized at 2.8. Cyclosporine plasma levels, which had been satisfactory, were noted to be elevated, so the dose was reduced accordingly.

At that time, the patient developed spiking fevers of 39°C (102°F) every morning. White blood count fell to 2500. She developed a pulmonary infiltrate bilaterally. A viral infection, specifically cytomegalic virus (CMV), was suspect. Open lung biopsy was performed for definitive diagnosis. Cultures taken at surgery grew CMV, as did blood cultures. The patient's respiratory status deteriorated to the point that ventilatory support was required. She was transferred to the intensive care unit and placed on a ventilator. Immunosuppression was greatly reduced. In fact, cyclosporine was discontinued, and methylprednisolone was reduced to 10 mg IV daily. Renal function showed further deterioration as the viral infection affected the kidney. Afer 5 days in the ICU and on a ventilator, the patient began to improve. The pulmonary infiltrate began to clear and the temperature elevations subsided. Renal function improved. The patient was extubated 2 days later and transferred from the ICU. One week later, her immunosuppressive regimen was changed to prednisone, 10 mg/day given orally, and low-dosage cyclosporine (6 mg/kg/day). The patient was discharged from the hospital 1 week later with a serum creatinine level between 1.9 and 2, without fever, and with normal respiratory function.

The need for nurses to be aware of drug actions such as those described cannot be overemphasized. Constant and thorough evaluation is mandatory in caring for this very complex group of patients. Because detailed information concerning the infectious complications, cardiovascular problems, and GI complications of the transplant recipient is not within the scope of this chapter, the reader is referred to the bibliography.

Hypertension

Hypertension is a common but often transitory complication following renal transplantation. Many patients requiring chronic antihypertensive therapy are hypertensive before the transplant, and their hypertension is made worse by posttransplant steroid therapy. Various factors are responsible for posttransplant hypertension.

Steroid-Induced Hypertension

Transplant recipients are placed on steroids, usually prednisone or methylprednisolone. Although these are glucocorticoids, they are converted into mineralocorticoids and cause sodium and water retention. Even for patients on a sodium-restricted diet, drug therapy is often necessary. Spironolactone, an aldosterone-blocking agent, is often useful in treating steroid-induced hypertension, along with the diuretics, hydrochlorothiazide and furosemide. Nurses must monitor for potential electrolyte imbalances (specifically, hyponatremia and hypokalemia) and instruct the patient and his family about the signs and symptoms of these imbalances and what to do if they occur.

The effect of these drugs does not occur immediately, and therefore electrolyte imbalances are usually not seen until several days after the medications are started. At this time, a brisk diuresis may follow, increasing the potential for both hypovolemia and electrolyte imbalances. Because rapid fluid loss will result in weight loss, the patient's weight should be carefully recorded.

Renin-Dependent Hypertension

Steroid treatment is only one mechanism that causes posttransplant hypertension. A second mechanism, excessive renin production, is seen rather frequently.

Immediately following the transplant procedure, the recipient may have markedly elevated blood pressure. Owing to the ischemic injury that occurs to the organ between time of removal and time of implantation, excessive amounts of renin may be released. Once adequate circulation has been established within the organ, this mechanism should "turn off," resulting in a return of the pressure to the preoperative level within a few days following the transplant.

Although renin itself is not a potent vasoconstrictor, its conversion to angiotensin I and angiotensin II causes vasoconstriction. The immediate postoperative period is not the only time in the progress of the transplant recipient's course that renin-dependent hypertension can occur.

Hypertension may be one of the first clinical manifestations of rejection. The basis of this hypertension is excessive renin production. Because rejection is an inflammatory response, vasculitis within the kidney impedes normal circulation and results in elevated renin levels. Renin levels are elevated in virtually all patients who have hypertension during an acute rejection episode. This phenomenon occurs in chronic rejection as well. Therefore, the nurse should pose the question of ensuing rejection when first detecting an elevated blood pressure.

Renal artery stenosis can also result in renin-dependent hypertension. The stenosis may cause a decrease in renal perfusion leading to increased renin production. When this occurs, an abdominal bruit may be auscultated lateral to the midline and medial to the kidney. The sudden appearance of a bruit or an increase in an abdominal bruit previously present is strongly suggestive of a renal artery stenosis.

Diagnosis of renal artery stenosis is made with angiography. Computer enhancement (digital subtraction angiography) allows a smaller amount of contrast material to be used. This is beneficial because the contrast material is potentially nephrotoxic. Once a transplant artery has been found to be stenotic, generally either surgical repair or balloon angioplasty is indicated to correct the problem. There is a risk of loss of some renal function or even of loss of the graft itself with either technique. However, the long-term adverse effects of uncontrolled hypertension resulting from an unrepaired renal artery stenosis are generally felt to be more serious threats to the patient than the risks of repairing the lesion. In fact, deterioration of renal function is more likely to occur if the stenosis is not corrected.

Drug Therapy. Metoprolol tartrate (Lopressor) and propranolol (Inderal) are often used to treat renin-dependent hypertension because they act as renin inhibitors. Because these drugs are cardiac depressants, congestive heart failure may result from prolonged use. The use of a diuretic may help prevent this complication. However, the use of catecholamine-depleting agents such as reserpine is unwise because the patient is unable to respond to a sympathetic drive, owing to the adrenergic blocking effects.

Minoxidil has been effective in treating renin-dependent hypertension that does not respond to therapy with a sympathetic blocker alone. A potent vasodilator, it is usually given with a diuretic such as furosemide because of the sodium and fluid retention it causes. A sympathetic blocker is also advisable to offset the tachycardia minoxidil creates. Hirsutism, the major obvious side effect of minoxidil, can be very distressing to the patient and may actually affect compliance with this therapeutic regimen.

Converting enzyme inhibitors (*e.g.,* captopril) are useful in the treatment of renin-dependent hypertension. A rapid drop in blood pressure can occur with even small doses of these medications. Patients must be closely monitored when drug therapy is initiated. The most serious side effect of such medications is bone marrow suppression. White blood counts and platelet counts must be watched carefully.

Volume-Dependent Hypertension
Volume-dependent hypertension is another problem for the transplant recipient. During rejection episodes or periods of acute tubular necrosis, the patient may become fluid-overloaded owing to inadequate fluid output from the kidney.

If the patient does not respond to diuretic therapy, the use of dialysis may be indicated for further control of the hypervolemic and hypertensive state until renal function recovers. The development of malignant hypertension precipitating hypertensive crisis is managed as with any other patient.

Drug Precautions
The aforementioned antihypertensive medications by no means constitute an inclusive list. Many other drugs are appropriate and useful, and those mentioned only represent examples. However, problems associated with antihypertensive therapy are not unique to the transplant patient. Lethargy, impotence, and orthostatic hypotension are just some of the untoward effects of such therapy. However, once renal function has become stable, the patient's steroid dose has been reduced, and his urine output is satisfactory, the need for antihypertensive medications is markedly reduced.

A PATIENT'S VIEW

How do patients who have experienced many complications view their decision to have a renal transplant? One patient received a cadaver transplant that chronically rejected after $3\frac{1}{2}$ years, underwent bilateral total hip replacements for aseptic necrosis, and had impaired vision resulting from cataracts. When asked if it had been worth it to him to be off dialysis and whether he would like to receive a new kidney graft, he responded without question or hesitation with an emphatic "Absolutely!"

People who have had successful renal transplantation, even in the face of complications, state unequivocally that they would not alter their decision to have received a renal graft. Both the success of such patients and their appreciation of new lives make transplantation a challenging and richly rewarding field.

REFERENCES

1. Hodgson S: Anemia associated with chronic renal failure and chronic dialysis. Nephrol Nurse 2:43–46, 1980
2. Schweizer R, Bartus S: Gastroduodenal ulceration in renal transplant patients. Conn Med 42:85–88, 1978
3. Archibald S, Jirsch D, Bear R: Gastrointestinal complications of renal transplantation, II: The colon. Can Med Assoc J 119:1301–1305, 1978
4. Welch J, Schweizer R, Bartus S: Management of antacid impactions in hemodialysis and renal transplant patients. Am J Surg 139:561–568, 1980
5. Salvatierra O Jr, Vincenti F, Amend W et al: Four-year experience with donor-specific blood transfusions. Transplant Proc 15, No. 1:924–931, 1983

6. Davis CK: Testimony presented before the Subcommittee on Investigations and Oversight. House Committee on Science and Technology, Washington, DC. April 27, 1983
7. A Report by the Task Force on Death and Dying of the Institute of Society, Ethics and the Life Sciences: Refinements in criteria for the determination of death: An appraisal. JAMA 221:48–53, 1972
8. Fulton J, Fulton R, Simmons R: The cadaver donor and the gift of life. In Simmons R, Klein S, Simmons R (eds): The Social and Psychological Impact of Organ Transplantation, pp 338–376, New York, John Wiley & Sons, 1977
9. Vincent C, Revillard JP, Pellet H, et al: B$_2$—Microglobulin in monitoring renal transplant function. Transplant Proc 11:438, 1979
10. Sandoz, Inc: Sandimmune (Cyclosporine) Clinical Experience Overview, pp 10–12. East Hanover, NJ, 1983

BIBLIOGRAPHY

Anderson RJ, Gambertoglio JD, Schrier RW: Clinical Use of Drugs in Renal Failure. Springfield, IL, Charles C Thomas, 1976

Blount M, Kinney AB: Chronic steroid therapy. Am J Nurs 74:1623–1631, 1974

Buszta C: The nurse, the transplant patient and the family. Nephrol Nurse 3, No. 6:4–8, 1981

Campbell J, Campbell A: The social and economic costs of end-stage renal disease. N Engl J Med 299:386–392, 1978

DeLuca H: Vitamin D metabolism. Clin Endocrinol (Suppl) 7:15s–17s, 1977

First International Congress on Cyclosporine, Houston, Texas, May 16–19, 1983. Transplant Proc (Suppl 1–2) 15, No. 4:2207–3187 December, 1983

Irwin BC: Renal transplantation. Crit Care Update 10, No. 2:28–35, 1983

Irwin BC: Renal transplantation: Advances in immunology—A nursing perspective. AANNT J 10, No. 4:11–15, 1983

Jett MF, Lancaster LE: The inflammatory-immune response: The body's defense against invasion. Crit Care Nurse 3, No. 5:64–84, Sept/Oct, 1983

Lamb J: Organ transplantation: Recognizing the donor. Am J Nurs 80:1600–1601, 1980

Lancaster LE: Renal failure: Pathophysiology, assessment, and intervention. Nephrol Nurse 4, No. 5:38–51, 1983; No. 3:30–38, 1983

Lancaster L (ed): The Patient with End-Stage Renal Disease. New York, John Wiley & Sons, 1979

Lane T, Stroshal V, Waldorf P: Standards of care for the CAPD patient. Nephrol Nurse 4, No. 5:34–45, 1982

Lazarus JM: Uremia: A clinical guide. Hosp Med 15:52–73, 1979

Luckenbaugh PR: An overview of nursing diagnosis and suggestions for use with chronic hemodialysis patients. Nephrol Nurse 5, No. 6:58–61, 1983

Mandell GL, Hook EW: Opportunistic infections. Hosp Med 4:40–48, 1968

Morris PJ (ed): Kidney Transplantation. New York, Grune & Stratton, 1979

Opelz G, Terasaki PI: Improvement of kidney graft survival with increased numbers of blood transfusions. N Engl J Med 299:799–803, 1978

Powers AM: Renal transplantation: The patient's choice. Nurs Clin North Am 16, No. 3:551–564, 1981

Richard AB, Robbins KC, Rovelli, MA: Nursing implications of ATG therapy in organ transplantation. AANA J 11, No. 5:20–24, 1984

Robbins KC, Richard AB, Rovelli, M: Donor-specific transfusions as pre-treatment for living related donor transplants and implications for nursing. Nephrol Nurse 5, No. 3:4–8, 1983

Sachs B: Renal Transplantation: A Nursing Perspective. Flushing, NY, Medical Examination Publishing Company, 1977

Southby JR, Moore JB: Nursing diagnoses for a child with end stage renal disease. AANNT J 10, No. 4:22–27, 1983

Stobo JD: Basic mechanisms of immunity. Hosp Med 16:22–32, 1980

Taylor J, Sadler B, Turk M: Thoracic duct lymph drainage as an adjunct to renal transplantation. Nephrol Nurse 1:12–16, 1979

Thomas FT, Lee HM: Factors in the differential rate of arteriosclerosis (A.S.) between long surviving renal transplant recipients and dialysis patients. Ann Surg 184:342–351, 1976

Veith FJ: Brain death and organ transplantation. Ann NY Acad Sci 315:417–441, 1978

Unit Four

Nervous System

23
Normal Structure and Function of the Nervous System

Barbara Brockway-Fuller

The nervous system traditionally is discussed in both anatomic and functional divisions. Anatomic components are the central nervous system (CNS) (brain and spinal cord) and the peripheral nervous system (spinal and cranial nerves). Functional divisions are the sensory, interpretive, and motor (somatic and autonomic) divisions.

Content will be ordered according to both divisions. First, however, cell anatomy and physiology and meninges will be discussed.

CELLS OF THE NERVOUS SYSTEM

The cellular units are the *neuron*—the basic functional unit—and its attendant cells, the *neuroglias* and *Schwann cells*. It may, perhaps, be easier to treat the attendant cells first and then proceed to neuronal functioning.

Neuroglial Cells

The neuroglial cells constitute the supportive tissue that lies within the CNS around the neurons. There are three types of glial cells: microglia, astrocytes, and oligodendroglia. These last cells are thought to produce the myelin that covers nerve fibers within the CNS.

Whereas neurons lose their ability to undergo mitosis early in the life of the individual, neuroglial cells seem to retain mitotic abilities throughout a person's life span. Because of this, nonmetastatic CNS lesions involve glial cells rather than neurons. As the glian tumor enlarges, however, it does adversely affect adjacent neurons early by exerting pressure and later by

promoting an inflammatory reaction along with the pressure. The counterpart of the myelin-producing oligodendroglial cell in the peripheral nervous system is the cell of Schwann.

Neurons

As stated earlier, the basic functional unit of the nervous system is the *neuron,* and all information and activity, whether sensory, motor, or integrative, is processed by it.

The precise characteristic of individual neurons is determined by their specific function. Some are extremely large and may give rise to extremely long nerve fibers. Transmission velocities in the long fibers may be as high as 100 m/second, whereas smaller neurons with very small fibers demonstrate velocities of 1 m/second. Some neurons connect to many different neurons in a "network," and still others have few connections to other cells of the nervous system.

It has been estimated that there are 12 billion neurons in the CNS. Three fourths of these neurons are located in the cerebral cortex, where information transmitted through the nervous system is processed. This processing, as already indicated, includes not only the determination of appropriate and effective responses but also the storage of memory and the development of associative motor and thought patterns.

Neuron Structure

The neuron is also termed a *nerve cell.* It consists of a nerve cell body that contains nuclear and cytoplasmic material and processes arising from this. These processes are functionally differentiated into axons and

413

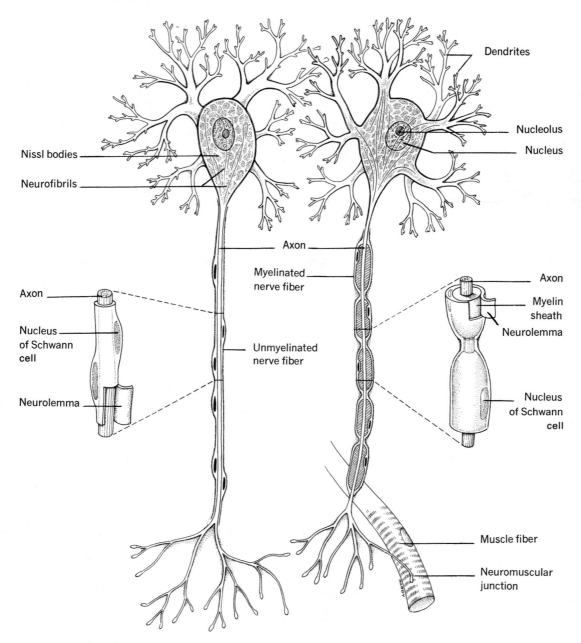

FIGURE 23-1
Typical efferent neurons. Left, unmyelinated fiber; right, myelinated fiber. (Chaffee EE, Lytle IM: Basic Physiology and Anatomy, 4th ed. Philadelphia, JB Lippincott, 1980)

dendrites (Fig. 23-1). *Axons* normally carry nervous impulses away from the cell body, whereas *dendrites* conduct the impulse toward the cell body. Axons and dendrites may be merely microscopic knobs or areas on the cell body surface, or they may be cylindrical processes that can, in certain cases, extend to over 1 m (4 ft) in length.

Neurons do not connect to one another. There are spaces between the axon (or axons) of one neuron and the dendrite (or dendrites) of another. This space is termed the *synapse*. Axons and dendrites may branch, enabling the axon of one neuron to synapse with dendrites of more than one other neuron. Similarly, axons from several neurons may synapse with a single neuron. The former is an example of divergence; the latter exemplifies convergence.

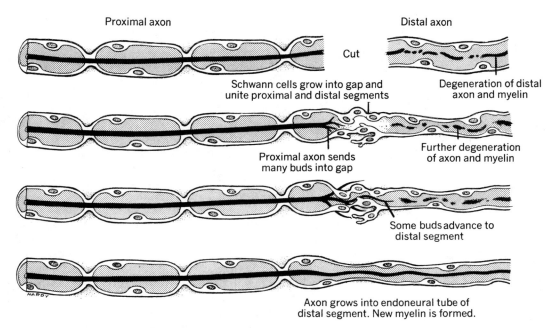

Proximal axon

Distal axon

Cut

Schwann cells grow into gap and
unite proximal and distal segments

Degeneration of distal
axon and myelin

Proximal axon sends
many buds into gap

Further degeneration
of axon and myelin

Some buds advance to
distal segment

Axon grows into endoneural tube of
distal segment. New myelin is formed.

FIGURE 23-2
Diagram of changes that occur in a nerve fiber that has been cut and then regenerates.
(Chaffee EE, Lytle IM: Basic Physiology and Anatomy, 4th ed. Philadelphia, JB Lippincott, 1980)

Nerves and Ganglia. Axons and dendrites are collectively referred to as *nerve fibers.* A bundle of nerve fibers together with their coverings is termed a *nerve.* A *ganglion* is a group of cell bodies.

Nerve Fiber Coverings. Within the CNS, some fibers are covered with a lipid-protein sheath termed the *myelin sheath.* This appears to be formed via the action of oligodendrocytes. Other fibers remain unmyelinated. Peripheral nerve fibers are all covered by a *neurilemma.* This is a sheath formed by the cells of Schwann, which wrap themselves around the fiber. The Schwann cells around some fibers also secrete myelin. Others do not (see Fig. 23-1). The neurilemma of myelinated fibers comes in contact with the fiber at periodic intervals. These periodic constrictions of the neurilemmal sheath are termed the *nodes of Ranvier.* Such nodes produce a faster impulse conduction.

Fiber Regeneration. If a nerve fiber is severed, the portion distal to the cell body will die. That part still attached to the cell body will regenerate. The neurilemma itself provides a channel that can be followed by a regenerating fiber so that it may become reattached to its original anatomical connection (Fig. 23-2). Regeneration occurs in the absence of a neurilemma, as in the case of CNS neurons. Because there is no channel to assure correct anatomical reconnection, most such regeneration does not produce recovered function. The regrowing stump may wind aimlessly among other structures or curl into a useless tangle. A bigger hindrance to functional regeneration within the CNS has been discovered, however—an overgrowth of neurological cells that occurs in response to injury. This produces a glial thicket that acts as a barrier to the reconnection of severed neuronal networks.

Nerve Impulse. The essence of the nerve impulse is the action potential and its self-propagated conduction, as described in the chapter on normal cardiac physiology. The neuronal membrane contains sodium pumps that keep the inside of the neuron more negatively charged than the outside interstitial fluid. As in cardiac tissue, the cytoplasm of the neuron contains anions (negatively charged particles) that are too large to leave the cell. These electrochemically attract, in part, positively charged postassium ions (potassium is also pumped into the neuron) and positively charged sodium ions as well. If this were all that happened, the influx of positively charged ions would counterbalance the negatively charged ones, electroneutrality would be established within the neuron, and nothing further could occur. However, the active transport enzyme system within the neuronal membrane pumps sodium out of the cell almost as fast as it enters. Even though potassium is pumped into the cell, this is insufficient to counterbalance the anions. Thus the inside of the neuron remains negative with respect to the outside as long as the sodium pumps are operating.

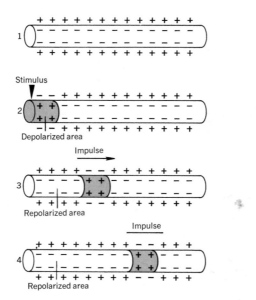

FIGURE 23-3
Propagation of impulses. (1) Resting membrane. (2) Action potential, first stage: stimulation of fiber results in depolarization. (3) Action potential, second stage: repolarization occurs as the resting potential is restored. (4) Propagation of impulses continues in direction of arrow. (Chaffee EE, Lytle IM: Basic Physiology and Anatomy, 4th ed. Philadelphia, JB Lippincott, 1980)

This, then, is the *resting polarity* of the neuron; it is typically −85 mv.

A stimulus acts locally to turn off sodium pumps. This causes a local influx of sodium and a consequent local *depolarization*. If enough pumps are temporarily inactivated, this can result in a depolarization that is large enough to inactivate sodium pumps in adjacent areas.

A depolarization of such self-propagating magnitude is termed an *action potential*. It is the essence of a nervous impulse. An action potential is a discrete temporary event because the sodium pump can be only temporarily inactivated. Once it turns back on, the electrical events reverse, and the resting potential is once again restored (Fig. 23-3).

The electrical activity embodied in the action potential can be monitored in certain clinical situations. For example, the electroencephalogram depicts multiple action potentials from surface neurons of the brain.

Synaptic Transmission. One neuron may stimulate or inhibit another by chemical transmission across the synapse. This involves the synthesis of the transmitter by the first neuron. Transmitter packets are then stored in the end (or ends) of its axon (or axons). As a nervous impulse passes down the axon, it triggers the release of a certain number of transmitter packets. These chemicals then diffuse across the synapse, where they

temporarily attach to receptor binding sites on the dendrite surface (Fig. 23-4).

While the transmitter is bound to the receptor site, the dendrite area is either stimulated (depolarized or hypopolarized) or inhibited (hyperpolarized). Most chemical transmitters are stimulators. Only one, gamma-aminobutyric acid (GABA), is known to hyperpolarize a neuron.

Within an extremely short interval (millionths of a second) the transmitter detaches from the binding site. It may then reattach or be inactivated. The latter occurs in two basic ways, depending on the chemical. In one way, the transmitter diffuses back into the axon to be reused another time (*e.g.,* norepinephrine). In the other way, the transmitter is destroyed by a chemical in the synapse. One example of this latter method is the destruction of acetylcholine by cholinesterase. In either case, the availability of a transmitter that can attach to the binding sites is temporally restricted. This enables rapid, repetitive, discrete stimulation (or inhibition) of neurons, a necessary factor in the functioning of the nervous system. From this picture we can see that synaptic transmission is a one-way street—from the axon across the synapse to the dendrite of the next neuron. It cannot proceed in the opposite direction. We also see that decreased destruction of transmitter can increase the effect of this transmitter on the postsynaptic membrane. Similarly increased destruction of transmitter reduces its postsynaptic effects.

The best known synaptic transmitters are acetylcholine and norepinephrine. Other transmitters include dopamine, serotonin, histamine, endogenous opiates, and gamma-aminobutyric acid (GABA). Most of these act to excite, or hypopolarize, the postsynaptic neuronal membrane. GABA and possibly some endogenous opiates act to inhibit, or hyperpolarize, the postsynaptic neuronal membrane.

Neuronal Thresholds. In the CNS (and sympathetic ganglia), the axons of several neurons may synapse with the dendrites or cell body of a single neuron. Some may release excitatory synaptic transmitters, whereas others may release an inhibitory transmitter. The excitatory transmitter released from a single axon is often insufficient to trigger an action potential in the postsynaptic neuron (*i.e.,* to excite the postsynaptic cell fully). Rather, it may be sufficient to depolarize, or excite, the postsynaptic membrane only partially. As such it is termed a *subthreshold stimulus*. The partial depolarization, or hypopolarization, it produces renders the postsynaptic neuron more easily excitable by subsequent excitatory transmitter stimuli from other axons, provided such transmitters arrive while the postsynaptic membrane is hypopolarized. Thus, this initial subthreshold excitatory stimulus is said to "lower the threshold" of the postsynaptic neuron for stimulation by another axon (presynaptic neuron).

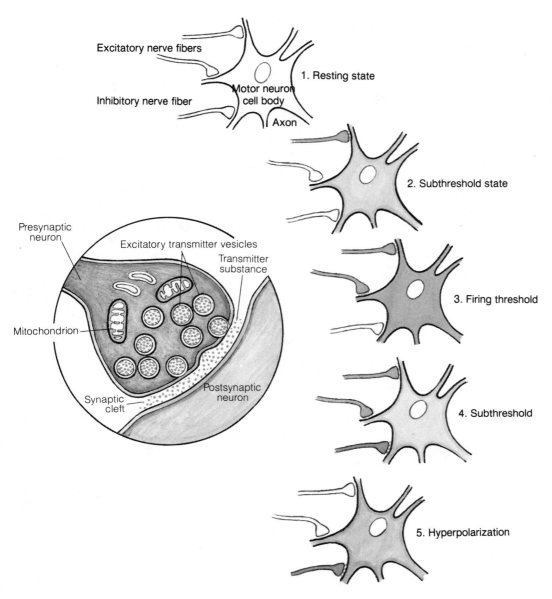

FIGURE 23-4

Conduction at synapses. Left, *enlarged view of liberation of chemical transmitter substance at a synapse;* right, *diagrams illustrating how a neuron may be excited or inhibited by transmitter substances liberated by presynaptic nerve fiber endings. Two excitatory and one inhibitory fiber are shown: (1) resting state; (2) subthreshold state; impulses from only one excitatory fiber cannot cause the postsynaptic neuron to fire; (3) firing threshold is reached by the addition of impulses from a second excitatory fiber; (4) subthreshold state is restored by impulses from an inhibitory fiber; (5) when the inhibitory fiber alone is carrying impulses, the postsynaptic neuron is in a state of hyperpolarization and is unable to fire. (Chaffee EE, Lytle IM: Basic Physiology and Anatomy, 4th ed. Philadelphia, JB Lippincott, 1980)*

Full excitation of a postsynaptic membrane is prerequisite to establishment of an action potential and thus the firing of a nerve impulse along the postsynaptic neuron. It may require the near simultaneous depolarization produced by excitatory transmitters from two or more presynaptic neurons.

If the synaptic transmitter is an inhibitory one (*e.g.,*

GABA), it will hyperpolarize, or "raise the threshold" of, the postsynaptic neuron. This renders it more difficult to be excited fully by excitatory transmitters. Figure 23-4 illustrates the action of three convergent presynaptic neurons on the threshold of a single postsynaptic neuron.

These principles underlie much of the normal functioning of cord internuncials and spinal reflexes. For example, certain descending fibers from the brain stem deliver a low-level subthreshold stimulation to certain cord neurons. Although this stimulation is insufficient to activate cord neurons, it is enough of a background stimulus to make it easier for other input to excite these neurons fully. Such subthreshold stimuli would be said to be *facilitatory*. When the cord is severed, the distal portion is also separated from receipt of such facilitatory brain stem influences. As a result, it takes greater stimuli to cause action potentials in the neurons in this part of the cord than before. Indeed, when initially separated from the brain, these cord neurons do not function noticeably at all for a few weeks. Such a condition is termed *cord shock*. In it, no reflexes are possible.

Neuronal thresholds can also be influenced by hormones. *Thyroxin* lowers thresholds of certain neurons, and one sign of hyperthyroidism is the presence of exaggerated cord reflexes, such as the knee jerk and ankle jerk.

MENINGES

The CNS is covered by three layers of tissue called, collectively, the *meninges* and consisting of the pia mater, the arachnoid layer, and the dura mater. The *pia mater* is the layer that lies next to the CNS. Next is the *arachnoid layer,* which contains a substantial vascular supply. Last is the *dura mater,* the thickest layer of all, lying next to the bones surrounding the CNS.

CEREBROSPINAL FLUID

Cerebrospinal fluid (CSF) functions as a fluid shock absorber, keeping the delicate CNS tissues from banging against surrounding bony structures and being mechanically injured. It also functions in the exchange of nutrients between the plasma and cellular compartments. CSF is a plasma filtrate that is exuded by the capillaries in the roofs of each of the four ventricles of the brain. As such, it is similar to plasma minus the large plasma proteins, which stay behind in the bloodstream. Most of this fluid is made in the lateral ventricles which are located in each cerebral hemisphere. It moves from there through ducts into the third ventricle of the diencephalon. From here it travels through the aqueduct of Sylvius of the midbrain and enters the fourth ventricle of the medulla. Then most of it passes through holes (foramina) in the roof of this ventricle and enters the subarachnoid space. (A small amount diffuses down into the spinal canal.) In this space, the CSF is reabsorbed back into the bloodstream at certain points called the *subarachnoid plexus.*

The formation and reabsorption of CSF are governed by the same hydrostatic and colloid osmotic forces that regulate the movements of fluid and small particles between the plasma and interstitial fluid compartments of the body. Briefly reviewed, the action of these forces is as follows. Two opposing teams of push-pull forces influence the movement of water and small particles through the semipermeable capillary membranes. One team is composed of plasma osmotic pressure and CSF hydrostatic pressure. It favors movement of water from the CSF compartment into the plasma. The movement of water in the opposite direction is influenced by the team of plasma hydrostatic pressure and CSF osmotic pressure. "Team influences" are exerted simultaneously and continually. In the ventricles, the flow of CSF reduces CSF hydrostatic pressure. This tips the collective team influence in favor of the movement of water and small particles from plasma to ventricles. The low plasma hydrostatic pressure of blood in the venous sinuses next to the arachnoid villi tips the scales in favor of the movement of water and solute from the CSF compartment back into the bloodstream. Death of cells lining the CSF compartment will spill proteins into the CSF. This elevates CSF osmotic pressure and retards reabsorption (while also hastening formation if the damage is in ventricle walls). Increased CSF proteins from this or other causes can provoke or exacerbate a condition of excess CSF called *hydrocephalus.*

CENTRAL NERVOUS SYSTEM

The purpose of this section is to consider major functions briefly so that their abnormalities can be associated with specific brain damage discussed in other chapters. The reader is referred to the bibliography for sources of in-depth discussions.

The CNS comprises the brain and spinal cord. It receives sensory input by way of sensory fibers (dendrites) within spinal and cranial nerves and sends out motor impulses by way of axons in these same nerves. The CNS also contains large numbers of neurons that are entirely contained within it. These neurons are termed *internuncial neurons,* or *interneurons,* and may exist within brain and cord or connect one with the other. Let us briefly examine each of the seven major parts of the brain and then the spinal cord.

Brain

Basic anatomy of the brain is illustrated in Figure 23-5. The parts of the brain in descending order are the cerebral hemispheres, diencephalon, midbrain, pons, medulla, and cerebellum. The general appearance of the brain can be viewed as a stem extending upwards from

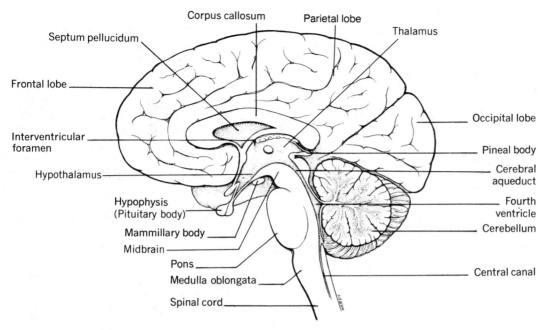

FIGURE 23-5
Midsagittal section of the brain.

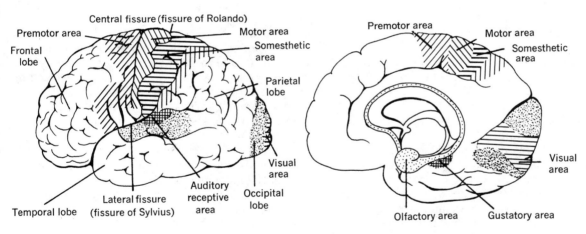

FIGURE 23-6
Diagram of the localization of function in the cerebral hemisphere. Various functional areas are shown in relation to the lobes and fissures: (left) *lateral view;* (right) *medial view.*

the spinal cord with an inferior small flowering overgrowth (cerebellum) covering the lower part of the stem and a large superior flowering overgrowth (cerebrum) covering most of the upper portion of the stem. The medulla, pons, and midbrain compose the brain stem. Some authors include the diencephalon.

Cerebrum
Each of the two (left and right) cerebral hemispheres contains a layer of cortex, six cells deep, covering the surface. Underneath this is white matter (nerve fibers). Deep within each hemisphere are several collections of nerve cell bodies termed the *basal ganglia* and a lateral ventricle containing cerebrospinal fluid. The left and right hemispheres are connected and communicate with each other by a transverse band of nerve fibers termed the *corpus callosum*. Each hemisphere has four lobes named for and generally underlying each of the following skull bones: frontal, parietal, temporal, and occipital. For the most part, each hemi-

sphere serves the contralateral side of the body (fibers cross over in the CNS).

One notable exception is Broca's speech area. This area of cortex subserves all motor speech functions and is located in a posterolateral area of the left frontal lobe for all right-handed and many left-handed persons. Damage to this area in an adult produces motor aphasia.

Cortex. The cortex is thought to operate in all higher mental functions such as judgment, language, memory, creativity, and abstract thinking. It also functions in the perception, localization, and interpretation of all sensations and governs all voluntary and especially discrete motor activities (Fig. 23-6). Various areas of the cortex have been identified as having different motor and sensory functions, but some of these areas are being implicated in other functions as well (*e.g.,* the occipital area is now known to function in some learning processes of blind individuals). Many areas of the cerebrum operate together to produce coordinated human function. Let us look at communication as an example.

Verbal communication depends on the ability to interpret speech and to translate thought into speech. Ideas are usually communicated between people by either spoken or written word. With the spoken word, the sensory input of information occurs through the primary auditory cortex. In auditory association areas, the sounds are interpreted as words and the words as sentences. These sentences are then interpreted by a common integrative area of the cerebral cortex as thoughts.

The common integrative area also develops thoughts to be communicated. Letters seen by the eyes are associated as words, thoughts, and sentences in the visual association area and integrated into thought in this area also. Operating in conjunction with facial regions of the somesthetic sensory area, the common integrative area initiates a series of impulses, with each representing a syllable or word, and transmits them to the secondary motor area controlling the larynx and mouth.

The speech center, in addition to controlling motor activity of the larynx and mouth, sends impulses to the respiratory center of the secondary motor cortex to provide appropriate breath patterns for the speech process.

Basal Ganglia. The basal ganglia function in cooperation with other lower brain parts in providing circuitry for basic and subconscious bodily movements. They provide (1) the necessary background muscle tone for discrete voluntary movements, (2) smoothness and coordination in functions of muscle antagonists, and (3) the basic automatic subconscious rhythmic movements involved in walking and equilibrium maintenance. Lesions of these basal ganglia will produce various clinical abnormalities such as chorea, hemiballismus, and Parkinson's disease.

Diencephalon

Below the cerebrum lies the next brain area, the diencephalon. This area contains the third ventricle and the thalamus. Below is the hypothalamus and above is the epithalamus or pineal gland (see Fig. 23-5). The diencephalon is the most superior portion of what most authors call the *brain stem* (diencephalon, midbrain, pons, and medulla).

The *thalamus* functions as a sensory and motor relay center. It relays sensory impulses, including those of sight and sound, up to the cortex. It also functions in a gross awareness of certain sensations, most notably pain. Discrete localization and the finer perceptual details are cortical functions, but the remaining awareness occurs at the thalamic and even midbrain areas.

The thalamus also has other cells, the axons of which travel to association areas of the cortex. The function of these cells and the cortical areas to which they attach are presently unknown.

Last, the thalamus possesses some of the fiber tracts of the reticular activating systems that function in promoting consciousness and possibly some aspects of attention.

The *hypothalamus* is the seat of neuroendocrine interaction. It is here that various neurosecretory substances are produced—hormones that were previously attributed to the posterior pituitary (antidiuretic hormone [ADH] and oxytocin) and that stimulate or inhibit the secretion of anterior pituitary hormones.

This area of the brain also contains centers for (1) coordinated parasympathetic and sympathetic stimulation, (2) temperature regulation, (3) appetite regulation, (4) regulation of water balance by ADH, and (5) regulation of certain rhythmic psychobiological activities (*e.g.,* sleep).

Limbic System

The hypothalamus, cingulate, gyrus of the cortex, the amygdala and hippocampus within the temporal lobes, and the septum and interconnecting fiber tracts among these areas compose a functional unit of the brain called the *limbic system.* This system provides a neural substrate for emotions (terror, intense pleasure, eroticism, etc.) Also, it is here that neural pathways provide a connection between higher brain functioning and endocrinologic-autonomic activities.

Midbrain

The midbrain lies between the diencephalon and the pons of the brain stem. It contains the aqueduct of

Sylvius, many ascending and descending nerve fiber tracts, and centers for auditory and visually stimulated nerve impulses. It is here that the *Edinger-Westphal nucleus* is located. This nucleus contains the autonomic reflex centers for pupillary accommodations to light. It receives fibers from the retina by way of cranial nerve II and emits motor impulses by way of sympathetic and parasympathetic (cranial nerve III) fibers to the smooth muscles of the iris. Impaired pupillary accommodation signifies that at least one of these inputs or outputs is damaged or that the midbrain itself is suffering insult (often from tentorial herniation or cerebral vascular accident [CDA].

Pons

The *pons varolli* lies between the midbrain and the medulla oblongata of the brain stem and has cell bodies of fibers contained in cranial nerves V, VI, VII, and VIII. It contains pneumotaxic and apneustic respiratory centers and fiber tracts connecting higher and lower centers, including the cerebellum.

Medulla

The *medulla* lies between the pons and the cord. It contains autonomic centers that regulate such vital functions as breathing, cardiac rate, and vasomotor tone as well as centers for vomiting, gagging, coughing, and sneezing reflex behaviors. It also contains the fourth ventricle. Cranial nerves IX to XII have their cell bodies in this area. Impairment in any of these vital functions or reflexes suggests medullary damage.

Cerebellum

The cerebellum is located just superior and posterior to the medulla. It receives "samples" of all ascending somesthetic sensory input as well as of all descending motor impulses. Use of these connections enables the cerebellum to match intended motor stimuli (before they reach the muscles) with actual sensory data. This ensures optimal match for voluntary motor "intention" with actual motor action, with time to alter the motor message in case of error. It sends its own messages up to the basal ganglia and cortex, as well as to parts of the brain stem, in order to perform three basic subconscious functions.

The cerebellum functions to (1) produce smooth, steady, harmonious, and coordinated skeletal muscle actions; (2) maintain equilibrium; and (3) control posture without any jerky or uncompensated movements or swaying.

Cerebellum disease can produce certain symptoms, the most prominent of which are disturbances of gait, equilibrium ataxia (overstability or understability of the walk), and termors.

Functionally Integrated Systems

There are three networks within the brain stem that bear mention here. They are the integrated systems responsible for consciousness, sleep, and posture-equilibrium.

Bulboreticular Formation. This is a network of neurons in the brain stem that function in maintaining bodily support against gravity and equilibrium. Figure 23-7 illustrates the anatomical location of the bulboreticular formation. This area receives information from a variety of sources that include all areas of the peripheral sensory receptors via the spinal cord, the cerebellum, the inner-ear equilibrium apparatus, the motor cortex, and the basal ganglia. The bulboreticular formation, then, is an integrative area for sensory information, motor information from the cerebral cortex, equilibrium information from the vestibular apparatus, and proprioceptive information from the cerebellum. Output from the bulboreticular formation travels down descending fibers to internuncial neurons in the cord. This output alters the tonus of muscles maintaining equilibrium and the positions of major body parts (trunk, appendages) necessary for the performance of discrete actions (*e.g.,* writing at a table, walking).

Reticular Activating System (RAS). The RAS is an ascending fiber system originating in the midbrain and thalamus (Fig. 23-7). Branches extend up to the cortex. In this way, the RAS can stimulate the cortex. The

FIGURE 23-7
Bulboreticular and reticular activating systems. Black area, *bulboreticular system;* striped area, *reticular activating system.*

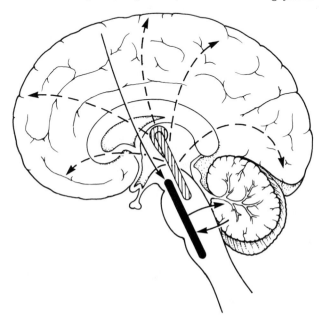

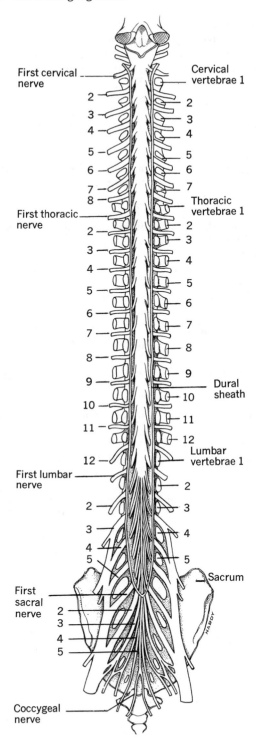

First cervical nerve
2
3
4
5
6
7
8
First thoracic nerve
2
3
4
5
6
7
8
9
10
11
12
First lumbar nerve
2
3
4
5
First sacral nerve
2
3
4
5
Coccygeal nerve

Cervical vertebrae 1
2
3
4
5
6
7
Thoracic vertebrae 1
2
3
4
5
6
7
8
9
Dural sheath
10
11
12
Lumbar vertebrae 1
2
3
4
5
Sacrum

FIGURE 23-8
Spinal cord lying within the vertebral canal. Spinous processes and laminae have been removed; dura and arachnoid have been opened. Spinal nerves are numbered on the left side; vertebrae are numbered on the right side. Note the site of origin of each spinal nerve in the cord and its point of exit from the vertebral column.

RAS is itself stimulated by the arrival of a variety of sensory impulses and chemical stimuli from various sources. These include input from the optic and acoustic cranial nerves, somesthetic impulses from the dorsal column and spinothalamic pathways, and fibers from the cerebral cortex. In addition, it is stimulated by norepinephrine and epinephrine.

The stimulation of the cortex by the RAS seems to be the major physiological basis for consciousness, alertness, and attention to various environmental stimuli. However, some of the aforementioned stimuli (*e.g.,* pain, noise) also can increase one's level of consciousness, at least temporarily. Decreased activity of the RAS produces decreased alertness or levels of consciousness including stupor and coma. Inactivation of the RAS can result from anything that interrupts the entry of a critical amount of sensory input or by any damage that prevents the RAS fibers from sending impulses to the cortex.

Sleep Centers. Two groups of neurons (nuclei) in the brain stem have been found to regulate different stages of sleep. One, the raphe, triggers the deeper stages of sleep. It may also play a role in sleep onset. The neurotransmitter substance from raphe fibers is serotonin. The other nucleus is the locus ceruleus. Its transmitter is norepinephrine. This nucleus is responsible for the events of "rapid eye movement" sleep (*i.e.,* dreaming). Neural mechanisms underlying the remaining stages of sleep, onset and cessation, have yet to be discovered.

Spinal Cord

The spinal cord lies within the neural canal of the vertebral column. It extends down and fills the neural canal to the level of the second lumbar vertebrae. A pair of spinal nerves exits between adjacent vertebrae the entire length of the vertebral column. Below the point at which the cord terminates, the neural canal is filled with spinal nerves, extending to their point of exit (Fig. 23-8). Because they occupy less space in the canal at these lower lumbar levels, it is here that spinal taps may most safely be performed. This anatomic fact also explains why injuries to lumbar and lower thoracic vertebrae can produce impairment at disproportionately lower body levels.

Within the cord lie interneurons, ascending sensory fibers, descending motor fibers, and the nerve cell bodies and dendrites of the second-order somatic (voluntary) and first-order autonomic motor neurons. The central area of the cord, the gray matter, contains nerve cell bodies and internuncial neurons (*i.e.,* nerve cells contained entirely within the cord). The gray matter has left and right dorsal and ventral projections, giving it an H-shaped appearance. Nerve cell bodies of motor neurons supplying skeletal muscles lie in the ventral horns. Left and right lateral projections or horns of gray matter exist in the thoracic, lumbar, and sacral cord. Within those lie the nerve cell bodies of autonomic neurons. Surrounding the gray matter is the white matter of the cord. It contains ascending and descending fiber tracts as well as fibers entering or leaving the cord. Its white color comes from the myelin that covers these fibers.

Spinal nerves contain both sensory and motor fibers. Each spinal nerve attaches to the cord via a dorsal and ventral root. The dorsal root houses the nerve cell bodies and fibers of sensory neurons. Motor fibers (whose nerve cell bodies lay within the gray matter) traverse the ventral root. Thus, damage to one root may impair sensory function without impairing motor function, or vice versa. A spinal nerve injury could damage both sensory function and motor functioning.

Sensory Division

The sensory division is composed of sensory receptors, sensory neurons, sensory tracts, and perceptive areas of the brain.

Sensations and Receptors

There is a wide variety of structures that respond to diverse stimuli. They range in structure and function from light-sensitive retinal cells to stretch-sensitive structures in muscles and tendons. Stimulation of a sensory receptor initiates an electrical change (generator potential), which in turn stimulates the sensory neuron synapsing with the receptor. A series of nerve impulses travel along the sensory neuron to the CNS, where they in turn stimulate neurons in either brain or cord tracts to carry impulses to the appropriate centers in the brain (thalamus and cortex), where the sensation may finally be consciously perceived.

Sensations are often divided into those of the major senses (*e.g.,* vision, hearing, and smell) and those termed somesthetic sensations (*e.g.,* pain, touch, and stretch). Somesthetic sensations provide information regarding such things as body position and conditions of the immediate external environment as well as conditions of the internal environment. These are called proprioceptive, exteroceptive, and visceral sensations, respectively. In this chapter, only somesthetic sensations will be discussed.

Proprioceptive sensations describe the physical position state of the body, such as tension in muscle, flexion or extension of joints, tendon tension, and deep pressure in dependent parts like the feet while one is standing or the buttocks while one is seated. *Exteroceptive sensations* monitor the conditions on the body surface. These include temperature and pain. *Visceral sensations* are like exteroceptive sensations except that they originate from within and monitor pain, pressure, and fullness from internal organs.

The sensory receptors for somesthetic sensations include both free nerve endings and specialized end organs. Free nerve endings are nothing more than small filamentous branches of the dendritic fibers. They detect crude sensations of touch, pain, heat, and cold. The precision is crude because there are many interconnections between the free endings of different neurons. However, they are the most profusely distributed and perform the general discriminatory functions, whereas the more specialized receptors discriminate between very slight differences in degrees of touch, heat, and cold.

Structurally, the special exteroceptive end organs for detection of cold, warmth, and light touch differ from one another and are quite specific in their function. The physiological basis for this specific function has not been determined but is presumed to be based on some specific physical effect on the organ itself.

There are three proprioceptive receptors. Joint kinesthetic receptors are found in the joint capsules and provide data concerning the angulation of a joint and the rate at which it is changing. Information from muscles concerning the degree of stretch is transmitted to the nervous system from the muscle spindle apparatus, whereas the Golgi tendon determines the overall tension applied to the tendons.

When a sensory receptor is stimulated, it responds with an increased frequency of firing (generator potential). At first there is a burst of impulses; if the stimulus persists, the frequency of impulses transmitted begins to decrease. All sensory receptors show this phenomenon of *adaptation* to varying degrees and at different rates. Adaptations to light touch and pressure occurs in a few seconds, whereas pain and proprioceptive sensation adapt very little, if at all, and at a very slow rate. The determination of the intensity of sensation is made on a relative rather than an absolute basis and follows a logarithmic response. Therefore, the intensity of a sensation increases logarithmically, whereas the frequency of response in the nerve ending increases linearly.

Although there are structurally different receptors for detecting each type of sensation, it is the area of the brain to which the information is transmitted that determines the *modality,* or type of sensation a person feels. The thalamus and somesthetic areas of the cortex operate together to attribute various sensory qualities and intensities to the nerve impulse information they receive.

Sensory Neurons

Stimulation of sensory receptors creates nerve impulses (action potentials) in sensory neurons. These neurons conduct such impulses to the CNS.

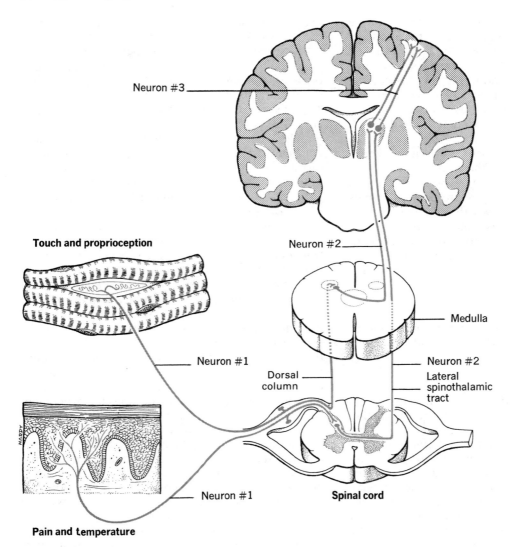

Touch and proprioception

Neuron #3

Neuron #2

Neuron #1

Dorsal column

Medulla

Neuron #2
Lateral spinothalamic tract

Neuron #1

Spinal cord

Pain and temperature

FIGURE 23-9
Diagrammatic representation of the decussation (crossing) of ascending tracts. First order neurons for touch and proprioception ascend in the dorsal columns to the medulla; here they synapse with second order neurons that cross to the opposite side before ascending to the thalamus. First order neurons for pain and temperature enter the dorsal gray matter of the cord; here they synapse with second order neurons that cross to the opposite side and ascend in the lateral spinothalamic tract to the thalamus. Third order neurons connect the thalamus with the cerebral cortex.

Sensory Pathways

Depending on the type of somesthetic receptor involved, fibers of sensory neurons may, upon entering the cord, do one of three things. They may travel the white matter of the cord on the same side of the body as the sensory receptor. There they will synapse with a second set of neurons that then cross over to the opposite side of the brain and travel to the thalamus. This pathway is termed the *dorsal column pathway* (Fig. 23-9) and is used for the conduction of impulses originating from stimulation of (1) muscle, tendon, and joint proprioceptors; (2) vibration-sensitive receptors; and (3) receptors in the skin involved in precise localization of touch.

Alternatively, the sensory neuron may synapse immediately upon entering the cord with a second neuron that then immediately crosses over to the opposite side of the cord. Fibers from this second neuron then travel up the white matter of the cord to the thalamus. This is called the *spinothalamic pathway* (Fig. 23-9). It conducts impulses concerned with pain, temperature, poorly localized touch, and sex organ sensations. In the thalamus, neurons of both the spinothalamic pathway and the dorsal column pathway synapse with other neurons that transmit impulses to the appropriate area of the somesthetic cortex. Because of this, impulses from either pathway give rise to consciously perceived sensations.

Last, certain sensory neurons may synapse with a neuron belonging to the *spinocerebellar* pathway. Spinocerebellar neurons do not cross over, and they carry impulses only as far as the cerebullum (and possibly lower brain stem). This pathway carries impulses originating from stimulation of muscle, tendon, and joint proprioceptors. Because this pathway ends at the cerebellum, it transmits sensory information that is never consciously perceived. These data is used in reflex postural adjustments.

Motor System

The motor system technically comprises the areas of the brain, descending fiber tracts, and the motor neurons involved in producing or altering movement or adjusting tonus of skeletal cardiac and smooth muscles and in regulating the secretions of the various exocrine and certain endocrine gland cells of the body. In practical terms, the heart is usually excluded from this system. Muscle and glandular tissues are referred to as the *effective organs* of this system.

The motor system can be divided on the basis of motor neurons and effector organs into *somatic* and *autonomic* subdivisions. The former involve skeletal muscles and motor neurons innervating them. The autonomic subdivision is composed of smooth muscle and gland cells plus the sympathetic and parasympathetic fibers innervating them.

Somatic Motor Division

Figure 23-10 depicts the major descending fiber tracts from motor areas of the cerebral cortex. Some of these fibers cross over to the opposite side of the body in the brain. Others cross over in the cord centers. Descending fibers from motor areas of the cortex ultimately stimulate somatic motor neurons, the nerve cell bodies of which lie in the anterior (ventral) horn of the gray matter in the cord. The axons of these motor neurons travel within spinal nerves and terminate adjacent to the membranes of skeletal muscle cells. The space between the somatic motor neuron axon and the muscle cell is termed the *myoneural junction*. When stimulated, somatic motor neurons conduct impulses to the ends of their axons. As the impulse arrives there, it triggers the release of a certain number of acetylcholine molecules that are stored in the terminal bouton. The acetylcholine diffuses across the myoneural junction and binds with receptor sites on a skeletal muscle cell. This triggers a chain of events leading to contrac-

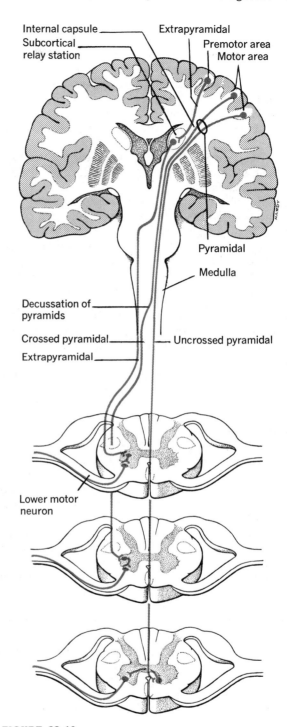

FIGURE 23-10
Diagram of motor pathways between the cerebral cortex, one of the subcortical relay centers and lower motor neurons in the spinal cord. Decussation (crossing) of fibers means that each side of the brain controls skeletal muscles on the opposite side of the body.

tion. Thus, willed intentional motor movements are enacted.

Not shown in Figure 23-10 are descending fiber tracts that stimulate motor neurons responsible for the movement of skeletal muscles of the head (*e.g.,* tongue, face, jaw). The general pattern and myoneural transmitter are the same, except the somatic motor neuron nerve cell bodies lay within certain areas of the brain.

Also not shown in Figure 23-10 are several extrapyramidal tracts that arise from brain stem centers (*e.g.,* bulboreticular formation, midbrain). Some of these cross over, whereas others do not. Fibers in these tracts descend the cord and ultimately stimulate either somatic motor neurons, which stimulate skeletal muscle cells, or other motor neurons (gamma efferent) that alter the tension of stretch receptor organelles (spindles) within the skeletal muscles. Alteration of spindle tension provokes a spinal reflex arc that efficiently and indirectly alters skeletal muscle tonus. These extrapyramidal pathways conduct impulses that produce the automatic coordinated alterations in skeletal muscle tonus and movement that are necessary for gross motor movements (*e.g.,* walking) and for appropriate posture for conduction of finer movements (*e.g.,* sitting at a desk with arm flexed in preparation for writing; standing).

Autonomic Division

This division comprises both *sympathetic* and *parasympathetic motor fibers.* They are responsible for contraction and relaxation of smooth muscle, rate of contraction of cardiac tissue, secretion of exocrine glands, and secretion of the adrenal medulla and islets of Langerhans in the pancreas.

The sympathetic and parasympathetic sections differ on the basis of (1) the anatomic distribution of nerve fibers, (2) the secretion of two different neural transmitters by the postganglionic fibers of the two divisions, and (3) the antagonistic effects of the two divisions on some of the organs they innervate. Figure 23-11 shows the anatomy of the sympathetic and parasympathetic nervous systems.

Both the sympathetic and parasympathetic motor pathways are essentially composed of a chain of two neurons carrying nerve impulses from the CNS to the effector organ. The first neuron in the chain is termed the *preganglionic neuron* and the second one is called the *postganglionic neuron.* Nerve cell bodies of preganglionic sympathetic neurons lay in the lateral horns of the gray matter of the thoracic and lumbar segments of the cord; those or preganglionic parasympathetic neurons lay either in certain areas of the brain or in the lateral horns of gray matter in the sacral cord.

Axons of preganglionic sympathetic neurons exit the cord and enter the ventral roots of spinal nerves.

They then leave the spinal nerve to enter a nearby sympathetic ganglion (via a connecting pathway termed a *ramus*). Within a ganglion, the preganglionic neuron synapses with a postganglionic one. The postganglionic sympathetic neuron then may reenter the spinal nerve or exit the ganglion via a special sympathetic nerve and travel to the effector organ.

Parasympathetic preganglionic axons leave the CNS via certain cranial or spinal nerves and travel to the effector organ. At or near the effector organ, they synapse with the postganglionic neuron, which in turn innervates the effector organ.

Acetylcholine is the neurotransmitter at *all* synapses between preganglionic and postganglionic autonomic neurons—both parasympathetic and sympathetic. It is also the transmitter secreted by the axons of postsynaptic parasympathetic neurons. For this reason, these axons are called *cholinergic fibers.* Sympathetic postganglionic fibers are called *adrenergic fibers* because they secrete noradrenalin (norepinephrine). The actions of these two arms of the autonomic division and their chemical transmitters are summarized in Table 23-1.

In addition to the two subdivisions of the autonomic motor division, there are three different actions of adrenergically (sympathetically) stimulated effector organs. These actions are determined by the type of receptor site in the effector organ. Receptor sites may be alpha, $beta_1$, or $beta_2$.

Patterns of autonomic function can be regulated or triggered by centers in the hypothalamus, medulla, and bulboreticular formations. However, autonomic functioning does not seem limited to the stem. Stimulation of certain cortical nerves can trigger both discrete and widespread autonomic changes. Exact mechanisms for these interactions await research. These centers in the CNS send impulses along descending fibers to the appropriate preganglionic autonomic neuron. In the cord, such fibers would travel via special descending tracts in the white matter until they reached the appropriate level of the cord. Thus, any interruption of these descending fibers (*e.g.,* transection of cervical tracts) would impede or prevent stimulation of preganglionic autonomic neurons in the thoracic, lumbar, and sacral regions of the cord.

Reflexes

Basically, a reflex is an instantaneous and automatic motor response to a sensory input. It arises from a special anatomical relationship among sensory receptors, sensory neurons, interneurons, somatic or autonomic motor neurons, and effector organs. The effector is the end organ that receives the motor impulse, such as skeletal, smooth, or cardiac muscles or an exocrine or endocrine gland.

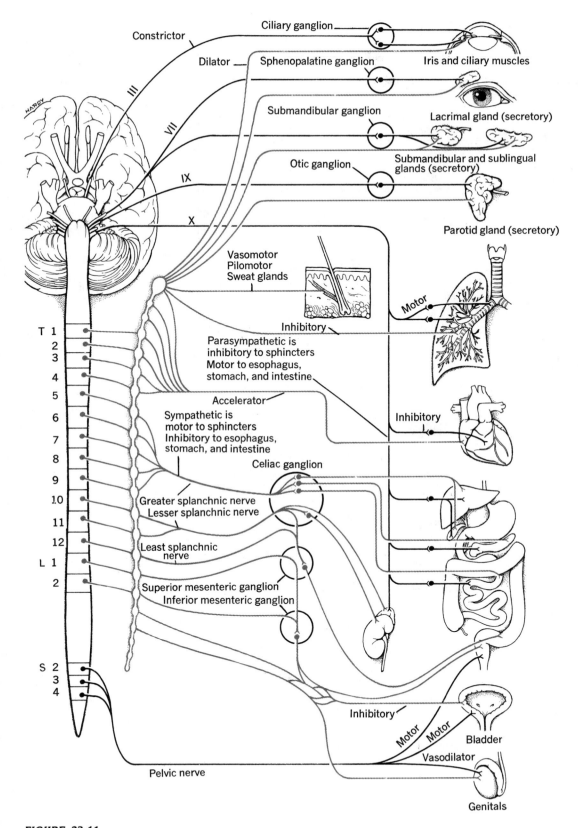

FIGURE 23-11

Diagram of the autonomic nervous system. Parasympathetic, or craniosacral, fibers are shown in black, and the sympathetic, or thoracolumbar, fibers are shaded. Note that most organs have a double nerve supply.

TABLE 23-1
RESPONSES OF EFFECTOR ORGANS TO AUTONOMIC NERVE IMPULSES AND CIRCULATING CATECHOLAMINES

Effector Organs	Cholinergic Impulses Response	Noradrenergic Impulses	
		Receptor Type	Response
Eye			
Radial muscle of iris	—	α	Contraction (mydriasis)
Sphincter muscle of iris	Contraction (miosis)		—
Ciliary muscle	Contraction for near vision	β	Relaxation for far vision
Heart			
S-A node	Decrease in heart rate; vagal arrest	β_1	Increase in heart rate
Atria	Decrease in contractility and (usually) increase in conduction velocity	β_1	Increase in contractility and conduction velocity
A-V node and conduction system	Decrease in conduction velocity; A-V block	β_1	Increase in conduction velocity
Ventricles	—	β_1	Increase in contractility and conduction velocity
Arterioles			
Coronary, skeletal muscle, pulmonary, abdominal viscera, renal	Dilatation	α β_2	Constriction Dilatation
Skin and mucosa, cerebral, salivary glands	—	α	Constriction
Systemic veins	—	α β_2	Constriction Dilatation
Lung			
Bronchial muscle	Contraction	β_2	Relaxation
Bronchial glands	Stimulation	?	Inhibition (?)
Stomach			
Motility and tone	Increase	α, β_2	Decrease (usually)
Sphincters	Relaxation (usually)	α	Contraction (usually)
Secretion	Stimulation		Inhibition (?)
Intestine			
Motility and tone	Increase	α, β_2	Decrease
Sphincters	Relaxation (usually)	α	Contraction (usually)
Secretion	Stimulation		Inhibition (?)
Gallbladder and ducts	Contraction		Relaxation
Urinary bladder			
Detrusor	Contraction	β	Relaxation (usually)
Trigone and sphincter	Relaxation	α	Contraction
Ureter			
Motility and tone	Increase (?)	α	Increase (usually)
Uterus	Variable*	α, β_2	Variable*
Male sex organs	Erection	α	Ejaculation
Skin			
Pilomotor muscles	—	α	Contraction
Sweat glands	Generalized secretion	α	Slight, localized secretion†
Spleen capsule	—	α β_2	Contraction Relaxation
Adrenal medulla	Secretion of epinephrine and norepinephrine		—
Liver	—	α, β_2	Glycogenolysis
Pancreas			
Acini	Secretion	α	Decreased secretion
Islets	Insulin and glucagon secretion	α	Inhibition of insulin and glucagon secretion
		β_2	Insulin and glucagon secretion
Salivary glands	Profuse, watery secretion	α β_2	Thick, viscous secretion Amylase secretion

TABLE 23-1 (Continued)

Effector Organs	Cholinergic Impulses Response	Noradrenergic Impulses	
		Receptor Type	Response
Lacrimal glands	Secretion		—
Nasopharyngeal glands	Secretion		—
Adipose tissue	—	β_1	Lipolysis
Juxtaglomerular cells	—	$\beta(\beta_1 ?)$	Renin secretion
Pineal gland	—	β	Melatonin synthesis and secretion

* Depends on stage of menstrual cycle, amount of circulating estrogen and progesterone, pregnancy, and other factors.
† On palms of hands and in some other locations ("adrenergic sweating").
(From Ganong WF: Review of Medical Physiology, 11th ed. Los Altos, Lange Medical Publications, 1983)

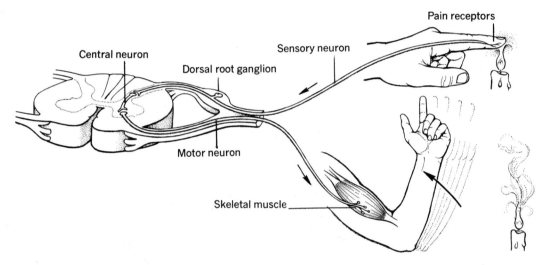

FIGURE 23-12
Diagram of withdrawal reflex.

Somesthetic sensory neurons involved in a reflex arc usually have branching axons: one branch participates in the arc (Fig. 23-12), whereas the other (not illustrated) travels up to the cerebrum via the dorsal column or spinothalamic tracts. This enables the person to perceive the sensation involved. However, such perception is not part of, nor requisite for, the operation of a reflex arc. Because it takes slightly longer for sensory data to reach the cortex than to reach an interneuron, a person often becomes aware of the sensation only during or following the occurrence of the reflex arc. Also, a cord reflex can occur even if the cord is transected above the level required for the reflex so that no sensory information can get to the brain. Reflexes may involve the cord or the brain. We will consider the former first.

Cord Reflexes

One type of common cord reflex is the *withdrawal reflex* (Fig. 23-12). Pain is the sensation that triggers this reflex. It stimulates sensory neurons, which in turn stimulate "central" interneurons, which stimulate motor fibers that innervate skeletal muscles. When contracted, the skeletal muscles will produce withdrawal of the body part (here, a hand) from the painful stimulus. Its occurrence depends on the appropriate anatomical connections, or "wiring," along sensory and motor neurons within the cord. If these become damaged (*e.g.,* cord shock or physical trauma), the reflex will not be possible.

Reflex withdrawal of one foot is associated with another reflex, the *crossed extensor reflex.* (Fig. 23-13). This reflex involves stimulation of various extensor

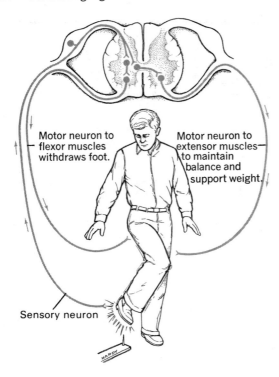

FIGURE 23-13
Diagram of flexor and crossed extensor reflexes.

Motor neuron to flexor muscles withdraws foot.

Motor neuron to extensor muscles to maintain balance and support weight.

Sensory neuron

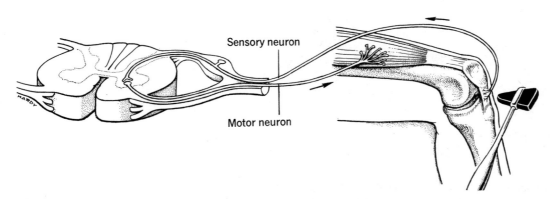

Sensory neuron

Motor neuron

FIGURE 23-14
Diagram of a stretch reflex.

muscles in the opposite leg so that the person's weight is fully supported while he withdraws one lower extremity from a painful stimulus. Such a reflex is very complex and involves many levels of the cord. Any imbalance, however slight, during the operation of this reflex in a normal person will trigger the occurrence of additional reflexes involving the bulboreticular formation, cerebellum, and various muscles of arms and trunk so as to maintain balance and posture.

Another cord reflex is the *stretch reflex,* most commonly illustrated via the clinical test of the knee jerk reflex (Fig. 23-14). Because of anatomical connections within the cord, the stimulation of stretch receptors in a muscle or a tendon automatically triggers an immediate contraction of the muscle. In the knee jerk reflex, the hammer blow stretches the tendon of the quadriceps. This reflexly causes contraction of the quadriceps, which causes the lower leg to "kick forward." Other stretch reflexes of clinical importance are the ankle jerk and the biceps and triceps reflexes. All involve stretching the muscle via a hammer tap of its tendon.

An important feature of all cord reflexes involving skeletal muscles is *reciprocal inhibition,* which occurs in the antagonist muscle of the one stimulated. For example, when a flexor reflex stimulates the biceps, it also inhibits its antagonist, the triceps, and provides for more efficient performance of motor activities in the upper arm.

Spinal cord activities also include reflex circuits, which aid in the *control of visceral functions of the body.* Sensory input arises from visceral sensory receptors and is transmitted to the spinal cord, where reflex patterns appropriate to the sensory input are determined. The signals are then transmitted to autonomic motor neurons in the gray matter of the spinal cord, which send impulses to the sympathetic nerves innervating visceral motor end organs. A most important autonomic reflex is the *peritoneal reflex.* Tissue damage in any portion of the peritoneum results in the response of this reflex which slows or stops all motor activity in the nearby viscera. Other autonomic cord reflexes are capable of *modifying local blood flow in response to cold, pain, and heat.* This vascular control by autonomic reflexes in the spinal cord can operate as a backup mechanism for the usual brain stem control patterns in patients with transectional injuries at the brain stem.

Also included in the autonomic reflexes of the spinal cord are those causing the *emptying of the urinary bladder and the rectum.* When the bowel or bladder becomes distended, sensory signals from stretch receptors in the bowel or bladder wall are transmitted via sensory neurons to the internuncial neurons of the upper sacral and lower lumbar segments of the cord. These neurons in turn stimulate parasympathetic motor neurons innervating the wall of the bowel or bladder and its internal sphincter. Somatic motor neurons innervating the extrinsic sphincter muscles are also reflexly stimulated by the internuncials. The net result of such motor neuron stimulation is a reflex contraction of bowel or bladder and an opening of the sphincters, thereby permitting defecation or micturition.

Descending fibers from the cerebral cortex also synapse with the internuncials. These fibers act to inhibit the reflex emptying of bowel or bladder at times or places deemed inappropriate by the individual. Toilet training of infants must await the functional maturation of these descending fibers. Cord transections or other damage above the level of the cord housing the neurons for the bowel or bladder evacuation reflexes will interrupt some or all of these descending fibers. This produces a condition wherein the patient cannot consciously control (*i.e.,* prevent) the emptying of his bowel or bladder or both. Damage to that level of the cord housing the anatomical neuronal connections for these reflexes (*e.g.,* spina bifida, cord shock, severe injuries to the sacral lower or lumbar cord) will prevent reflex evacuation of bowel or bladder or both. Such a patient may exhibit retention with overflow but will not possess any effective mechanism for emptying his bowel or bladder or both.

Brain Reflexes

Brain reflexes operate in the same way as do cord reflexes, except that the brain houses the connection, not the cord. Brain reflexes include those involving the *cardioregulatory and vasomotor centers* of the medulla, plus the pupillary adjustment center, which involves the midbrain. Because the sensory and motor arms of the heart rate and vasopressure reflexes are commonly known, we will discuss only the *pupillary reflex.*

Light in the retina causes stimulation of the optic nerve. Fibers in this nerve travel to the Edinger-Westphal nucleus in the midbrain. Here the sensory fibers synapse with interneurons. The result is outgoing autonomic motor impulses to the smooth muscles of the iris. Increases in parasympathetic impulses (by way of cranial nerve III) or decreases in sympathetic impulses cause pupillary constriction in response to the light. As the light stimulus of the retina decreases, this reflex causes pupillary dilation. Lack of this reflex signifies damage to the midbrain–optic fiber connection or to the oculomotor nerve (cranial nerve III).

Pain

The sensation of pain warrants special consideration because it plays such an important protective role for the body. Whenever there is tissue damage, nerve endings are stimulated and the sensation of pain is felt. This sensation is usually felt during the time that tissue is undergoing damage and ceases when the damage ends. This condition is due to the release of chemicals and metabolites such as histamine and bradykinin from damaged cells. Typical damaging stimuli are trauma (cutting, crushing, tearing), ischemia, and intense heat and cold.

In addition to these stimuli, acidity of the tissue fluid at the nerve fiber ending is now known to stimulate pain sensations that can be eliminated by making this fluid alkaline.

Variation in pain thresholds both among different people and within the same person at different times has been long known. (This is in addition to the wide variation in people's reactions to pain.) It was formerly thought that the sensation of pain depended in large part on the number of "pain receptor endings" that were simultaneously and continuously stimulated as well as on variations in cortical or brain stem thresholds.

Large Cutaneous Afferents

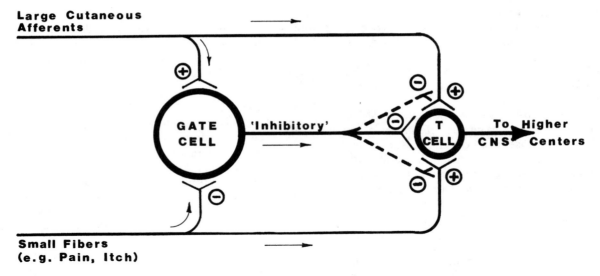

Small Fibers (e.g. Pain, Itch)

FIGURE 23-15
Spinal gate theory. (After Melzack R, Wall P: Pain mechanisms: A new theory. Science 150:971–979, 1965)

Gate Theory. More recent evidence, however, points to the existence of gating mechanisms in the substantia gelatinosa at all levels of the spinal cord, which are capable of regulating the amount of pain impulses that can enter the spinothalamic tract and travel to the brain. This cord level of pain regulation opens new avenues to the treatment of pain.

Briefly, two types of fibers are involved. One is a small diameter (S) fiber that carries impulses responsible for the sensation of pain (pain impulses). The other is a large diameter (L) fiber that carries impulses responsible for cutaneous tactile sensations. The S- and L-fibers each synapse with two other cells—a gate cell and a T-cell of the spinothalamic tract. The gate cell also synapses with the T-cell and acts to *inhibit* (by hyperpolarization) the T-cell. L-fiber impulses stimulate the gate cell, thereby hyperpolarizing the T-cell to a certain degree. S-fiber impulses inhibit the gate cell and stimulate the T-cell. Because the gate cell is inhibited, the T-cell is not. Thus, by itself, the S-fiber impulse readily gains access to the spinothalamic tract.

If tactile skin receptors *in the same dermatome* are stimulated simultaneously with S-fibers, the action of the L-fibers will (by way of the gate cell) hyperpolarize the T-cell and thereby make it more difficult for S-fiber impulses to stimulate the T-cell (gain access to the spinothalamic tract). Thus the relative S- to L-fiber activity can determine the degree of pain impulses that can enter the CNS at the level of the cord (Fig. 23-15).

Rubbing or other tactile sensation such as provided by transcutaneous nerve (skin) stimulation applied to a painful area may reduce the sensation of pain perceived by the patient.

Although much more remains to be learned, we know that primitive sensations of pain occur once the ascending impulses from the spinothalamic tract reach the midbrain, and more refined and somewhat localized perception occurs at the level of the thalamus. Most refined and localized sensations, as well as their significance to the person, occur at the level of the cortex.

Referred Pain. This type of pain is perceived as arising from a site that is different from its true point of origin. Well-known examples include the referring of pain from severe cardiac ischemia to the left arm or the referring of diaphragmatic pain to the neck and shoulder. The "true point of origin" for this type of pain is usually some visceral organ or deep somatic structure and the "point of reference" is some area of the body surface. A knowledge of the embryological development of various parts of the body provides an understanding of the physiological basis of referred pain. The true point of origin and its common referred-to areas were at one time, embryologically, close together and are innervated by sensory neurons that enter the same segment of the spinal cord. Even though the two areas move farther apart in the normal growth and development of a person, their innervation persists. Thus, sensory impulses originating from painful stimuli in either the "true" or "referred" body areas will enter the same level of the cord and synapse with the same neurons of the spinothalamic pathway at this level. There is no way for the cerebral cortex to "know" whether a given spinothalamic neuron was originally stimulated by pain from the true point of origin or the referred-to area. In localizing the source of the pain stimulus, the cortex relies on prior experience regarding the person's geographical knowledge of his own body. Because surface areas are more familiar to a person than the locations of his visceral or deep somatic structures, the referred-to locale is preferentially used over the more unfamiliar but true point of origin.

Endogenous Opiates. These are substances that in terms of molecular structure and action resemble opiate drugs. Two types are known: enkephalins and endorphins. Enkephalins are pentapeptides synthesized by certain CNS neurons. They appear to function as inhibitory neurotransmitters in pathways conducting impulses concerning pain (nociception). Stimulation of "enkephalinergic neurons" produces analgesia similar to that produced by opiate drugs. Enkephalins bind to opiate receptors on the postsynaptic membrane. In most cases, this inhibits (hyperpolarizes) the postsynaptic neuron by decreasing its sodium influx.

Opiate receptors and enkephalins have been discovered in various locations with the CNS. These locations function in the conduction of "pain impulses" up the cord and brain stem to the cortex, in areas associated with emotional effects produced by opiates, or in "analgesic centers" within the brain stem. One location is that part of the dorsal horn of gray matter housing the "spinal gate." Here, enkephalinergic neurons, which receive impulses from descending fibers of the nucleus raphe magnus in the medulla, in turn act on sensory neurons to inhibit the stimulation of T-cells by small fibers. This inhibits the entry of "pain impulses" into the spinothalamic tract. Enkephalins and opiate receptors exist in the medullary respiratory center. The latter perhaps explains the potent action of opiate drugs on respiration. They are also found in certain limbic system structures (*e.g.,* amygdala). This may explain the emotional effects produced by natural and synthetic opiate drugs. It also suggests that endogenous opiates may function in naturally evoked feelings of pleasure or well-being. The role of enkephalins and opiate receptors found in other brain centers, such as the basal ganglia and neocortex, is unclear at this time.

Enkephalins and opiate receptors are also richly distributed in three "central analagesic" areas of the brain stem: (1) the raphe magnus, (2) the periacqueductal gray matter of the midbrain, and (3) areas bordering the third ventricle in the thalamus. Electrical stimulation of these areas is known to produce varying but strong, widespread analgesic effects. Electrical stimulation of the first two areas produces a systemic analgesia that lasts for hours after the stimulation is stopped. It is one current modality for the treatment of intractable pain, but its effects are limited because (1) patients develop tolerance to therapy as they do to narcotics; and (2) there is cross tolerance between such "electrical-stimulation–produced analgesia" and narcotic drugs. The exact manner by which these areas produce analgesia is not currently known, but enkephalins are clearly involved as mediators because opiate blocking drugs such as naloxone will inhibit such electrical-stimulation–produced analgesia.

The raphe magnus (in the medulla) functions in regulating the spinal gates. Descending fibers from the raphe synapse at all levels of the cord with enkephalinergic internuncial neurons that regulate the ability of "pain-stimulated" sensory neurons to stimulate spinothalamic neurons. Thus, the raphe magnus controls the entry of pain impulses into the pain conduction system in the first place. What cannot enter cannot be perceived. It is not clear whether this raphe is, in turn, regulated by either of the two higher analgesic centers.

Opiate drugs exert their effects by binding with the opiate receptors in many or all of these areas — depending on dosage. Acupuncture and various "placebo analgesics" seem to act by causing a release of endogenous opiates because, in double blind studies, their analgesic effects are blocked by naloxone. Parts of the CNS involved in such analgesia are currently unknown. Differing levels of enkephalinergic neuron activity (especially in central analgesic areas) may provide a physiological basis for individual differences in pain reports and tolerances.

Endorphins are part of the pro-opiomelanocortin (POMC) molecule that is secreted by the corticotrop cells of the anterior pituitary (see Chap. 34). They consist of any segment of this POMC that also contains the five amino acid enkephalin sequence (represented by amino acids numbers 61 to 65). They bind to various opiate receptors in brain, especially the basal ganglia and the limbic system, and seem to function in endogenously produced analgesia. Their exact role or roles are unknown.

BIBLIOGRAPHY

Chaffee EE, Lytle IM: Basic Physiology and Anatomy, 4th ed. Philadelphia, JB Lippincott, 1980

Chusid JG: Correlative Neuroanatomy and Functional Neurology, 17th ed. Los Altos, Lange Medical Publications, 1979

Eccles JC: The Understanding of the Brain, 2nd ed. New York, McGraw-Hill, 1977

Eliasson SG et al: Neurological pathophysiology, 2nd ed. Oxford, Oxford University Press, 1978

Ganong WF: Review of Medical Physiology, 11th ed. Los Altos, Lange Medical Publications, 1983

Hickey J: The Clinical Practice of Neurological and Neurosurgical Nursing, Philadelphia, JB Lippincott, 1981

Hospital Practice, Special Report: Recent studies on the nature and management of acute pain. January, 1976

Melzack R, Wall PD: Pain mechanisms: A new theory. Science 150:971–979, 1965

Mountcastle VB: Medical Physiology. St Louis, CV Mosby, 1980

Nathan PW: The gate-control theory of pain: A critical review. Brain 99:213–258, 1976

Stephens G: Pathophysiology for Health Practitioners. New York, Macmillan, 1980

24
Assessment: Nervous System

Neurologic Nursing Assessment

Suzanne Provenzano*

For many critical care nurses, assessment and care of a patient with a neurologic problem constitute one of the biggest challenges—and one of the biggest headaches! In basic nursing education and in many critical care courses, an assessment of nervous system functioning is frequently covered last and not to the depth or complexity of other body systems. It is not uncommon, then, for even the experienced caregiver to feel confused when gathering data about the nervous system.

There are two major goals in the assessment of a patient with a real or potential neurologic problem. The first goal is to gather data about nervous system functioning in an objective and orderly manner. Data can be considered objective if several examiners, seeing the same phenomenon or behavior, would give similar descriptions. There should be a standard neurologic check sheet that is used by all the nursing staff, with clearly defined grading scales or terms to be used (*e.g.,* "stuporous" to one person may mean "lethargic" to another).

The second objective of neurologic assessment is to correlate the data over time. For such a correlation to be of value, the results of history, physical assessment, and diagnostic tests must be interrelated. Consideration of the information in a patterned format will help

* The author acknowledges the contribution of Corinne A. Cloughen, R.N., who prepared this material in the prevous edition.

in the establishment of both medical and nursing diagnoses and guide one in choosing and evaluating therapy.

HISTORY

Neurologic assessment by the nurse begins the moment she sees the patient. As she asks the patient routine questions about his problem, she should be alert for alterations in mental state, speech patterns, and thought processes. In reconstructing the story of the present illness, she should ask questions geared to detection of neurologic problems. It is helpful to have a family member or friend present who can confirm and clarify the patient's responses.

What to ask about

- Recent trauma that could affect the nervous system, (*e.g.,* a fall or an automobile accident).
- Recent infections, including sinusitis and ear or tooth infections.
- Recent headaches and problems with concentration and memory.
- Feelings of dizziness, loss of balance, "black-out" spells, tinnitus, and hearing problems.
- Clumsiness or weakness of the extremities and difficulty walking.
- Sensory distortions (*e.g.,* numbness, tingling, hypersensitivity, pain) or sensory loss in face, trunk, or extremities.
- Impotence or difficulty in urination.
- Recent difficulties in performing everyday activities.

A medical history is also important because it helps one ascertain evidence of vascular disease, diabetes, renal disease, anemia, cancer, and other metabolic dysfunctions that can complicate the neurologic picture. The patient's mental and emotional status as well as general intelligence should be noted. These aspects of the assessment may be delayed if the patient requires immediate medical attention.

LEVEL OF CONSCIOUSNESS

The quality of a patient's consciousness is the most basic and most critical parameter requiring assessment. The level of a patient's awareness of, and response to, his environment is the most sensitive indicator of nervous system dysfunction. Data about a patient's response to his internal and external environments should include information about orientation, recent and remote memory, judgment, reason, and social behavior.

In a critical care setting, where time for such in-depth data-gathering is limited, the Glasgow Coma Scale or a similar scale can provide a useful shortcut. Such a scale allows the nurse to grade objectively the patient's three major responses to the environment — eye opening, movement, and verbalization (Table 24-1). The patient's score is recorded as an eye, motor, verbal (EMV) sum, with a possible range of 3 to 15. An overall score of 8 or below is indicative of coma and, over time, is a predictor of a poor functional recovery.

An alternative to grading scales is to describe what stimulus is used and what the patient's response was. A suggested order of stimuli is as follows:

1. Call the patient by name.
2. Call his name louder.
3. Combine calling his name with light touch.
4. Combine calling his name with vigorous touch ("shake and shout").
5. Create pain.

When noxious stimuli are needed to evoke a response, the nurse should pay careful attention to where the painful stimulus is applied. It is not unknown to cause serious skin or tissue injury by a misplaced examiner's hand. Areas to avoid include the skin of the nipples and genital area. Instead, one should apply pain to the big toenail, the knuckles or nails of the fingers, the sternum, or the supraorbital ridge. When stimulating the last area, one should take care to not damage the eye itself.

MOVEMENT, STRENGTH, AND COORDINATION

Muscle weakness is a cardinal sign of dysfunction in many neurologic disorders. The nurse can test strength of extremities by offering resistance to various muscle groups, by using her own muscles, or by using gravity. As a quick test to detect weakness of the upper extremities, she can have the patient hold his arms straight out with palms upward, with his eyes closed. She should observe for any drift downward or pronation of the forearms. A similar test for the lower extremities includes having the patient raise his legs straight off the bed against the examiner's resistance. Weakness noted in any of these tests indicates damage to the upper or lower motor neuron pathways of the pyramidal system, which transmits commands for voluntary movement.

Assessment of muscle size, tone, and presence of tremors should also be made for each extremity. Dysfunctions noted here may be indicative of extrapyramidal tract disease in the diencephalon or midbrain. These pathways normally surpress involuntary movement by controlled inhibition.

The cerebellum is responsible for smooth synchronization, balance, and ordering of movements. It does *not* initiate any movements, so a patient with cerebellar dysfunction is not paralyzed. Instead, ataxia, dysmetria, and lack of synchronization of movement are common manifestations.

Some of the more common tests for cerebellar synchronization of movement with balance include the following:

• *Romberg test* — performed by having the patient stand with his feet together, first with his eyes

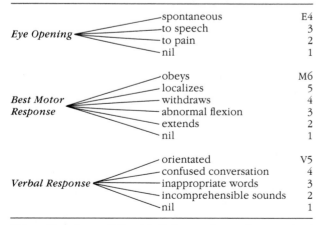

TABLE 24-1
GLASGOW COMA, OR RESPONSIVENESS, SCALE

Eye Opening	spontaneous	E4
	to speech	3
	to pain	2
	nil	1
Best Motor Response	obeys	M6
	localizes	5
	withdraws	4
	abnormal flexion	3
	extends	2
	nil	1
Verbal Response	orientated	V5
	confused conversation	4
	inappropriate words	3
	incomprehensible sounds	2
	nil	1

(Adapted from Jennett B, Teasdale G: Aspects of coma after severe head injury. Lancet 1, Pt 2:878, 1977)

open, then with eyes closed. Observe for sway or direction of falling and be prepared to catch the patient if necessary.

- *Tandem walking*—performed by having the patient walk heel to toe.
- *Finger to nose test*—performed by having the patient touch his finger to the examiner's finger, then touch his own nose. Overshooting or past-pointing the mark is called *dysmetria*. Both sides are tested individually.
- *Heel to shin test*—performed by having the patient run the heel of one foot down the shin of the other leg. This is done on both sides.
- *Rapidly alternating movement (RAM)*—checked on each side by having the patient touch each finger on one hand to his thumb in rapid succession or by performing rapid pronation and supination of

his hand on his leg. Inability to perform RAM is termed *adiadokokinesia*.

Assessment of movement and strength in a patient who cannot follow commands or is unresponsive can be difficult. For such a patient it is important to note what, if any, stimuli initiate a response and to describe or grade the type of response obtained.

Motor response in the comatose patient may be appropriate, inappropriate, or absent (Fig. 24-1, *A* to *E*). Appropriate responses, such as localization or withdrawal, mean that the sensory pathways and corticospinal pathways are functioning (Fig. 24-1, *A* and *B*). There may be monoplegia or hemiplegia, indicating that the corticospinal pathways are interrupted on one side.

Inappropriate responses include decorticate rigidity and decerebrate rigidity. *Decorticate* rigidity results

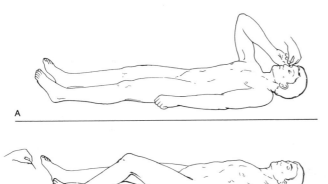

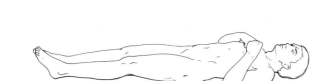

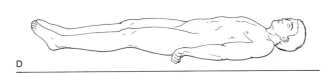

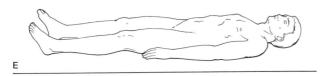

FIGURE 24-1

Motor responses to pain. When you apply a painful stimulus to your unconscious patient's supraorbital notch, he'll respond in one of these ways: (A) *Localizing pain. An appropriate response is to reach up above shoulder level toward the stimulus. Remember, a focal motor deficit such as hemiplegia may prevent a bilateral response.* (B) *Withdrawal. An appropriate response is to pull the extremity or body away from the stimulus. As brain stem involvement increases, your patient may respond by assuming one of the following postures. Each one shows more advanced deterioration.* (C) *Decorticate posturing. One or both arms in full flexion on the chest. Legs may be stiffly extended.* (D) *Decerebrate posturing. One or both arms stiffly extended. Possible extension of the legs.* (E) *Flaccid. No motor response in any extremity. An extremely ominous sign.*

TABLE 24-2

Deep Reflex Grades

4+— Very brisk response; evidence of disease and/or electrolyte imbalance; associated with clonus.
3+— A brisk response, possibly indicative of disease.
2+— A normal, average response.
1+— A response in low-normal range
0 — No response; possibly evidence of disease or electrolyte imbalance

(Reproduced with permission from Van Allen MW, Rodnitsky RL: Pictorial Manual of Neurologic Tests, 2nd ed. Copyright © 1981 by Year Book Medical Publishers, Inc, Chicago)

from lesions of the internal capsule, basal ganglia, thalamus, or cerebral hemisphere that interrupt corticospinal pathways. It is characterized by flexion of the arms, wrists, and fingers, by adduction of the upper extremities, and by extension, internal rotation, and plantar flexion of the lower extremities (Fig. 24-1, C).

Decerebrate ridigity consists of extension, adduction, and hyperpronation of the upper extremities and extension of the lower extremities, with plantar flexion of the feet (Fig. 22-1, D). Many times, the patient is also opisthotonic, with clenched teeth. Injury to the midbrain and pons results in decerebration. At times, the inappropriate responses of decortication and decerebration may switch back and forth. If there is no response to noxious stimuli or very weak flexor responses, the patient probably has extensive brain stem dysfunction (Fig. 24-1, E).

REFLEXES

A reflex occurs when a sensory stimulus evokes a motor response. Cerebral control and consciousness are not required for a reflex to occur. Superficial and deep reflexes are tested on symmetrical sides of the body and compared in relation with the strength of contraction elicited. Deep reflexes are commonly graded on a scale of 0 to 4, where grade 2 is indicative of normal response. (Table 24-2). Pathologic reflexes should be noted, including the presence of a Babinski sign (dorsiflexion of the big toe and fanning of the toes when the sole of the foot is stroked). This indicates pyramidal tract (upper motor neuron) dysfunction in a person over 2 to 3 years of age (Table 24-3).

PUPILLARY CHANGES

In conjunction with assessing the level of consciousness, one must check the pupils frequently. Pupils are best checked in a darkened room for size, shape,

equality, and reaction to light. Light directed into one eye should constrict the pupil in both eyes (consensual pupillary reflex). *Anisocoria* (unequal pupils) may be normal in a small percentage of the population or may be an indication of neural dysfunction. Ipsilateral dilation (dilation of the pupil on the same side as the injury) can be an indication of increasing intracranial pressure. Severe central or bilateral pressure at the tentorium may cause dilation and fixation of both pupils. Bilaterally constricted pupils may be due to damage to the pons and midbrain, which paralyzes the sympathetic fibers to the oculomotor nerve.

VITAL SIGNS

Classic signs of *increased intracranial pressure* (IICP) include an elevated systolic pressure in conjunction with a widening pulse pressure, slow bounding pulse, and respiratory irregularities.

Following any emergency treatment that may be indicated (*e.g.,* maintenance of the airway for adequate ventilation), vital signs should be taken immediately and followed frequently. Any indication of shock should alert one to search for signs of thoracic and intra-abdominal injuries. It must be remembered that vital signs are only signs and are not infallible in determining the patient's neurologic status (Fig. 24-2).

Hypoventilation following cerebral trauma can lead to respiratory acidosis. As the blood CO_2 increases and blood O_2 decreases, cerebral hypoxia and edema can result in secondary brain trauma. *Hyperventilation* following cerebral trauma produces respiratory alkalosis with increased blood O_2 and decreased blood CO_2 levels. This causes vasoconstriction of cerebral vessels and decreases oxygen consumption, resulting in cerebral hypoxia.

Because temperature elevation increases cellular metabolism, measures should be implemented to maintain temperature in the normal range, or hypothermia may be induced if indicated.

CRANIAL NERVES

I. Olfactory. The first cranial nerve contains sensory fibers for the sense of smell. This test is usually deferred unless the patient complains of an inability to smell. One tests the nerve, with the patient's eyes closed, by placing aromatic substances near his nose for identification. Fragrances that have a distinct smell (*e.g.,* soap, coffee, or cinnamon) should be used. Ammonia should not be used because the patient will respond to irritation of the nasal mucosa rather than the odor. Each nostril is checked separately. Loss of

TABLE 24-3
TESTS FOR REFLEX STATUS

		Deep Reflexes	
Reflex	Site of Stimulus	Normal Response	Pertinent Central Nervous System Segment
Biceps	Biceps tendon	Contraction of biceps	Cervical 5 and 6
Brachioradialis	Styloid process of radius	Flexion of the elbow and pronation of the forearm	Cervical 5 and 6
Triceps	Triceps tendon above the olecranon	Extension of elbow	Cervical 6, 7, and 8
Patellar	Patellar tendon	Extension of the leg at the knee	Lumbar 2, 3, and 4
Achilles	Achilles tendon	Plantar flexion of the foot	Sacral 1 and 2

	Superficial Reflexes	
Reflex	Normal Response	Pertinent Central Nervous System Segment
Upper abdominal	Umbilicus moves up and toward area being stroked	Thoracic 7, 8, and 9
Lower abdominal	Umbilicus moves down	Thoracic 11 and 12
Cremasteric	Scrotum elevates	Thoracic 12 and lumbar 1
Plantar	Flexion of the toes	Sacral 1 and 2
Gluteal	Skin tenses at gluteal area	Lumbar 4 through sacral 3

	Pathologic Reflexes	
Reflex	How Elicited	Response
Babinski	Stroke lateral aspect of sole of foot	In pyramidal tract disease, an extension or dorsiflexion of the big toe occurs — in addition to fanning of the toes
Chaddock	Stroke lateral aspect of foot beneath the lateral malleolus	Same type of response
Oppenheim	Stroke the anteromedial tibial surface	Same type of response
Gordon	Squeeze the calf muscles firmly	Same type of response

(DeJong RN, Sahs Al et al: Essentials of the Neurological Examination, pp. 39–47. Philadelphia, Smith Kline Corporation, 1976)

smell may be caused by a fracture of the cribiform plate or a fracture in the ethmoid area.

II. Optic. One checks gross visual acuity by having the patient read ordinary newsprint. The patient's preinjury need for glasses should be noted. One can test visual field by having the patient look straight ahead with one eye covered. The examiner will move a finger from the periphery of each quadrant of vision toward the patient's center of vision. The patient should indicate when he sees the examiner's finger. This is done for both eyes, and the results are compared with the examiner's visual fields, which are assumed to be normal. Damage to the retina will produce a blind spot. An optic nerve lesion will produce partial or complete blindness on the same side. Damage to the optic chiasm results in bitemporal hemianopsia, blindness in both lateral visual fields. Pressure on the optic tract can cause homonymous hemianopsia, half blindness on the opposite side of the lesion in both eyes. A lesion in the parietal or temporal lobe may produce contralateral blindness in the upper or lower quadrant of vision respectively in both eyes (this is known as *quadrant deficit*). Damage in the occipital lobe may cause homonymous hemianopsia with central vision sparing (Fig. 24-3).

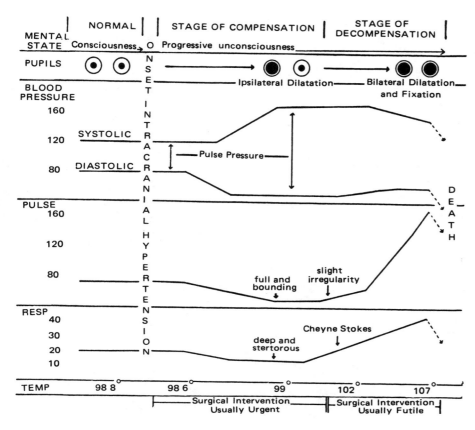

FIGURE 24-2

Chart showing changes in mental state, pupils, blood pressure, pulse rate, respiratory rate, and temperature before and after the onset of fatal increase of intracranial pressure.

An ophthalmoscopic examination should be performed, with close observation of the optic disc, the vessels, and the periphery of the retina.

III. Oculomotor; IV. Trochlear; VI. Abducens. These cranial nerves are checked together because they all innervate extraocular muscles. The parasympathetic fibers of the oculomotor nerve are responsible for lens accommodation and pupil size through control of the ciliary muscles. The motor fibers of the oculomotor nerve innervate the muscles that elevate the eyelid as well as those that move the eyes up, down, and medially, including the superior rectus, inferior oblique, inferior rectus, and medial rectus muscles. The trochlear nerve innervates the superior oblique muscle to move the eyes down and in. The lateral rectus muscle moves the eyes laterally and is innervated by the abducens nerve. Diplopia, nystagmus, conjugate deviation, and ptosis may indicate dysfunction of these cranial nerves. These nerves are tested by having the patient follow the examiner's finger with his eyes as it is moved in all directions of gaze (Fig. 24-4).

V. Trigeminal. The trigeminal nerve has three divisions: ophthalmic, maxillary, and mandibular. The sensory portion of this nerve controls sensation to the face and cornea. The motor portion controls the muscles of mastication. This nerve is partially tested by checking the corneal reflex; if it is intact, the patient will blink when the cornea is stroked with a wisp of cotton. Facial sensation can be tested by comparing light touch and pinprick on symmetrical sides of the face. The ability to chew or clench the jaw should also be observed.

VII. Facial. The sensory portion of this nerve is concerned with taste on the anterior two thirds of the tongue. The motor portion controls muscles of facial expression (Fig. 24-5). With a central (supranuclear) lesion, there is muscle paralysis of the lower half of the face on the side opposite the lesion. The muscles about the eyes and forehead are not affected. In a peripheral (nuclear or infranuclear) lesion, there is complete paralysis of facial muscles on the same side as the lesion.

The most common type of peripheral facial paralysis

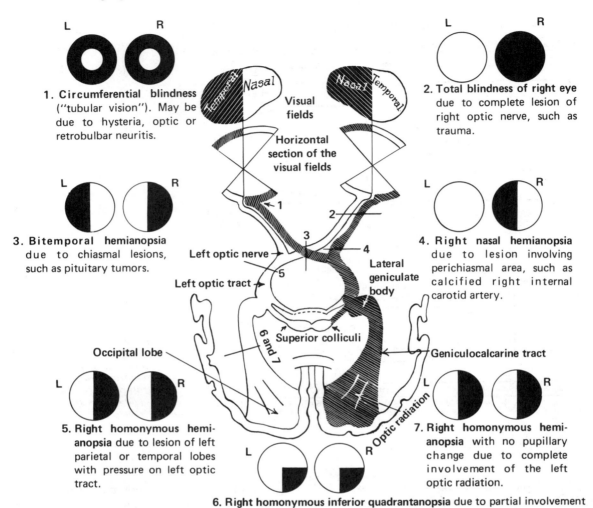

L R

1. **Circumferential blindness** ("tubular vision"). May be due to hysteria, optic or retrobulbar neuritis.

Visual fields

Horizontal section of the visual fields

L R

2. **Total blindness of right eye** due to complete lesion of right optic nerve, such as trauma.

L R

3. **Bitemporal hemianopsia** due to chiasmal lesions, such as pituitary tumors.

Left optic nerve →

Left optic tract →

Lateral geniculate body

L R

4. **Right nasal hemianopsia** due to lesion involving perichiasmal area, such as calcified right internal carotid artery.

Superior colliculi

Occipital lobe

Geniculocalcarine tract

L R

5. **Right homonymous hemianopsia** due to lesion of left parietal or temporal lobes with pressure on left optic tract.

Optic radiation

L R

7. **Right homonymous hemianopsia** with no pupillary change due to complete involvement of the left optic radiation.

L R

6. **Right homonymous inferior quadrantanopsia** due to partial involvement of optic radiations (upper portion of left optic radiation in this case).

FIGURE 24-3
Visual field defects associated with lesions of visual system. (Reproduced, with permission, from Chusid JG: Correlative Neuroanatomy & Functional Neurology, 17th ed, p 91. Copyright 1979, Lange Medical Publications, Los Altos, California)

is Bell's palsy, which consists of ipsilateral facial paralysis. There is drooping of the upper lid with the lower lid slightly everted, and facial lines on the same side are obliterated with the mouth drawn toward the normal side. Artificial tears and taping the eye closed may be indicated to prevent corneal abrasion and irritation.

VIII. Acoustic. This nerve is divided into the cochlear and vestibular branches, which control hearing and equilibrium, respectively.

The cochlear nerve is tested by air and bone conduction. A vibrating tuning fork is placed on the mastoid process; after the patient can no longer hear the fork,

he should be able to hear it for a few seconds longer when it is placed in front of his ear (Rinne's test). The patient may complain of tinnitus or decreased hearing if this nerve is damaged.

The vestibular nerve may not be routinely evaluated. The nurse should be alert, however, to complaints of dizziness or vertigo from the patient.

IX. Glossopharyngeal; X. Vagus. These cranial nerves are usually tested together. The glossopharyngeal nerve supplies sensory fibers to the posterior third of the tongue as well as the uvula and soft palate. The vagus innervates the larynx, pharynx, and soft pal-

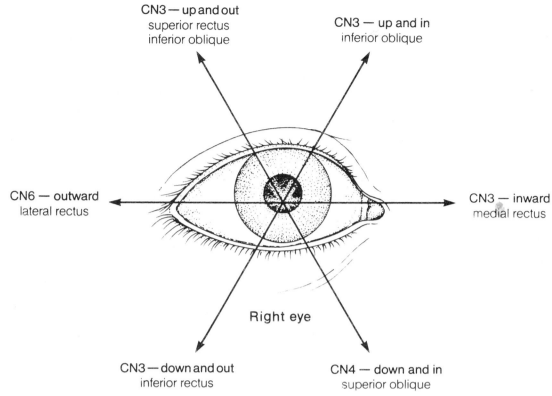

CN3 — up and out
superior rectus
inferior oblique

CN3 — up and in
inferior oblique

CN6 — outward
lateral rectus

CN3 — inward
medial rectus

Right eye

CN3 — down and out
inferior rectus

CN4 — down and in
superior oblique

FIGURE 24-4
Muscles used in conjugate eye movements in the six cardinal directions of gaze. (Adapted from Bates: A Guide to Physical Examination, 3rd ed, p 59. Philadelphia, JB Lippincott, 1983)

ate and conveys autonomic responses to the heart, stomach, lungs, and small intestines. Autonomic vagal functions are not usually tested because they are checked during the general physical examination. One can test these nerves by eliciting a gag reflex, observing the uvula for symmetrical movement when the patient says "ah," or observing midline elevation of the uvula when both sides are stroked. Inability to cough forcefully, difficulty with swallowing, and hoarseness may be signs of dysfunction.

XI. Spinal Accessory. This nerve controls the trapezius and sternocleidomastoid muscles. The examiner tests this nerve by having the patient shrug his shoulders or turn his head from side to side against resistance.

XII. Hypoglossal. This nerve controls tongue movement. It can be checked by having the patient protrude his tongue. Check for deviation from midline, tremor, and atrophy. If deviation is noted secondary to damage of the nerve, it will be to the side of the lesion.

OCULAR SIGNS IN THE UNCONSCIOUS PATIENT

Ocular position and movement are among the most useful guides to the site of brain dysfunction in the comatose patient. When observing the eyes at rest, it is not uncommon for one to note a slight divergency of gaze. If both eyes are conjugately deviated to one side, there is possible dysfunction either in the frontal lobe on that side or in the controlateral pontine area of the brain stem. Downward deviation suggests a dysfunction in the midbrain.

"Doll's Eyes" and Caloric Reflex

Although the unconscious patient cannot participate in the examination by moving his eyes through fields of gaze voluntarily, the examiner can still test his range of ocular movement using the oculocephalic ("doll's eyes") and oculovestibular (caloric) reflexes.

One can assess the oculocephalic reflex by quickly rotating the patient's head to one side and observing

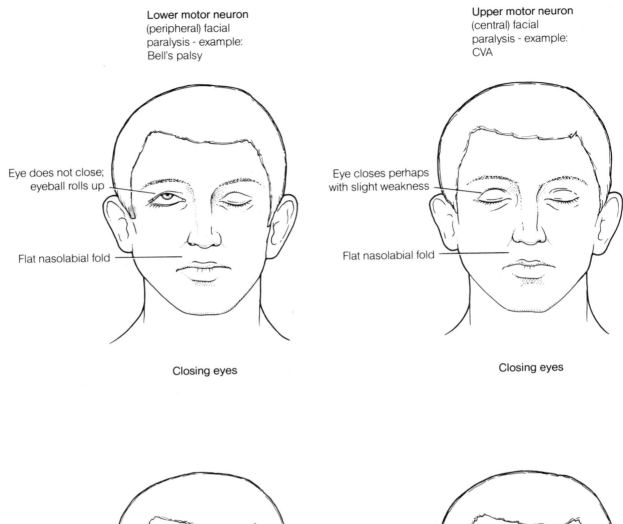

Lower motor neuron
(peripheral) facial
paralysis - example:
Bell's palsy

Upper motor neuron
(central) facial
paralysis - example:
CVA

Eye does not close;
eyeball rolls up

Eye closes perhaps
with slight weakness

Flat nasolabial fold

Flat nasolabial fold

Closing eyes

Closing eyes

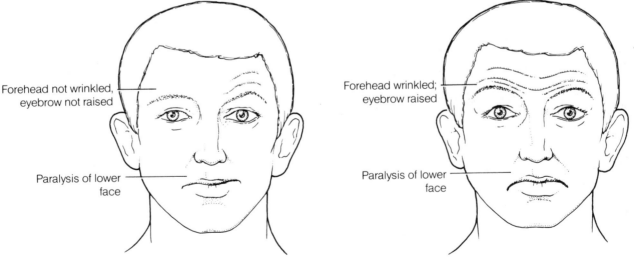

Forehead not wrinkled,
eyebrow not raised

Forehead wrinkled;
eyebrow raised

Paralysis of lower
face

Paralysis of lower
face

Raising eyebrows

Raising eyebrows

FIGURE 24-5
Facial movements with upper and lower motor neuron facial paralysis. (Adapted from Bates: A Guide to Physical Examination, 3rd ed, pp 416–417. Philadelphia, JB Lippincott, 1983)

the position of the eyes (Fig. 24-6). This maneuver must *never* be performed in a patient with possible cervical spine injury. A normal response consists of initial conjugate deviation of the eyes in the opposite direction then, within a few seconds, smooth and simultaneous movement of both eyes back to midline position.

An abnormal reflex response occurs when one eye does not follow the normal response pattern. Absence of any ocular movement when the head is briskly rotated to either side or up and down indicates an absent reflex and portends severe brain stem dysfunction.

The examiner tests oculovestibular reflex (caloric test) by elevating the patient's head 30° and irrigating each ear separately with 30 to 50 ml of iced water (Fig. 24-7). This test should never be performed in a patient who does not have an intact eardrum or who has blood or fluid collected behind it. In an unconscious patient with an intact brain stem, the eyes will exhibit horizontal nystagmus with slow, conjugate movement toward the irrigated ear followed by rapid movement away from the stimulus. When the reflex is absent, both eyes remain fixed in midline position, indicating midbrain and pons dysfunction.

SENSATION

The primary forms of sensation are evaluated first. These include light touch, superficial pain, temperature, and vibration. With the patient's eyes closed, multiple areas of the body are tested, including the hands, forearms, upper arms, trunk, thighs, lower legs, and feet.

The patient's ability to perceive the sensation should be noted, with distal areas compared with proximal areas and right and left sides compared at corresponding areas. One should determine whether sensory change involves one entire side of the body. Abnormal results may indicate damage somewhere along the pathways of the receptors in the skin, muscles, joints and tendons, spinothalamic tracts, or sensory area of the cortex.

Cortical forms of sensation should also be tested. Disturbances of these forms, when the primary forms of sensation are intact, indicate damage to the parietal lobe.

The inability to recognize objects by sight, touch, or sound is termed *agnosia.* The ability to recognize and identify objects by touch is called *stereognosis* and is a function of the parietal lobe. Identification of an object by the sense of sight is a function of the parieto-occipital junction. The temporal lobe is responsible for identification of objects by sound. Each of these senses should be tested separately. For example, a patient may not be able to identify a whistle by its sound but

may recognize it immediately if he holds it or looks at it.

Other cortical forms of sensation include the following:

- *Graphesthesia*—the ability to recognize numbers or letters traced lightly on the skin. Bilateral sides are compared.
- *Point localization*—the ability to locate a spot on the body touched by the examiner.
- *Two-point discrimination*—tested by using two sharp objects and determining the smallest area in which two points can be perceived.
- *Extinction phenomenon*—the inability to recognize that two areas have been touched when the examiner simultaneously touches two identical areas on opposite sides of the body.
- *Texture discrimination*—the ability to recognize materials such as cotton, burlap, and wool by feeling them.

DIAGNOSTIC TESTS

The complexity of the nervous system makes identification of specific dysfunction difficult. Modern diagnostic procedures now help unravel the mystery of neurologic structure and functioning (see following section).

OTHER OBSERVATIONS

- *Battle's sign,* bruising over the mastoid areas, suggests basal skull fracture.
- *Raccoon's eye,* or periorbital edema and bruising, suggests frontobasilar fracture.
- *Rhinorrhea,* drainage of cerebral spinal fluid (CSF) via the nose suggests fracture of the cribiform plate with herniation of a fragment of the dura and arachnoid through the fracture.
- *Otorrhea,* drainage of CSF from the ear, is usually associated with fracture of the petrous portion of the temporal bone.
- *Meningeal irritation* can be detected by the presence of nuchal rigidity in conjunction with pyrexia, headache, and photophobia. A positive Kernig's sign, pain in the neck when the thigh is flexed on the abdomen and the leg extended at the knee, also may be present.

Throughout the neurologic assessment, the examiner should note the patient's behavior for appropriateness, emotional status, cooperativeness, attention span and memory.

Following the neurologic examination, the nurse should record her findings, placing particular empha-

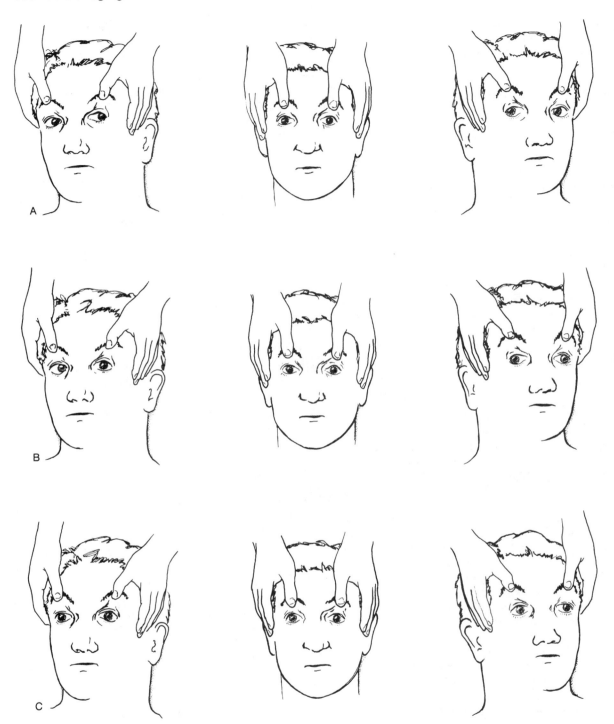

FIGURE 24-6

Test for oculocephalic reflex response (doll's eyes phenomenon). (A) Normal response — when the head is rotated, the eyes turn together to the side opposite to the head movement. (B) Abnormal response — when the head is rotated, the eyes do not turn in a conjugate manner. (C) Absent response — as head position is changed, eyes do not move in the sockets.

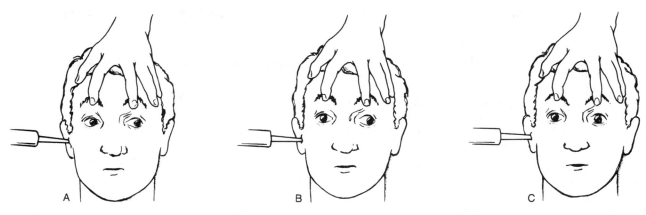

FIGURE 24-7
Test for oculovestibular reflex response (caloric ice water test). (A) *Normal response — ice water infusion in the ear produces conjugate eye movements.* (B) *Abnormal response — infusion produces dysconjugate or asymmetric eye movements.* (C) *Absent response — infusion produces no eye movements.*

sis on the abnormalities. Frequent reevaluation is necessary to ascertain change in the patient's condition.

BRAIN DEATH

The patient's condition may be so severe that brain death (Table 24-4) is the final outcome. The critical care nurse provides essential nursing care to such a patient as treatment is continued or as life-support measures are withdrawn. The nurse is involved in determining whether the patient has suffered brain death.

Many years ago, the common acceptable understanding of death was "total stoppage of the circulation of the blood and a cessation of vital functions such as respiration, pulsation, etc." In the 1960s, the advent of cardiopulmonary resuscitation measures made this criterion of death obsolete. In 1968, a landmark report was published by the Ad Hoc Committee of the Harvard Medical School to Examine the Definition of Death. This established the first widely accepted criteria to determine brain death. Finally, in 1979, the AMA House of Delegates passed a model bill on the following definition of death:

> "An individual who has sustained either (a) irreversible cessation of circulatory and respiratory functions, or (b) irreversible cessation of all functions of the entire brain, should be considered dead. A determination of death shall be made in accordance with accepted medical standards."*

* (From American Medical Association: Model Bill. Chicago, American Medical Association, 1979)

TABLE 24-4
POSSIBLE CLINICAL CRITERIA FOR BRAIN DEATH

Nature of the Comatose State Must be Determined

1. Drugs must be excluded as a possible cause of the coma.
2. The patient may not be hypothermic (*i.e.,* body temperature must exceed 33°C, or 91.4°F).
3. There must be an appropriate period of observation of patient in comatose state for adequate assessment.

Absence of All Cortical/Brain Stem Function Must Be Established

1. Absence of all cerebral responses to light, noise, motion, and pain.
2. Absence of all reflexes or muscle activity unless the reflex activity is determined to be of spinal cord origin.
3. Absence of spontaneous respirations with respirator disconnected for at least 3 minutes, with a PCO_2 of 55 mm Hg at least to stimulate respiratory response. Some institutions do not advocate arterial blood gases and do not recommend complete apnea for 3 minutes for fear of causing more neuronal death if viable brain function remains. In such institutions, high levels of oxygen are administered passively through endotracheal or tracheostomy tubes for rather prolonged periods without respiration for confirmation of apnea.
4. Absence of cranial nerve reflexes: fixed pupils that do not react to light and absence of oculovestibular reflex (caloric ice test response).

In addition, other tests may be required, for example:

5. Isoelectric electroencephalogram (EEG). Some institutions require only one isoelectric EEG; others require two, 12 hours apart.
6. Absence of intracranial blood flow, as demonstrated by angiography, radioisotope techniques, echo pulsation, or computed tomography scan after administration of contrast medium.

(From Rudy ER: Brain death. Dimens Crit Care Nurs 1, No. 3:183, 1982)

The first legal statute recognizing the concept of brain death was enacted in Kansas in the early 1970s. Since then, over 28 states have passed similar statutes. Today, the recognition of brain death is widespread, even in those states without such statutes. The adoption of clinical criteria to determine brain death has been facilitated by larger medical centers and by institutions actively involved in organ-transplant surgery.

The role of the nurse who is caring for a potentially brain dead patient is threefold:

- Question the possibility of brain death.
- Assist in gathering data necessary to determine brain death.
- Provide support, understanding, and empathy for the patient's family.

These tasks become even more difficult for the critical care nurse. It is often very hard to "switch gears" from fighting for a patient's life one day to accepting death the next day.

BIBLIOGRAPHY

Bates B: A Guide to Physical Examination, 3rd ed. Philadelphia, JB Lippincott, 1983
Demyer W: Technique of the Neurologic Examination, 3rd ed. New York: McGraw-Hill, 1980
King RC: Checking the patient's neurologic status. RN 45:57–62, 1982
Nursing Skillbook: Coping with Neurologic Problems Proficiently. Horsham, PA, Intermed Communications, 1980
Plum F, Posner JB: The Diagnosis of Stupor and Coma, 3rd ed. Philadelphia, FA Davis, 1980
Ricci MM (ed): Core Curriculum for Neuroscience Nurses, 2nd ed. Park Ridge, IL, American Association of Neuroscience Nurses, 1984
Rudy ER: Advanced Neurological and Neurosurgical Nursing. St Louis, CV Mosby, 1984
Smith BH: Differential Diagnosis, Neurology. New York, Arco Publishing, 1979
Snyder M, Jackle J: Neurologic Problems: A Critical Care Nursing Focus. Bowie, MD, Robert J Brady, 1981
Van Allen MW, Rodnitzky RL: Pictorial Manual of Neurologic Tests, 2nd ed. Chicago, Year Book Medical Publishers, 1981
Walleck CA: A neurologic assessment procedure that won't make you nervous. Nursing '82 12:50–58, 1982

Neurodiagnostic Techniques

Robert W. Hendee, Jr.

A number of modalities are now available to assist in the diagnosis of neurologic/neurosurgical problems. Owing to the proliferation and the overall accuracy of these technologies, there has been an unfortunate trend toward simplification of the basic clinical neurologic examination. However, the availability and diagnostic accuracy may benefit the patient in acute deterioration by shortening the time required to arrive at a diagnosis and institute a plan for treatment. Some of the older technology is now used less frequently (*e.g.,* pneumoencephalography and ventriculography), at least in the classic sense) but occasionally may still be very helpful. Modification of the older techniques also is now invaluable at times (*e.g.,* metrizamide ventriculography in conjunction with computed tomography). Table 24-5 summarizes some of the techniques that will be discussed and outlines nursing implications.

PLAIN RADIOGRAPHS OF THE SKULL AND SPINE

Plain radiographs of the skull and spine are used frequently to assess for fractures and dislocations in acute trauma. In addition, plain radiographs may be diagnostic when displacement of the calcified pineal gland is visible and therefore can be an immediate clue to the presence of a space-occupying lesion. The presence of pneumocephalus (air inside the calvarium) also allows diagnosis of an open skull fracture, which is most often via the cribiform plate (as in frontobasilar fractures) or via the petrous bone. Basilar skull fractures may be difficult to confirm on plain radiographs, regardless of whether they are in the anterior, middle, or posterior fossa, but they should be obtained when such fractures are suspected. The suspicion or frank presence of cerebral spinal fluid draining from the nose or ear or the presence of "raccoon sign" (biperiorbital ecchymoses) or "Battle's sign" (ecchymosis over a mastoid) should cause suspicion. If the clinical situation warrants, however, immediate evaluation by computed tomography should be carried out instead.

Plain radiographs of the skull may also demonstrate infection or neoplasm manifested by irregular or regular changes in the bone density or show other intracranial calcification suggestive of, for example, chronic subdural hematoma or calcification within a tumor such as an oligodendroglioma.

TABLE 24-5
NEURODIAGNOSTIC TESTS

Diagnostic Test	What it is	What it tells you	Nursing Implications
Lumbar puncture (invasive)	A hollow needle is positioned in the subarachnoid space at L_{3-4} or L_{4-5} level, and cerebrospinal fluid (CSF) is sampled. The pressure of the CSF is also measured. Normal pressure is 50 to 200 mm water.	The CSF is examined for blood and for alterations in appearance, cell count, protein, and glucose. The opening pressure is roughly equivalent to the intracranial pressure (ICP) for most patients.	This test is contraindicated in patients with suspected increased ICP because a sudden reduction in pressure from below may cause brain structures to herniate, leading to death. In preparation for this test, position the patient on his side with knees and head flexed. Explain to the patient that he may feel some pressure as the needle is inserted and that he must not move suddenly or cough. After this procedure, keep the patient flat for 8 to 10 hours to prevent headache. Encourage liberal fluid intake.
Cerebral angiography (invasive)	This is an x-ray contrast study in which radiopaque dye is injected via a catheter into the patient's cerebral arterial circulation. The contrast medium is directed into each common carotid artery and each vertebral artery and serial radiographs are then taken.	The contrast dye illuminates the structure of the cerebral circulation. The vessel pathways are examined for patency, narrowing, and occlusion as well as structural abnormalities (aneurysms), vessel displacement (tumors, edema), and alterations in blood flow (tumors, A-V malformations)	Exercise caution with patients who are dehydrated or have renal failure or diabetes. The radiopaque dye molecule is large enough to cause obstruction in the collecting tubules of the kidney if the glomerular filtration rate is sufficient to flush it downstream to the bladder. In preparation for this test, inform the patient as to the location of the catheter insertion (femoral artery is a common site) and that a local anesthetic will be used. Also warn him that a warm flushed feeling will occur when the dye is injected. After this procedure, assess the puncture site for swelling, redness, and bleeding. Also check the skin color, temperature, and peripheral pulses of the extremity distal to the site for signs of arterial insufficiency due to vasospasm or clotting.
Digital subtraction angiography (invasive)	In this test, a plain radiograph is taken of the patient's cranium. Then, radiopaque dye is injected into a large vein and serial radiographs are taken. A computer converts the images into digital form and "subtracts" the plain radiograph from the ones with the dye. The result is an enhanced radiographic image of contrast medium in the arterial vessels.	Extracranial circulation (arterial, capillary, and venous) can be examined. Vessel size, patency, narrowing, and degree of stenosis or displacement can be determined.	A large amount of contrast medium may be needed during this test, with resulting increased osmotic diuresis and risk of dehydration and renal tubular occlusion. There is less risk to the patient for bleeding or vascular insufficiency because the injection of dye is intravenous rather than intra-arterial. The patient must remain absolutely motionless during the examination (even swallowing will interfere with the results).
Computerized axial tomography, or CT scan (invasive and noninvasive)	A large scanner takes a series of x-ray images all around the same axial plane. A computer then creates a composite picture of various tissue densities visualized. The images may be enhanced with the use of IV contrast dye.	CT scans give detailed outlines of bone, tissue, and fluid structures of the body. They can indicate shift of structures due to tumors, hematomas, or hydrocephalus. A CT scan is limited in that it gives information only about structure of tissues, not about functional status.	Instruct the patient that he will lie flat on a table with the machine surrounding, but not touching, the area to be scanned. He must also remain as immobile as possible; sedation may be required. The scan may not be of the best quality if the patient moves during the test or if the x-ray beams were deflected by any metal object in or around the patient (*e.g.*, traction tongs, ICP monitoring devices).

(Continued)

TABLE 24-5
(Continued)

Diagnostic Test	What it is	What it tells you	Nursing Implications
Nuclear magnetic resonance (NMR) imaging (noninvasive)	A selected area of the patient's body is placed inside a powerful magnetic field. The hydrogen atoms inside the patient are temporarily "exited" and caused to oscillate by a sequence of radio-frequency pulsations. The sensitive scanner measures these minute oscillations, and a computer-enhanced image is created.	An NMR scan creates a graphic image of bone, fluid, and soft tissue structures. It gives a more defined image of anatomical details and may help one diagnose small tumors or early infarction syndromes.	Risk factors for this new technique are not well identified. This test is contraindicated in patients with previous surgeries where hemostatic or aneurysm clips were implanted. The powerful magnetic field can cause such clips to move out of position, placing the patient at risk for bleeding or hemorrhage. The patient (and any caregivers in the room) must remove all metal objects with magnetic characteristics (*e.g,* scissors, stethoscope).
Positron-emission tomography, or PET scan (invasive and noninvasive)	The patient either inhales or receives by injection radioactively tagged substances such as oxygen, nitrogen, and carbon. A gamma scanner measures the radioactive uptake of these substances, and a computer produces a composite image, indicating where the radioactive material is located, corresponding to areas of cellular metabolism.	This diagnostic test is the only one to measure physiological and biochemical processes in the nervous system. Specific areas can be identified as to functioning and nonfunctioning. Cerebral metabolism and cerebral blood flow can be measured regionally. PET scans help diagnose abnormalities (tumors, vascular disease) but also behavioral disturbances such as dementia and schizophrenia that may have a physiological basis.	The patient receives only minimal radiation exposure because the half-life of the radioisotopes used is from a few minutes to 2 hours.
Brain scan (invasive)	Brain scanning employs a technique in which a small amount of a radioactive isotope is injected intravenously. The gamma rays emitted by the isotope are then measured by a special scanner.	The scanner complies an image of the uptake and distribution of the isotope in the brain. Increased uptake may indicate hemorrhage. A-V malformation, hematoma, or tumor. Decreased distribution of the isotope may be evidence of an abscess or infarction.	Instruct the patient that the procedure may take from a few minutes to an hour or so, depending on how many cranial views are desired. Many patients may be concerned about the hazard of radiation. The amount of isotope used is minimal, and its radioactive half-life is short. The exposure is approximately equivalent to that received when a single routine radiograph is obtained.

Test	Description	Use	Nursing considerations
Myelography (invasive)	A myelogram is a radiographic study in which a contrast substance (either air or dye) is injected into the lumbar subarachnoid space. Fluoroscopy, conventional radiographs, or CT Scans are used to visualize selected areas.	The spinal subarachnoid space is examined for partial or complete obstructions due to bone displacements, spinal cord compression, or herniated intravertebral discs.	Instruct the patient as for a lumbar puncture. In addition, advise him that a special table will tilt him up or down during the procedure. After this procedure, the patient may be positioned flat or with the head of the bed elevated, depending on the contrast medium used.
Cortical evoked potentials (noninvasive)	In this test, a specialized device senses central or cortical cerebral electrical activity via skin electrodes in response to peripheral stimulation of specific sensory receptors. The sensory receptors stimulated can be those for vision, hearing, or tactile sensation. The signals are graphically displayed by a computer and characteristic peaks, and the intervals between them are measured.	Cortical evoked potentials provide a detailed assessment of neuron transmission along particular pathways. It has value in determining the integrity of visual auditory and tactile pathways in patients with multiple sclerosis and spinal cord injury. This test may also be used in the assessment of a sensory pathway before, during, and after surgery.	This test may be used in conscious as well as unconscious patients and can be performed at the bedside. The patient must be as motionless as possible during some phases of this test to minimize musculoskeletal interference. Depending on the sensory pathway being tested, the patient may be instructed to watch a series of geometric designs or listen to a series of clicking noises.
Electroencephalogram, or EEG (noninvasive)	An EEG is a recording of electrical impulses generated by the brain cortex that are sensed by electrodes on the surface of the scalp.	Analysis of the resulting tracings helps detect and localize abnormal electrical activity occurring in the cerebral cortex. It aids in seizure focus detection, localization of a source of irritation such as a tumor or abcess, and in the diagnosis of metabolic disturbances and sleep disorders.	Reassure the patient that he will not feel an electrical shock or pain during this test. You may also need to clarify for the patient that the machine cannot "read minds" or indicate the presence of mental illness. The patient's scalp and hair should be free of oil, dirt, creams, and sprays because they can cause electrical intereference and thus an inaccurate recording. Inform the EEG technician of electrical devices around the patient that may act as a source of interference during the procedure (*e.g.,* cardiac monitor, ventilator).

(Prepared by Suzanne Provensano, R.N., B.S.N., C.C.R.N., C.N.R.N.)

AIR STUDIES

Pneumoencephalography, which is performed by introduction of air via a lumbar puncture, and ventriculography, which is accomplished by direct introduction of air into the cerebral supratentorial ventricles, are now infrequently used because of the efficacy of computed tomography. The same techniques are not infrequently utilized, however, with iodinated contrast medium substituted for air and with computed tomography. The combination of metrizamide myelography with computed tomography of the spine is also very useful in assessing spinal cord abnormalities such as tumors, syringomyelia, and traumatic compression of the cord.

ANGIOGRAPHY

Angiography requires the introduction of contrast material directly into arteries supplying the brain or spinal cord and generally is used to supplement the study of abnormalities discovered during computed tomography. Digital subtraction angiography (DSN) is the process by which a fluoroscopic apparatus changes images from the standard fluoroscopy to digital information and is useful in study of the carotid arteries. Conventional film screen angiography is important in assessing vascular abnormalities such as aneurysms and arteriovenous malformations or highly vascular tumors such as meningiomas and choroid plexus papillomas. This technique is also very useful in evaluating vascular disease intracranially or the sequelae of such disease.

MYELOGRAPHY

Myelography, the roentgenographic study of the spinal cord, is now generally carried out by means of water-soluble iodinated compounds introduced with a small-gauge needle in the lumbar region. Occasionally, the introduction of air may be helpful, but the combination of myelography with computed tomography proves much more reliable and productive than myelography itself.

COMPUTED TOMOGRAPHY

Computerized axial tomography (CT, or CAT, scans) is a relatively new development in radiographic imaging that, owing to its speed, accuracy, and low-radiation dosage, has become the most important and widespread aid in diagnosis of central nervous system disease and abnormalities. CT scanning measures densities with radiation, providing a computerized picture. It has become invaluable because it permits rapid screening for hematomas and other traumatic or acute problems and has a high degree of accuracy in initial diagnostic efforts in vascular, neoplastic, infectious, congenital, and virtually all other abnormalities. As already noted, CT scanning allows highly accurate assessment of spinal lesions when used in conjunction with contrast myelography. The procedure is often performed both with and without enhancement (intravenous injection of iodinated contrast material) in serial fashion. Although CT scanning has not entirely eliminated the need for older and generally riskier and more uncomfortable procedures (*e.g.,* arteriography and air or metrizamide studies), it clearly is the screening method of choice at this time. Current limitations in the quality of CT scans are related to spatial and contrast resolution and to the speed of the scan.

NUCLEAR MEDICINE

Various radioactive substances with short half-lives in small amounts provide a different diagnostic method of evaluating for infectious processes, tumors, and problems in cerebral spinal fluid transport. In the last context, radionuclide cisternograms allow diagnosis of communicating hydrocephalus; when injected into shunt systems, radionuclides help one assess for the patency of the system diverting spinal fluid from the cerebral ventricles. In addition, radionuclide techniques may help one confirm the presence of a cerebral spinal fluid leak from a basilar fracture. More frequently, radioisotope studies are used to determine the presence or absence of cerebral blood flow in cases of suspected brain death.

As noted, a variety of radioisotopes are available. Computer techniques similar to CT scanning are being used to reconstruct images of the distribution of radioactive isotopes within the brain. These techniques, called *emission computed tomography,* will be discussed next.

EMISSION COMPUTED TOMOGRAPHY (ECT)

Two forms have been developed related to the type of radioactive materials and the detection system employed. Unlike CT scanning, positron emission tomography (PET) and single photon emission computerized tomography (SPECT) can measure some functional data such as cerebral metabolism and blood flow. Because these modalities are still largely experimental, they have very limited clinical application at present.

ULTRASONOGRAPHY

High-frequency sound waves are useful in establishing the presence of intraventricular hemorrhage and following the process of the clots and subsequent development and progression of hydrocephalus in premature infants. Real-time sonography also may be used through "windows" (through a patent anterior fontanelle or via a craniectomy or craniotomy) to assist in location of cerebral lesions intraoperatively and in guidance of the placement of ventricular catheters for shunts. Newer ultrasonographic devices (triple-frequency scanners) permit greater detail (at 7.5 mHz) of lesions. Ultrasonography is used frequently in assessment of fetal status, although there is some concern at present that the ultrasound may not be entirely benign.

NUCLEAR MAGNETIC RESONANCE (NMR)

This technique is also known as magnetic resonance imaging (MRI) and is now becoming more widely available, although it is still generally limited. This is an alternative to, or adjunct of, computed tomography and may soon surpass the use of CT when availability of the device increases. This modality uses nonionizing forms of energy to produce computerized sectional images in much the same fashion as CT. Signals from atomic nuclei in body tissues are induced by a strong magnetic field in conjunction with a radio-frequency oscillating magnetic field. In other words, this type of imaging is based on detection of the response of hydrogen protons to an applied radio-frequency pulse. The computer reconstructs this kind of information into sectional views.

One limitation is in evaluation of bone, wherein at least the cortex is essentially invisible because its hydrogen is immobile. Only time will reveal whether this technology has benefits—increased diagnostic clarity and avoidance of the ionizing radiation required for CT—and whether indeed there is no specific detrimental effect from the magnetic fields and radio frequency power densities being used at present.

ELECTRODIAGNOSIS

Electroencephalography (EEG) With electroencephalography, a record is made of the brain's electrical activity. This method is probably most valuable in the investigation and management of seizures. Additionally, it may help in localization of structural abnormalities such as tumor, vascular anomalies, and abscesses. Although electroencephalography does not give information about the nature of underlying pathology, it may, in people with established seizures, help one classify the nature of the disorder and monitor the efficacy of anticonvulsant therapy. Direct recordings of electrical activity made either from the brain's exposed surface (electrocorticography) or by implanted electrodes (depth electrography) may help one extirpate a focus of intractable seizure activity during surgery.

Electromyography (EMG). This is the study of the electrical activity of muscles and may allow localization of a lesion to muscular, neural, or junctional components of the motor nerve units involved. EMG abnormalities, as is true in EEG, do not define specific disease states. Electromyography may, however, provide baseline information that will help one choose subsequent modalities (*i.e.,* myelography or spinal CT) which then, with classical information, allows specific diagnosis.

Management of peripheral nerve lesions may be helped by EMG in conjunction with nerve conduction studies in which the time of passage of an electrical impulse between two points is measured and compared with norms. Prognostic information can be derived in this fashion.

Visual Evoked Potentials, or Visual Evoked Responses (VEP, or VER). This method involves recording of electrical activity from the visual (occipital) cortex in response to stimulation of the retina. This allows evaluation of the structural integrity of the visual pathway. One of two general types of visual stimuli may be used: patterned stimuli or unpatterned flashing lights. The resulting VEP waveform is primarily dependent on the type of stimulus.

Brain Stem Auditory Evoked Potentials (Responses) (BAER). This method is similar to VER except that a stimulus is presented to the auditory nerve, following which one normally sees a series of potentials or responses correlating with sequential activation of peripheral, pontomedullary, pontine, and midbrain portions of the auditory pathway. Information is thus gained about the auditory function and also about the intactness of certain brain stem and cerebral areas. This technique has been most helpful in assessment of possible posterior fossa lesions, the cause and potential reversibility of coma, the diagnosis of multiple sclerosis, the value of shunting in hydrocephalus, and in localizing brain stem lesions, other than multiple sclerosis.

Somatosensory Evoked Potentials (Responses) (SER, or SEP). This technique involves stimulation of the upper or lower extremities with recordings from the scalp overlying the contralateral somatosensory cerebral cortex. Lesions of peripheral nerves and within the spinal cord, brain stem (diencephalon), and cerebral hemispheres may be assessed by this technique. Like the other methods, it may be used to monitor possible injury to nervous structures during intraoperative manipulations and may be helpful in localization of neurologic lesions. This is again, however, nonspecific information.

Invasive Neurologic Assessment Techniques

Rae Nadine Smith

Harvey Cushing, a pioneer in blood pressure measurement, is said to be the first neurosurgeon to introduce a form of instrument monitoring. We have progressed from this early, intermittent, and limited pressure monitoring into advanced techniques for continual pressure measurement. In 1951, Guillaume and Janny published the first report on continuous monitoring of intracranial pressure. Today, invasive techniques are frequently used for accurate and continuous assessment of system arterial blood pressure (BP), pulmonary artery pressure (PAP), intracranial pressure (ICP), and cerebral perfusion pressure (CPP) of the neurologic patient.

Correlation of invasive measurements with noninvasive clinical assessment frequently reduces the amount of time required to diagnose the problem accurately, increases the amount of time available for treatment, provides continual feedback on the patient's response to selected treatments, and assists with prognosis. Aggressive management of critically ill neurologic and neurosurgical patients has reduced mortality without increasing the incidence of vegetative or severely disabled patients.

INVASIVE PRESSURE MEASUREMENTS

Determination of invasive pressures requires the use of a transducer and monitor. A transducer can be defined as a device used to change varying pressures into proportionately varying signals that can be displayed on an oscilloscope, meter, or recorder. A variety of transducers, including unbonded strain gauge, solid state, differential transformer, quartz crystal, and disposable transducers, are currently available for clinical application.

Blood Pressure

Direct, or invasive, blood pressure (BP) measurements of critically ill patients provide a variety of advantages over indirect, or noninvasive, techniques. These include accuracy (indirect or cuff pressures are particularly inaccurate during hypotensive episodes because of decreased cardiac output and increased vascular resistance); ability to monitor the mean arterial pressure (MAP); provision of a continual reading with an alarm system; access for blood sampling; and more efficient use of nursing time. Neurologic conditions in which accurate and continual blood pressures are important include increased intracranial pressure, vascular lesions, strokes, and spinal cord injury. These conditions will be discussed subsequently.

Increased Intracranial Pressure (IICP)

Both hypoxia and hypercarbia contribute to alterations of ICP. An increased PCO_2 results in cerebral vasodilation, thereby increasing blood volume and ICP. Serial blood gases are necessary if PCO_2 is to be regulated by a method such as controlled hyperventilation. The majority of patients with severe head injuries develop hyperventilation with respiratory alkalosis.

Early changes in respiratory patterns are usually too subtle for bedside detection. Serial blood gases obtained by an indwelling arterial cannula provide a safer, more efficient technique of blood sampling and certainly one more comfortable for the patient than repeated arterial punctures. The continual monitoring of the pressure between blood gas samplings protects the patient from the risk of bleedback and clotting of the cannula.

In patients with IICP or the potential to develop it, direct mean blood pressure measurement is compared with the mean ICP to determine the cerebral perfusion pressure (MAP minus mean ICP). A normal CPP is at least 50 to 60 mm Hg.

A drop in CPP may activate the medullary vasomotor center, resulting in an increase in blood pressure.

Irritation or depression of the parasympathetic nervous system may induce bradycardia and hypotension.

Patients being managed with induced barbiturate coma often demonstrate spontaneous and unstable fluctuations in blood pressure, requiring continuous systemic arterial BP monitoring.

Vascular Lesions

It is well established that an elevation of blood pressure is a cause of aneurysm rerupture. Aneurysms and subarachnoid hemorrhages are frequently treated by induced hypotension. Just as blood pressure is continuously monitored on a patient in shock being treated with vasopressors to increase pressure, it should likewise be monitored on the patient being treated with hypotensive agents to reduce pressure. In this situation, both hypertension and severe hypotension must be avoided.

Strokes

MAP must be maintained at a level above 60 to 70 mm Hg to prevent the loss of autoregulation mechanisms in areas of focal cerebral ischemia.

Spinal Cord Injury

During a laminectomy, increased blood pressure is often considered a warning sign of pressure on the spinal cord.

Clinically, acute cervical cord injuries are often associated with hypotension. In this situation, blood pressure monitoring is often accompanied by blood volume monitoring, such as pulmonary artery and central venous pressure (CVP) monitoring.

During the hypotensive stage, patients with acute spinal cord injury have a low CVP. As sympathectomized muscles gradually regain tone, the blood-containing space contracts.

If the patient has been receiving vigorous fluid replacement to correct his low blood pressure and low CVP, pulmonary edema may result.

Increased fluid volume causes increased venous pressure on the left side of the heart that frequently is not manifested in CVP readings taken on the right side of the heart. Therefore, pulmonary artery pressures (PAPs) are routinely measured in these patients.

Blood Pressure Measurements

The basic system for blood pressure measurement consists of a transducer that is connected by a tubing system directly to the patient's artery, usually the radial or femoral. Other sites include brachial, axillary, superficial temporal, central aorta, and dorsalis pedis arteries. Pressure from the artery is transmitted to the transducer by a column of fluid and converted to a pressure tracing that can be read on a monitor.

Clotting of the arterial cannula is avoided by administration of a mildly heparinized flush solution, such as normal saline, at a continual rate of 3 to 6 ml/hour. To prevent bleeding back, one maintains the flush solution at a pressure higher than the patient's systolic arterial pressure. The complication of sepsis is minimized by maintenance of a sterile system between the transducer and the patient.

Pulmonary Artery Pressures (PAPs)

PAPs reflects pressures from the left side of the heart and gives an accurate determination of fluid volume as affected by intravenous fluid replacement or diuresis.

Conditions in which accurate blood volume monitoring is indicated include cord injury, head injury, multiple trauma, and increased intracranial pressure.

Cord Injury

Pulmonary edema usually develops within 11 to 24 hours after cord injury. Death from pulmonary edema is not uncommon in acute quadriplegia.

Head Injury

Pulmonary edema develops rapidly after head injury.

Multiple Trauma

The blood volume picture is further complicated in the trauma patient who presents with acute cervical spinal cord injury with associated injury, particularly of the chest. It is often difficult for one to determine whether the patient is hypotensive secondary to the sympathectomy effect or to the blood loss.

IICP (Increased Intracranial Pressure)

Management techniques such as osmotherapy and induced barbiturate coma lead to cardiovascular instability and hypovolemia. Affected patients require frequent measurements of cardiac index.

Pulmonary Artery Pressure Measurement

To determine right atrial, right ventricular, pulmonary artery, and wedge pressures and, in selected patients, cardiac output and continuous mixed venous oxygen saturation ($S\bar{v}o_2$) measurements, one inserts a balloon-tipped catheter.

The catheter is inserted percutaneously or by venous cutdown into the antecubital, jugular, subclavian, or femoral vein. It is then advanced through the vein into the right atrium, to the right ventricle, and into the pulmonary artery.

The progress of the catheter through the right side of the heart is followed by distinctive waveform changes on the oscilloscope or recorder. With the balloon inflated, the catheter wedges into a distal branch of the pulmonary artery. This pulmonary artery wedge pressure reflects pressure from the left side of the heart. PAWs are taken intermittently; with the balloon deflated, continuous PAPs are obtained.

The basic system for setting up and maintaining the PA catheter is the same as that described for blood pressure measurement, using a continual flush rate of 3 ml/hour.

Intracranial Pressure (ICP)

ICP monitoring used in conjunction with other invasive and noninvasive assessment techniques, such as CT scanning, proton NMR, emission tomography (SPET, PET), and evoked potentials, has significantly aided in the diagnosis, treatment, and prognosis of patients with a potential for developing intracranial hypertension.

ICP measurement usually provides an indication of

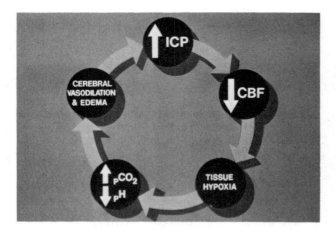

FIGURE 24-8
Cycle for malignant progressive brain swelling. As the ICP increases, cerebral blood flow (CBF) decreases, leading to tissue hypoxia, a decrease in pH, an increase in PCO₂, cerebral vasodilation, and edema, thus leading to further pressure increases. This malignant cycle continues until herniation occurs.

changes in ICP dynamics before such changes are clinically evident, facilitating the initiation of measures to reduce increased intracranial pressure (IICP).

The classic syndrome of IICP, which includes increased pulse pressure, decreased pulse, and decreased respirations with pupillary changes, usually occurs only in association with posterior fossa lesions and seldom with the more commonly observed supratentorial mass lesions, such as subdural hematoma. When these classic Kocker-Cushing signs do accompany a supratentorial lesion, they are associated with a sudden pressure increase and usually herald a state of decompensation. Brain damage is usually irreversible at this point, and death is imminent.

Between the onset of IICP and herniation is a stage in which a wide variety of treatments are available to reduce ICP. Measures such as hyperventilation, the drainage of CSF, hypothermia, and the use of corticosteroids, barbiturates, and hypertonic solutions have proved valuable adjuncts to surgery. Because these techniques are usually most effective before the patient becomes clinically symptomatic, the need for pressure-reducing measures is best determined by direct pressure measurement (Fig. 24-8).

The usual duration for ICP monitoring is 3 to 5 days. The diagnostic and therapeutic benefits of ICP monitoring far outweigh the minimal risk.

Indications for ICP Monitoring

The Monro-Kellie hypothesis states that the volume of the intracranium is equal to the volume of the brain plus the volume of the blood plus the volume of the cerebrospinal fluid (CSF). Any alterations in the volume of any of these components of the cranial vault, as well as the addition of a lesion, may lead to an increase in ICP (see boxed data).

The brain can accommodate or compensate for minimal changes in volume by partial collapse of the cisterns, ventricles, and vascular systems. During this compensatory period, the ICP remains fairly constant. When these compensatory mechanisms have been fully used, pressure increases rapidly until herniation occurs, and the blood supply to the medulla is cut off (Fig. 24-9). The ability of the intracranial contents to compensate depends on the location of the lesion and the rate of expansion.

Conditions that may be indications for ICP measurement include head injury, subarachnoid hemorrhage, pediatric problems, brain tumors, cardiac arrest, PEEP, strokes, and surgery. Discussions of these conditions follow.

Head Injury
Diagnosis. Patients who develop intracranial mass lesions after head injury almost universally develop intracranial hypertension. Uncontrollable elevation of ICP is the cause of death in approximately half the fatally injured patients. Ischemic brain damage has been documented in more than 90% of patients with fatal head injuries. Increased morbidity is associated with patients exhibiting moderate elevations of ICP. Brain electrical dysfunction and disturbances of cerebral blood flow are frequently associated with intracranial pressures greater than 40 mm Hg. ICP monitoring has proved valuable in detection of cerebral edema and hematoma formations. In a 1983 study conducted by Obrist and colleagues,[1] closed head injury patients with ICPs greater than 20 mm Hg had poorer outcomes and a higher incidence of subdural hematomas. Various diagnostic studies, such as computerized axial tomography (CT scans) and cerebral angiography, are then used to differentiate between the two. ICP monitoring also facilitates differentiation of brain stem dysfunction secondary to increases in ICP from primary brain stem injury, which is associated with a normal ICP.

In addition, it has been recommended that continued monitoring be carried out for all patients with burr holes, patients who fail to regain consciousness within 48 hours after injury, and patients whose level of consciousness deteriorates, unless the patient has meningitis or a brain abscess.

Becker[2] has established the following criteria for selection of head-injured patients for ICP monitoring:

- Inability to obey commands or utter recognizable words despite cardiopulmonary stabilization
- Abnormal CT scan
- Multimodality evoked potentials

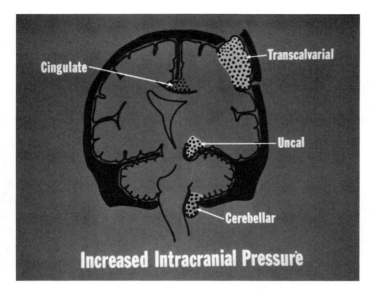

FIGURE 24-9
The major types of cerebral herniation are (1) herniation of the cingulate gyrus under the falx; (2) herniation of the uncus of the temporal lobe beneath the free edge of the tentorium; (3) downward displacement of the midbrain through the tentorial notch; and (4) sometimes, with an open head injury, transcalvarial herniation.

Eisenberg and associates[3] monitor ICP in head injury patients with a Glasgow coma scale less than 7 or an abnormal CT scan or both.

Treatment.   Therapy for IICP is as follows:

- *Diuretics and dehydration.* The amount and frequency of drugs used to treat IICP are titrated by continual monitoring.
- *Intermittent positive pressure ventilation (IPPV).* The control of PCO_2 levels may require drugs such as chlorpromazine or morphine sulfate to optimize the patient's response to the ventilator. Increases in ICP secondary to muscle tremors may be treated with paralytic agents such as pancuronium bromide (Pavulon), necessitating dependence on artificial ventilation. Because neurologic response is suppressed by these drugs, ICP, blood pressure, PA, and cerebral perfusion pressure (CPP) monitoring become mandatory for safer patient care.

Iatrogenic increases in pressure secondary to therapeutic measures such as chest physiotherapy, suctioning, and positioning are quickly identified.

Prognosis.   Miller and Sullivan[4] reported on a series of 160 consecutive, severely head-injured patients. They determined that patients with intracranial mass lesions following head injury often develop early, severe intracranial hypertension. Patients with acute subdural hematomas seem to be most prone to IICP. In patients with diffuse brain injury, ICP is usually elevated but not to the same degree. It was reported that patients who maintained ICPs of 45 to 60 torr within

Indications for ICP Monitoring

Increased volume of brain
Cerebral edema
Trauma
Surgery
Stroke
Tumor
Increased volume of blood
Hematomas
A-V malformations
Aneurysm
Stroke
Increase in PCO_2
Increased volume of CSF
Decreased CSF reabsorption
Congenital hydrocephalus
Lesions
Tumors
Abscesses

the first 48 hours after injury, despite all therapeutic intervention, had a mortality rate approaching 100%.

In patients with diffuse brain injury, any elevation above 10 torr on admission resulted in progressively worsening prognoses. Miller and Sullivan believe that this suggests that the initial level of ICP is to some degree an indication of the extent of diffuse brain damage. Recurrent or persistent intracranial hypertension was more frequently a problem with intracerebral lesions, contusion, hematoma, and brain swelling than with discrete extracerebral hematomas, whether epidural or subdural. Recurrent or persistent intracranial hypertension was associated with a poorer outcome.

Subarachnoid Hemorrhage

Preoperative Considerations. The level of ICP correlates well with the clinical grade of the hemorrhage. The ICP is of value in determining the best time for surgery, predicting and detecting rebleeding, and determining the etiology of neurologic deterioration. ICP monitoring facilitates the use of various drugs and other management techniques such as hyperventilation and continuous ventricular fluid drainage or a permanent shunt to compensate for CSF absorption impairment.

Pediatrics

Neonates and Infants. Noninvasive anterior fontanelle monitoring has proved useful in hyaline membrane disease, intracranial hemorrhage, meconium aspiration syndrome, meningitis, and hydrocephalus.

Head Injury. Children are particularly prone to cerebral edema, but if successfully managed they have a good prognosis.

Reye's Syndrome. The mortality and morbidity of this disease have been substantially reduced by the measurement of ICP, usually by intraventricular catheter or subarachnoid screw, and the subsequent control of cerebral edema and maintenance of adequate cerebral perfusion. When continuous monitoring is used, the frequent A waves seen in these children can be detected and treated. This has proved particularly useful in stage 3 or 4 coma.

During exchange transfusions, marked alterations in ICP have been observed. In patients with diminished brain compliance or impairment of cerebral vascular autoregulation, exchange transfusion may have an adverse effect on ICP. The use of ICP monitoring reduces this risk.

Brain Tumors

ICP tends to remain normal, with episodic increases seen particularly at night. Elevations in ICP tend to occur when the mass has enlarged to the point at which the patient is demonstrating neurologic deterioration with papilledema, headache, and vomiting. Metastatic tumors can cause massive edema. Patients may be monitored preoperatively to determine their response to the preoperative therapeutic regimen and to assist in determining the optimal time for surgery. Postoperatively, they may be monitored to assist with the diagnosis and treatment of diffuse generalized cerebral edema secondary to extensive manipulation of the brain during surgery.

Cardiac Arrest

Of long-term cardiac arrest survivors, 10% to 20% suffer permanent severe brain damage ranging from intellectual changes to vegetative states following global ischemic-anoxic insults. ICP measurement has been of value in the development of new specific neuron-saving therapies for "postresuscitation disease" to assist in the restoration of mentation.

Post End Expiratory Pressure (PEEP)

The use of PEEP can increase ICP or reduce arterial blood pressure, thereby reducing CPP and decreasing cerebral blood flow (CBF). This may be because PEEP causes a rise in intrathoracic pressure, which reduces cardiac filling pressure, leading to a decrease in cardiac output. The circulatory compensation is incomplete and the blood pressure falls, causing a reduction in CPP. ICP may be increased by impedance to cerebral venous outflow. In one study, significant increases in ICP occurred in approximately 50% of the patients given PEEP. Patients with baseline ICPs greater than 25 mm Hg showed the most significant increases in ICP.

For optimal titration of PEEP in the patient who may develop intracranial hypertension, it is recommended that ICP and blood pressure be monitored continuously and measurements be made of neurologic status and intracranial and pulmonary compliance. Volume pressure responses (VPRs) and arterial blood gases are therefore indicated.

Strokes

Increases in ICP are common with spontaneous intracerebral hemorrhage and routinely present in comatose patients. In ischemic stroke, high ICP is likely after cerebral infarction has progressed to coma with midline brain shift. ICP monitoring has been effective in the initiation and maintenance of therapeutic intervention. It has also provided valuable information for research on the mechanisms and amelioration of focal brain ischemia.

Surgery

During surgery, ICP monitoring provides assistance in determining the optimal position for the patient and his responses to various anesthetic agents and ventilatory support.

ICP Measurement

There are basically three techniques for measuring ICP: (1) intraventricular, (2) subarachnoid (subdural), and (3) epidural (extradural). All three methods require strict aseptic technique during insertion and maintenance.

Intraventricular Technique

The intraventricular technique of ICP measurement was first reported in 1951 and remains the most frequently used method. It consists of placement of a catheter into the lateral ventricle. A twist drill hole is placed lateral to the midline at the level of the coronal

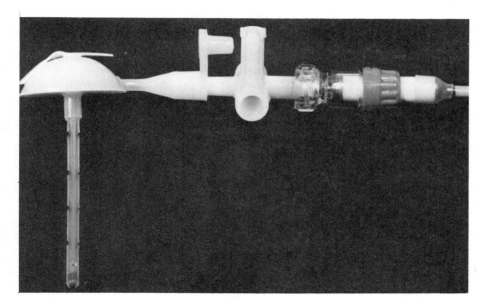

FIGURE 24-10
Intraventricular cannula with subminiature transducer.

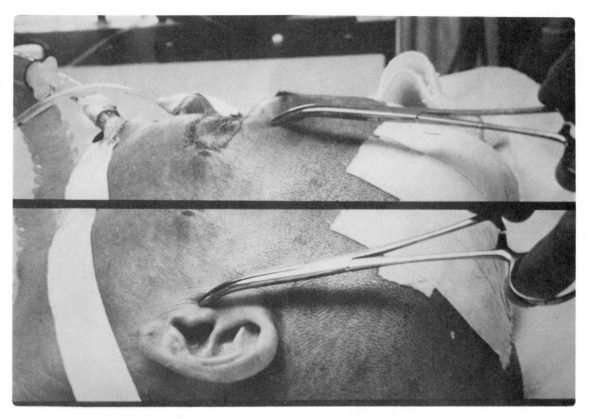

FIGURE 24-11
Zero reference points for lining up venting port of transducer with the level of the foramen of Monro.

suture, usually on the nondominant side. A catheter is placed through the cerebrum into the anterior horn of the lateral ventricle. On occasion, the occipital horn is used. Connected to the ventricular catheter by a stopcock or pressure tubing is a pressure transducer (Fig. 24-10). Sterile saline or Ringer's lactate solution is used to provide the fluid column between the CSF and diaphragm of the transducer. A continuous flush device is not used for ICP measurement.

The miniature transducer may be positioned directly on the patient's head. A standard size transducer is mounted at the bedside, with the venting port positioned at the level of the foramen of Monro (Fig. 24-11). External landmarks for this position are the edge of the brow or the tragus of the ear. For every 1 inch of discrepancy between the level of the transducer and the pressure source, there is an error of approximately 2 torr.

Advantages
- Direct measurement of pressure from the CSF
- Access for CSF drainage or sampling
- Access for determining VPRs
- Access for instillation of drugs

Disadvantages
- Need to puncture the brain
- Difficulty in locating the lateral ventricle following midline shifting of the ventricle or collapse of the

FIGURE 24-12
Disposable subarachnoid screw kit. (Codman Disposable ICP Kit, Codman J Shurtleff Inc, Randolph MA)

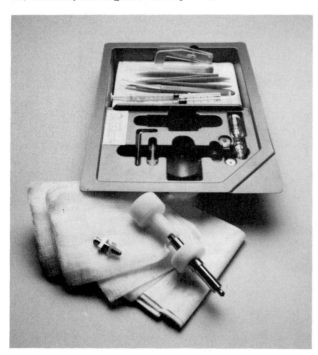

ventricle as a normal compensatory mechanism for increases in pressure
- Risk of infection. Becker reported no infection in patients monitored 3 days or less, with a 6% infection rate in patients monitored more than 3 days. Becker also reported a hemorrhage complication rate of 1.4%.[2]

Subarachnoid Technique
The measurement of ICP by means of a subarachnoid screw (Figs. 24-12 and 24-13) was first reported in 1973. The screw device is inserted through a twist drill hole and extends into the subdural or subarachnoid space. Although the cerebrum is not penetrated, pressures, as with the intraventricular technique, are measured directly from the CSF. A transducer filled with saline or Ringer's lactate solution may be fastened directly to a stopcock on the screw or connected by pressure tubing. As with any technique for monitoring ICP, a continuous flush device is contraindicated.

An alternate technique for monitoring subarachnoid pressure is the ribbon-shaped cup catheter, available in both adult and pediatric sizes. The catheter is usually used in conjunction with a craniotomy procedure and is inserted through a subcutaneous tunnel and burr hole. Volume pressure responses have been determined with these techniques. Subarachnoid pressures usually correlate well with intraventricular pressures.

Advantages
- Direct pressure measurement from CSF
- No need to penetrate cerebrum to locate ventricle
- Access for determining volume pressure responses
- Access for CSF drainage and sampling
- Ease of insertion

Disadvantages
- Risk of complications comparable to those associated with intraventricular technique
- Need for closed skull
- Greater difficulty in VPR studies and with CSF drainage than ventricular catheters
- Possible blockage of the measuring devices from high ICP
- Possible underestimation of ICP when it is elevated

Epidural Technique
This technique involves placement of an epidural device such as a balloon with radioisotopes, a radio transmitter, or a fiberoptic or pneumatic transducer between the skull and the dura. Some researchers feel that dural compression and surface tension, as well as thickening of the dura during prolonged monitoring, tend to cause inaccuracies in the pressure readings. Although subarachnoid and intraventricular pressures

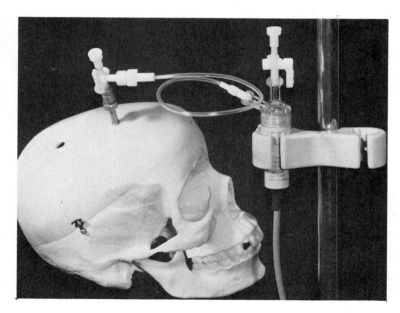

FIGURE 24-13
Measurement of ICP by means of subarachnoid technique with standard size transducer.

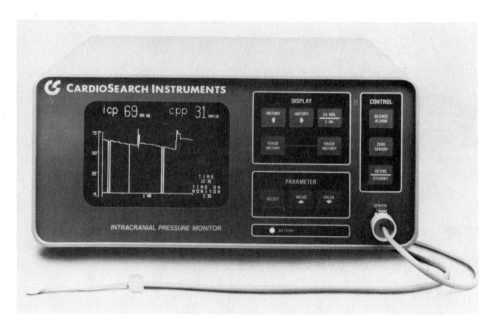

FIGURE 24-14
ICP monitor. Utilization of a pneumatic epidural transducer and a standard pressure transducer permits CPP monitoring. (Courtesy of CardioSearch Tampa, Fl)

correlate well with each other, there have been inconsistent correlations between direct CSF pressure and pressure measurement using various epidural techniques. At this time, the pneumatic epidural system looks promising (Figs. 24-14 and 24-15, *A* and *B*).

Certain fiberoptic and solid state transducers have proved of value for noninvasive anterior fontanelle pressure monitoring of neonates and infants. A special holder is used to attach the transducer to the anterior fontanelle. A normal ICP is less than 10 mm Hg. These pressures have correlated well with intraventricular pressures.

Advantages
- Less invasive
- Usefulness of selected tranducers for anterior fontanelle monitoring

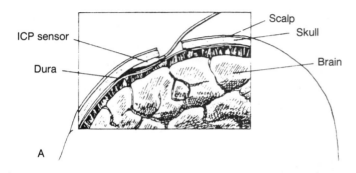

A

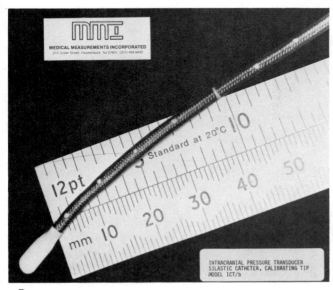

B

FIGURE 24-15
(A) *Epidural monitoring. Note placement of pneumatic transducer between dura and skull. (Courtesy of CardioSearch, Tampa FL) (B) Intracranial pressure transducer, silastic catheter, calibrating tip, Model ICT/b. (Courtesy of Medical Measurements Inc, Hackensack NJ)*

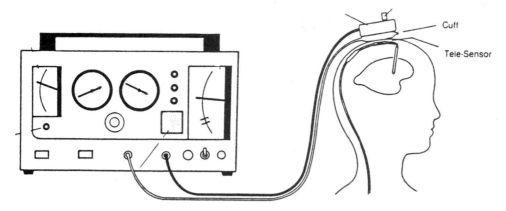

FIGURE 24-16
ICP telemetry. This system may be used for monitoring an intraventricular catheter and shunt. (Courtesy of Radionics, Burlington, MA)

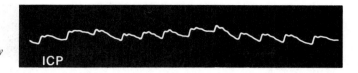

FIGURE 24-17
ICP waveform demonstrating hemodynamic and respiratory oscillations.

Disadvantages

- Questionable reflection of CSF pressure. With high ICPs, epidural pressures may considerably over-read ventricular pressures.
- Slow response time. Many systems are unable to pick up transient peaks caused by Valsalva maneuvers and respiratory changes.
- No route for CSF drainage and sampling
- Infeasible volume pressure responses
- Inability to zero and calibrate some systems after measurement is initiated
- Transducer placement. Transducer must touch but not indent the dura and must be paralled to, or coplanar with, the dura. If the dura is stretched, the pressure recording will be affected by dural compliance.

Telemetry Technique

Telemetry systems have been reported with both epidural and intraventricular devices. Its two major uses are reduction of the risk of infection and long-term monitoring. The latter is helpful in follow-up evaluation in long-term patients, such as those with hydrocephalus, some with metabolic encephalopathies, and those with brain tumors who are undergoing chemotherapy (Fig. 24-16).

ICP Ranges and Waveforms

Range. Normal ICP ranges between 0 and 10 mm Hg, with an upper limit of 15 mm Hg. ICP is routinely monitored as a mean pressure. During coughing or straining, a normal ICP may increase to 100 mm Hg. In acute situations, patients frequently become symptomatic at pressures ranging from 20 to 25 mm Hg.

The patient's tolerance of a change in ICP varies with the acuteness of its onset. Patients with a slower buildup of ICP, as occurs with certain brain tumors, are more tolerant of elevations in the ICP than patients in whom pressure changes rapidly, as seen in those with acute subdural hematoma. Uncontrolled ICP between 20 and 25 mm Hg is considered the "kiss of death" for the head-injured patient. Sustained intracranial hypertension greater than 60 mm Hg is usually fatal.

ICP may rise to the level of the MAP. The greater the variations in the mean ICP, the more nearly exhausted are the compensatory mechanisms for intracranial volume increases.

Although protocols vary, measures to reduce ICP are usually initiated if the patient shows neurologic deterioration, such as a score of 7 or less on the Glasgow Coma Scale or an ICP of 16 mm Hg or greater.

Although ICP is routinely monitored as a mean pressure, systolic and diastolic pressures should be noted. Because there is a linear relationship between pulse pressure (PP) and ICP, PP may be utilized to estimate intracranial elastance, particularly in the patient with cerebral vasoparalysis.

Waveforms. ICP waveforms provide an index of ICP dynamics. The appearance of ICP waveforms varies according to the technique of measurement being used and the patient's pathology. Hemodynamic and respiratory oscillations can be observed in ICP traces. Sometimes, the waveforms closely resemble arterial pressure waveforms; other times, they resemble CVP waveforms. To varying degrees, oscillations corresponding to the arterial pulsations are seen.

At times, a small "a" wave is superimposed on diastole, reflecting right atrial pressure.

Alterations in arterial driving force, disturbance of venous outflow, and cerebral vasodilation have been correlated with changes in waveform appearances.

In patients with ICP less than 20 mm Hg, a slower waveform, synchronous with respiration and caused by changes in intrathoracic pressure, can be seen (Fig. 24-17).

Some patients exhibit waveform variation, most commonly A, B, and C waves. *A waves,* also known as *plateau waves,* are spontaneous, rapid increases of pressure between 50 and 200 mm Hg, occurring at variable intervals (Fig. 24-18). They tend to occur in patients with moderate elevations of ICP, last 5 to 20 minutes, and fall spontaneously. The plateau waves are usually accompanied by a temporary increase in neurologic deficit. Although the mechanism of A waves has not been firmly established, it is felt that they indicate decreased intracranial compliance, and measures should be used to prevent their occurrence. They may result from an increase in blood volume with a simultaneous decrease in blood flow. The sudden reversal of high pressure may be caused by increased CSF absorption with reduction of CSF pressure. In a study involving patients with aneurysm, Nornes correlated an increased frequency of plateau waves with a tendency to rebleed (Safar, 1981).[5] Falls in CPP with intact autoreg-

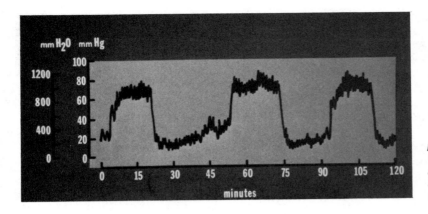

FIGURE 24-18
"A", or plateau, waves. Associated with decreased intracranial compliance, they may be secondary to an increase in blood volume with a simultaneous decrease in blood flow.

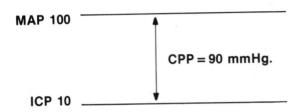

FIGURE 24-19
Cerebral perfusion pressure. CPP = MAP − ICP. For adequate cerebral blood flow, CPP should exceed 50 mm Hg.

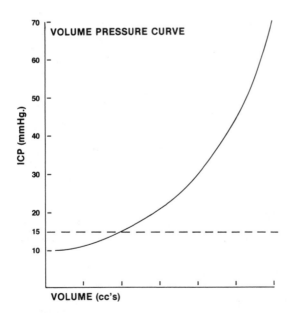

FIGURE 24-20
Volume pressure curve. Volume pressure response (VPR) provides a method of estimating the compensatory capacity of the intracranial cavity.

ulation and low intracranial compliance have been correlated with the initiating plateau waves.

B waves are small, sharp rhythmic waves with pressures up to 50 mm Hg, occurring at a frequency of 0.5/minute to 2.0/minute. They correspond to changes in respiration, providing clues to periodic respiration related to poor cerebral compliance or pulmonary dysfunction. B waves are often seen with Cheyne-Stokes respirations. At times, they occur in patients with normal ICP and no papilledema. They may be secondary to oscillations of cerebral blood volume.

C waves are small, rhythmic waves with pressures up to 20 mm Hg, occurring at a rate of approximately 6/minute. They are related to the blood pressure. Like A waves, they indicate severe intracranial compression, with limited remaining volume residual within the intracranial space.

Cerebral Perfusion Pressure
One calculates CPP by subtracting the mean ICP from the mean systemic arterial pressure (MAP) (Fig. 24-19):

$$CPP = MAP - ICP.$$

Cerebral perfusion pressure (CPP) provides a clinical estimate of cerebral blood flow.

Normal cerebral blood flow (CBF) is provided by a CPP in the range of 40 to 130 torr. The autoregulation system for maintenance of constant blood flow does not function at pressures less than 40 torr. When the CPP is zero, there is no CBF. In other words, when ICP equals MAP, CPP equals zero and CBF is zero. CBF may totally cease at pressures somewhat above zero.

If CPP decreases secondary to a decreased blood pressure, CBF begins to drop at 50 to 60 torr. If CPP decreases secondary to increased ICP, CBF is maintained until the CPP falls to 40 mm Hg in adults and 30 mm Hg in newborns. A severe reduction in CPP is accompanied by an absence of brain stem auditory evoked potentials, indicating changes in brain stem function.

TABLE 24-6
TROUBLESHOOTING ICP LINES

Problem	Cause	Action
No ICP waveform	Air between the transducer diaphragm and pressure source	Eliminate air bubbles with sterile saline or Ringer's lactate.
	Occlusion of intracranial measurement device with blood or debris	Flush intracranial cath or screw as directed by physician: 0.25 ml sterile saline is frequently used.
	Transducer connected incorrectly	Check connection and be sure the appropriate connector for amplifier is in use.
	Incorrect gain setting for pressure or patient having plateau waves	Adjust gain setting for higher pressure range.
	Trace turned off	Turn power on to trace.
False high-pressure reading	Transducer too low	Place the venting port of the transducer at the level of the foramen of Monro: For every 2.54 cm (1 inch) the transducer is below the pressure source, there is an error of approximately 2 mm Hg.
	Transducer incorrectly balanced	With transducer correctly positioned, rebalance. Transducer should be balanced every 2 to 4 hours and prior to the initiation of treatment based on a pressure change.
	Monitoring system incorrectly calibrated	Repeat calibration procedures.
	Air in system: Air may attenuate or amplify pressure signal	Remove air from monitoring line.
High-pressure reading	Airway not patent: An increase in intrathoracic pressure may increase PCO_2	Suction patient. Position. Initiate chest physiotherapy.
	Ventilator setting incorrect	Check ventilator settings.
	PEEP	Draw arterial blood gases, since hypoxia and hypercarbia cause increases in ICP.
	Posture	Head should be elevated 15° to 30° unless contraindicated by other problems such as fractures.
	Head and neck	The head should be positioned to facilitate venous drainage.
	Legs	Limit knee flexion.
	Decerebrate	Muscle relaxants or paralyzing agents are sometimes indicated.
	Excessive muscle activity during decerebrate posturing in patients with upper brain stem injury may increase ICP	
	Hyperthermia	Initiate measures to control muscle movement, infection, and pyrexia.
	Excessive muscle activity	
	Increased susceptibility to infection	
	Fluid and electrolyte imbalance secondary to fluid restrictions and diuretics	Draw blood for serum electrolytes, serum osmolality. Note PAP. Evaluate I & O with specific gravity.
	Blood pressure: Vasopressor responses occur in some patients with IICP	Use measures to maintain adequate CPP.
	Low BP associated with hypovolemia, shock, and barbiturate coma may increase cerebral ischemia	
False low-pressure reading	Air bubbles between transducer and CSF	Eliminate air bubbles with sterile saline or Ringer's lactate.
	Transducer level too high	Place the venting port of the transducer at the level of the foramen of Monro. For every 2.54 cm (1 inch) the transducer is above the level of the pressure source, there will be an error of approximately 20 mm Hg.
	Zero or calibration incorrect	Rezero and calibrate monitoring system.
	Collapse of ventricles around catheter	If ventriculostomy is being used there may be inadequate positive pressure. Check to make sure a positive pressure of 15 to 20 mm Hg exists. Drain CSF slowly.

(Continued)

TABLE 24-6
(Continued)

Problem	Cause	Action
	Otorrhea or rhinorrhea	These conditions cause a false low-pressure reading secondary to decompression. Document the correlation between drainage and pressure changes.
	Leakage of fluid from connections	Eliminate all fluid leakage.
	Dislodge of catheter from ventricle into brain	Contact physician regarding appropriate diagnostic studies and intervention. Use soft catheter designed for intraventricular measurement.
	Occlusion of the end of a subarachnoid screw by the necrotic brain	In most cases, remove screw.

When brain damage is severe, as with widespread brain edema or when blood flow has been arrested in the brain, CBF may be reduced at relatively normal levels of CPP. This is due to impedance to the flow of blood across the cerebrovascular bed. CBF may not increase despite increases in CPP if autoregulation is impaired. This condition is referred to as *pressure-flow dissociation,* or *vasomotor paralysis.*

Volume-Pressure Curve

The relationship between changes in volume and changes in pressure is critical in patient management. This is demonstrated by the volume-pressure curve, which relates supratentorial ICP to the volume of the increasing mass lesion. When the intracranial lesion begins to develop, there is little initial increase in pressure because of the compensatory shifts of blood and CSF. Once these compensatory mechanisms have been fully used, the curve becomes steeper or nonlinear. This usually occurs at approximately 15 torr. Uniform increments of volume now cause progressively larger increases in ICP. This is due to a decrease in intracranial compliance. The cranial contents become stiffer, and free communication of CSF between the lateral ventricles and infratentorium is lost. Drastic increases in ICP may result from hypercarbia, hypoxia, rapid eye movement (REM) sleep, pyrexia, or the administration of certain anesthetics.

One can test intracranial compliance and elastance clinically by obtaining a volume pressure response (VPR). A technique used by Miller[4] consists of injecting 1 ml of sterile saline into the intraventricular catheter or 0.1 ml into the subarachnoid screw. If the ICP increases less than 2 torr with a 1-ml injection given over an interval of 1 second, the patient is not undergoing compensatory changes. A response of at least 3 torr/ml is considered a sign of altered compensation or compliance. A VPR of 5 torr/ml or more is an urgent indication for repeat study of the patient. Intracranial mass lesions, extracerebral hematomas, and intracerebral hematomas and swelling have been correlated with such readings and may be confirmed by CT scan. It is recommended that VPRs be done by way of an intraventricular cannula. In select cases, intraventricular fluid is withdrawn after the study (Fig. 24-20).

Troubleshooting ICP

When the monitor indicates a change in ICP, one must first determine whether the reading is accurate. If the reading is accurate, an attempt is then made to determine the reason for the pressure change. Table 24-6 provides a guide to troubleshooting ICP lines.

REFERENCES

1. Obrist WD et al: Factors relating to intracranial hypertension in acute head injury. In Ishii S et al (eds): Intracranial Pressure V. New York, Springer-Verlag, 1983
2. Becker DP: Selecting patients for intracranial pressure monitoring in severe head injury. In Ishii S et al (eds): Intracranial Pressure V. New York, Springer-Verlag, 1983
3. Eisenberg HM et al: The effects of three potentially preventable complication on outcome after severe closed head injury. In Ishii et al (eds): Intracranial Pressure V. New York, Springer-Verlag, 1983
4. Miller JD: Significance and management of intracranial hypertension in head injury. In Ishii S et al (eds): Intracranial Pressure V. New York, Springer-Verlag, 1983
5. Safar P: Cardiopulmonary Cerebral Resuscitation. Philadelphia, WB Saunders, 1981

BIBLIOGRAPHY

Chapman, PH et al: Telemetric ICP monitoring after surgery for posterior fossa and third ventricular tumors. J Neurosurg 60:649–651, 1984
Saul TG et al: Effect of intracranial pressure monitoring and aggressive treatment on mortality in severe head injury. J Neurosurg 56:498–503, 1982
Shapiro H et al: Intracranial pressure responses to PEEP in head injured patients. J Trauma 18, No. 4:254–256, 1978
Trauner D et al: Treatment of elevated intracranial pressure in Reye syndrome. Ann Neurol 4, No. 3:275–278, 1978

25
Management Modalities: Nervous System

Interventions for the Patient with Increased Intracranial Pressure (IICP)

Rae Nadine Smith

Cerebral blood volume and CSF circulation are the two major mechanisms responsible for the regulation of intracranial pressure. Therefore, most management techniques for IICP are oriented toward control of these two regulatory mechanisms to keep ICP below 23 mm Hg. When possible, treatment is initiated when ICP elevates to between 16 and 20 mm Hg.

Surgical decompression, ventricular drainage, low PCO_2, massive steroids, osmotic diuretics, and induced barbiturate coma are among the measures used to treat intracranial hypertension. Although no one therapeutic regimen has been universally accepted, the goals in treatment of the patient with IICP remain the same:

• To reduce ICP
• To improve CPP
• To reduce brainshift and distortion and the systemic effects that they induce

The following discussion covers measures currently used in the management of IICP.

Surgical Decompression. Intracranial mass lesions are evacuated as early as possible, usually with replacement of the bone flap.

Ventilation. Endotracheal intubation is usually used with a tracheostomy performed by the third day if ventilation is still required. Intermittent positive pressure ventilation (IPPV) is indicated in head-injured patients in coma, patients with ICPs greater than 30 torr after postcranial surgery, patients with chest injuries, and patients with decerebrate spasms or uncontrolled seizures secondary to brain damage. Reducing the arterial PCO_2 causes cerebral vasoconstriction, which reduces cerebral blood volume.

Ventilation is usually done at a slow rate (approximately 10 to 12 cycles/minute) with a high tidal volume (15 ml/kg body weight) to moderate hypocapnia (25 to 35 torr). If necessary, small doses of chlorpromazine or morphine sulfate are often used to phase the patient with the ventilator. For selected patients, paralyzing agents such as pancuronium bromide are used. When paralyzing or tranquilizing drugs are used, ICP monitoring is mandatory. With normally reacting blood vessels, a drop in PCO_2 from 40 to 20 torr is associated with a reduction in elevated ICP of approximately 30%. Reduction of PCO_2 below 20 mm Hg causes no further vasoconstriction. Lowering PCO_2 below 25 may increase lactic acid and dysrhythmias.

Arterial PO_2 is maintained over 70 mm Hg.

PEEP is used at levels up to 20 cm of water to improve oxygenation in patients with pulmonary dysfunction and requires ICP monitoring. Hyperbaric oxygenation to produce mild cerebral vasoconstriction as a mechanism of reducing ICP is being studied.

Position. The head is elevated 15° to 30° unless contraindicated by limb fractures. Flexion of the knees is

465

contraindicated. Rotation of the head should be avoided.

Hypothermia. Although hypothermia decreases the cerebral metabolic rate of oxygen consumption, used alone it may cause a reduction of cerebral blood flow. Except in cases involving patients in induced barbiturate coma, normothermia is usually used. Temperature elevations are promptly treated.

Hypothermia has been successfully used in conjunction with induced barbiturate coma. The combination may offer synergistic protection, acting through different mechanisms to control IICP.

Blood Pressure Control.

Blood Pressure Reduction. IICP and neurologic dysfunction can be aggravated by systemic vasodilator drugs such as sodium nitroprusside (Nipride). With a normal PCO_2, Nipride causes a significant increase in ICP with only a slight decrease in blood pressure. The use of hyperventilation attenuates but does not obliterate the ICP effect.

When induced hypotension is needed in the patient with IICP, Nipride administration should be carefully titrated. Ideally, the drug should be used in surgery only after the skull is opened.

Although high arterial blood pressure may be detrimental in patients with IICP, in patients with a very high ICP, a reduction in blood pressure may further reduce cerebral blood flow. Reduction of arterial blood pressure is contraindicated in patients with brain edema when CBF is already reduced.

Blood Pressure Elevation. Postoperative intracranial aneurysm patients with cerebral ischemia secondary to severe intracranial vascular spasm have demonstrated marked clinical improvement following short periods of induced arterial hypertension.

CSF Drainage. In situations involving impaired absorption of CSF, such as after a subarachnoid hemorrhage, impaired circulation of CSF as with hydrocephalus and certain brain tumors, or IICP without total collapse of the ventricles, controlled CSF drainage may facilitate a reduction in ICP. Ventricular drainage should always be against a positive pressure of 15 to 20 torr to prevent ventricular collapse. Best results are obtained when there is bilateral dilatation of the ventricles. Decompression should be gradual, particularly in children. Although CSF drainage is routinely done by intraventricular catheter (ventriculostomy), in selected patients CSF can be drained by a subarachnoid screw. (Figs. 25-1 and 25-2, *A* and *B*).

FIGURE 25-1
Holter-Hausner fifth ventricle external CSF drainage system. (Courtesy of Holter-Hausner International, Bridgeport, PA)

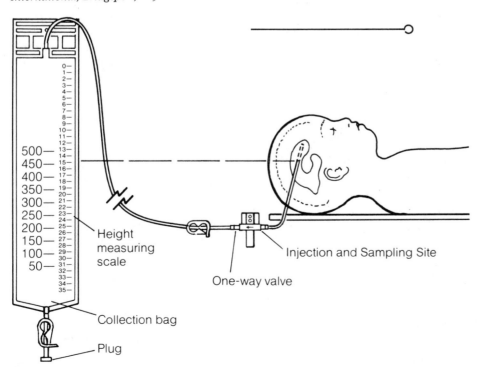

Steroids. Glucocorticoids such as dexamethasone, betamethasone, and methylprednisolone have proved effective in reducing brain edema and ICP and in improving neurologic status, particularly in brain tumor patients with peritumoral edema. Clinical improvement is usually seen within 24 hours. An elevated resting ICP is not usually reduced until the second or third day of treatment. Steroid therapy has proved most effective in patients with focal chronic lesions. Standard doses of steroids have not been effective in reducing IICP associated with acute head injury, but higher doses of dexamethasone may be of value. In head-injured patients, steroids may be given for 3 days and, if improvement is seen, extended to 7 to 10 days.

Osmotherapy. Osmotic agents such as mannitol, urea, and glycerol, and isosorbide may be used to assist in the management of IICP. They may decrease ICP by decreasing CSF volume and increasing CPP and seem most effective in managing ICP elevations that have occurred within the previous hour. At times, loop diuretics such as Lasix (furosemide) are used in conjunction with osmotherapy, requiring even more careful consideration of fluid and electrolyte balance. Although the osmotics have long been considered to introduce the risk of rebound, with ICP returning to or becoming higher than the pressure initially being treated, this phenomenon is now being questioned. Some investigators feel that rebound is unlikely when the drugs are properly managed. With diffuse head injury, an increase in CBF secondary to increased CPP may increase ICP. The effect of mannitol varies with the type of injury. Regardless of which agent is used, the optimal dose is the lowest dose that reduces ICP. Because the absolute effect of any drug cannot be determined in advance, continual monitoring of ICP is required to determine the correct dosage for a given patient. By titrating drug administration by means of ICP monitoring, one can avoid the problem of increased osmolarity resulting from too high or too frequent dosages.

The hyperosmotic agent most commonly used is 20% mannitol. Intravenous urea is seldom used because of the problem with severe local reaction if leakage occurs at the injection site. Mannitol therapy is often initiated if the patient's ICP has exceeded 20 to 15 mm Hg for at least 10 minutes. A dose of 0.25 to 1.00 g/kg of body weight is administered intravenously over a 10- to 15-minute period. Both bolus and continuous infusion techniques are utilized. The use of barbiturates reduces the mannitol requirement. Results should be evident within 15 minutes of completion of administration. Osmotherapy may increase CBF even when ICP is not reduced. In extremely ill patients, the administration of mannitol may cause parallel increases in blood pressure and ICP, with clinical deterioration.

Garritson and colleagues[1] state that the four variables related to ICP response to mannitol are (1) the level of ICP 1 hour before administration, (2) the level of ICP at the time of administration, (3) the cumulative dose given over the preceding 6 hours, (4) the current mannitol dose.

Low normovolemia is maintained, usually two thirds of daily fluid requirements. Serum osmolarities are often maintained between 290 to 310 mOsm/ml. With IICP, colloid fluids such as albumin make maintenance of an adequate circulating volume possible. Solutions such as normal saline may promote brain edema secondary to a reduction in colloid osmotic pressure.

Calcium Antagonists (Blockers). The effect of various calcium channel blockers such as nimodipine, nifedipine, verapamil, and diltiazem on the prevention and management of cerebral ischemia secondary to cerebral vasospasm are being investigated. It is hypothesized that these drugs inhibit large cerebral arteries from contracting by blocking the influx of extracellular calcium, resulting in the prevention of neurologic deficits secondary to cerebral arterial spasm. Because systemic arteries remain capable of contracting, calcium antagonists do not produce significant systemic hypotension.

Alkalyzing Agents. The effects of alkalyzing agents such as THAM and Meylon (sodium bicarbonate) in ICP reduction via suppression of brain swelling are being investigated. These agents may improve tissue acidosis, recover vascular tone, or act as hyperosmolar agents, preserving CBF in the ischemic lesion.

Induced Barbiturate Coma. Although somewhat controversial, induced barbituate coma has been documented as increasing survival and decreasing morbidity, particularly in patients with head injuries and Reye's syndrome.

Mechanism. The mechanism by which ICP is reduced in barbiturate coma has not been firmly established. The barbiturate appears to have a direct, restrictive effect on cerebral vasculature, diverting small amounts of the blood from well-perfused areas to ischemic areas, thereby improving cerebral pressure and collateral circulation. Vascular spasms are reduced, improving CBF. It lowers the systemic blood pressure, thereby decreasing blood-brain barrier disruption. Effects of noxious stimuli such as critical care unit noise are blunted, and patients are more tolerant of positioning and suctioning. The total muscle relaxation and immobilization reduce cerebral venous pressure. Both blood pressure and ICP become less labile.

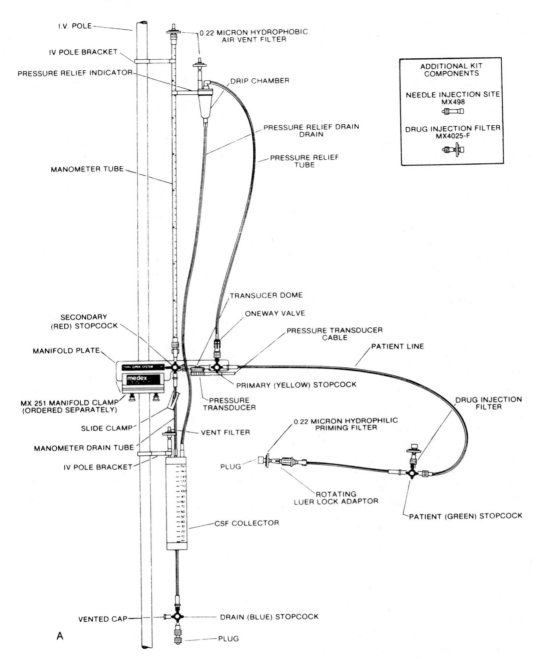

FIGURE 25-2
ICP and CSF drainage systems. Various systems are commercially available for measuring ICP
and draining CSF. (A) Courtesy of Medex Inc., Hilliard OH. (B) Courtesy of PS Medical, Santa
Barbara CA.

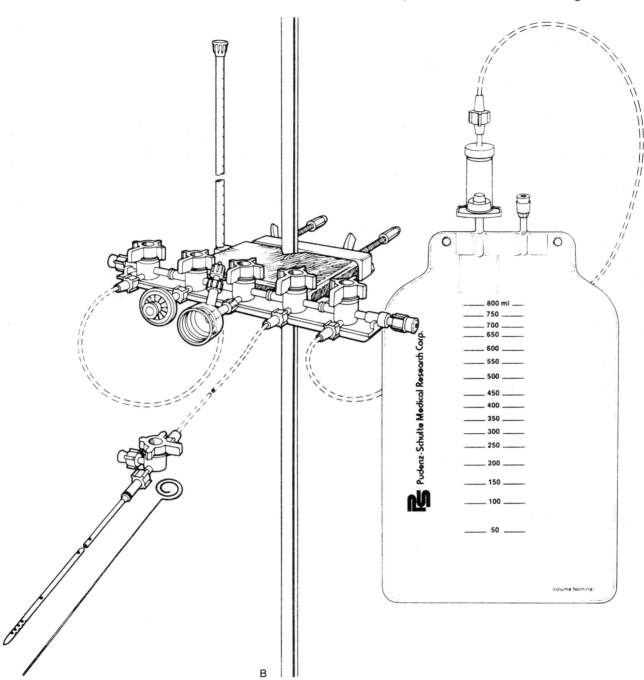

B

Indications. Criteria vary extensively. In one published protocol, barbiturate coma was initiated on head-injured patients with a Glasgow Coma Scale Score of 7 or less and in whom the ICP reached 25 mm Hg for longer than 10 minutes with the patient at rest while being treated with hyperventilation, steroids, mannitol and CSF drainage.

Procedure. Prior to administration of the barbiturate (usually pentobarbital), ICP, blood pressure, PAP, and electrocardiogram (EGG) monitoring with assisted ventilation are initiated. Baseline electroencephalogram (EEG) and brain stem–evoked responses (BAER) recordings are taken. An EEG is taken prior to initiation of barbiturate coma so that spontaneous electrocortical activity can be documented, and BAER are recorded so that brain stem integrity can be assessed. Although high serum barbiturate levels will totally suppress electrocortical activity, BAER will remain as long as there is brain stem function.

Dosage. To place the patient in a light coma, one administers a loading dose of 3 to 5 mg/kg of pentobarbital by slow intravenous push. The expected response is a drop in ICP of at least 10 torr within 10 minutes. If the patient responds to the loading dose, a maintenance dose of 1 to 3 mg/kg hour is given so that barbiturate levels will be maintained at 2.5 to 3.5 mg/dl and EEG activity will be maintained at 2 to 5 Hz for several days. Impaired liver or kidney function will affect serum barbiturate levels. If the patient does not respond to the first loading dose, a second loading dose is given 2 hours later. The onset of action of intravenous pentobarbital is 1 minute. It has a half-life of 4 hours. The usual techniques for reduction of ICP continue to be used in conjunction with barbiturates. Mannitol doses are reduced. High-dose pentobarbital therapy is initiated with a loading dose of 10 mg/kg/hour IV for 4 consecutive hours, followed by a continuous maintenance infusion of 1.6 mg/kg/hour. If ICP falls, CSF drainage and mannitol infusion are gradually discontinued.

Nursing Management. The patient in barbiturate coma becomes dependent. Clinical neurologic evaluation is almost impossible, making extensive, accurate monitoring of physiological responses to therapy mandatory. Artificial ventilation is required, and all vital functions must be maintained by the critical care team. Table 25-1 summarizes the management of the patient in induced barbiturate coma.

Indications for Discontinuing Barbiturate Coma. Barbiturate coma should be discontinued if any of the following exist: an ICP less than 15 torr for 24 to 72 hours; a normal VPR (less than 3 torr/ml); a systolic blood pressure less than 90 torr despite the use of vasopressors such as dopamine; lack of ICP response; progressive neurologic impairment such as deterioration of auditory BAER; abolition of the need for vasodilator therapy to reduce systolic blood pressure below 160 torr; cardiac arrest.

TABLE 25-1
MANAGEMENT OF PATIENTS IN INDUCED BARBITURATE COMA

Problem	Outcome	Management
Uncontrolled IICP (ICP > 20 torr for > 30 minutes and unresponsive to usual Rx methods)	ICP maintained at less than 15 torr CPP at least 60 to 70 torr Temperature between 37°C and 38°C rectally	Monitor ICP continuously. Calculate CPP (MAP − ICP) every hour; notify physician if 50 torr or less. Restrict fluids to 80 ml/hour or as ordered. Administer diuretics (*e.g.,* mannitol, Lasix) as ordered. Maintain normothermia with hypothermia-hyperthermia blanket or antipyretic agents.
Adequate barbiturate level to control ICP	Serum barbiturate level maintained at about 3 mg/dl ICP at less than 15 torr	Administer pentobarbital every hour slowly intravenously as ordered (rate 10 minutes/100 mg). Monitor daily serum barbiturate levels
Hypotension due to cardiovascular instability and hypovolemia	Arterial systolic pressure maintained above 90 torr Urinary output at least 30 ml/hour CVP and PAP within normal limits Normal sinus rhythm	Continuously monitor arterial pressure, PAP, CVP, ECG pattern. Check cuff pressure every shift and prn. Administer vasopressor (*e.g.,* dopamine if systolic <90 torr). (One dose of pentobarbital may be held.) Check urinary output every hour.

TABLE 25-1
Continued

Problem	Outcome	Management
Respiratory depression (unable to breathe spontaneously, absence of cough reflex)	Arterial blood gases — PCO_2: within normal limits or 22 to 25 torr PO_2: 100/torr Normal breath sounds bilaterally	Maintain on ventilator at 10 to 14/minutes and sigh 10 : 2 ratio or as ordered. Insert endotracheal tube or give tracheostomy care. Monitor cuff pressure continuously. Suction and bag every hour and prn. Irrigate tube with normal saline prn. Suction nasopharyngeal secretions every 2 hours and prn. Check arterial blood gases daily and prn. Check breath sounds every 1 to 2 hours.
Fluid and electrolyte imbalance 2° to fluid restriction, diuretics, and GI suction	Serum osmolality <320 mOsm Serum electrolytes within normal limits (*e.g.,* NA, K) Normal sinus rhythm Absence of T-wave depression and U waves BUN, creatinine, and hematocrit within normal limits Absence of clinical signs of dehydration	Serum osmolality twice a day (hold mannitol, Lasix if >320 mOsm and notify physician). Electrolytes, BUN, creatinine, Hct daily and prn. Monitor PAP and ECG pattern continuously. Check urinary output and specific gravity every hour. Monitor total intake and output every 24 hours and cumulatively. Observe skin and mucous membranes for evidence of dehydration.
GI depression (absence of bowel sounds, inability to assimilate)	Absence of vomiting Absence of impaction Absorption of tube feedings	Use Salem-sump or nasogastric tube for gravity drainage or intermittent suction. Measure gastric output every shift. Auscultate for bowel sounds every shift and prn Palpate abdomen for distention. Check for impaction. Check gastric contents for assimilation when tube feedings are initiated after bowel sounds have returned.
Loss of gag, swallow, and corneal reflexes	Absence of aspiration Absence of trauma to cornea	Suction oropharynx every hour and prn. Position on each side; avoid placing on back as much as possible. Cleanse eyes and apply liquid tears or Lacri-Lube S.O.P. every 4 hours and prn. Tape eyelids closed prn.
Susceptibility to infection	WBC within normal limits Cultures negative	Practice strict aseptic technique. Culture questionable sites prn.
Inadequate nutrition due to catabolic state	Minimal weight loss	Give multivitamins daily as ordered. Provide parenteral hyperalimentation as ordered.
Immobility	Absence of atelectasis Absence of skin breakdown Absence of thrombophlebitis and pulmonary embolism Absence of contractures	Institute appropriate preventive measures (specific details of care are beyond the scope of this chapter).
Inability to cope and lack of understanding by the family/significant others	Verbalization of realistic expectations Verbalization of an appropriate understanding of the patient's condition and the therapy	Allow the family members to vent their feelings and ask questions. Answer questions. Give appropriate information without generating unrealistic expectations.

(Reproduced with permission from Ricci M: Intracranial hypertension: Barbiturate therapy and the role of the nurse. J Neurosurg Nurs 11, No. 4:247–252, 1979)

The barbiturates are gradually tapered over a period lasting from 24 hours to several days. Arousal is gradual and prolonged, even after blood levels have been zero for several days. Patients must be weaned slowly and carefully from the respirator because of muscle weakness resulting from the therapy.

Patients have vacuous facial expressions for several days despite normal blood barbiturate levels. Occasionally, during the first 24 hours, they develop slow, abnormal movements that appear athetotic in nature. Dysarthria is common. Anticonvulsants are used for control of withdrawal seizures. Status epilepticus has been reported.

NURSING ASSESSMENT AND INTERVENTION

Extracranial Causes of IICP. Assess the patient for extracranial causes and potential causes of IICP and provide appropriate interventions to prevent elevations in ICP and/or decrease ICP (see Table 25-2).

Position of Neck, Head, and Hips
• Avoid rotation of head.
• Position head and neck to promote optimal venous drainage, reducing risk of distention of cerebral blood vessels.
• Avoid flexion of hips.
• Assess tracheotomy ties to ensure that they are not interfering with venous outflow.
• Check for neck swellings due to masses, infections, or hematomas.

Cardiovascular Instability
• Maintain accurate invasive lines.
• Maintain normotension. Continual arterial hypertension eventually leads to IICP, particularly in patients with cerebral contusions or impaired cerebrovascular resistance. Hypotension may result in cerebral ischemia secondary to reduced CPP.
• Maintain normothermia. Pyrexia causes vascular dilation, which may increase cerebral edema.
• Maintain CPP, CO, BP, and PAP within acceptable ranges.

TABLE 25-2
EXTRACRANIAL CAUSES OF IICP

• Position of neck, head, and hips
• Cardiovascular instability
• Increased intrathorcic pressure
• Increased abdominal distention
• Decerebrate posturing and agitation
• Metabolic abnormalities
• Nontherapeutic touch and painful procedures
• Extraneous sounds

Increased Intrathoracic Pressure
• Confirm airway patency. Suctioning may cause an increased PCO_2 with a Valsalva maneuver, resulting in increased intrathoracic pressure and a decrease in cerebral venous outflow.
• Avoid too vigorous hyperventilation prior to suctioning.
• Check ventilator for incorrect settings or excessive PEEP and adjust.
• Auscultate the chest to confirm air entry into both lungs. Aspirated gastric contents and pneumomediastinum have been documented as causes of IICP (Zegeer, 1984).[2]
• Measure cardiac outputs and SvO_2.
• Obtain arterial blood gases.
• Avoid foot boards.

Metabolic Abnormalities
• Maintain fluid and electrolyte balance.
• Hyponatremia may result from administration of hyperosmotic agents. If serum sodium concentration falls below 120 mEq/liter, there is an increased risk of brain swelling secondary to osmotic edema.
• Monitor arterial blood gases, electrolytes, mixed venous oxygen saturations, PAPS, and cardiac output.

Nontherapeutic Touch: Painful Procedures and Extraneous Sounds
• Minimize noxious stimuli. Significant ICP elevations as well as the triggering of A waves have been documented during consecutive suctioning, pupillary light checks, indirect cuff blood pressure measurements, injection of drugs, insertion of nasogastric tubes, turning, painful stimulation, oral or skin hygiene, and discussion of the patient's condition at bedside (Walleck, 1983[3]. Stewart, 1984[4]).
• Use theraputic touch, family voices, and music.

Patients with IICP. Nursing care activity can compound the primary and secondary intracranial insults, contributing to rapid deterioration in the unstable patient who has lost intracranial compliance, autoregulation, and vasomotor tone.

Management of the patient with IICP or the potential for intracranial hypertension includes the following:

• Eliminate extracranial causes of intracranial pressure elevations.
• Maintain accurate ICP and CPP measurements.
• Space patient care activities to avoid cumulative effects.
• Minimize interruptions in osmotherapy and ventilator support.

CONCLUSION

Numerous medical and nursing interventions are available for reducing the mortality and morbidity associated with IICP. Clinical assessment alone does not provide adequate information for giving optimal care to the critically ill patient with IICP.

Monitoring ICP, CPP, BP, and PAP and correlating these measurements with other clinical assessments often reduce the time required to obtain an accurate diagnosis, increase the time available for treatment, and provide continual feedback on the patient's response to selected treatments.

REFERENCES

1. Garritson HD et al: Effectiveness of fluid restriction, mannitol and furosemide in reducing ICP. In Ishii S et al (eds): Intracranial Pressure V. New York, Springer-Verlag, 1983
2. Zeeger LJ: Systemic cardiovascular effects of intracranial disorders: Implications for nursing care. J Neurosurg Nurs 16, No. 3:161–167, 1984
3. Walleck C: The effect of purposeful touch on intracranial pressure. NTI Res Abstr Heart Lung 12, No. 4: 428–429, 1983
4. Stewart E: The effect of nursing procedures on ICP. Abstract in Hitchens M (ed): Proceedings of the 11th Annual National Teaching Institute of the American Association of Critical Care Nurses, Dallas, 1984

BIBLIOGRAPHY

Allen GS: Comparison of calcium antagonists in cerebral vascular disease. In Battye (ed): New Perspectives in the Diagnosis and Management of Subarchnoid Hemorrhage. New York, Science & Medicine, 1984
Belleguarrigue R et al: Control of intracranial pressure in severe head injury. In Ishii S et al (eds): Intracranial Pressure V. New York, Springer-Verlag, 1983
Ricci M: Intracranial hypertension: Barbiturate therapy and the role of the nurse. J Neurosurg Nurse 11, No. 4:247–252, 1979
Tyler DC et al: Increased intracranial pressure: An indication to decompress a tension pneumomediastinum. Crit Care Medi 12, No. 5:467–468, 1984

Hypothermia

Carolyn M. Hudak

INDICATIONS

The use of hypothermia (lowered body temperature) in clinical situations ranges from treatment of gastric hemorrhage to attempts to prevent irreversible cerebral damage. Decreased body temperature reduces cellular activity and consequently the oxygen requirement of tissues. Hypothermia is therefore induced in situations involving interrupted or reduced blood flow to vital areas to minimize tissue damage due to diminished oxygen delivery. This is the rationale for using hypothermia during open heart and neurosurgical procedures.

The presence of fever (hyperthermia) in any patient produces greater cellular oxygen requirements because of the increased rate of metabolism. Each degree of temperature elevation above normal increases metabolism approximately 7%. This fact becomes especially significant in the patient whose vital centers may already be compromised because of cerebral edema that is surgically induced or the result of another form of insult such as hypoxia from cardiac arrest. It is to provide some margin of safety in these situations until injured tissue can recover that the body temperature is lowered or maintained at normothermic levels. Current emphasis is on prevention of marked elevations in body temperature as opposed to marked reduction of the temperature. Physiological responses to cold remain the same, and there are occasions when actual hypothermia is desirable.

Because the critical care nurse is usually responsible for inducing the hypothermic state and monitoring the patient during this therapy, it is important for her to be aware of the physiological manifestations of the various phases of body cooling.

PHASES OF HYPOTHERMIA

1. Cooling Phase

For the conscious patient, reduction of body temperature is at best an unpleasant experience. It goes without saying that adequate explanation and support for the patient and his family are integral parts of nursing care.

Methods. Although the method of inducing hypothermia will depend on the situation and the equipment available, there are essentially two ways to proceed—surface cooling and the more direct method of bloodstream cooling.

Surface cooling, which involves the use of blankets that circulate a refrigerant, is the method usually employed in critical care units. The cooling blanket may be placed directly against the patient, or, more esthetically, a sheet can cover the blanket and be tucked under the mattress to hold the blanket in place. (This should not negate turning the blanket with the patient to maintain skin contact with the cooling device.) The important point here is to avoid placing any degree of thickness between the patient and the blanket, as this will serve as an insulator and impede the cooling process.

When cooling is initiated, one blanket may be placed under the patient and another placed on top to hasten the cooling process. If a top blanket is used, one must exercise care in observing the patient's respiratory status because the weight of the cooling blanket may limit chest excursion. Keeping the blanket in contact with areas of superficial blood flow such as the axilla and groin will also expedite cooling. In the event that a cooling device is not available, one can apply ice bags to initiate the cooling process, using these same principles.

Bloodstream cooling is the method employed during open heart surgical procedures when the blood passes through the cooling coils in the cardiopulmonary bypass machine.

Assessment and Intervention. The body's initial reaction to cold exposure is an attempt to conserve body heat and to increase heat production. *Skin pallor* that occurs is due to a vasoconstrictor response that limits superficial blood flow and thus loss of body heat. Intense activity in the form of *shivering* occurs to maintain body heat. The effects of these compensatory responses will be reflected in the vital signs, and it is important that the nurse understand these transient variations and consider them in evaluating the patient.

During the first 15 to 20 minutes of hypothermia induction, all *vital signs* increase. Pulse and blood pressure rise in response to the increased venous return produced by vasoconstriction. Respiratory rate increases to meet the added oxygen requirements of increased metabolic activity produced by shivering and to eliminate the additional carbon dioxide produced. If the patient hyperventilates with shivering, respiratory alkalosis can develop. The initial rise in temperature is a reflection of this increased cellular activity (Table 25-3).

TABLE 25-3
PHYSIOLOGICAL REACTIONS DURING THE FIRST 15 TO 20 MINUTES OF HYPOTHERMIA INDUCTION

Parameter	Response
Skin	Pallor
Motor activity	Shivering
Pulse	Increased
Blood pressure	Increased
Respiratory rate	Increased
Temperature	May increase initially owing to increased cellular activity

Because the patient requiring hypothermia usually has an existing cellular oxygenation problem, the increased oxygen consumption induced by shivering is undesirable. For this reason, chlorpromazine (Thorazine) may be given at the beginning of induction to reduce hypothalamic response. *Hypoglycemia* is a potential occurrence during vigorous shivering because increased glucose is required for the increased metabolic activity.

After approximately 15 minutes, the vasoconstrictor effect is broken by means of a negative feedback loop, and warm blood flow to the body surface is reestablished. This accounts for the reddened skin color following initial skin pallor. (One can demonstrate this same phenomenon by holding an ice cube in the hand for a short period of time.)

As superficial warm blood flow is reestablished, body heat is lost and body temperature begins to drop. The temperature can be monitored by a rectal probe taped in place, which allows for frequent or continuous readings. Fecal material should be removed before the probe is inserted. Because blood cooled at the body surface continues to circulate through the body core, downward drift of the temperature usually continues for approximately 1°F after the cooling blanket is turned off. In the obese patient, a greater degree of drift may be experienced. For this reason, the cooling device should be turned off before the desired hypothermic level is actually attained. One must monitor temperature closely to determine whether the trend remains downward or whether an increase in temperature occurs, requiring use of the blanket again.

Skin care becomes particularly crucial owing to the presence of cold and its circulatory effects. One can change the patient's position to eliminate pressure points, taking care to move the blanket with the patient so that body contact is maintained with the cooling device. Experience has indicated that the skin can be protected by application of a thin coating of lotion followed by talcum powder; this does not appear to impede the cooling process. The application can be repeated in accordance with the skin care program, but the skin should be gently washed at least every 8 hours so that the accumulated coating is removed.

2. Hypothermia

Assessment and Intervention. When the desired level of hypothermia is achieved, usually around 32°C (89.6°F), a number of other physiological changes become apparent. The vital signs at this stage are all diminished. The development of respiratory acidosis is a real possibility because, at deeper levels of hypothermia, ventilation falls off more rapidly than does reduced carbon dioxide production. Also, with increasing hypothermia the oxygen dissociation curve shifts to the left, and at lower tensions oxygen is not readily released by hemoglobin to the tissues. Because of the developing circulatory insufficiency and increased metabolic activity due to shivering, metabolic acidosis also is a possibility.

Secretion of antidiuretic hormone is inhibited, and an increase in urine output may be noted with a drop in the specific gravity. During hypothermia, water shifts from the intravascular spaces to the interstitial and intracellular spaces. This results from movement of sodium into the cell in exchange for potassium and movement of water with it. This fluid shift produces hemoconcentration, and nursing measures must be taken to prevent embolization. Such measures include passive range of motion exercises and frequent change of position.

In hypothermic states, for every degree of temperature below normothermic levels, cerebral metabolism is decreased 6.7%. At 25°C (77°F) the brain volume is reduced 4.1%, and extracellular space increases about 31.5%. The sensorium fades at 34° to 33°C (93° to 91.4°F). For the neurologic patient who already has a depressed sensorium, other measures for evaluation of changes in the patient's level of response must be relied on, such as assessment of purposeful or nonpurposeful movements in response to painful stimuli and the degree of painful stimuli necessary to elicit a response.

Because all cellular activity diminishes with hypothermia, cerebral activity decreases and hearing fades at approximately 34° to 33°C (93° to 91.4°F) owing to reduced cochlear response. At 18° to 30°C (82° to 86°F) there is no corneal or gag reflex, and pulse irregularities may be noted as the result of myocardial irritability, which probably occurs because of the movement of potassium into the cell.

Ventricular fibrillation is a common occurrence at this level, and consequently the patient is usually maintained at a hypothermic level around 32°C (89.6°F) so that cardiac problems are avoided.

Drugs tend to have a cumulative effect in the hypothermia patient. Decreased perfusion at the injection site and decreased enzyme activity result in slower chemical reactions. Therefore the intravenous route is preferred, and intramuscular or subcutaneous injections should be avoided. If a drug must be given hypodermically, it should be given deeply intramuscularly, and vigilance must be maintained during the rewarming phase for cumulative effects.

Another potential occurrence during hypothermia is that of *fat necrosis*. This results from prolonged exposure to cold and decreased circulation, which allows crystals to form in the fluid elements of the cells, leading to necrosis and cellular death. Nursing measures

TABLE 25-4
PHYSIOLOGICAL EFFECTS OF THE HYPOTHERMIC STATE

Parameter	Response	Possible Complications
Skin	Decreased circulation leading to crystal formation in cells	Fat necrosis
Vital signs	Diminished	Respiratory acidosis Metabolic acidosis
Urinary output	Increased	
Fluid volume	Hemoconcentration	Embolization
Sensorium	Fades at 34°C to 33°C	Increased difficulty in determining mental status
Hearing	Fades at 34°C to 33°C	
Cardiac rhythm	Myocardial irritability below 28°C	Dysrhythmias

that can minimize fat necrosis include turning the patient frequently, massaging the skin to increase circulation, and avoiding prolonged application of cold to any one area (Table 25-4).

When the patient has reached the desired hypothermic level, vital signs will also level out at reduced values. Changes in vital signs must therefore be evaluated in light of the patient's hypothermic state. For example, if the nurse is caring for a neurosurgical patient cooled to 32°C (89.6°F) and if his vital signs have decreased as she would normally expect, an increase in pulse, respirations, or blood pressure to "normal levels" must be interpreted in view of the hypothermic state. Is an infectious process present? Are changes occurring in the patient's neurologic status? Is intracranial pressure increasing?

If the patient is to be maintained at the hypothermic level for a prolonged period of time, this can be accomplished in a number of ways. The patient (after his temperature has risen several degrees) may need to be placed on the cooling blanket periodically and returned to the desired hypothermic level.

One should perform nursing measures gently, with a minimal degree of activity to the patient to prevent an increase in body heat, such as when providing passive range of motion exercises. The nurse should bathe the patient with tepid or cool water to avoid increasing temperature in this manner.

It cannot be overemphasized that prevention of pulmonary problems in the hypothermic patient is almost entirely dependent upon nursing care. Change of position allowing for postural drainage, measures to promote adequate ventilation, and suctioning to remove accumulated secretions are all extremely important in this patient.

Rewarming

Methods. Once it is determined that the patient no longer requires the hypothermic state, rewarming can be accomplished by a number of methods, including surface rewarming, bloodstream rewarming, and natural rewarming. The last is the preferred method. The cooling device is removed. A blanket may be used to cover the patient, but no artificial heat is used, and the patient is allowed to warm at his own rate. As the patient approaches normothermic levels, it is to be anticipated that vital signs will return to precooling levels owing to reversal of the physiological events.

Assessment and Intervention. One of the hazards of artifically induced rewarming is that the skin and muscles may be warmed before the heart. The heart remains in a cooled state and is unable to maintain a sufficient cardiac output to meet the oxygen demands of the superficial areas. Further warming increases the dilatation of peripheral vessels and blood pools, resulting in decreased circulating volume, decreased venous return, and therefore decreased cardiac output. This sequence of events can be avoided if the heart is warmed first, as in the bloodstream method, or if the body is allowed to rewarm naturally.

Other complications that may occur during the rewarming process are hyperpyrexia, shock (for reasons just cited), and acidosis. The acidosis occurs as a result of the increase in metabolic activity in those areas already warmed and an insufficient circulation to meet the metabolic requirements of this increased activity. Oliguria may also result, probably because of antidiuretic hormone secretion.

During this rewarming phase, the patient must be monitored closely for indications necessitating recooling. With the patient's normothermic status used as a baseline, these indications would include a fading sensorium, greater increase in pulse and respirations than would normally be expected with the warming process, and a drop in the blood pressure. Another important facet to be monitored is the cumulative effect of drugs given previously.

The necessity for interpretion of clinical changes in the patient on the basis of the physiological changes brought about through cooling and then rewarming cannot be overemphasized. The nurse must anticipate changes and findings based on the patient's pathology and other variables present that would alter those findings. When those findings that are anticipated do not occur, and when there is a deviation from the anticipated, the critical care nurse must be prepared to ask the question *Why?* and go about systematically determining the reason that the anticipated change is not present. Only when the nurse is able to do this can optimal nursing care be rendered.

BIBLIOGRAPHY

Alexy B: Problems due to cold. J Emerg Nurs 6:22–24, 1980

Balderman SC et al: The optimal temperature for preservation of the myocardium during global ischemia. Ann Thorac Surg 35, No. 6:605–614, 1983

Koht A: Serum potassium levels during prolonged hypothermia. Intens Care Med 9, No. 5:275–277, 1983

Levy LA: Severe hypophosphatemia as a complication of the treatment of hypothermia. Arch Intern Med 140, No. 1:128–129, 1980

Levy WJ: Hypothermia and the electroencephalogram. Anesthesiology 58, No. 4:396–397, 1983

Southwick FS et al: Recovery after prolonged asystolic cardiac arrest in profound hypothermia: A case report and literature review. JAMA 243, No. 12:1250–1253, 1980

26
Spinal Cord Injury

Marilynn Mitchell

SOCIETAL IMPLICATIONS

There are approximately 12,000 spinal cord injuries in the United States every year. About 4000 patients die before reaching a hospital, and about 1000 die during hospitalization.

The worldwide etiologic factors in spinal cord injury (SCI) are, in order of decreasing incidence, as follows: vehicular accidents, falls, and sports injuries (particularly diving accidents). Males are more often the victim of SCI than females. The average age at the time of injury ranges from 15 to 35 years.

Advances have been made in the care and rehabilitation of patients with SCI. The increasing worldwide incidence of SCI, along with better medical care and longer survival, may contribute to the strain on the medical economy of all nations. Average first-year hospital costs for patients with acute cervical SCI range from $35,000 to $75,000, and the average lifetime expenses of a paraplegic in the United States are more than $750,000.

One solution to the social, emotional, and financial catastrophies associated with SCI seems to be prevention of such injuries — primarily through education of the public in safety measures. Better vehicular design, more industrial safety measures, and reduction of the number of drunk drivers all are important in preventing a rise in the number of victims of spinal cord injuries.

FUNCTIONAL ABILITIES AT DIFFERENT LEVELS OF INJURY

Spinal cord injury is one of the most devastating of all traumatic injuries. Nursing care must be directed toward the concomitant physical, emotional, and so-cial problems. With alertness to changes, close observation, and ongoing assessment of these patients by the critical care nurse, many complications of cord injury no longer occur, or at least are recognized early so that appropriate treatment is implemented.

Realistic goal-setting is determined by the level and extent of the injury. The higher the injury on the spinal cord, of course, the greater the loss of motor activity and sensation. The level of spinal cord injury is defined by the number of the most distal uninvolved segment of the cord.

C1 – C4 Lesions. With a C1 – C4 lesion, the trapezius, sternomastoid, and platysma muscles remain functional. Intercostal muscles and the diaphragm are paralyzed, and there is no voluntary movement (physiological or functional) below the spinal transection. Sensory loss for levels C1 through C3 includes the occipital region, the ears, and some regions of the face. Sensory loss is illustrated by a diagram of the dermatomes of the body (Fig. 26-1, *A* and *B*).

A patient with a C1, C2, or C3 quadriplegia requires full-time attendance because of his dependency on a mechanical ventilator. This person is also dependent in all activities of daily living, such as feeding, bathing, and dressing. A person with this level of injury is able to operate an electric wheelchair (which should have a high back for head support) with chin or breath control. A mouthstick can be used to operate a typewriter or a telephone.

A C4 quadriplegic usually needs a mechanical ventilator too, but he may be removed from it intermittently. The patient is usually dependent on others for the activities of daily living, although he may be able to feed himself with the aid of feeding devices. This patient still needs an electric wheelchair, although be-

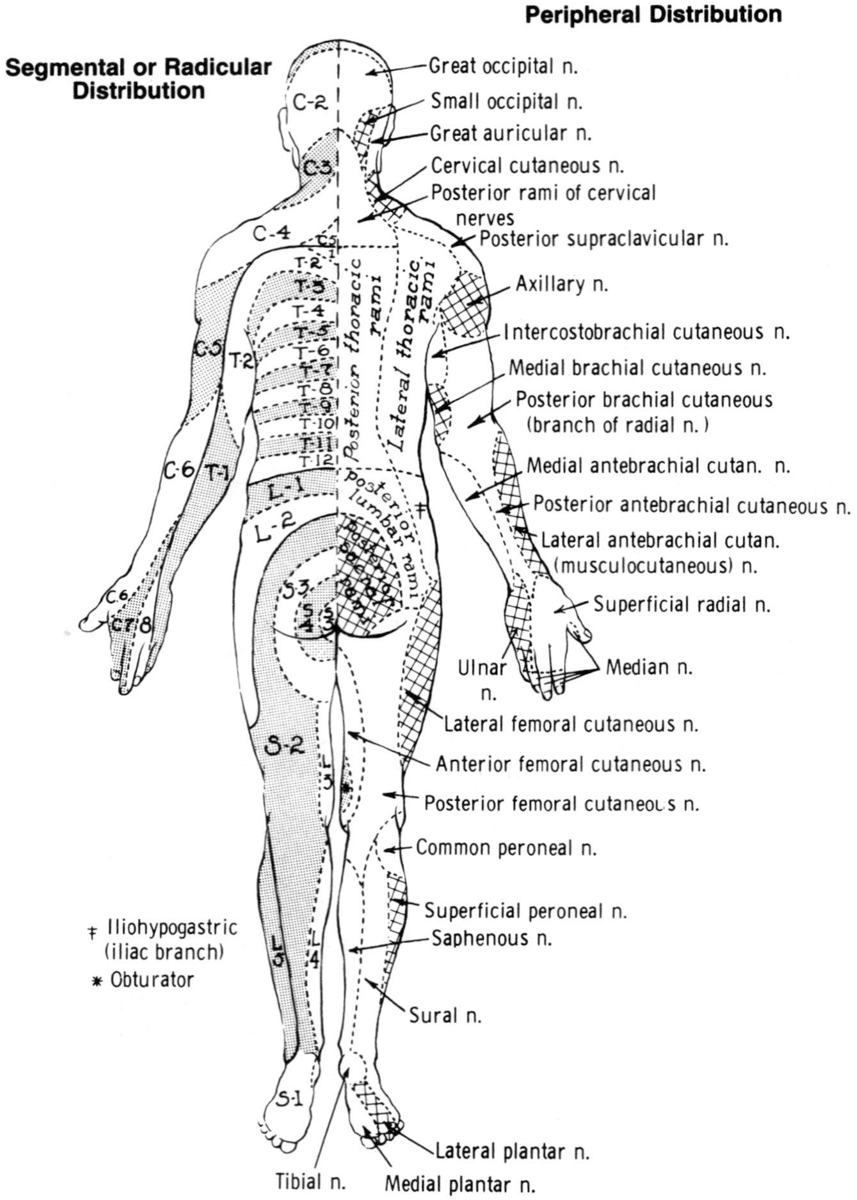

Peripheral Distribution
Segmental or Radicular Distribution
Great occipital n.
Small occipital n.
Great auricular n.
Cervical cutaneous n.
Posterior rami of cervical nerves
Posterior supraclavicular n.
Axillary n.
Intercostobrachial cutaneous n.
Medial brachial cutaneous n.
Posterior brachial cutaneous (branch of radial n.)
Medial antebrachial cutan. n.
Posterior antebrachial cutaneous n.
Lateral antebrachial cutan. (musculocutaneous) n.
Superficial radial n.
Ulnar n.
Median n.
Lateral femoral cutaneous n.
Anterior femoral cutaneous n.
Posterior femoral cutaneous n.
Common peroneal n.
Superficial peroneal n.
Saphenous n.
Sural n.
Lateral plantar n.
Tibial n.
Medial plantar n.
Posterior thoracic rami
Lateral thoracic rami
Posterior lumbar rami
C-2
C-3
C-4
C-5
T-2
T-3
T-4
T-5
T-6
T-7
T-8
T-9
T-10
T-11
T-12
C-6
T-1
C-7
C-8
L-1
L-2
S-3
S-2
L-5
L-4
S-1
ǂ Iliohypogastric (iliac branch)
* Obturator

FIGURE 26-1A
Cutaneous innervation. (Reproduced, with permission, from Chusid JG: Correlative Neuroanatomy & Functional Neurology, 17th ed, p 206. Copyright 1979, Lange Medical Publications, Los Altos, California)

cause of better head control, a high-backed chair is not essential.

C5 Lesions. When the C5 segment of the cord is damaged, the function of the diaphragm is impaired secondary to posttraumatic edema in the acute phase. Intestinal paralysis and gastric dilatation may compound the respiratory distress. The upper extremities are outwardly rotated from impairment of the supraspinous and infraspinous muscles. The shoulders may be markedly elevated owing to uninhibited action of the levator scapulae and trapezius muscles. Following the acute phase, reflexes below the level of the lesion are exaggerated. Sensation is present in the neck and the triangular area of the anterior aspect of the upper arms.

A C5 quadriplegic is usually dependent for activities such as bathing, shaving, and combing of hair, but he has better hand-to-mouth coordination, allowing him to feed himself with the aid of a feeder or brace. These aids permit him to brush his teeth and to dress his upper extremities. With the use of mechanical aids, this patient can usually write.

Assistance is needed, as with higher level quadriplegia, in transfers from wheelchair to bed or vice versa.

Peripheral Distribution

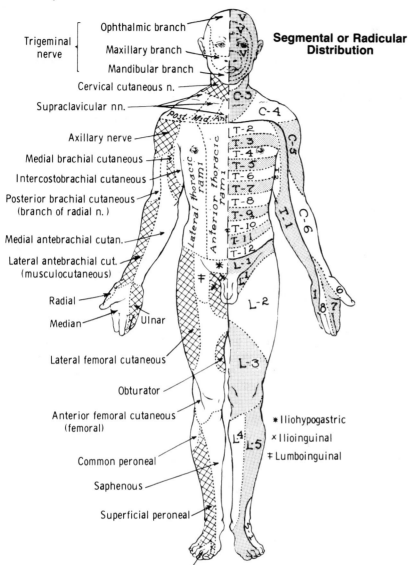

Segmental or Radicular Distribution

Trigeminal nerve
- Ophthalmic branch
- Maxillary branch
- Mandibular branch

Cervical cutaneous n.

Supraclavicular nn.

Axillary nerve

Medial brachial cutaneous

Intercostobrachial cutaneous

Posterior brachial cutaneous (branch of radial n.)

Medial antebrachial cutan.

Lateral antebrachial cut. (musculocutaneous)

Radial

Median — Ulnar

Lateral femoral cutaneous

Obturator

Anterior femoral cutaneous (femoral)

Common peroneal

Saphenous

Superficial peroneal

Deep peroneal

* Iliohypogastric
× Ilioinguinal
‡ Lumboinguinal

FIGURE 26-1B
Cutaneous innervation. (Reproduced, with permission, from Chusid JG: Correlative Neuroanatomy & Functional Neurology, 17th ed, p 205. Copyright 1979, Lange Medical Publications, Los Altos, California)

An electric wheelchair is still preferable with a C5 quadriplegic, although a manual wheelchair may be managed if it has quad pegs (projections on the hand rim that allow for greater ease of movement of the wheelchair). A person with this level of injury may find that manual manipulation of a wheelchair is very tiring.

C6 Lesions. In a C6 segment lesion, respiratory distress may occur because of intestinal paralysis and ascending edema of the spinal cord. The shoulders are usually elevated, with arms abducted and forearms flexed. This is due to the uninhibited action of the deltoid, biceps, and brachioradialis muscles. Functional recovery of the triceps depends on correct positioning of the arms (forearm in extension, arm in adduction). Sensation remains over the lateral aspect of the arms and dorsolateral aspect of the forearm.

A C6 quadriplegic is independent in most of his own hygiene and is sometimes successful in lower extremity dressing and undressing. He is independent in feeding with or without mechanical aids. Light housework can be accomplished, and he is able to drive a car with hand controls.

C7 Lesions. Cord lesions at the level of C7 allow the diaphragm and accessory muscles to compensate for the affected abdominal and intercostal muscles. The upper extremities assume the same position as in C6 lesions. Finger flexion is usually exaggerated when the reflex action returns.

A C7 quadriplegic has the potential for independent living without the care of an attendant. Transfers are independent, as are upper and lower extremity dressing and undressing, feeding, bathing, light housework, and cooking.

C8 Lesions. The abnormal position of the upper extremities is not present in C8 lesions because the adductors and internal rotators are able to counteract the antagonists. The latissimus dorsi and trapezius muscles are strong enough to support a sitting position. Postural hypotension may occur when the patient is raised to the sitting position owing to the loss of vasomotor control. One can minimize this postural hypotension by having the patient make a gradual change from the lying to the sitting position. The patient's fingers usually assume a claw position.

A C8 quadriplegic should be able to live independently. He is independent in dressing, undressing, driving a car, homemaking, and self-care.

T1–T5 Lesions. Lesions in the T1–T5 region may cause diaphragmatic breathing. The inspiratory function of the lungs increases as the level of the thoracic lesion descends. Postural hypotension is usually present. A partial paralysis of the adductor pollicis, interosseous, and lumbrical muscles of the hands is present, as is sensory loss for touch, pain, and temperature.

T6–T12 Lesions. Lesions at the T6 level abolish all abdominal reflexes. From the level of T6 down, individual segments are functioning, and at the level of T12, all abdominal reflexes are present. There is spastic paralysis of the lower limbs. Patients with lesions at a thoracic level should be functionally independent.

The upper limits of sensory loss in thoracic lesions are as follows:

Level of Lesion	Upper Limit of Sensory Loss
T2	Entire body to inner side of the upper arm
T3	Axilla
T5	Nipple
T6	Xyphoid process
T7, T8	Lower costal margin
T10	Umbilicus
T12	Groin

Bowel and bladder function may return with the reflex automatism.

L1–L5 Lesions. The sensory loss involved in L1 through L5 lesions is as follows:

Level of Lesion	Sensory Loss
L1	All areas of the lower limbs, extending to the groin and back of the buttocks
L2	Lower limbs, except the upper third of the anterior aspect of the thigh
L3	Lower limbs and saddle area
L4	Same as in L3 lesions, except the anterior aspect of the thigh
L5	Outer aspects of the legs and ankles and the lower limbs and saddle area

Patients with these lesions should attain total independence.

S1–S6 Lesions. With lesions involving S1 through S5, there may be some displacement of the foot. From S3 through S5, there is no paralysis of the leg muscles. The loss of sensation involves the saddle area, scrotum, glans penis, perineum, anal area, and the upper third of the posterior aspect of the thigh.

Adaptive Devices. Paraplegics vary in the amount of adaptive equipment that is useful in helping them be functionally independent: this depends on the level of injury. A T4 paraplegic may be able to stand up and walk with the aid of long leg braces and forearm crutches, although performance of this requires a great deal of physical energy.

T10 paraplegics are often more successful in ambulation with long leg braces and forearm crutches because there is more musculature preserved at this level than at the T4 level. L2 paraplegics can often accomplish ambulation with short leg braces and forearm crutches.

ORTHOPAEDIC VERSUS NEUROLOGIC LEVEL OF INJURY

These generalized goals for functioning at the different levels of spinal cord injury are not hard and fast for every patient. Functional performance may vary among patients, depending on whether one has a complete or an incomplete lesion. When an injury to the spinal cord is incomplete, there may be segments distal to the lesion that are still intact, although the orthopaedic level of injury is higher. For instance, the orthopaedic level of injury may be a C5 fracture, but the patient may be neurologically intact to C6. Because it is important to know what level of performance a patient can achieve, the neurologic level to which he can perform is really more significant than knowledge of the location of orthopaedic injury.

When one is speaking of a complete cord injury, the orthopaedic level of injury may be the same as the neurologic level of injury. No segments distal to the injury are preserved. A person with complete cord injury will closely follow the dermatome chart for his level of sensory loss.

INCOMPLETE CORD TRANSECTIONS

Incomplete cord transections often fit into recognizable neurologic syndromes.

FIGURE 26-2

Cross-section of the spinal cord to show the area involved in the central cord syndrome. Sensory loss typically is slight, and weakness is greater in the arms and hands than in the legs because of the distribution of nerve fibers in the corticospinal tracts. (L) descending lumbar nerve fibers; (T) thoracic nerve fibers; (C) cervical nerve fibers. (Redrawn from Ernest, MP: Neurologic Emergencies. New York, Churchill-Livingstone, 1983)

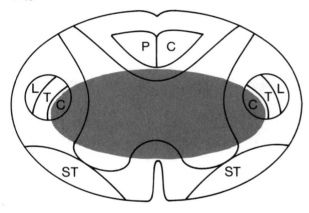

FIGURE 26-3

Cross-section of the spinal cord to show the area involved in the Brown-Séquard syndrome. There are hemiparesis and loss of position and vibratory sense on the side of the lesion, with contralateral loss of pain and temperature. (PC) Posterior columns; (CS) Corticospinal tract; (ST) Anterolateral spinothalamic tract. (Redrawn from Ernest MP: Neurologic Emergencies. New York, Churchill-Livingstone, 1983)

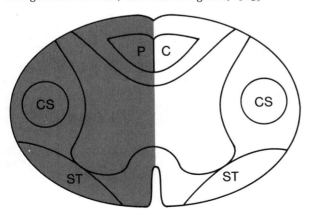

Central Cord Syndrome. Damage to the spinal cord in this syndrome is centrally located. Hyperextension of the cervical spine is often the mechanism of injury, and the damage is greatest to the cervical tracts supplying the arms. Clinically, the patient may present with paralyzed arms but with no deficit in the legs or bladder (Fig. 26-2).

Brown-Séquard Syndrome. The damage in this syndrome is located on one side of the spinal cord, such as a hemisection from a stab wound. The clinical presentation is one in which the patient has either increased or decreased cutaneous sensation of pain, temperature, and touch on the same side at the level of the lesion. Below the level of the lesion on the same side, there is complete motor paralysis. On the patient's opposite side, below the level of the lesion, there is loss of pain, temperature, and touch sense because the spinothalamic tracts cross soon after entering the cord. The posterior columns will be interrupted ipsilaterally, but this does not cause a major deficit because some fibers cross instead of running ipsilaterally. Clinically, the patient's limb with the best motor strength has the poorest sensation. Conversely, the limb with the best sensation has the poorest motor strength (Fig. 26-3).

Anterior Cord Syndrome. The area of damage in this syndrome is, as the name suggests, the anterior aspect of the spinal cord. Clinically, the patient usually has complete motor paralysis below the level of injury (corticospinal tracts) and loss of pain, temperature, and touch sensation (spinothalamic tracts), with preservation of light touch, proprioception, and position sense (posterior columns) (Fig. 26-4).

INITIAL EVALUATION AND TREATMENT

From 25% to 65% of patients with SCI have injuries associated with the spinal cord trauma. Head injuries are the most common and usually accompany a cervical cord injury. Chest injury often accompanies a thoracic spinal cord injury. A complete neurologic examination should be performed, with special attention given to ventilatory status. The chest, head, and abdomen should be examined. Appropriate radiographs of the chest, skull, abdomen, and long bones may be indicated. Placement of a nasogastric tube and urinary catheter can also help one evaluate the patient for other injuries.

There is some controversy about whether certain spinal cord injuries should be managed surgically or

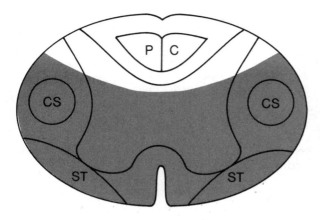

FIGURE 26-4
Cross-section of the spinal cord to show the area involved in the anterior cord syndrome. There are paraparesis and loss of pain and temperature to the level of the lesion (or just below it), but position and vibratory sense are relatively spared. (Redrawn from Ernest MP: Neurologic Emergencies. New York, Churchill-Livingstone, 1983)

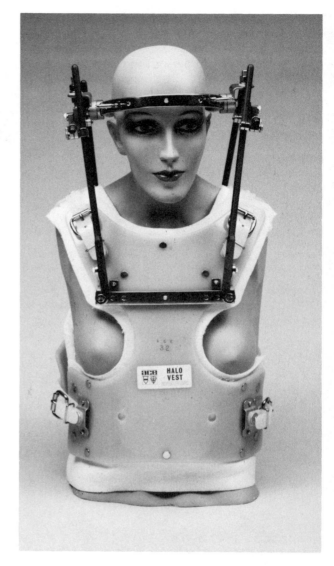

FIGURE 26-5
Halo brace. (Courtesy of Ace Medical Company, Los Angeles, CA)

nonsurgically. One clear indication for surgical intervention is an open injury, such as a gunshot or stab wound. Another indication is gross or late instability of the fracture site. Immobilization of unstable injuries is especially important in incomplete lesions, where further cord injury may result in further neurologic deficits.

Surgical stabilization is accomplished by placement of Harrington rods, by laminectomy and fusion, or by anterior fusion. Bone used for fusion is usually taken from the iliac crest, tibia, or ribs.

Nonsurgical management of cervical injuries involves use of skull tongs, halo traction, or a halo brace. Because use of a halo brace has the advantage of earlier mobilization, it is becoming the method of choice in many areas (Fig. 26-5).

The injury must be stable before a halo brace is applied. Sometimes, halo traction is used until the fracture is reduced or stability is achieved, then the halo brace is applied.

A patient in a halo brace should be moved as a unit so that strain on any one area of the brace is avoided. The upright bars should never be used as a handle to move the patient. Skin inspection should be done daily by the nurse. Extra padding may be added if the skin shows signs of breaking down under the vest. A pillow case can be slid between the skin and the sheepskin liner; if it comes out with signs of serosanguinous drainage, there is definitely an area of skin breakdown.

Nurses should also be aware of how to remove the anterior part of the halo vest in the event that access to the chest is needed, as for CPR. A wrench should always be taped to the cross bar on the front of the vest. The wrench will undo the two bolts that attach the uprights to the front vest. Four buckles are then unbuckled (two at the shoulders and two at the sides). One can then lift the anterior vest off without altering the alignment of the neck.

A rather new psychological phenomenon has been observed in patients who are having their halo brace removed for the first time, after 12 to 16 weeks. Although patients may have been told repeatedly during the period preceding removal of the brace that their deficits are permanent, many patients seem to attribute the deficits to their halo brace. Perhaps unconsciously, they believe that after the halo is removed, they will improve. When removal of the halo brace does not improve their deficits, they may experience significant depression and begin to grieve for a loss that actually occurred several months earlier. This has been termed *post-halo depression,* and it can be a significant problem. Intervention with psychological support may be necessary at this time.

IMMOBILIZATION

Most of the injury to the spinal cord occurs at the time of the accident. Secondary injury may occur from movement of an unstable spine, which causes further cord compression or cord damage from bony fragments. It is vitally important that the rescue crew at the scene of the accident and the emergency department personnel have as their primary goal prevention of further neurologic damage. They must also recognize impending complications of a spinal cord injury, such as respiratory distress, which is the primary early cause of death in patients with cervical cord injuries.

Because elapsed time from injury significantly affects prognosis, the patient with a spinal cord injury should be transported as rapidly as possible to a specialized unit or a hospital with adequate diagnostic and treatment facilities to handle such trauma. Some sort of neck immobilization is necessary before transport is possible. A long back board may be effectively used to keep the spine rigid, and sandbags and tape will secure the head.

If there will be some delay in removing the injured person from the accident scene, a soft collar may be applied temporarily. It still allows some movement of the head so should be used only until a more stable device can be applied.

Four-poster braces also are used in the field. If rescuers have good access to the victim, this brace provides better immobilization than a soft collar.

ACUTE PHASE OF SPINAL CORD INJURY

Assessment

During the initial assessment of a spinal cord–injured patient, a *digital rectal examination* is important in the determination of whether the injury is incomplete or complete. The lesion is incomplete if the patient can feel the palpating finger or if he can contract the perianal muscles around the finger voluntarily. Sensation may be present in the absence of voluntary motor activity. Sensation is seldom absent when voluntary perianal muscle contraction is present. In either case, the prognosis for further motor and sensory return is good. Preservation of sacral function might be the only finding that indicates an incomplete lesion, and significant neurologic recovery may occur in the patient with an incomplete cord injury.

Rectal tone by itself, without the criteria of voluntary perianal muscle contraction or rectal sensation, is not evidence of an incomplete cord injury. Some rectal tone may be accounted for by local reflexes.

Spinal Shock

Spinal shock can be seen with either complete or incomplete motor and sensory deficits. Spinal shock differs from traumatic shock in several ways. In cord lesions above the sympathetic outflow (T5), there is an initial fall in blood pressure. This *hypotension* is more pronounced in cervical injuries. The blood pressure returns to normal a few days after the injury, but the reflex depression remains for a long period.

The reduced peripheral resistance and consequent pooling of blood in spinal shock are due to the vasomotor paralysis that occurs in spinal injury above the level of T6 and produce hypotension. In this instance, the hypotension is like that of neurogenic shock. The low blood pressure in uncomplicated cord injury is accompanied by bradycardia due to reflex vagal activity. When other injuries are present, there may be hypovolemia and tachycardia. Cardiac arrest is a potential danger in spinal shock because of this vasomotor instability. There also is the potential for deep vein thrombosis in the spinal shock phase because of venous pooling of blood, but it is more likely to occur after reflex activity has returned.

Hypothermia and absence of sweating below the injury level may also be seen in the spinal shock stage. Initially, flaccid paralysis is seen below the level of injury with bowel and bladder atony. Sacral reflexes and priapism may be present in patients with upper motor neuron lesions.

The appearance of involuntary spastic movement indicates that the spinal shock is resolving. Reflex activity returns over several days in patients with upper motor neuron lesions. Reflex perianal muscle contraction often returns before the deep tendon reflexes (DTRs). One can test for the reflex perianal muscle contraction during a digital rectal examination by pinching the glans or the base of the penis (bulbocavernous reflex) or by pulling on the Foley catheter. In a female, squeezing of the clitoris will stimulate the reflex, if present. Absence of this spinal reflex arc implies that there is no physiological continuity between the lower spinal cord and supraspinal centers.

NURSING INTERVENTIONS

Respiratory Care

Possible nursing diagnosis: Potential for ineffective breathing patterns related to reduced muscular innervation.

Hypoventilation from inadequate innervation of respiratory muscles is a common problem after spinal cord injury. It is important for one to assess whether the intercostal muscles are functioning or whether the patient has only diaphragmatic breathing. The diaphragm, the major respiratory muscle, is innervated by the phrenic nerve, which travels through the third, fourth, and fifth cervical segments of the cord.

Any time a patient has a cervical cord injury, *respiratory failure* should be anticipated. Even though the patient may initially have what appears to be adequate diaphragmatic breathing (the intercostals would not be functioning because they are innervated from the thoracic region of the cord), cord edema can act like an ascending lesion and may compromise function of the diaphragm. Frequent checks of tidal volume and vital

FIGURE 26-6
Quad coughing technique. These positions are for diaphragmatic quad coughing only. (Top) *To push the diaphragm, place one hand flat in the middle of the torso above the stomach and below the ribs.* (Middle) *Front view of the ribs; diaphragm indicated by heavy line.* (Bottom) *To compress the chest, place both hands flat and position on both sides of the chest. Do not move on top of the rib cage because this could cause damage.*

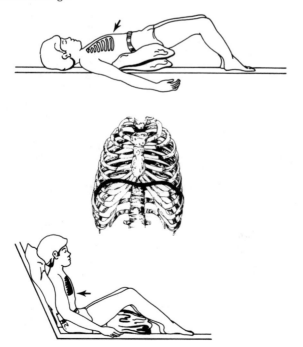

capacity and frequent auscultation of breath sounds should be routine.

The spinal cord–injured patient may have further respiratory compromise because of preexisting pulmonary disease or coexistent chest injuries. Alveolar ventilation may be directly affected by the pulmonary collapse or by consolidation from *retained secretions* or aspiration of vomitus. *Pulmonary edema* may also result from incorrect management of intravenous fluids. Paralytic ileus and gastric dilatation may increase the pressure on the diaphragm and cause further respiratory embarrassment. Interference with the cough reflex and fluid imbalance may combine to obstruct the airways.

Assisting the patient with the *quad coughing technique* may help him clear his airways more effectively despite weakness or loss of the respiratory muscles that produce the automatic cough reflex. With this quad coughing technique, the sides of the patient's chest (if he is on his side or abdomen) or the diaphragm (if he is supine) are compressed during exhalation (Fig. 26-6). This technique is often most helpful following postural darainage or clapping of the chest.

When turning a patient to a *prone position* on a Stryker frame, the nurse needs to remain at the bedside for the first few turns to evaluate the patient's respiratory tolerance of the turn. High quadriplegics can experience respiratory arrest in the prone position because movement of the diaphragm is compromised. Bradycardia in the prone position also is common.

Metabolic Considerations

Possible nursing diagnoses: Potential for fluid volume deficit and alterations in nutrition related to specific metabolic changes from spinal cord injury.

The patient with spinal cord injury demonstrates a surprisingly florid metabolic response to an injury that is usually associated with little tissue damage. If the injury is uncomplicated, the metabolic derangement reaches a peak within 48 to 72 hours post injury. A return to normal may be anticipated between 10 and 14 days post injury.

When the spinal injury is complicated by other factors such as surgical intervention or other medical problems, the metabolic response is greater and more prolonged. This metabolic response is characterized by a marked retention of sodium and water, increased potassium excretion, breakdown of body protein, and an oliguric period followed by diuresis. A reduced glomerular filtration rate secondary to hypotension compounds the sodium and water retention.

Starvation also is a factor in the metabolic disturbance because the majority of cord-injured patients are unable to tolerate oral food or fluid for at least a week following the injury. This can lead to a negative nitrogen balance in the body.

Because it may be difficult for one to ascertain the patient's state of hydration on admission owing to the vasodilatation, *monitoring of fluid intake and output* is necessary for prevention of pulmonary edema, tubular necrosis, electrolyte imbalance, and congestive heart failure.

The intravenous caloric intake should be approximately 2000 calories/24 hours. It may be necessary for one to give the patient *hyperalimentation* to accomplish this. Patients with spinal cord injury tend to lose weight easily because of the increased catabolic activity.

Research on metabolic and endocrine changes in patients with spinal cord injuries has provided some interesting data. Apparently, body areas that have become insensitive as a result of the cord injury do not secrete anti-inflammatory steroids in adequate amounts. This lack of secretion may play a role in the genesis of pressure sores in the SCI patient. During surgical procedures, this attenuation of the normally expected rise in corticosteroid levels is also seen. Because excessive inflammation of the surgical site may occur as a result of the minimal cortisol release, this must be kept in mind if the patient undergoes surgery.

Cord-injured patients also have a decrease in testosterone levels that is significant enough to contribute to the negative nitrogen balance seen in these patients. Thus, careful positioning and turning of the SCI patient are necessary for prevention of pressure sores, and exercising and sitting are necessary for avoidance of excessive bone loss.

Both the sudden absence of muscular activity and sensations in the SCI patient and the mental state of helplessness appear to alter central nervous system metabolism. Depression coincides with a fall in a brain metabolite excreted in the urine as tryptamine. Thus, it is important for the nurse to understand that depression in some SCI patients might have a metabolic basis and that a trial of pharmocologic therapy might be beneficial to such patients.

Gastrointentinal Considerations

Possible nursing diagnosis: Potential alteration in nutrition due to interruption of bowel innervation.

Cord-injured patients often have gastrointestinal difficulties. This complication is seen most frequently in the patient whose lesion is in the cervical or thoracic region of the cord. The pathophysiology of this complication is thought to involve an imbalance between parasympathetic and sympathetic innervation of the bowel caused by interruption of the supraspinal control of sympathetic centers in the thoracic and upper areas of the spinal cord.

The cessation of smooth muscle function lasts for about 5 to 7 days. There is an accumulation of fluid in the stomach and intestines with vomiting and *abdominal distension.* Acute gastric dilatation frequently occurs in patients with high cord lesions with or without paralytic ileus. When the distention compresses the vena cava or elevates the diaphragm, there may be an exacerbation of the hypotension or hypoventilation associated with cervical cord injury.

Acute gastrointestinal *hemorrhage* may also occur secondary to a stress ulcer. Signs of a *stress ulcer,* which is due to an abnormal release of catecholamines, often occur between 6 and 14 days after injury. The problem may be aggravated by steroid therapy. The nurse should be alert if the quadriplegic patient complains of sudden unexplained shoulder pain. It may be referred pain from the gastrointestinal tract. One may instill a small amount of antacid medication into the patient's stomach whenever the *p*H of the gastric aspirate is below 3 in order to prevent the complication of stress ulcer. Cimetidine also may be prescribed in an attempt to prevent stress ulcers.

The combination of starvation and gastrointestinal and metabolic changes may precipitate ketosis, dehydration, and other electrolyte and acid-base imbalances. Because of the gastrointestinal complications, a nasogastric tube should be inserted and bowel sounds monitored. The *nasogastric tube* prevents vomiting and probably aids in earlier resolution of the ileus. *Oral fluids* may be started at 25 to 50 ml/hour after bowel sounds have returned. If there is no evidence of residual gastric aspirate, oral fluids may be gradually increased. Food intake may begin when the patient can tolerate 75 to 150 ml of fluid each hour. Chances are great that the patient initially will have a poor appetite, partly because of depression and partly because of sensory loss.

Skin Care

Possible nursing diagnosis: Potential for impairment of skin integrity related to loss of sensation.

Pressure is a common cause of structural damage to a muscle and its peripheral nerve supply. There is a definite time/pressure relationship in the development of *pressure sores.* Skin can tolerate minute pressure indefinitely, but great pressure for a short time is disruptive. Microscopic tissue changes secondary to local ischemia occur in less than 30 minutes. Pressure interferes with arteriolar and capillary blood flow.

When the pressure is prolonged, there is a definite damage to superficial circulation and tissue. The damage may be associated with congestion and induration of the area or blistering and loss of superficial epidermal layers of skin. As the pressure continues, the deeper skin layers are lost, leading to necrosis and ulceration. Serous drainage from such an ulceration can constitute a continuous protein loss of as much as 50 g/day. Prolongation of the pressure results in deep penetrating necrosis of the skin, subcutaneous tissue, fascia, and muscle. The destruction may progress to gangrene of the underlying bony structure. Pressure necrosis can begin from within the tissue over a bony prominence, where the body weight is greatest per square inch.

A *turn schedule* for the patient is obviously important. Turning should be carried out at least every 2 hours. Use of an air mattress does not preclude the need to turn. The condition of the skin should be checked before and after the position change. Patients should be encouraged to check their own skin condition with a mirror, when possible, to recognize their skin's tolerance to pressure, that is, the amount of time one can lie or sit in the same position without redness that does not fade within 15 minutes.

Numerous automated beds are now on the market that provide the patient with continuous motion. Many of these beds can be helpful in minimizing pulmonary skin complications.

Patients should also be taught how to do *weight shifts,* especially when they are getting up in their wheelchair for long periods during the day. A weight shift is a means of relieving pressure from any bony prominence. When the patient is in the sitting position, the main bony prominences are the ischial tuberosities and the sacrum.

There are several methods of accomplishing a weight shift. There is a *full recline,* in which the patient is reclined in his wheelchair to relieve the ischial pressure, and the weight is thereby distributed throughout his entire dorsal surface. The patient accomplishes the *side-to-side* weight shift by hooking his forearm around one push-handle of the wheelchair and then leaning sideways over the opposite wheelchair tire. The patient performs the *half push-up* weight shift to relieve pressure from one ischium by leaning on one elbow and pushing off the opposite wheelchair tire or armrest. He repeats this process in the other direction to relieve pressure from the opposite ischium. With the *full push-up* weight shift, the patient relieves ischial pressure by pushing up with his arms from the tires or armrests of the wheelchair. Which of these weight shifts a patient can accomplish will of course depend on his motor ability.

To avoid skin breakdown, one should protect the skin from perspiration, stool, and urine. Use of incontinence pads tends to hold the perspiration next to the skin and thus should be avoided. A bedpan does not work well with a spinal cord–injured person. It is so hard that it can cause a pressure area over the coccyx, it does not allow access to the anus for digital stimulation, and it can upset the spinal alignment necessary for proper healing.

Contractures

Possible nursing diagnosis: Impaired physical mobility related to loss of innervation to muscles.

Prevention of contractures should be initiated on admission. Muscle shortening from disuse of an extremity can occur within 3 days. A paralyzed extremity is more likely to contract to a flexed position because the muscles used to flex an extremity are stronger than those used to extend it. If contractures are allowed to develop, the patient's recovery cannot be optimal. He will not be able to recover full motor use of a contracted extremity.

Cardiovascular Care

Possible nursing diagnosis: Potential for decreased cardiac output related to loss of vasomotor tone and pooling of blood in periphery.

During the spinal-shock phase, vasomotor tone is lost and blood pools in the periphery, lowering blood pressure because of the decreased circulating volume. *Orthostatic hypotension* may also occur because the patient is unable to compensate for changes in position. The vasoconstricting message from the medulla cannot reach the blood vessels because of the cord lesion.

Deep vein thrombosis is a silent complication in spinal cord–injured patients and carries with it the hazard of *pulmonary embolism.* The development of a thrombosis is influenced by stasis in the venous system, local trauma, continuous contact of the patient's calves and thighs with the bed, prolonged immobilization, and the patient's inability to sense pain.

With the development of venous thrombosis, there is swelling of the involved limb, local redness, increased skin warmth, and a slight systemic temperature rise (which may be masked if the patient is receiving steroids).

The *routine turn schedule* for skin maintenance mobilizes the patient sufficiently to help prevent venous thrombosis. Thigh-high *elastic stockings* or bandages properly applied also have prophylactic value. They should be removed for about 30 minutes each 8-hour period.

Other preventive measures include *determination of the patient's leg circumference* 20 cm above and below the upper border of the patella on admission, for a baseline, and then daily thereafter. *Passive range of motion exercises* for lower extremities should be carried out at least twice a day. *Anticoagulant therapy* also may be considered. If there is no contraindication, such as concomitant head injury, the patient should be placed in *Trendelenburg's position* (about 15°) for a minimum of 1 hour every 8 hours so that the blood can more easily return to the heart from the lower extremities.

Because of the spinal cord lesion and the lack of sympathetic control, the patient may become poikilothermic, a condition in which the body tends to assume the temperature of the environment. This makes the patient especially vulnerable to hypothermia.

Bowel Program

Possible nursing diagnosis: Alterations in bowel elimination related to paralytic ileus and gastric dilatation during spinal shock, later related to imbalance between parasympathetic and sympathetic innervation of the bowel.

Smooth muscle peristalsis begins as soon as the paralytic ileus secondary to spinal shock resolves. The nurse must keep in mind that bowel impaction frequently occurs during the period of ileus. The defecation reflex remains intact with lesions above the sacral segments. The reflex is interrupted with lower motor neuron lesions, but the autonomous bowel has an intrinsic contractile response. Bowel training is based on a fixed time pattern that takes the place of the cerebrally monitored urge. For the patient with a lower motor neuron lesion, continence is assured by regular evacuation of the bowel.

Peristalsis should be stimulated as soon as bowel sounds are present. This is safely done with stool softeners, mild laxatives, or suppositories. Enemas, other than the oil-retention type, should be avoided because the risk of intestinal perforation is high.

The actual bowel program may be based on bowel habits prior to the injury. The time of day should be established in relation to the patient's future social needs. A bowel program can be used in conjunction with digital stimulation.

Once a pattern is established, *digital stimulation* may be used alone. While the pattern of evacuation is being established, digital stimulation should be used after any involuntary bowel movement so that complete evacuation of the rectum is assured. There may be patients who will not tolerate digital stimulation without having an episode of autonomic dysreflexia. Dibucaine (Nupercaine) can be used for insertion of the suppository or for digital stimulation in those patients prone to this phenomenon.

A bowel program may be modified according to individual need, as determined by stool consistency. A high fluid intake should be maintained.

Urinary Management

Possible nursing diagnosis: Alteration in pattern of urinary elimination related to loss of innervation to bladder and loss of reflex arc.

Acute tubular necrosis may occur during the first 48 hours post injury as a result of hypotension. In the acute phase of injury, the urine output should be measured hourly. An indwelling catheter is necessary for this procedure. One should test the urine for specific gravity, blood, protein, bile, and sugar to help monitor electrolyte balance.

The long-range objective of bladder management, regardless of the level of the lesion, is to achieve a means whereby the bladder consistently empties, the urine is sterile, and the patient remains continent. The ultimate goal is to have the patient catheter free, with consistent low residual urine checks, no urinary tract infection, and no evidence of damage to the upper urinary tract structures.

Intermittent Catheterization. One method of bladder management is accomplished by intermittent catheterization, and it may begin in the early recovery phase after the spinal shock has resolved. The purpose of this program is to exercise the detrusor muscle, with the goal again being to have the patient catheter-free. The advantage of this method is that no irritant remains in the bladder; consequently, the risk of urinary tract infection, periurethral abscess, and epididymitis is reduced.

With this method, the patient is initially catheterized every 4 to 6 hours. A record is kept of voided amounts and residual amounts. If there is a residual of over 500 ml, the frequency of catheterization should be increased until residuals are under that amount. A urine specimen is obtained for culture and sensitivity at the start of the program. The fluid intake between catheterizations is limited to 600 to 800 ml. The number of catheterizations can be decreased as voided amounts increase or as residual amounts decrease. When a male patient begins to void between catheterizations, an external collector can be used to maintain continence.

Prior to the catheterization procedure, the patient should be assisted to empty the bladder by Créde, Valsalva, and dilatation, or any other method that will trigger voiding. These methods stimulate the sacral reflex arc. The objective is to achieve a repeatable residual urine volume of 10% of the voided volume. The catheterizations may be stopped when the residuals become less than 150 ml.

Factors that may hinder efforts to achieve urinary continence include bowel impactions, cystitis, bladder stones, pressure sores, systemic infections, and anxiety.

Indwelling Catheter. Another urinary protocol that can be followed involves an indwelling bladder catheter. This catheter can be a urethral or suprapubic. The catheter is attached to a gravity drainage system at all times. High fluid intake is encouraged. The catheter insertion site should be washed once or twice daily with soap and water. Betadine swabs also may be used to cleanse the insertion site. These catheters should not be changed routinely, but only if they become plugged or develop granulation inside. Male urethral catheters should be taped up on the abdomen so that urethral-scrotal fistulas are prevented. Female urethral catheters should be taped to the inside of the thigh.

A male urethral catheter should not be larger than a size 16, 5-ml inert catheter. A female urethral catheter should not be larger than a size 20, 5-ml inert catheter. A suprapubic catheter should not be larger than a size 24, 5-ml inert catheter.

The method of clamping an indwelling catheter with intermittent release and drainage of the bladder is no longer used in many spinal cord rehabilitation facilities. If the patient should have a large residual volume between the times the bladder is drained, the urine can do nothing except reflux back into the kidneys. This situation can be very detrimental to the patient's kidneys. Overdistention also destroys the detrusor muscle's ability to contract, thereby jeopardizing the return of automatic functions.

For management of a neurogenic bladder, various techniques have been tried in an attempt to produce contractions of the detrusor muscles. Tapping on the suprapubic area, massaging and stimulating the perigenital regions, pulling the pubic hair, applying cold water to the genitalia, and dilating the rectal sphincter are among the methods used to manage this problem.

The Mayo Clinic has developed a nonmanual triggering technique that involves an electrical tapping device that can be strapped over the suprapubic region. The tapping device is used only for induction of bladder detrusor contraction and is removed after urination is accomplished. Its purpose is to retrain the detrusor muscle that does not contract enough to initiate micturition. Of the eight SCI patients used in the trial, six no longer needed the device after 3 to 4 weeks of bladder retraining. Owing to ongoing research, more such devices are becoming available to patients with SCI.

Medications

Possible nursing diagnosis: Potential for alteration in tissue perfusion related to lack of muscle tone.

Some medications are commonly used in patients with spinal cord injuries, whereas others are contraindicated. *Cortisone* (dexamethasone MSD) may be used initially for a short period to relieve the physiological stress phenomenon. Intravenous therapy *(hyperalimentation)* may be indicated during the spinal-shock phase or possibly for longer periods, depending upon coexistent complications. The intravenous site of choice is the subclavian vein because in this area there is less chance of thrombosis secondary to the vasomotor paralysis. For this reason, the veins of the lower extremities should never be used for intravenous administration. Low-dose *heparin* may be used

prophylactically against venous thrombosis, although there is much contradictory literature regarding its worth.

Subcutaneous and intramuscular injections are not absorbed well because of the lack of muscle tone. Sterile abscesses may result, causing autonomic dysreflexia or an increase in spasms. *Injection sites* are the deltoid area, the anterior thigh, and the abdominal area. These sites should be rotated, and the volume injected should not exceed 1 ml at any one site.

As a rule, sensation in cord-injured patients is limited. Intractable pain may be present after spinal shock and is due to nerve root damage. Abnormal sensation may occur at the level of the lesion in injuries causing diverse nerve root damage, such as with gunshot wounds or knife wounds. Narcotics are not favored because of the high probability of addiction. Attention to position and other comfort measures, along with the use of mild analgesics such as aspirin or acetaminophen, is a more acceptable approach.

Tranquilizers can be used to dull the environment during the initial stage following cord injury; however, behavioral problems are not relieved by tranquilizers. The psychological stages of the recovery process must be resolved, and this cannot be accmplished if the patient remains sedated. As reflex automatism returns, relief of spasms can be achieved with *diazepam*.

Physical Therapy

Possible nursing diagnosis: Impaired physical mobility related to loss of innervation to muscles.

A program of physical therapy and rehabilitation should be organized shortly after the patient's hospital admission. Realistic short- and long-term goals must be set jointly with the patient. Rehabilitation is often a very protracted process. The patient must be aware that results from the program will not be seen overnight. Thus, it is important that the patient and his family be part of the rehabilitation conference when goals are discussed.

A myriad of problems can surround the patient with a spinal cord injury. Each person responds differently and adjusts to his injury in a different way. When a patient's whole life must be changed because of a spinal cord injury, the emotional and social problems, as well as the physical ones, can seem overwhelming. Patients need the support of the family and significant others at this time. The critical care nurse assumes a major role in helping both patient and family to cope with the problems. Rehabilitation of cord-injured patients can be slow and tedious and psychologically draining for the nurse, but it also offers great rewards in terms of the personal satisfaction that comes from meeting the challenges.

Sexuality

Possible nursing diagnosis: Potential for sexual dysfunction related to loss of innervation distal to level of spinal cord lesion.

After a cord injury, patients are concerned about their ability for sexual function, although many may not verbalize this concern for quite a time. When the questions do come, it is helpful if the nurse can respond in an informed way instead of telling the patient to ask the physician. Failure of professionals to inquire about the patient's sexual concerns tends to confirm his fears that his sexual life is over.

Most male cord-injured patients believe that their total sexuality is tied to erection and ejaculation. There are three general types of erection in men: psychogenic, reflexogenic, and spontaneous.

A *psychogenic erection* can result from sexual thoughts. The area of the cord responsible for this type of erection is between T11 and L2. Therefore, if the lesion is above this level, the message from the brain cannot get through the damaged area.

Reflexogenic erections are a direct result of stimulation to the penis. Some patients may get this type of erection when changing their catheter or pulling the pubic hairs. The length of time the erection can be maintained is variable; thus, its usefulness for sexual activity is variable. Reflexogenic erections are better with higher cervical and thoracic lesions. Damage to lumbar and sacral regions may destroy the reflex arc.

The third type of erection is *spontaneous.* This may occur when the bladder is full, and it comes from some internal stimulation. How long the spontaneous erection lasts will determine its usefulness for sexual activity. The ability to achieve a reflexogenic or spontaneous erection comes from nerves in the S2, S3, and S4 segments of the cord. Male penile implants are now available for patients whose erections are very brief or not present at all.

Not many men with a complete cord injury have ejaculations. Sometimes retrograde ejaculation into the bladder will occur. Some male patients remove their urethral catheter prior to intercourse. Others leave their catheter in place and fold it back over the penis. Despite the physical side effects of the spinal cord injury, the patient's sex drive should not change from what is was before the injury.

Women with spinal cord injury may find they need to use a lubricating jelly such as KY jelly (water soluble) prior to intercourse. If the woman was practicing birth control before the injury, it should still be a concern after the injury. Fellatio and cunnilingus are practices many patients find satisfying.

The nursing role is to help encourage the SCI patient with whatever counseling is needed. The sexuality of an individual involves the total person, not just sexual behavior. It includes what one thinks about himself in general. Cord-injured patients need to be made aware that meaningful, loving relationships are still attainable. Sexual counseling is often needed to communicate these messages.

Some centers are meeting the needs of early legitimization of sex-related concerns by employing a sexual health care clinician in acute SCI units. This clinician is a nonphysician specialist trained to diagnose and treat sexual dysfunctions of disabled persons. The clinician is under medical supervision and is part of the rehabilitation team. Experience has indicated that sexual assessment, diagnosis, and management constitute a technical specialty that requires in-depth training. Creation of such a role is a new and exciting idea.

AUTONOMIC DYSREFLEXIA

Autonomic dysreflexia, or hyperreflexia, is a syndrome that sometimes occurs in patients with a spinal cord lesion at T7 or above and constitutes a medical emergency. The syndrome presents quickly and can precipitate a seizure or a stroke. Death can occur if the cause is not relieved.

The syndrome can be triggered by bladder or intestinal distention, spasticity, decubitus ulcers, or stimulation of the skin below the level of the injury. Ejaculation in the male can initiate the reflex, as can strong uterine contractions in the pregnant female.

These stimuli produce a sympathetic discharge that causes a reflex vasoconstriction of the blood vessels in the skin and splanchnic bed below the level of the injury. The vasoconstriction produces extreme hypertension and a throbbing headache.

Vasoconstriction of the splanchnic bed distends the baroreceptors in the carotid sinus and aortic arch. They in turn stimulate the vagus nerve, resulting in a bradycardia, which is the body's attempt to lower the blood pressure. The body attempts to reduce the hypertension also by superficial vasodilatation of vessels above the cord injury. As a result, there is flushing, blurred vision, and nasal congestion. Because the spinal cord injury interrupts transmisson of the vasodilatation message below the level of the lesion, the vasoconstriction continues below the level of the lesion until the stimulus is identified and interrupted. The vasoconstriction results in pallor below the level of the lesion, whereas flushing occurs above the lesion.

When autonomic dysreflexia is recognized, there are several things the alert nurse can do quickly and can teach the patient to do. The head of the bed should be elevated, and frequent checks of the blood pressure should be made. The bladder drainage system can be quickly checked for kinks in the tubing. The urine collection bag should not be overly full. Some protocols for checking the patency of the urinary drainage system include irrigation of the catheter with 10 to 30 ml of irrigating solution. The nurse should make sure that absolutely no more than that amount is used because the addition of the fluid may aggravate the massive sympathetic outflow already present. If the symptoms persist after these checks are made, the catheter should be changed so that the bladder can empty. If the patient did not have a catheter in place when the hyperreflexia began, one should be inserted.

If the urinary system does not seem to be the cause of the stimulus, the patient should be checked for *bowel impaction*. The impaction should not be removed until the symptoms subside. Dibucaine (Nupercaine) or lidocaine (Xylocaine) ointment can be applied to the rectum to anesthetize the area until symptoms subside. Patients prone to autonomic dysreflexia use these ointments routinely with their bowel program.

If the patient's blood pressure does not return to normal, the use of a *sympathetic ganglionic blocking agent* such as atropine sulfate, guanethidine sulfate (Ismelin), reserpine (Serpasil), or methyldopa (Aldomet) may be used. Hydralazine (Apresoline) and diazoxide (Hyperstat) also are sometimes used.

PSYCHOLOGICAL PROCESSES

Different authors have different names for the stages of loss and grief a patient with spinal cord injury goes through on the road to rehabilitation. The psychological adjustment to the loss of one's previous physical abilities is unique to each individual. The rate at which a person works through this process varies, and none of the stages is static. A person can move back and forth between stages. The emotions felt and displayed by a patient with a cord injury are no different from the emotions felt by all of us at one time or another, and recognition of that fact may help one empathize with the patient's feelings.

Whatever names we give to the stages of grief, there are certain emotions that are felt by the patient following a cord injury. These will be discussed next.

Stage I — Shock and Disbelief. During this phase, the patient does not request an explanation of what has happened to him. He is overwhelmed by the injury. There may be more concern with whether he will live than with whether he will walk again. This period may result in extreme dependence on the staff members. Staff members at the same time may feel that the patient does not understand the ramification of his injury. The staff may identify with his feelings of being overwhelmed because they themselves are often overwhelmed with the acute medical management of this catastrophic illness.

Stage II — Denial. The process of denial is an escape mechanism for the patient. Generally, the whole disability is not denied, but particular aspects of it are. For instance, the patient may say he cannot walk now, but in 6 months he will be able to. Bargaining, instead of being a separate stage, can be considered a form of denial. Bargains with God may be in the form of offering Him the legs if He will just return function of the arms. Staff often find it difficult to deal with patients in this stage.

A helpful approach is to focus on the here and now instead of trying to break down the denial. For instance, when a patient refuses to go to physical therapy or refuses certain aspects of his care because this is not a permanent disability, the staff can say that *today* he cannot walk; therefore, these treatments are necessary.

Focus on the present problems. This is not the stage to talk to the patient about long-term changes, such as ordering a wheelchair or making modifications on his home. More appropriate matters to deal with would be bladder training, skin care, and range of motion exercises.

Stage III — Reaction. During this stage, instead of denying the impact of the injury, the patient expresses this impact. There may be severe depression and loss of motivation and involvement. Previous hobbies or interests lose their meaning. There is great helplessness during this period, and there may be suicidal statements.

Staff members can help at this stage by listening to the patient as he works through his feelings. The staff should avoid setting up failure situations, which could happen if they push the patient too fast. Because the patient tends to withdraw during this stage, staff may help by introducing diversional activities.

Another type of reaction seen is *acting out,* which may include anger or sexual, drug, or alcohol abuse. Anger may be expressed verbally or physically. The patient feels no one can do anything right — including family and staff. This kind of behavior makes staff want to avoid contact with the patient. Some limits do need to be set with the patient to protect himself and the staff if he becomes truly abusive.

Stage IV — Mobilization. Problem-solving behavior can be seen during this stage. The patient is looking toward the future and wants to learn about his self-care. In fact, he may become very possessive of his therapist or nurse and resent the time she spends with other patients. This is a time of sharing and planning between patient and staff.

Stage V — Coping. It is felt by some in the field of rehabilitation that people do not accept the disability *per se* but instead learn to cope with it. Disability is still an inconvenience, but it is no longer the center of their lives. Life is again meaningful to the person, and he is again involved with others.

SPINAL CORD INJURY RESEARCH

It seemed for several years that there was not much new or dramatic in SCI research. Hopes were raised briefly in the mid 1970s when Soviet scientists claimed that introduction of enzymes into transected spinal cords of rats resulted in recovery of up to 80% of hind limb locomotion in as many as 50% of these animals. American scientists were unable to reproduce the Russians' results, which were thought to have been obtained on rats with incomplete spinal transections. The enzymatic approach has now been abandoned.

Hyperbaric oxygenation research has been in progress for several years. The hypothesis is that it might stimulate regeneration of the spinal cord. Most of the continued research into hyperbaric oxygenation concerns the acute stage of SCI; it is not thought to have much value in the chronic situation.

Some studies continue in the area of traditional therapies. One multicenter study is evaluating whether steroids should be administered in conventional doses or megadoses in order to reduce the cord's swelling immediately after injury. The question of whether cooling the spinal cord to lower metabolic activity prevents further cord destruction has been debated since the 1960s. There is some belief that if cooling is applied to the cord in the first 4 to 6 hours after injury, further destruction will not occur. This investigation continues, and the results are still inconclusive.

Dimethyl sulfoxide (DMSO) has been used in animals in an attempt to reduce spinal cord edema in an acute SCI. A few investigators are looking at this possibility in humans. A newer line of study involves the use of an opiate antagonist and at this time looks rather promising. Use of the drug is based on the fact that the spinal cord goes into shock after injury. Because endorphins (opiate family) may be involved in the production of shock, blocking endorphin action may perhaps prevent shock. Researchers have studied the opiate antagonist, naloxone, in cats with SCI. When naloxone is administered within 1 hour of injury, approximately 80% of the cats exhibit functional recovery and are walking within a few weeks, and they show increased blood flow to the spinal cord.

Prosthetic research has been emphasized over the past few years. There are studies involving artificial control of the bladder through electrical stimulation. The idea is to allow a patient with a spinal cord injury and no natural bladder control to void by pushing a button that triggers electronic release of the urinary bladder sphincter through sacral nerve root stimulation. An implanted device such as this does not seem unreasonable.

Dr. Jerrold Petrosky at Wright State University in Ohio is working on a process involving implantation of a microprocessor near paralyzed muscles. Electrodes detect nerve signals that are interrupted on the way to the paralyzed muscles and repeat these signals to the microprocessor. The small computer then generates signals of its own and passes them along to the muscles.

Advances in electronics have contributed to prosthetic developments. These advances have facilitated miniaturization of devices and lower costs. Wheelchairs were, until recently, generally accepted as the only realistic means of mobility for most SCI patients. Many environmental barriers might be overcome if some degree of non-wheelchair mobility could be restored to these patients. Today, standing, rising from a sitting position, and gaiting are not unrealistic goals thanks to the research on functional electrical stimulation (FES), particularly that done with paraplegics. This stimulation restores a biped gait in these patients. FES is said to restrenghten disused, atrophied, and upper motor neuron–lesioned muscles. FES uses natural bone support of body weight and existing joints, ligaments, and muscle power. There are no external braces or orthopedic devices. The muscle provides a self-regenerating energy supply, and electrical stimulation is used only for triggering, so FES orthotic devices have low battery needs. FES, when delivered by means of an implanted stimulator, becomes virtually an integral part of the patient and thus enhances patient acceptance.

Another area of research is monitoring of the spinal cord with computer-averaged cortical-evoked potentials. Early results suggest that incomplete cord injuries due to contusion or mechanical compression will recover, depending on the amount of initial force or energy applied and the length of time for which compression is applied.

Current clinical methods of spinal cord monitoring use cortical-evoked potentials that travel through the ascending posterior columns after a peripheral nerve is stimulated. It is uncertain whether this method actually demonstrates cord dysfunction caused by anterior cord compression or whether it is a measure of damage to the central gray matter. It is not feasible to monitor descending or efferent (motor) tracts in the clinical setting because this requires insertion of extradural electrodes into the spinal canal.

There does not yet seem to be a standardized method of evaluating somatosensory-evoked responses with incomplete SCI. One hypothesis is that rapid anterior compression of the spinal cord will cause an incomplete paralysis that will not recover if maintained chronically and that removal of the chronic compression will allow recovery of the cord to varying degrees. A key question is whether spinal cord monitoring involving averaged cortical-evoked potentials resulting from peripheral nerve stimuli will be able to predict the type and degree of incomplete injury accurately. It is suggested by some that such a monitoring system may help predict recoverable lesions and also indicate when surgical decompression should be performed to obtain recovery of neurologic function. This monitoring should also be helpful during spinal cord surgery.

Prosthetic devices for spinal cord–injured patients may not be the ultimate answer, but they certainly can improve the quality of life for those with neurologic deficit.

Advances in rehabilitation techniques and shortening of hospital stays are making an impact. Active research continues in the area of the pathophysiology of the injury and how to reverse the damage to neural tissue. The SCI patient rarely loses hope that a cure may be the next great discovery of medical science, and researchers in this field have the same goal.

BIBLIOGRAPHY

Adelstein, W, Watson P: Cervical Spine Injuries. J Neurosurg Nurs 15, No. 2:65–71, 1983

American Association of Neuroscience Nurses: Core Curriculum for Neuroscience Nurses, 2nd ed. Park Ridge, IL, 1984

Bohlman H, Bahniuk, Raskulinecz G: Spinal cord monitoring of experimental incomplete cervical spinal cord injury. Spine 6, No. 5:428–436, 1981

Carol M, Ducker T, Byrnes D: Acute care of spinal cord injury: A challenge to the emergency medicine clinician. Crit Care Q 2, No. 1:7–21, 1979

Earnest MP: Neurologic Emergencies. New York, Churchill-Livingstone, 1983

Feustel D: Autonomic hyperreflexia. Am J Nurs 76:228–230, 1976

Howard M, Corbo-Pelaia S: Psychological aftereffects of halo traction. Am J Nurs Dec, 1982, pp 1839–1840

Hummelgard A, Martin E: Management of the patient in a halo brace. J Neurosurg Nurs 14, No. 3:113–119, 1982

Kelly E: Orthopedic management of the patient with a spinal injury. Curr Probl Surg No. 17, 4:205–215, 1980

Kralj A, Bujd T et al: Gait restoration in paraplegic patients: A feasibility demonstration using multichannel surface electrode FES. J Rehab R D, 20, No. 1:3–20, 1983

Medical News: From regeneration to prosthesis: Research on spinal cord injury. JAMA 245, No. 13:1293–1303, 1981

Milazzo V, Resh C: Kinetic nursing—A new approach to the problems of immobilization. J Neurosurg Nurs 14, No. 3:120–124, 1982

Miller S, Szasz G, Anderson L: Sexual health care clinician in an acute spinal cord injury unit. Arch Phys Med Rehab 62:315–320, 1981

Rudy E: Advanced Neurological and Neurosurgical Nursing. St Louis, CV Mosby, 1984

Shoemaker W, Thompson W, Holbrook P: Textbook of Critical Care. Philadelphia, WB Saunders, 1984

Sinaki M, Caskey P, Anders Ness: Bladder retraining device for handicapped persons. Arch Phys Med Rehab 63:587, 1982

Solomon J: Sex and the spinal cord injured patient. J Neurosurg Nurs 14, No. 3:125–127, 1982

Taggi J, Manley MS: A Handbook of Sexuality After Spinal Cord Injury. Denver, Craig Hospital, 1978

Walker JR, Halstead L: Metabolic and endocrine changes in spinal cord injury: III. Less quanta of sensory input plus bedrest and illness. Arch Phys Med Rehab 63:628–630, 1982

27
The Brain-Injured Patient

Nursing Diagnoses and Interventions

Suzanne Provenzano*

Brain injuries are among the most devastating and lethal catastrophes among humans. The critical care nurse is in a central position to understand the psychological and physiological changes that brain-injured patients undergo in the acute care setting. The nursing process uniquely helps the nurse identify and focus on nursing diagnoses and interventions based on the consequences of the patient's pathology.

PROBLEMS WITH BREATHING

Ineffective Breathing Patterns

Because the neurophysiology of respiration is so complex, a neurologic insult could produce problems at any number of levels. The highest level of respiratory control is found in the brainstem structures of the pneumotaxic center, the nucleus solitarius, and the medulla oblongata. The brain stem centers can be injured by increased intracranial pressure and hypoxia as well as by direct trauma or interruption of blood supply. Cerebral trauma that alters the level of consciousness usually results in alveolar hypoventilation due to shallow respirations. These factors can ultimately lead to respiratory failure, which accounts for a high mortal-

* We wish to acknowledge the contributions of Marilynn J. Washburn, R.N., and Cary Lou Martinson, R.N., who prepared this section in previous editions of the book.

ity rate among head-injured patients. Different respiratory patterns can be identified when there is an intracranial dysfunction (Fig. 27-1).

Cheyne-Stokes breathing is periodic breathing in which the depth of each breath increases to a peak and then decreases to a state of apnea. The hyperpneic phase usually lasts longer than the apneic phase. Cheyne-Stokes respiration usually indicates bilateral lesions located deep in the cerebral hemispheres. With traumatic brain injury, the onset of Cheyne-Stokes breathing might be due to herniation of the cerebral hemispheres through the tentorium, indicating a deteriorating neurologic condition. This herniation can also cause compression of the midbrain, and *central neurogenic hyperventilation* will be observed. This hyperventilation is sustained, regular, rapid, and fairly deep. It is usually caused by a lesion of the low midbrain or upper pons.

Apneustic breathing indicates respiration with a pause at full inspiration and full expiration. The etiology of this pattern is usually occlusion of the basilar artery, which causes infarction of the lateral portions of the brain stem.

Cluster breathing may be seen when the lesion is high in the medulla or low in the pons. This pattern of respiration is seen as gasping breaths with irregular pauses.

The real centers of inspiration and expiration are located in the medulla oblongata. Any rapidly expanding intracranial lesion, such as cerebellar hemorrhage, can compress the medulla, and *ataxic breathing* will result. This is totally irregular breathing consisting of both deep and shallow breaths associated with irregular pauses. When this pattern of respiration occurs, a ventilator should be made available to the patient be-

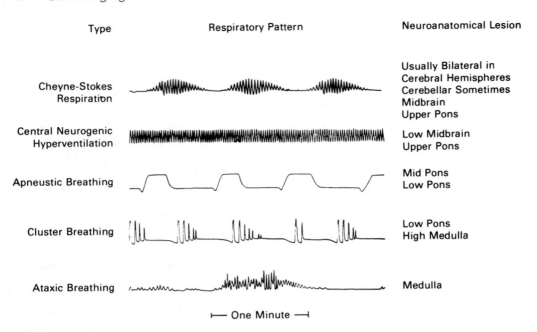

Type	Respiratory Pattern	Neuroanatomical Lesion
Cheyne-Stokes Respiration		Usually Bilateral in Cerebral Hemispheres Cerebellar Sometimes Midbrain Upper Pons
Central Neurogenic Hyperventilation		Low Midbrain Upper Pons
Apneustic Breathing		Mid Pons Low Pons
Cluster Breathing		Low Pons High Medulla
Ataxic Breathing		Medulla

⊢— One Minute —⊣

FIGURE 27-1
Abnormal respiratory patterns associated with coma. (Gifford RRM, Plaut MR: Abnormal respiratory patterns in the comatose patient caused by intracranial dysfunction. J Neurosurg Nurs 7, No. 1:58, 1975)

cause neither respiratory rhythm nor continuation of respiration can be predicted.

Interference with some cranial nerves also can influence respiration. The brain stem centers receive information from chemoreceptors in the carotid artery and aorta and from stretch receptors in the lungs by way of the glossopharyngeal (IX) and the vagus (X) nerves. Outgoing information from the brain stem then travels by way of the phrenic nerve, which leaves the spinal cord with the third cervical nerve and activates the diaphragm. The intercostal muscles that expand the chest wall are activated by the intracostal nerves of the thoracic spinal cord. Even if the brain stem centers, the cranial nerves, and the thoracic nerves all are intact, the patient may still develop respiratory problems if pulmonary hygiene is inadequate.

The nurse must be alert to subtle changes in the patient's respiratory pattern to prevent a secondary hypoxic insult to an already injured patient.

Impaired Gas Exchange

A number of brain-injured patients will have perfectly normal respiratory rates and patterns but still suffer pulmonary complications. These may be related to retained secretions, obstructed airways, and pulmonary edema.

The patient should be positioned on his side or in the coma position (Fig. 27-2). One must take care to avoid extreme neck flexion because both the airway and intracranial pressure may be compromised. An oral airway may be used to prevent obstruction of the upper airway by the tongue. Frequent position changes or use of a roto kinetic bed will help prevent pooled secretions in dependent lung fields.

The nurse should assess the patient's respiratory rate and effort, as well as skin color, breath sounds, and chest expansion. If an abnormality is encountered, arterial blood gases should be measured to evaluate the effectiveness of ventilation. When suctioning is required, the patient should be hyperoxygenated before, during, and after the procedure so that secondary brain injury due to hypoxia and increased intracranial pressure is minimized. In addition, suctioning via the nasopharynx should be avoided in a patient with suspected basilar skull fracture.

A serious pulmonary complication of head-injured patients is pulmonary edema. It may be primarily neurogenic in origin or result from adult respiratory distress syndrome (ARDS). Pulmonary edema may result from an injury to the brain that causes the Cushing reflex. An increase in systemic arterial pressure occurs as a sympathetic nervous system response to increasing ICP. This increase in general body vasoconstriction causes more blood to be shunted to the lungs. Altered permeability of the pulmonary blood vessels contributes to the process by allowing fluid to move into the alveoli. The impaired diffusion of oxygen and carbon dioxide from the blood can lead to further increases in ICP (Fig. 27-3).

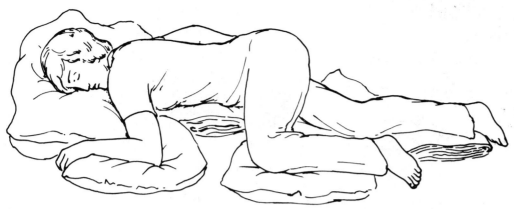

FIGURE 27-2
Coma position. Shoulders are turned almost prone for better drainage of the oral and nasal passages.

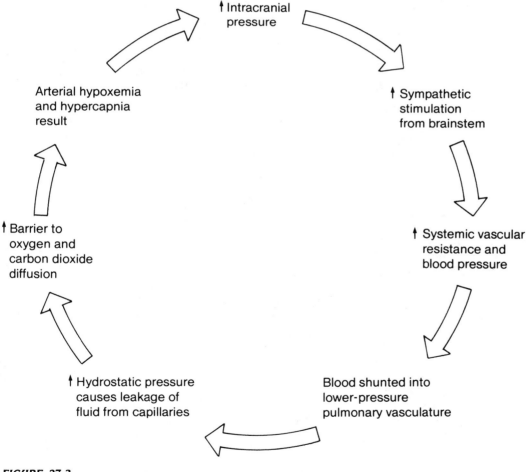

FIGURE 27-3
Mechanism of neurogenic pulmonary edema in brain-injured patients.

PROBLEMS WITH MOVEMENT

Impaired Physical Mobility

A major result of severe brain injury can be its effect on body movement. Hemiparesis or hemiplegia may occur as a result of damage to the motor areas of the brain. In addition, an unconscious patient may have no voluntary control of movement, depending on the depth of coma. Nursing interventions are based on an assessment of the patient's degree and type of motor functioning present.

Movement occurs as a result of the synapsing of two large groups of neurons. Nerve cells in the first group originate in the posterior portion of each frontal lobe called the precentral gyrus, or "motor strip." Axons from these "upper" motor neurons terminate either in the brain stem or in the anterior gray horns at various levels in the spinal cord. Here they synapse with "lower" motor neurons, which travel from the brain stem or spinal cord to specific muscles. Each of these neuron groups transmits particular information regarding movement. Thus, the patient will exhibit specific symptoms if either of these two neuron pathways is injured (Table 27-1).

Bed Positioning. With damage at the brain stem level, tonic reflexes are released, resulting in the assumption of abnormal postures. Abnormal muscle tone is reinforced by these reflexes and, in time, can create complications such as increased spasticity, scoliosis, contractures, and hip subluxation. It is easier to "mold" a patient's posture and muscle tone early post injury. Proper positioning helps inhibit abnormal tone and allows for easier handling by the physical and occupational therapists and nurses who are helping the patient maintain full range of motion.

Countering Abnormal Posturing. Most common in the brain-injured patient is opisthotonic posturing. This is a forward arching of the back and hyperextension of the head with all extremities rigid and straight or hyperextended. This posturing is exaggerated when the patient is supine. Trunk rotation and flexion of the lower extremities will help break up this posturing (Fig. 27-4). If the patient is left flat on his back with legs out straight, one will see an increase in extensor muscle tone. Turning the hips to a side-lying position and flexing the knees will relax the tone.

Head positioning is important because of an asymmetric tonic neck reflex. This reflex is demonstrated when the extremities on the same side to which the head is turned extend and the opposite extremities flex. Therefore, one who is attempting to do range of motion on a tightly drawn up arm should try turning the head to that side and see whether the muscle tone decreases.

Each brain-injured patient will have different reflexive positioning, and the nurse must evaluate what positions can be accomplished. The goal of effective positioning is to break up reflexive patterns and decrease abnormal muscle tone.

Preventing Contractures. Passive range of motion is used to stretch muscles and to maintain joint mobility. With the immobile patient, the nurse should move

---

TABLE 27-1
A COMPARISON OF UPPER AND LOWER MOTOR NEURON FUNCTION

Neuron	Pathway/Names	Functions	Signs of Dysfunction

Neuron group no. 1, or "upper" motor neurons	From motor area of cerebral cortex to brain stem (corticobulbar tracts) or to spinal cord (corticospinal tracts)	Carries commands for voluntary movement of specific body parts
		Carries inhibition commands to control the response of the next neuron pathway
			Loss of voluntary muscle control
			Loss of inhibition of lower motor neurons, resulting in:
			  Preservation of reflex arcs
			  Pathologic reflex responses
			  Spastic muscles
			  Increased muscle tone
			  Little or no muscle atrophy

Neuron group no. 2, or "lower" motor neurons	From brain stem or spinal cord to specific muscle groups; names end in the word "nerve" (*e.g.,* femoral nerve, radial nerve).	Relays commands from the upper motor neurons to effect voluntary muscle movement
		Forms the effector response branch of the reflex arc
			Loss of voluntary muscle movement
			No reflex arc activity, resulting in:
			  Flaccid muscles
			  No pathological reflex responses
			  Decreased muscle tone
			  Significant muscle atrophy

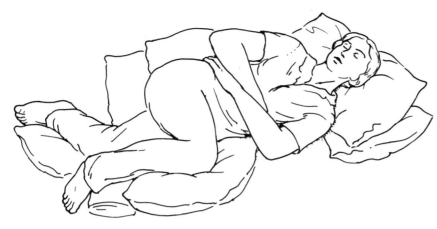

FIGURE 27-4
Bed positioning for reflex inhibition in brain-injured patients. This position uses trunk rotation and lower-extremity flexion to relax abnormal muscle tone.

each joint through its normal range of motion on a regular basis. The activity is accomplished easily during a bath. When tightness does occur, splinting may help the patient regain lost range of motion.

Pillow splinting is an easy and effective way to splint an extremity. The nurse places one or two pillows along the patient's outstretched arm and secures them tightly with an Ace bandage. The pillow splint can be left in place for approximately an hour at a time if skin pressure points are not a problem. With proper use of pillow splints, range of motion in the elbow joint can be increased and maintained.

With a tight hand grip, either voluntary or involuntary, a cone can be used to decrease the development of hand contractures. Pressure on the insertion of a muscle inhibits muscle contraction; thus, use of a hand cone instead of a soft wash cloth can actually cause relaxation of the hand and maintain normal functioning.

Alteration in Skin Integrity
Related to Prolonged Immobility

With loss of motor function, the brain-injured patient is vulnerable to skin breakdown. The unconscious patient, and anyone who is immobilized is prone to skin problems because of pressure, moisture, shearing forces, and diminished sensation.

There is one major rule that one must follow to maintain skin integrity: Prevent pressure. With current technology, there are numerous tools that can help one achieve this goal. Beds are available that distribute the patient's body weight evenly over the skin while supporting him on a cushion of air blown through fine glass beads (Clintron bed). There are beds designed to change pressure areas constantly by keeping the patient in continual motion from side to side (Roto-Rest bed). There are beds designed to facilitate turning while maintaining body alignment, such as the Stryker frame, the circle electric bed, and the Stoke-Edgerton bed. There also are numerous items to be placed on a bed to make pressure less of a problem, such as alternating pressure air mattresses, water mattresses, gel-foam pads, and sheepskins. The fact remains, however, that an immobile patient who is not turned regularly can develop pressure sores in time, no matter what mattress is used. Each patient must be evaluated individually as to his skin tolerance (how fast his skin turns red without his being turned). The average skin-pressure tolerance time for an acutely ill patient is 2 hours.

Another technique that can help prevent pressure problems is the use of padding above and below prominent bony processes. For example, when the patient is on his side, the nurse can place a rectangular foam pad or small pillow above and below the hip trochanter and above the lateral malleolus of the ankle. Padding should also be placed between bony pressure points such as the knees (Fig. 27-5). The nurse should place her hand under the bony processes to confirm that pressure has been relieved. When the patient is on his back, she should place a pad above and below the sacrum and above the heels (Fig. 27-6). Circular pads called "doughnuts" may actually impair circulation by causing circular pressure around the protected area. Use of rectangular pads allows for collateral circulation while relieving pressure.

Skin massage with lotion is helpful in stimulating circulation to a pressure area, but the skin should be dried carefully because moisture can lead to irritation.

Another prime cause of a breakdown in skin integrity is the shearing effect of linen against skin. The patient should be placed on a lift sheet (folded drawsheet or bath blanket), on which one can maneuver him in the bed. To shield the patient's elbows and heels, one should use soft foam or sheepskin protectors.

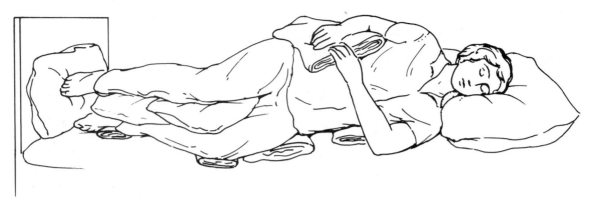

FIGURE 27-5
Side lying position. Pads are used above and below the trochanter and lateral malleolus to relieve pressure.

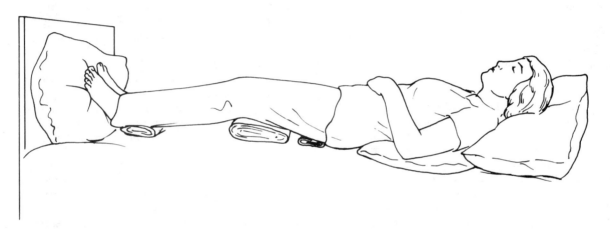

FIGURE 27-6
Supine position. Pads are used above and below the sacrum and above the heels to relieve pressure. A pad above the knees prevents hyperextension of the knees and relieves pressure on the popliteal space.

PROBLEMS WITH SECONDARY INJURY

Potential Injury Related to Seizures

Seizures occur in approximately 10% of head-injured patients during the acute stage. The nurse should make preparations for the possibility of seizures by having a padded tongue blade or oral airway at the patient's bedside and suction equipment close at hand. The bed siderails should be kept up; padding the rails with bath blankets or foam cushions may minimize the risk of secondary injury from a seizure. During a seizure, the nurse should focus her attention on maintaining a patent airway while observing the progression of seizure events (see Chap. 28, Table 28-8) and preventing further injury to the patient. If there is enough time before muscle spasticity begins, and the jaws clench, a padded tongue blade, an oral airway, or a plastic bite stick should be inserted between the patient's teeth. This will prevent the patient from biting his tongue and will keep the airway clear. One must *never* try to force *anything* between the teeth or pry the jaws open. The patient should be turned on his side to allow secretions to drain or to be suctioned more easily. The patient's movements should be restrained only enough to prevent him from hitting objects, causing bruising or injury.

The only medical treatment for seizures is drug therapy. Diazepam is the most widely used drug and is given slowly IV. Because the drug depresses respirations, the patient's respiratory rate and rhythm should be carefully monitored. Once the seizure has been terminated, one may order phenobarbital or phenytoin (Dilantin) to maintain seizure control. Because phenytoin is a cardiac depressant, the nurse should pay careful attention to the patient's cardiac rate and rhythm. This drug should be given intravenously, no faster than 50 mg/minute (see discussion of seizure disorders, Chap. 28).

Potential Infection Related to Leak of Cerebrospinal Fluid

It is not uncommon for some head-injured patients with a skull fracture to have a leak of cerebrospinal fluid (CSF) from the ears or nose. It may result from a fracture in the anterior fossa near the frontal sinuses or from a basilar skull fracture of the petrous portion of the temporal bone. One can detect the presence of CSF by testing the clear, watery drainage for sugar with a dextrostix. CSF will be positive for sugar; mucus will not. Blood-tinged drainage should be collected on a sterile gauze pad and observed for the "halo" sign of blood surrounded by a clear or yellow-colored ring of spinal fluid.

When CSF rhinorrhea or otorrhea has been detected, the draining areas should not be cleaned, irrigated, or suctioned. A sterile pad may be placed under the nose or over the ear and should be changed when damp. The nurse must instruct the awake patient not to blow his nose or sniff and not to put his finger in his nose or ear. Drainage usually slows down quickly, and the dural tear closes without any problem.

PROBLEMS WITH HYDRATION, NUTRITION, AND ELIMINATION

Potential Fluid Volume Imbalances

Nearly all severely head-injured patients will have a problem with maintenance of a balanced hydration state. For some patients, it will be a self-limiting response to the stress of trauma. In a physiological stress state, more antidiuretic hormone (ADH) and more aldosterone are produced, resulting in fluid and sodium retention. The process usually reverses itself within a day or two when diuresis occurs.

In some patients with neurologic trauma—especially those with skull fractures, damage to the pituitary or hypothalmus, or increased intracranial pressure—the clinical picture may be complicated by *diabetes insipidus (DI)*. In this condition, there is a dysfunction in the production and storage of ADH, with a subsequent decrease in the amount of ADH present in the blood. Without ADH, the kidneys excrete too much water, leading to dehydration (Table 27-2). The same cerebral pathology sometimes leads to an opposite problem of too much ADH being produced in excess of the body's needs. This *syndrome of inappropriate ADH (SIADH)* is characterized by fluid retention and consequent hemodilution (Table 27-2).

Accurate measurement of intake and output and evaluations of changes in patient weight from day to day are essential to the assessment of fluid balance. The nurse should also assess the patient's skin and mucus membranes for drying and cracking, which predispose to further injury. Close observation of the patient's cardiovascular status is required with evaluation of the trends in vital signs, CVP, PAP, and cardiac output. In view of the alterations in fluid balance from trauma and the added effect of diuretic therapy, the critical care nurse must be vigilant for problems that could lead to a secondary neurologic injury.

Inadequate Nutrition

Adequate nutrition plays a primary role in recovery from illness and is often neglected. A state of catabolism and negative nitrogen balance is a common finding in head-injured patients. Standard intravenous solutions are generally inadequate to prevent this problem. In addition, the body's demand for energy

---

TABLE 27-2
A COMPARISON OF DIABETES INSIPIDUS AND THE SYNDROME OF INAPPROPRIATE ADH SECRETION

	Diabetes Insipidus (DI)	*Syndrome Inappropriate ADH (SIADH)*
Clinical Manifestations	Increased thirst drive in the awake patient Polyuria, usually more than 5 liters/day Urine specific gravity 1.001 to 1.005 Volume depletion, as evidenced by slightly elevated hematocrit and serum sodium levels	Lethargy and confusion, leading to coma and seizures Decreased urine output, usually less than 500 ml/day Urine specific gravity usually greater than 1.025 Hemodilution, as evidenced by decreased hematocrit and hyponatremia
Medical Therapy	Appropriate fluid replacement PO and/or IV Supplemental ADH therapy using injectable pitressin or nasal spray solutions of desmopressin (DDAVP)	Fluid restriction Furosemide diuretics Drug therapy with demeclocycline hydrochloride (Declomycin), which blocks the effect of ADH on the kidney

and substrates for repair and growth can cause breakdown of body proteins at an accelerated rate.

The nurse should assess the patient's ability to chew, swallow, and protect the airway before initiating an oral feeding program. She can elicit the swallow and gag reflexes by pressing down on the patient's tongue with a tongue blade, then touching the back of the throat with another. Putting a small amount of semi-solid ice cream, Jello, or custard in the patient's mouth is a more specific test of swallowing. The nurse should make sure that suction equipment is near to prevent aspiratioin in case the reflexes are weak or absent. Chewing involves a different pattern of neuromuscular coordination and should be tested with soft foods such as bread or mashed potatoes.

For the unconscious patient or one for whom aspiration is a hazard, nutritional support in the form of tube feeding or parenteral hyperalimentation should be started early. Enteral feedings are suitable as long as peristalsis is present. They may be given through a nasogastric tube or via surgically implanted gastrostomy or jejunostomy tubes. Whether the feedings are intermittent or continuous, the nurse should aspirate gastric/bowel contents to assure correct tube placement and check for excessive residual remaining. A small amount of vegetable dye food coloring added to the feeding helps one assess for regurgitation and aspiration. The more acutely injured patient may need parenteral nutrition until normal bowel function returns.

Alteration in Bowel Elimination: Incontinence

Monitoring bowel elimination and facilitating normal defecation are time-consuming nursing responsibilities. In the acute stage in the care of a severely head-injured patient, other responsibilities take priority, such as the prevention of increased intracranial pressure. Later, however, spending time to establish a good bowel program will enable the patient to concentrate on other aspects in his rehabilitation program.

The actual mechanism of emptying the bowel is basically a reflex activity at the spinal cord level. With brain injury, the voluntary control of stimulating or inhibiting the reflex is impaired. The reflex may be stimulated by the nurse on a routine basis to establish a predictable, controlled bowel program. The stimulation may be accomplished with a finger, a small-volume enema, or a chemical stimulant such as a Dulcolax suppository.

Digital stimulation involves insertion of a gloved, lubricated finger into the external rectal sphincter. With a slow circular motion against the sphincter, the spinal cord reflex will be initiated. Both internal and external rectal sphincters will open, peristalsis will increase, and a normal evacuation can occur. If done too vigorously, digital stimulation can cause discomfort.

For patients who are too alert to tolerate this procedure, an enema or a suppository may be preferable.

All these methods, along with attention to diet and judicious use of stool softeners and laxatives, enable the nurse to facilitate regular bowel habits for the patient. Establishing a regular routine for daily bowel movements prevents constipation and impaction as well as accidental bowel movements or continuous small stools and avoids embarrassment for the patient and family members.

Altered Patterns of Urinary Elimination

In the acutely brain-injured patient, fluid management is essential, and a Foley catheter is necessary for accurate measurement of urinary output. Too often, the Foley catheter is forgotten as a source of irritation and of potential infection. Even though a brain-injured patient has lost voluntary control of his bladder, the reflexes for normal voiding may be intact. The bladder muscle, like other muscles in upper motor neuron disease, may become hypertonic and spastic. The patient may experience bladder spasms, frequency, incontinence, and residual collections of urine.

Management of urinary elimination without the use of an indwelling catheter is the objective of bladder management in the brain-injured patient. Once the acute phase of injury has passed and the patient's clinical condition is stable, one may perform diagnostic tests to evaluate the extent of bladder function. Such tests include an intravenous pyelogram (IVP) and cystometric studies for measurement of bladder capacity and pressure. When the evaluation is complete, a decision can be made about which approaches to achieving urinary control will be of benefit to the patient. Techniques such as intermittent catheterization, frequent toileting, and the use of external collectors require skillful nursing care to be effective. For those patients who cannot safely be managed without a catheter, an indwelling suprapubic cystostomy tube may provide effective bladder drainage with less risk of infection.

PROBLEMS WITH BEHAVIOR AND COMMUNICATION

Neurologic damage does not occur without effecting some change in a person's behavior response. His personality and entire characteristic behavior pattern will undergo some changes, either temporary or permanent, depending on the locus and severity of the injury.

Impaired Communication

The patient with cerebral trauma who presents with a breakdown in communication abilities is not alone. This dysfunction is the most frequently occurring handicap in head-injured patients. Such an impairment results from the combined effects of disorganized and confused language processing and specific aphasic disorders, if present. The patient cannot process his internal and external environment using the abilities of alertness, selective attention, discrimination, memory, and the association, integration, and analysis of sensory stimuli with internal thoughts. As a result, the patient's communication can become

- *Disoriented*—not appropriate to the situation, question, or discussion
- *Disorganized*—Fragmented and lacking in comprehension
- *Confused*—confabulatory, overelaborate, or at odds with the situation
- *Stimulus-bound*—relevant to a part but not the whole concept of a statement or question
- *Reduced in initiation*—reliant on others to stimulate and structure language responses
- *Reduced in inhibition*—lacking in specificity and precision in relationship to the original statement or question

The true impact of a communication disorder is that it isolates patients from their surroundings. Because the nurse has more frequent contact with the patient than any other health professional, the manner in which the nurse handles the patient's communication attempts is a critical factor in helping him remain in contact with the environment. The nurse should be aware that the hospitalized patient usually wants to communicate something within the following categories:

- *States of being*—pain; need for food, warmth, fluid, or rest
- *Feelings*—either the patient's feeling or his perception of others' feelings toward him
- *People*—family, friends, hospital personnel
- *Places*—inside or outside the hospital

Knowledge of what the patient's major concerns are and use of alternate channels of communication (*e.g.,* facial expressions, gestures, body posture, pictures) will aid in the exchange of information between nurse and patient. (See discussion that follows: Communication Disorders in the Brain-Injured Patient.)

Alteration in Thought Processes

Cognition involves the ability to perceive, integrate, and interpret both internal and external environmental stimuli appropriately. In this way, we regulate and control our behavior. The brain-injured patient will perceive, integrate, and interpret his surroundings in a disorganized fashion. Consequently, his behavioral response can seem inappropriate, confused, hostile, or apathetic. Nursing assessment of the patient's cognitive abilities will aid in formulating the best way to approach a brain-injured patient at various stages during recovery (Table 27-3).

TABLE 27-3
COGNITIVE BEHAVIOR OF BRAIN-INJURED PATIENTS AND NURSING APPROACHES

Cognitive Behavior Level	Nursing Approaches
1. *No response* to any stimuli 2. *Generalized response:* stimuli response is inconsistant, limited, nonpurposeful with random movements or incomprehensible sounds. 3. *Localized response:* responses to stimuli are specific but inconsistent. Patient may withdraw or push away, may make sounds, follow some simple commands, or respond to certain family members.	Levels 1, 2, and 3 A. Assume that patient can understand all that is said. Converse *with* the patient, not *about* him. B. Do not overwhelm the patient with talking. Leave some moments of silence between verbal stimuli. C. Manage the environment to provide only one source of stimulation at a time. If talking is taking place, the radio or TV should be off. D. Encourage the family to provide short, random periods of sensory input that is meaningful to the patient. A favorite TV programor tape recording or 30 minutes of music from the patient's favorite radio station will provide more meaningful stimulation than constant radio accompaniment, which becomes as meaningless as the continual bleep of the cardiac monitor.

(Continued)

TABLE 27-3
(Continued)

Cognitive Behavior Level	Nursing Approaches
4. *Confused-agitated:* response is primarily to internal confusion with increased state of activity; behavior may be bizarre or aggressive; patient may attempt to remove tubes or restraints or crawl out of bed; verbalization is incoherent or inappropriate; patient shows minimal awareness of environment and absent short-term memory.	Level 4 A. Be calm and soothing in manner when handling the patient. Approach with gentle touch to decrease the occurrence of defensive emotional and motor reflexes. B. Watch for early signs that the patient is becoming agitated (*e.g.,* increased movement, vocal loudness, resistance to activity). C. When the patient becomes upset, do not try to reason with him or "talk him out of it." Talking will be an additional external stimulus that the patient cannot handle. D. If the patient remains upset, either remove him from the situation or remove the situation from him.
5. *Confused, inappropriate, nonagitated:* Patient is alert and responds consistently to simple commands; has short attention span and easily distracted memory impaired with confusion of past and present events; can perform previously learned tasks with maximal structure but is unable to learn new information; may wander off with vague intention of "going home." 6. *Confused-appropriate:* Patient shows goal-directed behavior but still requires external direction; is able to understand simple direction; is able to understand simple reasoning; follows simple directions consistently and requires less supervision for previously learned tasks; has improved past memory depth and detail and beginning immediate awareness of self and surroundings.	Levels 5 and 6 A. Present the patient with only one task at a time. Allow him to complete it before giving further instructions. B. Make sure that you have the patient's attention by placing yourself in view and touching the patient before talking. C. If the patient becomes confused or resistant, stop talking. Wait until he appears relaxed before continuing with instruction or activity. D. Use gestures, demonstrations, and only the most necessary words in giving instructions. E. Maintain the same sequence in routine activities and tasks. Describe these routines to the patient and relate them to time of day.
7. *Automatic-appropriate:* Patient is able to complete daily routines in structured environment; has increased awareness of self and surroundings but lacks insight, judgment, and problem-solving ability.	Level 7 A. Supervision is still necessary for continued learning and safety. B. Reinforce the patient's memory of routines and schedules with clocks calendars and a written log of activities.
8. *Purposeful-appropriate:* Patient is alert, oriented, able to recall and integrate past and recent events; responds appropriately to environment; still has decreased ability in abstract reasoning, stress tolerance, and judgment in emergencies or unusual situations.	Level 8 A. The patient should be able to function without supervision. B. Consideration should be given to job-retraining or return to school.

(Reprinted with permission from Hagen C, Malkmus D, Durham P: Levels of cognitive functioning. In Rehabilitation of the Head Injured Adult: Comprehensive Physical Management. Downey, CA, Professional Staff Association of Rancho Los Amigos Hospital, Inc, 1979, pp. 87–88.)

Communication Disorders in the Brain-Injured Patient

Carole K. Hahn

Because the brain contains centers for all thought processes, a patient who has sustained brain injury is likely to demonstrate some kind of communication disorder. Areas that may be affected include speech, language, memory, visual perception, cognitive abilities, problem-solving, concentration, and thought organization. The site of the injury and etiology determine the type of problem, its severity, and prognosis.

APHASIA

Patients who have sustained injury to certain areas of the dominant cerebral hemisphere may evidence aphasia. The left hemisphere of the brain is usually dominant for speech, regardless of handedness. Specific areas of the left hemisphere that have been defined as most important for speech and language function are (1) the posterior temporoparietal region (Wernicke's area); (2) the three gyri anterior to the precentral face area (Broca's area); and (3) the supe-

rior, supplementary area, which appears to be dispensable but is probably important if other areas of speech are destroyed (Fig. 27-7).

Aphasia is a term used to describe an acquired loss of language, with reduction of available language in all modalities. It is important to understand the difference between speech and language. Language is the entire system of symbols that we learn as children to communicate efficiently with one another. This language system consists of our ability to interpret what sounds we hear as words, of the letters and numbers we learn to read and write to communicate without drawing detailed pictures of our environment, and of our ability to produce certain sounds to convey thoughts to other people. Speech is merely the sounds we make with our mouths to convey language.

Language encompasses all aspects of the learned symbols we use to communicate — listening, reading, writing, numbers. An aphasic patient may have difficulty thinking of the correct word or may say inappropriate or meaningless jargon words. He is usually not aware of his errors. Because all language modalities are usually about equally impaired, an alphabet board or language board will not be helpful to this type of patient because he will have difficulty recognizing letters and words also.

When communicating with an aphasic patient, it is best to use simple language and ample gestural and environmental cues. Pointing to the desired object, tone of voice, facial expression, time of day, and hospital routine all contribute to the patient's understand-

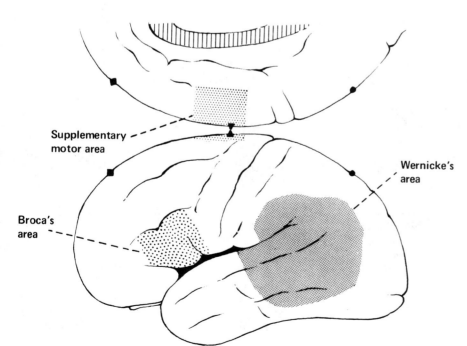

Supplementary motor area

Wernicke's area

Broca's area

FIGURE 27-7
Three speech areas of dominant cerebral hemisphere: (1) the posterior, or parietotemporal, area (Wernicke's area) is most important; (2) the anterior, or Broca's, area is next most important but is dispensable in some patients at least; (3) the superior, or supplementary motor, area is dispensable but may be important after damage to other speech areas. (Redrawn after Fig. IV-8 in Penfield W, Roberts L: Speech and Brain-Mechanisms, p 80. Princeton, Princeton University Press, 1959. Reprinted by permission of Princeton University Press)

ing. One should use pantomime and encourage the patient to do the same to aid communication.

Aphasic patients quickly become adept at "filling-in the blanks" when they do not understand completely. It is easy to overestimate their level of auditory comprehension and to assume that the aphasic patient understands everything that is being said. It is important to check this level of understanding fairly. The nurse should ask the patient to point to objects in the room, being careful not to nod or point in the correct direction. This is often difficult for a tester to do, because we all use gesture naturally. The questions that are asked of the patient should be modified because he will learn quickly what responses are expected of him. Getting a clear picture of the patient's level of understanding is not only important clinically but will alleviate frustration and confusion for the staff. The patient may be labeled as uncooperative, cross, or irrational when the staff believes he understands, but he behaves as if he does not.

A normal tone of voice should be used. Aphasic patients are not deaf (unless they were pre onset) but merely have difficulty understanding the meaning of what they hear. Short sentences should be used; the patient may forget the beginning of a long sentence by the time you finish saying it. Useless chatter that may confuse him should be avoided.

APRAXIA

Apraxia is the inability to carry out, on request, a complex or skilled movement that cannot be accounted for by muscle weakness or paralysis, sensory deficits, or lack of understanding. *Ideational apraxia* is the inability to formulate the ideational concept to perform complicated motor acts, even though the patient knows what he wants to do. *Ideomotor praxia* is the state in which the patient can perform an act spontaneously or habitually but not on command. *Limb-kinetic (motor) apraxia* is the loss of memory patterns needed to perform a movement. *Oral apraxia* and *verbal apraxia* refer to apraxia affecting the volitional positioning of the oral musculature to speak or perform oral movements.

Performance of an apraxic patient is inconsistent and variable. In speech, he may be able to say words spontaneously but cannot repeat them when he wants to. He may spontaneously pick up his spoon to eat his soup but cannot demonstrate its function when the soup is removed. Apraxia may be seen in any voluntary movement such as pointing, swallowing, talking, walking, or dressing.

If apraxia is present, the nurse should avoid giving the patient a command to follow. Instead of saying,

"Take a drink of water," she should simply give him the glass and let him perform the act automatically.

DYSARTHRIA

Dysarthria is a group of speech disorders resulting from disturbances in muscular control of the speech mechanism (weakness, slowness, poor coordination, or altered muscle tone) due to damage to the central or peripheral nervous system. Motor processes of speech that may be affected include respiration, phonation, resonance, articulation, and prosody. Specific types of dysarthria have been defined and can be a valuable diagnostic tool to determine the site of the neurologic lesion.

Patients who are difficult to understand because of slurred, dysarthric speech should be encouraged to reduce their rate of speaking and to "overemphasize" speech movements. These patients are likely to have swallowing difficulties, also because of muscle weakness or poor coordination.

VISUAL PERCEPTION DEFICITS

The right hemisphere of the brain is the center of visual-spatial functions. It controls the ability to judge distance, size, position, rate of movement, form, and the relation of parts to wholes. A patient who has sustained right hemisphere damage, usually resulting in left hemiplegia, is likely to speak in complete sentences but evidences problems in visual perception and spatial planning. Even with concentration, he may be unable to roll over in bed, feed himself, or discriminate the inside or outside of his clothes. He may have difficulty judging distances from an object or determining when he is sitting upright or leaning. This type of patient often has difficulty reading because he "loses his place" continually.

These difficulties often go undiagnosed because the patient is highly verbal and appears to be functioning normally. Because of his behavior, it is easy to overestimate this patient's abilities. He acts as if his deficits are not present. He tends to make excuses for his errors, such as, "I never was much of a reader." "I have a calculator to add and subtract." "My husband does all of the driving; he could push this wheelchair." The left hemiplegic is often a poor judge of his own abilities and safety.

These patients respond best to verbal cuing. Excess visual input, such as cluttered room, large number of people, gesturing to patient, may be more confusing than helpful. The nurse should try talking a patient through an activity and encourage him to describe each step himself at the same time. These patients benefit from repetition for new learning.

VISUAL FIELD DEFICITS

Homonymous hemianopsia is a visual field deficit that often occurs with cerebral vascular accident (CVA). Because neural pathways for vision cross at the chiasm, lesions occurring in the occipital area (visual cortex) produce blindness in half of both eyes on the opposite side of the lesion (see Fig. 24-3 in Chap. 24).

Most right hemiplegics who have right field cuts learn to compensate for this deficit quickly by turning their heads slightly. This enables them to use the intact visual field of both eyes. Formal testing can be performed when the patient can understand testing directions and can maintain his focus on a midline point. However, the nurse can clinically detect visual field deficits by observing functional activities such as eating, response to staff and visitors approaching from both sides, and personal hygiene activities.

Left hemiplegic patients typically have more difficulty compensating for left visual field deficits because their visual perception is also impaired. These patients may deny that objects exist to their left even when attention is called to them. This left ignoral generally makes the rehabilitation process difficult.

Left *aversion, neglect,* or *ignoral* can be observed in reading. Typically, a patient can spell a word aloud but does not see all the letters when asked to read a word. He may mistake the word *women* for *men* because he does not see the letters *wo.* He may mistake numbers by omitting the left side. Thus he may mistake *$24.99* for *$4.99.* When writing, the patient typically writes only on the right side of the page (Fig. 27-8). Because the spatial organization center is also affected, this patient has difficulty recognizing these deficits, much less compensating for them.

COGNITIVE DEFICITS

Patients who sustain brain injury from trauma are likely to exhibit language disorders that are symptoms of generalized cognitive disorganization. Basic speech and language skills may be intact but may reflect problems in short-term memory, thought organization, concentration, initiation, and orientation. Coma or decreased level of response may persist for several weeks or months. Patient responses may be limited in nature (reflex movements, increased gross body movement, opening eyes) and may be noted only when stimulation is present. When left alone, the patient may remain quiet and still. As level of awareness increases, he

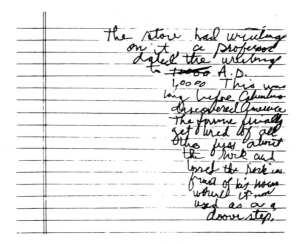

FIGURE 27-8
Example of patient's writing demonstrating left visual ignoral.

may begin to respond to discomfort by pulling at his nasogastric or tracheostomy tube or by becoming restless or agitated. Although he is apparently unresponsive to environmental stimulation, he does respond to his own internal agitation and stimulation, often in a nonpurposeful manner.

With increased awareness, the patient begins to respond to things around him, although he has difficulty maintaining selected attention for any length of time. Short-term memory is extremely impaired, although long-term memory may be intact. The patient may begin to wander with the intention of going home. Agitation may persist but is more goal-directed and aimed at external stimuli. The patient may be able to tolerate irritations (catheter, nasogastric tube, etc.) once they have been explained to him.

As the patient's ability to concentrate increases, improvements in short-term memory and learning will be evident. He will begin to show carry-over for old learning tasks (dressing, hygiene, etc.); new learning tasks show little carry-over. He may have difficulty organizing his thoughts to perform an activity. Because a great deal of retraining is based on language and reasoning, the speech pathologist can often provide guidance in improving the patient's cognitive organization.

BIBLIOGRAPHY

American Association of Neuroscience Nurses: Core Curriculum for Neuroscience Nursing, 2nd ed. Park Ridge, IL, 1984

DeYoung S: The Neurologic Patient. Englewood Cliffs, NJ, Prentice-Hall, 1983

Doenger ME et al: Nursing Care Plans: Nursing Diagnoses in Planning Patient Care. Philadelphia, WB Saunders, 1982

Farber SD: Neurorehabilitation—A Multisensory Approach. Philadelphia, WB Saunders, 1982

Saul TG: Intensive care of the brain-injured patient. Crit Care Q 5, No. 4:82–89, 1983

Snyder M et al: Neurologic Problems: A Critical Care Nursing Focus. Bowie, MD, Robert J Brady, 1981

Reestablishment of Oral Intake

Cynthia Johnson Dahlberg

NORMAL SWALLOWING FUNCTION

Knowledge of normal swallowing function is essential before an oral intake program is initiated for a brain-injured patient. Swallowing is primarily a reflexive action and is usually described in three stages.

Prior to the initiation of the swallowing reflex, there is volitional preparation of the food or liquid as it is introduced in the oral cavity. Solids are masticated and mixed with saliva to a softer consistency. In the oral stage, the tongue controls a bolus of food or liquid by pressing it against the soft palate and forming a seal around it. There is a respiratory pause on inspiration as the larynx moves up and forward to close and protect the airway. The seal around the bolus is broken as the soft palate elevates and closes the nasopharynx to prevent nasal regurgitation. The oral stage may include some volitional tongue movements but is primarily a reflexive action.

In the pharyngeal stage, with the soft palate elevated and the airway occluded, the tongue propels the bolus back against the posterior pharyngeal wall with anterior to posterior rippling motions. The muscles of the pharynx then contract sequentially to move the bolus down through the pharynx. The cricopharyngeal sphincter relaxes and opens in the esophageal stage as the bolus of food enters the esophagus. Peristaltic waves carry the bolus down the esophagus and into the stomach.

The swallowing reflex can be initiated by sensory stimulation of three cranial nerves. The glossopharyngeal nerve (IX) innervates the posterior tongue, the mucosa of the oropharynx, and the soft palate, and the tonsillar area. The vagus nerve (X) provides sensory innervation to the mucosa of the larynx above the level of the vocal cords, the epiglottis, portions of the pharynx, and the esophagus. The trigeminal nerve (V) provides sensory innervation to the mucosa of the palate, the uvula, and the tonsillar area. Sensory stimulation to initiate a swallow is conveyed to the cranial nuclei in the medulla of the brain stem, which coordinates the simultaneous inhibition of respiration and the motor act of swallowing.

Over 20 different muscle pairs are involved in the swallowing process, and they are innervated by six cranial nerves and the motor neurons of the first three cervical levels of the spinal cord. The cranial nerves involved include the hypoglossal (XII) for tongue movements; the vagus (X) for movement of the larynx, pharynx, and esophagus; the glossopharyngeal (IX) for pharyngeal muscle contractions and elevation of the soft palate; the facial (VII) for portions of the laryngeal action; and the trigeminal (V) to activate the tensor muscle of the soft palate. Swallowing is the most complex "all-or-none" reflex that results in an integrated, synchronized pattern that is individually constant and occurs below the level of consciousness.

FACTORS TO BE CONSIDERED BEFORE INITIATION OF ORAL INTAKE

Medical Condition. The patient's medical condition should be stable before oral intake is initiated. Conditions that contraindicate oral intake include fever (which may mask signs of aspiration pneumonia), the necessity of frequent suctioning, respiratory insufficiency, and other acute medical problems. Aspiration pneumonia can seriously complicate the patient's condition, especially in the presence of other medical problems.

Level of Consciousness. The level of consciousness should at least allow for generalized responses to noxious stimulation, such as grimaces, restlessness, or pushing away. Sleep and wake cycles should be present with periods of consistent eye opening, but maintenance of eye contact or eye tracking is not necessary.

Swallowing Ability. Swallowing ability should be evaluated and determined to be adequate without danger of aspiration. The most effective evaluation technique is fluoroscopy of a barium swallow recorded on video tape (videofluoroscopy) or movie film (cinefluoroscopy), with the patient in an upright position. Anteroposterior and lateral views of the passage of barium in the swallowing sequence can easily reveal swallowing dysfunctions, such as poor tongue control, difficulty in initiation of the swallow, nasopharyngeal regurgitation, pharyngeal retention, inadequate relaxation of the cricopharyngeal area, or aspiration into the larynx. If cine- or videofluoroscopy demonstrates significant aspiration, an oral intake program is contraindicated.

Swallowing function is evaluated by subjective observation as well, and in some settings this may be the only method available. Many patients will reflexively swallow with tactile stimulation around the mouth or larynx when swallowing saliva. The action of the tongue, the upward movement of the larynx, and the respiratory pattern are observed for rate, duration, and sequence and are compared with normal function. Observation of lip closure and tongue mobility will provide information about the adequacy of the oral stage of swallowing. Drooling is indicative of poor tongue control or decreased oral sensation or both. Slurred speech or a weak voice or both are indications of impairment in the oral/laryngeal musculature, which may impair swallowing ability as well.

Some patients also demonstrate primitive oral reflexes with stimulation of the oral area. These are the same reflexes that a newborn has and are usually controlled by higher brain centers by the age of 1 year. The patient's brain injury has removed the inhibitory control mechanisms of the higher brain centers, and, consequently, the primitive brain-stem reflexes are released.

The most easily observed primitive oral reflexes are a suckling pattern (a repetitive forward, upward, and backward movement of the tongue usually followed by a swallow), chewing (rhythmical chewing motions without jaw closure), and biting (jaw closure and holding when the area between the teeth or the gums is stimulated).

Respiratory Status. Another major consideration before the beginning of oral intake is the patient's respiratory status. Respiratory function should be adequate with a small metal Jackson tracheostomy tube (size 4 or below), a Kistner button, or a normal airway.

If the patient's respiratory function is such that a cuffed tracheostomy tube or a Jackson, size 5 or larger, is required, ideally the oral intake program should be postponed because a large tracheostomy gives the patient an artificial airway that alters the normal coordination of respiration and swallowing. It is impossible to cough through the vocal cords with an inflated cuff. Even with the cuff deflated, cough strength through the cords is significantly decreased owing to the large diameter of the tracheostomy tube. The tracheostomy tube can limit upward and forward movement of the larynx because the tube itself anchors the trachea to the muscles and skin of the neck. Regurgitation and aspiration into the larynx may result from compression of the cervical esophagus by the tracheostomy tube.

The larger tracheostomy tubes with inflated cuffs cause even more compression of the esophagus; food or secretions may overflow and rest above the inflated cuff, and pressures from the swallow itself force liquids and even semisolids around the cuff into the trachea.

Consequently, larger tracheostomy tubes are a negative factor in attempts to reestablish swallowing function. However, in many settings the physician prefers establishing a safe swallow prior to the removal of the cuffed tracheostomy tube. If this is the case, evaluation is preferred with the cuff deflated. For patients with tracheostomy tubes, a saliva test can be done bedside to rule out aspiration. A small amount of food coloring is given by mouth (blue is preferred). If colored mucus appears through the tracheostomy tube, aspiration is present and the patient cannot safely begin oral intake.

Cough Strength. The final consideration is evaluation of cough strength. The patient should demonstrate a cough reflex adequate for protection of the airway. A weak cough will not clear the airway in the event of aspiration, and thus the patient should not be started on oral intake.

Overall Criteria. The patient is ready to initiate an oral intake program if the aforementioned five factors are met: Medical condition is stable; at least generalized responses to noxious stimuli are present; swallowing function is present; respiratory function is adequate; and the cough reflex is strong. Most severely brain-injured patients require at least a few weeks post injury before all these requirements are met.

PROCEDURE

Removal of Nasogastric Tube. If the patient has a nasogastric tube, it should be removed at least a few hours before food is introduced orally. The nasogastric tube can cause nasal and pharyngeal irritation, esophagitis, and laryngeal edema. The irritation and inflammation produce excessive secretions that are difficult to remove and interfere with the swallowing process. The presence of a foreign object passing through the nasal, oral, pharyngeal, and esophageal areas only interferes with swallowing efficiency. In some cases, the swallowing evaluation must be done with the nasogastric tube in place. If so, a small silastic tube is preferred.

Positioning. The patient is best positioned in bed or in a chair from 45° to 90° upright, with the neck slightly flexed. Care should be taken not to extend the neck, as this makes upward movement of the larynx (to protect the airway from aspiration) more difficult. The ideal environment is free from distracting noises and movements for more effective concentration on the swallowing process.

Food Selection. Often the physician will order clear liquids for the initial oral trial. Thin liquids are easily affected by gravity, and they flow through the mouth and pharynx quickly, before the patient is able to initiate a swallow. Consequently, solids with a clear liquid base, such as gelatin and popsicles, are a better choice because they can more easily be controlled in the mouth. Small ice chips can be used to provide stimulation to the oral cavity and swallowing reflex.

Food should be chosen to provide maximum stimulation in temperature, taste, color, and texture when possible. Bland tastes and lukewarm temperatures (*e.g.,* tepid tap water) provide minimal stimulation to the patient and should be avoided in the initial stages, especially for patients with a reduced level of awareness. Milk products and sweets should be avoided as well because they cause excess mucus production.

Pureed foods are introduced if the patient demonstrates adequate control of the clear solids. Thick liquids are preferred to thin ones for patients with poor oral control or delayed initiation of swallowing. The diet expands as the patient gains swallowing efficiency and control. From pureed foods, the patient progresses to foods that require minimal chewing, such as finely chopped meat, fruit, and vegetables. As chewing ability and tongue control improve, foods are chopped in larger pieces until the patient is able to tolerate a regular diet. Foods the patient did not enjoy prior to injury are to be avoided. Close contact should be maintained with the dietary department to provide nutritious and attractive meals within the patient's swallowing ability. The dietitian also can be helpful in recommending various protein or caloric supplements if indicated.

Techniques. Techniques used during an oral intake session depend on the patient's individual swallowing pattern, but some *general suggestions* apply to most patients. It is important to verbalize the entire process to the patient, even if understanding is questionable. The food or liquid should be described in terms of taste, smell, and appearance. The swallowing process is emphasized with comments such as "Move your tongue," "Push that food back," "Hold your breath," and "Swallow." The food is introduced as far posteriorly in the mouth as possible with firm downward pressure from the spoon. Metal spoons should always be used because plastic spoons can easily break and shatter, especially if the patient has a biting reflex.

In *hemiplegic patients* with unilateral sensory or motor impairment of the face, food and liquid should be placed in the mouth on the intact side. Also, swallowing efficiency can be improved if the patient's head is tilted slightly to the intact side so gravity will direct the food or liquid to the area of normal sensory and motor function. "Pocketing" of food in the impaired side of the mouth is characteristic of hemiplegic patients, and they need to be reminded to clear food from the mouth on both sides. Following a meal, it is important for one to check the oral cavity carefully and clear any residual food that may have lodged in the impaired side.

The *amount per swallow* is initially small, approximately 5 ml or less. Patients with poor tongue control lose food in the sides of the mouth. The food or liquid can also drop into the airway prior to the initiation of the swallow, causing choking. Large amounts may not be completely evacuated after the first swallow. The food remaining in the oral cavity can easily slide down the pharynx after the swallow is completed and cause choking. Many patients have greater difficulty with liquids than with solids; consequently, liquids of a thicker consistency should initially be given carefully in small amounts, with gradual progression to thin liquids.

If the introduction of food or liquid into the mouth fails to set off the reflexive swallow, *additional stimulation* is provided. Firm upward pressure under the chin, light upward stroking of the larynx, or light tactile stimulation around the mouth may provide the stimulation necessary to trigger the swallowing reflex.

Staff members who feed the severely brain-injured patient must be carefully observant of the patient's swallowing behaviors. The staff member provides external control of the swallowing process with the introduction of food into the mouth, the amount per swallow, and the stimulation of the swallowing reflex. Too much food given too quickly greatly increases the likelihood of aspiration.

Intake Goals. Goals are established for the total amount of fluid and caloric intake needed in 24 hours. All caregivers participating in the oral intake program should use a consistent feeding technique and accurately record the amount of fluid and caloric intake.

Supplemental methods of intake are used when the patient is unable to maintain adequate nutrition orally. These supplemental methods may include intravenous feeding or gastrostomy. Reinsertion of the nasogastric tube should be avoided, if possible, owing to the irritation of the swallowing mechanism and interference with the swallowing process. However, some patients may be able to reestablish oral intake with the presence of a small silastic nasogastric tube. If short-term (*i.e.,* a few days to a few weeks), leaving the nasogastric tube in during oral intake can be an appropriate method of maintaining supplemental intake. In cases of significant swallowing dysfunction with slow improvement in swallowing ability, a gastrostomy is ideal; the patient can continue on a consistent feeding program, and adequate nutrition can be maintained.

Careful monitoring of oral intake to maintain adequate nutrition is essential, especially in the initial stages. Periodic serum electrolytes and nitrogen balance checks are indicated. Weight should be charted on a regular basis.

WHEN TO DISCONTINUE ORAL INTAKE

Oral intake should be discontinued if the patient shows evidence of aspiration pneumonia. A sudden spike in temperature, a chest roentgenogram showing right lower lobe infiltration, or increased right lower lobe sounds after feeding are all indicative of aspiration.

Aspiration pneumonia is most frequently found in the right lower lobe of the lung owing to the effect of gravity and the relatively straight downward course of the right bronchus as compared with the more acute angle of the left bronchus. The oral intake program should also be discontinued if the patient develops other complications that require priority treatment. Any significant decrease in the patient's level of consciousness may indicate neurologic complications, and the oral intake program should again be terminated.

BIBLIOGRAPHY

Best CH, Taylor NB: The Physiological Basis of Medical Practice, 10th ed. Baltimore, Williams & Wilkins, 1979

Ganong WF: Review of Medical Physiology, 9th ed. Los Altos, Lange Medical Publications, 1979

Logemann J: Evaluation and Treatment of Swallowing Disorders. San Diego, CA, College-Hill Press, 1983

28
Common Neurologic Disorders

Robert W. Hendee Jr.
Marilynn Mitchell

General Considerations

Nurses in a critical care unit caring for patients who have acute nervous system injury or illness serve as the patient's first line of defense. In order to ensure superior care, a multitude of routine supportive acts must be performed in repetition.

Concomitantly, the nurse must carry out frequent neurologic and (in cases of multiple systems injuries) other evaluations with constant vigil for subtle changes in blood pressure, pulse rate and regularity, respiratory activity, sensorial status (level of consciousness), and motor and sensory function. Alterations, when they occur, may be the initial indication of impending deterioration, leading to rapid demise unless immediate action is taken to alleviate the underlying pathology. An example may be helpful:

CASE STUDY

A 19-year-old right-handed woman was seen in the emergency room following a vehicular-induced closed head injury. During the initial neurosurgical evaluation her arousal mechanism was moderately depressed, but she responded purposefully and uniformly upon request. No focal or lateralizing signs were evident except for tendency for enlargement of the left pupil (pupillary inequality is termed *anisocoria*). One hour later, following repair of facial lacerations and with stability of sensorial status, she was moved to the critical care unit for further observation. The patients condition was discussed with the receiving nurse by the neurosurgical resident.

Soon thereafter the nurse noted definite, persistent anisocoria, with diminished reaction to light of the dilating pupil and more difficulty in arousing the patient. Immediately the resident was called, and in the interim mannitol was prepared for intravenous administration. This was begun upon the physician's arrival because a deteriorating situation was apparent. The patient was transferred to the operating room, by which time her respiratory condition required external assistance, both pupils had dilated, and she was unresponsive to painful stimuli. Emergency trephinations revealed an acute subdural hematoma over one cerebral hemisphere and an epidural hematoma over the opposite hemisphere.

Fortunately the young woman recovered with minimal neurologic damage. Her life was undoubtedly saved by the awareness and prompt action of the critical care nurse.

Opportunity for the nurse to discover other interesting and extremely important findings is ever present. Serosanguineous drainage from ears, nose, or scalp wound, even when it has been debrided and repaired but incompletely explored in the emergency unit, will represent cerebrospinal fluid (CSF) leak until proved otherwise. Progressive urinary output of abnormally high levels following injury or certain types of intracranial and facial surgery may represent diabetes insipidus (DI). Neither of these conditions necessarily need cause concern about the immediate demise of the patient. If unobserved too long, however, they may result in unnecessary intracranial infection or hypovolemia and severe electrolyte imbalance. These in turn will lead to new problems of care and worsened condition of the patient, possibly precluding complete recovery or ultimately leading to death.

Experience aids the nurse in sharpening her powers of observation to recognize the slight changes that may be the precursors of the full constellation of signs of increased intracranial pressure or brain herniation. The same holds for alterations in lower-extremity motor and sensory function after incomplete spinal cord injury. Experience also imparts confidence to the nurse, as does knowledge of the more common patterns of deterioration, in assisting her to determine whether additional observation is warranted or whether she should seek the physician's reevaluation immediately.

Physicians rendering quality care in the treatment of critically ill patients should always allocate time to discuss with the nurse, even briefly, the particulars of each new patient upon his arrival in the critical care unit. At that time, the nurse must establish *precise* baseline information to her own satisfaction and seek clarification if necessary.

In these days of vehicular abuse, exposure to dangerous equipment, and use of complex mechanical recreational devices, many patients in any large and active critical care unit are those with acute cranial or spinal injuries. Intracranial abscesses, aneurysms, arteriovenous malformations and tumors, and nontraumatic spinal cord lesions also continue to require neurosurgical care. The following section will discuss some of the common problems that may arise in the general neurosurgical population.

Neurosurgical Problems

INCREASED INTRACRANIAL PRESSURE

Elevated intracranial pressure may be acute, subacute, or chronic, depending on the duration, severity, and rapidity with which it develops. The magnitude of the effects is determined by the extent to which the intracranial structures adapt and the time allowed for the process. It then refers to a situation wherein the normal central nervous system contents are obliged to compete for space within the bony confines of the cranium. Additional limitations are imposed by the sensitivity of the brain in general to trauma and of the cranial nerves and vessels to stretch and compression. The fibrous partitions between parts of the brain (falx cerebri, tentorium cerebelli) also act as intrinsic barriers to displacement of the cranial contents and may result in pressure against the nervous and vascular structures.

Competition with the normal intracranial contents may arise extrinsic to the brain—for example, from epidural or subdural hematomas or tumors arising from the covering of the brain (meningiomas), all of which may exert pressure against any of the brain's surfaces. Intrinsically, hydrocephalus (due to tumors located in the posterior fossa or elsewhere, subarachnoid hemorrhage, or congenital anomalies), intracere-

bral or intracerebellar hematomas (due, for example, to hemorrhage from aneurysms), malformations, and cerebral edema all may create abnormal intracranial pressure.

A focal or diffuse intracranial lesion of sufficient size, regardless of the etiology or whether extracerebral or intracerebral, imparts a mass effect, the result of which is an obligatory shift of the normal contents. If the pressure is acute and the mass significantly large, dramatically rapid adverse effects will be noted, as in the case of most epidural hematomas. These are usually due to temporal bone fracture and laceration of the middle meningeal artery, implying more rapid hemorrhage than that which is venous in origin, unless large venous structures such as the major venous sinuses are involved. Such structures are the origin of major venous bleeding, which may lead to early tragedy.

The ultimate result, even in the case of long-standing, slowly evolving subdural hematomas, is some degree of impingement on the superficial cerebral substance and secondary distortion of the cranial nerves, vessels, and brain stem.

Pressure of the medial aspect (uncus) of the medially displaced temporal lobe on the superior part of the third cranial (oculomotor) nerve results in progressive pupillary dilatation on the same side because of interference with the pupilloconstrictor fibers carried by that nerve. Occasionally, the opposite oculomotor nerve will be compressed against its ipsilateral cerebral peduncle, with false lateralization of the abnormal (enlarged) pupil.

A sign of early increased intracranial pressure may be seen in injury to the sixth cranial (abducens) nerve, which is manifested by impaired abduction of the appropriate globe. The abducens nerve traverses the greatest distance between sites of origin and function and thereby has the greatest theoretic chance of injury by compression or stretch.

Compression of the cerebral hemispheres or distortion of or injury to the brain stem will result in alterations in arousal. In the latter structure, the reticular activating system is involved. Interference with the cardiorespiratory centers will be evidenced by depression and perhaps irregularity of pulse rate and concomitant elevation of blood pressure, as well as abnormalities visible on the cardiac monitor suggestive of primary cardiac disease. In addition, there will be abnormalities of respiratory depth, rate, and regularity. Pupillary abnormality, decreased spontaneous movement, and weakness of the opposite limbs, and, where the dominant side of the brain is involved, speech dysfunction (dysphasia) also will be apparent. It should be noted, however, that lateralizing signs (hemiparesis, speech disorders, pupillary changes) may not be present initially; rather, headache, progressively severe nausea, emesis, and sensorial depression leading to obtundation will be the most striking symptoms and findings.

It is helpful for both nurse and physician to have concise understanding of the terminology used for the various pathologic levels of consciousness. It is burdensome to rely on more categories than those that follow:

- *Stuporous/very lethargic*—sleepy or trancelike but can still be aroused to respond with volitional, well-defined, and purposeful acts, whether or not the acts are socially acceptable
- *Semicomatose*—does not perform volitional acts on request but does have individual, purposeful movements (defensive withdrawal) or motor activity that is categorized as
- *Decerebrate*—extension of lower extremities; extension and inward rotation of upper extremities
- *Decorticate*—extension of lower extremities; flexion and internal or external rotation of forearms
- *Opisthotonic*—extension of extremities, neck, and trunk
- *Coma*—implies no spontaneous or induced response except that noted, for example, in the pulse and respiratory rate when nociceptive (painful) stimulation is used

Continuous monitoring techniques that allow instantaneous readings of intracranial pressure are becoming universally used in the care of critically ill patients regardless of the cause of the increased pressure. Such monitors may be of the kind that measure surface pressure (epidural or subdural), or they may record central pressure by means of catheters placed within a lateral ventricle. The former generally require insertion in an operating theater environment, whereas the latter may be easily installed via a twist drill hole placed through the calvarium with the patient remaining in the intensive care unit bed. Although the ventricular catheter technique is most invasive, it also serves as a ventriculostomy, allowing for removal of CSF, which at times, even in small quantities, may help to reduce intracranial pressure significantly. Both devices allow for more rapid therapeutic response to patients having increased intracranial pressure and are valuable additions to the total monitoring of the patient (see Chap. 24).

CEREBRAL CONCUSSION AND CONTUSION

A *cerebral concussion* is the transient stage in which consciousness is lost after a blow to the head. Implied or inherent therein is interruption of normal neural activity. The loss of consciousness is "usually reversible." Retrograde amnesia (loss of memory of events prior to the injury, varying in severity depending on the degree of injury.

It is obvious that severe head injuries may be sustained without cerebral concussion by the strict definition—that is, without loss of consciousness, even briefly. Moreover, patients with injuries that consist purely of concussion should be expected to recover without any neurologic sequelae. Patients who remain unconscious for more than 1 hour must be suspected of having suffered more than a simple concussion.

It is worth emphasizing that loss of consciousness is not mandatory for a diagnosis of severe head injury, at the same time recognizing that a certain percentage of patients with a clinical diagnosis of "simple" cerebral concussion will upon observation be found to have or develop significant injury.

This is well illustrated in the "classic" case of epidural hematoma, in which the patient is initially rendered unconscious, perhaps only for a minute or so, and appears to recover, refusing medical assistance. A short time afterward the patient becomes drowsy, eventually obtunded, hemiparetic, and develops anisocoria. Unless neurosurgical intervention occurs, virtually all victims will die. This is the reason that head-injured patients must be observed so closely in the critical care unit even though they may at the onset and, for the great percentage, later, appear quite normal.

Cerebral contusion *per se* is usually more serious and refers to injury resulting in bruising of the brain. This may be minimal or a widespread, massive, and fatal nerve tissue insult.

Contusions in general carry a higher risk than concussions regarding permanent damage and significant lesions. Contusions may be accompanied by brain lacerations and hematomas and may lead to depressing problems of intractable, fatal cerebral edema. Individuals with focal or lateralizing neurologic signs are evaluated by specific neurodiagnostic procedures (computerized axial tomography [CT] if available and if time permits, or cerebral angiography) to differentiate brain contusion, a nonoperative problem, from traumatic space-occupying lesions that may be surgically remediable.

Treatment for contusion without accompanying surgical injury consists of excellent general supportive care and usually steroids to preclude or reduce concomitant cerebral edema.

CEREBRAL EDEMA AND SWELLING

A frequent and frustrating situation arising as a consequence of cerebral trauma is the appearance of cerebral edema and swelling. Cerebral edema is the existence of excess cerebral fluid (intracellular and intercellular), whereas swelling results from increased blood flow and volume (*i.e.,* hyperemia of the brain). The former causes increased bulk in which the white matter is more vulnerable than the gray and occurs frequently in association with cerebral tumors, abscesses, vascular abnormalities (A-V malformations, etc.) and hematomas (intracerebral or extracerebral).

Cerebral edema and swelling occur concomitantly most commonly in contusions caused by impact forces. Cerebral edema may be present in association with thrombosis of cortical veins or the sagittal sinus, hypoxia (following near-drowning, aborted sudden infant death syndrome), Reye's syndrome, water intoxication, vascular inflammation, exposure to cold, tin poisoning, and hormonal imbalance. These result in "benign" intracranial hypertension or pseudotumor cerebri wherein the presence of a tumor is mimicked.

Both surgical and medical modalities have been directed at cerebral edema, albeit the former has had limited success. Medical techniques for edema and swelling are virtually the same and include adequate respiratory care (airway and ventilation) to preclude or reduce hypoxia, which may lead to further edema. In addition, dehydrating agents that are hyperosmolar in nature (*e.g.,* mannitol), which attract fluids into the vascular space for transport to the kidneys, are used. Diuresis may also be created by agents such as furosemide. Mannitol appears to be less associated with a rebound phenomenon than urea. In this situation, plasma osmotic pressure becomes lower than tissue osmotic pressure, inducing a return fluid shift to the interstitial compartment with resultant edema.

Steroids such as dexamethasone act to reduce edema, probably by a stabilizing effect on membrane permeability, and have a slower onset of action but reduce the rebound of dehydrating agents when used in conjunction with them.

Other methods include relative dehydration of the body *in toto* by restriction of replacement fluid and use of salt-containing fluids to maintain the patient on the low or dry side of fluid maintenance; hypothermia to decrease the metabolic needs of the injured cerebral tissue; elevation of the head, when feasible, to promote venous return from the brain to the heart; and cautious use, when deemed necessary, of intermittent positive pressure breathing techniques, which, although beneficial to pulmonary care, may increase intracranial pressure.

Barbiturates have been progressively used to induce artificial coma in nonoperative or postoperative cases of trauma, in Reye's syndrome, and in other situations. These agents apparently reduce cerebral metabolism and, in conjunction with paralytic agents, create a totally restful environment for the patient and allow accurate control of ventilation in intubated individuals. Significant problems with hypotension may negate the benefits, however, and require additional agents to maintain adequate peripheral pressure and cerebral perfusion. Another obvious drawback is the loss of many parameters that otherwise may be measured as a sign of clinical status.

Experience proves that, in general, younger patients tend to show higher rates of recovery following cerebral contusions and edema than patients do past the second or third decade.

The signs of cerebral edema and swelling are those of any space-occupying situation if the intracranial pressure is sufficiently elevated. Severe, intractable edema and swelling may be present from the onset or appear later (by hours or days), even acutely, despite the appearance of a relatively stable course and the use of the entire spectrum of preventive or therapeutic measures.

Because of the importance of observing these patients without the effect of outside influences (the exception being persons in elective barbiturate coma), sedatives and analgesics are rarely used; if required to allay severe pain from associated injuries (*e.g.,* fractures), they should be utilized only in a most judicious manner and with close observation for stability of vital and neurologic signs. Paraldehyde seems to be efficacious when the patient is severely confused or combative and thus threatening more harm to himself by thrashing.

If the patient shows more depression in sensorial status at any time, squeezing the trapezius or discreet use of a safety pin in the sole will assist in determining whether arousal is possible, as from an exhausted slumber that is known to occur when a patient is exposed to a critical care unit environment for several days. If the patient is severely ill to begin with, recognition of changes indicative of deterioration becomes more difficult because there is less room for physiological change.

CSF FISTULA

Fistulas that allow leakage of CSF are dangerous because they may predispose to meningeal infection, cerebritis, and death. They frequently follow injuries causing basilar skull fractures and meningeal tear or depressed skull fractures in which the irregular bone edge interrupts the meningeal integrity. CSF leak may occur spontaneously without antecedent trauma in situations of chronic, progressive elevated intracranial pressure.

Fracture at the base involving the posterior or middle cranial fossa may allow drainage of the bloody or serosanguineous fluid by way of the external auditory canal. Eventually the fluid becomes xanthochromic, then clear, and if infected may be purulent.

Drainage from the nares by way of the paranasal or frontal sinuses is seen in basilar or low frontal fractures in the frontal fossa. Patients who are sufficiently alert may complain of fluid trickling into the oropharynx when reclining or partially seated. Often discharge through the nares is noted by a spurt or flow of fluid when the patient sits or stands and leans forward.

A specimen of the discharge should be obtained in any case for evaluation by the physician. If the fluid does not contain blood or its disintegration products, a positive glucose test (qualitative) confirms the suspicion of the fluid as CSF.

It is important to be more vigilant for CSF leaks if basilar skull fracture is identified on examination of the skull radiographs, if the patient has Battle's sign (ecchymosis, edema, and tenderness over the mastoid bone), or if there are periorbital or nasal discoloration and edema.

Suspicion should be raised promptly whenever dressings covering a scalp wound become stained with watery, usually serosanguineous, fluid. There may exist a previously undetected fracture with underlying meningeal laceration. Postoperative staining of a craniotomy dressing will indicate inadequate meningeal closure or elevated intracranial pressure decompressing itself by CSF leak through the meningeal suture line.

In any case, it is of utmost importance that prophylactic antibiotics be administered until the fistula heals spontaneously (with the assistance of lumbar punctures to lower the CSF pressure, if necessary) or correction of wounds or operative closure is carried out.

It is usual to maintain as far as possible, with appropriate right- or left-sided dependent posturing, a head-up position to allow better drainage. This lowers the intracranial CSF "pressure head" and precludes pooling of CSF in, for example, the paranasal sinuses, whereby bacterial organisms then have a better chance to congregate for access through the fistula to the intracranial fluid.

In the presence of CSF leak, one should not try to clear the nose by blowing because this allows forceful retrograde displacement of organisms into the fistula.

DIABETES INSIPIDUS (DI)

DI represents a pathologic state wherein abnormally great quantities of dilute urine are excreted, at times up to 20 liters/day. The kidneys have lost ability to control the amount of fluid output because of absence or deficit in antidiuretic hormone (ADH), which is produced in the supraoptic and paraventricular nuclei of the hypothalamus. The hormone is eventually released by the neurohypophysis (posterior pituitary) and appears to act on the distal renal tubules to promote reabsorption of water. Approximately 85% of the hypothalamic nuclei involved in production of the hormone must be impaired before insufficient ADH is available.

The excessive urinary output is matched by excessive thirst in persons alert enough to recognize it, requiring increased fluid intake. This contrasts with the situation found in psychogenic polydipsia, in which excess water is consumed, resulting secondarily in excess output.

Patients with depressed arousal and inability to regulate their own intake will eventually lose enough fluid to lead to hypovolemia and death unless replacement in proper amounts is supplied for them. Replacement of water and glucose alone without appropriate electrolytes will result in water intoxication and cerebral edema because electrolytes accompany the water lost by the kidneys.

Control of water balance is more complicated than one may be led to believe based on the preceding information alone. The entire complex mechanism is not fully understood, but it incorporates not only ADH but osmoreceptors and baroreceptors and one additional hormone at least, aldosterone. In general, however, if the water available to the body is decreased, the secretion of ADH is increased, leading to water retention. In states of excess body water, ADH secretion is normally diminished, allowing for loss of the excess fluid.

DI is usually expected, transiently at least, but at times it occurs in florid and permanent fashion following open procedures for pituitary and parasellar lesions (craniopharyngioma) and in transphenoidal approaches using cryotherapy for pituitary ablation. It is hoped that newer transphenoidal microsurgical techniques, where applicable, will preclude leaving a postoperative pituitary cripple and reduce the chances for DI.

DI may also be seen in other surgical procedures performed in the region of the hypothalamus and in head injuries with basilar fractures involving the sphenoid bone, gunshot wounds of the head, hypothalamic tumors, hydrocephalus, maxillofacial injuries with displaced fractures, nasopharyngeal tumors invasive of the base of the skull, aneurysms encroaching upon the sellar or suprasellar space, and the like. Of course, some patients without traumatic lesions may have DI among other symptoms or as the sole presenting symptom.

In cases of DI it is essential that evaluation be carried out for concomitant anterior pituitary insufficiency. This is usually manifested initially as adrenal crisis with hypotension, generalized weakness, anorexia, depressed arousal, hypothermia, and psychotic symptoms.

Recognition of DI in the early postoperative period may be difficult if cerebral dehydrating agents have been used before or during surgery because the diuresis created by them may continue for the first postoperative day or so. Use of steroids may also cause increased urinary output. If the patient is awake, however, he will complain of progressively severe thirst if DI is present. Urine output will increase and persist despite the amount of fluid intake (which is usually maintained below normal replacement levels after cranial neurosurgery), and urine specific gravity will fall or remain below about 1.007 to 1.008. Suspicion of the entity is confirmed by serum and urine electrolyte and osmolality determinations (see Chap. 19).

The presence of persistent DI will result in exhaustion of the alert patient, who is unable to rest for long because of the frequent need to micturate and replenish fluids, with replacement fluids consisting of iced juices and other electrolyte-containing liquids. In this case, vasopressin (Pitressin) will eventually be required, just as in severe, continuing DI in patients unable to replace their losses voluntarily.

It should be reemphasized that patients developing florid DI may lose enormous amounts of urine in a relatively short period of time, leading to hypovolemia, unless a diagnosis is surmised or established and treatment is undertaken. When the diagnosis is secure, it is most efficacious to allow the patient to satisfy his replacement needs by drinking according to his thirst. It is more difficult in those requiring intravenous therapy, but, especially in the latter cases, meticulous quantitation of intake and output is mandatory.

It should also be noted that transient, manageable DI may occur and then undergo spontaneous total remission even after a florid initial course. The use of vasopressin, unless as a short-acting form, coincident with the spontaneous remission might lead to relative renal insufficiency and oliguria until effects of the extrinsic vasopressin are completed.

INTRACRANIAL HEMORRHAGE

Intracranial hemorrhage not related to trauma is encountered most frequently secondary to rupture of cerebral aneurysms. It may also occur from vascular malformation, rupture of weakened vessels under the strain of systemic hypertension, or occasionally in relation to cerebral neoplasms *per se* or leukemic infiltrates or aggregates.

More common than generally recognized are hemorrhages during periods of anticoagulation therapy for previous myocardial infarction, because of vascular insufficiency, and as prophylaxis of pulmonary embolus in phlebitis of the lower extremities. Admittedly there is usually an antecedent minor head injury or episode of severe straining in anticoagulated patients.

Massive, rapid hemorrhages also may occur in diffuse intravascular coagulopathy (DIC), whatever the basic cause. The hemorrhage may be confined to the spaces associated with the meningeal layers or involve the intracerebral substance.

In ruptured aneurysms, unless there is a space-occupying lesion that necessitates emergency surgery, such as subdural or intracerebral hematoma, the patient is frequently too ill for immediate surgery because of severe spasm in the cerebral vessels. He generally does not become a candidate for direct attack on the aneurysm unless the neurologic situation improves markedly and repeat arteriography confirms remission of vascular spasms.

This holds true despite the knowledge that a significant percentage may be expected to have a recurrent hemorrhage that could prove fatal in the interval while awaiting sufficient improvement to allow surgery.

Headache (frequently severe), nausea, emesis, stiff and tender neck, and photophobia are common complaints if the patient is adequately alert.

SYNDROME OF INAPPROPRIATE SECRETION OF ANTIDIURETIC HORMONE (SIADH)

This phenomenon was initially described by Schwartz[1] and colleagues and further defined by Bartter.[2] The features are hyponatremia and hypotonicity of the plasma in conjunction with excretion of urine, which is hypertonic to plasma and which contains appreciable amounts of sodium. In addition there is absence of hypokalemia and edema; normal cardiac, renal, and adrenal function; and normal or expanded plasma and extracellular fluid volumes (*i.e.,* no evidence if dehydration or hypovolemia). The presence of low serum blood urea nitrogen and uric acid levels assists in confirming the diagnosis.

The secretion of ADH (vasopressin) is "inappropriate" in that it continues despite the decreased osmolality of the plasma.

Some neoplastic conditions (carcinoma of the lung, duodenum, pancreas, or thymomas) may produce a chemical substance that is similar to or identical with the arginine vasopressin produced in the hypothalamo-pituitary system but that is independent of normal physiological controls. Thus, an aberrant secretion is the factor in these cases.

In other conditions such as hemorrhage, trauma, central nervous system infection or disease, and pulmonary disease and in the postoperative period, abnormal secretion of endogenous ADH is the etiology. Use of medications such as vincristine, chlorpropamide, hydrochlorothiazide, and carbomazepine (Tegretol) may also result in the syndrome.

The symptomatology of SIADH is basically that of

water retention at one end of the spectrum proceeding to water intoxication at the other end. In this regard, I have seen definite symptoms that subsequently cleared with the usual therapy, even with a serum sodium reduced no more than the range of 120 to 125.

Bartter[2] states that water retention (and concomitant dilution of the serum sodium concentration) occurring slowly or when not severe causes headache, asthenia, somnolence, lethargy, and confusion. More rapidly occurring dilution, or water intoxication *per se,* is associated with anorexia, nausea, and emesis, proceeding to delirium, fits, aberrant respirations, hypothermia, and coma. Prior to coma, the stretch reflexes may disappear, the presence of Babinski's sign is noted, and pseudobulbar palsy may occur.

One can establish the diagnosis by readily available laboratory procedures, although radioimmunoassay of plasma ADH might be the most confirmatory method. The serum sodium concentration and serum osmolality are the best routine indices.

Treatment consists of restriction of fluid intake (even limited to perhaps 500 ml/day maximum in severe cases) and where applicable the treatment of underlying disorders (*e.g.,* administration of cortisone in Addison's disease) or the discontinuation of carbomazepine or other causative medications. Administration of salt (sodium chloride solutions) is usually of only transient benefit, but one may consider its use in cases in which water intoxication is severe in order to attempt to increase serum osmolality acutely.

REFERENCES

1. Schwartz WB, Bennet W, Curelop S et al: A syndrome of renal sodium loss and hyponatremia probably resulting from inappropriate secretion of antidiuretic hormone. Am J Med 23:529–542, 1957
2. Bartter FC: The syndrome of inappropriate secretion of antidiuretic hormone. Disease-A-Month, Year Book Medical Publishers, November 1973

BIBLIOGRAPHY

Merritt HH: A Texbook of Neurology, 6th ed. Philadelphia, Lea & Febiger, 1979
Rosenberg RN (ed): Neurology. New York, Grune & Stratton, 1980

Cerebrovascular Disease

INTRODUCTION

Cerebrovascular disease is the most frequent neurologic disorder of adults. It is the third leading cause of morbidity and mortality in the United States, after heart disease and cancer. Although statistics indicate that the number of people having strokes in the United States has been declining since the late 1950s, there are still over 500,000 strokes ("cerebrovascular accidents") each year. Only one third of patients are able to return to a fully functioning life after the stroke.

Cerebrovascular disease (CVD) includes any pathological process that involves the blood vessels of the brain. Most CVD is due to thrombosis, embolism, or hemorrhage (Fig. 28-1). The mechanism of each of these etiologies is different, but the result is the same —ultimate ischemia or hypoxia to a focal area of the brain. Ischemia may lead to brain necrosis (infarction).

Cerebral thrombosis is often associated with atherosclerosis. Conditions such as sickle cell disease and polycythemia may predispose a person to cerebral thrombosis. Infectious processes and inflammation may produce cerebral thrombophlebitis.

Strokes due to embolus may be a result of blood clots, fragments of atheromatous plaques, lipids, or air. Emboli to the brain most often come from the heart, secondary to myocardial infarction or atrial fibrillation.

If hemorrhage is the etiology of a stroke, hypertension is often a precipitating factor. Vascular abnormali-

FIGURE 28-1
Vascular changes preventing blood flow. (From Brunner LS, Suddarth DS: Textbook of Medical-Surgical Nursing, 5th ed. Philadelphia, JB Lippincott, 1984.)

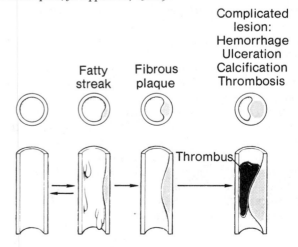

Fatty streak · Fibrous plaque · Complicated lesion: Hemorrhage Ulceration Calcification Thrombosis · Thrombus

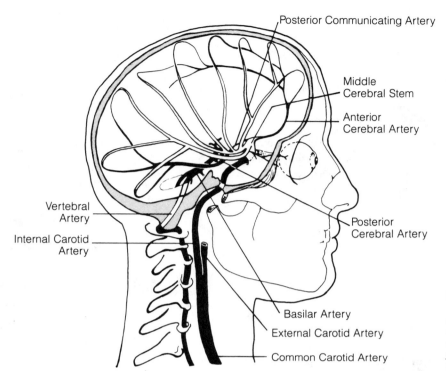

Posterior Communicating Artery

Middle
Cerebral Stem

Anterior
Cerebral Artery

Posterior
Cerebral Artery

Vertebral
Artery

Internal Carotid
Artery

Basilar Artery

External Carotid Artery

Common Carotid Artery

FIGURE 28-2
The major vessels to the brain. The internal carotid, anterior, and middle cerebral arteries constitute the anterior circulation. The vertebral, basilar, and posterior cerebral arteries and branches compose the posterior circulation.

ties such as arteriovenous malformations (AVMs) and cerebral aneurysms are more prone to rupture and cause hemorrhage in the presence of hypertension. In children, however, subarachnoid hemorrhage and intracerebral hemorrhage suggest trauma, aneurysms, or AVM rather than hypertension as the cause.

ANATOMY OF BRAIN VASCULATURE

The brain is supplied with blood from two major sets of vessels: the carotid, or anterior, circulation and the vertebral, or posterior, circulation (Fig. 28-2). Each system comes off the aortic arch as a pair of vessels: the left and right common carotids and the left and right vertebrals. Each carotid bifurcates to form the internal and external carotid artery. The vertebral arteries arise from the subclavian arteries. The vertebrals join to form the basilar artery, and that in turn divides to form the two posterior cerebral arteries, which supply the medial and inferior surfaces of the brain as well as the lateral portions of the temporal and occipital lobe (Fig. 28-3).

The circle of Willis is the area in which the branches of the basilar and internal carotid arteries unite. The circle of Willis is composed of the two anterior cerebral arteries, the anterior communicating artery, the two posterior cerebral arteries, and the two posterior communicating arteries (Fig. 28-4). This circular net-

FIGURE 28-3
Arterial supply areas in the brain.

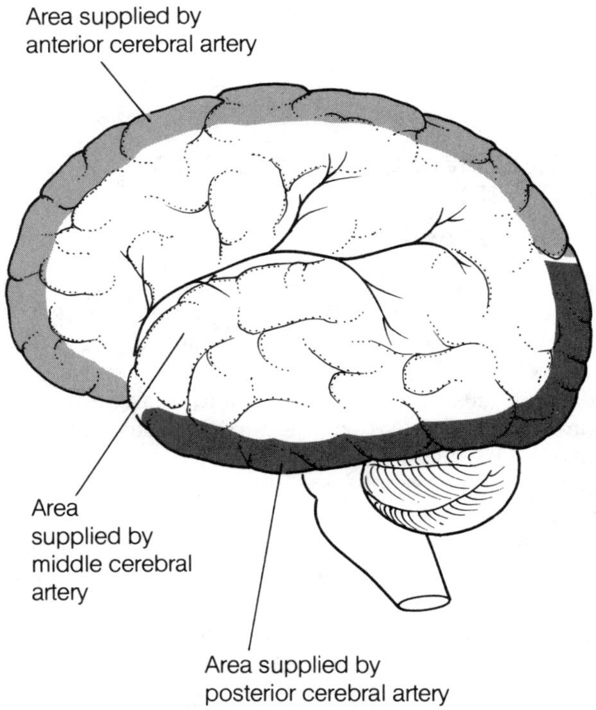

Area supplied by
anterior cerebral artery

Area
supplied by
middle cerebral
artery

Area supplied by
posterior cerebral artery

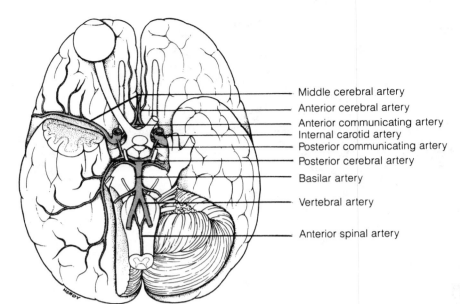

Middle cerebral artery
Anterior cerebral artery
Anterior communicating artery
Internal carotid artery
Posterior communicating artery
Posterior cerebral artery
Basilar artery
Vertebral artery
Anterior spinal artery

FIGURE 28-4
The Circle of Willis seen from below the brain.

work permits blood to circulate from one hemisphere to the other and from the anterior into the posterior areas of the brain. It is a system that allows for collateral circulation if one vessel is occluded. It is not unusual, however, for some vessel within the circle of Willis to be atrophic or even absent. This accounts for different clinical presentations among patients with the same lesion. For example, an occluded carotid artery in a patient with a fully patent circle of Willis may be totally asymptomatic, but a patient in whom the circle of Willis is incomplete may demonstrate a massive cerebral infarction.

CEREBROVASCULAR ACCIDENT (STROKE)

Classification

A stroke may be defined as a neurologic deficit that has a sudden onset and lasts over 24 hours resulting from cerebrovascular disease. Approximately three fourths of strokes are due to vascular obstruction (thrombi or emboli), resulting in ischemia and infarction. About one fourth of strokes are hemorrhagic, resulting from hypertensive vascular disease (which causes an intracerebral hemorrhage), a ruptured aneurysm, or an arteriovenous malformation.

Each of the three types of stroke has a fairly typical time course. Thrombotic strokes may be subdivided into transient ischemic attacks (TIAs), stroke in evolution, or completed stroke. Thrombotic strokes may occur suddenly and be complete early, or they may

progress over a period of time, depending on how much blood is able to get through the vascular lumen. Both embolic and hemorrhagic strokes typically present suddenly and progress rapidly over minutes or hours. There is usually little or no warning.

Sixty percent of thrombotic strokes occur during sleep. If the stroke is not complete at the time of the initial attack, symptoms may evolve over several hours or days. There may be some temporary improvement in clinical deficits, but then there follows a rapid progression of permanent deficits. This symptom development is referred to as stroke-in-evolution.

The most frequent neurovascular syndrome seen in thrombotic and embolic strokes is due to involvement of the middle cerebral artery. This artery mainly supplies the lateral aspects of the cerebral hemisphere. Infarction to that area of the brain may cause contralateral motor and sensory deficits. If the infarcted hemisphere is dominant, speech problems result, and aphasia may be present.

Pathophysiology

When blood flow to any part of the brain is impeded as a result of a thrombus or embolus, oxygen deprivation of the cerebral tissue begins. Deprivation for 1 minute can lead to reversible symptoms, such as loss of consciousness. Oxygen deprivation for longer periods can produce microscopic necrosis of the neurons. The necrotic area is then said to be infarcted.

The initial oxygen deprivation may be due to general ischemia (from cardiac arrest or hypotension) or hypoxia from an anemic process or high altitude. If the neurons are only ischemic, and have not necrosed yet, there is a chance to save them. This situation is analogous to the focal injury caused by a myocardial infarction. An occluded coronary artery can produce an area of infarcted (dead) tissue. Surrounding the infarcted zone is an area of ischemic tissue, which has been marginally deprived of oxygen. This ischemic tissue, as in the brain, may be either salvaged with appropriate treatment or killed by secondary events.

Clinical Manifestations

A patient with vascular disease may present with a TIA. This is a neurological deficit that totally resolves within 24 hours. Its average duration is 10 minutes, after which the symptoms completely disappear. A patient may also present with a reversible ischemic neurologic deficit (RIND). This event may persist beyond the 24-hour duration of a TIA, but it eventually will clear completely. The third possible clinical presentation is a completed stroke, which leaves the patient with a permanent deficit.

Of those patients who have TIAs, one third will have a major stroke, one third will continue to have TIAs but will not have a major stroke, and one third will have a resolution of their TIAs.

Symptoms seen with TIAs depend a great deal on the vessels involved. When the carotid and cerebral arteries are involved, the patient may have blindness in one eye, hemiplegia, hemianesthesia, speech disturbances, and confusion. When the vertebrobasilar artery is involved, dizziness, diplopia, numbness, visual defects in one or both fields, and dysarthria can be seen. Table 28-1 is a list of common deficits seen with cerebrovascular disease and of suggested nursing interventions.

Some generalizations can be made about the probable disabilities of a patient if one knows both the side of the brain in which the stroke occurred and the "handedness" of the patient. Ninety-three percent of people are right-handed. This means that their left hemisphere is dominant. Of the 7% of the population who are left-handed, about 60% have their dominant speech center in their left hemisphere, as do right-handed people.

TABLE 28-1
COMMON DEFICITS AND EMOTIONAL REACTION TO STROKE WITH GENERAL NURSING INTERVENTION

Common Motor Deficits

1. Hemiplegia (side of the body opposite the cerebral episode)
   Hemiparesis (side of the body opposite the cerebral episode)
2. Dysarthria (muscles of speech impaired)
3. Dysphagia (muscles of swallowing impaired)

Nursing Intervention

1. Position in proper body alignment, use a hand roll to keep the hand in functional position.
   Provide frequent passive range of motion.
   Reposition every 2 hours.
2. Provide for an alternate method of communication.
3. Test the patient's palatal and pharyngeal reflexes before offering nourishment.
   Elevate and turn the patient's head to the unaffected side
   If the patient is able to manage oral intake, place food on the unaffected side of his mouth.

Common Sensory Deficits

1. *Visual deficits* are common because the visual pathways cut through much of the cerebral hemispheres)
   a. Homonymous hemianopsia (loss of vision in one half of the visual field on the same side)

Left   Right

   b. Double vision (diplopia)
   c. Decreased visual acuity
2. Absent or diminished response to superficial sensation (touch, pain, pressure, heat, cold)

Nursing Intervention

   a. Approach patient from the unaffected side; remind him to turn his head to compensate for visual deficits.

   b. Apply eye patch to affected eye.
   c. Provide assistance as necessary.
2. Increase the amount of touch in administering patient care.
   Protect the involved areas from injury.
   Protect the involved areas from burns.
   Examine the involved areas for signs of skin irritation and injury.
   Provide the patient with the opportunity to handle various objects of different weight, texture, and size.
   If pain is present, assess location, type, and duration of pain.

(Continued)

TABLE 28-1
(Continued)

3. Absent or diminished response to proprioception (knowledge of position of body parts)
4. *Perceptual deficits* disturbance in correctly perceiving and interpreting himself or his environment)
   a. Body scheme disturbance (amnesia or denial for paralyzed extremities)

   b. Disorientation (to time, place, and person)

   c. Apraxias (loss of ability to use objects correctly)
   d. Agnosias (inability to identify the environment by means of the senses)
   e. Defects in localizing objects in space, estimating their size, and judging distance
   f. Impaired memory for recall of spatial location of objects or places

   g. Right-left disorientation

Language Deficits
1. *Expressive aphasia* (difficulty in transforming sound into patterns of understandable speech): Can speak in single-word responses
2. *Receptive aphasia* (impairment of comprehension of the spoken word): Able to speak, but uses words incorrectly and is unaware of these errors
3. *Global aphasia* (combination of expressive and receptive aphasia): Unable to communicate at any level

4. *Alexia* (inability to understand the written word)

5. *Agraphia* (inability to express ideas in writing)

Intellectual Deficits
1. Loss of memory
2. Short attention span
3. Easily distractable
4. Poor judgment
5. Inability to transfer learning from one situation to another
6. Inability to calculate, reason, abstract

Emotional Deficits
1. Emotional lability (exhibits reactions easily or inappropriately)
2. Loss of self-control and social inhibitions
3. Reduced tolerance to stress
4. Fear, hostility, frustration, anger
5. Confusion and despair
6. Withdrawal, isolation
7. Depression

Bowel and Bladder Dysfunction

Bladder: Incomplete upper motor neuron lesion

1. Unilateral lesion from the stroke results in partial sensation and control of bladder so that the patient experiences frequency, urgency, and incontinence
2. If stroke lesion is in the brain stem, there will be bilateral damage, resulting in an upper motor neuron bladder with loss of all control of micturition.

---

3. Teach the patient to check the position of his body parts with his eyes.

   a. Protect the involved area.
      Accept patient's perception of himself.
      Position patient to face the involved area.
   b. Control the amount of change in patient's schedule.
      Reorient the patient as necessary.
      Talk to patient; tell him about his environment.
      Provide a calendar, clock, pictures of family, and so forth.
   c. Correct misuse of objects and demonstrate proper use.
   d. Correct misinformation.

   e. Reduce any stimuli that will distract the patient.

   f. Place necessary equipment where patient will see it, rather than tell the patient something such as, "It is in the closet."
   g. Use instructions like "Lift this leg." (Point to the leg.)

Nursing Intervention
1. Ask patient to repeat individual sounds of alphabet as a start at retraining.

2. Speak clearly and in simple sentences; use gestures as necessary.

3. Evaluate what language skills are intact, speak in very simple sentences, ask patient to repeat individual sounds, and use gestures or any other means to communicate.
4. Point to written names of objects and have the patient repeat the name of the object.
5. Have the patient write words and simple sentences.

Nursing Intervention
1. Provide necessary information as necessary.
2. Divide activities into short steps.
3. Control any excessive environmental distractions.
4. Protect patient from injury.
5. Repeat instructions as necessary.
6. Do not set unrealistic expectations for patient.

Nursing Interventions
1. Disregard bursts of emotions; explain to the patient that emotional lability is part of the illness.
2. Protect the patient as necessary so that his dignity is preserved.
3. Control the amount of stress experienced by the patient.
4. Be accepting of the patient; be supportive.
5. Clarify any misconceptions; allow the patient to verbalize.
6. Provide stimulation and a safe, comfortable environment.
7. Provide a supportive environment.

Nursing Intervention

Do not suggest insertion of an indwelling catheter immediately after the stroke.

1. Observe patient to identify characteristics of voiding pattern (frequency, amount, forceful, or constant dribbling).

2. Maintain accurate intake and output record.

Nursing note: Incontinence after consciousness is usually due to urinary tract infection caused by a urinary catheter that has been in place.

TABLE 28-1
(Continued)

3. Possibility of establishing normal bladder function is excellent	3. Try to allow patient to stay catheter-free: Offer the bedpan or urinal frequently; take the patient to the commode frequently; assess the patient's ability to make his need for help with voiding known. If a catheter is necessary, remove as soon as possible and implement a bladder training program.
Bowel	
1. Impairment in stroke patient due to deterioration in the level of consciousness, dehydration, or immobility	1. Develop a bowel training program: Provide dietary foods known to stimulate defecation (prune juice, roughage); institute suppository and laxative regimen.
2. Constipation with potential impaction most common problem	2. Give enemas as necessary.

(From Hickey P: The Clinical Practice of Neurological and Neurosurgical Nursing, pp. 364–366. Philadelphia, JB Lippincott, 1981)

Based on the preceding information and the clinical picture demonstrated, the following summarizes the probable disabilities associated with stroke:

Left Hemispheric Stroke
- Right-sided hemiparesis or hemiplegia
- Slow and cautious behavior
- Right visual field defect
- Expressive, receptive, or global aphasia

Right Hemispheric Stroke
- Left-sided hemiparesis or hemiplegia
- Spatial-perceptual deficits
- Poor judgment
- Distractibility
- Impulsive behavior
- Apparent unawareness of deficits of affected side and therefore susceptibility to falls or other injuries
- Left visual field defect

Diagnostic Information

Diagnosis of a stroke is based on physical examination and history. The age of the patient is useful because strokes are more likely to occur in older people. It is helpful to know the type of onset of symptoms from the patient. If the symptoms began suddenly and were severe within an hour, the most likely diagnosis is embolic ischemic brain infarction or intracranial hemorrhage. Nonvascular diseases such as tumors, abscesses, subdural hematomas, and encephalitis rarely progress that quickly.

If atrial fibrillation or a carotid bruit is found on physical examination, it may suggest the diagnosis of stroke. It is important to note the level of consciousness when the patient presents. Ischemic cerebrovascular disease usually does not cause a depression in the level of consciousness. Nonvascular processes and intracranial hemorrhage must be considered if the patient has a depressed level of consciousness.

A CT (computerized axial tomography) scan may be useful in differentiating between cerebrovascular le-

sions and nonvascular lesions. For example, a subdural hemorrhage, brain abscess, tumor, or intracerebral hemorrhage will be visible on the CT scan. An area of infarction may not show on CT scan for 48 hours.

A brain scan has limited value in the acute setting but may be helpful if it is positive. A brain scan will show major infarcted areas, but not as early as the CT scan.

Angiography was done more often before the CT scan was available to distinguish cerebrovascular lesions from nonvascular ones. Early angiography in a stroke patient is often performed if an intracranial hemorrhage is suspected, if the patient is rapidly deteriorating neurologically, or if the patient has a suspected acute carotid occlusion.

One may perform a lumbar puncture to look for blood in the cerebrospinal fluid (CSF). The CT scan may not show low concentrations of blood in the CSF. It is important to know whether hemorrhage is present because this information may help the physician decide whether or not to anticoagulate the patient.

Management

Nursing Assessment and Intervention
As mentioned earlier, with a cerebral infarction there is a central core of brain tissue that is irreversibly lost. Around this dead zone is an area of tissue that may be salvageable. It should be the focus of initial treatment to save as much of the ischemic area as possible. Three ingredients necessary to that area are oxygen, glucose, and adequate blood flow. The oxygen level can be monitored through arterial blood gases, and oxygen can be given to the patient if indicated. Hypoglycemia can be evaluated with serial checks on blood glucose.

Cerebral perfusion pressure is a reflection of the systemic blood pressure, the intracranial pressure, the autoregulation still functioning in the brain, and the heart rate and rhythm. The parameters most easily controlled externally are the cardiac rhythm, rate, and blood pressure. Arrhythmias can usually be corrected.

Causes of tachycardia, such as fever, pain, and dehydration, can be treated.

Patients with moderate hypertension are usually not treated acutely. If their blood pressure is lowered after the brain is accustomed to the hypertension for adequate perfusion, the brain's perfusion pressure will fall along with the blood pressure. If the diastolic blood pressure is above about 105 mm Hg, it may need to be lowered gradually. This may be accomplished very effectively with nitroprusside.

If intracranial pressure is elevated in a stroke patient, it usually occurs after the first day. Although this is a natural response of the brain to some cerebrovascular lesions, it is destructive to the brain. The destructive response, such as edema or arterial vasospasm, can sometimes be treated or prevented. The usual methods of controlling increased intracranial pressure may be instituted, such as hyperventilation, fluid restriction, head elevation, avoidance of neck flexion or severe head rotation that would impede venous outflow from the head, use of osmotic diuretics such as mannitol, and perhaps administration of dexamethasone, although its use remains controversial. Anticoag-ulation may be initiated if the stroke was not hemorrhagic.

Rehabilitation should be started as early as possible. Physical therapy, occupational therapy, and speech therapy all may be needed, depending on the patient's deficits.

Diligent nursing observations are necessary, especially during the acute phase, when the stroke may be evolving. Any deterioration in the patient's neurologic status should be reported immediately.

The nurse must provide optimal care to prevent the many complications possible after stroke, such as urinary tract infection, aspiration pneumonia, decubitus ulcers, contractures, and thrombophlebitis. Discharge planning should begin early during the hospitalization. Patient and family teaching can begin upon admission to the hospital (see Table 28-2).

Psychological Assessment and Intervention

Stroke victims may display emotional problems, and their behavior may be different from the prestroke baseline. Emotions may be labile; for example, the patient may cry one moment and laugh the next, with-

TABLE 28-2
NURSING CARE PLAN: STROKE

Potential Problem	Goal	Nursing Action
Left hemisphere: Possible speech involvement, right hemiplegia; aphasia (expressive-receptive); slow, cautious, disorganized behavior; right visual field cut	Return to optimal level of function with neurologic rehabilitation	1. Participate in neurologic rehabilitation consultation, including occupational therapy, physical therapy, speech. 2. Use facilitative equipment to improve communication (*e.g.*, writing board, picture board, letter board). 3. Position affected side properly.
Right hemisphere: left hemiplegia; spatial perceptual deficits, memory deficits; emotional lability; left hemianopsia; apraxia; poor judgment	Return to optimal functional level; support of patient and family in dealing with new body image	1. Participate in neurologic rehabilitation consultation. 2. Promote awareness of body and environment on affected side. 3. Divide tasks into simple steps; elicit return demonstration of skills. 4. Use verbal clues to enhance patient understanding. 5. Use slow minimal movements and avoid clutter in area around patient. 6. Provide emotional support to patient and family. 7. Position patient in bed to prevent his falling. Consider posey restraint.
Pulmonary embolus/deep vein thrombosis	Prevention of pulmonary embolus and deep vein thrombosis	1. Participate in rehabilitation consultation. 2. Elastic stockings. 3. Check passive/active range of motion. 4. Tilt table (if necessary). 5. Institute heparin therapy (contraindicated with hemorrhagic stroke). 6. Measure thigh and calf circumferences every day. 7. Observe lower extremities frequently for tenderness, redness, warmth, pain. 8. Observe patient for signs of restlessness, anxiety, fever, chills, dyspnea, hypotention.

TABLE 28-2
(Continued)

Potential Problem	Goal	Nursing Action

Seizures	Elimination or control of seizure activity	1. Take precautions against seizures:
		  a. Side rails up and padded
		  b. Bed in low position
		  c. Tongue blade available
		  d. O_2 and suction at bedside
		2. Administer antiseizure agents.
		3. Accurately observe and record seizure activity.
		4. Maintain electrolyte balance through proper nutrition and IV therapy.

Nutritional deficiency	Nutritional balance, electrolyte balance	1. Initially, make frequent assessment of swallow and gag reflexes. 2. Monitor fluid and electrolyte status (*e.g.,* SMA-6 every morning, weight every other day, intake and output). 3. Institute tube feeding when bowel sounds are present. 4. Initiate neurologic bowel and bladder protocol. 5. Consider gastrostomy if patient is on prolonged tube feedings.
Contractures, foot drop, muscle atrophy	Patient with complete range of motion in all extremities	1. Participate in neurologic rehabitation consultation. 2. Check passive/active range of motion. 3. Provide space boots. 4. Provide splints if needed for physical therapy. 5. Position patient up in chair ASAP. 6. Position patient correctly with pillows while he is in bed.
Skin decubitis ulceration	Prevention of decubiti	1. Provide air mattress or kinetic bed. 2. Turn patient every 2 hours. 3. Provide sheep skin. 4. Provide heel and elbow pads. 5. Ensure adequate nutrition. 6. Administer decubitis care.
Increase in ICP secondary to cerebral edema or hemorrhage	Absence of complications; control of ICP	1. Check neurologic signs per routine. 2. Observe for increased systolic BP with widening pulse pressure, change in level of consciousness, bradycardia, headache, vomiting, papilledema. 3. Prevent constipation (bowel program). 4. Raise head of bed. 5. Ensure that intake and output is accurate. 6. Insert Foley catheter. 7. Avoid flexion, extension, or severe rotation of patient's head.

out being able to explain why or to control himself. Tolerance to stress may be reduced. A minor stress in the prestroke state may be perceived as a major problem after the stroke. Families may not understand the behavior. Stroke victims may use loud profanity with the nursing staff or with their family members, yet the family cannot understand it because the patient may never have used any profanity before the stroke. It is the nurse's role to help the family understand these behavioral changes. There is much that the nurse can help do to modify the patient's behavior, such as controlling stimuli in the environment, providing rest periods throughout the day to prevent the patient from becoming overtired, giving positive feedback for acceptable behavior or positive accomplishments, and providing repetition when the patient is trying to relearn a skill.

Surgical Intervention

TIAs are often viewed as a warning of impending stroke due to occlusion of a vessel. Some patients with atherosclerotic disease of extracranial or intracranial vessels may be good surgical candidates. Carotid endarterectomy may be beneficial to a patient with narrowing of the vessels.

Cranial bypass surgery involves anastomosing an extracranial artery that perfuses the scalp to an intracranial artery distal to the occluded site. The procedure often used when there is intracranial involvement is the superior temporal artery anastomosis to the middle cerebral artery (STA-MCA). Collateral circulation is thus provided to areas of the brain supplied by the middle cerebral artery. Many STA-MCA anastomoses are performed with the hope of preventing a future stroke in patients with unilateral focal cerebral ischemia who present with TIAs.

Pharmacologic Management

There are some drugs being used experimentally in the management of strokes. Trental (pentoxifylline) is a drug that has been approved for use in England, West Germany, France, Japan, and other European, Asian, and Latin American countries in treating chronic and acute obstructive arterial disease. It is still being tested in the United States. Trental is an analogue of theobromine (a methylxanthine). It is thought that the drug increases the microcirculatory capillary blood flow, thus improving perfusion and oxygenation to ischemic brain tissue. If this is in fact what happens, perhaps with its use some of the ischemia zone surrounding the area of infarction can be salvaged, thus minimizing the stroke victim's deficits.

Stroke Prognosis

With a thrombotic or embolic stroke, the amount of brain ischemia and infarction that might occur is difficult to predict. There is a chance that the stroke will extend after the initial insult. There can be massive cerebral edema and an increase in intracranial pressure to the point of herniation and death following a large thrombotic stroke. The prognosis is influenced by the area of the brain involved and the extent of the insult. Because thrombotic strokes are often due to atherosclerosis, there is risk of a future stroke in a patient who has already suffered one. With embolic strokes, patients may also have subsequent episodes of stroke if the underlying cause is not treated. If the extent of brain tissue destroyed from a hemorrhagic stroke is not excessive and is in a nonvital area, the patient may recover with minimal deficits. If the hemorrhage is large or in a vital area of the brain, the patient may not recover. About 30% of intracerebral hemorrhages are less massive, making survival possible.

The Aphasic Patient

Expressive and Receptive Aphasia

Stroke victims may demonstrate much frustration with their deficits. Probably no deficit produces more frustration for the patient and those trying to communicate with him than the one involving the production and understanding of language. Aphasia can involve motor abilities or sensory function or both. If the area of brain injury is in or near the left Broca's area, the memory of motor patterns of speech are affected (see Chap. 27, Fig. 27-7). This results in an expressive aphasia, in which the patient understands language but is unable to use it appropriately.

Receptive aphasia is usually a result of injury to the left Wernicke's area, which is the control center for recognition of spoken language. The patient is thus unable to understand the significance of the spoken word. Presence of both expressive aphasia and receptive aphasia is referred to as global aphasia. Table 28-3 summarizes differences between expressive and receptive problems.

It is important for the nursing staff to remember to tell families that just because a person has an aphasia does not mean that he is intellectually impaired. Communication at some level should be attempted, whether it is by writing, pointing at alphabet charts, or with gestures. Nurses should involve the family in speaking slowly and allowing the patient time to answer questions. Speech therapy should begin as early as possible.

ARTERIOVENOUS MALFORMATIONS (AVMs)

Pathophysiology

AVMs also can be included in the discussion of cerebral vascular disease. These congenital developmental defects in the capillaries may occur at any site in the central nervous system but are frequently found in the area of the middle cerebral artery. An AVM is composed of a mass of arterial and venous channels, with many dilated areas. The capillaries in an AVM have failed to develop normally between the arterial and venous blood supplies, so the channels of the two blood supplies are connected by abnormally thin vessels.

There is degeneration of the brain parenchyma around and within the malformation. Blood is shunted directly from the arterial to the venous system. This pathway offers less resistance to blood flow than the normal capillary bed, so the AVM consequently receives a large blood flow. Arteries dilate to handle the increased perfusion of the AVM, and veins enlarge to drain the additional blood away. Collateral vessels may dilate in an attempt to carry the additional load, adding to the mass of the lesion.

Large AVMs may cause an "intracerebral steal" situation whereby arterial blood is diverted away from one area of the brain because of lowered vascular resistance in another. It is thought that AVMs can steal

TABLE 28-3
COMPARISON OF EXPRESSIVE AND RECEPTIVE APHASIA

Expressive Aphasia	*Receptive Aphasia*
1. Hemiparesis is present because motor cortex is near Broca's area.	1. Hemiparesis is mild or absent because lesion is not near motor cortex. Hemianopsia or quadrantanopsia may be present.
2. Speech is slow, nonfluent; articulation is poor; speaking requires much effort. Total speech is reduced in quantity. Patient may use telegraphic speech, omitting small words.	2. Speech is fluent; Articulation and rhythm are normal. Content of speech is impaired; wrong words are used.
3. Patient understands written and verbal speech.	3. Patient does not understand written and verbal speech.
4. Patient writes aphasically.	4. Content of writing is abnormal. Penmanship may be good.
5. Patient may be able to repeat single words with effort. Phrase repetition is poor.	5. Repetition is poor.
6. Object naming is often poor, but it may be better than attempts to use spontaneous speech.	6. Object naming is poor.
7. Patient is aware of deficit, often experiencing frustration and depression.	7. Patient is often unaware of deficit.
8. Curses or other ejaculatory speech may be well articulated and automatic. Patient may be able to hum normally.	8. Patient may use wrong words and sounds.

enough blood from adjacent areas of the brain to cause ischemic damage in the otherwise normal area. The neurologic signs and symptoms seen in the patient correlate with the area of the brain that is deprived of blood flow. The size, shape, and location of the AVM also determine the deficits seen.

Signs and Symptoms

The onset of symptoms may occur in childhood or early adult life. In many patients, the chief complaint is headache, which is often unilateral. Seizures may be another initial symptom: first focal, then developing to generalized. Hemorrhage occurs in about 50% of patients before they are admitted to the hospital. An AVM that has bled once has a 1 : 4 chance of bleeding again within 4 years. An AVM that has bled more than once has a one in four chance of bleeding again within a year. Hemorrhage associated with an AVM can be intracerebral, subdural, or subarachnoid.

Alteration of brain tissue within the AVM and depletion of blood perfusion to adjacent areas may cause the patient to exhibit paresis, mental deterioration, or aplasia of an extremity. There may be transient episodes of dizziness, syncope, sensory deficits or tingling, visual deficits (usually hemianopsia), and confusion. If the bleeding is severe, there may be elevation of intracranial pressure with brain stem compression and unconsciousness.

Management

Two available management modalities for AVMs are artificial embolization and surgical excision. The embolization technique involves the introduction of small silastic beads into the internal carotid artery where they subsequently enter the AVM. This results in thrombosis and destruction of the lesion (Fig. 28-5). This technique is useful when the AVM is not in a surgically accessible area and excision is impossible. It is effective for AVMs supplied by the middle cerebral artery because the silastic beads tend to follow the flow pattern of the middle cerebral artery.

The primary danger of this procedure is that a bead may dislodge from the AVM and migrate to the capillaries of the lung. Sometimes the AVM may appear occluded after the procedure, but collateral circulation redevelops, providing a new vascular supply to the area and reactivating the AVM.

Complete surgical excision eliminates the possibility of recurrent bleeding. Surgery is usually performed after the patient has stabilized from the hemorrhage — about 2 to 3 weeks. Sometimes the artificial embolization procedure is performed first, followed by surgical excision 4 weeks later.

Nursing Intervention

The severity and duration of any postoperative disability will depend largely on the location and extent of the vascular lesion and the resultant ischemia. Imme-

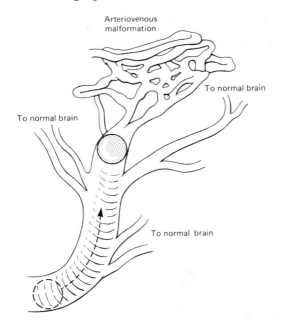

FIGURE 28-5
Small silastic beads or spheres are introduced into artery to block blood flow to the arteriovenous malformation. (Hickey J: The Clinical Practice of Neurological and Neurosurgical Nursing, p 393. Philadelphia, JB Lippincott, 1981)

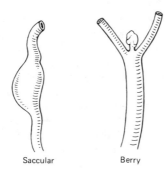

FIGURE 28-6
Saccular and berry aneurysms. (Hickey J: Clinical Practice of Neurological and Neurosurgical Nursing, p 377. Philadelphia, JB Lippincott, 1981)

diately postoperatively, the patient should be watched for a change in neurologic status, especially a change in level of consciousness. The nurse must be alert for the development of new deficits or for a worsening of those present preoperatively. Cerebral edema may develop after surgery, causing a change in neurologic status.

Obviously, a patent airway is required, and mechanical hyperventilation may be necessary to reduce intracranial pressure. Management of fluids and electrolytes is very important, with a careful watch for hyponatremia, which can cause an increase in the cerebral edema. Accurate intake and output records are important.

Monitoring of vital signs is crucial. The goal is to avoid any significant change, especially in blood pressure. One must treat hypotension immediately to prevent a drop in cerebral perfusion. Cardiac dysrhythmias may be present, especially if there was bleeding into the subarachnoid space. Many dysrhythmias cause a drop in cardiac output, and consequently the cerebral perfusion falls. For this reason, dysrhythmias should be treated.

The critical care nurse may help awaken an unconscious patient by talking directly to him. However, research indicates that even in an unconscious patient, talking *about* him around the bed causes a rise in intracranial pressure. There should be no talk in the patient's presence that would not be said directly to the patient if he were awake. One cannot be sure whether an unconscious patient has an intact brain stem and is comprehending everything that is said in his environment.

Preoperative education of patient and family will make the postoperative period less stressful. Rehabilitation for specific deficits should begin early, and family participation in the rehabilatation program should be encouraged.

CEREBRAL ANEURYSMS

Pathophysiology

A major type of cerebrovascular disease in addition to stroke and AVM is cerebral aneurysm. An aneurysm is a round, saccular dilation of the arterial wall that develops as a result of weakness of the wall. Arterial vessels are composed of three layers: the endothelial lining, the smooth muscle, and the connective tissue. A defect in the smooth muscle layer allows the endothelial lining to bulge through, creating an aneurysm.

Description and Location

Some aneurysms are called "berry aneurysms" because they look like a berry, having a stem and neck. Saccular aneurysms do not have a neck but resemble a ballooning of the vessel (Fig. 28-6).

Most aneurysms arise from larger arteries around the anterior section of the circle of Willis. The most frequent site of occurrence is the juncture of the posterior communicating artery and the internal carotid artery. Other common aneurysm sites include the basilar artery, anterior cerebral artery, anterior communicating artery, and middle cerebral artery (see Fig. 28-4). Only about 15% of aneurysms occur within the vertebrobasi-

TABLE 28-4
CLASSIFICATION OF CEREBRAL ANEURYSMS

Category	Criteria
Grade I (minimal bleed)	Asymptomatic; alert with minimal headache, slight nuchal rigidity, and no neurological deficit
Grade II (mild bleed)	Alert, mild to severe headache, nuchal rigidity, minimal neurological deficit (as third nerve palsy)
Grade III (moderate bleed)	Drowsy or confused, nuchal rigidity; may have mild focal deficits
Grade IV (moderate to severe bleed)	Stupor, mild to severe hemiparesis, nuchal rigidity, possible early decerebration
Grade V (severe bleed)	Deep coma, decerebrate rigidity, moribund appearance

(From Hickey J: The Clinical Practice of Neurological and Neurosurgical Nursing, p 380. Philadelphia, JB Lippincott, 1981)

lar system. Aneurysms most often form at the bifurcation of arteries.

Because aneurysm-forming vessels usually lie in the space between the arachnoid and the brain, hemorrhage from an aneurysm usually occurs in the subarachnoid space. Sometimes, however, the force of the rupturing vessel can be so great that it pushes blood through the pia and into the brain substance, causing an intracerebral hemorrhage, or through the arachnoid into the subdural space, causing a subdural hemorrhage.

Signs and Symptoms

Many aneurysms are silent and never cause a problem but may be discovered on postmortem examination. If an aneurysm does cause problems, they will usually occur in the 35- to 60-year age group.

Before an aneurysm bleeds or ruptures, about half the patients will have some warning signs. These may include headaches, lethargy, neck pain, a "noise in the head" (a bruit), and optic, oculomotor, or trigeminal cranial nerve dysfunction.

After an aneurysm has bled or ruptured, the patient usually complains of an explosive headache. There is a decrease in the level of consciousness, cranial nerve dysfunction, visual disturbances, perhaps hemiparesis or hemiplegia, and often vomiting. All these signs are related to an increase in intracranial pressure. With a subarachnoid hemorrhage, there will be signs of meningeal irritation, such as a stiff and painful neck, photophobia, blurred vision, irritability, fever, and positive Kernig's and Brudzinski's signs. Exactly which deficits are present depends on the location of the aneurysm, the subsequent hemorrhage, and the severity of the bleeding.

The actual amount of blood loss through an aneurysm is usually quite small because of the severe vasoconstriction of vessels in the area of the aneurysm. This vasospasm may help stop the bleeding, but it can also cause ischemia to parts of the brain, resulting in localized neurologic deficits.

When there is blood in the subarachnoid space, it irritates the brain stem, causing abnormal activity in the autonomic nervous system centers, often with cardiac dysrhythmias and hypertension. Another complication of blood in the subarachnoid space is hydrocephalus. This may occur as the result of obstruction of the narrow channels through which the CSF flows (*e.g.,* the aqueduct of Sylvius) by red cells in the cerebrospinal fluid. The blood in the subarachnoid space also may impede reabsorption of the CSF from the arachnoid villi. Both these situations will cause hydrocephalus, with enlargement of the lateral and third ventricles.

Diagnosis, Classification, and Prognosis

The diagnosis of a cerebral aneurysm is usually made on the basis of the history, physical examination, lumbar puncture, cerebral arteriogram, and often a CT scan. Aneurysms are graded according to their severity. A classification system is shown in Table 28-4.

Between 20% to 40% of patients die at the time of the initial bleed of their aneurysms. Rebleeding is the leading cause of death in patients with a history of ruptured aneurysm. Of those who survive the first hemorrhage, 35% to 40% bleed again, with a mortality rate of about 42% at that time. Rebleeding most often occurs around the seventh day post original bleed.

Management

Management of a patient with a ruptured or leaking aneurysm includes bedrest in a dark environment to minimize the photophobia, often sedation, and a quiet room with minimal stimulation to reduce meningeal irritation.

Some physicians include the use of aminocaproic acid (Amicar) in their management of the patient with an aneurysm. This is an antifibrinolytic agent that delays the lysis of blood clots. At the time of hemorrhage from an aneurysm, about 10 to 20 ml of blood escapes from the vessel. Loss of 30 to 50 ml of blood would be a massive hemorrhage, and the patient would probably not survive. A blood clot normally forms over the bleeding vessel, then dissolves several days later. Aminocaproic acid may be used to prevent the breakdown of the clot over the aneurysm.

Precautions must be observed in patients receiving aminocaproic acid because there may be clot formation in other areas, such as a pulmonary embolus or a deep vein thrombosis (DVT). The patient should receive passive range of motion exercises to the legs, and thigh and calf circumference should be measured daily, 20 cm above and 20 cm below the upper patella, so that any early signs of DVT can be detected. Some physicians encourage use of elastic hose or stockings.

Stool softeners are often used in the management of the aneurysm patient to prevent straining. Mild analgesics may be used for relief of headache; acetaminophen or codeine can be used without masking neurologic signs. If hypertension is present, a drug that can control it is employed, such as hydralazine hydrochloride (Apresoline) or methyldopa (Aldomet).

Blood in the subarachnoid space will cause an elevated temperature. An antipyretic, usually acetaminophen, and hypothermia blankets are used if necessary. Steroids are controversial, but if used, dexamethasone (Decadron) is the steroid of choice. Fluids are often restricted to prevent cerebral edema.

Nursing Assessment and Intervention

Nurses caring for a patient with a subarachnoid hemorrhage should be aware of the patient's baseline neurologic status and be alert to changes. Patients are sometimes difficult to assess clinically when they are receiving sedation. A change in level of consciousness (LOC) is probably the first clinical sign that will be seen if the patient is deteriorating, unless an intracranial monitoring device is in place, in which case increasing intracranial pressure (ICP) may be recognized immediately. Size and reactivity of the patient's pupils are important to document, along with changes in motor and sensory function. Sudden appearance of a cranial nerve defect or increasing severity of headache should be reported immediately. Blurred vision and aphasia also may be present, along with other neurologic deficits.

One may intubate and hyperventilate the patient with a subarachnoid hemorrhage to keep the PCO_2 low and thus keep intracranial pressure low. Hypocarbia causes vasoconstriction of the cerebral vessels, which reduces the volume of blood flow to the head, thus reducing ICP.

Maintenance of an adequate airway is vital. If suctioning is necessary, it is important that the suction catheter go in and out quickly so that a buildup of PCO_2 is avoided and sustained coughing by the patient is prevented.

Conversation over the unconscious patient's bed should be limited to what would be said if the patient was fully awake. One can never be sure when the patient's brain stem is intact and conversation is being perceived, regardless of whether there is motor response to demonstrate this. The critical care nurse should talk to the patient about what is going to be done to or for him, even if his level of consciousness is impaired. This applies to all patients with a neurologic problem that affects the LOC.

Aneurysm Surgery

Surgical excision of the aneurysm may be considered if it is in an accessible area. Aneurysms of the vertebrobasilar system often present a problem of surgical inaccessibility. Some aneurysms may be wrapped in a gauzelike material and coated with an acrylic substance that gives the aneurysm support. There is some controversy about when to surgically intervene in an aneurysm. Some physicians believe in stabilizing the patient after the hemorrhage for 7 to 10 days. Others believe that surgery should be performed immediately following the hemorrhage. At this point, neither group is showing significantly improved results with one or the other method of treatment.

Vasospasm: A Complication

Vasospasm can occur postoperatively as well as preoperatively in the aneurysm patient. In fact, 30% to 50% of patients develop vasospasm preoperatively. Postoperatively, 65% develop vasospasm. The aneurysm may have been successfully clipped, but owing to this challenging complication, the patient may end up with a large area of ischemic or infarcted brain and severe deficits.

None of the pharmacologic attempts to control vasospasm has been very successful thus far. Papaverine hydrochloride, which has spasomolytic effect on smooth muscle and the vascular system, has been tried without much success. A regimen of aminophylline and isoproterenol (Isuprel) has been used, based on the theory that these drugs inhibit enzymes that are active in vasomotor contraction. Another hypothesis implicates elevated serotonin levels in vasospasm, so serotonin antagonists such as reserpine (Serpasil) and kanamycin (Kantrex) have been recommended by some. In the laboratory setting, nitroprusside has proved somewhat effective in relieving cerebrospasm through its relaxation of smooth muscle, but it has some limitations in the clinical setting. Currently, calcium blocking agents are being investigated for their possible use in relieving cerebral vasospasm.

The critical care nurse must be acutely aware of the possibility of vasospasm in the patient with an aneurysm. It is especially important to observe the patient for signs of deterioration in LOC, hemiparesis, visual problems, and possible seizure activity.

BIBLIOGRAPHY

Blanco K: The aphasic patient. J Neurosurg Nurs 14, No. 1:34–37, 1982

Dean JM, Rogers M: Cerebrovascular disease. In Shoemaker W, Thompson W, Holbrok P: Textbook of Critical Care, pp 961–968. Philadelphia, WB Saunders, 1984

Doolittle N: Arteriovenous malformations: The physiology, symptomatology, and nursing care. J Neurosurg Nurs 2, No. 4:221–226, 1979

Earnest M: Neurologic Emergencies. New York, Churchill-Livingstone, 1983

Hickey J: The Clinical Practice of Neurological and Neurosurgical Nursing. Philadelphia, JB Lippincott, 1981

Houston C: Hypothermia and cardiac arrest in the treatment of giant aneurysms. J Neurosurg Nurs 16, No. 1:15–22, 1984

Nicholson C: Cranial bypass — A case study. J Neurosurg Nurs 15, No. 3:136–139, 1983

Peck S: Calcium blocking agents for treatment of cerebral vasospasm. J Neurosurg Nurs 15, No. 3:123–127, 1983

Polhopek M: Stroke: An update on vascular disease. J Neurosurg Nurs 12, No. 2:81–87, 1980

Shoemaker W, Thompson WL, Holbrook P: Textbook of Critical Care. Philadelphia, WB Saunders, 1984

Snyder N, Jaekle M: Neurologic Problems, A Critical Care Nursing Focus. Bowie, MD, Robert Brady Co, 1981

Stephens G: Pathophysiology for Health Practitioners. New York, Macmillan, 1980

Stroker R: Impact of disability on families of stroke clients. J Neurosurg Nurs 15, No. 6:360–365, 1983

Seizure Disorders

A seizure is a sudden discharge of a group of neurons resulting in a transient impairment of consciousness, movement, sensation, or memory. The term *epilepsy* is usually reserved for a chronic disorder involving recurrent seizures. The term *seizure disorder* may refer to one isolated occurrence or to a recurrent situation. There seems to be less social stigma associated with the term *seizure disorder* than with *epilepsy*.

Seizures may be caused by a variety of pathological conditions, including brain tumors, trauma, blood clots, meningitis, encephalitis, electrolyte disorders, alcohol and drug overdose and withdrawal, metabolic disorders, uremia, overhydration, toxic substances, and cerebral anoxia. Some seizures are idiopathic (*i.e.,* of unknown etiology).

Between 5% and 50% of patients with head trauma develop posttraumatic seizures. When trauma is the cause, the seizures occur within 2 years of the injury in 90% of the cases. Craniotomies may leave scar tissue, which can be a future site for seizure activity.

Seizures develop in 10% to 20% of patients with strokes. Central nervous system infections result in 17% to 34% of those patients having seizures. Lesions of the brain can be produced by degenerative CNS diseases, such as multiple sclerosis, Alzheimer's disease, and Huntington's chorea, and these can be a site for seizure activity. Seizures usually are a symptom of some cerebral pathology, and not a disease entity in themselves, as is demonstrated in the following case study:

CASE STUDY

The patient, a 50-year-old business executive, had been having right-sided headaches intermittently for approximately 4 weeks. During a business luncheon, he got up from the table and walked in circles for about 5 to 6 minutes, after which he fell to the floor and lost consciousness.

At the hospital the patient had no recall of what had happened. He did recall a metalic, bitter taste in his mouth prior to the incident, along with a throbbing right-sided headache. When the patient was examined, a left hemiparesis and left visual field cut were noted. EEG demonstrated some abnormal right temporal spikes. A CT scan revealed a lesion in the same temporal lobe, which at the time of surgery proved to be a low-grade glioma.

DIAGNOSIS

An often invaluable piece of information in the diagnosis of seizure disorders is a description of the attack by an eyewitness. The patient also may be able to help in the description of the event, especially if he felt an aura prior to the attack.

A CT scan is usually part of the seizure diagnostic workup. Such pathology as tumor, edema, infarct, congenital lesion, hemorrhage, arteriovenous malformation, or ventricular enlargement can be seen on CT scan.

Skull radiographs are not usually of much help in the diagnostic workup of seizures, except perhaps to rule out a fracture. The CT scan is more inclusive.

A metabolic work-up may be useful. Tests for blood glucose, electrolytes, calcium, and hepatic and renal function are often obtained. Presence of infection may be searched for. Platelet count, sedimentation rate, and serological or immunological tests also may be ordered. A lumbar puncture may help determine presence of an infection, such as meningitis. The CSF (cerebrospinal fluid) also is examined for cells, protein, glucose, and cultures. In the presence of a central nervous system infection, there may be an elevation of WBCs and protein and a decrease in the glucose level, as compared with the serum value. Normally, the serum glucose is one-half to two-thirds the serum value.

Electroencephalography (EEG) is often beneficial in confirming the seizure diagnosis and in localizing a lesion if one exists. EEGs show neurologic function, whereas CT scans demonstrate anatomy. Most EEGs are done during a time when the patient is not actively seizing, however, so it may not be too informative unless the patient happened to be seizing during the EEG recording. Sometimes, photic stimulation and hyperventilation can provoke a generalized seizure of the absence type. These stimuli are usually included during the routine EEG recording. If a patient appears to be clinically seizing and the concurrent EEG is normal, the possibility of hysterical seizures or pseudoseizures should be considered.

A complete neurologic examination should be included in a seizure work-up. A focal finding may help one determine the origin of some seizure activity. Along with the neurologic examination, should be a history elicited. Often the history will reveal precipitating factors that may have provoked the seizure, even in usually well-controlled patients. Some common precipitating factors may be fever, injury, menses, sleep deprivation, drug use, physical exhaustion, and hyperventilation. Emotional stress from the home or work environment is also a possible precipitating factor.

TABLE 28-5
INTERNATIONAL CLASSIFICATION OF EPILEPTIC SEIZURES

I. Partial seizures
  A. Simple partial (consciousness retained)
    1. Motor
    2. Sensory
    3. Autonomic
    4. Psychic
  B. Complex partial (consciousness impaired)
    1. Simple partial, followed by impaired consciousness
    2. Consciousness impaired at onset
  C. Partial seizures with secondary generalization
II. Generalized seizures
  A. Absences
    1. Typical
    2. Atypical
  B. Generalized tonic-clonic
  C. Tonic
  D. Clonic
  E. Myoclonic
  F. Atonic
III. Unclassified Seizures

(From ILAE: Proposal for revised clinical and electroencephalographic classification of epileptic seizures. Epilepsia 22:489, 1981. New York, Raven Press. Reprinted with permission)

CLASSIFICATION

Seizures are classified according to clinical and electrographic (EEG) criteria established by the Commission on Classification and Terminology of the International League Against Epilepsy. The two main categories are generalized and focal, or partial, seizures (Table 28-5). Generalized seizures are those that show synchronous involvement of all regions of the brain in both hemispheres. Partial seizures are those that show clinical or electrographic evidence of a focal onset, involving one particular part of the brain.

Partial Seizures

There are two types of partial seizures: simple and complex. Partial seizures of either type may progress to a generalized seizure if the abnormal electrical discharges spread from the initial focus to involve the remainder of the brain.

Differentiation of the two types of partial seizures is based on whether consciousness is retained or impaired. When there is no impairment of consciousness, the attack is termed a simple partial seizure, which may be motor, sensory, autonomic, or psychic in nature, depending on the seizure focus. If the focus is in the posterior frontal lobe near the motor cortex, there will be motor involvement of the contralateral side of the body.

The old jacksonian classification is an example of a simple partial seizure with motor involvement. Clinically, there are repetitive, usually unilateral involuntary contractions of a specific muscle group, such as thumb flexors. Adjacent muscle groups are progressively affected, often until one entire side of the body is involved. In the individual patient, the seizure almost always begins in the same area and migrates in the same pattern, called the jacksonian march.

If the focus is in the anterior parietal lobe, which is involved with the sensory cortex, no clinical evidence of seizure may appear. The patient may describe sensory phenomena related to the focus in the contralateral side of the brain. Partial seizures with psychic symptoms are rare.

Complex partial seizures (also known as temporal lobe, psychomotor seizures or automatisms) often have their focus in or near the temporal lobe, although sometimes the focus is in the frontal lobe. There is always an impairment in the level of consciousness. Clinical manifestations with this type of seizure are varied, and the behavior exhibited may be quite bizarre. There may be visual, auditory, or olfactory hallucinations (*e.g.,* seeing things not really in the environment, hearing voices telling the patient to do something, or smelling an odor, such as that of brewing coffee). A bisceral sensation such as nausea, vomiting, or profuse sweating may precede the seizure.

The patient may demonstrate automatisms, or automatic behaviors, such as playing with buttons on clothing or becoming preoccupied with some other motor activity. During the seizure, the patient is usually not combative, but if he is provoked or if someone attempts to restrain him, he may become agitated and asocial. After the seizure episode, the patient has no recall of the behavior that was displayed. Such a patient may be misdiagnosed as a psychiatric problem because behaviors are often similar in both situations.

Generalized Seizures

In a generalized seizure, the entire brain is activated at once, synchronously, without a focal onset (Fig. 28-7). There is no aura or prodromal warning unless it is a partial seizure that has generalized.

Typical absence seizures, formerly called petit mal, are diagnosed by 3-second spike wave activity on EEG (*i.e.,* 3 cycles/second Hz). These seizures usually occur in children and are often outgrown by puberty.

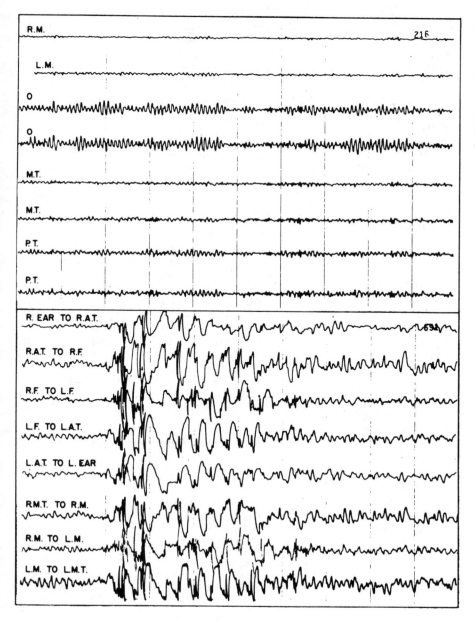

FIGURE 28-7
Contrast of a normal electroencephalogram with that of an epileptic patient during a generalized tonic-clonic seizure. Note the sharp, spiky waves recorded during the seizure. (Hickey J: The Clinical Practice of Neurologic and Neurosurgical Nursing, p 413. Philadelphia, JB Lippincott, 1981)

After puberty, the patient may not have any further seizure activity, or the type of seizure may change to a generalized type of activity.

Clinically, a typical absence seizure does not involve any violent involuntary movements or incontinence. There may be minor motor manifestations such as eye-blinking. There is a transient, often unnoticed loss of consciousness or contact with the environment. The behavior, with vacant staring, may resemble day-dreaming and is over within a few seconds. Teachers may report to parents that their child daydreams when in fact the child may be having several typical absence seizures during the day. There are no postictal symptoms.

Atypical absence seizures clinically resemble the typical absence seizures. The primary difference is demonstrated on EEG. Only the typical absence seizure demonstrated 3-second spike wave activity. Atypical absence seizures may be seen in both children and adults. There may be minor automatisms, and the patient usually has other types of seizures also, which are often refractory to medical therapy. Atypical absence seizures are frequently associated with mental retardation.

Generalized tonic-clinic seizures were, in the old classification, called grand mal, or major motor, seizures. These seizures involve a bilateral tonic extension of the extremities followed by synchronous bilateral jerking movements. There may be a cry, incontinence of stool or urine or both, tongue-biting, and foaming at the mouth. There is a sudden loss of consciousness. The seizure is followed by a postictal period, during which the patient is exhausted and extremely difficult to arouse. As the patient awakens, he may experience diffuse muscle soreness and initial confusion.

Tonic or clonic generalized seizures exhibit only one phase of the previously described tonic-clonic activity.

Myoclonic seizures are typified by synchronous, asymmetrical rapid jerking of one of more extremity, the trunk, or a specific muscle group. They may be seen with metabolic encephalopathies such as hepatic failure, with infectious processes, and with degenerative processes. There is no loss of consciousness associated with myoclonic seizures.

Atonic seizures, previously classified as "drop attacks," or akinetic seizures, are another type of generalized seizure. There is usually loss of consciousness, but the episode may be so brief that the patient is unaware of the blackout. The patient is aware of the sudden loss of muscle tone as he falls to the ground.

Unclassified Seizures

Some seizures do not fit any of the aforementioned classifications, perhaps because clinically or electro-graphically they do not meet the criteria of the established categories. Sometimes the diagnosis of a seizure disorder needs to be confirmed with observation and in-hospital monitoring, rather than on an out-patient basis.

STATUS EPILEPTICUS

Status epilepticus is a medical emergency characterized by a series of seizures without recovery of the baseline neurologic status between the seizures. Most authorities agree that clinical, or EEG, seizure activity that lasts 30 minutes or more constitutes status epilepticus. The newer classification of status epilepticus is shown in Table 28-6.

Convulsive status includes muscle twitching, generalized tonic-clinic seizures, simple partial seizures, and myoclonic seizures. The non-convulsive category includes absence seizures and complex partial seizures. An example of absence status is demonstrated in the following case study.

CASE STUDY: ABSENCE STATUS

The patient, a 12-year-old girl, was sent home from school one hot day by the school nurse. It was thought that the girl had become overheated while playing volleyball during gym class.

Her behavior was described as "weird" by her classmates all day. She had had several episodes of staring out the classroom window that morning, with a vacant look on her face. During a later class she was only intermittently responsive, answering a few questions with "yes" or "no." Her answers were somewhat delayed. Occasionally, she played with the buttons on her dress and exhibited brief periods of lip-smacking.

The patient did not recall the behavior when questioned by her mother. The girl's mother took her to a physician, where an EEG showed somewhat irregular, generalized spike waves at 3 Hz. The EEG became normal following injection of 5 mg of diazepam IV. Also, the patient immediately became more responsive.

The most serious and most common type of status epilepticus is the generalized tonic-clonic type, which is associated with a mortality rate of about 10%. One should institute medi-

---

TABLE 28-6
CLASSIFICATION OF STATUS EPILEPTICUS

I. Convulsive status
   A. Generalized tonic-clonic status
   B. Partial motor status ("epilepsia partialis continua")
II. Non-convulsive status
   A. Absence status (petit mal status)
   B. Complex partial status (psychomotor status)
   C. Partial sensory status

(From Earnest M: Neurologic Emergencies. New York, Churchill-Livingstone. [Modified from ILAE: Proposal for revised clinical and electroencephalographic classification of epileptic seizures. Epilepsia 22:489, 1981. New York, Raven Press. Reprinted with permission])

cal therapy promptly, within 30 minutes from time of onset, to prevent the brain from becoming hypoxic and depleting the metabolic substrates of the brain, which may lead to irreversible brain damage. Thus, the medical goals are to control the seizure immediately and to provide for effective long-term management.

The initial nursing goals are to monitor vital signs and to ensure that there is a patent airway. Suction and oxygen should be available. A patient with the known potential for seizure activity should have an oral airway or padded tongue blade at the bedside along with padded bedrails. Nonconvulsive status may be present with a "twilight period," during which there would be time to insert an oral airway. Intravenous access will be an immediate need when status epilepticus occurs.

Treatment

Treatment of status epilepticus usually involves the use of diazepam, phenytoin, phenobarbital, or any combination of these drugs. Diazepam, a rapid-acting drug with short duration, may stop all types of status activity immediately. Because of the rapid onset of action, it can be dose-regulated according to the effects it has. The dosage of diazepam is 5 to 20 mg, injected IV at a rate of 5 mg or less per minute while one watches for respiratory depression. Because the duration of action of diazepam is short, 10% to 50% of patients treated with this drug alone experience recurrent seizure activity.

It is recommended that diazepam be accompanied by another drug, such as phenytoin. Phenytoin provides long-term control in about 80% of the cases of status epilepticus. The dose of phenytoin is 12 to 18 mg/kg. A loading dose of 1 to 1.5 g is given to most adults. The drug should be administered at a rate of 40 to 50 mg/minute while the patient is on a cardiac monitor. If the drug is given too rapidly, there may be a widening of the QRS complexes, cardiac conduction disturbances, bradycardia, hypotension, and cardiac arrest.

Phenytoin is highly alkaline and will precipitate easily in any IV solution that contains dextrose. It should be given in normal saline or lactated Ringers solution. The onset of action is 10 to 20 minutes. When given with diazepam, which acts immediately, the phenytoin will be effective by the time the diazepam is beginning to wear off. Phenytoin is not usually effective against typical absence seizures.

One may give phenobarbital intravenously to stop status epilepticus or may administer the drug to treat seizures on a long-term basis. The dose is 5 to 8 mg/kg, and the effects are seen in 5 to 25 minutes. The rate of injection is 40 to 60 mg/minute. When phenobarbital is given along with diazepam, the respiratory depression effect of each may be compounded, so respirations should be carefully monitored.

Once the status epilepticus is under control, the etiology should be searched for because seizures are often a sign of underlying pathology and not the disease entity in itself.

DRUG MANAGEMENT OF SEIZURE DISORDERS

Drug management of any seizure activity, whether status epilepticus or other types, should be systematic (Table 28-7). Patients may be admitted to the critical care unit having received a little diazepam, some phenytoin, and some phenobarbital in the emergency department. No drug is therapeutic, and it is difficult to know how to treat the patient.

Typically a patient should be started on one drug, and it should be pushed until it reaches a therapeutic

---

TABLE 28-7
PRINCIPLES OF TREATMENT OF SEIZURES

I. Establish the diagnosis and rule out underlying cerebral pathology.
II. Classify seizure type, using clinical and EEG criteria.
III. Select AED of first choice for seizure type.
IV. Increase dose slowly till end-point is reached:
    A. Complete seizure control,
    B. Optimum plasma drug level, or
    C. Toxic side effects appear
V. If poor seizure control, gradually withdraw first drug while replacing with second drug of choice for seizure type; monotherapy is preferable to polypharmacy.
VI. If improvement is only partial, other drugs may be necessary.
VII. Adjust dose gradually according to plasma levels, keeping in mind:
    A. Pharmacokinetics of each drug
    B. Potential drug interactions
VIII. If best medical therapy is unsuccessful, refer to specialized epilepsy center for intensive monitoring and possible surgical therapy.

(From Earnest M: Neurologic Emergencies. New York, Churchill-Livingstone. [Modified after Meinardi H, Rowan AJ, (eds): Advances in Epileptology, p 211. Amsterdam, Swets and Zeitlinger, 1978, with permission])

blood level. If the patient continues to seize, a second drug should be added to the regimen until it is at therapuetic levels and so on until the seizures are controlled.

Different types of seizures respond better to specific drugs. Partial seizures (simple or complex) and generalized seizures of the tonic-clonic type respond to carbamazepine, phenytoin, primidone, and phenobarbital. Some studies suggest that valproate, chlorazepate, clonazepam, and methsuximide are useful in some refractory cases of complex partial seizures.

Ethosuximide is the drug of choice for simple absences, and phenobarbital usually is the second choice. Valproate or clonazepam is useful in atypical absences, atonic seizures, and myoclonic seizures. Myoclonic seizures may be treated with ACTH or a ketogenic diet or both.

Therapeutic blood levels should be checked periodically. Drug screens can identify patients who are not compliant with their treatment, those who may metabolize the drugs at different rates, or those who are not absorbing it. It is generally agreed that most anticonvulsive drugs may be taken once or twice daily, and still maintain therapeutic levels, because of the long halflife of these drugs.

RHABDOMYOLYSIS AND MYOGLOBINURIA

Myoglobin is an iron-containing pigment found in skeletal muscle, especially in those specialized for sustained contraction. There is muscle damage with seizure activity, as with many other activities. Severe exercise, such as jogging, performing military calisthenics, marathon running, and riding mechanical bulls, can cause the same type of muscle breakdown. Patients who are found after lying unconscious for a period of time, those who present with amphetamines or heroin overdoses (with the accompanying shaking chills), and those who demonstrate phencyclidine (PCP, angel dust) abuse when there is unusual muscular hyperactivity may develop profound rhabdomyolysis.

The protein from the destroyed tissue turns the patient's urine red or cola-colored. The muscle cell breakdown releases myoglobin into the bloodstream, which is rapidly filtered by the kidneys, producing the dark red or brown urine. The myoglobin can occlude the kidneys, and renal failure may result. The critical care nurse may be the first to recognize the signs of this serious complication.

Treatment or rhabdomyolysis involves flushing the kidneys. Extensive skeletal muscle necrosis may be associated with massive loss of arterial volume into necrotic muscle and subsequent shock. The large volume replacement necessary for these patients approximates that seen in extensively burned patients. Furosemide or mannitol or both are sometimes used for diuresis, along with volume replacement. The hyperkalemia due to the cellular breakdown and renal dysfunction may also require treatment.

NURSING ASSESSMENT

The critical care nurse who witnesses an actual seizure can help the physician diagnose the type of seizure and localize the focus. A specific description of the seizure should include the following:

Onset. The nurse should determine whether the seizure had a sudden onset or whether it was preceded by a warning aura.

Duration. Timing of the seizure from onset to end is important. What was the frequency of seizures?

Motor Activity. The nurse should note the parts of the body involved and determine whether both left and right sides were involved. In what part of the body did the seizure begin, and how did it progress? Was rigidity, jerking, or twitching observed?

Eyes and Tongue. The nurse should notice whether there was any deviation of the eyes or tongue to one side or the other.

State of Consciousness. Arousability is important. Was the patient arousable during the seizure or immediately after it? If there was unconsciousness, the duration of that period should be timed. Was there confusion or awareness and clear memory of the event after the seizure?

Distractability. The nurse should determine whether the patient responds to the environment during the seizure, such as when his name is called. Some patients, often drug abusers, may try to feign seizures, which will be revealed when they respond to their names.

Pupils. The nurse should note any change in size, shape, or equality of the pupils and their reaction to light or any deviation to one side.

Teeth. The nurse should observe whether the teeth were clenched or open.

Respirations. The rate, quality, or absence of respiration and the presence of cyanosis should be observed.

TABLE 28-8
OBSERVATIONS OF A SEIZURE

Parameter	Observations
Time	1. Length of entire seizure
	2. Length of various phases
Movement	3. Part of body affected first
	4. Progression of movement to other parts
	5. Type of movement (spastic, clonic, tremors)
	6. Movement of eyes to one side
	7. Movement after seizure (flaccid?)
Respiratory status	8. Apnea (duration)
	9. Cyanosis
	10. Secretions (amount, color, need for suctioning)
Level of consciousness	11. Loss of consciousness or decrease in level of consciousness and duration
	12. Changes in postictal period
Pupils	13. Size
	14. Change in reactivity
Behavior	15. Automatisms
	16. Bizarre behavior
	17. Behavior in postictal period
Elimination	18. Incontinence (urine or stool)
Mouth condition	19. Postictal condition of tongue and mucous membranes (note bloody sputum)

(From DeYoung: The Neurologic Patient: A Nursing Perspective, p 168. Englewood Cliffs, NJ, Prentice-Hall, 1983)

Body Activities. Incontinence, vomiting, salivation, bleeding from the mouth or tongue should be reported.

After the Seizure. Sometimes after a seizure there can be a transient paralysis, weakness, numbness, tingling, aphasia, other injuries, a postictal period, or amnesia regarding the seizure and events prior to and following it.

Precipitating Factors. By talking to the patient, the nurse may uncover a precipitating factor. Fever, emotional or physical stresss, and anticonvulsant noncompliance all may precipitate a seizure.

Observational Guidlines

An example of one observational guide is shown in Table 28-8. The purpose of the guide is to standardize the process of observation and the recording of data.

Seizure activity charts are very helpful for describing seizures of hospitalized patients. An example is shown in Fig. 28-8.

If a nurse encounters a patient who is seizing, she should stay with him and protect him from his environment. A seizing patient should never be restrained. Any tight or restrictive clothing can be loosened. If the patient already has his teeth clamped, the nurse should not attempt to insert an oral airway or tongue blade because such action may break off teeth, which the

patient may aspirate. A patent airway should be maintained during the seizure. It may help to turn the patient on his side to prevent aspiration. The nurse should reassure and reorient the patient if the seizure has left him disoriented and frightened.

PSEUDOSEIZURES

Pseudoseizures are psychologically based. They have no associated abnormal discharges from the brain. They may closely resemble epileptic seizures, thus making the diagnosis difficult. Some patients may have both disorders present, pseudoseizures and a real seizure disorder.

Pseudoseizures are frequent in children and adolescents (the mean age range is 18.5 to 27.5 years), and the incidence is twice as high in women as in men. The onset of a pseudoseizure may be gradual or sudden, and it is usually longer than an epileptic seizure. Pseudoseizures occur more often around witnesses. Environmental influences can affect the course of a pseudoseizure and may precipitate it. Patients may follow commands and focus their eye contact on a witness. When one woman was asked if she would allow her seizure to be filmed, she immediately began seizing. The investigator asked her to wait until he got his camera, and she stopped the seizure immediately.

There is abnormal motor activity with pseudosei-

SEIZURE ACTIVITY SHEET

Patient's Name _____

Room No. _____ Age _____

Physician _____

Date	Time	Before		During								After				Nurse's Initials
		Warning Signs	Part of Body Where Seizure Began	General or Localized	Type of Movement	Duration of each Phase		Level of Consciousness	Pupils	Other	Behavior	Paralysis	Location of Paralysis	Sleep	
						Tonic	Clonic								

FIGURE 28-8
An example of a seizure activity chart. (Hickey J: The Clinical Practice of Neurological and Neurosurgical Nursing, p 427. Philadelphia, JB Lippincott, 1981)

zures. One unusual type is opisthotonus, in which the head and legs are bent backward and the trunk arches forward. The protective mechanisms we have to prevent us from harming ourselves, such as breaking a fall with our arms and protecting our head from hitting the ground, are present in patients who have pseudoseizures but not in those who have real seizures.

With pseudoseizures, there is no tongue-biting, incontinence, or dilated pupils, the corneal reflex is present, and there is response to painful stimulation. Confusion after the pseudoseizure is usually absent.

Table 28-9 distinguishes epileptic seizures from pseudoseizures.

Because the nurse spends more time with a patient than most other personnel do, it is important that she develop skills in differentiating pseudoseizures from true seizures through clinical observations. Once the patient is diagnosed, the nurse should be aware of the stigma that family and society may associate with his condition. The nurse can help by promoting use of the more objective term *pseudoseizure* rather than the judgmental term *hysterical seizure,* which some people use to describe the condition.

The treatment plan usually involves the use of psychotherapy. Hypnosis also has been a helpful intervention, especially in determining the precipitating cause of the pseudoseizure. Often, the cause can be abolished by hypnotic suggestion.

TABLE 28-9
CRITERIA FOR DISTINGUISHING EPILEPTIC SEIZURES FROM PSEUDOSEIZURES

Description	Epileptic	Pseudoseizure
Apparent cause	Absent	Emotional disturbance
Warning	Varies, but more commonly unilateral or epigastric aura	Palpitation, malaise, choking, bilateral foot aura
Onset	Commonly sudden	Often gradual
Scream	At onset	During course
Convulsion	Rigidity followed by "jerking"; rarely rigidity alone	Rigidity or "struggling"; throwing limbs and head about
Biting	Tongue	Lips, hands, or more often other people and things
Micturation	Frequent	Never
Defecation	Occasional	Never
Duration	A few minutes	Often half an hour or several hours
Restraint needed	To prevent self-injury	To control violence
Termination	Spontaneous	Spontaneous or artificially induced (water, etc.)

(From Konikow N: Hysterical seizures or pseudoseizures. J Neurosurg Nurs 15, No. 1:22–26, 1983)

PSYCHOLOGICAL IMPLICATIONS

The psychological reaction of a patient with a known seizure disorder is varied. One response to the feelings of dependency and loss of self-esteem that seizures may precipitate is social withdrawal. This may seem to the patient to be an adequate coping mechanism, but it can foster feelings of depression.

People with long histories of seizures may develop personality disorders. They may be manipulative, hostile, and aggressive. Children may demonstrate personality disorders through temper tantrums, hyperactivity, or antisocial behavior. The reaction of others to people with seizure disorders must be one of acceptance and support. Therapeutic interaction can help the patient achieve resocialization.

Denial is another psychological coping mechanism that may be displayed by patient or family. If the interval between seizures is long, this mechanism is easier to use. When a patient uses denial, there may be concurrent noncompliance with medical therapy.

Often family members, especially parents, feel guilty about the seizure disorder. This can result in overprotection and prevent the person from developing independence. Conversely, the person with the seizure disorder may become the scapegoat for the family, and all the family troubles may be attributed to him.

Epilepsy has had a negative connotation throughout history. At one time it was thought that people with "fits" were controlled by evil spirits. Insanity and mental deficiency also have been linked with this disorder.

Today, although people are better informed, many still avoid a person with epilepsy. A seizure is viewed as a form of deviant behavior and can be very frightening to onlookers because of the unexpectedness and unpredictability of the episodes. Much of the social stigma of seizures could be alleviated by improvement of society's understanding of the problem. Public education is very important because general reaction to the disorder can influence how a person copes with his disorder.

BIBLIOGRAPHY

Earnest MP: Neurologic Emergencies. New York, Churchill-Livingstone, 1983

Hawken M: Seizures: Etiology, classification, intervention. J Neurosurg Nurs 2, No. 3:166–170, 1979

Hickey J: The Clinical Practice of Neurological and Neurosurgical Nursing. Philadelphia, JB Lippincott, 1981

Konikow N: Hysterical seizures or pseudoseizures. J Neurosurg Nurs 15, No. 1:22–26, 1983

Lovely, M: Identification and treatment of status epilepticus. J Neurosurg Nurs 12, No. 2:93–96, 1980

Ozuna J: Psychosocial aspects of epilepsy. J Neurosurg Nurs 2, No. 4:242–246, 1979

Woodward E: The total patient: Implications for nursing care of the epileptic. J Neurosurg Nurs 14, No. 4:166–169, 1982

Unit Five

Metabolic System: Gastrointestinal and Endocrine Systems

29
Normal Structure and Function of the Gastrointestinal System

Barbara Brockway-Fuller

Body cells require nutrients (fats, carbohydrates, and minerals) in order that they may obtain the energy that they require to fuel their normal operations and the materials that they need to synthesize cell structures, systems, and products. Most nutrients are present in the environment in forms that cannot enter the bloodstream to reach tissue cells (*e.g.,* complex large molecules). The functions of the digestive system are to receive these nutrients, to break them down into molecules that are small enough to reach and enter the bloodstream (digestion), and to enable these molecules to enter the bloodstream (absorption) so that they can be delivered to all tissues. Accessory operations include the movement of ingested food along the digestive system, the recycling of materials utilized in digestion (colonic reabsorption of water, bicarbonate, potassium, bile salts, etc.), and the elimination of the undigested food residue from the body (defecation).

STRUCTURE

Macrostructure

Alimentary Canal. The general structure of the digestive system is shown in Figure 29–1. It is composed of the alimentary canal (a tube about 8m [25 feet] long that begins at the oral cavity and ends at the anus) and the accessory glands (salivary) and organs (liver and pancreas) that empty their products into this tube at certain points.

The oral cavity opens into the pharynx, a structure that allows the passage of both nutrients and air. The anterior pharynx is divided into an oropharynx and nasopharynx, connecting to the oral and nasal cavities,

respectively. The posteroinferior end of the pharynx (at about the level of the sixth cervical vertebrae) connects to the esophagus and larynx. A thin cartilaginous flap covered by soft tissue reflexly covers the larynx during swallowing and the passage of food and water to the esophagus.

The esophagus is a 25-cm (10-inch) tube that leads to the stomach. The walls of the upper third of this tube are composed of skeletal muscle, as are the walls of the mouth and pharynx. The remaining esophageal walls contain smooth muscle, as does the remainder of the alimentary canal until the external anal sphincter, which again is composed of skeletal muscle. The lower esophageal sphincter (LES), which is the muscle between the stomach and esophagus, is thickened and has more tonus than other esophageal muscle, and it prevents reflux of gastric contents up into the esophagus. The other end of the stomach opens into the small intestine. This opening is surrounded by the pyloric sphincter, a structure that minimizes intestinal reflux. The first 25 to 30 cm (10 to 12 inches) of the small intestine is called the duodenum. The next 2 to 2.5m (7 to 8 feet) is the jejunum, and the remaining 3 to 3.6m (10 to 12 feet) consists of the ileum. The opening of the terminal ileum into the first part of the colon (cecum) is guarded by the ileocecal valve, which prevents reflux of colonic contents back into the ileum. Protruding inferiorly from the cecum is a blind-ended 2.5- to 20-cm (1 to 8 inch) tube called the vermiform appendix. The ascending colon extends superiorly from the cecum to a point just inferior to the lower border of the liver. The colon then flexes transversely and crosses to the left side of the abdominal cavity to a point just inferior to the stomach, where it curves again

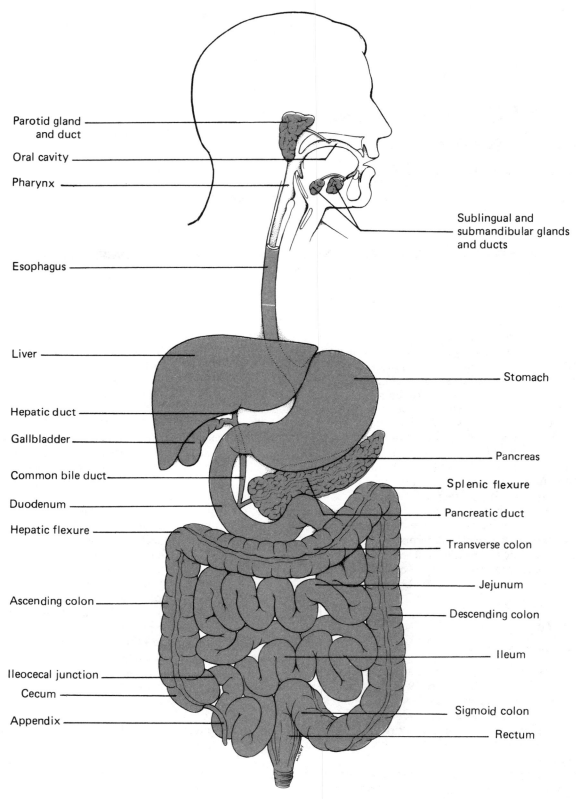

FIGURE 29-1
Diagram of the digestive tract.

to become the descending colon. This part of the colon passes down on the left side of the abdomen to the level of the iliac crest, where it becomes the sigmoid colon. This S-shaped portion of colon bends first toward the right side of the abdomen, but almost immediately it sharply bends posteriorly and upward toward the sacrum. Just as abruptly it curves anteriorly again, completing its S shape, and then continues downward to the pelvic floor as the rectum. The last 2.5 cm (1 inch) or so of the rectum, the anal canal, passes between the levator and muscles of the pelvic floor and opens to the exterior body surface as the anal orifice. Two sphincters guard this orifice: an internal one composed of smooth muscle and an external one composed of skeletal muscle.

Pancreas. This organ contains both exocrine tissue and endocrine tissue. The latter constitutes the islets of Langerhans, which will be discussed in a later endocrine metabolic section. The exocrine (acinar) cells are arranged in lobules and empty their secretions into an internal pancreatic ductal system (Fig. 29-2). These internal ducts drain into an external pancreatic duct (duct of Wirsung) that joins the common bile duct to form a shared short duct called the ampulla of Vater. This ampulla, carrying both bile and pancreatic secretions, opens into the duodenum. It is encircled by a smooth muscle ring, the sphincter of Oddi. Because of the anatomical arrangements between the common bile duct and the duct of Wirsung, a gallstone

that obstructs the ampulla of Vater can obstruct both the normal flow of bile and pancreatic secretions. (Such obstruction, although rare, can lead to a stasis of pancreatic secretion resulting in acute pancreatitis.) Some persons have a second external pancreatic duct (duct of Santorni) that opens into the duodenum near the pylorus.

Innervation. The gastrointestinal tract is supplied with both somatic motor and autonomic motor fibers. The former innervate the skeletal muscles of the oropharyngeal cavity, the first few centimeters of the esophagus, and the external anal sphincter. This enables voluntary control of such activities as chewing, initiation of swallowing, and defecation. Autonomic fibers supply the remainder of the digestive system, including salivary glands, pancreas, and liver (Fig. 29-3).

Autonomic fibers function in the regulation of (1) the secretions from the exocrine cells of the salivary glands, pancreas, stomach, and intestines; (2) tonicity of sphincter muscles; and (3) motility of the gastrointestinal tract in general. The operations are not usually voluntary controlled, although they may be reflexly altered by pschosocial factors operating under the neuronal influence of higher brain centers. Thus, fear can decrease the volume and increase the viscosity of salivary gland secretions, resulting in the sensation of a dry mouth. Merely the sight or smell of a meal may trigger gastric secretions. Emotions may increase or

FIGURE 29-2
Liver and biliary system, showing connections of the ducts of the liver, gallbladder, and pancreas.

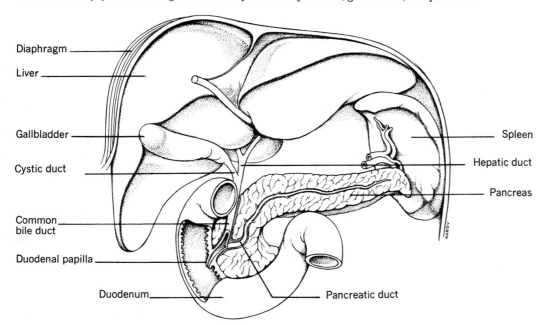

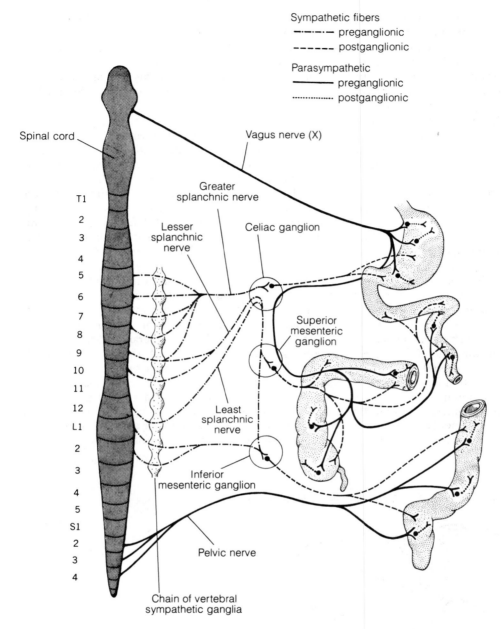

FIGURE 29-3
Diagram showing the autonomic innervation of the gastrointestinal tract. (Drawing by Edith Tagrin, reproduced from Human Design by William S. Beck, © 1971 by Harcourt Brace Jovanovich, Inc. by permission of the publisher.)

decrease gastrointestinal mobility, thereby promoting diarrhea or constipation.

Note that in Figure 29–4, most parts of the gastrointestinal tract receive both sympathetic and parasympathetic fibers. In general, these two types of autonomic fibers have contrasting influences. Sympathetic stimulation results in decreased motility, increased sphincter tonicity (closure), and decreased exocrine secretions. Parasympathetic stimulation results in increased motility, opening of sphincter, and increased exocrine secretions. Note also that in Figure 29–4 a *cranial* nerve (vagus) carries parasympathetic fibers to most of the gastrointestinal tract.

Circulation. The upper esophagus receives blood from the esophageal artery branching from the tho-

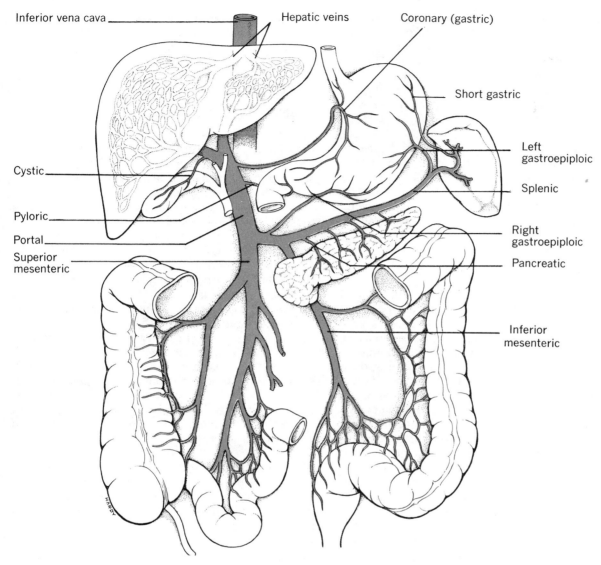

FIGURE 29-4
The portal circulation. Blood from the gastrointestinal tract, spleen, and pancreas travels to the liver by way of the portal vein before moving into the vena cava for return to the heart. (Chaffee EE, Lytle IM: Basic Physiology and Anatomy, 4th ed. Philadelphia, JB Lippincott, 1980)

racic aorta. The celiac artery, branching from the abdominal aorta, supplies blood to the lower esophagus, stomach, duodenum, gallbladder, and pancreas. The next aortic branch, the superior mesenteric, supplies blood to the intestine from the jejuneum to the transverse colon. The next branch from the abdominal aorta, the inferior mesenteric artery, supplies blood to the descending and sigmoid colon and rectum.

Venous drainage of the majority of the gastrointestinal tract is illustrated in Figure 29–4. Two points bear mention. First, all blood from the alimentary canal from the stomach to and including the inner portion of the rectum drains into the hepatic portal vein. This blood contains all absorbed nutrients, reabsorbed water, electrolytes, and bile salts and any products from commensal colonic bacteria. Thus, this material from the gastrointestinal tract is subject to "hepatic processing" before being mixed with blood in the general circulation. This hepatic processing removes potentially harmful materials before they can reach the rest of the body. For example, ammonia produced by the protein catabolizing action of colonic bacteria can be hepatically removed, thereby preventing ammonium encephalopathy. The second important point is that blood from the lower two thirds of the rectum bypasses the hepatic portal system, instead draining via the middle and inferior rectal veins and the external iliac vein into the inferior vena cava. Similarly, although not illustrated here, blood from the lower esophagus is drained via the hemizygous and azygous veins directly into the inferior vena cava. In the event of hepatic portal hypertension (*e.g.,* cirrhosis of the liver), collateral channels develop in both the esophagus and the rectum between veins that drain into the hepatic portal vein and veins that drain into the systemic circulation. Such collaterals can then provide an increased shunting of blood directly from the gastrointestinal tract into the general circulation. Pressure increases in these collaterals also cause esophageal and rectal varices.

Microstructure

The alimentary tract is basically composed of a central hollow tube, the lumen, through which food passes. It is surrounded by five layers of tissue. Proceeding from the lumen outward, they are the mucosa, submucosa, circular smooth muscle, longitudinal smooth muscle, and serosa. The mucosal layer contains cells responsible for gastrointestinal secretions and those sensitive to chemical and mechanical stimuli. In parts of the gastrointestinal tract in which absorption occurs, this layer is more convoluted or possesses finger-like projections (villi). Such structural modifications increase the surface area per unit volume, thereby facilitating absorption. The submucosa contains blood vessels, nerve network, and areolar connective tissue. In the process of absorption, molecules in the lumen of the gastrointestinal tract must pass through the mucosa and connective tissue before entering the capillaries of the submucosa. The two smooth muscle layers function in the two major types of gastrointestinal motility: propulsive motion and blood-mixing movements. The stomach has an additional layer of smooth muscle to facilitate its food-mixing movements. The outer serosa layer is continuous with the mesenteries and forms part of the visceral peritoneum.

There are two nerve networks that extend the length of the gastrointestinal tract: the submucosal plexus and the myenteric plexus (located between the two smooth muscle layers). The submucosal network is composed of neurons that receive stimulation from the sensory cells in the mucosal layer. The myenteric plexus is a network of motor neurons that stimulate the smooth muscles of the gastrointestinal tract. It receives sensory input from the submucosal plexus. Together, these two plexes function in locally coordinated regulation of gastrointestinal motility (*e.g.,* peristalsis) and secretion (*e.g.,* certain gastric secre-

tions). These networks are often called "intrinsic" because their operations can proceed even if extrinsic nerves to the gut are severed.

FUNCTIONS

Oropharyngeal Cavity

Secretions. The majority of saliva is produced by three pairs of salivary glands: submaxillary, sublingual, and parotid. Saliva is composed of mucus, which serves primarily as a lubricant to facilitate swallowing, and salivary amylase, a starch-digesting enzyme. Stimuli eliciting salivation include sight, smell, and thoughts of food as well as a pleasant taste and smooth texture of food in the mouth. (Rough, bad-tasting, unpleasant-smelling foods reduce salivary gland secretion.) These stimuli activate the two salivary centers in the medulla of the brain stem. These centers then send "autonomic motor impulses" to the salivary glands via the seventh and ninth cranial nerves (parasympathetic fibers) and branches from the first and second thoracic nerves (sympathetic fibers). Parasympathetic stimulation or the administration of drugs that mimic such stimulation (cholinergics) or enhance it (neostigmine) will promote a copious secretion of watery saliva. Sympathetic stimulation or sympathomimetic drug administration will produce a scanty output of thick saliva. Cholinergic blockers (*e.g.,* atropine) also will produce scanty salivation.

Motility. Food in the mouth is initially subject to mechanical breakdown by the act of chewing. This produces a bolus of food held together and lubricated by saliva that then can be swallowed. Swallowing has two phases: (1) an initial voluntary phase, described here and including the first third of the esophagus, and (2) an involuntary phase described under the discussion of the esophagus.

Swallowing is triggered by the presence of food or fluid in the pharynx. This presence mechanically stimulates pharyngeal sensory receptors that cause impulses to be sent along sensory fibers in the fifth cranial nerve to the swallowing center in the medulla. The arrangement of neurons in this center is such that the arrival of "sensory impulses" reflexly triggers the outflow of impulses down motor fibers in the ninth and tenth cranial nerves to pharyngeal and laryngeal structures. This causes the following coordinated events, which propel the solid or fluid substance into the esophagus: (1) pull of the soft palate upward to seal off the nasopharyngeal area; (2) closure of the epiglottis down over the opening into the larynx; (3) relaxation of the muscles of the upper esophagus; and (4) contraction of pharyngeal muscles, which moves

TABLE 29-1 FACTORS INFLUENCING LOWER ESOPHAGEAL SPHINCTER (LES)* TONUS	
Increased Tonus	*Decreased Tonus*
Gastrin	Secretin
Proteins in chyme	CCK-PZ
Prostaglandin F_2	Glucagon
Moclepramide	Fats in chyme
	Nicotine
	Alcohol
	Prostaglandins E, E_2, A_2
	Anticholinergic drugs

*The LES is a modified portion of esophagus, not a true sphincter *per se.* Thus, its autonomic stimuli alter the motility and normal tone of the smooth muscles in the wall of the gastrointestinal tract.

the food or fluid into the opened esophagus. Damage to sensory or motor fibers (in cranial nerves 5, 9, or 10) or to the swallowing center in the brain stem may weaken or eliminate the ability to swallow or produce malcoordinated swallowing wherein food or fluid enters the nasopharynax or larynx or both.

Esophagus

Secretions. Cells of the mucosal layers in the esophagus secrete only mucus. This protects the esophageal lining from damage by gastric secretions or food substances and acts as a lubricant, thus facilitating the passage of food.

Motility. Once food or fluid enter the esophagus, it continues to still be propelled through the first third of the lumen by reflexes involving the swallowing center and the ninth and tenth cranial nerves. In these reflexes, food or fluid stimulates pressure or stretch receptors in the wall of the esophagus. Stimulation of these receptors causes impulses to be conducted along sensory fibers to the swallowing center. Reflex output from the swallowing center, or muscle (down motor fibers in the ninth and tenth cranial nerves) produces a pattern of esophageal relaxation ahead of the food or fluid and esophageal muscle contraction behind it, thereby propelling the matter being swallowed through this first part of the esophagus.

In contrast, propulsion of food or fluid along the remainder of the esophagus is accomplished by local reflexes involving sensory receptors and the two nerve plexes in the wall of the esophagus. This process, peristalsis, occurs as follows: Food or fluid distends the esophageal area. This distention stimulates stretch receptors that reflexly (by the two plexes) promote both

relaxation of the esophageal muscles ahead of the area of distention and contraction of the esophageal muscles in and behind it. This squeezes the food or fluid ahead into the newly relaxed area, which then becomes the distended one. Thus, the peristalsis reflex repeatedly recurs until the food or fluid arrives at the lower esophageal sphincter (LES). The LES is the last centimeter ($\frac{1}{2}$ inch) or so of the esophagus whose smooth muscles remain normally in a contracted state. This prevents the reflux of gastric contents in the esophagus and subsequent damage to the esophageal lining by gastric acid and enzymes. The wave of peristalsis causes the LES to relax, thereby allowing food to enter the stomach. Tonus of the LES can be altered by a variety of agents (Table 29-1). Thus, some people may suffer from a hypertensive LES that impedes esophageal emptying (which could lead to overdistention of the lower esophagus), whereas others have a hypertensive LES that results in repeated episodes of gastric reflux (which may lead to lower esophageal strictions).

Stomach

Secretions. In addition to mucus-secreting cells, three types of secretory cells are contained in the gastric mucosa: parietal cells, which secrete hydrochloric acid (HCl) and intrinsic factor; chief cells, which secrete digestive enzymes; and G cells (in antrum only), which secrete the hormone gastrin. The luminal surface membranes of the gastric mucosal cells and their tight fit against one another provide a protective barrier against damage caused by the HCl. This barrier can be disrupted by a variety of agents, including bile salts, alcohol, aspirin, and steroids.

The digestive enzymes are secreted as an inactive precursor, pepsinogen, which is activated by HCl in the gastric lumen to provide three pepsins that digest the ingested proteins. The chemical action of HCl also breaks down food molecules. Intrinsic factor is necessary for the intestinal absorption of vitamin B_{12}. Gastrin stimulates secretion by the chief and parietal cells and promotes the growth of the gastric mucosa.

Three classes of factors operate by neural or hormonal means to regulate gastric secretions. These factors are cephalic, gastric, and intestinal. In the cephalic phase, sight, smell, and thoughts of food—as well as the presence of food in the mouth—act on brain stem centers, reflexly prompting parasympathetic (vagal) stimulation of gastric secretions by the chief and parietal cells. Although G cells also are innervated by vagal fibers, such parasympathetic influences are not important in the regulation of human gastrin secretion. The stomach also receives sympathetic innervation. Such neural pathways provide the mechanisms whereby emotions may influence gastric secretions. Fear and depression seem to decrease gastric secretions, whereas anger and hostility increase them.

The gastric phase refers to the stimulation of gastric secretions by the presence of food (chyme) in the stomach. Distention of the stomach wall by the food stimulates stretch receptors in the wall of the stomach. Chemicals, mainly proteins, in the chyme stimulate chemoreceptors in the mucosa. Both types of receptors in turn activate neurons in the submucosal plexus, which then stimulate neurons in the myenteric plexus, which in turn stimulate secretion by the parietal and chief cells. Proteins in the chyme promote gastrin secretion, which provides an additional stimuli for parietal and chief cell secretion. These secretions are eventually halted by a combination of events. The stretch receptors and chemoreceptors in the wall of the stomach become refractory to stimulation, and the acidity of the chyme inhibits further gastrin secretion.

Events in the intestinal phase further inhibit gastric secretions. This phase begins when the chyme reaches the duodenum. The fats, carbohydrates, and HCl in the chyme stimulate certain intestinal mucosal cells to secrete the hormones GIP and CCK-PZ. These hormones (discussed further on) inhibit secretions by the parietal and chief cells. Removal of a part of the duodenum that secretes these hormones leads to gastric hypersecretion.

Histamine is a strong stimulus for gastric HCl secretion. The gastric mucosa possess H_2 histamine receptors. Although the exact sites of these receptors are not currently known, evidence suggests that hormonal and possibly neural factors that promote HCl secretion do so via histamine. H_2 receptor blockers (*e.g.,* cimetidine) are known to reduce gastric acid secretion markedly. Another drug, omeprazole, inhibits an intracellular step in the HCl secretion process in parietal cells. If approved for used by the FDA, it will be valuable in treating patients who are unresponsive to H_2 blockers. Other factors that stimulate gastric secretions are alcohol, caffeine, and hypoglycemia. The first two factors act directly via gastric chemoreceptors and the intramural nerve plexes in the stomach wall. Hypoglycemia acts by way of the brain stem and vagal fibers.

Motility. The passage of food from the esophagus into the stomach reflexly initiates receptive relaxation. After the stomach has thereby filled with food, peristaltic contractions mix the food and repeatedly squirt small amounts of it at a controlled rate into the duodenum. The pyloric sphincter plays only a minor role in gastric emptying. Its main function is to prevent duodenal reflux. Mild peristaltic contractions that persist after the stomach has completely emptied are called hunger contractions. They play no obligatory role in appetite regulation.

Gastric emptying can be retarded by vagotomy or by factors stemming from current "unreadiness" of the duodenum to receive additional gastric chyme. Among these are fats, proteins, or HCl in the duodenal chyme; duodenal distention; and CCK-PZ and GIP hormones.

Pancreas

Secretions. The exocrine acinar cells secrete both a watery alkaline (sodium bicarbonate and potassium bicarbonate) and digestive enzymes. They enter the duodenum by way of the sphincter of Oddi. The bicarbonate neutralizes the highly acidic chyme just recently arrived in the duodenum from the stomach. The pancreatic enzymes digest proteins (trypsin, chymotrypsin, elastase, and carboxypeptidase), fats (lipase and esterase), nucleic acids (nucleases), and starch (amylase). These are secreted from the pancreas in inactive forms. Once the pancreatic secretions arrive in the duodenum, inactive trypsin is activated by an intestinal mucosal enzyme, enterokinase. Active trypsin then activates the other pancreatic enzymes. Regulation of pancreatic secretion occurs by both neural and hormonal means. Vagal stimulation causes the secretion of an enzyme-rich pancreatic juice. Hormonal regulation will be discussed later.

Small Intestine

Secretions. Chyme in the duodenum is mixed with thick alkaline mucus and digestive enzymes secreted by the intestinal mucosal cells and pancreas and bile from the liver. Intestinal enzymes digest nucleic acids and complete the protein and carbohydrate digestion begun by the other enzymes. They break disaccharides into monosaccharides (maltose, lactose and sucrase) and polypeptides into amino acids (peptidases).

Intestinal lactose levels are high at birth. In most Western European populations and in a few African tribes, these levels remain high throughout life. In other populations, the lactose levels of most people fall in childhood and remain low or negligible throughout life. This causes lactose intolerance in these persons. It is estimated that 70% of blacks and 20% of whites in the United States are lactose-intolerant. Deficiency of this or any other intestinal enzyme that digests disaccharides can lead to diarrhea, bloating, and flatulence following ingestion of sugars.

Enzyme, bicarbonate, and bile secretions are regulated primarily by chemical factors, specifically hormones. Neural influences play less of a role. Food, which stimulates intestinal stretch or chemoreceptors, is thought to initiate local reflex areas involving the two intramural plexes. This results in the secretion of mucus and enzymes from the intestinal mucosa. Pancreatic enzyme secretions and the outflow of bile from the gallbladder are triggered by the hormone CCK-PZ. This is secreted by cells of the intestinal mucosa in response to acid and partially digested proteins and fats in duodenal chyme. Alkaline secretions from the pancreas are triggered by the hormone secretin. This is produced by intestinal mucosal cells in response to acid in duodenal chyme. The actions of both enzyme and alkaline pancreatic secretions eventually eliminate the stimuli for the secretion of the CCK-PZ and secretin. Reduction in the secretion of secretin and CCK-PZ in turn reduces the stimulus for pancreatic secretions. They gradually cease until another meal or fresh gastric chyme enters the duodenum.

Other hormones (*e.g.,* vasoactive intestinal peptide, bombesin, somatostatin, and substance P) and endorphins also are produced by the small intestine. Because their role in normal human digestion is unclear, they will not be discussed.

Motility. The small intestine has two types of movement: mixing and peristaltic contraction. The intramural plexes are primarily responsible for these movements, but they may be enhanced or retarded by extrinsic autonomic stiumulation, as discussed previously. Peristalsis operates here, just as it did in the esophagus and stomach, to propel food along. During mixing movement, intestinal distention provokes (via the intramural reflex arcs) constrictions at intervals along its length. This makes the distended area resemble links of sausage. These constrictions then relax, and new areas become constricted. Repetition of this process continually kneads the chyme, thereby eventually exposing all molecules of this material to the absorptive surfaces of the intestinal mucosa.

Emptying of the small intestine into the colon occurs in the same way as gastric emptying does. Peristaltic waves build up pressure in the ileum behind the ileocecal valve and push the chyme through the valve into the colon. The valve then acts to prevent backflow. Ileal emptying can be retarded by intramural reflexes, which are initiated by a full (distended) colon.

Absorption. The mucosal layer of the small intestine has many folds covered with many finger-like projections (villi). The luminal surface of each villa is covered with microvilli. These vastly increase the absorptive area of the small intestine.

Fluid, digestive end products, vitamins, bile salts, and secretions from mouth, stomach, pancreas, and intestines are absorbed in the small intestine. Both active transport and passive diffusion processes are involved. Some products of fat digestion enter the lymphatics in the submucosa. The remainder of these products and all other absorbed materials enter the

hepatic portal circulation through submucosal capillaries. Bile and pancreatic bicarbonate are recycled for reuse. By reducing transit time, diarrhea can decrease bicarbonate reabsorption, thereby predisposing a patient to acidosis. Fat-soluble vitamines (A, D, E, and K) require bile salts to facilitate their absorption. Gastric HCl helps dissolve iron and convert it to an absorbable (ferrous) form. Absorption occurs by active transport in the upper half of the small intestine. Iron absorption is increased when body stores are depleted or erythropoiesis is enhanced.

Large Intestine

Secretions. The mucosal cells of the colon secrete mucus, which lubricates the passage of chyme.

Motility. Colonic movements include mixing and peristaltic movements. These operate as described for the small intestine. A third movement, which only the colon possesses, is the mass movement. This consists of simultaneous contractions of colonic smooth muscle over large portions of the descending and sigmoid portions of the colon. This movement rapidly moves the undigested food residue (feces) from these areas into the rectum.

Filling of the rectum triggers the defecation reflex by stimulating stretch receptors in the rectal wall. Stimulation of the stretch receptors causes sensory (afferent) nerve fibers to transmit impulses to the lower part of the spinal cord. Because of anatomical arrangements of neurons in this part of the cord, these afferent impulses reflexly cause nerve impulses to travel out of the cord along parasympathetic motor fibers that innervate the smooth muscles of the descending and sigmoid colon, the rectum, and the internal anal sphincter. These afferent impulses also reflexly cause nerve impulses to be sent out of the cord along somatic motor neurons that innervate the skeletal muscle of the external anal sphincter. The total effect of these events is to produce (1) coordinated contractions of the colon and rectum, (2) relaxation (opening) of the sphincters, and (3) the output of feces from the anus. Blocking of this reflex in "continent" individuals is obtained by transmission of impulses from higher brain centers down fibers in the spinal cord to the somatic motor neurons that innervate the external sphincter. These descending impulses inhibit the activity of these particular motor neurons. This prevents them from causing the external sphincter to relax. Inappropriate defecation is thus prevented. After a few minutes, the defecation reflex ceases, but it usually returns a few hours later.

Humans cannot digest the cellulose, hemicellulose, or lignin from plant tissues. Thus, these plant materials form a large portion of the undigested food residue.

They are usually termed "vegetable fiber" or "dietary bulk." These fibers attract and "hold" water, thereby promoting a larger, softer stool. Low quantities of bulk result in a relatively inactive colon and infrequent or smaller dryer, and harder bowel movements. Tantalizing epidemiological reports suggest that high-fiber diets are associated with a decreased incidence of diverticulitis and colonic cancer. However, any causal relationship between dietary fiber and the incidence of disease remains to be discovered.

Absorption.   It is in the large intestine that most of the water and potassium are absorbed from the chyme. This produces a semisolid residue of undigested food (feces) that can be eliminated from the body. Diarrhea can reduce the transit time for chyme, thereby limiting such potassium and water reabsorption. This can result in hypokalemia and dehydration. Diarrhea also can be caused by materials that "hold" water in the chyme (*e.g.*, $MgSO_4$), resulting in a semiliquid, fast-moving bowel movement.

Commensal bacteria.   At birth, the colon is sterile, but large colonic bacterial populations become established soon afterward. Some of these organisms manufacture vitamin K and a number of B vitamins. For a long time, such bacterially produced vitamins were thought to be absorbed by the colonic mucosa. This is now known to be untrue for vitamin K and most of the B vitamins. Only bacterially produced folic acid is colonically absorbed. Other bacteria produce ammonia, which is colonically absorbed. Normally, this is removed from the blood once it reaches the liver. However, in persons with seriously impaired liver function or with collateral circulatory routes that bypass the liver (usually the result of portal hypertension), such ammonia can remain in the circulation and lead to encephalopathy.

Vomiting (Emesis).   Vomiting results from the relaxation of the LES and the rest of the esophagus combined with simultaneous strong contractions of abdominal muscles and diaphragm and closure of the epiglottis over the airway. The contractions squeeze the stomach and force its contents up the esophagus and out the mouth. In addition, irritation of the small intestine (either by materials in the chyme, by inflammation, or by disease process) can cause special movements that constitute reverse peristalsis. These movements, identical with peristalsic movement, move chyme toward the pyloric valve. They can be sufficiently strong to force open the pyloris and enter the stomach. This is how intestinal contents are vomited. If golden-yellow bile from the duodenum spends any appreciable time in the stomach, acids will turn it green. Occasionally, vomiting of intestinal contents

can be so rapid that bile spends hardly any time in the stomach. Then the vomitus will contain golden yellow bile. If blood is allowed time in the stomach, acids will turn it brownish-black (coffee-ground color). If vomiting does not allow sufficient time for this acid action to occur, blood in the vomitus will have its normal red color.

Liver

Microscopic Structure.   The functional unit of the liver is a cylindrically shaped lobule that measures approximately 1.5 mm in diameter and 8 mm in length. Each lobe of the liver contains between 50,000 and 100,000 lobules. Microanatomy of the lobules is shown in Figure 29–5. Rows of liver cells (hepatocytes) radiate from a central venule, as do spokes of a wheel. Branches of both the hepatic artery and hepatic portal vein lie at the periphery of the wheel. Blood from these branches is poured into open channels (hepatic sinuses) that run between alternate rows of hepatocytes. These sinuses drain into the central venule, which in turn carries blood to the hepatic vein. Approximately 400 ml of blood, held within the venous sinuses, can be made available in emergencies to compensate for hypovolemia. Blind-ended bile canaliculi arise between the other rows of hepatocytes. They carry newly secreted bile to larger ducts located at the periphery. These smaller ducts eventually drain into the common bile duct. Bile that is leaving the liver is concentrated and stored in the gallbladder. Fluid and electrolyte reabsorption in the gallbladder can increase the concentration of bile salts, cholesterol, and bilirubin 12-fold. Thus, the gallbladder with a maximum capacity of 50 ml can hold a 24-hour output of bile (600 ml) from the liver. The intestinal hormone CCK-PZ stimulates gallbladder contraction. CCK-PZ and local reflexes initiated by duodenal peristalsis open the sphincter of Oddi. These events permit an outflow of bile down the common bile duct into the duodenum.

Function of Hepatocytes.   The liver cells perform many functions (Table 29–2). They degrade steroid hormones, thereby preventing excess blood levels of estrogen, testosterone, progesterone, aldosterone, and glucocorticosteroids.

Another hepatic function concerns protein metabolism. Hepatocytes deaminate proteins and synthesize nitrogenous wastes (*e.g.*, uric acid). They also convert ammonia manufactured by colonic bacteria into another waste, urea. They also synthesize plasma proteins (*e.g.*, albumin and globulin). The albumins maintain normal plasma colloid osmotic pressure. A fall in this pressure leads to edema and can contribute to ascites.

Cross section of liver lobule

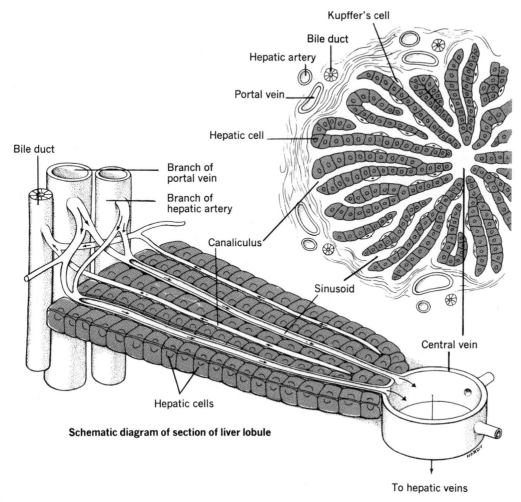

Schematic diagram of section of liver lobule

FIGURE 29-5
A section of liver lobule showing the location of the hepatic veins, hepatic cells, liver sinusoids, and branches of the portal vein and hepatic artery. (Chaffee EE, Lytle IM: Basic Physiology and Anatomy, 4th ed. Philadelphia, JB Lippincott, 1980)

The globulins bind to a certain portion of the daily hormonal output from the thyroid and adrenal cortex glands. Binding inactivates these hormones, thereby keeping blood levels low. Bound hormones can be released during the day to maintain normal plasma levels of those hormones. Decreased hepatic protein levels can lead to a clinical excess of these hormones.

Hepatocytes also make bile, which contains water, bile salts, cholesterol, bilirubin gluconate, and inorganic acids. Bile salts aid digestion by emulsifying dietary fats and fostering their absorption and the absorption of fat-soluble vitamins through the intestinal mucosa. They also prevent the cholesterol in the bile from precipitating out of solution and forming calculi

(stones). Over 90 percent of the daily output of bile salts is reabsorbed for recycling by an active transport process of the ileal mucosa. There are two sources of biliary or plasma cholesterol: dietary production and hepatic manufacture. Certain genetic conditions cause the liver to manufacture supernormal amounts of cholesterol.

Another hepatic function is elimination of bilirubin from the body. Old or defective erythrocytes are phagocytosed by large reticuloendothelial cells lining the large veins and the sinuses of the liver and spleen. These phagocytes degrade the hemoglobin of these cells into biliverdin, iron, and globulin molecules. The last two components are recycled by the body in

---

TABLE 29-2
HEPATOCYTE FUNCTIONS

- Steroid (hormone and drug) catabolism
- Degradation of certain drugs
- Production of bile
- Elimination of bilirubin
- Synthesis of coagulation factors I (fibrinogen), II (prothrombin), V (proaccelerin), VII (proconvertin), IX (plasma thromboplastin component), and X (Stuart factor)
- Mineral and vitamin storage
- Protein metabolism, including synthesis of plasma proteins, conversion of ammonia to urea, deamination, and transamination.
- Fat metabolism, including lipoprotein synthesis, cholesterol synthesis, and conversion of protein and carbohydrates into fat.
- Carbohydrate metabolism, including glycogen storage, gluconeogenesis, and release of glucose into plasma

---

future erythropoiesis. The biliverdin is almost immediately converted to free bilirubin. Because this is an insoluble compound, it is transported bound to plasma albumin molecules. The hepatocytes convert this insoluble bilirubin into a soluble (and thus excretable) form by conjugating it with glucuronic acid to form bilirubin gluconate. This soluble form of bilirubin is then added to the bile and is eliminated from the body via the feces. Bilirubin gluconate gives the bile its normal golden-yellow color. Commensal organisms in the intestines convert most of the bilirubin gluconate into a darker brown compound, urobilinogen, which gives the feces its natural brown color. Because it is soluble in water, urobilingen can also be absorbed from the colon back into the bloodstream and be excreted by way of the kidneys. Excess plasma levels of either the conjugated or unconjugated (insoluble) bilirubin produce jaundice. Excess unconjugated bilirubin can cross the immature or damaged blood brain barrier and bind with the basal ganglia, resulting in kernicteris.

The liver buffers plasma glucose levels. This "hepatic glucostatic function" involves two mechanisms. When plasma glucose levels are high, hepatocytes remove glucose from the plasma. This glucose is stored in polymer form as glycogen. As plasma glucose levels decline, the hepatocytes convert the glycogen back into glucose molecules (glycogenolysis) and release them into the bloodstream. Although many body tissues have the requisite cellular enzymes for glycogenolysis, hepatocytes are one of the few cell types that can release this intracellular glucose into the bloodstream. Hepatocytes do not simply respond directly to plasma glucose. These glucostatic functions are mediated by several hormones; some (*e.g.,* insulin) promote hepatic glucose uptake, and others (*e.g.,* glucagon, growth hormone, and epinephrine) stimulate glycogenolysis and the release of glucose from liver cells.

The liver does not contain enough glycogen reserves to be able to buffer plasma glucose during prolonged fasting or severe exercise. During these times, low plasma glucose levels stimulate the secretion of one or more hormones (glucagon, glucocorticoids, or thyroxine) that trigger the biochemical conversion of intracellular fatty and amino acids into glucose (gluconeogenesis), which the liver cell can then release into the bloodstream or store as glycogen. Only hepatocytes possess the enzyme that is critical for gluconeogenesis. Glycogen storage is important for other functions of liver cells. A glycogen-rich hepatocyte conjugates bilirubin at a faster rate and is more resistant to toxins and infectious agents.

Hepatocytes possess a "mixed-function-oxidase system" (MFOS) of enzymes that degrade certain drugs, among which are alcohol, benzodiazepines, tranquilizers, phenobarbital, phenytoin (Dilantin), and sodium warfarin (Coumadin). This system operates in addition to other intracellular systems that also degrade some of these drugs. Its clinical significance lies in the nature of the drugs that this system catabolizes and in the fact that MFOS activity can be either inhibited or augmented ("induced") by these same drugs, depending *when* they are taken. Administration of two MFOS catabolized drugs within a few hours of one another or together will cause each agent to act competitively, slowing down the degradation of the other. Thus, simultaneous ingestion of diazepam alcohol and (Valium) can result in slower degradation of each drug. This will result in higher blood levels of both chemicals for a longer time after administration. The repeated administration of one MFOS-catabolized drug for several days will cause the MFOS system to enlarge physically and to possess more enzymes. This is called "induction." Once induced, the MFOS degrades drugs more rapidly (including the drug that initiated the induction). If administration of a second MFOS-catabolized drug is begun after MFOS induction, a larger dose of this drug will be required to produce a given effect. For example, induction of the MFOS by diazepam would increase the dosage of Coumadin needed to produce a given therapeutic effect. Other drugs are degraded by various hepatic systems.

BIBLIOGRAPHY

Ganong WF: Review of Medical Physiology, 11th ed. Los Altos, Lange Medical Publications, 1983

Porth C: Pathophysiological Concepts of Altered Health States. Philadelphia, JB Lippincott, 1982

Mountcastle VB: Medical Physiology. St Louis, CV Mosby, 1980

30
Assessment: Gastrointestinal System

Nursing History and Physical Assessment

Helen C. Busby

Differentiation of the signs and symptoms of a gastrointestinal disorder challenges an inquisitive mind. One must determine whether the assessment findings are related to a known condition or whether they herald a new complication. Is the comatose patient's respiratory distress due to a pulmonary disorder or to a mucous plug lodged in the nasopharynx? Is the bright red blood in the stool due to a gastrointestinal bleed or to bleeding from external hemorrhoids? Is the complaint of abdominal pain due to the trauma of recent bowel surgery or to a distended stomach? With a careful assessment of the gastrointestinal system, the nurse can obtain information that will clarify specific patient problems.

NURSING HISTORY

Excluding emergency conditions that require immediate action to preserve life, an assessment of the gastrointestinal system begins with the nursing history. The patient should be questioned about any past problems with anorexia, indigestion, dysphagia, nausea, vomiting, pain, jaundice, constipation, gas, diarrhea, bleeding, or hemorrhoids. It is necessary for the nurse to follow through and expand on positive responses. She should determine when the problem appeared, whether medical treatment was sought, what precipitated the symptom, what relieved it, what made it

worse, and whether the problem is current. Questions should be asked regarding food allergies, food intolerance, special diets, antacids, laxatives, alcohol, caffeine, and medications presently being taken, especially aspirin, steroids, antibiotics, and anticoagulants. The patient should be asked about recent weight gain or loss, bowel habits, recent surgeries (including dental work), and any family history of ulcers, colitis, or cancer. The patient should be instructed to point to any area of pain, describe the pain in his own words, and relate what he does to relieve it. The most common complaints about the gastrointestinal system are pain, dysphagia, nausea, vomiting, diarrhea, and constipation. A review of the gastrointestinal system focuses on the following five features:

General Appearance. Motor activity, body position, nutritional state (thin or obese), recent changes in weight, eating habits, and apparent state of health.

Skin. Color (jaundice, cyanosis, pallor), turgor, edema, texture (oily, dry), and dermatologic conditions.

Head. Color of sclerae, sunken eyes, breath odor, condition of teeth (dentures, caries), condition of tongue, and condition of buccal mucosa.

Abdomen. Size, shape, visible protrusions, scars, fistulas, limited respiratory excursion, and excessive skin folds (indicates muscle wasting).

Psychological Factors. Recent emotional upsets, depression, and anxiety.

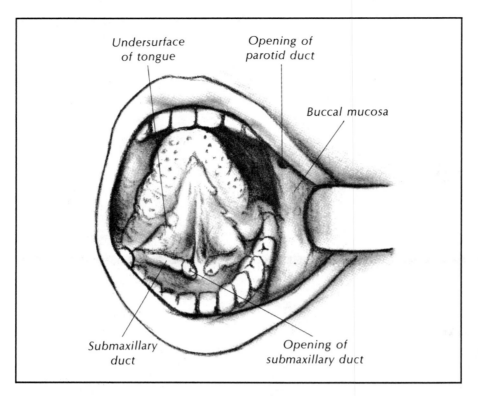

Undersurface of tongue

Opening of parotid duct

Buccal mucosa

Submaxillary duct

Opening of submaxillary duct

FIGURE 30-1
Structures in the mouth. (Bates B: A Guide to Physical Examination, 3rd ed, p 64. Philadelphia, JB Lippincott, 1983)

EXAMINATION

Examination of the oral cavity is accomplished by inspection and palpation. A good light source, a tongue depressor, and an examining glove are needed. The patient should be placed in a comfortable position, preferably sitting upright. The nurse should explain the procedure to the patient and obtain his cooperation. The first step is inspection of the lips and jaw for abnormal color, texture, lesions, symmetry, and swellings. The temporomandibular joint is palpated bilaterally for mobility, tenderness, and crepitus. The bite is inspected for malocclusion by having the patient clench his teeth. The upper incisors and canine teeth slightly overlap the lower ones; otherwise, the upper and lower teeth would meet. The lips should be retracted to allow adequate visualization during the inspection. If the patient has dentures, the nurse should inspect how well they fit, then have the patient remove them. The inside of the mouth should be inspected with a good light source. Missing, broken, loose, and decayed teeth should be identified. Redness, pallor, white patches, plaques, ulcers, bleeding, and masses of the gums and entire buccal mucosa should be

noted. The parotid ducts and the submaxillary ducts should be located (Fig. 30-1).

Any suspicious area should be palpated with a gloved finger for tenderness or induration. The patient should be asked to stick out his tongue, which is checked for symmetry of movement, swellings, lesions, and an abnormal coating. The tongue blade is used to depress the tongue, and the movement of the soft palate and uvula is observed as the patient says "ah"; these structures should rise symmetrically. The hard and soft palates, the uvula, the tonsils, the pillars, and the posterior pharynx, are inspected for redness, pallor, patches, lesions, and petechiae. Any unusual breath odor should be described.

If there are no contraindications to the performance of an examination of the abdomen, the patient should be instructed to empty his bladder, and then should be placed in the supine position with his arms at his sides and his knees slightly bent. This position will relieve tension on the abdominal wall. The need for an abdominal examination should be evaluated if the patient is experiencing pain. An abdominal examination should not be performed if the patient has appendicitis, dissecting abdominal aortic aneurisym, or poly-

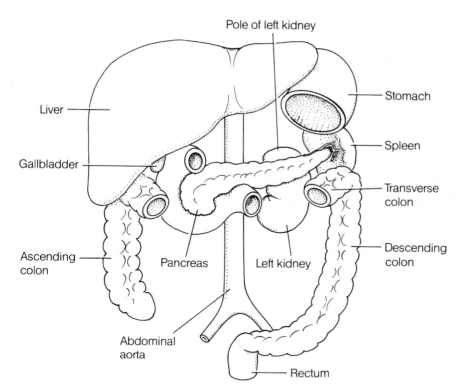

FIGURE 30-2
A map of abdominal organs.

cystic kidneys or if he has had an organ transplantation. The abdominal examination must be stopped at any time the procedure becomes too uncomfortable for the patient or increases the intensity of the pain or when findings indicate one of the aforementioned diagnoses.

The abdominal examination is performed by inspection, auscultation, percussion, and palpation, in that order. The examination should always be performed with a systematic approach. The patient should be draped in a manner that will expose the abdomen while protecting the patient's modesty. The abdomen is divided into its four sections (RUQ, LUQ, LLQ, RLQ), and visualized are the underlying structures (Fig. 30 – 2). The nurse stands at the foot of the patient and inspects for symmetry of the abdomen, visible masses, and visible pulsations. She then moves to the patient's side, positions herself to obtain an eye-level view across the abdomen, and inspects for abdominal movement from respirations, peristalsis, pulsations, any exaggerated movement, and an eversion of the umbilicus. Normal peristalsis is not visible, even in a very thin person. Pulsation of the aorta is normally seen in the epigastric area. In a thin person, the femoral pulses may be visible. The color of the skin should be observed. Signs of edema (*e.g.,* tense, shiny skin) and the presence of a hernia (becomes visible with a cough) should be recorded. Any rashes, striae, ecchy-

moses, lesions, scars, and dilated veins should be noted. A blue-tinged umbilicus is known as "Cullen's sign" and may be an indication of intra-abdominal bleeding.

Next, the four quadrants of the abdomen are auscultated with the diaphragm of the stethoscope. To prevent contraction of the abdominal muscles (which will obscure other sounds), the examiner lifts the stethoscope completely off the abdominal wall when changing its location. One should use only light pressure on the diaphragm and listen for a full 3 minutes in one location to confirm the absence of sound. The frequency and character of sounds heard should be described. Normal bowel sounds are irregular bubbly sounds and occur every 5 to 15 seconds. Hyperactive bowel sounds are rapid, high-pitched (tinkling), and loud. Edema of the abdominal wall can be detected by observation of any imprint of the diaphragm. The bell of the stethescope is used to auscultate over the abdominal aorta, the renal arteries, and the femoral arteries for bruits (a continuous purring, blowing, or humming sound). If a bruit is heard neither percussion nor palpation should be performed. The physician must be notified of this finding if it was not previously heard.

Following auscultation, percussion should be performed in all four quadrants. The sound that will be percussed depends on the underlying structure. A dull

TABLE 30-1
CLINICAL RECORDING OF GASTROINTESTINAL ASSESSMENT

Wears upper and lower dentures. Lips are cyanotic; no ulcers or cracking. Buccal mucosa bright red; no ulcers or nodules. Tongue, gums, and floor of mouth cyanotic. Unable to identify parotid and submaxillary ducts. Tonsils absent. No lesions, plaques, or exudates.

No complaints of abdominal pain. Appetite good. No difficulty swallowing; no nausea or vomiting. Has indigestion when eating while stressed. Bowel movement every day. No diarrhea or constipation. No history of jaundice, gallbladder, or liver disorders.

Abdomen is flat and symmetrical with good muscle tone and without visible pulsations or peristalsis. Frequent borborygmi in all quadrants. Renal and femoral arteries not auscultated because of overriding bowel sounds. No palpable areas of tenderness or masses. Liver span percusssed at 4 cm. Spleen not palpable. Pole of right and left kidney palpated in respective upper outer quadrants approximately 2 cm below costal margin. Aortic and femoral pulses 4$^+$.

TABLE 30-2
CONDITIONS THAT PRODUCE INTRA-ABDOMINAL PAIN AND TENDERNESS

1. Perforated peptic ulcer
2. Dissecting or ruptured aneurysm
3. Pancreatitis
4. Cholecystitis
5. Regional enteritis
6. Ulcerative colitis
7. Diverticulitis
8. Appendicitis
9. Occlusion of mesenteric artery
10. Ruptured ectopic pregnancy
11. Acute renal infections
12. Pelvic inflammatory disease
13. Hepatitis
14. Extra-abdominal causes:
    (a) Myocardial disease
    (b) Respiratory disease
    (c) Diabetic or thyroid crisis
    (d) Spinal cord lesion
    (e) Acute intermittent porphyria
    (f) Pneumonia
    (g) Acute glaucoma

sound will be heard over solid organs, such as the liver or a stool-filled colon. A tympanic sound will be heard over air, as in the gastric bubble. Percussion is done to check the size of an organ and to detect excessive amounts of fluid or air in the abdomen. Percussion for determination of the size of the liver should be performed along the right midclavicular line. One method is to begin at the iliac crest and work upward. The point at which the sound becomes dull is marked, then percussion is performed from the clavicle down. A dull sound represents a rib, which must not be mistaken for the superior edge of the liver. The superior edge is marked and is measured in centimeters. The normal liver will measure 6 to 12 cm.

One begins palpation of the abdomen by using a light touch to identify muscular resistance and abdominal tenderness in all four quadrants. One or two fingers are used to depress the abdominal wall 1 cm ($\frac{1}{2}$ inch). Skin temperature, muscle resistance, tender areas, and masses are noted. The femoral artery is palpated bilaterally. One must always palpate a symptomatic area last to assure patient cooperation and relaxed muscles.

Deep palpation is used for localization organs and large masses. The tips of the fingers are used to depress the abdominal wall firmly to a depth of 7.5 cm (3 inches). One palpates for an enlarged spleen, for the lower edge of the liver, and for the pole of the right and

TABLE 30-3
GASTROINTESTINAL NURSING DIAGNOSES

General Nursing Diagnoses	Associated Nursing Diagnoses
Pain	Fear of serious illness
	Alteration of rest/activity pattern
Dysphagia	Alteration in nutrition (less)
	Fluid volume deficit
Nausea and vomiting	Fluid and electrolyte deficit
	Alteration in nutrition (less)
	Alteration in comfort
Diarrhea	Potential for impaired skin integrity
	Possible fluid and electrolyte deficit
Constipation	Alteration in comfort
	Knowledge deficit related to proper nutrition and bowel habits

left kidney. Palpation is performed in the epigastric area for the pulse of the aorta. If an area of tenderness is found with light palpation, one should check it for rebound tenderness by quickly withdrawing the fingertips following depression. Rebound tenderness usually indicates an inflammation of the peritoneum. If there is ascites, tests should be performed to determine whether a fluid wave is present.

The rectum is assessed by inspection and palpation. The skin around the rectum is normally darker than the surrounding area. One should inspect for inflammation, lesions, fissures, and hemorrhoids palpate with a well-lubricated rubber-covered finger for outpouching, nodules, tenderness, irregularities, and a fecal impaction.

The final step in an assessment of the gastrointestinal system is the documentation of findings. The documentation should be concise and informative. Pertinent negative findings are indicated. Table 30-1 provides a typical example of documentation of an assessment.

A complete assessment of the gastrointestinal system is not performed at regular intervals. However, an alert nurse will always be assessing for changes in the system that requires a more detailed examination. Table 30-2 outlines conditions that may produce the symptoms of pain and tenderness in the abdomen.

The recommended nursing diagnoses for disorders of the gastrointestinal tract are outlined in Table 30-3.

Assessment of the gastrointestinal system is important in the determination of the causes of nutritional disorders, acid-base imbalances, bleeding episodes, and pain within the system. It is also performed to monitor therapy, to determine the necessity of preventive health teaching, and to monitor an abnormality in another system that is reflected in the gastrointestinal system. A new finding must never be disregarded.

BIBLIOGRAPHY

Bates B: A Guide To Physical Examination, 3rd ed. Philadelphia, JB Lippincott, 1983

Given B, Simmons S: Gastroenterology in Clinical Nursing, 3rd ed. St Louis, CV Mosby, 1979

Malkiewicz J: For a Really Thorough Abdominal Exam. RN 45, No. 10: 59–63, 1982

Potter D (ed): Assessment, Nurses Reference Library. Springhouse, PA, Intermed Communications, 1982

Roberts A: Systems and signs—digestive system: The acute abdomen. Nursing Times 77, No. 27: 79–86, 1981

Schwarz T: Is it "acute abdomen"? RN 45, No. 70: 29–31, 94–96, 1982

Diagnostic Techniques for the Gastrointestinal System

William Seiffert

A variety of diagnostic tests can be used to help in the diagnosis of gastrointestinal and abdominal abnormalities in the critical care setting.

Radiographs of the abdomen (the abdominal series, or three-way view of the abdomen, consisting of films of the flat abdomen, films of the upper abdomen and upper chest with the patient erect, and films obtained with the patient lying on his side [decubitus]) help delineate free air in the abdomen from a problem such as a perforated viscus or possibly a ruptured abscess. Bowel obstructions as indicated by dilated loops of bowel with air fluid levels or intestinal volvulus can be seen on these films. Decubitus films help determine the presence of ascites.

Upper GI and barium enema contrast studies can be performed to help define the presence of peptic ulcers, sites of bleeding, tumors, and inflammatory processes such as Crohn's disease and ulcerative colitis.

Gastrointestinal endoscopy is an important adjunct to the barium studies in that it allows direct visualization of portions of the intestinal tract. Sites of bleeding can be noted, and tumors and inflammatory processes can be biopsied.

Arteriography of the intestinal tract can be useful in defining the sites of bleeding that are otherwise difficult to determine. The catheter is placed in either the superior or inferior mesenteric artery, and contrast is injected. If the patient is actively bleeding at that time, the site may visualize well as a blush of contrast within the intestinal tract. If bleeding continues, the surgeon has the exact site localized for surgical excision. Arteriography is also extremely helpful in defining aneurysms of the aorta.

Ultrasonography has been useful in defining aneurysm of the aorta, tumors within various solid structures in the abdomen, abscesses and abnormalities of the biliary system (*e.g.,* cholelithiasis and dilated biliary ducts), and cholecystitis.

Paracentesis, or peritoneal tap with lavage of the peritoneal cavity, can be most useful in trauma cases in which intra-abdominal hemorrhage must be defined. It can also help determine whether pancreatitis is present by measurement of the amylase and lipase in the fluid aspirated and whether tumors are present by cytology studies.

Computerized axial tomography scans also are useful in defining tumor masses and abscesses.

31
Management Modalities: Gastrointestinal System

Helen C. Busby
William Seiffert

Nutritional Support of the Critically Ill Patient

Adequate nutritional support of the critically ill patient is one of the most important advances in patient care since the development of antibiotics.

Historically, it has long been recognized that health and nutrition go hand in hand. As the fund of knowledge of normal metabolism increased, the effects of stress (e.g., injury and infection) also were being investigated. For example, in 1936 it was found that among patients who were undergoing surgical treatment for peptic ulcer, there was a 33% mortality rate in those with a preoperative loss of more than 20% of their body weight. This compared with a 3.5% mortality rate for those who were in a better nutritional state.[1] Similarly, Cahill noted that a loss of one third of the total body protein by a previously normal person was fatal.[2] It became readily obvious that significant stress increased mortality and morbidity by reducing body mass, delaying wound healing, and altering the normal immune responses.

This chapter will present a basic overview of the physiology and pathophysiology of stress on the nutritional state of the patient. Following this, the methods of assessment and nutritional support will be discussed.

For good homeostasis, there must be a balance between energy supply and energy expenditure. The total expenditure of energy by the body is the sum of physical activity, growth, and basal metabolic rate (BMR). The BMR is the energy that a person requires to perform the essential physiological processes at rest. If the BMR is increased by 10% to 15%, the resting metabolic expenditure (RME) is calculated. RME takes into account the energy for minimal physical activity to the BMR.

The importance of stress on energy balance is illustrated by the following considerations: Fever increases the RME by 7% for each degree Fahrenheit, the postoperative state increases the RME by 10% to 15%, infection increases the RME by 20% to 50%, and thermal burns raise the RME by as much as 125%. It is evident that maintenance of an energy balance in those states would require a tremendous amount of calories.[3]

Besides requiring energy balance, the body must also maintain nitrogen balance. This is crucial because nitrogen represents the building blocks of protein. If the body is building protein, a state of anabolism exists and protein balance is said to be positive. If, however, the body is breaking down protein, a state of catabolism exists and the balance swings to negative.

The catabolic state is seen in trauma, sepsis, and certain disease states. It represents the breakdown of protein for energy purposes. When protein is lost in this manner, it represents a loss of essential body function. Protein molecules represent such structures as enzymes, cell membranes, contractile protein in muscle, and blood proteins. Their loss is critical to the outcome of a patient during a catabolic state.

METABOLIC RESPONSE TO INJURY

A traumatic event, regardless of its cause, triggers a complex series of hormonal responses that significantly alter the body's metabolism. The major effect of this is an increase in protein and fat catabolism with a retention of water and sodium and a loss of potassium. The pituitary hormone, ADH, is released in response to such factors as hypovolemia, pain, stress, and drugs. By acting on the collecting ducts of the kidney, ADA reduces free water excretion, thus correcting the hypovolemic state. ACTH also is released from the pituitary and stimulates the adrenal gland to secrete mineralocorticoids and glucocorticoids. The mineralocorticoid aldosterone causes sodium retention and potassium excretion by its action on the kidney. This function, along with the action of ADH, is the major volume regulatory system by which the body maintains blood pressure in the face of trauma.

The glucocorticoids, of which cortisol is the most important, act in several ways to produce energy substrate for the body during stress. They act on the liver to stimulate gluconeogenesis but also are catabolic in that they cause muscle protein breakdown to aminoacids and decreased protein synthesis. They also release free fatty acids from lipid stores.

The catecholamines, epinephrine and norepinephrine, are released from the adrenal medulla during stress. They also set into motion a series of reactions aimed at increasing energy substrate for the body.

Lipolysis results from increased catecholamine secretion. Free fatty acids are then available as an energy source by the liver, kidney, lung, heart, and skeletal muscle. Ketone bodies are formed from fatty acids by the liver. These also are used as an energy source.

Catecholamines cause a hyperglycemia to develop during stress, called "stress diabetes." This clinical state arises through a variety of mechanisms. Liver and glycogen and muscle glycogen are converted to glucose. Insulin released from the pancreas is suppressed, and glucagon is released. Uptake of glucose in the peripheral tissues also is reduced.

Both ACTH and catecholamines act to release glucagon. Glucagon then acts on the liver to promote gluconeogenesis. It also helps break down skeletal muscle glycogen to glucose and aids in oxidation of fat.

The hormonal reactions of ACTH, catecholamines, glucagon, insulin, and growth hormone act in synergism to supply the body with energy substrate and to control blood volume to help ensure survival during stress. This stress can be either starvation or trauma. However, in starvation, the levels of cortisol and catecholamines are not elevated to the magnitude of those seen in severe trauma. This may account for the fact that there is a rise in metabolic rate in the posttraumatic state rather than the fall that occurs in starvation. In starvation, the body tends to preserve lean body mass and protein, but following trauma, protein becomes the major source of calories. The mechanisms for this is not well understood.

During the initial phase of stress, the body utilizes carbohydrates in the form of glycogen. These stores may last as long as 8 to 12 hours. Following this, amino acids from protein and to some degree fatty acids make up the bulk of energy substrate.

Nitrogen, a major component of amino acids, helps form the building blocks of protein. One gram of nitrogen equals 6.25 g of protein, which is equal to about 30 g of lean body mass. If losses of 15 to 25 g day occur, as is often seen in major trauma (*i.e.,* burns, major fractures, and sepsis), as much as 7.5 kg (16 lb) of lean body mass can be lost.[4]

Although these drastic losses cannot be eliminated, they can be offset by an adequate supply of calories and amino acids. If the nutritional substrate is supplied and other factors of support such as blood pressure and respiratory status are maintained, the body will enter a phase of "available opportunity." During this time, the levels of catecholamines, cortisol, and glucagon drop and insulin rises. Protein breakdown is curtailed, and protein resynthesis is favored.

If catabolism is allowed to continue without the support of calories and amino acids, wound healing cannot take place. At this point, there is direct competition for the necessary substrates by the rest of the body. The patient must be evaluated continuously for determination of metabolic needs because his clinical status is constantly changing.

NUTRITIONAL ASSESSMENT

The assessment of the patient who needs nutritional assistance is multifactorial and includes dietary history, anthropometric measurements, biochemical studies, immunological responses, and nitrogen balance studies.

The dietary history, often obtained by a dietitian, can help one determine nutritional state before illness onset. It can also help in directing further needs during the illness. However, the history is often not obtainable or does not fit the prevailing clinical picture. The other four parameters therefore become especially important.

Anthropometric measurements involve physical measures of the body and provide a rough estimate of body fat percentage. Skin fold and muscle circumferences of the arms are often used to make these measurements. Biochemical studies pertain to rapid turnover proteins such as prealbumin, albumin, and transferrin. The levels of these various proteins reflect the rapidity of protein synthesis and breakdown.[5]

Immunological studies help ascertain nutritional status by allowing evaluation of the recall antigens to TB, mumps, and *Candidia*. These are applied as skin tests, and, if no reaction is seen, a state of altered immunocompetency may exist. It has been documented that normal lymphocyte response to skin tests is not seen in malnourished people. Also, reduced lymphocyte counts are seen in these patients.

One very important parameter of protein synthesis and metabolism is the measure of nitrogen balance. This balance is calculated from the amount of nitrogen intake against that which is excreted in the urine as urea. The normal adult turns over about 300 g of protein in 24 hours and excretes the equivalent of 50 to 65 g of protein during that time.

Nitrogen balance is calculated with the following equation:

$$\text{Nitrogen balance} = \frac{\text{Protein intake}}{6.25} - \text{Urinary urea nitrogen} + 4$$

If the number derived is zero, nitrogen balance is present. If the number is positive, protein synthesis is occurring. A negative number indicates that protein catabolism exists. The amino acid and nitrogen needs of the patient can be calculated by this measurement.

TOTAL PARENTERAL NUTRITION (HYPERALIMENTATION)

Because administration of total parenteral nutrition (TPN) is feasible, the acutely ill patient's nutritional status is considered early in the illness and treated aggressively. By means of hyperalimentation, sufficient calories and nitrogen to sustain life can be supplied to the body. Any patient who has lost the ability to absorb nutrients from the gastrointestinal tract should be considered for this therapy. Enteral hyperalimentation (tube feeding) should be utilized if the gastrointestinal tract is intact and functional.

The patient with a long-term postoperative course, the patient with multiple trauma, the patient receiving chemotherapy, and the patient being treated with acute hemodialysis are but a few candidates for this sophisticated therapy (Table 31–1). The increased energy required by the body to handle the stresses imposed on it by these conditions will lead to the starvation state without nutritional support.

Protein-sparing nutrition alone may be used for short-term therapy in persons with no nutritional deficiencies and little change in their metabolic rate (*i.e.,* elective surgery). The administration of isotonic amino acid solutions by way of a peripheral vein will preserve body protein by supplying amino acids for normal protein synthesis. It will not assist in tissue repair. If the person progresses to protein/calorie malnutrition, as in hypermetabolic states or faulty nutrition, TPN should be instituted.

Solution Admixture

The solution of TPN therapy begins as an admixture containing 20% to 30% glucose and 3.5% to 5.0% amino acids. The ratio of the calories (glucose) to the nitrogen (amino acid) should be 200:1. This ratio will preserve the nitrogen balance of the body; the hypertonic glucose will be used for calories, allowing the amino acids to be used for protein synthesis. If this ratio is not preserved, excess amino acids will be lost in the urine when adequate glucose is present, or amino acids will be used for calories if adequate glucose is not present. Optimal therapy requires 200 calories to each 1 g of nitrogen.

Daily additions to the base solution should include potassium, sodium, and chloride. The daily requirements of these elements are greatly increased because of the increased volume of water intake and output. With the increased intake of glucose and amino acids, hypokalemia will soon result if additional potassium is not administered in sufficient quantities to maintain normal serum potassium levels. Potassium is also nec-

TABLE 31–1
INDICATIONS FOR TOTAL PARENTERAL NUTRITION

Malnutrition	Diverticulitis
Malabsorption	Alimentary tract fistula
Chronic diarrhea	Alimentary tract anomalies
Chronic vomiting	Reversible liver failure
Failure to thrive	Acute and chronic renal failure
Gastrointestinal obstruction	Burns
Ulcer disease	Hypermetabolic states
Granulomatous enterocolitis	Complicated trauma or surgery
Ulcerative colitis	Short bowel syndrome
Pancreatitis	Protein-losing gastroenteropathy
Severe anorexia nervosa	Nonterminal coma
Indolent wounds and decubitus ulcers	Malignant disease (adjunctive therapy)

(From Dudrick SJ: Total intravenous feeding: When nutrition seems impossible. Drug Therapy, Hospital Edition 1, No. 2:92, 1976)

TABLE 31-2
TESTS THAT MAY BE ON A HYPERALIMENTATION PANEL

Chemistry	Normal Ranges	Results
pH	7.35-7.45	
Sodium	135-149 mEq/liter	
Potassium	3.5-5.3 mEq/liter	
Chlorides	100-109 mEq/liter	
Calcium	4.5-5.7 mEq/liter	
Phosphorus	1.45-2.76 mEq/liter	
Magnesium	1.5-2.4 mEq/liter	
Glucose	70-115 mg/dl	
BUN	8-22 mg/dl	
Creatine	0.8-1.6 mg/dl	
Bicarbonate	22-26 mEq/liter	
Total protein	5.5-8.0 g/dl	

essary for the transport of glucose across the cell membrane. Magnesium, calcium, phosphorus, and other trace elements are added as deficiencies occur. Because cations are poorly absorbed in the intestinal tract, the intravenous requirements of these elements are less than one would suspect. A multiple vitamin preparation is usually mixed in 1 liter of base solution per day. A unit of albumin also may be included daily to supplement protein intake.

Decisions concerning the amount of additives necessary to maintain the patient's electrolyte balance are ascertained from serial blood tests. Positive nitrogen balance is monitored by serial blood urea nitrogen (BUN) and creatinine levels. A hyperalimentation panel (Table 31-2) is done daily until the electrolytes are stabilized. Once stabilization is achieved, the serum levels may be checked every other day to once a week.

Glucose intolerance may occur at the onset of treatment if the pancreas does not respond to the increased glucose load. Blood glucose levels can be easily monitored with a finger stick and a blood glucose reagent strip. Parenteral insulin, either by continuous intravenous infusion or by intermittent subcutaneous injections, should be administered when necessary to maintain the quantitative urine glucose at the 2% level.

Flow Rate and Volume

The rate of infusion of the hypertonic solution must be constant over a 24-hour period to achieve maximum assimilation of the nutrients and to prevent hyperglycemia or hypoglycemia. One cannot increase the flow rate to compensate for interruptions or slowing of the infusion because glycosuria with osmotic diuresis (diuresis from body compartments and cells leading to dehydration) can occur. Headache, nausea, and lassitude are early symptoms of too rapid an infusion. Too slow an infusion results in the administration of fewer

nutrients, and hypoglycemia with a rebound of insulin may occur.

The aim of treatment is a continuous infusion that meets the caloric requirements of the patient by allowing maximum use of the carbohydrate and protein substrates with minimal renal excretion. The flow rate must be checked faithfully every 30 to 60 minutes. If a slowing does occur (as from an obstruction in the infusion line from a kink in the tubing), an increase of flow not to exceed 10% of the original rate may be instituted to bring the caloric intake back to the desired level. An infusion pump will help ensure continuous accurate infusion. However, because such pumps are mechanical devices subject to malfunctions, the nurse must keep a close watch on the flow rate.

Volume is given according to established water metabolism levels (2500 ml/24 hr in adults and 100 ml/kg/24 hr in infants) and carbohydrate metabolism (0.5 g/kg/hr). The initial intake is 1000 to 2000 ml/24 hours, with a gradual increase according to the patient's tolerance, as established by careful clinical and chemical monitoring. Generally, the maximum daily volume is 3 liters. However, patients undergoing massive catabolism, such as that occurring in severe or extensive burns or severe traumatic injuries, often require 4 to 5 liters/day.

If there is a problem with the integrity of the kidneys or heart, one must carefully calculate fluid volume to prevent cardiopulmonary overload. A special hypertonic solution, nephramine, may be used in this setting. This solution provides the eight essential amino acids in 250 ml and, when diluted with the 500 ml of the hypertonic glucose solution, provides the necessary calories and proteins for 24 hours without an excess of water.

With these severe nutritional deficiencies, in which excess calories are required, the intravenous infusion of lipids in adjunct with the hyperalimentation solution may be employed. The 10% fat emulsion delivers a fat particle comparable to a chylomicron (normally digested fat particle) and provides 1:1 calorie/m of solution. These calories do not require insulin for use by the body; therefore, the danger of hyperinsulinemia or rebound hypoglycemia is eliminated.

Intralipids are isotonic and can be infused in a peripheral line. One can monitor fat clearance from the blood by observing the serum for turbidity 4 to 6 hours post infusion. Tolerance to the infusion of intralipids is very good, and the use of this solution for supplying calories is increasing. As much as 60% of the required caloric intake may be supplied with intralipids.

If the patient is receiving adequate nutrition, his weight gain should be 100 to 300 g/day($\frac{1}{4}$ to $\frac{1}{2}$ lb/day). If he is gaining much more, it is probably due to water retention and not tissue gain, and the volume infused needs to be adjusted downward.

Infusion Sites

Knowing the nature of the hyperalimentation solution, one can easily understand that the usual normal intravenous routes are not used because this hypertonic solution would rapidly cause thrombosis at the tip of the intravenous catheter. Because this high caloric nitrogen solution must be rapidly diluted and dispersed within the blood vessels, the superior vena cava is an excellent site. Figure 31–1 indicates the different routes that can be used. Passage of the intravenous

catheter into the superior vena cava by way of the subclavian vein is the route of choice because it allows the patient the greatest freedom of movement without disturbing the injection site and because the incidence of infection at this level of the body is lower. Jugular veins may be used but are not as comfortable for the patient. Basilic vein routes are too susceptible to irritation and infection for long-term therapy. The femoral vein as a route to the inferior vena cava is rarely selected because it is highly susceptible to contamination from body pathogens, such as abdominal wound drainage, urine, and stool.

Infection Potential

Two key factors are involved in the success of hyperalimentation therapy: (1) the long-term presence of the indwelling catheter directly in the superior vena cava, and (2) the hypertonic solution. Both are prime sites for the source of infection.

Insertion Site. The puncture site is a potential portal of entry of organisms, and the solution is an excellent culture medium for many species of bacteria and fungi. Meticulous asepsis in the care of the line and in the preparation of the solution cannot be overstressed.

Asepsis starts with the insertion of the indwelling catheter. This is performed under strict sterile technique, and a sterile dressing is applied to the site. This

FIGURE 31-1
Venous anatomy for hyperalimentation routes.

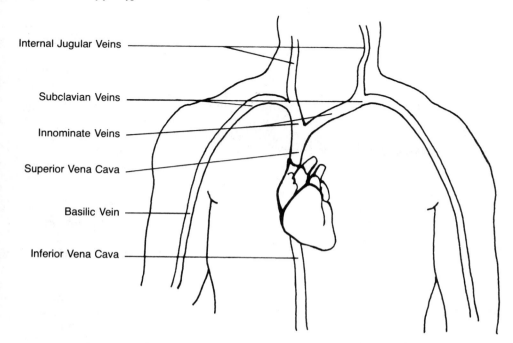

Internal Jugular Veins

Subclavian Veins

Innominate Veins

Superior Vena Cava

Basilic Vein

Inferior Vena Cava

dressing should be changed every 24 to 72 hours. At the time of the dressing change, the site should be examined for signs of leakage, edema, and inflammation, and the catheter should be checked for any kinking of the tube. One should cleanse the skin with a solvent such as acetone to remove surface skin fat that harbors pathogenic organisms and adhesive tape, which, if allowed to accumulate, will cause irritation and skin breakdown. A large area surrounding the catheter is cleansed with an antibacterial solution (*e.g.,* an iodine preparation), and a broad-spectrum antibiotic ointment is applied to the puncture site. An occlusive "op site" dressing is applied over the area. The presence of a tracheostomy or open and draining wounds near the insertion site requires special precautions to maintain sterility of the site. A transparent plastic waterproof surgical drape over the entire dressing will help prevent contamination from fluid or exudates if the op site dressing is not used. With infection control procedures, the sterility of the insertion site can be maintained for the length of the treatment, even if the treatment lasts for months.

Solution Sterility. Maintaining sterility of the solution is mandatory. As already stated, the solution is an excellent culture medium for pathogens. It should be prepared in the pharmacy by a pharmacist. The nurse should combine additives in the solution under a laminar air-flow hood to assure a particle-free environment. If the nurse must add electrolytes and other elements to the base solution, she must be aware of any contamination that may occur from syringes, needles, medication vials, and so forth. A new solution hung every 8 hours (with disposal of any solution left in the container after 8 hours) may be employed. Solutions are inspected for clouding or particular matter when the flow rate is checked every 30 to 60 minutes.

All of the intravenous tubing should be changed every 24 to 72 hours, at the time a new solution is hung. The new tubing, the new solution, and the dressing change should be correlated to take place at the same time. If dressings are changed every 48 to 72 hours and the tubing is changed daily, the indwelling catheter and tubing connection sites should be situated so that a change of tubing does not interfere with the integrity of the dressing. The tubing change is made with the patient in a low Fowler's position or flat in bed to prevent an air embolism from occurring with a deep inspiration.

Drug Administration Precautions. No intravenous push or piggyback medications should be given in the same line as the hyperalimentation solution. No steroids, pressor drugs, antibiotics, or other parenteral drugs are ever added to the base solution because they may interact with the fibrin hydrolysate or with one another, forming a precipitate that would not be visible to the naked eye. In addition, the mixing of drugs (other than the electrolytes) in the solution could necessitate adjusting the flow rate according to their requirements rather than those of the nutritional hypertonic solution. If any intravenous medication or blood transfusions are necessary, an alternate route should be started for their administration. Only the hyperalimentation solution with its electrolyte additives added under aseptic conditions should be administered through the central line. The subclavian catheter should not be used to draw blood samples, either. Any break in the system is an entrance for infection; maintenance of the sterility is of the utmost importance.

The introduction of the three-way subclavian and Hickman catheters has greatly facilitated the care of patients who are receiving hyperalimentation therapy. These catheters provide three separate infusion channels with exits in three different sites in the central vein. Therefore, one channel can be utilized for the hyperalimentation solution, one for intravenous antibiotics and other medications, and one for the infusion or withdrawal of blood.

NURSING ASSESSMENT AND INTERVENTION

Nursing care is based on the patient's individual requirements. The degree of illness may vary from that of the severely burned, critically ill person to that of the postoperative gastrectomy patient who is up and about, progressing satisfactorily. The patient relies on the nurse for management of the hyperalimentation therapy. The goals of nursing care are maintenance of fluid and electrolyte balance fulfillment of nutritional requirements, prevention of infection, and provision of comfort. Interventions required of the nurse include the following:

- Measuring the patient's weight every day at the same time with the same scale.
- Accurately measuring the intake and output to provide a picture of the patient's fluid balance.
- Monitoring blood studies for abnormal glucose and electrolyte levels.
- Monitoring flow rate of solution.
- Observing for signs of solution infiltration and reporting any pain or swelling in the area of the catheter insertion.
- Monitoring vital signs according to the patient's status.
- Monitoring body temperature, reporting an elevation, changing the intravenous tubing and solution if an elevation occurs, culturing discarded tubing and solution, discontinuing therapy (including removing the catheter, if indicated), and

culturing the tip of the catheter at time of removal. An elevated temperature may be due to an allergic reaction to the nutrients, an infection around the catheter, contamination of the fluid or infusion tubing with resulting septicemia, or the person's own disease process.

- Using strict aseptic technique when changing solution, tubing, and dressings.
- Encouraging activity and ambulation to decrease the risks of phlebitis, cardiopulmonary problems, and muscle wasting. Lack of exercise and muscle inactivity also lead to a catabolic state with protein breakdown and excretion.
- Providing psychological support with frequent patient contact and verbal reassurance.

Essential to the fulfillment of the physical, physiological, and psychological needs of the patient is an expert team approach that involves the nurse, the physician, and the pharmacist.

REFERENCES

1. Nutrition in Trauma and Stress — Reference Manual. Minneapolis, Minnesota, The Doyle Pharmaceutical Company, 1980
2. Cahill G: Starvation in man. N Engl J Med 282: 669, 1970
3. Griggs BA: Energy and Protein Requirements in Stress and Trauma. Critical Care Nursing Currents, Ross Laboratories, Vol. 2, No. 2, April–June, 1984
4. Bivins BA, Rosenberg IH, Weinberg RB et al: Balanced Parenteral Nutrition. Chicago, Abbot Laboratories, 1982
5. Goldman DR, Brown FH et al: Medical Care of the Surgical Patient. Philadelphia, JB Lippincott, 1982

BIBLIOGRAPHY

Kaminski Jr: Complications of hyperalimentation during the management of the critically ill. In Summary Proceedings 22nd Annual Symposium on Critical Medicine. Los Angeles, University of California, March, 1984, pp 170–172

Larson: Complications of intravenous therapy. In Summary Proceedings 22nd Annual Symposium on Critical Medicine. Los Angeles, University of California, March, 1984, pp 66–72

O'Keefe SJ et al: The influence of intravenous nutrition on protein dynamics following surgery. Metabolism 30:1150–58, 1981

Priestnal KW et al: Parenteral nutrition by a subclavian line. Nursing Times, January, 1980, pp 78–81

32
Acute Gastrointestinal Bleeding

Helen C. Busby
William Seiffert

PATHOPHYSIOLOGY

Bleeding in the gastrointestinal tract is caused primarily by gastric ulcers or gastritis. However, duodenal ulcers, esophageal varices, carcinoma, ulcerative colitis, polyps, diverticuli, hemorrhoids, and hypercoagulable states can erupt in a bleeding eipsode. Because bleeding that occurs from the lower gastrointestinal tract usually either is not severe enough to warrant the person's admission to a critical care unit or is treated surgically, the following discussion concentrates on upper gastrointestinal tract bleeding.

The appearance of the person presenting with upper gastrointestinal tract bleeding varies considerably, depending on the amount and rapidity of blood loss. Gastrointestinal bleeding that is the result of an erosion through an artery will be profuse and will not stop with medical management. Bleeding that is caused by gastritis or oozing from granulation tissue at the base of an ulcer will be smaller in quantity, transient in nature, and will usually respond to medical management.

Hematemesis. The patient who is vomiting blood is usually bleeding from a source above the ligament of Treitz (at the duodenojejunal junction). Reverse peristalsis is seldom sufficient to cause hematemesis if the bleeding point is below this area. The vomitus may be bright red or coffee-ground in appearance, depending on the amount of gastric contents at the time of the bleeding and the length of time the blood has been in contact with gastric secretions. Gastric acid converts bright red hemoglobin to brown hematin, accounting for the coffee-ground appearance of the drainage.

Bright red blood results from profuse bleeding and little contact with gastric juices.

Melena. Tarry stools will consistently occur in all persons who accumulate 500 ml of blood in their stomach. A tarry stool may be passed if as little as 60 ml of blood has entered the intestinal tract. Massive hemorrhage from the upper gastrointestinal tract, along with the increased intestinal motility that occurs, may result in stools containing bright red blood. It will take several days after the bleeding has stopped for melena stools to clear.

MEDICAL MANAGEMENT

The immediate medical care of the person admitted with gastrointestinal bleeding includes four steps:

1. *Assessing* the severity of the blood loss
2. *Replacing* a sufficient amount of blood to counteract shock
3. *Diagnosing* the cause of bleeding
4. *Planning* a definitive type of treatment

A decision for surgical intervention is based on many factors in the medical history and the physical examination. A person who has repetitive bleeding episodes, a history of a gastric ulcer, or sclerotic blood vessels will likely require surgery as soon as possible.

NURSING PROCESS

The nursing care plan presented in Table 32-1 is an example of the nursing management of a patient who is experiencing an upper gastrointestinal bleed.

TABLE 32-1
NURSING CARE PLAN FOR PATIENT WITH GASTROINTESTINAL BLEEDING

Nursing Diagnosis	Goals	Nursing Intervention
1. Fluid volume deficit related to blood loss. (a) Shock management	• Prevention of shock	• Monitor vital signs frequently. • Administer replacement fluids and blood. • Administer specific therapy to control bleeding. • Measure urine output hourly. • Measure gastric bleeding. • Place patient on complete bedrest. • Provide verbal reassurance. • Provide a calm atmosphere. • Monitor blood studies for abnormal hematology. • Measure intake and output.
(b) Intravenous infusion management	• Maintenance of a patient, stable intravenous route • Prevention of infection • Achievement of patient comfort • Maintenance of fluid and electrolyte balance	• Regulate fluid infusion as indicated. • Monitor system for patency, infiltration, inflammation, and signs of infection. • Use aseptic technique when changing dressings and tubings. • Anchor intravenous appliance and tubing securely. • Monitor fluid and electrolyte balance. • Administer prescribed intravenous medications. • Monitor blood studies for abnormal electrolytes.
(c) Blood transfusion management	• Administration of the correct product at the proper flow rate • Recognization of a transfusion reaction • Minimization of patient anxiety regarding safety of blood transfusion.	• Follow policy and procedure for blood and blood product administration. • Check intravenous line for patency prior to connecting blood or blood product. • Check that product container is correct for the patient. • Monitor vital signs. • Observe for signs and symptoms of transfusion reaction. • Provide verbal reassurance. • Provide frequent patient contact.
(d) Nasogastric tube management	• Maintenance of tube function • Patient comfort • Prevention of damage to the nares	• Irrigate gastric tube with saline to maintain patency. • Check function of drainage system. • Anchor tube securely. • Cleanse nares and change position of tube every 8 hours. • Provide oral hygiene every 4 hours. • Monitor blood studies for abnormal electrolytes.
2. Potential for anxiety related to sight of blood and fear of death	• Prevention of psychological threat	• Demonstrate calmness, competency, and efficiency when performing procedures. • Explain procedures and provide reassurance. • Provide an atmosphere of acceptance. • Attend constantly during potential anxiety-producing procedures. • Encourage expression of feelings. • Listen to patient • Provide quiet, restful environment.
3. Potential for airway obstruction related to placement of Sengstaken-Blakemore tube	• Prevention of airway obstruction	• Provide constant surveillance. • Elevate head of bed. • Place pair of scissors at bedside. Cut entire tube and remove if respiratory distress occurs. • Maintain prescribed pressure in balloons and prescribed traction. • Sedate patient as necessary to keep him at rest. • Restrain patient's arms when he is agitated and restless. • Suction nasopharynx frequently. • Irrigate nasogastric tube to maintain patency of tube. • Cleanse and lubricate nares.

Assessment of Blood Loss and Shock

To assess the severity of blood loss and to prevent or correct deterioration into hypovolemic shock, the nurse must assess the patient frequently. In the first stage of bleeding—less than 500 ml of blood loss—the person may show signs only of weakness, anxiety, and perspiration. Following a significant bleed, the body temperature will elevate to 38.4° to 39°C (101° to 102°F) in response to the bleeding, and bowel sounds will be hyperactive owing to the sensitivity of the bowel to blood.

If the intravascular volume decreases because of continued blood loss, a sympathetic nervous system response will cause a release of the catecholamines, epinephrine and norepinephrine. These will initially cause an increase in heart rate in an attempt to maintain an adequate blood pressure. Following a blood loss of 500 to 1000 ml (1 to 2 pints), the signs and symptoms will begin to present a picture of shock.

As the shock syndrome progresses, the release of catecholamines triggers the blood vessels in the skin, lungs, intestines, liver, and kidneys to constrict, thereby increasing the volume of blood flow to the brain and heart. Because of the decreased flow of blood in the skin, the person's skin will be cool to the touch. With decreased blood flow to the lungs, hyperventilation will occur to maintain adequate gas exchange. As blood flow to the liver decreases, metabolic waste products accumulate in the blood. This, combined with the absorption of decomposed blood from the intestinal tract and a decrease of blood flow through the kidneys, causes an increase in the blood urea level. In fact, the blood urea nitrogen (BUN) may be used to follow the course of a gastrointestinal bleed. A BUN above 40—in the setting of a gastrointestinal bleed and a normal creatinine level—indicates a major bleed. The BUN will return to normal approximately 12 hours after the bleeding has stopped.

An excellent parameter in assessing shock is urinary output, which *must* be measured hourly. As the intravascular volume decreases, urine output decreases owing to the reabsorption of water by the kidneys in response to the release of antidiuretic hormone (ADH) by the posterior lobe of the pituitary gland (see Chapter 21 on the effects of hypovolemic shock on the kidneys).

A drop in the person's blood pressure is an advanced sign of the shock syndrome and indicates that the body's own protective mechanisms have been overwhelmed.

Every nurse must always be alert for changes in this patient's condition. The patient must be monitored closely, assessed with knowledge and skill, his events anticipated, and significant changes reported immediately. The nurse must also allay the fears and apprehension of the patient. The sight of the blood alone is very upsetting to him, as he probably sees it in larger quantities than it really is, and he may well feel that he is going to bleed to death. If the nurse displays competency, efficiency, and the ability to answer his questions satisfactorily, she will provide a calming effect while the necessary procedures are carried out.

Blood Transfusion and Gastric Intubation

The patient admitted with gastrointestinal bleeding needs an immediate intravenous infusion route by means of a large-caliber intracatheter or cannula. Blood is typed and crossmatched, and transfusion treatment is based on the presence of shock as well as on the blood count and blood volume levels. A central venous line may be placed to facilitate monitoring intravascular volume (see Chapter 8 on hemodynamic pressure monitoring).

One may insert a Levin tube into the person's stomach to assist with the diagnosis, to assess the rate of bleeding, to remove irritating gastric secretions, to prevent gastric dilatation, and to lavage with an iced solution to decrease bleeding tendencies by reducing blood flow.

Iced Saline Irrigation. If the person is presenting with hematemesis, the stomach is irrigated with iced saline until the returned solution is clear. It is important to keep accurate records of the amount of fluid used for irrigation so that this fluid can be subtracted from the total amount of aspiration to ascertain the true amount of bleeding.

Another method that may be used to control gastric bleeding is a continuous irrigation of the stomach with iced saline containing levarterenol (Levophed). The usual dilution is two ampules of levarterenol per 1000 ml of normal saline. The principal action of this agent is vasoconstriction. Following absorption in the stomach, levarterenol is immediately sent to the liver by way of the portal system, where metabolism of the drug takes place; thus, a systemic reaction is prevented.

Instillation of Topical Thrombin. If continuous irrigation with iced saline does not decrease the amount of bleeding, the instillation of topical thrombin into the stomach may be ordered. Thrombin clots blood at the site of bleeding by acting directly with fibrinogen. Because of this action, topical thrombin is used only on the surface of bleeding tissue and is never injected into blood vessels where extensive intravascular clotting would result.

The speed with which thrombin clots blood depends on its concentration; for example, 5000 units of topical thrombin in 5 ml of saline is capable of clotting 5 ml of blood in 1 second. One must remember that to clot the site of bleeding in the stomach, the topical thrombin must come in contact with the capillary that is bleeding. This may not be possible; therefore, topical thrombin will not be beneficial in every case of upper gastrointestinal tract bleeding.

The procedure for instillation of topical thrombin is more time consuming than difficult:

1. Aspirate stomach contents and measure.
2. Instill per nasogastric tube 60 ml (2 oz) of a buffer solution and clamp the tube. Dilute acid is detrimental to thrombin activity; therefore, stomach acids must be neutralized prior to administration of thrombin. Milk may be used until the pharmacy can prepare a buffer solution. Because this phosphate buffer solution is stable only for 48 hours, solutions cannot be stored for future use.
3. After 5 minutes, instill another 60 ml of the buffer solution, containing 10,000 units of topical thrombin. Clamp tube.
4. After 30 minutes, aspirate the stomach. If no fresh bleeding is evident, instill 60 ml of the buffer and clamp the tube.
5. Repeat instillation of 60 ml of the buffer solution every 1 to 2 hours for 24 to 48 hours.
6. If bleeding is not controlled after the 30 minutes or if bleeding begins again, repeat steps 1 through 4. Repeat this procedure until bleeding is stopped.
7. Remember to total the aspiration and mark as output. Because the buffer solution is absorbed, mark this amount as intake.

Administration of Pitressin

Intravenous vasopressin (Pitressin) may be instituted, especially if the bleeding is due to esophageal varices or gastritis. This drug lowers portal hypertension and therefore decreases the flow of blood at the site of bleeding. It is sometimes infused by means of selective arterial catheter placement. Pitressin needs to be used with caution because it can cause a hypertensive state. It may also affect the urinary output by its ADH properties.

Correction of a Hypocoagulable State

It is not unusual to find a patient with severe gastrointestinal bleeding who is having a hypocoagulable state that is due to a variety of clotting factor deficiencies. Certainly, one of the foremost problems in this category is liver failure in a patient who is unable to manufacture the factors. Another common clinical situation is one of prolonged intravenous feedings in patients who have been on multiple antibiotics and who are

subsequently vitamin K–deficient. Regardless of the cause, one must correct this situation to try to reduce the amount of bleeding. Vitamin K can be given in the form of phytonadione (AquaMEPHYTON), 10 mg intramuscularly or, very carefully and slowly, intravenously, in an attempt to restore the prothrombin time to normal. If other major factor deficiencies are thought to exist, one can give fresh frozen plasma in order to correct the abnormality.

Sengstaken-Blakemore Tube

Esophageal varices should be suspected in the patient who has been addicted to alcohol and who presents with upper gastrointestinal bleeding. To control the hemorrhage from the varices, pressure is exerted on the cardia of the stomach and against the bleeding varices by a double-balloon tamponade (the Sengstaken-Blakemore tube) (Fig. 32-1).

Once the tube is positioned in the stomach, the stomach balloon is inflated with no more than 50 cc of air. The tube is then slowly withdrawn until the gastric balloon fits snugly against the cardia of the stomach. Once it is determined by radiograph examination that the gastric balloon is in the right place, at the cardia and not in the esophagus, the gastric balloon can be further inflated—up to the desired amount without surpassing the balloon's capacity. Traction is then placed on the tube where it enters the patient and is achieved by means of a piece of sponge rubber, as shown in Figure 32-1. This procedure may be sufficient to control the bleeding if the varices are in the cardia of the stomach. In fact, a Linton tube may be tried before the Sengstaken-Blakemore tube is inserted (Fig. 32-2).

If bleeding continues, the esophageal balloon is inflated to a pressure of 25 to 40 torr and maintained at this pressure for 24 hours. Pressure for longer than 24 hours could cause edema, esophagitis, ulcerations, or perforation of the esophagus.

If bleeding persists after this, traction is applied to the end of the balloon. This may consist of suspending a weight from the end of the tube or putting a football helmet on the patient and securing the tube, under traction, to the face bar.

The potential dangers of this treatment require constant observation and intelligent care. It is essential that the three tube openings be identified, correctly labeled, and checked for patency prior to insertion. The pressures in the balloons must be maintained, and the balloons must be kept in their proper position. If the gastric balloon ruptures, the entire tube may rise into the nasopharynx and completely obstruct the airway. A pair of scissors should be readily available at the bedside. The tube should be cut immediately to deflate the balloons rapidly, and the entire tube should

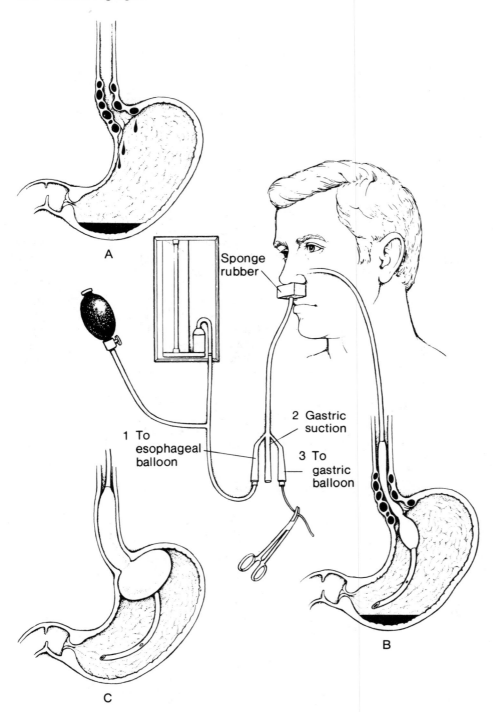

Sponge
rubber

1 To
esophageal
balloon

2 Gastric
suction

3 To
gastric
balloon

A

B

C

FIGURE 32-1
*Diagram showing esophageal varices and their treatment by a compressing balloon tube
(Sengstaken-Blakemore). (A) Dilated veins of the lower esophagus. (B) The tube is in place in
the stomach and the lower esophagus but is not inflated. (C) Inflation of the tube and the
compression of the veins that can be obtained by inflation of the balloon. (Brunner LS,
Suddarth DS: Textbook of Medical-Surgical Nursing, 5th ed. Philadelphia, JB Lippincott, 1984)*

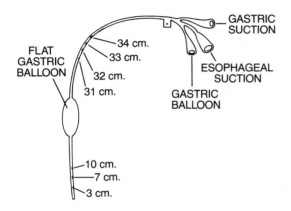

FIGURE 32-2
Linton tube. (Courtesy of Davol, Inc)

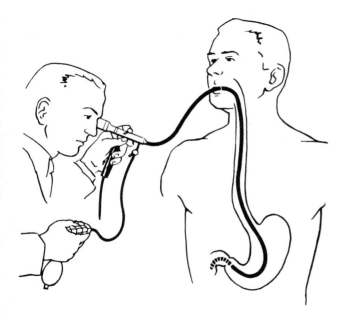

FIGURE 32-3
Patient undergoing gastroscopy. Note the extreme flexibility of the tube with the patient in the sitting position. (Adapted from McNeer G, Pack GT: Neoplasms of the Stomach. Philadelphia, JB Lippincott, 1967)

be removed whenever a question of respiratory insufficiency or aspiration occurs. It is wise to restrain the patient's arms prophylactically if he is agitated and restless to prevent him from dislodging the tube.

Nursing care of a patient with a Sengstaken-Blakemore tube in place involves skillful application of knowledge.

• The person is kept at complete rest because exertion, such as coughing or straining, tends to increase intra-abdominal pressure that predisposes to further bleeding.
• The head of the bed is kept elevated to reduce the flow of blood into the portal system and to prevent reflux into the esophagus.
• Because the person is unable to swallow, saliva must be suctioned frequently from the upper esophagus.
• The nasopharynx also needs frequent suctioning owing to the increased secretions resulting from irritation by the tube. A nasogastric tube may be inserted into the esophagus to the top of the esophageal balloon to control these secretions and to prevent their aspiration into the lungs.
• The nasogastric tube should be irrigated every 2 hours to ensure its patency and to keep the stomach empty.
• The nostrils are checked frequently, cleansed, and lubricated to prevent tube-caused pressure areas.

Persons with liver damage tolerate the breakdown products of blood in the intestinal tract very poorly. Therefore, it is imperative that blood *not be* allowed to remain in the person's stomach because it will migrate into the intestinal tract. Bacterial action on the blood in the intestinal tract produces ammonia, which is absorbed into the bloodstream. The ability of the liver to convert ammonia to urea is impaired, and ammonia intoxication ensues (see Chapter 33).

After the crisis is reversed, surgery for a portal systemic shunt may be indicated. If not, medical management continues.

Reducing Gastric Acid

Because gastric acid is extremely irritating to bleeding sites in the upper gastrointestinal tract, it is necessary to decrease the acidity of the gastric secretions. With the introduction of the drugs cimetidine (Tagamet) and ranitidine hydrochloride (Zantac), it is possible to decrease the production of gastric acid. At a gastric pH of 2, the mechanism for stimulating gastric secretions is totally blocked. Cimetidine raises the gastric pH by inhibiting the action of histamine. A single dose will decrease acid secretion for up to 5 hours. To neutralize the remaining gastric acid, one can give the patient antacids in sufficient quantity and often enough to be effective (*i.e.,* Maalox, 60 ml every 2 hours).

Diagnostic Studies

Diagnostic studies are performed as soon as possible for the purpose of establishing a definite diagnosis.

A prothrombin time is performed to rule out (1) the presence of long-term anticoagulant therapy (which may not immediately be made known in the excitement of admitting a patient during an episode of gastrointestinal bleeding) and (2) liver disease. A prolonged prothrombin time may be indicative of liver disease.

As soon as the person's clinical condition stabilizes, an upper gastrointestinal series or gastroscopy may be performed (Fig. 32-3). Both are of immense value to the physician in deciding definitive treatment.

Summary

Treatment of the upper gastrointestinal bleeding episode is continued until there is no further evidence of active bleeding. The nurse will probably experience many frustrations while caring for such patients; however, constant observation and expert nursing care are essential to both stabilization and a return to wellness.

BIBLIOGRAPHY

Boyer T: Bleeding esophageal varices: differential diagnosis and emergency medical and surgical management. In Summary Proceedings 22nd Annual Symposium on Critical Care and Medicine. Los Angeles, University of California, March, 1984, pp 341–342

Brunner LS, Suddarth DS.: Textbook of Medical-Surgical Nursing, 54th ed. Philadelphia, JB Lippincott, 1984

Given BA, Simmons SJ: Gastroenterology in Clinical Nursing, 3rd ed. St Louis, CV Mosby, 1979

Guyton AC: Basic Human Physiology. Philadelphia, WB Saunders, 1977

Holvey DN (ed): Merck Manual of Diagnosis and Therapy, 13th ed. Rahway, Merck & Co, 1977

Jeejeebhoy KN: Life-threatening gastrointestinal bleeding: differential diagnosis and acute management. In Summary Proceedings 22nd Annual Symposium on Critical Care and Medicine. Los Angeles, University of California, March, 1984, pp 275–278

Jones EA, Schafer DF: Fulminant hepatic failure. In Zakim D, Boyer TD (eds): Hepatology. Philadelphia, WB Saunders, 1982

Macdougall, BRD et al: H_2 Receptor antagonists and antacids in the prevention of acute gastrointestinal hemorrhage in fulminant hepatic failure. Lancet 1:617, 1977

Warren J, et al: Is intravenous administration of branched chain amino acids effective in the treatment of hepatic encephalopathy? A multicenter study. Hepatology 3:475, 1983

Watson, JE: Medical-Surgical Nursing and Related Physiology, 2nd ed. Philadelphia, WB Saunders, 1979

33
Hepatic Failure

Helen C. Busby
William Seiffert

Liver function is essential to life. The production and storage of certain essential elements and the detoxification of many harmful substances occur within the liver. Fortunately, this organ has an exceptional functional ability and regenerative capacity. Liver disease may be acute or chronic, and dysfunction may be reversible or irreversible, depending on the amount of tissue involved and the nature of the insult.

ANATOMY

The liver is the largest glandular organ in the human body. This two-lobed (right and left lobes) organ lies just below the diaphragm, with its greatest portion located to the right side of the body. Its superior (rounded) surface fits into the curve of the diaphragm and is in contact with the anterior wall of the abdominal cavity. The inferior surface is molded over the stomach, the duodenum, the pancreas, the hepatic flexure of the colon, the right kidney, and the right adrenal gland.

In keeping with its function as a gland, the liver removes certain elements from the blood and converts them into forms the body can use. The functional unit of the liver is called a *lobule.* In the tissues surrounding each lobule are found the terminal branches of the portal vein, the hepatic artery, and the bile ducts (see Chap. 29, Fig. 29-11).

The *portal vein* is formed behind the head of the pancreas by the union of the superior mesenteric and the splenic veins. At its entrance to the liver, the portal vein divides into two trunks, which supply both lobes of the liver. The branches of the portal vein then disperse throughout the tissue of the liver and become the interlobular veins as they encircle each lobule. The blood sinusoids then pass toward the center of each lobule, where they unite and form the central veins, which in turn form the sublobular veins, which then become the hepatic veins. The two hepatic veins drain into the inferior vena cava.

The *hepatic artery* supplies the liver with nutrients. This artery, along with the left gastric and splenic arteries, is the terminal branch of the celiac artery. The branches of the hepatic artery within the lobule of the liver form capillaries that communicate with the sinusoids from the interlobular veins.

The *bile ducts,* which carry the bile secreted by the liver cells to the duodenum to aid in the digestion of fats, originate within the liver cells as bile canaliculi. They anastomose to each other and then pass to the periphery of the lobule, where they form the primary bile ducts. These bile ducts from both lobes of the liver then unite to form the hepatic duct. The hepatic duct becomes the common bile duct after its connection with the cystic duct (see Chap. 29, Fig. 29-2).

The *cystic duct* and the *gallbladder* are just an enlargement in the biliary system in which excess bile secretion may be stored. The gallbladder concentrates bile and then empties its contents, by way of the common bile duct, into the duodenum during digestion.

The common bile duct and the main duct from the pancreas usually unite just before the duct enters the lumen of the duodenum. There is often a dilation of the tube after this junction (the ampulla of Vater). The opening of the common bile duct in the duodenum is about 8 to 10 cm from the pylorus.

PHYSIOLOGY

The physiological processes that occur in the liver are multiplex. This is probably due to the extremely high permeability of the cell membranes in the hepatic sinusoids and to the large volume of blood that is exposed to these sinusoids. In this area, the large protein molecule diffuses almost as easily as the smaller fluid molecule; thus, a rapid exchange of substances between blood and liver cells occurs.

A vast array of biochemical reactions that are vital for continuation of the metabolic process occur in the liver. We will not undertake the explanation of these chemical reactions but rather will concentrate on four major functions of the liver that we have labeled (1) storage and distribution, (2) conversion, (3) secretion, and (4) detoxification.

Storage and Distribution

The liver very efficiently stores essential elements needed by the body and releases them according to bodily needs. In addition to storing glucose and protein, the liver stores trace metals such as iron and copper and the vitamins B_{12}, A, D, and many of the B-complex group.

Whenever we think of vitamins that are concerned with the liver, we must include vitamin K. Although vitamin K is not stored in the liver, it is closely related to liver function. This fat-soluble vitamin is absorbed from the intestinal tract, and adequate absorption is dependent upon the liver's ability to secrete bile into the intestinal tract. More importantly, vitamin K is a vital coenzyme in the liver's ability to produce the plasma proteins: prothrombin and Factors IX and X. These two proteins are necessary for blood coagulation (see Chap. 12).

The liver plays a major role in replenishing the blood's supply of glucose when the blood concentration falls below normal. Liver cells are highly permeable to glucose (digested carbohydrate) and will absorb 75% of all excess glucose entering the blood. This is accomplished by the enzyme glucokinase, which accelerates the rate of glucose uptake by the liver cell. Glucokinase production is regulated by levels of insulin in the bloodstream. The absorbed glucose is stored in the liver as glycogen.

The liver is the largest storehouse for amino acids in the body. The amino acids derived from protein digestion travel to the liver by way of the portal vein. Intracellular enzymes in the parenchymal cells of the liver convert the excess amino acids into cellular proteins. These proteins are then stored in the liver and released as needed to maintain equilibrium between the body's cellular and plasma proteins. The rate at which the liver converts its cellular proteins into plasma proteins depends on metabolic needs. In the normal body, approximately 30 g of stored protein are used every day. However, if large amounts of plasma proteins are being lost, as in severe burns, the liver can increase its production of plasma proteins to as much as 4 g/hour, or 100 g/day.

Conversion

The liver plays an active role in the conversion of carbohydrates, proteins, and fatty acids into energy. Energy is required for all chemical reactions to occur. The compound adenosine triphosphate (ATP) is the basic source of energy at the cellular level. The energy released from the metabolism of carbohydrates, proteins, and fatty acids is eventually oxidized into ATP. All three nutrients are progressively degraded to acetylcoenzyme A (acetyl-CoA), which is further degraded to ATP, CO_2, and H_2O. ATP contains high-energy phosphate bonds that when hydralized provide the energy for cellular work (secretory processes, muscle contraction, nerve conduction, etc.). The supply of these nutrients into the body depends on a functioning liver.

Glucose. Glucose is the end product of digested carbohydrates and is the main source of energy for the body. The liver closely monitors the level of glucose in the bloodstream and releases stored glucose as necessary to maintain a normal blood level. When the concentration of blood glucose falls below normal, the concentration of blood insulin also falls. The low blood level of insulin has an inhibitory effect on glycogenesis, allowing glucose to remain in the bloodstream.

If this action alone is not sufficient to raise the blood glucose level to normal, the glycogen stored in the liver is converted back into glucose by the enzyme glucose 6-phosphatase and released into the bloodstream. Glucose 6-phosphatase is activated by blood levels of epinephrine and glucagon. The liver can also increase blood glucose concentration by the process of gluconeogenesis, which is conversion of certain amino acids into glucose.

Protein. The end product of protein digestion circulates in the blood as amino acids. These amino acids are resynthesized by the liver to form the three major plasma proteins: albumin, fibrinogen, and the globulins. *Albumin* is necessary to maintain the colloid osmotic pressure throughout the body, thereby preventing excess loss of fluid from blood capillaries. *Fibrinogen* is necessary in the coagulation process, and the *globulins* are necessary for the formation of antibodies. Of these three major plasma proteins, the liver produces all the body's albumin and fibrinogen and 50% of the body's globulins. In addition, the liver, with the help of vitamin K, synthesizes all the body's prothrombin and blood factors V, VII, IX, and X which are essential to the activation of fibrinogen.

Fatty Acid. When cellular and plasma proteins are in equilibrium and the protein storage cells are saturated, certain amino acids are degraded by the body and stored as fat. These amino acids are ketogenic, and when the amine radical is split from the carbon skeleton in the degradation process, ammonia is released (deamination). The liver converts this ammonia into urea and releases it into the bloodstream. It is then secreted into the urine by the kidneys. The fatty acids that remain after deamination are synthesized into triglycerides.

Triglycerides, phospholipids, and cholesterol are the principal lipids, or fats, of the body. A large portion of the triglycerides, most of the phospholipids, and essentially all of the cholesterol are formed in the liver. *Triglycerides* are composed of one, two, or three fatty acid molecules bound to one glycerol molecule. Triglycerides become the body's source of energy when glucose is not available. After the initial breakdown of the triglyceride molecule to fatty acids and glycerol, the liver degrades the fatty acid molecule to acetyl CoA. The final conversion to ATP, CO_2, and H_2O follows the same pathway as acetyl CoA derived from the metabolism of glucose.

Phospholipids are complex triglyceride compounds. They are a component of the myelin sheath and are used in the formation of thromboplastin, in chemical reactions requiring the phosphate radical, and in the formation of elements necessary for the structure of cells.

Cholesterol is a sterol formed from the degradation products of a fatty acid and is the main component of bile. It is an important element in maintaining the permeability of cell membranes throughout the body and in forming certain steroid hormones such as aldosterone and cortisol.

Secretion

The only substance actually secreted by the liver is bile. The bile solution contains bile salts, cholesterol, bilirubin, fatty acids, and plasma electrolytes. The secretion occurs in the canaliculi of the lobule and produces about 1000 ml of bile per day. Hepatic bile is diverted into the gallbladder, where water and electrolytes are reabsorbed. The final solution of bile in the gallbladder is five to ten times more concentrated than that originally secreted by the liver. The bile is stored in the gallbladder and is emptied into the intestine whenever the gallbladder muscle is stimulated to contract by the hormone cholecystokinin. Cholecysto-

kinin is released from the intestinal mucosa following the ingestion of fat into the intestine.

Bile salts are formed from bile acids that occur in the liver during the degradation of fatty acids. The bile salts create a detergent effect on the fat globules in the intestine, which causes them to break up into small globules that are more easily attacked by the fat-splitting enzymes. More importantly, bile salts increase the solubility of the digested fats, thereby allowing their passage through the intestinal wall. If bile salts are absent, the fat globules are excreted in the stool, and a metabolic deficit of lipids will occur. The bile salts themselves are mostly reabsorbed along with the fat and recirculated through the liver and into the bile. A small amount of bile salt is lost in the feces, but the liver will replace this.

Cholesterol in the bile is probably due to the fact that it is a by-product of bile salt secretion; its presence in bile performs no known function. Normally insoluble in water, cholesterol is held in solution in the bile by the hydrotropic action of the fatty acids and the bile salts. Under abnormal conditions it may precipitate and form gallstones. The amount of cholesterol present in bile depends on the amount of cholesterol in the diet. The more cholesterol ingested, the higher the concentration of it in bile. The cholesterol in solution is readily reabsorbed from the intestinal tract.

Bilirubin is the end product of metabolism of the heme portion of the hemoglobin molecule. When worn out or defective erythrocytes are phagocytized, the resultant bilirubin attaches itself to a plasma protein, mainly albumin. This bilirubin circulates in the plasma until it comes in contact with a liver cell that absorbs it; separates it from its protein; conjugates (joins) it with glucuronic acid, which makes it highly soluble; and secretes it into a bile canaliculus. When the bile is in transit through the intestines, the bilirubin glucuronide is converted into urobilinogen by intestinal bacteria. Most of this urobilinogen makes its exit from the body in the feces. Some urobilinogen is reabsorbed into the bloodstream, and some of this is excreted by the kidneys into the urine. The remaining urobilinogen is reconverted by liver cells back into bilirubin and secreted in the bile.

Detoxification

The detoxification process that occurs in the liver protects the body from many harmful substances that enter the bloodstream. Each sinusoid of the liver is lined with a layer of reticulum cells called *Kupffer's cells*. These phagocytic cells are very efficient in digesting bacteria, viruses, and other foreign matter that are brought to them by the blood flow. They are also capable of forming antibodies against the invader, if necessary. These cells are particularly important because they destroy bacteria that are constantly entering the portal blood flow directly from the gastrointestinal tract. Over 99% of the bacteria entering the body in this manner are destroyed before they can do any harm. The Kupffer's cells also destroy other particulate matter in the bloodstream (*i.e.,* worn-out red blood cells).

The liver also absorbs most drugs that enter the bloodstream. Because the liver is the body's center for chemical reactions, it is not surprising that drugs entering the liver will be modified and excreted in a different form. There are several mechanisms by which the liver accomplishes this process, including oxidation reduction, hydroxylation, sulfoxidation, deamination, and dealkylination. By these processes, many substances can be altered in such a way that they may be either utilized by the body in the altered state or excreted in a variety of intermediate forms. In addition to this, conjugation reactions occur that produce water-soluble derivatives that can be more easily excreted in the bile and urine. The time required for the drug to be cleared from the bloodstream depends upon the rate of blood flow through the liver and the absorption efficiency of the liver cells.

It is crucial for the nurse to remember the role of the liver in drug metabolism. If the patient has significant liver disease, impaired drug metabolism may result, and, subsequently, reduced doses of many medications may be required. This is especially true with morphine derivatives, barbiturates, and sedatives. These medications should be used with extreme caution in patients with liver disease because reduced detoxification processes can lead to significant buildup of the drug within the body.

PATHOPHYSIOLOGY

As previously discussed, the liver is made up of four major components: the parenchyma, Kupffer's cells, bile ducts, and blood vessels. All are suspended in a fibrous stroma. Disease processes can affect these components and, if severe enough, can lead to liver failure. Knowledge of the pathophysiology creating the clinical situations helps the nurse care for persons with liver disease.

Hepatitis

Diffuse inflammation of the liver (hepatitis) can be caused by infections from viruses and by toxic reactions from drugs and chemicals. When this occurs, the parenchymal cells are injured, and various intracellular enzymes called *transaminases* are released into the blood. The most common of these transaminases are the serum glutamic-oxaloacetic transaminase (SGOT) and serum glutamic-pyruvic transaminase

(SGPT). Obviously, if enough liver cells are injured, the important metabolic and detoxifying processes of the liver are lost.

The viral infections of the liver parenchyma have been classified according to their specific infecting agent. There are three types of acute viral hepatitis: A, B, and non A–non B.

Type A Hepatitis. Type A, often referred to as *infectious hepatitis,* is transmitted by the fecal–oral route. It has a high prevalence in low socioeconomic regions. It can be epidemic in nature, and shellfish are often implicated in its transmission. The clinical course of type A hepatitis usually runs 1 to 3 months. Recovery is usually complete and does not lead to chronic hepatitis or cirrhosis. However, in rare instances type A hepatitis may lead to fulminating liver failure.

The diagnosis of type A hepatitis is made by observation of high transaminase levels (Table 33-1) and the presence of rising hepatitis A antibody (anti-HAV) in the serum. It is important to note that by the time the patient presents with symptoms of hepatitis, he is no longer shedding the virus in his stool and is generally not infective.

Type B Hepatitis. Type B hepatitis is usually spread by a parenteral route. Some of the more common mechanisms of transmission are blood transfusions, needle-stick accidents in medical personnel, and the use of contaminated needles by drug addicts. However, there are a significant number of patients who contract type B hepatitis from nonparenteral routes. The antigen has been identified in body secretions such as semen, mucus, and saliva, and exposure to a person with type B hepatitis can result in infection. There is a high incidence of type B hepatitis among male homosexuals. It appears that a break in the skin or the mucous membrane is necessary for the transmission to occur.

There are three antigens identified with type B hepatitis: surface antigen, core antigen, and E antigen.

Hepatitis B surface antigen (HBSAG) is the first antigen to rise in the patient's blood and is usually present at the time the transaminase levels are rising. As the patient improves, the transaminase levels and the level of HBSAG decrease. Chronic active hepatitis is seen in 10% of the patients who have type B hepatitis. They continue to have levels of HBSAG and can be infective to others. The degree of liver impairment in chronic active hepatitis is variable from mild to serious and can progress to cirrhosis. This type of hepatitis is the leading cause of fulminant liver failure and is implicated in approximately 60% of all cases. Usually, as the patient's clinical condition improves, the surface antigen titer falls, and the antibody to the surface antigen rises. Because of a persisting antigen-antibody re-

TABLE 33-1
LIVER FUNCTION TESTS

Tests	Normal Values	Comments
Protein Studies	*g/100 ml*	
Total (Serum)	6.5–8	
Albumin	4–5.5	Albumin is a major part of total blood proteins. It is important in the maintenance of osmotic pressure between blood and tissue.
Globulins	2–3	Globulins are needed for the production of antibodies as well as helping maintain osmotic pressure.
Fibrinogen	0.2–0.4	Fibrinogen is necessary in the coagulation process.
Electrophoresis	*Percent of 100% total protein*	
Albumin	53%	Electrophoresis separates the various protein fractions by an
Alpha globulins	14%	electric current. In parenchymal liver cell disease, the
Beta globulins	12%	amounts of serum proteins will be depressed, or the ratio of
Gamma globulins	20%	the proteins to each other will be altered.
Prothrombin Time	12–15 seconds	Prothrombin is synthesized to thrombin (in the absence of vitamin K) by the liver. This test is a good index of prognosis, as a prolonged pro-time is indicative of severe functional loss.
Enzyme Studies		
SGOT	10–40 units	Transaminases are a catalyst in the breakdown of amino acids.
SGPT	5–35 units	SGPT is the specific enzyme released by damaged liver cells.
LDH	165–300 units	LDH is present in large amounts in liver tissue.
Alkaline phosphatase	2–5 Bodansky units	This enzyme hydrolyzes phosphate esters and is useful in differential diagnosis if jaundice is present. It is excreted through the biliary tract. If it is elevated, nucleotidase and leucine amino peptidase will determine whether elevation is due to biliary obstruction.
Gamma glutamyle transferase	0–30 IU	Endothelia enzyme is found in the liver and closely follows elevations in alkaline phosphatase.
Bilirubin		
Total	0.9–2.2 mg/100 ml (0.8 mg/dl)	This test measures the ability of the liver to conjugate and
Conjugated (direct)	0.5–1.4 mg/100 ml (0.6 mg/dl)	excrete bilirubin. If the conjugated bilirubin is low and the
Unconjugated (indirect)	0.4–0.8 mg/100 ml (0.2 mg/dl)	unconjugated high, a preliver block is indicated. If the conjugated bilirubin is high and the unconjugated normal or low, a postliver block is indicated.
Isotope Liver Scans		Isotope scanning of the liver helps define liver cell function and replacement of active liver cells with nonfunctioning tissue, such as scar tissue secondary to cirrhosis, tumors, and abscesses.
CT Liver Scanning		CT scanning is an adjunct that helps define space-occupying lesions within the liver, such as tumors and abscesses. It may be more specific for the finding of tumors and less helpful than the isotope scanning in the determination of liver cell function.

action taking place, these patients may develop an immune complex disease such as glomerulonephritis.

E antigen may be very helpful in determining who is the most infective. Patients with high E antigen tend to be much more infective than those with high antibody to E antigen. Patients with E antigens usually have very active liver disease, which may be either acute or chronic. Those with high antibody to E antigen may have a tendency to be carriers for a long time.

Core antigen and core antibody titers are becoming more useful as they become more readily available to the practitioner. Core antibody titers may in fact be helpful in determining a previous infection with type B hepatitis after the surface antigen has become negative.

Non A – Non B Hepatitis. The third type of hepatitis is designated *non A – non B hepatitis.* When type A and type B hepatitis have been ruled out by the various blood tests and the patient has an acute episode of hepatitis, especially following blood transfusions, non A–non B hepatitis is the most likely diagnosis. There are no specific tests for this, and it often becomes a diagnosis of exclusion. Its transmission and clinical course are similar to type B hepatitis. However, patients with non A–non B hepatitis tend to develop chronic hepatitis with a greater frequency than patients with type B hepatitis. A significant percentage of patients with non A–non B hepatitis develop fulminant hepatitis, but the percentage is somewhat less than patients with type B hepatitis.

Drug-Induced Hepatitis. The picture of viral hepatitis can be mimicked both clinically and pathologically by a drug-induced hepatitis. This actually results from a toxic reaction to the liver cells from either the drug itself or one of its metabolites.

The major drugs involved in toxic reactions include the halogenated anesthetic agents such as halothane, the antihypertensive medication methyldopa, the antituberculous medication isoniazid, and the phenytoins such as phenytoin (Dilantin). Most of these medications cause their toxicity through intermediate metabolites of the drug and rarely by their direct effect on the hepatocytes. There also may be a hypersensitivity reaction to the drug or to one of its metabolites. Acetaminophen and aspirin are other medications that can cause some degree of hepatic toxicity. The acetaminophen toxicity can be overwhelming and fatal owing to the toxic effect of its metabolites on the liver cells (see Chap. 36).

"Fatty Liver"

Toxic effects on the liver, or multiple nutritional deficiencies in the diet, may cause an increase in fat accumulation within the parenchymal cells. The net result is an enlarged liver referred to as *fatty metamorphosis,* or a *fatty liver.* The cause of the fatty changes in the parenchymal cells is unclear, but it may be a response to alterations in enzymatic function responsible for normal fat metabolism.

Alcoholism. One of the more classic examples of fatty infiltration of the liver, and subsequent hepatitis, is seen with alcohol ingestion. Initially, the response of the liver to alcohol ingestion is one of fatty metamorphosis. If the alcohol ingestion is discontinued, the fatty metamorphosis decreases and the liver normalizes. This happens in nutritionally deficient, as well as in nutritionally normal, patients. However, if the alcohol ingestion continues, further toxic effects occur, leading to necrosis of liver cells. Interestingly enough, this necrosis occurs around the central vein

rather than the portal triads as seen in viral hepatitis and other toxic reactions.

The patient with alcoholic hepatitis also shows elevated transaminase levels. His prothrombin time may also begin to elevate, and he may have a very low albumin due to significant loss of liver function (see Table 33-1). The loss of function may progress to cirrhosis as long as the toxic effect of alcohol is present, and this may eventually lead to liver failure.

The exact nature of the toxic effect of alcohol is unknown, but it appears to be related to the quantity of alcohol ingestion over a significant period of time. Other factors, such as nutrition, do not seem to play a part. It has been reported that the alcohol may induce immunologic response with a secondary inflammatory reaction. Continued exposure to the alcohol simply prolongs and propagates this immune response with its attendant inflammatory reaction.

Other Liver Disorders and Symptoms

Jaundice. Jaundice is often the presenting clinical sign of liver disease. It can occur from the liver cells' inability to excrete bile (intrahepatic cholestasis) or from obstruction of the bile ducts (obstructive jaundice). Drugs and sepsis are often implicated in intrahepatic cholestasis, whereas stones and tumors may cause obstructive jaundice.

Tumors. The liver parenchyma can be disrupted extensively by either primary tumors, such as hepatomas, or by metastatic tumors. This extensive replacement of liver tissue can lead to hepatic failure. Remaining hepatocytes are unable to carry on normal metabolic processes, and hypoprothrombinemia and hypoproteinemia often result. These patients may also present with severe obstructive jaundice due to tumor infiltration and subsequent compression of the bile ducts.

Arterial Insufficiency. Blood flow to the liver generally protects the hepatocytes from anoxic injury. Portal venous blood has a high oxygen concentration and, coupled with the arterial supply, provides good protection against anoxic injury. However, in the event of traumatic or surgically induced arterial insufficiency, previously injured hepatocytes are extremely susceptible to anoxic insults.

With progressive inflammatory injury to the parenchyma, the normal architecture of the liver becomes deranged by fibrous bands of scar tissue. In between these bands of fibrous tissue are regenerating liver cells. The result of this architectural derangement is impaired blood flow to the sinusoids of the liver. The portal blood is unable to flow through the liver; thus, portal vein pressures rise. With sufficient back pres-

TABLE 33-2
NURSING CARE PLAN FOR THE PATIENT WITH HEPATIC FAILURE

Nursing Diagnosis	Goals	Nursing Intervention
Potential for Fluid and Electrolyte Imbalance* This problem may be related to replacement therapy, malnutrition, gastric suctioning, paracentesis, diuretics to reduce water retention, vomiting, diaphoresis, inadequate fluid intake, elevated aldosterone levels, and diarrhea induced by enemas, laxatives and antibiotics. The patient may complain of headache, weakness, numbness and tingling of extremities, muscle twitching, thirst, nausea, muscle cramps, and confusion. The nurse may observe an increase or decrease in urinary output, profuse perspiration, prolonged vomiting, frequent liquid stools, poor skin turgor, muscle tremors or spasms, edema, irritability, changes in mental status, stupor, coma, and cardiac arrhythmias. The patient relies on the nurse for patency of the infusion line, correct administration of intravenous fluids and medications, supervision of flow rate, and prevention of infection.	Maintenance of fluid and electrolyte balance and prevention of physical harm and infection	Accurately measure intake and output, monitor vital signs, monitor blood studies for abnormal findings, measure body weight every day, inspect for dryness of mucous membranes and subcutaneous edema, and administer replacement therapy. Maintain a large, stable intravenous line, regulate flow rate of infusions, check patency of line, maintain sterility of the system, observe site for inflammation and infiltration, and change intravenous sites as indicated.
Potential for Infection This diagnosis may result from the general state of poor health, which lowers body resistance.	Maintenance of nutrition to all cells, promotion of rest, achievement of good hygiene, and prevention of infection	Provide hygiene, provide periods of rest, monitor vital signs, assess nutritional needs, observe aseptic technique when performing procedures, and administer antibiotics as ordered.
Potential for Impaired Gas Exchange This problem is related to generalized weakness, prolonged bed rest, prolonged immobility, and lethargy.	Maintenance of an oxygen supply to all cells and prevention of pulmonary disturbances	Change the patient's position frequently, encourage coughing and deep breathing, suction the airway as needed, provide respiratory exercises such as the use of an inspiratory spirometer, request adjunct Ventilatory therapy when indicated, administer oxygen as indicated, assess lung sounds, monitor vital signs, monitor blood gas values, and assess for cyanosis and dyspnea.
Potential for Impaired Tissue Perfusion and Skin Breakdown This diagnosis is related to prolonged bedrest, immobility, subcutaneous edema, and poor nutrition.	Improvement of circulation and prevention of decubitus ulcers	Change the patient's position, keep the skin clean and dry, maintain a dry, wrinkle-free bed, provide range of motion exercises, provide frequent massage to bony prominences, use an antipressure mattress, prevent skin irritation (from tape, excessive pressure, powder granules, foreign objects, drainage, etc.) ambulate the patient as indicated, and provide nutritional requirements.
Self-Care Deficit and Alteration in Oral Mucous Membranes This problem is related to the debilitation caused by the disease state. The patient relies on the nurse for a bath, hair care, mouth care, and skin care.	Achievement of good hygiene and comfort	Anticipate the patient's needs, brush teeth, clean dentures, brush hair, remove thick oral secretions, lubricate lips and skin, and provide privacy, warmth, cleansing baths, and mouth rinses.

(Continued)

TABLE 33-2
(Continued)

Nursing Diagnosis	Goals	Nursing Intervention
Potential for Drug Intoxication This diagnosis is related to the diseased liver's inability to detoxify drugs.	Prevention of drug intoxication	Observe for signs and symptoms of a cumulative drug reaction from drugs the patient is receiving; use physical restraint rather than sedation whenever possible.
Potential for Complications Related to Drug Therapy This problem is related to the patient's reliance on the nurse to provide the correct drugs in the appropriate doses at specific times, to observe drug side effects, and to prevent overdosage.	Prevention of patient dependence	Administer medications as prescribed and assess for cumulative effects, side effects, and adverse reactions.
Potential for Bleeding This diagnosis is related to deficiencies of clotting factors.	Prevention of loss of blood volume	Assess for signs of bleeding, test stool, examine urine and nasogastric drainage for the presence of blood, administer clotting factors as prescribed, monitor coagulation studies, estimate blood volume loss, and monitor vital signs.
Alteration in Neurologic Status This condition is related to hepatic encephalopathy.	Lowering of the level of ammonia in the blood in order to prevent progression of neurologic changes	Cleanse the bowel with strong cathartics and high colonic enemas, maintain an empty bowel with nasogastric suctioning, administer oral, nonabsorbable antibiotics such as neomycin to lower the bacterial count in the colon, administer lactulose (Cephulac) to decrease the intestinal pH and increase ammonia excretion, and observe for asterixis ("liver flap"), loss of spatial orientation, and apraxia (inability to write).
Emotional Shock This diagnosis may be related to intense anxiety, nightmares, thought disorganization, and poor concentration ability.	Promotion of comfort, rest, sleep, and relaxation; prevention of emotional injury	Acknowledge and accept a temporary period of dependency, restrict visitors, establish routines, allow choices whenever possible, decrease sensory overload, encourage use of the patient's family's strengths, involve and support the family, establish therapeutic communication, and provide a calm, unhurried approach, an atmosphere of acceptance, verbal reassurance, frequent patient contact, and rest periods.
Skin Discomfort This condition is due to excessive bilirubin pigments in the blood that infiltrate and irritate the skin.	Provision of comfort by decreasing dryness and itching of the skin	Bathe the skin with cool water, maintain a cool environment, maintain fluid intake, lubricate the skin, and apply antipruritic medication as indicated.

sure on the portal system, collateral circulation develops and allows blood flow to go from the intestines directly to the vena cava. The increased blood flow to the veins of the esophagus leads to esophageal varices; of the spleen, splenomegaly; of the hemorrhoidal veins, hemorrhoids.

Ascites. Another consequence of portal and sinusoidal hypertension is ascites. This entity represents a large collection of hepatic lymph within the abdominal cavity. In patients with portal hypertension, the production of hepatic lymph is increased and frequently is produced at a greater rate than can be reabsorbed by the thoracic duct. Two other factors are involved in the formation of ascites:

1. Elevated venous pressures in the portal system increase the transudation of fluid into the abdomen. This is often potentiated by hypoproteinemia, which causes a decreased osmotic pressure in the blood.
2. Elevated aldosterone levels increase sodium retention, and this tends to aggravate ascites and edema.

Hepatic Failure.   When extensive damage to the liver parenchyma occurs, regardless of its etiology, the patient may develop hepatic failure. These patients may present with high fevers and severe abdominal pain. Their liver cells often necrose to such an extent that the liver shrinks in size. Hepatic encephalopathy may develop, and drowsiness, irritability, confusion, and finally stupor and coma may be seen. Laboratory studies often reveal elevated prothrombin times and elevated blood ammonia levels. Such patients may also be significantly hypoglycemic owing to loss of the liver's crucial role in glucose metabolism.

The hypoglycemia may well add to the neurologic signs of delirium and confusion—seizures may even occur. Decreased clotting factor production may lead to a disseminated intravascular coagulopathy (DIC) (see Chap. 12).

An interesting phenomenon called *hepatorenal syndrome* also may develop in fulminant liver failure. In this entity, the kidneys no longer function, and the patient becomes uremic. There is an oliguric renal failure. However, the kidney morphology is normal, and if these kidneys are transplanted into a person with a normal liver, they begin to function immediately and normally.

Hepatic Encephalopathy.   Patients with severe liver disease may progress to hepatic encephalopathy. Clinically, they start with a quiet delirium or stupor and then may progress to profound coma. Sometimes they become very agitated and difficult to manage. Often they have a characteristic hyperventilation syndrome with a respiratory alkalosis.

The etiology of the hepatic encephalopathy and the hyperventilation syndrome is probably related to toxic agents absorbed from the intestinal tract. Elevated serum ammonia and some amino acids have been implicated as these agents. The amino acids may act as false neurotransmitters and contribute to the encephalopathic state.

Those with portal systemic shunts may develop hepatic encephalopathy quite rapidly, and they often hemorrhage from esophageal varices or other sites in their gastrointestinal tract. The hemorrhage produces a significant nitrogenous load to the intestinal tract in the form of blood, in which bacterial deamination produces the ammonia. Normally, this ammonia is detoxified to urea by the liver. When the liver is unable to perform this detoxification or when a good portion of the portal blood is shunted around the liver, the circulating level of ammonia rises. If ammonia and the other toxic agents can be reduced through effective therapy, the encephalopathy will gradually clear.

MANAGEMENT

The liver cells have a remarkable capacity for regeneration following injury. There is very little that can be done therapeutically to enhance this natural healing process. In general, patients with liver disease require careful supportive care during their illness and recovery, and care of the patient with severe liver disease often becomes the responsibility of the critical care nurse. These patients require careful attention and nursing care that is based on sound judgment because they often arrive in some state of unconsciousness. The skin and sclera will be jaundiced. Coagulation times will be prolonged, and bleeding is apt to occur from many sources. Mild sores, if not present, may develop owing to the debilitated state of the patient.

Treatment of these patients consists of the following:

- Maintaining those bodily functions not impaired by the disease (*i.e.,* respirations)
- Intervening when assistance is required to maintain specific function (*i.e.,* fluid balance)
- Taking over the function of those systems in which failure may be complete (*i.e.,* replacement of clotting factors)

NURSING PROCESS

Nursing care of the patient with hepatic failure is determined by a careful assessment that includes a nursing history, a physical examination, laboratory results, and the medical regimen. The plan of care must consider fluid and dietary requirements, replacement therapy, prevention of infection, caution in drug administration, potential for bleeding disorders, potential for neurologic changes, possible bowel cleansing requirements, and prevention of respiratory, circulatory, and skin complications. The nurse must continuously assess her interventions to evaluate their effectiveness. The plan of care should be changed whenever interventions are no longer necessary or effective or when new problems arise requiring new interventions. We have included nursing diagnoses, goals, and interventions in Table 33-2 as a guide to planning the care for a patient with hepatic failure.

Recovery from hepatic failure is neither rapid nor easily accomplished. There are frequent setbacks and periods of no apparent improvement. The nursing staff must receive support so that they can deal effectively with the frustrations and intensity of the required care. Survival for the patient with hepatic failure greatly depends on optimal nursing and medical management.

BIBLIOGRAPHY

Beeson PB, McDermott W, Wyngaarden JB: Cecil Textbook of Medicine. Philadelphia, WB Saunders, 1979

Boyer JL et al: Patient care goes to a liver symposium. Patient Care 13, No. 18–19, 1979; 14, No. 4, 1980

Boyer T: Acute (infectious) hepatitis: an update including immunization and delta agent. In Summary Proceedings, 22nd Annual Symposium on Critical Care Medicine. Los Angeles, University of California, March, 1984

Boyer T: Management of acute hepatic failure and hepatic coma: facts and fantasies. In Summary Proceedings, 22nd Annual Symposium on Critical Care Medicine. Los Angeles, University of California, March, 1984

Brunner LS, Suddarth DS: Textbook of Medical-Surgical Nursing, 5th ed. Philadelphia, JB Lippincott, 1984

Campbell C: Nursing Diagnosis and Intervention in Nursing Practice. New York, John Wiley & Sons, 1978

Fredette S: When the liver fails. Am J Nurs 84, No. 1, 64–67, 1984

Guyton AC: Basic Human Physiology. Philadelphia, WB Saunders, 1977

34
Normal Structure and Function of the Endocrine System

Barbara Brockway-Fuller

Communications between subsystems in the body are accomplished by way of three modalities. One is the nervous system, which is discussed in Unit 4. Another is the cellular secretions of chemicals that are locally contributed in interstitial fluid. Examples of such chemicals include those that trigger a local inflammatory response and prostaglandins. The third modality is the cellular secretion of chemicals that are circulated through the bloodstream. This last modality of communication is known more commonly as the *endocrine system*. The secretions of endocrine cells are termed *hormones*.

Until the mid 1950s, the boundary between the endocrine and nervous system was quite clear. Then, with the discovery of hypothalamic neurons that secreted blood-borne chemicals, the line of demarcation between these blurred. Now, hormones identical with these produced by established endocrine glands (*e.g.,* insulin, ACTH, and CCK-PZ) are known to be secreted by various other parts of the brain, where it is postulated they may function as neurotransmitters. Table 34-1 lists the more commonly recognized endocrine glands and their secretions. This chapter, however, will consider only those major glands whose pathology can provoke crisis situations relevant to critical care nursing (*e.g.,* water intoxication, hypertensive crises, hypocalcemic tetany, thyroid storm, addisonian crisis, and diabetic ketoacidosis).

As a preface to the discussion of individual glands, let us review commonalities regarding hormone production, secretion, transport, metabolism, and modality of action. Basic principles concerning all but the last of these are illustrated in Figure 34-1. From this we see that the level of hormonal activity in the body depends on the relation between production and degradation. In the case of a protein-bound hormone (*e.g.,* thyroid hormones and cortisol), the level of activity also depends on the level of free as opposed to bound plasma hormone. Hormones act on target cells in one of three ways. They may act to increase intracellular levels of cyclic AMP, which in turn acts as a second messenger within the cell to produce the hormonally triggered response of the target cell. Examples of hormones that increase cyclic AMP are calcitonin, adrenocorticotropic hormone, glucagon, catecholamines bound to beta receptors, parathormone, vasopressin, and thyroid-stimulating hormone. Other hormones, such as epinephrine and norepinephrine, when bound to alpha receptors act by increasing intracellular levels of calcium. Steroid hormones from the adrenal cortex, testes, and ovaries act by entering the nucleus of the target cell and binding to the genetic material, DNA. This binding triggers the target cell to produce certain enzymes, which in turn cause the typical hormonally induced response of the target tissue.

HYPOTHALAMUS

This inferior portion of the diencephalon of the brain has many functions. Our concern here will be limited to two of these: (1) the production of the hormones ADH and oxytocin, which are stored in the posterior pituitary, and (2) the regulation of anterior pituitary hormone secretion. The anatomical interrelationship between the hypothalamus and pituitary is depicted in Figure 34-2.

TABLE 34-1
ENDOCRINE SYSTEM IN SUMMARY

Endocrine Gland and Hormone	Principal Site of Action	Principal Processes Affected
Hypothalamus		
Corticotropin-releasing factor	Anterior pituitary	Release of adrenocorticotropin
Thyrotropin-releasing factor	Anterior pituitary	Release of thyrotropin
Luteinizing hormone-releasing factor	Anterior pituitary	Release of luteinizing hormone
Follicle-stimulating hormone-releasing factor	Anterior pituitary	Release of follicle-stimulating hormone
Growth hormone-releasing factor	Anterior pituitary	Release of growth hormone
Growth hormone-release inhibiting factor	Anterior pituitary	Inhibition of release of growth hormone
Prolactin-releasing factor	Anterior pituitary	Release of prolactin
Prolactin-release inhibiting hormone	Anterior pituitary	Inhibition of release of prolactin
Pituitary Gland		
Anterior Lobe		
Growth hormone	General	Growth of bones, muscles, and other organs
	Liver	Somatomedin
Thyrotropin	Thyroid	Growth and secretory activity of thyroid gland
Adrenocorticotropin	Adrenal cortex	Growth and secretory activity of adrenal cortex
Follicle-stimulating	Ovaries	Development of follicles and secretion of estrogen
	Testes	Development of seminiferous tubules, spermatogenesis
Luteinizing or interstitial cell–stimulating	Ovaries	Ovulation, formation of corpus luteum, secretion of progesterone
	Testes	Secretion of testosterone
Prolactin or lactogenic	Mammary glands	Secretion of milk
Melanocyte-stimulating	Skin	Pigmentation (?)
Posterior Lobe		
Antidiuretic (vasopressin)	Kidney	Reabsorption of water; water balance
	Arterioles	Blood pressure (?)
Oxytocin	Uterus	Contraction
	Breast	Expression of milk
Pineal Gland		
Melatonin	Gonads	Sexual maturation
Thyroid Gland		
Thyroxine and triiodothyronine	General	Metabolic rate; growth and development; intermediate metabolism
Thyrocalcitonin	Bone	Inhibits bone resorption; lowers blood level of calcium
Parathyroid Glands		
Parathormone	Bone, kidney, intestine	Promotes bone resorption; increased absorption of calcium; raises blood calcium level
Adrenal Glands		
Cortex		
Mineralocorticoids (*e.g.,* aldosterone)	Kidney	Reabsorption of sodium; elimination of potassium
Glucocorticoids (*e.g.,* cortisol)	General	Metabolism of carbohydrate, protein, and fat; response to stress; anti-inflammatory
Sex hormones	General (?)	Preadolescent growth spurt (?)
Medulla		
Epinephrine	Cardiac muscle, smooth muscle, glands	Emergency functions: same as stimulation of sympathetic system
Norepinephrine	Organs innervated by sympathetic system	Chemical transmitter substance; increases peripheral resistance

TABLE 34-1
(Continued)

Endocrine Gland and Hormone	Principal Site of Action	Principal Processes Affected
Islet Cells of Pancreas		
Insulin	General	Lowers blood sugar; utilization and storage of carbohydrate; decreased gluconeogenesis; increased lipogenesis
Glucagon	Liver	Raises blood sugar; glucogenolysis and gluconeogenesis
Testes		
Testosterone	General	Development of secondary sex characteristics
	Reproductive organs	Development and maintenance; normal function
Ovaries		
Estrogens	General	Development of secondary sex characteristics
	Mammary glands	Development of duct system
	Reproductive organs	Maturation and normal cyclic function
Progesterone	Mammary glands	Development of secretory tissue
	Uterus	Preparation for implantation; maintenance of pregnancy
Prostaglandins	General smooth muscle, cell membranes	Contraction–relaxation, enzyme activation
Kidney		
Calcitrol	Intestine	Calcium absorption
	Bone	
	Renal tubules	
Thymus		
Thymosin	Lymphatic tissue	Cellular immunity, T-lymphocytes
Gastrointestinal Tract		
Gastrin	Stomach	Production of gastric juice
Enterogastrone	Stomach	Inhibits secretion and motility
Secretin	Liver and pancreas	Production of bile; production of watery pancreatic juice (rich in $NaHCO_3$)
CCK-PZ	Pancreas	Production of pancreatic juice rich in enzymes
CCK-PZ	Gallbladder	Contraction and emptying

(From Chaffee EE, Lytle IM: Basic Physiology and Anatomy, 4th ed. Philadelphia, JB Lippincott, 1980)

Antidiuretic Hormone (ADH or Vasopressin) and Oxytocin

Production. These hormones are produced by nerve cells originating from areas (nuclei) just above the optic chiasma (supraoptic) and lateral to the third ventricle (paraventricular). They "drip" from the axonal ends of these nerve cells into the tissue of the posterior pituitary, where they are stored. Neural impulses from these hypothalamic cells cause the posterior pituitary to release these hormones into the bloodstream. Because of their neuronal production, these hormones are sometimes termed *neurosecretory material.*

Metabolic Fates. The half-life of ADH is 18 minutes. It is degraded principally by the liver and kidneys.

Actions. Basically ADH acts on the cells of the renal collecting ducts to increase their permeability to water. This results in increased water reabsorption un-accompanied by and independent of any electrolyte reabsorption. This reabsorbed water increases the volume of and decreases the osmolarity of the extracellular fluid. At the same time, it decreases the volume of and increases the concentration of the urine excreted. The term *vasopressin* originated from the observation that large, supraphysiological dosages of ADH act on arteriole smooth muscle to elevate blood pressure. Although this pressor action of ADH does not appear to play a role in the normal homeostasis of blood pressure, some researchers think that it may play a role in counteracting the fall in blood pressure that results from hemorrhagic or other drastic hypovolemic states.

Regulation of ADH. There are three major stimuli for the regulation of ADH secretion. The first is plasma osmolality. This is monitored by osmoreceptors in the anterior hypothalamus. An increase above the normal osmolality of the plasma (290 mOsm/kg) results in

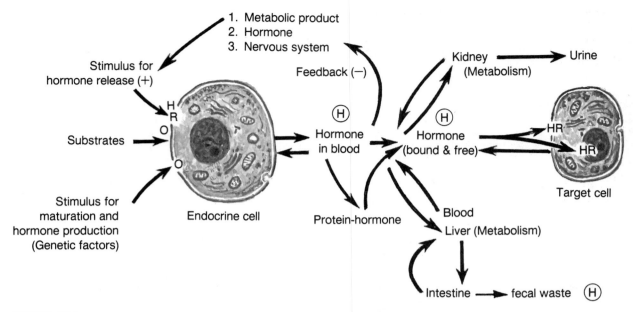

FIGURE 34-1
Diagram of the complex cellular interactions required to maintain an effective balance of hormones within the blood to regulate cellular functions. Specific cell receptors (R) will react to hormones (H) or other substances (O) in the blood that can act as stimuli for cellular mechanisms. (Chaffee EE, Lytle IM: Basic Physiology and Anatomy, 4th ed. Philadelphia, JB Lippincott, 1980)

neural stimuli from these receptors to the ADH-secreting cells, reflexly increasing ADH secretion. This in turn increases water retention, thereby diluting the extracellular fluid (ECF) and lowering the plasma osmolality back to normal. Similarly, a fall in plasma osmolality reflexly triggers a decrease or cessation in ADH secretion. This allows more water excretion, thereby raising the ECF osmolality again. ADH secretion can be altered by changes in osmolality of less than 1%. This osmoreceptor-mediated reflex arc functions in maintaining normal osmotic homeostasis of the ECF.

The second stimulus consists of changes in ECF volume. Stretch receptors in the low pressure portion of the cardiovascular system (*e.g.*, vena cavae, right side of the heart, and pulmonary vessels) monitor blood volume. Stimuli from these receptors are conducted by afferent fibers to the hypothalamus (by way of the brain stem). A decrease in blood volume reflexly stimulates ADH secretion. The resultant increase in water retention elevates the blood volume without affecting arterial blood pressure. A rise in blood volume reflexly stops ADH secretion. This halts water retention, thereby restoring the normal volume of the ECF compartment. This mechanism operates to alter ADH secretion in response to changes in body position. Movement from the recumbent to the upright position causes a temporary decrease in the stimulation of volume receptor because blood pools in the legs. This results in an increase in ADH secretion. Recumbency

increases venous return from the legs. The increased volume reflexly triggers a decrease in ADH secretion, thereby increasing the volume of urine excreted. Such recumbent diuresis is especially notable in persons with edema of the lower extremities.

The third stimulus, changes in arterial blood pressure, also can reflexly regulate ADH secretion. The hypothalamus receives information from pressure receptors, located in the carotid sinuses and aorta. A fall in arterial pressure reflexly increases ADH secretion. The water retention thereby produced increases the plasma volume and pressure. A rise in arterial pressure produces the opposite effect. This mechanism may play more of a role in compensating for large changes in arterial blood pressure (*e.g.*, impending or actual shock).

Various other stimuli have been shown to influence ADH secretion. Increased ADH secretion can be prompted by angiotension II, pain, "stress," opiates, nicotine, clofibrate, chlorpropamide, and barbiturates. ADH secretion is inhibited by alcohol and certain opiate antagonists.

Actions and Regulation of Oxytocin Secretion.
This hormone stimulates contraction of the myoepithelial cells that line the milk ducts of the breast. This causes milk to be squeezed into the sinuses leading to the nipple surface (*i.e.,* milk ejection, or "let-down"). Oxytocin secretion is reflexly triggered by the hypo-

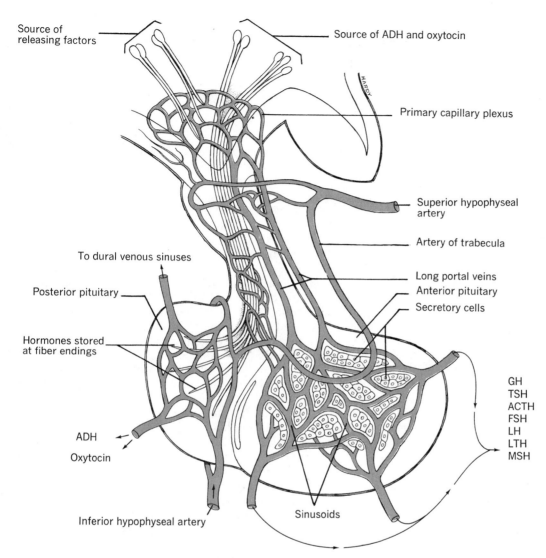

FIGURE 34-2
Highly diagrammatic and schematic representation of hypophyseal nerve fiber tracts and portal system. Releasing factors produced by cell bodies in hypothalamus trickle down axons to proximal part of stalk, where they enter the primary capillary plexus and are transported via portal vessels to sinusoids in adenohypophysis for control of secretions. ADH and oxytocin, produced by other cell bodies in hypothalamus, trickle down axons for storage in neurohypophysis until needed. (Chaffee EE, Lytle IM: Basic Physiology and Anatomy, 4th ed. Philadelphia, JB Lippincott, 1980)

thalamic receipt of afferent impulses from touch receptors around the nipples. Thus, suckling by the infant or manual stimulation can trigger milk let-down. Ocytocin also causes contraction of the smooth muscles of the uterus. Such contractions play a role in labor and may facilitate the transport of sperm from the cervix to the fallopian tubes. During pregnancy, oxytocin secretion is stimulated by cervical dilation and estrogen and inhibited by progesterone and alcohol.

Hypophysiotropic Hormones

Other hypothalamic neurons produce "hypophysiotropic" hormones that stimulate or inhibit hormonal secretion by the anterior pituitary (adenohypophysis). These hormones are secreted into a capillary plexus (near the median eminence) that supplies blood to the anterior pituitary. A given hypophysiotropic hormone regulates the secretion of one or two anterior pituitary

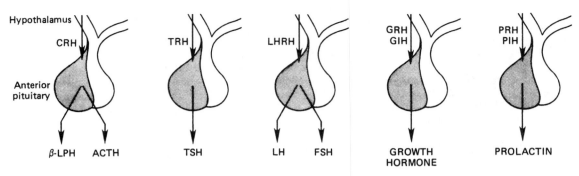

FIGURE 34-3
*Effects of hypophysiotropic hormones on the secretion of anterior pituitary hormones. (Ganong
WF: Review of Medical Physiology, 11th ed. Los Altos, CA, Lange Medical Publications, 1983)*

hormones. Both growth hormone (somatotropin) and prolactin are dually controlled by both a stimulatory and an inhibiting hypophysiotropic hormone. Figure 34-3 illustrates the hypophysiotropic regulation of adenohypophyseal secretions.

Such hypothalamic regulation of pituitary functioning can be disrupted by hypothalamic lesions. This can lead to over- or undersecretion of one or more hormones released from the anterior or posterior pituitary. The hypothalamus also receives input from various higher and lower brain centers. These neural connections together with the influence of the hypothalamus on the pituitary provide a beginning biological basis for the construction of conceptual models that describe how stress, emotions, environmental stimuli, and perceptions may affect endocrine functions.

ANTERIOR PITUITARY (ADENOHYPOPHYSIS)

This organ contains five morphologically different types of cells that secrete polypeptide hormones: (1) somatotrops, which secrete growth hormone (somatotropin); (2) mammotrops, which secrete prolactin (luteotropic hormone, or LTH); (3) thyrotrops, which secrete thyroid-stimulating hormone (TSH); (4) corticotrops, which secrete adrenocorticotropic hormone (ACTH), beta lipotrophin (BLPH), beta endorphin, and gamma malanophore–stimulating hormone (MSH); and (5) gonadotrops, which secrete luteinizing hormone (LH) and follicle-stimulating hormone (FSH). Each type of cell is separately regulated via hypophysiotropic hormones (see Fig. 34-3). LTH, LH, and FSH act on cells of the gonads (ovaries and testes) to regulate gamete (sperm and egg) and hormone production.

TSH stimulates cells of the thyroid gland to produce and secrete the two thyroid hormones. This and the manner by which these hormones alter TSH output

will be discussed later. The corticotrops manufacture a long polypeptide chain, 265 amino acids long, called *pro-opiomelanocortin (POMC)*. Before secretion, POMC is separated into shorter fragments. Three of these are readily identified as ACTH, gamma MSH, and BLPH. Part of the BLPH molecule can be further split off to form an endogenous opiate called *beta endorphin*. Endogenous opiates are further discussed in the chapter on the normal physiology of the nervous system. The role of this opiate from the pituitary is not yet known.

Melanin is a dark pigment contained in special structures called *melanophores* within the cells of the skin of lower vertebrates (*e.g.,* fish, amphibians, and reptiles). MSH stimulates the dispersion of the melanin granules within these melanophores. This darkens the animal temporarily. Birds and mammals (including humans) have melanin, but it cannot be dispersed and is not contained within melanophores. The normal function of MSH in humans is not known, although there is some evidence that it can cause a darkening of certain areas of skin in humans with Addison's disease. In this condition, excess CRH stimulates corticotrops to secrete ACTH. Along with this, the other fragments of POMC, including MSH, are released. The role and regulation of ACTH will be discussed later in the section on the adrenal cortex. This leaves only growth hormone to be discussed here.

Growth Hormone (Somatotropin)

The production and secretion of this polypeptide hormone have already been discussed.

Metabolic Fate. Somatotropin is degraded primarily in the liver. Other metabolic sites have yet to be uncovered. The half-life of plasma somatotropin is approximately 25 minutes.

Actions. This hormone acts both directly on target cells and indirectly by stimulating the liver and other as yet unidentified tissues to secrete various growth factors termed *somatomedins.*

Direct actions include (1) increasing the breakdown of fats (lipolysis) in adipose cells and the release of the fatty acids produced by lipolysis into the bloodstream (this is termed its *ketogenic effect*); (2) increasing hepatic glycolysis and thereby increasing plasma glucose levels (this is often called an *anti-insulin action*); (3) increasing the sensitivity of insulin-producing cells to certain stimuli; (4) increasing the cellular uptake of amino acids; and (5) stimulating erythropoiesis.

The various somatomedins seem to exert growth-promoting activity in different types of tissues. Normally, the net result of somatomedin-mediated growth hormone activity consists of (1) an increase in the formation of cartilage in the epiphyseal plates, which fosters the growth in length of long bones; (2) an increase in other skeletal growth; and (3) the growth of all other parts of the body (*e.g.,* soft tissue and viscera).

All growth hormone actions operate together to produce growth (*e.g.,* by cell division) and to provide the materials needed for this growth (*i.e.,* amino acids for synthesis of protein cell structure, such as membranes and enzymes as well as fatty acids and glucose to provide energy for the cell growth and erythrocytes to increase the availability of oxygen to growing tissues).

Regulation. The secretion of growth hormone is regulated by two hypothalamic hormones. One, somatotropin-releasing hormone (SRH), stimulates the somatotropin to secrete growth hormone. The other, somatotropin-inhibiting hormone (somatostatin, SIH), suppresses somatotrop secretion. One somatomedin acts in a negative-feedback ''loop' to regulate growth hormone secretion by stimulating the hypothalamic output of SIH, which in turn decreases further growth hormone secretion.

Other stimuli that influence the secretion of growth hormone are varied. Age is the most important overriding variable, and the actions of many of these other stimuli are influenced by it.

In general, factors that, at the appropriate age, may stimulate the secretion of growth hormone include hypoglycemia, fasting, exercise, protein meal, glucagon, stress (both physiologic and psychologic), deeper stages of sleep, and drugs that bind to dopamine receptors. Major stimuli that decrease the output of growth hormone include REM sleep (dreaming), elevated plasma levels of glucose or fatty acids, and cortisol.

THYROID

This gland is a bilobed, richly vascularized structure. The lobes lay lateral to the trachea just beneath the larynx and are connected by a bridge of thyroid tissue, called the *isthmus,* that runs across the anterior surface of the trachea. Microscopically, the thyroid is composed primarily of spheroid follicles, each of which stores a colloid material in its center. The follicles produce, store, and secrete the two major hormones: T_3 (triiodothyronine) and T_4 (thyroxine). When the gland is actively secreting, the follicles are small and contain little colloid. Inactive thyroid tissue contains large follicles, each of which possesses a large quantity of stored colloid. Other cells, the parafollicular cells (C-cells), are scattered between the follicles. Parafollicular cells secrete the hormone calcitonin. It and two other hormones influence calcium metabolism. They will be discussed later.

Thyroid Hormones

Manufacture and Secretion. The follicular cells absorb tyrosine (an amino acid) and iodide from the plasma and secrete them into the central colloid portion of the follicle, where they are used in the synthesis of T_3 and T_4. Two iodide molecules are attached, first one and then the other, to each tyrosine molecule. Two such doubly iodinated tyrosines are combined to form T_4. (The subscript refers to the number of iodide molecules that this substance contains.) T_3 is formed by the combination of a doubly iodinated tyrosine with a singly iodinated one. These hormones are then stored in the colloid until they are needed. When they are to be secreted, the follicle cells transport them from the colloid to the plasma. Because of the role of iodine in the manufacture of thyroid hormones, the uptake (from the plasma), storage, and release of small amounts of radioactive iodine by the thyroid can be used to measure the activity of this gland. Because the thyroid gland is virtually the only tissue of the body that absorbs and stores iodine, larger amounts of radioactive iodine can be utilized to destroy portions of the thyroid gland as a treatment for hyperthyroidism.

Transport and Metabolic Fate. Less than 1% of the secreted T_3 and T_4 remain free and physiologically active in the plasma. The remainder is bound to plasma proteins. Most is bound to thyroxine-binding globulin (TBG), a molecule manufactured by the liver, and the remainder is bound to two types of plasma albumin. Such protein-bound hormone serves as a reservoir to replace free T_3 and T_4 that has been degraded, thereby maintaining stable blood levels of thyroid hormones. An earlier index of thyroid secretion, the protein bound iodine (PBI) index, utilized the protein-bound fraction of secreted thyroid hormones. It measured the iodide contained in the T_3 and T_4 attached to plasma proteins. This index is still used occasionally, although now plasma T_3 and T_4 are measured directly by radioimmunoassay. The plasma proteins involved in transporting T_3 and T_4 are manufactured in the liver. Consequently, liver damage that decreases the plasma levels of these proteins can produce a condition resembling thyroid hormone excess (*i.e.,* hyperthyroidism). Plasma levels of these proteins also can be depressed by glucocorticoids, androgens, and L-asparaginase (an antineoplastic drug). They are elevated by estrogens, opiates, clofibrate, and major tranquilizers.

Thyroid hormones are deiodinated and catabolized by the liver, kidneys, and various other tissues. A small amount of degraded hormone is added to the bile secreted by the liver and is excreted in the stool.

Actions.   Thyroid hormones enter the cells, where they (primarily T_3) bind with receptors on the cell nucleus. Through this interaction with the nucleus, these hormones can alter the cellular synthesis of various enzymes and thereby modify cellular operations. Interestingly enough, the iodine in these hormones does not seem requisite for their actions: Several synthetic noniodine-containing thyroid hormone analogues exist. Some endocrinologists view T_4 as a prohormone form of T_3 because of the following considerations: (1) T_3 is more potent and acts more rapidly than T_4; and (2) about 35% of all plasma T_4 is converted intracellularly (by removal of an iodide molecule) into T_3.

The actions of thyroid hormones are widespread and apparently stem from their stimulation of the basal metabolic rate (BMR) of most tissues (excluding brain, anterior pituitary, spleen, lymph nodes, testes, and lungs). The exact manner whereby these hormones act on cell metabolism is not yet clear. Evidently, T_3 and, to a lesser extent, T_4 act to increase the mitochondrial enzyme systems involved in the oxidation of foodstuffs. The energy released by such oxidation is not efficiently stored in the high-energy bonds of ATP. Much is lost in the form of heat. This increases O_2 consumption of and heat production by these tissues (*i.e.,* the BMR). This is also termed the *calorigenic action.*

Effects secondary to calorigenesis include an increased cellular need for vitamins, increased nitrogen excretion, catabolism of protein and fat stores if the supply of carbohydrates is insufficient, and weight loss.

T_3 and T_4 have other effects that are independent of their calorigenic ones. The ways in which these effects are produced are even less well understood than calorigenesis. Thyroid hormones are essential for the normal growth and development of many body systems, the most notable of which are the skeletal and nervous systems. These hormones may stimulate the secretion of growth hormone and potentiate its effect on various tissues. The effect of thyroid hormones on the nervous system is best illustrated by the cretinism resulting from congenital thyroid insufficiency. Thyroid hor-

mones are also necessary for normal levels of neuronal functioning. Thyroid insufficiency leads to slowed reflexes and mentation, and decreases in level of consciousness (by way of decreased levels of reticular-activating system activity).

Regulation.   The secretion of T_3 and T_4 by the thyroid gland is primarily regulated by the secretion of thyroid stimulating hormone (TSH) from the anterior pituitary gland. TSH stimulates the manufacture and secretion of T_3 and T_4. A negative-feedback regulatory loop exists whereby increased levels of free (unbound) T_3 and T_4 suppress TSH secretion. Decreased plasma TSH results in decreased thyroid function, which causes a fall in free plasma T_3 and T_4. Low T_3 and T_4 levels act to stimulate TSH secretion. If, for some reason, a TSH-induced increase in thyroid activity does not raise the plasma levels of free T_3 and T_4, the continued high levels of TSH will eventually cause an increase in the size of the thyroid gland (nontoxic goiter). In this case, an enlarged thyroid is not associated with overproduction of hormone.

This feedback loop maintains homeostasis of the daily secretion of TSH and thyroid hormones. In addition to being influenced by circulatory T_3 and T_4 levels, TSH secretion is regulated by a hypothalamic neurosecretory material termed *thyrotropin-releasing hormone (TRH).* The hypothalamic regulation of TSH and, consequently, of thyroid function seems to function in infant thermoregulation. In this process, TRH output is increased in response to cold and decreased in response to heat. The elevated thyroid hormone production presumably increases calorigenesis, which raises the body temperature of the "cold" infant. Similarly, a heat-provoked decrease in TRH causes a decrease in TSH and thyroid activity. This is thought to decrease calorigenesis, thereby decreasing the temperature of the "hot" infant. The effect of TRH in thermoregulation of adults is negligible.

HORMONAL INFLUENCES ON CALCIUM METABOLISM

Three hormones exert a major influence on calcium metabolism. Two of these, calcitrol and parathormone, elevate plasma calcium levels; one, calcitonin, decreases blood levels of calcium.

Calcitrol

Manufacture.   This hormone is produced by the action of both the liver and kidneys on vitamin D. Ultraviolet light changes certain provitamins in the skin to a group of compounds, collectively referred to as *vitamin D.* One of these, D_3, can also be obtained from vitamin D–enriched and other foods. The liver converts D_3 to 25-hydroxycholecalciferol (calcidiol), which is then altered by kidney cells to a more active form, 1,25-dihydroxycholecalciferol (calcitrol).

Transport and Metabolic Fate. Details are not known.

Action. Calcitrol acts on intracellular enzymes of intestinal mucosal cells to increase calcium absorption. To a lesser extent, it also increases the active transport of calcium out of osteoblasts into the bloodstream. Both these actions elevate plasma calcium levels. In vitamin deficiency states, the effect of decreased intestinal absorption outweighs any decrease in the mobilization of calcium from bone so as to produce an overall hypocalcia and poor mineralization of bone.

Regulation. Plasma calcium and phosphate levels operate in a negative-feedback loop to influence the activity of the renal enzyme system, which catalyses the conversion of metabolically inactive calcidiol to the metabolically active calcitrol. High plasma calcium levels decrease calcitrol formation, whereas low levels increase it. The formation of calcitrol is also facilitated by parathormone and decreased by metabolic acidosis and hypoinsulinemia (diabetes mellitus). The hypocalcemia seen in chronic renal disease results from a calcitrol deficiency.

Parathormone

This hormone is produced by the parathyroid glands. Each lobe of the thyroid gland typically contains two parathyroid glands: one in its superior pole and one in its inferior pole. Variation exists among individuals with respect to the number and distribution of parathyroid glands. Some persons have more or less than four. Others have parathyroid tissue in the mediastinum.

Manufacture and Secretion. Parathormone is a polypeptide produced and secreted by the chief cells of the parathyroid glands.

Transport and Metabolic Fate. Parathormone is transported free (unbound) in the plasma, has a half-life of less than 20 minutes, and is metabolically degraded by cells in the liver.

Action. Parathormone acts upon two target tissues: bone cells and kidney tubules. In bone, it stimulates osteoclast activity and inhibits osteoblast activity. This results in bone reabsorption with consequent mobilization of calcium and phosphate from the bony matrix into the bloodstream. In the kidney, parathormone increases the reabsorption of calcium by distal tubule

cells and decreases the reabsorption of phosphate by proximal tubule cells. The net effect of these multiple actions is elevation of plasma calcium levels and lowering of plasma phosphate levels. At the cellular level, parathormone produces these effects by activating adenyl cyclase, thereby increasing the intracellular levels of cyclic AMP in the target tissues.

Regulation. Plasma calcium levels alter parathormone secretion by way of a negative-feedback loop. Secretion is inhibited by high plasma calcium levels and stimulated by low blood levels of calcium. Indeed, the calcitrol-deficiency–induced hypocalcemia, which occurs in chronic renal failure, typically produces a secondary hyperparathyroidism. Parathyroid gland secretion also is stimulated by hypomagnesemia.

Calcitonin

Manufacture and Secretion. This polypeptide hormone is produced by the parafollicular cells (C-cells) of the thyroid gland. It may also be secreted by nonthyroidal tissue (*e.g.,* lung, intestine, pituitary, and bladder).

Transport and Metabolic Fate. Calcitonin seems to be transported unbound in the plasma. It has a half-life of less than 10 minutes.

Actions. Calcitonin lowers plasma calcium and phosphate levels by (1) inhibiting osteoclastic bone reabsorption, and (2) increasing urinary phosphate and calcium excretion. Calcitonin levels are elevated during pregnancy and lactation. This suggests that it may be helpful to protect the mother's skeleton from excess calcium loss during these periods of calcium drain by the infant.

Regulation. Calcitonin does not seem to function in the normal daily homeostasis of plasma calcium levels. It appears to serve more of an "emergency function" in that it is secreted only when the plasma calcium level exceeds 9.3 mg/dl. At high blood calcium levels, calcitonin secretion is stimulated by increased levels of plasma calcium.

Other Hormones That Influence Calcium Metabolism. Four hormones bear mention here. T_3 and T_4 are thought by some workers to produce hypercalcemia, but the mechanism of action is unknown. Estrogens prevent parathormone from raising plasma calcium by mobilizing calcium from bone. Growth hormone increases urinary calcium excretion while also increasing intestinal calcium absorption. These two effects counterbalance each other, thereby producing no net change in plasma calcium levels. Glucocorticoids tend to lower plasma calcium levels by (1) decreasing intestinal absorption of calcium, and (2) increasing renal calcium excretion.

ISLETS OF LANGERHANS

This name refers to the more than one million ovoid islands (clusters) of cells that are scattered throughout the pancreas, predominantly in the tail. Owing to this distribution of islet cells, acute attacks of pancreatitis, which generally spare the tail, usually spare the islets. Episodes of chronic recurrent pancreatitis, however, typically involve all of the pancreas. Consequently, they cause islet cell destruction and diabetes. Each cell cluster is richly supplied with capillaries, into which its hormones are secreted. The islets are composed of four types of cells (1) alpha cells, which secrete glucagon; (2) beta cells, which secrete insulin; (3) delta cells, which secrete somatostatin; and (4) F cells, which secrete pancreatic polypeptide. Let us examine the hormones secreted by each of these cell types in more detail.

Insulin

Manufacture and Secretion. The precursor of insulin, proinsulin, is manufactured in the granular endoplasmic reticulum, as are all cell proteins. Proinsulin is a "necklace" of amino acid beads that has one end folded over the other, so that it resembles a squashed figure nine. It subsequently leaves the reticulum to be stored as secretory granules in another cell structure. Here, two ends of the folded proinsulin "necklace" become attached to one another (by way of disulfide bands) to form two parallel chains resembling railroad tracks. The two ends are then separated from the "center of the necklace." This center chain of amino acids is termed *C-peptide*. Proinsulin can be found in the plasma as a result of certain islet tumors or over-stimulation of the beta cells. C-peptide is secreted into the bloodstream along with insulin. Because there is a 1:1 ratio between C-peptide and insulin, plasma C-peptide levels can be used to measure endogenous insulin secretion or degree of beta cell activity.

Metabolic Fate. Insulin is currently known to act only on a few types of tissues. However, the membranes of nearly all types of body cells possess insulin receptors. The possession of insulin receptors by cells on which insulin does not act may be explained by the discovery of five circulating peptide growth factors (somatomedins) that appear to have insulin-like action. The insulin receptors possibly may be found to serve as receptors for these growth factors as well as for insulin.

Once a molecule of insulin binds to an insulin receptor, both are taken into the cytoplasm of the cell by endocytosis. Binding of insulin to receptors initiates the physiological action of insulin upon the cell. After binding, the insulin–receptor complex is "absorbed" by indocytosis into the cell and destroyed within 14 to 15 hours by lysosomal enzymes. New receptors replace the destroyed one in the cell membranes. Plasma insulin has a half-life of approximately 5 minutes. About 80% of all circulating insulin is catabolized by liver and kidney cells.

Actions. The mechanism by which insulin exerts its action is currently unknown. It is known only that insulin does not activate adenyl cyclase. The actions of insulin are summarized in Table 34-2.

In addition, insulin is known to facilitate glucose uptake by connective tissue, leukocytes, mammary glands, lens of eye, aorta, pituitary, and alpha islet cells. In general, insulin enables glucose to be readily available for aerobic oxidation by the Krebs citric acid cycle in muscle, adipose, and connective tissue cells. Facilitation of the preferential use of glucose as cellular fuel means that the cells do not need to oxidize (burn) fatty or amino acids. Instead, these can be con-

---

TABLE 34-2
MAJOR ACTIONS OF INSULIN UPON FAT AND MUSCLE CELLS

Muscle Cells	Adipose Cells
Increased glucose entry	Increased glucose entry
Increased K^+ uptake	Increased K^+ uptake
Increased glycogen synthesis	Increased fatty acid entry and synthesis
Increased amino acid entry	Increased fat deposition
Increased protein synthesis	Increased conversion of glucose to fatty acids
Decreased protein catabolism	Inhibition of lipolysis
Increased ketone entry into cells	

TABLE 34-3
FACTORS AFFECTING INSULIN SECRETION

Stimulators	*Inhibitors*
Glucose	Somatostatin
Mannose	2-Deoxyglucose
Amino acids (leucine, arginine, others)	Mannoheptulose
Intestinal hormones (GIP, gastrin, secretin, CCK, glucagon, others?)	α-Adrenergic–stimulating agents (norepinephrine, epinephrine)
β-Keto acids	β-Adrenergic–blocking agents (propranolol)
Acetylcholine	Diazoxide
Glucagon	Thiazide diuretics
Cyclic AMP and various cyclic AMP– generating substances	Phenytoin
β-Adrenergic stimulating agents	Alloxan
Theophylline	Microtubule inhibitors
Sulfonylureas	Insulin

(Reproduced, with permission, from Ganong WF: Review of Medical Physiology, 11th ed. Copyright 1983 by Lange Medical Publications. Los Altos, California)

served. Protein synthesis and fat storage are increased in liver, muscle, and adipose tissue. Breakdown of fats and proteins is decreased. Hepatic gluconeogenesis also is decreased or halted, and glycogen synthesis is increased.

Regulation. Insulin secretion is influenced by a variety of factors (Table 34-3). Monosaccharides serve as the primary regulatory mechanism for insulin secretion. Elevated plasma levels of glucose, fructose, and mannose act in a negative-feedback loop to increase the secretion of insulin. Lower levels of these sugars decrease insulin output. Other monosaccharides (*e.g.,* galactose, xylose, and arabinose) have no effect on insulin secretion. Glucagon and beta adrenergic–stimulating chemicals increase insulin secretion by stimulating adenyl cyclase, an enzyme that elevates levels of cyclic AMP within beta cells. Theophylline, which inhibits the degradation of beta cell cyclic AMP, also promotes production. Beta cells are also stimulated to secrete insulin by tolbutamide and other sulfonurea derivatives, acetylcholine or impulses from vagal nerve branches to the islets, selected amino acids such as arginine, and beta ketoacids. The mechanism of action of these stimuli is currently unclear. Insulin production is inhibited by the following: (1) alpha adrenergic–stimulating agents, (2) beta adrenergic–blocking agents, (3) diazoxide, (4) thiazide diuretics, (5) phenytoin, (6) alloxan, (7) agents that prevent glucose metabolism (2-deoxyglucose or mannoheptose), (8) somatostatin, and (9) insulin itself.

Chronic stimulation of beta cells, such as by a high carbohydrate diet for several weeks, can cause a limited amount of hypertrophy and subsequent increase in the insulin-producing capacity. Overstimulation, however, will produce beta cell exhaustion. Stimula-

tion of these exhausted cells produces beta cell death and a depletion in the beta cell reserve. Beta cell activity is also decreased by the administration of exogenous insulin. Such decreased activity enables the cells to "rest" and results in their being temporarily hyperproductive following the withdrawal of exogenous insulin. The quantity and activity of insulin receptors also can be regulated by various factors. Increased amounts of insulin, obesity, acromegaly, and excess glucocorticoids decrease the receptors' number or activity or both. Exercise and decreased circulating levels of insulin increase the activity of insulin receptors.

Glucagon

Secretion. This polypeptide hormone is manufactured and secreted by the alpha islet cells.

Metabolic Fate. The half-life of plasma glucagon is 5 to 10 minutes. This hormone is degraded mainly by the liver.

Actions. The major function of glucagon is to elevate blood sugar levels by influencing enzyme systems within liver, fat, and muscle cells and then to enable this plasma glucose to enter and be utilized by body cells (*e.g.,* muscle) by stimulating the secretion of insulin. By this function, glucagon prevents hypoglycemia between meals, during exercise, during the first few days of fasting, and following a high-protein meal (the protein stimulates an increase in plasma insulin, which causes a rapid cellular uptake of absorbed dietary carbohydrates).

In order to perform this function, glucagon stimulates liver cells to perform glycogenolysis and gluconeogenesis. This increases the glucose concentration within liver cells, and, because they can dephosphorylate intracellular glucose, this glucose can be released from the liver into the bloodstream. The fatty acids and amino acids needed for gluconeogenesis are supplied by the glucagon-stimulated breakdown of fats in adipose cells and the release of fatty acids into the bloodstream. If the supply of fatty acids is not sufficient, glucagon also stimulates the breakdown of proteins into amino acids in muscle cells and the release of amino acids into the plasma. These fatty acids and amino acids are then taken up by hepatocytes and used as raw materials in gluconeogenesis. Glucagon also elevates plasma ketone levels by increasing hepatic ketone production and promotes the secretion of somatostatin and growth hormone.

Although glucagon opposes the effects of insulin on blood sugar levels, it also stimulates the secretion of insulin. This apparent contradiction is actually a logical "second step" in the biological function of this hormone. It enables the increased plasma glucose to enter and be used by various tissues. To be certain, an elevated plasma glucose level will itself stimulate insulin secretion, but this takes a while. The direct action of glucagon on beta cells simply is faster.

At the cellular level, the actions of glucagon on cell enzyme systems are mediated by glucagon-induced elevations in intracellular cyclic AMP. This chemical then acts as a "second messenger" to alter the enzyme activity of the cell to produce the "actions of glucagon." Because of this effect on intracellular cyclic AMP, large amounts of exogenous glucagon will increase the ionotropic capacity of myocardial tissue. However, lower levels of endogenous glucagon do not seem to have this effect.

Regulation. As is the case with beta cells, alpha cells are stimulated by beta adrenergic agonists, theophylline, elevated plasma levels of dietary amino acids (primarily those used in gluconeogenesis), and vagal (cholinergic) stimulation. Glucagon secretion is also prompted by glucocorticoids (*e.g.,* cortisol, CCK-PZ, and gastrin). Exercise, physical stress, and infections also increase alpha cell activity. Whereas the effects of exercise on glucagon secretion seem to be mediated by increased beta adrenergic activity, stress and infection probably operate by increasing plasma glucocorticoid levels. Dietary amino acids are believed to enhance glucagon secretion by their effects on CCK-PZ or gastrin or both because intravenous amino acids exert little or no effect on alpha cells.

Elevated plasma glucose operates by a negative-feedback loop to retard or halt the output of glucagon; however, plasma insulin must be present for this mechanism to operate. Like beta cell secretion, alpha

cell secretion is inhibited by alpha adrenergic agonists, phenytoin, and somatostatin. Fatty acids and ketone bodies in the plasma can inhibit glucagon secretion, but this inhibition must be weak because plasma glucagon levels can be quite elevated during diabetic ketoacidosis.

Somatostatin

Manufacture and Secretion. This ubiquitous tetradecapeptide is produced not only by the delta cells of the pancreas but also by (1) the hypothalamus, where it functions as an inhibitor of anterior pituitary growth hormone secretion; (2) neurons of the CNS, where it probably functions as a synaptic neurotransmitter agent; and (3) delta cells in the gastric mucosa, where it inhibits the secretion of gastrin and other lesser known gastrointestinal hormones. Islet cell somatostatin is secreted into the bloodstream and thus functions as a hormone.

Metabolic Fate. This is currently not known.

Actions. Pancreatic somatostatin inhibits the activity of all other islet cells. The biological significance of this action is not yet known. The only current clinical data of relevance concern delta cell tumors. These produce a clinical picture that resembles diabetes mellitus but that is reversible with tumor ablation.

Regulation. The secretion of somatostatin from islet cells is increased by glucose, certain amino acids, and CCK-PZ. Factors that may inhibit islet somatostatin secretion are currently unknown.

Pancreatic Polypeptide

Not much is known about this islet hormone in humans. Its secretion in humans is enhanced by dietary protein, exercise, acute hypoglycemia, and fasting. Somatostatin and elevated plasma glucose levels decrease the secretion of this polypeptide. No definite actions of this hormone have been established for humans.

ADRENAL GLANDS

An adrenal gland lies at the superior pole of each kidney. Each gland is composed of an inner core, the medulla, surrounded by an outer layer, the cortex. Although they are structurally related, the medulla and cortex are derived from different embryological tissue and function as separate entities.

Adrenal Medulla

This gland is basically a modified sympathetic ganglion. The axons of preganglionic sympathetic neurons arrive from the thoracic cord by way of splanchnic nerves (see Fig. 23-11 and Table 23-1). They synapse in the adrenal medulla with modified postganglionic cells that have lost their axons and secrete chemicals directly into the bloodstream. Thus, the adrenal medullas may appropriately be viewed as endocrine extensions of the sympathetic arm of the autonomic nervous system.

Manufacture and Secretion. Four chemicals are produced and secreted by two morphologically different cell types: (1) dopamine, a precursor of norepinephrine; (2) norepinephrine, the typical product of postganglionic sympathetic neurons; (3) epinephrine, a methylated version of norepinephrine; and (4) opioid peptides (enkephalins). The first three chemicals are collectively termed *catecholamines*. They are stored in granules with the medulla cells. Their secretion is triggered by stimulation of the preganglionic neurons that innervate the medulla. This causes them to release acetylcholine, which in turn prompts the formerly postganglionic medulla cells to secrete. The stimulus for the secretion of opioid peptides has not yet been identified.

Metabolic Fate. The half-life of plasma catecholamines is approximately 2 minutes. These compounds are rapidly degraded by plasma renal and hepatic catechol O-methyl transferase enzymes into vanillylmandelic acid (VMA), metanephrine, and normetanephrine, which are excreted in the urine. Only a very small quantity of nondegraded catecholamines are found in the normal urine. The metabolism and fate of the medullary enkephalins are unknown.

Actions. Predictably, the epinephrine and norepinephrine secreted by the adrenal medulla mimic the effects of mass discharge from sympathetic neurons (see Table 23-1). Apart from this, however, they produce several metabolic actions. First, they elevate blood sugar levels by activating an enzyme, phosphorylase, which promotes hepatic glycogenolysis. Because liver cells possess the enzyme glucose 6-phosphatase, the glucose produced by this glycogen breakdown is able to diffuse out of hepatocytes and into the bloodstream. These hormones also induce muscle cells to participate in elevating blood sugar levels, although this process is less direct. Phosphorylase in muscle cells also is activated by these catecholamines. However, the intracellular glucose thereby produced is unable to exit the muscle cells because they do not possess glucose 6-phosphatase. Instead, this glucose is catabolized to lactate, which can leave the muscle cells. Lactate then circulates to the liver, where it is converted to glucose that can enter the bloodstream by way of stimulation of beta adrenergic receptors on islet cells. These hormones can also elevate plasma glucose levels by stimulating the secretion of glucagon and increase the uptake of glucose by body tissues by stimulating the secretion of insulin. Epinephrine and norepinephrine can also produce the opposite effects by stimulating alpha adrenergic receptors on islet cells. Because of differential effects of both hormones on alpha and beta adrenergic receptors, the net result is that epinephrine elevates plasma glucose much more than does norepinephrine.

A second metabolic effect of catecholamines is promotion of lipolysis in adipose tissue. This elevates plasma free fatty acid levels and provides an alternative energy source for many body cells. Circulating catecholamines also increase alertness by stimulating the reticular activating system (see Chap. 23).

Lastly, these hormones produce an increase in the metabolic rate of the body and a cutaneous vasoconstriction, both of which result in an elevation in body temperature. However, the accelerated metabolism requires the presence of the thyroid and adrenal cortex hormones.

The physiological actions of both adrenal medullary dopamine and the enkephalins are currently unknown. Exogenous dopamine is useful in combating certain shocks because it has a positive ionotropic effect on the heart (by way of B_1 receptors) and produces renal vasodilation and peripheral vasoconstriction. The overall effect of moderate dosages is elevation of systolic blood pressure (without an appreciable increase in diastolic blood pressure) together with retention or restoration of renal output. In order to understand and compare the actions of drugs that mimic adrenal medullary hormones, one must learn which receptors are stimulated by these agents (a_1, a_2, b_1, b_2) and determine what effects these receptors mediate (see Table 23-1).

Regulation. Stimulation of the adrenal medulla glands is part of a general sympathetic-adrenal medulla (SAM) response to exercise and to perceived threats to one's biopsychological integrity and survival (Cannon termed the latter the "fight or flight" response). Hypoglycemia also stimulates increased adrenal medulla secretion.

The results of the SAM response enable the body to perform vigorous physical exertion optimally. The heart rate and blood pressure are increased (increasing perfusion), and blood flow is shunted away from the skin and gastrointestinal tract to more "vital" organs for exertion, such as skeletal muscles, brain, and heart. The reticular activating system is stimulated, fostering alertness. Blood glucose and fatty acid levels are raised, thereby increasing the available energy sources for cells. Pupils are dilated, increasing the field of peripheral vision and the amount of light entering the eyes. Sweat glands are stimulated, providing cooling of the body in advance of and during the time that the body temperature is elevated as the result of the physical exertion. The majority of this SAM response is mediated by sympathetic nerve fibers to various body structures. Circulating catecholamines play only a minor role. Furthermore, many of the tissue responses (*e.g.,* muscle cells) to such sympathetic demands require the presence of glucocorticoids to enable the tissues to meet the demands of the SAM response, and indeed the SAM response often accompanies the stress-induced secretion of adrenal steroids discovered by Seyle (this and the endocrine response to both physical and psychological stress will be discussed in the section on the adrenal cortex).

The SAM response is initiated by the perception of a stimulus or situation that a person evaluates on the basis of past experience and current resources to be a threat to his well-being. This response involves the cerebral cortex. Impulses from the cortex may travel by way of nerve fibers to the limbic system, where they are involved in generating an emotional response. Additional impulses from both the cortex and limbic system stimulate sympathetic centers in the diencephalon. These centers in turn discharge a specific pattern of impulses down descending fibers to various sympathetic neurons in the cord, bringing about the SAM response.

Adrenal Cortex

This gland is composed of three histologically different layers. Its exterior is covered by a capsule. The outermost layer, the zona glomerulosa, lies just beneath the capsule. It produces and secretes primarily mineralocorticoids, such as aldosterone. The inner two layers, the zona fasciculata and zona reticularis, manufacture and secrete glucocorticoids (cortisol and corticosterone) as well as adrenal androgens and estrogens. If these inner cortical layers are destroyed, they can be regenerated from zona glomerulosa cells. Because the biosynthetic pathways and metabolic fates for all adrenocortical hormones are interrelated, these will be discussed together for all hormones. Actions and regulation will be considered separately for mineralocorticoids, glucocorticoids, and sex steroids.

Manufacture and Secretion. Figure 34-4 depicts the metabolic pathways for synthesis of all adrenocortical hormones. Each of these metabolic steps is gov-

FIGURE 34-4
Biosynthetic pathways for adrenal cortical hormones. Cells in all three layers contain all pathways except that from corticosterone to aldosterone: only cells of the zona glomerulosa can perform this step (*).

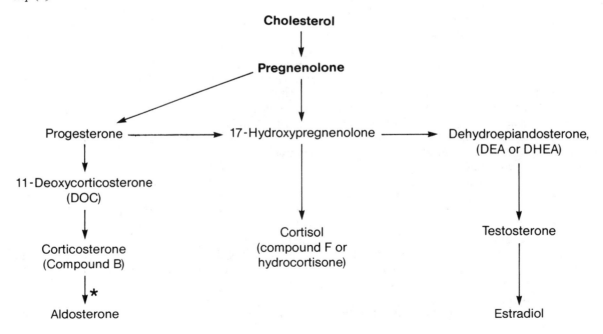

erned by a specific enzyme. Genetic deficiencies in one or more of these enzymes produce syndromes involving the underproduction and/or overproduction of various cortical hormones. Drugs that act to inhibit specific enzymes are used clinically to assess cortical function. One such drug is metyrapone, which inhibits cortisol synthesis.

Metabolic Fate. Following secretion, plasma cortisol and, to a lesser extent, corticosterone are bound to a plasma globulin called *corticosteroid-binding globulin (CBG)*, or *transcortin*. Only the unbound hormones are physiologically active. The bound glucocorticoids serve as a hormone reservoir that is used to replace degraded unbound hormone. The half-lives of plasma corticosterone and cortisol are roughly 50 and 80 minutes, respectively. CBG is manufactured by liver cells. Thus, decreased hepatic function (*e.g.,* cirrhosis) can lead to subnormal quantities of plasma CBG, which in turn result in excess quantities of circulating unbound, active glucocorticoids.

Only a small amount of aldosterone is bound to plasma proteins. Its half-life is approximately 20 minutes.

Adrenal steroids are degraded by the liver. Their metabolites are converted to a soluble form by the same enzyme system that conjugates bilirubin (*i.e.,* the glucuronyltransferase system). The adrenal steroids and bilirubin compete for this system, and an excess of one type of substance may potentially inhibit the degradation of the others. Depressed hepatic function also can retard the degradation of adrenal steroids, thereby producing a clinical picture of hormone excess. The soluble degraded steroid metabolites are excreted by the kidneys.

Actions of Glucocorticoids. The effects of pharmacological dosages of these hormones will be considered separately from those of normal physiological levels. As the name "glucocorticoid" suggests, cortisol and corticosterone influence glucose metabolism. They elevate plasma glucose levels by promoting hepatic gluconeogenesis and glycogenolysis. To facilitate gluconeogenesis, these hormones cause the breakdown of fat in adipose tissue and proteins in connective, lymphatic, and muscle tissue and the release of fatty and amino acids into the bloodstream, which carries them to the liver.

Glucocorticosteroids also enable tissues to respond to glucagon and catecholamines; they also prevent rapid fatigue of skeletal muscle. The mode by which glucocorticoids produce these effects is not currently understood, and they go unnoticed in the normal person. One can best appreciate them by noting the result of their absence in adrenalectomized and untreated

people who are exposed to perceived threat or stress. As such, these "enabling" and metabolic effects possibly constitute a major portion of the "stress resistance" provided by the glucocorticosteroids.

Cortisol and corticosterone also act on the kidneys to permit the excretion of a normal water load in one of three ways: (1) Glucocorticoids make distal or collecting tubules more permeable to the reabsorption of water independently of sodium reabsorption; (2) glucocorticoids increase the glomerular filtration rate; or (3) glucocorticoids reduce the output of antidiuretic hormone (ADH).

The effects of glucocorticosteroids on plasma components are mixed. They decrease the numbers of plasma eosinophils and basophils while increasing the numbers of circulating neutrophils, platelets, and erythrocytes. By both suppressing production and increasing destruction, glucocorticoids decrease the numbers of lymphocytes. They also decrease the size of lymph nodes. A major function of lymphocytes is to provide either humoral immunity (with antibodies) or cell-mediated immunity. Stress-induced elevations in glucocorticoid secretion and the resulting decrease in lymphocytes may explain the decrease in immunocompetence that so often occurs in people who are under psychological or physical stress.

Other effects of physiological levels of glucocorticoids include decreasing olfactory and gustatory sensitivity: People with adrenal insufficiency can detect various chemicals (*e.g.,* sugar, salt, urea, and KCL) by either taste or smell with a sensitivity that is 40 to 120 times greater than normal.

In pharmacological dosages, glucocorticoids possess immunosuppressive anti-inflammatory and antihistaminic activity. They inhibit various parts of the inflammatory response, including edema, the influx of phagocytes, the activation of complement, and the formation of prostaglandins and leukotrienes. This can be very dangerous to patients with infections because the inflammatory response prevents the spread of invading microorganisms and serves as a sign that damage is present. Conversely, glucocorticoids can be of great benefit in the treatment of certain noninfective inflammatory conditions (*e.g.,* rheumatoid arthritis and systemic lupus erythematous). Glucocorticoids can also be beneficial in the treatment of certain allergies (*e.g.,* asthma, hives, and minimal change glomerular disease) because they prevent the release of histamines from mast cells. Of course, their use as immunosuppressives that enable patients to receive organ transplants is well known. In any case, the potentially deleterious side effects of glucocorticoids usually require that they be utilized after other treatments (*e.g.,* nonsteroidal anti-inflammatory drugs or antihistamines) have failed or when the benefits clearly outweigh the risks (*e.g.*, in renal disease or with organ transplants). In addition to allowing the spread of infections and immunosuppression, glucocorticoids trigger the development of all or part of Cushing's syndrome (*e.g.*, diabetes, hypertension, protein-wasting, and osteoporosis) and inhibit growth in infants and children.

Regulation of Glucocorticoid Secretion. The secretion of glucocorticoids is triggered by the release of corticotropin-releasing factor (CRF), a neurosecretion released by the hypothalamus, which in turn stimulates the cells of the anterior pituitary to secrete adrenocorticotropic hormone (ACTH). Without the stimulus of ACTH, the cells of the zona fasciculata and zona reticularis do not secrete glucocorticoids. Elevated plasma glucocorticoid levels function in a negative-feedback loop to decrease or halt the secretion of CRF and thereby indirectly ACTH as well.

There is a diurnal rhythm to the secretion of CRF that causes a similar rhythm in the output of ACTH and glucocorticoids. The net result is that maximal glucocorticoid secretion occurs between 6:00 and 8:00 A.M. in persons sleeping from midnight to 8:00 A.M. in a 24-hour day. Tumors that secrete CRF, ACTH, or glucocorticoids do not demonstrate such a rhythm, a fact that is useful in their diagnosis. The "biological clock" that regulates this and other diurnal, or circadian, rhythms is located in the hypothalamus, just above the area where the optic nerves cross (optic chiasma). Presumably, fibers from this area send impulses to the CRF-secreting area of the hypothalamus to regulate this neurosecretion.

The hypothalamic neurosecretion of CRF is also triggered by neural impulses from higher brain centers (*e.g.*, cerebral cortex) in responses to psychological stress. This type of stress is defined according to Lazarus' cognitive-phenomenological theory as a situation in which demands exceed the coping resources of the individual. This can occur slowly and deliberately or instantaneously and without the person's being precisely aware that such a phenomenon has occurred. Prior to the mid 1970s, Selye's proposed general adaptation syndrome was the only existing model for physiological responses to stress. According to this theory, any type of stress, physical or psychological, would trigger the release of glucocorticoids by the CRF-ACTH mechanism. Then, in an elegant series of experiments on monkeys that separated psychological from purely physical stressors, Mason and coworkers discovered that glucocorticosteroids were typically released only in response to psychological stress. These researchers found that physical stressors (cold, starvation, etc.) each induced a different pattern of responses from almost all the endocrine glands. Each type of stressor studied produced a different profile of endocrine responses that continued to change over several days following exposure of the animal to the stress-provoking agent. This work was later confirmed in humans. Thus, the physiological responses to stress can no longer be attributed only to the glucocorticoids.

Now we can conceptualize the perception of a potential physical or psychological threat to one's well-being as triggering a SAM response. If the demands of this or any other situation are evaluated as exceeding one's current resources, the CRF-ACTH-glucocorticosteroid mechanism is activated. The beneficial functions of normal levels of glucocorticoids in enabling tissues to respond to glucagon and catecholamines are more than adequate to meet the needs of the SAM mechanism for a short time. When these needs continue, additional stress-induced glucocorticoid secretion is required. Eventually, if the stress continues unameliorated, exhaustion of the adrenal cortex occurs, glucocorticoid levels drop, tissues are no longer able to meet the demands of the SAM mechanism, muscle fatigue occurs, readily available cell energy sources (*e.g.*, plasma glucose and fatty acid) are depleted, and vascular collapse and death may result.

Actions of Mineralocorticoids. Aldosterone and glucocorticoids that have some mineralocorticoid function (*e.g.*, DOCA) increase sodium reabsorption by the cells of the collecting ducts and distal tubules of the nephrons. Because of the cation exchange system in the distal tubule cells (see Chap. 18), such sodium reabsorption can increase potassium secretion, thereby fostering potential hypokalemia. The reabsorption of sodium osmotically causes water reabsorption. This expands the volume of extracellular fluid (ECF). The increase in blood volume causes an elevation in blood pressure. Edema does not usually result, however, because above a certain level of aldosterone-induced sodium reabsorption, the expansion of the ECR compartment may trigger (1) the secretion of natriuretic hormone, or (2) decreased sodium reabsorption in the proximal tubule. Either of these effects will oppose the action of aldosterone and sodium excretion.

Regulation of Mineralocorticoid Secretion. The primary mechanism for this is the renin-angiotensin system. Pituitary ACTH does not stimulate zona glomerulosa cells under normal conditions. Cells of the juxtaglomerular apparatus (JGA) are wedged between the renal afferent arteriole as it enters the glomerulus and the distal tubule as it passes by this area. The JGA has baroceptor cells that monitor the afferent arteriole blood pressure and other cells that monitor the sodium and chloride concentration in the urine within the distal tubule (the less the concentration, the slower the formation of filtrate, if all other factors are equal). A fall either in blood pressure or in the concentration of electrolytes stimulates the JGA to secrete the glycoprotein hormone renin. Thus, the major classes of stimuli that trigger renin secretion are (1) decreased renal perfusion (*e.g.,* hypotension, dehydration, hemorrhage, and constriction of renal artery), and (2) low ECF salt concentrations (*e.g.,* from excessive use of diuretics).

Renin converts a circulating plasma globulin into angiotensin I. As the blood passes through the lungs (and to a lesser extent in other parts of the circulatory system), angiotensin I is converted to angiotensin II. This physiologically active chemical acts on (1) the zona glomerulosa to promote aldosterone secretion, which leads to retention of salt and water, and (2) the vascular smooth muscle, thereby stimulating profound vasoconstriction. The net result of both actions of angiotensin II is elevation of systemic blood pressure, which will, among other things, improve renal perfusion.

The JGA contains B_2 receptors and can also be stimulated by sympathetic fibers. Prostaglandins also stimulate the JGA. Thus, the secretion of renin can now be pharmacologically decreased by beta$_2$ blockers (*e.g.,* propranolol). Prostaglandin inhibitors (aspirin, nonsteroidal anti-inflammatory agents, or indomethacin) may be found to exert a similar action. Captopril prevents the conversion of angiotensin I to angiotensin II. These effects have made captopril and beta$_2$ blockers very useful as antihypertensive agents.

Aldosterone secretion is also stimulated by an increase in plasma potassium, but not sodium, levels. The potassium seems to act by facilitating the conversion of cholesterol to aldosterone in zona glomerulosa cells. Another regulating factor for aldosterone secretion is posture. An upright body position increases aldosterone levels by increasing production and decreasing degradation. How this works is unclear, but because of this, aldosterone levels of bedridden patients are slightly subnormal. There also is a poorly understood diurnal rhythm of aldosterone secretion, with highest levels occurring in the early morning hours just prior to the person's awakening. This rhythm is not due to the diurnal CRF-ACTH rhythm because that affects only glucocorticoid secretion.

BIBLIOGRAPHY

Cannon WB: The Wisdom of the Body. New York, Norton, 1931

Ganong WF: Review of Medical Physiology. Los Altos, Lange Medical Publications, 1983

Gerich JE: Role of growth hormone in diabetes mellitus. N Engl J Med 310, No. 13:848–849, 1984

Mason JW: Emotion as reflected in patterns of endocrine integration. In Levi L (ed): Emotions: Their Parameters and Measurement. New York, Raven Press, 1975

Roth J, LeRoith D, Shiloach J et al: The evolutionary origins of hormones, neurotransmitters and other extracellular messengers. N Engl J Med 306, No. 9:523–426, 1981

Selye H: The Stress of Life. New York, McGraw-Hill, 1975

35
Diabetic Emergencies

Frank Davidoff

Diabetes: A Disease of Disordered Nutrition

Critically ill diabetic patients present a bewildering array of signs and symptoms: stupor, hyperventilation, vomiting, falling urine output, and unstable blood pressure all may be present and clamoring for attention. The number and complexity of laboratory measurements flashing past may be intimidating. Yet there is a basic coherence to all this metabolic "violence." The route to understanding the disorder lies in an understanding of the physiology of nutrition because diabetes is a disease of disordered nutrition.

FEEDING AND FASTING

The body faces two different nutritional challenges every day: nutrient storage and the release of nutrient from storage depots. The first arises because ingested nutrients are absorbed from the gastrointestinal (GI) tract over a relatively brief period of time. Under the usual circumstances of daily living, for example, glucose absorption occupies roughly a 3-hour period following each meal, or about one third of the 24 hours. Most tissues, however, use nutrients fairly constantly, particularly for energy, over the 24 hours. The body must therefore jealously guard the excess nutrient being absorbed, storing it away for use in between feeding times, in order to maintain a relatively constant internal environment. Preventing wastage of ingested nutrient must have been extremely important

for survival during evolution because it led to extraordinarily efficient storage mechanisms. Nutrient storage in the feeding phase of nutrition is appropriately referred to as an *anabolic* state.

After storing incoming nutrient, the body faces an entirely different nutritional task: feeding the tissues from stored reserves. This task is a delicate one. Nutrients must be released from storage depots at exactly the right rate. If release is too slow, other tissues may "starve in the midst of plenty." If release exceeds consumption by even a small amount, nutrients are lost, primarily in urine, leading to accelerated depletion of body reserves. If release becomes totally uncontrolled, both consumption and excretion mechanisms become swamped; nutrients accumulate in extracellular fluid, distorting and disfiguring the physiochemical environment that bathes every cell, leading to physiological malfunction, symptoms, and ultimately death.

A key concept in understanding the physiology of the fasting state is the dynamic balance that regulates the release of nutrients. Thus, in general, nutrient release from tissue storage sites does not depend on a positive signal, such as a hormonal trigger, to call it into action. Rather, the storage tissues left to themselves (*i.e.*, isolated tissues deprived of both nutrient [substrate] input and hormonal signals) spontaneously break down and release their stored nutrients; that is, they are in a *catabolic* state, almost as though it were their fundamental condition to sacrifice their own constituents for "more important" functions elsewhere. Control of this process is achieved by a second, negative hormonal signal, which restrains the rate of nutrient release, setting it precisely to meet the required rate of nutrient demand. It should now be clear why

600

the dynamic balance between spontaneous tissue nutrient release and hormonally controlled damping down of this release in the fasting phase of nutrition is sometimes referred to as an *anticatabolic* state.

It is apparent from our discussion of nutritional physiology so far that at any one moment in the course of a normal 24-hour day the human body can almost never be said to be in nutrient balance. Rather, balance shifts from hour to hour, from moderately positive to moderately negative, and it is only over the course of the entire day that the sum of these positives and negatives begins to approach balance (zero). Indeed, in free-living, healthy adults, energy balance probably approximates zero only in the course of 1 to 2 weeks.[1]

The two basic nutritional tasks are as follows:

- Storage of excess nutrient during food absorption.
- Re-release of nutrient from storage tissues between meals.

THE "BIG HEAD PROBLEM" AND THE CENTRAL ROLE OF GLUCOSE

Apart from understanding the feeding-fasting duality and its control, one must have a knowledge of another major concept to make sense of diabetes and diabetic catastrophes, namely, the unique metabolic role of the brain. In humans, the brain is not only disproportionately large but also virtually completely dependent on glucose for its energy supplies, in contradistinction to most other large organs that can easily switch to long-chain free fatty acids and indeed do so in preference to glucose when both substrates are presented together.

The large size of the human brain and its continuous dependence on glucose as an energy source, sometimes referred to as the *big head problem,* is compounded by the fact that, at least in adults, the brain stores almost no glucose (as glycogen).[2] As a result, normal brain function depends from minute to minute on a supply of glucose from the bloodstream, as evidenced by the almost immediate appearance of cerebral dysfunction when blood sugar falls below normal levels and equally dramatic restoration to normal when blood sugar rises again. The brain also needs its glucose-derived energy at the same rate day and night, waking and sleeping, working and resting, at a rate of about 5 g (1 tsp)/hour, which represents about half of the average daily adult glucose intake.

A number of other tissues also are either relatively dependent (*e.g.,* white blood cells, kidney medulla) or totally dependent (*e.g.,* red blood cells) on glucose-derived energy, although glucose deprivation does not have such immediate, obvious, or potentially harmful consequences for them as it does for the brain. The problem of feeding the brain thus looms as a task of central importance in human nutritional physiology. In the course of evolution, preservation of brain function has emerged as a development of highest priority, as indicated by the number and importance of the physiological mechanisms directed at providing energy to the brain, sometimes at the expense of other organs.

In point of fact, the brain, as we will see, can use one other major energy source, namely *ketone bodies.* These are not a normal dietary constituent but are generated within the body from its own fat stores as a kind of emergency fuel especially adapted to the fasting state. An understanding of the changing tissue fuel requirements and fuel sources over time (from the fully nourished condition during a meal, through the three phases of increasingly stringent adaptation to prolonged fasting) provides a high-power view of the physiological mechanisms involved in the maintenance of normal nutrition and fleshes out the metabolic scenario that one needs to understand diabetes.

The Big Head Problem
- In humans the brain is disproportionately large.
- The brain requires glucose continuously for energy, at 5 g/hr
- Without its energy supply, brain function deteriorates in minutes.

THE FOUR PHASES OF NUTRITION

The Fed State

From the first mouthful of a meal through the absorption of the last of the ingested nutrients from the gastrointestinal tract, the fed state is characterized by a condition of metabolic plenty. Because most meals for free-living subjects contain a mixture of the three macronutrients, with carbohydrates usually predominating, three different physiological mechanisms are required to store these nutrients, which enter the body in several-fold excess of minute-to-minute need. A limited fraction of carbohydrate not burned immediately is stored as glycogen, both in liver and in muscle; the remainder is promptly converted to fatty acids and glycerol and ultimately packed away as triglyceride in the fat droplets of adipose tissue. Feeding the brain its requisite ration of glucose is obviously no problem under these circumstances.

Dietary fat enters the circulation as chylomicrons, a complex microdroplet fat emulsion, which is cleared primarily for storage directly into adipose tissue. Amino acids are taken up into most tissues in proportion to their need, and amino acids in excess of immediate need are probably stored at least temporarily in a depot of skeletal muscle proteins.[3]

If the meal contains even small quantities of carbohydrate, the metabolic storage response to feeding results in a shutting down of nutrient release from storage depots, and a more or less complete switchover, therefore, to a carbohydrate economy (*i.e.,* primary dependence on glucose for the energy needs of nearly all tissues). As measured by studies of glucose influx rates, this tide of nutrient influx appears to end about 3 hours after the meal is started.[4]

The Postabsorptive State

The term *postabsorptive* is well chosen not only because it describes the timing of this nutritional phase but also because it clearly marks this condition as a normal or physiological daily event, a condition of "noninput" of nutrients, to be distinguished from the rigorous and stressful condition of more prolonged fasting. Once glucose is no longer entering the circulation from the GI tract, the brain must be fed from glucose stored in a tissue that can release it into the circulation for use elsewhere in the body. Liver glycogen is the only such store, and because the glycogen content of the whole liver amounts to only about 75 g, at a utilization rate that decreases slowly from its initial 5 g/hour, this source lasts only about 18 hours. Defined in terms of reliance on liver glycogen, the 15-hour period, from 3 to 18 hours after the last meal, constitutes postabsorptive metabolism.

During these 15 hours, long-chain free fatty acids are released at an increasing rate from adipose tissue and, when presented to most tissues (other than brain, red cells, renal medulla, etc.), are metabolized for energy in preference to glucose. Over the period of the postabsorptive state the body progressively makes the switch from a predominantly carbohydrate to a primarily fat economy. Although this change is in part brought about by the decrease in available glucose supplies, it also has the secondary effect of "sparing" glucose from use by most tissues other than the brain.

Short Fasting

Gluconeogenesis. As fasting progresses beyond the point of liver glycogen depletion, the brain must rely on an alternative glucose supply, one in which new glucose is created from precursor substances. The details of this process of *gluconeogenesis* (*neo* = new; *genesis* = creation) and its regulation are extraordinarily complex, but the essentials can be outlined fairly briefly. Glucose, a 6-carbon molecule, can be created anew only from 3-carbon fragments. In mammalian metabolism, this structural constraint has important nutritional and physiological consequences because such 3-carbon compounds can be supplied only from sources other than fatty acids. The 2-carbon units that form the basic structure of fatty acids cannot be combined or rearranged to make new glucose.

Therefore, despite the abundant fat stores in fasting humans, gluconeogenesis must depend on three nonfat sources for these 3-carbon building blocks: (1) lactate, from partial breakdown of glucose in several peripheral tissues; (2) glycerol, from the degradation of triglyceride stored in adipose tissue; and (3) certain amino acids derived ultimately from tissue proteins. All these are brought centrally to the liver, the only organ capable of converting these smaller precursors back into glucose and rereleasing it into the bloodstream.

Gluconeogenesis from the first two of the 3-carbon precursors, lactate and glycerol, represents a strict recycling of carbons without a net loss to the body because these 3-carbon molecules are derived in the first place from peripheral glucose metabolism. In contrast, that portion of gluconeogenesis that uses amino acids puts a net drain on body protein stores because the nitrogen is not reused for the most part but converted to urea in the liver and excreted in the urine. The overall result of the amino acid–to–glucose conversion is the sacrifice of structural and functional tissue proteins for the primary purpose of providing the brain with its obligatory glucose substrate.

Ketogenesis. The reassembly of 3-carbon fragments to glucose within the liver requires energy, which the liver, like the other tissues, at this point finds most easily available by oxidizing fatty acids from the abundant supply present in the circulation. During fasting, however, the liver uniquely and progressively alters its fatty acid metabolizing mechanism. It no longer oxidizes fatty acids all the way to CO_2 and water, but rather to their constituent 2-carbon fragment, acetate. These acetate molecules recombine, still in the liver, into 4-carbon fatty "by-products," the ketone bodies, acetoacetate and hydroxybutyrate. The ketones then leave the liver and enter the circulation, representing a kind of water-soluble fat, which is used very efficiently for energy by most peripheral tissues. The rate of ketone body consumption by most tissues, particularly the brain, increases in proportion to their level in the circulation.

Ketogenesis and gluconeogenesis are thus seen to be critically important physiological adaptations to the metabolic stress of fasting, and under the usual conditions of fasting the two processes are tightly coupled. The net result of these adaptations is the increasing flow of lactate, glycerol, amino acids, and long-chain fatty acids into the liver and the net release from the liver of glucose, ketone bodies, and urea.

As fasting progresses beyond 18 hours, the time at which liver glycogen is depleted, the rates of both gluconeogenesis and ketogenesis increase rapidly, reaching a maximum at about 48 to 72 hours following the meal. The circulating level of ketone bodies at this point has risen 10- to 20-fold, from its "fed state" level of about 0.1 mEq/liter to a level of about 1 to 2 mEq/liter, high enough to exceed the renal threshold and produce the characteristic *ketonuria* of fasting. Beyond this time, ketogenesis continues at a steady, rapid rate in the liver, but the consumption of ketone bodies by muscle and adipose tissues diminishes slowly and progressively. As a result, the circulating ketone level continues to rise, reaching 6 to 7 mEq/liter if fasting is prolonged to 3 weeks, a rise of some 50- to 75-fold above its initial fed level.

Prolonged Fasting

After about 3 weeks of total fasting, the level of circulating ketone bodies plateaus and remains relatively constant thereafter. Metabolism then enters the phase of prolonged fasting, a more- or-less steady state of adaptation to the most serious metabolic challenge of all, starvation. This adaptation is characterized by its extremely tight regulation, directing itself to maximal preservation of body stores while not permitting the composition of nutrients circulating in blood to become too greatly displaced from normal.

The most important result of the great increase in circulating ketones is that an energy alternative to glucose is made available to the brain. After 3 to 4 weeks of complete fasting, ketones provide about 60% of the brain's energy supply. The demand for glucose production in the liver is thus lessened by at least this amount, which in turn reduces the drain on body protein stores. As a result, urinary nitrogen excretion drops progressively from 10 g/day in the postabsorptive state to about 3 g/day after prolonged fasting. This spares about 42 g of tissue protein or 150 g of lean tissue weight per day, an adaptation that is obviously critical to prolonged survival. In addition to this specific drop in gluconeogenic requirement, the body adapts to fasting in a more general way by lowering its overall resting metabolic energy requirement about 20%, further sparing endogenous energy and protein reserves.

The circulating level of free fatty acids, which rises to a maximum during the period of short fasting, remains quite constant thereafter, supplying a greater and greater proportion of energy needs in muscle and most visceral tissues other than the brain. Blood glucose levels, in contrast, fall during the first 3 to 4 days of fasting and then remain constant thereafter. The

blood sugar levels may go remarkably low during fasting, generally somewhat lower in women than in men, sometimes as low as 25 to 30 mg/dl, without any accompanying symptoms of cerebral disturbance. This is presumably because ketone bodies have partially replaced glucose as the energy supply to the brain.[5,6]

> ### The Four Phases of Nutrition
>
> - *Fed state.* Glucose is available for tissue energy needs.
> - *Postabsorptive.* Liver glycogen provides limited glucose supplies.
> - *Short fasting.* Fatty acids provide most tissue energy; glucose for the brain comes from gluconeogenesis; ketogenesis develops.
> - *Prolonged fasting.* Tightly regulated gluconeogenesis and ketogenesis provide brain nutrient, sparing body protein breakdown; maximal switch to a "fat economy."

HORMONAL CONTROL OF NUTRITIONAL PHYSIOLOGY

Insulin. Understanding the control of nutritional balance is very much simplified by the realization that both feeding and fasting metabolism are primarily regulated by a single hormone, *insulin*. After a meal, insulin levels rise rapidly into the anabolic range of 50 μU to 100 μU/ml, then decline as the surge of entering nutrients is stored (Fig. 35-1, *A*). At its tissue target sites, these large amounts of insulin directly stimulate a variety of important biochemical storage steps including the rate of glucose entry into insulin-sensitive cells across the plasma membrane and the rate of glycogen, fatty acid, and protein synthesis.

As the postabsorptive state draws on, insulin levels fall into their anticatabolic range of 5 μU to 10 μU/ml, about tenfold below the anabolic range, passing through a "null-point" poised between these two different insulin actions (see Fig. 35-1, *A*). In the anticatabolic range, insulin no longer stimulates storage mechanisms but provides the negative signal that suppresses the otherwise self-sustaining breakdown of glycogen, triglycerides, and protein in a variety of tissues and gluconeogenesis in liver. Of course, insulin in its higher, anabolic range maximally suppresses these catabolic events at the same time it turns on storage mechanisms.

Other Hormones. Besides insulin, there are other hormones that play some role in the "fine tuning," or modulation and smoothing, of metabolic control. In particular, *glucagon* provides a counterregulatory

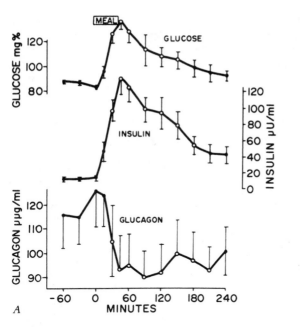

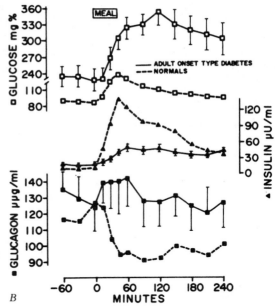

FIGURE 35-1
Insulin and glucagon responses to eating a large carbohydrate meal. (A) Normal subjects. Note the large, early, rapidly rising increase in insulin level, the simultaneous drop in glucagon level, and the moderate, well-damped excursion of blood glucose level. (B) Comparison of normal versus moderate diabetic subjects. Insulin level rises late, sluggishly, and relatively little; glucagon level increases paradoxically, and blood glucose remains at abnormally high levels for a long time in diabetic subjects. (Muüller W et al: Abnormal alpha cell function in diabetes. N Engl J Med 283:109–115, 1970, with permission)

"pull" to insulin's "push" because glucagon directly stimulates. The breakdown of glucose stored as glycogen (glycogenolysis), of fat stored as triglyceride (lipolysis), and the synthesis of new glycose (gluconeogenesis) in the liver. On a minute-to-minute basis, then, the rates of the major opposing nutrient storage and release processes are regulated by the balance between insulin versus glucagon levels. Moreover, glucocorticoids from the adrenal cortex, catecholamines from the adrenal medulla and peripheral adrenergic neurons, and growth hormone (somatotropin) from the anterior pituitary provide "permissive" control of metabolism by both direct effects on tissues and indirect effects on insulin/glucagon release. As a group, these other hormones, like glucagon, all work to stimulate tissue breakdown and nutrient release, in essence, a part of the "stress response."

Despite the importance of these catabolic, or counterregulatory, hormones in normal physiology, the absence of one or another of them seems to be well tolerated, apparently because the presence of the others can compensate for the loss. In contrast, insulin emerges as the only "storage hormone" and thus is uniquely important as the prime regulator of metabolism. Insufficiency of insulin produces a series of disruptions in metabolism collectively referred to as *diabetes mellitus.*

Hormonal Control of Nutritional Physiology

- Insulin is the "storage hormone."
- High insulin levels cause nutrient storage (anabolism).
- Low insulin levels regulate release of stored nutrient (anticatabolism).
- Glucagon promotes nutrient release, gluconeogenesis, and ketogenesis.
- The "stress hormones" hydrocortisone, catecholamines, and growth hormone all oppose insulin action.

THE TWO FORMS OF DIABETES: MILD AND SEVERE

The Basic Disturbance

When insulin secretion becomes slightly impaired, the insulin-secreting β-cells of the pancreatic islets have no difficulty providing the low levels of insulin required to regulate fasting metabolism. Thus, in the mildest forms of diabetes (various terms for this form of diabetes include *type II diabetes, chemical diabetes, adult onset–type diabetes,* and *noninsulin-de-*

pendent type diabetes), fasting blood sugar may be *normal.* It is only when the challenge of feeding calls for anabolic levels of insulin that the insulin secretory mechanism of the β-cells is insufficient to a degree. The rate of glucose (and other macronutrient) storage therefore is diminished, and it is this lag in storage that permits glucose to rise to *higher* levels and to return to baseline levels more *slowly* than normal.

These alterations characterize an abnormal glucose tolerance test, the major diagnostic tool for detecting mild diabetes, standing in sharp contrast to the brief, tightly damped excursions of blood sugar in nondiabetic subjects (Fig. 35-1, *B*).[7] In the mildest diabetics, all these nutrients are retained within the body and ultimately taken up into tissues. Overall glucose utilization rates remain normal, and many of these patients therefore can, and do, continue to gain weight.

As insulin secretion capacity declines further, the β-cells cannot even supply the small amounts required in the postabsorptive or fasting states. Fasting metabolism becomes progressively unregulated, resulting not only in loss of nutrient storage capacity but also in uncontrolled catabolism. Thus, even in the absence of any ingested food, blood sugar rises above normal owing to inappropriately accelerated glycogenolysis and gluconeogenesis. Concomitantly, the rates of lipolysis and ketogenesis become uncontrolled, leading to spiraling levels of ketones in the circulation. As the concentrations of glucose and ketones rise above the renal threshold, these nutrients are lost into the urine, imposing a calorie drain on the body and giving rise first to the glycosuria characteristic of moderate diabetes and, ultimately, to the ketonuria of severe diabetes.

In the most severe diabetes (other terms for which include *type I diabetes, insulin-dependent diabetes, juvenile onset–type diabetes, and ketosis-prone diabetes*), body weight may not be maintained, despite large calorie and protein intakes, and the flesh may be literally melted down and lost through the siphon of the urine (the word *diabetes,* from the Greek word meaning "siphon," was first applied to the disease several thousand years ago).

In summary, insulin possesses both anabolic and anticatabolic functions. The anabolic functions of insulin seem to be widely appreciated because it is intuitively obvious that a storage regulator would be needed to control nutritional physiology during the feeding phase. In contrast, the anticatabolic effects of insulin, which prevent excessive mobilization of stored glucose, fat, and protein, as well as excessive glucose and ketone production during fasting, are generally more difficult to conceptualize. It is therefore somewhat ironic that a defect in secretion of feeding phase insulin produces relatively minimal disruptions in metabolism, whereas loss of the unimpressive, basal, fasting insulin levels permits the intrinsic cata-

bolic processes of the body to become so unregulated that body substance is lost, distorting the amount and composition of body fluids to the point at which serious illness or even death results. This most extreme form of diabetic abnormality, ketoacidosis, represents the major diabetic emergency.

Mild Vs. Severe Diabetes

- Mild (type II) diabetes represents insufficient insulin for nutrient storage.
- Severe (type I) diabetes occurs when even the low levels of insulin needed to regulate fasting metabolism are not maintained.

Diabetic Ketoacidosis

For reasons that should now be obvious, diabetic ketoacidosis is sometimes referred to as a state of "accelerated fasting" or "superfasting." Although there are many metabolic complications of this state,[8, 9, 10] the major damage to the patient occurs through pathophysiological changes in three distinct areas: (1) hyperosmolarity, (2) ketoacidosis, and (3) volume depletion (Fig. 35-2, *A*). These three disturbances interact with one another in certain ways that will soon become apparent (Fig. 28-2, *B*, *C*, and *D*). Initially, however, they can and should be understood separately, not only because each affects the patient in a highly specific manner, but because in any one patient the degree of severity of each disturbance may vary separately from very slight to very severe. Indeed, certain patients exhibit a severe abnormality in one area but none at all in the others. Although these patients represent metabolic conditions separate and distinct from diabetic ketoacidosis, their conditions overlap diabetic ketoacidosis very closely. They will be discussed at the end of this section to highlight each of the component parts of the diabetic ketoacidosis syndrome.

The following case study illustrates many of the key features of diabetic ketoacidosis.

CASE STUDY

M. O., a 41-year-old man, was admitted to the hospital on March 29, 1984, with the chief complaint of fatigue, cough, nausea, and vomiting for 4 days.

The patient had been diagnosed as having diabetes mellitus $1\frac{1}{2}$ years prior to admission. Since that time, he had been

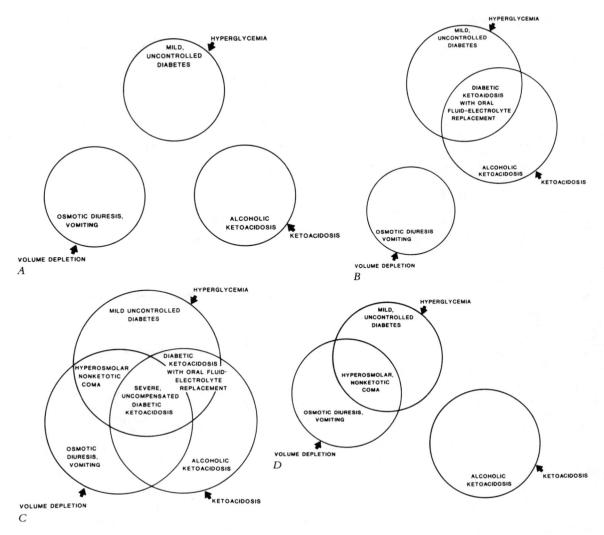

FIGURE 35-2
*The pathophysiological components of diabetic ketoacidosis and their several interactions. (A)
The three major pathophysiological components, viewed as distinct elements. (B) Modified
diabetic ketoacidosis: hyperglycemia and ketoacidosis are present, but volume depletion is
minimal. Volume depletion may be prevented either because oral water and electrolyte intake
have been sufficient to replace losses or because the syndrome developed very rapidly. Blood
sugar and ketone levels can rise quickly, but it takes considerable time for osmotic diuresis to
deplete the body of water and electrolytes. Therefore, patients seen early may be less volume-
depleted than those who have been developing the condition for many days or even weeks. (C)
Full-blown diabetic ketoacidosis. All three pathophysiological elements make major contribution. (D) Hyperosmolar nonketotic coma: hyperglycemia, hyperosmolality, and volume
depletion always are present, often to extreme degree, but ketosis is absent or trivial, by definition.*

maintained without incident on 48 units of NPH insulin in the
morning and 16 units of NPH in the evening. Four days before admission, the patient began to cough, raising first clear,
then brownish, sputum. He soon became fatigued, then experienced some nausea and intermittent vomiting. Two days
before admission, he omitted his evening insulin, then took
no further insulin the day before and day of admission "because he was not eating anything." On the day of admission,
the patient's wife noted that he had become "less responsive

and was breathing fast and deeply" and brought him to the
emergency room.

On admission, the patient's rectal temperature was 27°C
(97°F), pulse was 132, respirations were 24 and deep, and
blood pressure was 108/72. Physical examination demonstrated him to be oriented but lethargic, with coarse rales at
both lung bases, but was otherwise negative.

Admission laboratory work revealed a hematocrit of 51.6,
white blood cell count of 36,400, and 4+ glucose and ketones

on urinalysis. Admission laboratory work included glucose 910 mg/dl, Na+ 128, K+ 6.7, Cl− 90, HCO3− 4, BUN 43, creatinine 2.3 mg/dl, serum ketones 4+ at 1:2 dilution, and trace to 1:32 dilution. Arterial blood *p*H was 7.06, PO2 112, PCO2 13, and HCO3− 2.5. The admission chest film was negative, but sputum cultured on admission ultimately grew out *Haemophilus influenza* and *Streptococcus pneumoniae*.

Initial therapy consisted of an intravenous infusion of normal saline and 20 units of regular insulin by IV push, followed by an infusion of insulin at 5 units/hour during the first 9 hours. The patient's mental status and sense of well-being improved rapidly. The following flow sheet summarizes the biochemical changes over the first 15 hours.

The patient remained afebrile and was not treated with antibiotics. By the time of discharge 4 days later (April 2, 1984) he was eating well, his blood sugars were controlled on his usual doses of NPH insulin, and his cough had improved.

BIOCHEMICAL FLOWSHEET INDICATING DIABETIC KETOACIDOSIS IN PATIENT M. O.

Time	Sugar	pH	Na+	K+	Cl−	HCO3−	BUN/ Creatinine
13:00	910	7.06	128	6.9	90	4	43/2.3
15:00	492		132	6.8	101	6	41/1.7
17:15	375	7.25	137	4.1	106	8	45/1.4
22:00	303		139	4.7	114	15	27/1.2
04:00	304		143	4.3	113	22	22/1.1

PRECIPITATING EVENTS

Although diabetic ketoacidosis can and does occur in patients who have completely lost their capacity to secrete insulin without other obvious triggering or precipitating factors, it is quite common for stressful events, most commonly infection (as in the previous case study), sometimes emotional turmoil, to provide the "last straw" that sets the process in motion. The hormonal responses to stress include release of glucagon, glucocorticoids, and catecholamines, all of which, as indicated, drive catabolic processes at accelerated rates. The mechanism by which stress operates to initiate diabetic ketoacidosis is therefore not difficult to conceptualize. Indeed, even in the virtual absence of insulin secretion it is unusual for diabetic ketoacidosis to develop if these other hormones also are lacking, as in diabetic patients who have undergone hypophysectomy (thereby removing growth hormone and adrenocorticotropic hormone [ACTH]) or those rendered diabetic by complete pancreatectomy (thereby removing glucagon).

Of course, when a patient's own capacity to secrete insulin has been completely lost, the patient then becomes completely dependent on injected insulin.

Stopping or skipping insulin injections, particularly in the setting of stress or infection, is therefore often a major precipitating event in ketoacidosis. About half the time, however, no specific precipitating cause for episodes of ketoacidosis is identified.

Diabetic ketoacidosis is often precipitated by one of the following:

- Infection
- Emotional or other stress
- Withdrawal of insulin therapy

HYPERGLYCEMIA AND HYPEROSMOLARITY

In contrast to normal subjects, whose blood sugars never rise above about 150 mg/dl, or even mild diabetics, in whom the level rarely exceeds 350 to 400 mg/dl, patients in diabetic ketoacidosis not uncommonly exhibit blood sugars of 1000 to 1500 mg/dl. It is clear that the mechanisms that usually protect the body from such catastrophic rises in blood sugar must have broken down completely in such patients. The central mechanism that protects against hyperosmolarity turns out to be renal glucose excretion, the very same mechanism that causes the second type of abnormality in diabetic ketoacidosis, volume depletion (Fig. 35-3).

As long as the circulating blood volume remains relatively normal, glucose is filtered at the kidney glomerulus into the renal tubules; as long as the filtered glucose load remains relatively small, all of this glucose is reabsorbed into the bloodstream. When the filtered load increases above a certain level, however, as when the blood sugar exceeds the normal threshold of about 180 mg/dl, glucose begins to escape into the urine because the reabsorption capacity of the tubules is exceeded. As the filtered load increases further, urinary glucose loss increases very rapidly, and nearly all extra glucose put into the circulation thereafter is lost into the urine. This renal "escape valve" serves as a very powerful protective device to prevent extreme accumulation of glucose in blood. Indeed, in diabetic subjects whose circulating blood volume is well maintained, it is extremely unusual to find blood sugar levels in excess of 500 mg/dl because of the intense glucose diuresis.[11] Conversely, *any patient whose blood sugar is higher than this level must be suspected of having either a severely reduced circulating blood volume, renal damage, or both.*

As we shall see, it is glycosuria itself that is largely responsible for volume depletion. In a diabetic patient who is badly out of control and in whom oral replace-

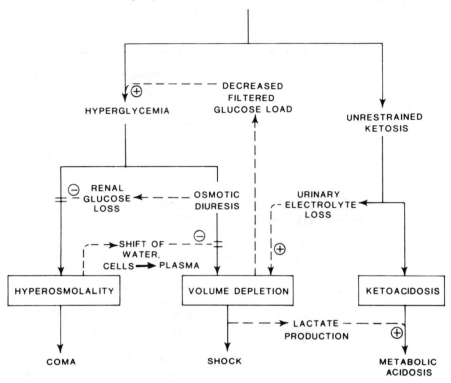

Severe Insulin Deficiency

(Excess of: Glucagon, Catecholamines, Glucocorticoids, Growth Hormone)

FIGURE 35-3
*The metabolic consequences of severe insulin deficiency and their interrelations leading to
diabetic ketoacidosis. Dashed arrows represent secondary interactions that reduce (−) or
aggravate (+) the severity of primary disturbances.*

ment of sodium and water has been sufficient to compensate for urinary losses, a vicious cycle is set up in which hyperglycemia leads to volume depletion, which, uncompensated, in turn reduces urinary glucose losses, which again permits the blood sugar to rise even higher.

It appears to be the hyperosmolarity of body fluids itself, resulting from this upward spiral in blood sugar, rather than ketosis, acidosis, or volume depletion, that primarily accounts for the lethargy, stupor, and, ultimately, coma that occur as diabetic ketoacidosis worsens. The evidence for this conclusion rests on the general correlation between degree of hyperosmolarity and degree of coma, in contrast to preserved mental function in states in which pure ketoacidosis exists without hyperosmolarity.[12, 13]

CASE ANALYSIS

Our patient presented with the chemical findings of extreme hyperglycemia. As expected in this situation, the BUN and creatinine were elevated, indicating that renal perfusion was reduced, permitting less glucose to escape into the urine, and allowing the blood sugar to reach these high levels. The patient's lethargic mental state was consistent with the moderately severe hyperosmolality.

The development of hyperglycemia, hyperosmolarity, and coma in diabetic ketoacidosis is schematically outlined in the left and center portions of Figure 35-3.

KETOSIS AND ACIDOSIS

The second major consequence of severe insulin deficiency is uncontrolled ketogenesis. As ketoacids enter the extracellular fluid, the hydrogen ion is stripped from the molecule (Equation 1) and neutralized by combining with bicarbonate ion buffer, thus protecting the *p*H of extracellular fluids and leaving behind ketoacid anion residues. The resultant carbonic acid (see Equation 2) breaks down into water and CO_2 gas, which literally "fizzes" out through the lungs.

Equation 1:

$$\left.\begin{array}{l} H^+\text{-acetoacetic acid} \\ H^+\text{-}\beta\text{-hydroxybutyric acid} \end{array}\right\} + HCO_3^- \rightarrow H_2CO_3^- \left\{\begin{array}{l} \text{acetoacetate}^- \\ \beta\text{-hydroxybutyrate}^- \end{array}\right.$$

Equation 2:

$$H_2CO_3 \rightarrow H_2O + CO_2 \text{ gas}(\uparrow)$$

Therefore, as ketoacid anions accumulate, they progressively displace bicarbonate from extracellular fluid. The usual laboratory determination of electrolytes does not measure ketoacid concentrations directly. However, an excess of total measured cations (sodium plus potassium) over total measured anions (chloride plus bicarbonate) provides a clue to the presence of these so-called unmeasured anions. This excess, sometimes referred to as the *anion gap,* can serve as an indirect measure of the quantity of ketoacids present.

A total of 6 to 7 mEq/liter of ketoacids, which would reduce serum bicarbonate from its usual 25 mEq/liter to 18 to 19 mEq/liter, seems to be well tolerated by most diabetic patients. Because, as we have seen, prolonged fasting alone can cause a physiologic starvation ketosis of this degree, it seems logical to consider this a *mild* degree of ketoacidosis when it is produced by uncontrolled diabetes rather than by starvation.

In the range of 6 to 15 mEq/liter of ketone bodies, with corresponding bicarbonate levels of 10 to 19 mEq/liter, the buffering and acid-compensating mechanisms of the body become more seriously stressed, but in this range pH usually remains at least partially protected. Ketoacidosis of this degree is never physiologic, and when due to diabetes it can therefore be considered to be *moderate* in degree. Once the bicarbonate level falls below 10 mEq/liter owing to ketoacid accumulations greater than 15 mEq/liter, the protection against acidosis rapidly reaches its outer limit, and even slight interference with compensating mechanisms can send body pH plummeting to very low levels. Ketoacidosis of this degree (15 mEq/liter of ketoacid accumulation) is obviously severe and life-threatening.

Hyperventilation

The neutrality of body fluids is primarily protected by the bicarbonate buffering system, which determines the pH at all times by the ratio of bicarbonate anion to CO_2 gas in plasma. If bicarbonate anion is lost owing to its displacement by ketoacid anions, extra CO_2 gas must be driven off at the lung by hyperventilation in order to keep the ratio at or close to its usual value of

20:1 and to maintain pH close to its physiologic value of 7.4. Hyperventilation, gradual at first, then rapidly more vigorous and more obvious as arterial pH drops below 7.2, is therefore a characteristic physical finding in diabetic ketoacidosis. This dramatic increase in ventilation, which occurs more by an increase in the *depth* than in the *frequency* of breathing, is known as *Kussmaul breathing*. The presence of clear-cut Kussmaul breathing is therefore a signal that extracellular fluid pH is at or below 7.2, a relatively severe degree of acidosis.[14]

The outer limit of compensation for a declining bicarbonate buffer reserve is imposed by the maximal rate of hyperventilation that the lungs can achieve. At the usual rates of total CO_2 production by the body, the lungs breathe fast enough to drive the total CO_2 gas level in blood down to about one fourth its normal value but not lower. Hyperventilation can therefore compensate, at least partially, for bicarbonate levels as low as 6 to 8 mEq/liter, one fourth its normal range of 24 to 32 mEq/liter. As bicarbonate drops below that level, however, CO_2 gas remains disproportionately high relative to bicarbonate, and pH then drops at an alarming rate. It is for this reason that bicarbonate levels below 10 mEq/liter are taken as an indicator of severe acidosis and call for more aggressive therapy.

Testing For Serum Ketones

Serum ketones can be measured semiquantitatively at the bedside by testing progressive dilutions of serum with *nitroprusside reagent* (powder or crushed tablets).[15] This maneuver serves several important purposes: (1) It rapidly helps confirm the *diagnosis* of diabetic ketoacidosis once it has been suggested by history, physical examination, and urine testing; (2) it is possible to make a rough assessment of *degree* of ketoacidosis, at least to the extent of categorizing it as mild, moderate, or severe; and (3) a major discrepancy between the amount of ketones estimated by the serum nitroprusside procedure and the total anion gap calculated from the electrolytes determined in the laboratory suggests that a *second unmeasured anion,* usually lactate, is contributing to the acidosis in addition to ketoacids.

Kidney Action

Finally, because ketoacids are excreted in the urine largely as their sodium, potassium, and ammonium salts, the loss of ketones through the kidneys contributes to the problems of water and electrolyte losses, the third important category of physiological damage in diabetic ketoacidosis. The development of metabolic acidosis in diabetic ketoacidosis is outlined on the right side of Figure 35-3.

In our patient M. O., the extremely low initial serum bicarbonate concentration of 2.5 to 4 signalled the consumption of nearly all the available buffering capacity of plasma, indicating the presence of *severe* metabolic acidosis. This conclusion was reinforced by the anion gap of $(128 + 7) - (90 + 3) = 42$, about 30 mEq above the usual anion gap upper limit of 12, thus indicating the presence of 30 mEq of "unmeasured anions." The semiquantitative serum ketones were strongly positive at a dilution of 1:2, confirming the presence of a large quantity of ketone bodies, which could account for most of the unmeasured anion. The diagnosis of diabetic ketoacidosis of severe degree is thus firmly established.

The patient's deep, rapid respirations represented Kussmaul breathing, a critically important compensating mechanism that had reduced his arterial CO_2 level (PCO_2) to about one fourth its usual level, which had helped keep his blood *p*H from falling below its already very low level of 7.06.

FLUID AND ELECTROLYTE LOSSES: VOLUME DEPLETION

Osmotic Diuresis

Although glucose loss through the kidneys helps protect against the ravages of extreme hyperosmolarity, the diabetic patient developing ketoacidosis pays a price for this glycosuria. Glucose remaining in the glomerular filtrate, after the renal tubules have reabsorbed all they can, forces water to remain in the tubules. This glucose-rich filtrate then sweeps out of the body, carrying with it water, sodium, potassium, ammonium, phosphate, and other salts. The resulting rapid urine flow and obligate loss of water and electrolytes that would otherwise be reabsorbed is known as an *osmotic diuresis*. Salts of ketone bodies, as well as the urea resulting from rapid protein breakdown and accelerated gluconeogenesis, also contribute to the solute load in the renal tubule, further aggravating the diuresis.

Salt And Water Loss

The average amounts of salts and water lost to the body through osmotic diuresis during the development of diabetic ketoacidosis have been measured directly. These numbers serve as important markers for understanding the degree of physiological damage done to the patient.[16] Overall water loss in a 70-kg adult patient presenting in diabetic ketoacidosis amounts to about 6 to 7 liters or 15% of total body water.

One can determine that of this, about 3 liters are derived from the extracellular compartment, judging from the accompanying average loss of 420 mEq of *sodium* and assuming that the sodium concentration of normal extracellular fluid is 140 mEq/liter. This represents a loss of at least 20% of extracellular water, which is a very major insult to the integrity of the body fluids. Another 3 liters is derived from the intracellular space, as indicated by the loss of 300 mEq of *potassium*, the major intracellular cation, because the potassium concentration within cells is normally about 100 mEq/liter.

The fluid lost to the body is slightly hypotonic, meaning that it contains a slight excess of water as compared with the volume of salts, as would be expected from an osmotic diuresis due to glucose and urea. These figures, as noted, represent averages. The *net* losses found in any particular patient will be the result of many different factors, among them the intensity and duration of the hyperglycemia and thus the intensity of osmotic diuresis; the amount of water and electrolyte replaced by mouth during this time; the presence of other fluid and electrolyte losses such as vomiting, diarrhea, or sweating; and the integrity of renal function (see Fig. 35-2, *B*).

Compensatory Mechanisms

Sodium and water make up the central structure of the extracellular fluid, including the vascular volume. Removal of these large quantities of sodium and water from the body is therefore perceived as a serious threat to the maintenance of the circulation, and a variety of compensatory mechanisms are called into play to prevent vascular collapse and shock. For example, an increase in pulse rate usually occurs that helps maintain cardiac output in the face of shrinking intravascular volume.

At least as important, however, is a protective shift in body fluid brought about by the hyperglycemia itself. Because free glucose is limited almost entirely to the extracellular water, an osmotic pressure gradient is set up across the cell membrane, between the extracellular compartment and the interior of the cells. Therefore, the higher the blood sugar, the more water is drawn out of cells and into the extracellular space. Thus, as sodium and water are lost into the urine, shrinking the extracellular fluid, they are, in effect, "replaced" (at least as to their osmotic effect) by glucose entering from the liver and by water entering from all cells, which reexpand the extracellular fluid again (see Fig. 35-3, *left*).

The very hyperosmolarity that produces damaging central nervous system (CNS) effects and osmotic diuresis therefore provides at least a partial and temporary mechanism for preventing vascular collapse, an important "prop" to the structure of the extracellular fluid in ketoacidosis. It is, however, a rather shaky one because of its rapid reversal when blood glucose is lowered again.

Adverse Effects

Despite these efforts at compensation, circulatory integrity is progressively compromised as diabetic ketoacidosis progresses, leading ultimately to a series of secondary pathologic changes, some of which in turn develop into self-perpetuating, vicious spirals.

Decrease in Glomerular Filtration. First, loss of vascular volume produces a fall in glomerular filtration, which is why the usual measures of renal function, including blood urea nitrogen (BUN) and creatinine levels, are characteristically elevated in ketoacidotic patients. We have already seen how decreasing renal function permits blood glucose levels to spiral to extreme values (see Fig. 35-3, *center*), but other consequences, particularly difficulty in controlling potassium excretion, also result from this change. Because the excretion of potassium by the kidney occurs by the exchange of potassium for sodium, adequate sodium must be present at the exchange site in the kidney for the rate of potassium excretion to keep pace with the need for excretion. When vascular volume is diminished and renal perfusion is consequently reduced, not enough sodium may be available for this exchange. Despite a total body depletion of potassium, the serum potassium level may therefore rise above normal, even to dangerous or lethal levels.

Decrease In Tissue Perfusion. A second major consequence of diminished vascular volume is a generalized decrease in tissue perfusion. Well before the drop in volume has reached the point at which blood pressure actually falls and full-blown shock is said to be present, blood is shunted away from many tissues, and the perfusion of nearly all tissues suffers. The resultant decrease in oxygen delivery causes those tissues to shift to some degree of anaerobic glucose metabolism, resulting in the increased production of lactic acid. The release of this second organic acid into the circulation simply lowers the bicarbonate further, aggravating the already existing metabolic acidosis (see Fig. 35-3, *right*). A combined lactic acidosis and ketoacidosis is not an uncommon finding, therefore, in patients with diabetic ketoacidosis.

Phosphate Loss. Tissue hypoxia due to decreased tissue perfusion may be aggravated indirectly in ketoacidosis as the result of urinary loss of another electrolyte, phosphate. As body phosphate stores are depleted, circulating phosphate levels fall quite low in plasma, depriving the red cells of an essential reactant used to form a variety of organic phosphate compounds. Under these circumstances, red cells become depleted of certain key phosphate derivatives, which in turn increases the tightness of oxygen binding to the

hemoglobin within those cells. As these cells pass through the poorly perfused tissues, less oxygen is given up than from red cells with a normal complement of phosphate compounds, and tissue hypoxia is worsened.

Shock. Finally, if vascular volume falls low enough, compensation mechanisms fail, blood pressure drops, and true shock supervenes. A rapidly worsening cycle of acidosis, tissue damage, and deepening shock may then occur, leading ultimately to irreversible vascular collapse and death. The full-blown syndrome of diabetic ketoacidosis is characterized by major contributions from all three major pathophysiological disruptions (see Fig. 35-2, *C*), each of which is primarily responsible for one of the major clinical features: coma, shock, and metabolic acidosis (see Fig. 35-3).

CASE ANALYSIS

The history of increasing symptoms over at least 4 days in our patient M. O. suggested that this episode of ketoacidosis had been developing for a substantial period of time, sufficient for the osmotic diuresis to produce extensive salt and water losses. The development of nausea prevented volume replacement by mouth, and vomiting further aggravated the losses.

The rapid pulse and low blood pressure on admission were further clues to the presence of significant hypovolemia, which was confirmed by the elevated BUN and creatinine, reflecting inadequate circulating blood volume to maintain renal perfusion. Finally, the elevated serum potassium ($K^+ = 6.7$ mEq/liter, normal = 3.5 to 4.8 mEq/liter) indicated that not enough sodium was being filtered in the kidney to permit adequate potassium exchange and potassium excretion.

The three major disturbances of physiology in diabetic ketoacidosis are

- Hyperosmolality, due to hyperglycemia
- Metabolic acidosis, due to accumulation of ketoacids
- Volume depletion, due to osmotic diuresis

Each of these three disturbances

- May be more or less severe in any single patient
- May interact to aggravate or compensate for the other disturbances

---

THERAPY

Rational, effective therapy for diabetic ketoacidosis must be based on an understanding of the mechanisms of metabolic damage, both primary and secondary, as already outlined. Each therapeutic maneuver is directed primarily at one of the three areas of physiological disruption. However, it should be clear by now (see Figs. 35-2 and 35-3) that none of these disruptions exists completely separate from the others. Thus, therapy that reverses one abnormality may also have important *benefits and risks* in other areas because of their interlocking nature.

Volume: Salt And Water Replacement

The most immediate threat to life in a critically ill ketoacidotic patient is *volume depletion.* Once the diagnosis is even seriously considered, the first priority is always to get a large, secure intravenous line in place. A cutdown may be necessary in a severely dehydrated patient almost in shock because veins may be collapsed and hard to find. As soon as this line is established, 0.9% (normal) saline is rapidly infused. The goal is to reverse the worst of the extracellular volume depletion as soon as possible. Infusing the first liter in 1 hour is not too fast a rate because this will replace only one third of the extracellular loss in the average patient and even less in others who are more dehydrated. Other plasma expanders, such as albumin and plasma concentrates, may be necessary if low blood pressure and other clinical signs of vascular collapse do not respond properly to saline alone.

Rapid infusion of saline in diabetic ketoacidosis may not be without its own complications. The rapid dilution of plasma proteins during saline infusion lowers the oncotic (osmotic) pressure of plasma. The lowered oncotic pressure in turn allows fluid to leak out of the vascular space through the capillary walls and is suspected of contributing to the development of pulmonary edema or cerebral edema in some patients during therapy, particularly children and the elderly.[17, 18] Even though they are improving biochemically, patients should therefore be carefully observed during the first 24 to 36 hours for the clinical signs of pulmonary edema: increasing cough, frothy sputum, dyspnea, cyanosis and rales, and failure to awaken from stupor or coma, which could represent the development of cerebral edema.

Assessment. Once volume replacement is initiated, there is time to plan the remainder of therapy in a somewhat more considered fashion. At this point, an assessment of the severity of total volume depletion can be made. The history, intensity, and duration of symptoms; amount of oral intake; presence of other fluid losses through vomiting and so forth; and documentation of the amount of weight actually lost all will provide important clues to the seriousness of volume depletion. The physical examination provides additional information: Decreased tissue turgor (sometimes even to the extent of softened consistency of the eyeballs in severely dehydrated patients), tachycardia, decreased sweating, and postural or supine hypoten-

sion all help confirm the extent of volume loss. A numerical estimate of total body fluid loss is extremely valuable in planning phased therapy (*e.g.,* the fraction of loss to be replaced over each time interval).

Goals Of Volume Replacement. Volume replacement is not only critical in preserving the integrity of the circulation but also instrumental in treating hyperglycemia, preventing hyperkalemia, and reducing lactic acidosis. Because any patient with a blood sugar significantly above 450 to 500 mg/dl became that way in large part because of volume depletion severe enough to prevent compensatory renal glucose loss, it makes physiological sense to rely on volume replacement for restoration of that glucose excretory mechanism. It has been conclusively demonstrated that the fall in blood sugar during treatment of diabetic ketoacidosis is about 80% attributable to glucose loss into the urine, rather than being primarily the result of insulin-induced changes in glucose production and consumption.[19] This is not to say that insulin effects are trivial in treating ketoacidosis, but rather that in the earliest phases of treatment insulin therapy *complements* proper fluid and electrolyte replacement.

Finally, one should remember that volume losses will continue throughout the first several hours of therapy as long as glycosuria and the osmotic diuresis are not completely controlled. Volume replacement must therefore restore not only the deficits that *exist* at the time of the patient's arrival but also those that continue to be *created* during therapy, before full metabolic control is achieved.

Insulin

Because the primary deficit leading to diabetic ketoacidosis in the first place is severe insulin deficiency, insulin obviously stands as a key component of successful therapy. Indeed, until the advent of insulin, diabetic ketoacidosis was almost never fully reversible and was usually fatal.

Several metabolic effects of insulin are of special importance in the treatment of ketoacidosis. First, insulin promptly shuts off the supply of free fatty acids emerging from adipose tissue, thereby restricting the production of ketones at its source. Second, insulin directly inhibits hepatic gluconeogenesis, preventing further addition of glucose to an already overburdened extracellular fluid. Simultaneously, hepatic ketogenesis is further reduced, which assures the ultimate reversal of the ketoacidosis itself. Third, insulin restores cellular protein synthesis. Although this effect occurs more slowly, it in turn permits the restoration of normal potassium, magnesium, and phosphate stores within tissues.

Insulin induces a relatively limited increase in tissue glucose uptake during the therapy of diabetic ketoacidosis.[20] It is therefore primarily the *anticatabolic* effects of insulin, the reduction of glucose and ketone *inflow,* that are important in the early part of therapy. When glucose and ketones are no longer entering the extracellular fluid, the body is in a position to reduce hyperglycemia and ketonemia by both urine losses and continuing tissue consumption. The *anabolic* effects of insulin have little role early in the therapy of ketoacidosis, becoming much more important in later phases.

Cautions. The extremely high glucose values found initially in patients with diabetic ketoacidosis are psychologically distressing to contemplate. It is always tempting, therefore, to choose a course of therapy that will reduce the blood sugar as quickly as possible. However, there are two good reasons to avoid dropping the blood sugar too fast or too far, particularly if the approach to its lowering is primarily to rely on insulin without sufficient simultaneous volume replacement.

In the first instance, recall that large quantities of glucose in the extracellular space draw water out of cells; glucose and water together partially reexpand the volume lost from osmotic diuresis of sodium and water (see Fig. 35-3). Sudden and rapid lowering of the blood sugar with insulin, through a combination of increased tissue uptake plus decreased gluconeogenesis, allows water to move very rapidly back into cells, withdrawing the prop to extracellular volume and provoking potentially catastrophic vascular collapse.[21] The sequence of events highlights in yet another way *the importance of early volume replacement with sodium and water,* preceding or concurrent with insulin therapy.

The second problem arises in patients with prolonged, severe hyperglycemia, in whom large quantities of glucose (or glucose-derived compounds) accumulate slowly within the brain.[22] Compared with water, these compounds are only poorly permeating. Thus, if the blood sugar is lowered too fast and too far (below about 250 mg/dl), particularly without sufficient electrolyte replacement in extracellular fluid, water is freed up to move into the brain, drawn by the accumulated intracerebral glucose metabolites. The result may be cerebral edema, with a worsening of coma instead of the expected improvement as the blood sugar falls.

High vs. Low Dosage. In the past, insulin was used in relatively large doses, such as 200 to 400 units in the first 24 hours, usually in intravenous bolus doses, in treating diabetic ketoacidosis; this was based on the theory that "insulin resistance" was present. Although some work indicates that all ketoacidotic patients are indeed insulin-resistant[23] and although such high-dose insulin therapy was generally quite successful, it has become apparent with further experience that lower doses are often equally effective. Low-dose insulin is generally given by continuous intravenous infusion or intramuscular injection rather than by the conventional intravenous bolus or subcutaneous doses.[24] As the trend toward ever lower doses has grown, considerable controversy has developed concerning the optimal dose and route of insulin therapy.[25]

Perhaps the most useful position at this point is to be aware of the pitfalls of both the high- and low-dose approaches and to adopt general guidelines to therapy of ketoacidosis that are necessary to avoid the worst of these. When regarded in this fashion, the controversy appears to be somewhat of a "tempest in an IV bottle."

One may apply the following set of principles when attempting to achieve optimal therapy:

- It is rational to give an initial loading dose of insulin to fill tissue insulin-binding sites and to assure initiation of insulin action.
- The major drawback of low-dose insulin therapy is the possibility of undertreating: Some patients are much less responsive to insulin than others, and at the outset there is no way to distinguish those who will be, in fact, somewhat more insulin-resistant. It therefore cannot be assumed that all patients will respond appropriately to low doses. Moreover, there is no intrinsic virtue to using the lowest possible dose: Insulin is cheap and nontoxic.
- The major drawbacks of high-dose therapy, which have already been listed, are less a function of excessive insulin *per se* than of insufficient recognition of volume depletion and insufficiently aggressive volume replacement. Although late hypoglycemia is also somewhat more likely with high-dose insulin, hypoglycemia is easily prevented if intravenous glucose is added to the regimen at the appropriate time; it is easily detected if the patient is carefully watched, and it is easily treated.
- Whatever insulin dose and route are chosen, changes in blood sugar and clinical state should indicate a clear-cut, beneficial response before it can be assumed that the chosen therapy is effective. If blood sugar does not drop and blood pressure and urine output do not stabilize, insulin or fluid therapy may not have been adequate. There is *no* substitute for the ancient and honorable practice of close patient monitoring.

Potassium And Phosphate Replacement

All patients in diabetic ketoacidosis are deficient in total body potassium stores to a greater or lesser degree. Many other factors conspire to affect the circulating plasma potassium level in patients with diabetic ketoacidosis, however, and most of these factors tend to raise the plasma level. Thus, insulin deficiency itself, hyperchloremic acidosis,[26] and hyperosmolality[27] all allow potassium to shift out of cells and into the extracelluar space. Moreover, the renal excretion of potassium, which usually serves as the major minute-to-minute regulator of plasma potassium, also is impaired in diabetic ketoacidosis because hypovolemia reduces renal perfusion and intrinsic kidney function is often reduced owing to diabetic renal disease. These last two factors prevent potassium excretion from the plasma. Depending on the balance between total body potassium losses versus rises in plasma potassium, the initial plasma potassium in patients with ketoacidosis may range from very low to very high. Potassium replacement must therefore be withheld until an accurate measurement of this level is reported back from the laboratory. Beginning intravenous K^+ therapy in the presence of unrecognized hyperkalemia and inadequate renal mechanisms for handling potassium loads can rapidly lead to a fatal outcome. Although the electrocardiogram (ECG) can provide bedside clues to the presence of high or low K^+ levels, there is enough room for error in its interpretation to discourage a decision about K^+ therapy based on the ECG alone.

If the initial serum potassium level is low, intravenous K^+ is generally begun right away. This is particularly important because both insulin and saline can be predicted to drive the K^+ even lower, possibly to dangerously low levels at which skeletal muscle paralysis and cardiac arrest may occur. If the initial K^+ is normal or high, intravenous K^+ is generally withheld until it is clear that the level has begun to drop *and* that urine flow is established.

Failure of the K^+ to fall can occur because of (1) persistent, uncorrected acidosis (which drives K^+ out of cells and into extracellular fluid): (2) hyperosmolality itself; (3) intrinsically impaired renal function; or, perhaps most importantly, (4) insufficient restoration of circulating volume.

Phosphate levels generally also drop during therapy, aggravating any preexisting tendency of red cells to bind oxygen more tightly. Although in most patients this is not thought to be an effect of major importance,[28] limited phosphate replacement seems reasonable. Therefore, many patients now receive phosphate in the middle and later phases of therapy, usually combined with K^+ replacement, in the form of potassium phosphate salts added to the intravenous infusion. Patients who are receiving phosphate therapy intravenously should be watched carefully for signs of tetany: tingling around the mouth or in the hands, neuromuscular irritability, carpopedal spasm, or even seizures. Tetany may occur because the phosphate lowers the level of circulating calcium.

Bicarbonate: Pro And Con

Patients with mild or moderate ketoacidosis who are properly and promptly treated with salt, water, and insulin will eventually excrete and metabolize the ketone bodies remaining in extracellular fluid. As this process continues, bicarbonate anions are increasingly reabsorbed from the renal tubules to replace the disappearing unmeasured anions, and the bicarbonate deficit is slowly repaired. This self-induced recovery is quite satisfactory in the majority of ketoacidotic patients.[29] Sometimes the large amounts of chloride administered along with the sodium in intravenous saline may produce a confusing but transient hyperchloremia and delay for several days the full return of the bicarbonate level to normal.

For patients with the most severe degrees of acidosis, whose bicarbonate levels are initially 10 mEq/liter or lower, concern arises about a relatively sudden decompensation of buffering capacity when CO_2 gas cannot be driven any faster from the body by hyperventilation, with resultant rapid worsening of the acidosis. In these patients it makes sense to infuse bicarbonate intravenously early in the course of therapy. The deficit in bicarbonate can be calculated quite exactly and an appropriate amount given intravenously over several hours to raise the level at least to the 10 to 12 mEq/liter range.[30]

Possible CNS Acidosis. The major risk to rapid correction of the acidosis by bicarbonate replacement arises from yet another imbalance, or disequilibrium, between the extracellular fluids of the body and those surrounding the brain, resulting from unequal rates of movement of certain molecules across the blood-brain barrier. In this instance, bicarbonate moves into the brain-associated fluids much more slowly than CO_2 gas (plus H_2CO_3). As a result, the expected and desired parallel rise of both HCO_3^- and CO_2 that occurs elsewhere in the body during treatment does not occur in the cerebral compartment, but CO_2 (and H_2CO_3) rises more quickly than HCO_3^-. The net result is a shift in the HCO_3^-: CO_2 ratio that drives the cerebral fluid *p*H down, producing a paradoxical, although again transient, worsening of cerebral acidosis. This CNS acidosis may then be manifested clinically by deepening stupor or coma in a patient whose arterial *p*H seems to be improving. Fortunately, a major degree of cerebral impairment due to this *p*H disequilibrium is unusual, and the central acidosis corrects itself with time if the patient is otherwise supported.

CASE ANALYSIS

Despite evidence of severe hyperglycemia, metabolic acidosis, and volume depletion, our patient M. O. responded promptly to standard and fairly conservative therapy that included volume replacement with saline and low-dose intravenous insulin. Clinical and chemical signs indicated steady and progressive improvement over the first 15 hours of treatment:

- The falling blood sugar from 910 to 304 mg/dl over this time reflected continued renal glucose loss with concomitant insulin-induced decrease in hepatic glucose production.
- The falling BUN and creatinine indicated that volume replacement had restored renal perfusion.
- Even without the use of intravenous bicarbonate, the serum bicarbonate level rose from 4 to 22 mEq/liter as the production of ketones was turned off by insulin and ketones were metabolized to bicarbonate, which was reabsorbed by the kidney.
- Arterial blood *p*H was restored from its initial very low level of 7.06 to 7.25 as the bicarbonate buffer reappeared in plasma.
- Serum potassium fell from 6.9 into the normal range as insulin drove potassium back into cells, *p*H improved, osmolality returned to normal, and improved renal perfusion permitted exchange of potassium for sodium.
- Finally, the rise in serum chloride from the low initial value of 90 mEq/liter (normal range: 96 to 103 mEq/liter) to the abnormally high level of 114 mEq/liter is not entirely understood but reflects in part the intravenous infusion of large amounts of chloride.

Principal Concerns in Biochemical Therapy for Diabetic Ketoacidosis

- Volume replacement, primarily salt and water
- Insulin
- Potassium and phosphate replacement
- Bicarbonate

General Care

Looking for Precipitating Causes

Proper metabolic management alone does not assure a favorable outcome in patients with diabetic ketoacidosis because a number of aspects of general care are at least as critical. First, a careful search for precipitating causes is always necessary, not only because one must take care to prevent future episodes but also because the ketoacidosis may not respond well (even to aggressive metabolic therapy) if an underlying problem, particularly infection, remains undetected and untreated.

Two of the most difficult and confusing areas in clinical assessment are the frequent occurrence of abdominal symptoms (nausea, vomiting, abdominal pain, tenderness, and rigidity) and the interpretation of stupor or coma.

Abdominal Symptoms And Coma

Gastric motility is greatly impaired as diabetic ketoacidosis develops; gastric distention with stagnant, dark, heme-positive "crankcase oil" fluid is therefore quite common. Vomiting, with the ever-present threat of aspiration, particularly in the stuporous patient, can be a significant problem. Nasogastric intubation for decompression may therefore be very useful, both in reducing discomfort and in minimizing the risk of aspiration, as long as one performs it with proper care to avoid aspiration during passage of the tube.

Conscious patients are often *extremely* thirsty, but it is a mistake to give in initially to their pleas for water because adding fluid to an already distended stomach inevitably leads to worsening of abdominal distress and usually to vomiting. Reassurance that the thirst will pass as therapy progresses and provision of ice chips to minimize the sensation of thirst are more humane and appropriate in the long run.

Severe abdominal pain, tenderness, and ileus frequently prove to be due to the ketoacidosis itself, but this clinical picture initially may be difficult to distinguish from an intra-abdominal catastrophe such as perforated viscus, which may have precipitated the ketoacidosis. A similar problem arises in interpreting stupor or coma: Did intracerebral bleeding or infection precipitate both the acidosis and the coma, or did the acidosis produce coma? Lumbar puncture may be the only way by which reassurance on this point can be obtained, primarily by permitting one to look for evidence of infection — meningitis, encephalitis, or brain abscess. Blood, urine, and throat cultures are almost always appropriate in the general search for infection.

Coma Care

The principles of coma care are really no different for the severely ill ketoacidotic person than for any other patient. The primary point of emphasis during this care is the concern for vomiting and aspiration. Proper positioning on the side, continuous close observation, and the ready availability of a nasopharyngeal suctioning apparatus are the keys to avoidance of aspiration. Nasogastric intubation may safely be carried out in patients who are conscious and who have a good gag reflex, but for stuporous or comatose patients a cuffed endotracheal tube should be in place before one makes any attempts to pass a nasogastric tube.

Managing Bladder Function

A similarly knotty problem arises in the management of bladder function in ketoacidotic patients. On the one hand, early access to bladder urine is of extreme importance: First, it may be of tremendous help in making the earliest possible diagnosis; second, urinary tract infection is not uncommonly the trigger event, and must be sought; third, knowing that urine flow is established is critical to assessment of circulatory competence and to the decision for potassium therapy. Later in treatment, monitoring of urine flow, sugar, and acetone levels is a very useful complement to measurements of plasma metabolites and fluid balance.

On the other hand, catheterization of the bladder always introduces the risk of urinary infection and may not be necessary for achieving the aforementioned goals. In the conscious patient who can voluntarily void, catheterization is not actually necessary. Therefore, one should make every effort to obtain urine samples from such patients without catheterization, recognizing that in long-standing diabetes a neurogenic bladder with incomplete bladder emptying is commonly present. Urine specimens in such patients may provide imperfect sampling of their metabolic condition, and interpretation of volumes or tests should be performed with appropriate caution.

If catheterization is absolutely necessary, an indwelling catheter connected to closed drainage is perfectly acceptable and certainly useful. Its presence should never be ignored, however, and one should make a conscious effort to remove it at the earliest possible opportunity because the longer it remains in place, the greater the risk of bladder sepsis. Repeated straight catheterizations may provide the requisite information with less risk of infection, but whatever catheterization program is chosen, scrupulous aseptic technique for insertion is of prime importance.

Flow Sheets

It should be apparent by now that management of diabetic ketoacidosis depends on an unusually large and complex amount of numerical information. Measurements are needed in many separate but interacting areas. These measurements must be expressed in fairly precise numbers and must be repeated over time. Important therapeutic decisions depend on trends in these numbers and their response to treatment.

There is no way in which information of this amount and importance can properly be handled if it is kept largely in the physician's head, on the individual laboratory reports, or even in the progress notes in the body of the record. A separate flow sheet must be set up that displays the key data, including vital signs, blood chemistries, urine tests, fluid balance, and medications, in neat and orderly fashion according to time. The flow sheet serves a more general secondary function as well by focusing attention on the *need for continuous monitoring until the patient is clinically and chemically improved.*

Phases of Care

Although there are no sharp lines between them, the course of management of diabetic ketoacidosis naturally divides itself into several phases.

First Phase. The first phase consists of the immediate effort to establish the diagnosis and, once ketoacidosis is even strongly suspected, to assure that life-preserving therapy is begun. An abbreviated history from family or friends of an unconscious patient, a search for a diabetic identification card or jewelry, a rapid assessment for clinical clues of volume depletion and Kussmaul respiration, and blood-drawing for initial chemistries should not take more than a few moments. Blood sugar by glucose oxidase strip (Dextrostix) and serum ketone measurements at the bedside may be all that one needs to clinch the diagnosis. While these preliminaries are being performed, the best possible intravenous line is established, and volume replacement is begun.

Second Phase. Once this first phase is completed, a second phase of more considered assessment and therapy begins. Details of the history and physical examination, including the careful search for precipitating causes, should be obtained while the more complete laboratory assessment is awaited. Cultures, ECG, and appropriate roentgenograms are performed at this point. The flow sheet is set up, and decisions are made about coma care, intubation, and catheterization.

Third Phase. A third phase is then entered in which the worst of the metabolic damage is repaired. This phase lasts roughly 8 to 24 hours, depending on how sick the patient is on admission and how responsive he proves to be to therapy. The goal during this phase is *not* to achieve complete correction of all the abnormalities. Indeed, as we have seen, excessive speed of correction can be hazardous, particularly in patients in whom ketoacidosis has been developing gradually over a long period of time, because the body's adaptations to the metabolic insults are not all immediately reversible and overly agressive therapy may actually make some problems worse.

The key difficulties to be watched for during this phase are as follows:

- *Worsening Stupor or Coma.* Aside from the possibility of CNS infection or stroke, the major concerns are for osmotic or *p*H disequilibrium from excessively rapid correction of blood sugar or bicarbonate. The most important clue here is clinical worsening of mental state in the face of "chemical" improvement.
- *Hypotension.* Certainly sepsis, myocardial infarction, and other causes of shock must be looked for, but again, rapid reducion of blood sugar without sufficient sodium and water replacement may be responsible.
- *Hyperkalemia.* Early occlusion of the arterial supply to a limb (not rare in diabetics with severe peripheral vascular disease and easily overlooked in a

comatose, hypotensive patient) can permit leakage of large amounts of potassium into the circulation, producing or aggravating hyperkalemia. The limbs should therefore be monitored for asymmetric pallor, coldness, rubor, and so forth. More often, hyperkalemia results from premature K^+ infusion, persistent acidosis, and insufficient volume replacement.

Fourth Phase. Finally, a fourth phase arrives in which the patient's clinical state is stable or improving and the majority of the metabolic abnormalities are reversed. The completion or recovery then occurs over a period of about 12 days and includes repletion of body stores of many nutrients, including magnesium, protein, phosphate, and so forth, as cell constituents are resynthesized.[31]

Once it is clear that gastrointestinal tract function is restored, oral replacement is not only desirable but also necessary to provide all of the complex nutrition required for recovery; however, oral feedings should be withheld until gastric distention is gone and intestinal motility is clearly present. It is during this phase that attention should be directed at *preventing* future recurrences of diabetic ketoacidosis.

Prevention

Often overlooked, prevention is really one of the most important aspects of diabetic ketoacidosis management. In fact, it can easily be argued that diabetic ketoacidosis is not only unpleasant, dangerous, and expensive but also unnecessary because, in theory, it should always be preventable. In practical terms, of course, there is probably no way in which all episodes can be prevented, particularly in previously undiagnosed diabetics in whom the disease is not even suspected. In many other patients, however, the recurrence of ketoacidosis represents an admission of failure in management.

Prevention of diabetic ketoacidosis breaks down into two aspects: outpatient and inpatient.

Ambulatory Care

In outpatient settings, there are no great mysteries to successful prevention. What is needed is not sporadic application of complicated measures but consistent use of a few simple rules. The most important of these are discussed subsequently.

Patient Education. Ideally, patients and their families should understand enough about the mechanism and meaning of ketoacidosis to be able to avoid those things that are likely to bring it about, to recognize its approach, to slow it down or minimize its development, and to seek help fast, if it does begin to happen.

Perhaps the most common avoidable mistake arises from lack of appreciation of the importance of insulin's *anticatabolic effects*. Most ketosis-prone patients easily and intuitively accept the need for insulin injections if they are hungry and eating well but have considerable difficulty in recognizing their insulin need when they are ill, anorectic, not eating, or actually vomiting.

Every such patient needs to be instructed repeatedly that

- His body, like that of any nondiabetic person, *must have insulin, even if no food is being taken in.*
- The amount of insulin required in the postabsorptive or fasting state alone is about half of the total he would need if he were eating, although when he is fasting, it must be spread out as an insulin "trickle" rather than given in insulin "bursts."
- Illness generally increases insulin need, so that even if not eating, he may actually require more than 50% of his usual daily dose.
- If insulin is taken in restricted doses (two split doses of intermediate-acting insulin in 24 hours), insulin reactions are unusual.

An "illness" regimen should be planned ahead of time, discussed, and rehearsed, and it should include the following:

- Religious injection of reduced-dose, intermediate-acting insulin at least once, possibly twice a day
- A call to the patient's nurse or physician early rather than late
- Urine testing for ketones
- Injections of small, supplemental doses of short-acting insulin several times daily if necessary, according to the results of the urine tests, until glucose levels come under control

Refills. The second most frequent communication problem is a misunderstanding about insulin refills and logistic problems in obtaining refills or the necessary advice about crisis management. Most pharmacies now will sell insulin to patients without a rigid requirement for a current prescription, but "Murphy's Law" (If something can go wrong, it will) seems to apply to insulin regimens. Accordingly, it is not unheard of for a patient to miss several days of insulin therapy and to explain the situation with any of a variety of excuses: "I ran out and my doctor's appointment was only a few days away"; "In the excitement of the horse show, I skipped a few doses". . . the examples go on and on. Similarly, difficulty in reaching a medical person for advice by phone or limited access to a medical care facility may interfere with timely therapy in such a way as to permit unnecessary episodes of ketoacidosis. A relatively simple measure such as establishment of a "diabetes hot-line" can have a dramatic impact in reducing the number of episodes.[32]

Individual Patterns. Beyond these general causes, certain diabetic patients seem to develop their own individual patterns for recurrent episodes of ketoacidosis: the patient who is mentally incompetent and without an adequate caretaker network; the alcoholic patient who develops ketoacidosis during sprees; the adolescent patient in whose battle with his parents, neglect of his diabetes has become his "ultimate weapon"; the patient who has denied the existence of his diabetes so firmly that its care is viewed with utmost lack of concern. These patients challenge the ingenuity, persistence, and professionalism of the entire health-care team, but many patients will eventually respond.

Inpatient Settings. Prevention of diabetic ketoacidosis in inpatient settings is a different matter entirely. Here the key is close monitoring in patients known to be ketosis-prone and a high index of suspicion in patients not previously known to be diabetic. Regular urine testing in known diabetics will always permit ketoacidosis to be prevented, as long as the materials for testing of sugar and acetone are known to be fresh and active, the testing is properly done, and abnormal results are promptly reported. Of course, not all urinary ketosis is diabetic ketosis because fasting regularly produces ketonuria. The main differential clue is, of course, the absence of concurrent glycosuria with fasting ketonuria, but if there is any doubt, the matter should be investigated immediately with the proper confirmatory blood testing.

In hospitalized patients not known to be diabetic who develop unexplained extreme thirst, negative fluid balance, stupor, or hyperventilation, diabetic ketoacidosis is a part of the differential diagnosis, particularly in those with obvious triggering stresses such as severe infection, trauma, CNS bleeding, and so forth. A high index of suspicion and proper testing will exclude or make the diagnosis, and in the latter instance may be lifesaving.

CASE ANALYSIS

The precipitating causes of the episode of ketoacidosis in our patient M. O. were classic: (1) the onset of an episode of respiratory infection and possibly some initial gastroenteritis; and (2) failure of this totally insulin-dependent patient to understand the continuing need for insulin even in the absence of food intake. This episode of ketoacidosis could probably have been prevented if the patient had continued to take insulin, at perhaps one half to two thirds his usual dose, with supplemental short-acting insulin as needed. If the nausea and vomiting had been controlled early, he might also have been able to continue oral fluid and sodium replacement. This case makes obvious the value of a "diabetes illness plan" and early contact during an acute illness with a physician or a nurse familiar with diabetes management.

Fortunately, despite the patient's severe chemical abnormalities, he was only lethargic, not comatose, perhaps because he was young and otherwise healthy and ketoacidosis had developed over a short time. He thus avoided the need for intubation or catheterization and tolerated very well the rapid shifts in volume, *p*H, and osmolality induced by therapy. His management was materially aided by the *flow chart* that was taken directly from his medical record (reproduced in the case study, which was presented earlier in this chapter). The patient's rapid response allowed his hospitalization to be brief, particularly compared with the practice of earlier days, a consideration of increasing importance in the "DRG era." The slow repletion of body constituents and readjustment of diabetic regimen, the "fourth phase" of therapy, could thus be safely completed in this patient outside the hospital, but for many patients, particularly older and sicker ones, such early discharge could be a major mistake.

General and Nursing Care Concerns in the Therapy of Diabetic Ketoacidosis

- Help in the search for precipitating causes
- Thirst, vomiting, and preventing aspiration
- Care for coma and bladder function
- Flow sheet monitoring of intake, output, and medications
- Prevention by education for outpatients and early recognition of high-risk inpatients

---

HYPEROSMOLAR COMA

Not infrequently, patients develop the marked hyperglycemia and hyperosmolarity of diabetic ketoacidosis, but without the ketoacidosis—the syndrome of so-called hyperosmolar nonketotic coma (see Fig. 35-2, *D*). The syndrome is important because of (1) its similarities to and its differences from full-blown diabetic ketoacidosis, (2) the differential diagnosis, and (3) the differences in management.

Manifestations

Characteristically, such patients are elderly and not previously known to have diabetes. They become a bit drowsy, take in less and less by mouth, are noted over several days to slip ever deeper into stupor, and are finally brought to the hospital in a state of extreme volume depletion. Blood sugar in these patients is more or less by definition over 600 mg/dl, and in addition to the total extracellular sodium and water losses, a large additional "free water" deficit exists, probably because of failure of the thirst mechanism and consequent lack of oral intake. These patients therefore often have very high serum levels of both sodium and glucose, with the latter sometimes in excess of 2000 mg/dl, and extraordinarily high serum osmolarities.

From our discussion of the mechanism of extreme hyperglycemia, one might expect that poor renal function must contribute even more greatly to the development of the hyperosmolar nonketotic syndrome than to diabetic ketoacidosis itself and, indeed, renal function is generally much worse in the former. As in most things related to diabetes, the hyperosmolar syndrome is not always "pure": Some patients have a degree of ketosis as well. However, it seems logical to consider the diagnosis to be the hyperosmolar syndrome only if the anion gap attributable to ketoacids is less than about 7 mEq/liter and to diagnose full-blown ketoacidosis if this anion gap is greater than 7 mEq/liter.

Causes

Although the reason that some patients develop hyperosmolar coma without acidosis is very intriguing, it is usually not known. In experimental animals, a combination of mild diabetes, large doses of glucocorticoids, and extreme water deprivation is required to produce a model of the disease.[33] The model may have important similarities to the human situation because the patient's history frequently includes extremely poor water intake in the face of continuing insensible and urinary water loss and because upon recovery the patient's diabetes is usually mild and does not require insulin.

In some patients, it is clear that the syndrome is iatrogenic, induced by one of a variety of medications (*e.g.,* glucocorticoids, diazoxide, and diuretics), by dialysis against hyperosmolar glucose solutions, or by prolonged intravenous hypertonic glucose infusion (*e.g.,* in central hyperalimentation regimens).

Management

In a general way, therapy for the hyperosmolar syndrome is very similar to those aspects of therapy for diabetic ketoacidosis that are directed at the hyperglycemia and volume depletion. The major difference is the extent or degree of the volume depletion, which is, on the whole, considerably greater in the hyperosmolar syndrome and which calls for extremely vigorous replacement. Moreover, these patients not only seem to require less insulin to control their hyperosmolar state but also are even more vulnerable to sudden loss of circulating blood volume with rapid, insulin-induced blood-sugar reduction than are ketoacidotic patients. It has even been suggested, therefore, that the hyperosmolar nonketotic syndrome be treated with saline alone, with insulin omitted altogether, but small doses of insulin are generally given.

Prognosis

Patients who develop the hyperosmolar nonketotic coma syndrome do not do very well. Complications are frequent, and mortality rates may be 25% to 50%.

The multiplicity of associated diseases in what is mostly an elderly population, the inability of the cardiovascular system to handle the rapid volume shifts during the development and treatment of the syndrome, and the intravascular thrombosis and the focal seizures (presumably due to extreme hyperconcentration of blood and poor local blood flow) all seem to contribute to this rather bleak outlook.

Hyperosmolar coma is a complication of diabetes characterized by the following:

- Extreme hyperosmolality and water losses
- Lack of acidosis
- Frequent coma and focal seizures
- Occurrence primarily in the elderly
- High mortality rate
- Mild diabetes in those who recover

ALCOHOLIC KETOACIDOSIS

At the opposite metabolic extreme from patients with diabetic hyperosmolar nonketotic coma are an entirely different group with severe ketoacidosis but no hyperglycemia (see Fig. 35-2, *A*). These latter ketoacidotic patients do not actually belong in this discussion because they do not have diabetes; rather, their ketoacidosis is induced by heavy alcohol intake, and their glucose tolerance is quite normal. They are nonetheless important to the discussion for the light they shed on pathogenesis and on clinical manifestations of diabetic ketoacidosis and because alcoholic ketoacidosis may figure prominently in the differential diagnosis of certain patients. Moreover, because the therapy of the two conditions is very different, the distinctions must be clearly recognized.[34]

Manifestations

Patients who develop alcoholic ketoacidosis are almost invariably women. They are usually chronic drinkers who, just before they become ill, suddenly increase their drinking, then just as suddenly begin vomiting and stop drinking. Vomiting usually then continues, abdominal pain develops, and 2 or 3 days later they seek care—awake, alert, only slightly dehydrated, often with Kussmaul breathing, and usually with a silent, tender, distended, and resistant abdomen. Urinalysis initially shows strongly positive ketones but no sugars, and the blood sugar is usually normal or low, although it may be *slightly elevated.* However, the anion gap is very large, serum ketones are positive at higher dilutions, and arterial *p*H is decreased, sometimes to extremely low values.

Management

In striking contrast to diabetic ketoacidosis, the most effective therapy for alcoholic ketoacidosis consists initially and primarily of simple intravenous dextrose and water, without insulin. Modest amounts of saline may be added to the regimen if vomiting has been severe and volume depletion is significant. During therapy, serum phosphate may drop to an extremely low concentration. The level should be monitored, and phosphate salts administered accordingly, lest a "low phosphate" syndrome develop.[35]

Causes

The development of alcohol ketoacidosis seems to depend on a combination of several factors whose relative importance and mechanism remain speculative. Certain biologic "host" characteristics are probably required because only a small minority of all alcoholic patients develop the syndrome, and, more importantly, if they later resume drinking, ketoacidosis often develops repeatedly in these same patients. Moreover, the striking predominance of female over male patients suggests that the hormonal milieu may contribute. In addition, several environmental factors are so constant that they almost certainly play a role. Alcohol is obviously involved, although alcohol by itself is necessary but not sufficient. Vomiting may also be a cause rather than a result of the syndrome, possibly by provoking a marked release of stress hormones including catecholamines, and as suggested by the rapid and complete response to glucose therapy, glucose deprivation also may figure into production of the syndrome.

Alcoholic ketoacidosis may be confused with diabetic ketoacidosis but is a distinct syndrome characterized by the following:

- History of heavy drinking
- Occurrence primarily in women
- Lack of significant hyperglycemia, hyperosmolality, or volume deficits
- Prompt response to therapy with dextrose and water

HYPOGLYCEMIA

Although it may be apparent to medically trained people that of the two diabetic emergencies ketoacidosis is actually far more life-threatening than hypoglycemia, the patient usually perceives even mild hypoglycemia as a much greater problem.

Manifestations

First, hypoglycemia in diabetics, although most prevalent in the insulin-dependent group, is much more common than ketoacidosis. Second, the onset of hypoglycemia is much more rapid and its manifestations are much more variable, often occurring in such subtle ways as to evade the victim's notice until he is unaware of what is happening and unable to seek the proper remedy. Insulin-induced hypoglycemia reactions therefore often occur in the midst of the patient's daily life, which can be, at the very least, embarrassing and at worst highly dangerous. Third, even though measurable recovery from hypoglycemia is rapid and complete within minutes after proper treatment, many patients remain emotionally (and possibly physiologically) shaken for hours or even days following insulin reactions. Finally, in extreme, severe situations, prolonged or recurrent hypoglycemia, although uncommon, does have the potential to cause permanent brain damage and can even be fatal.

Preventing, treating, and generally coping with each of the diabetic emergencies are difficult enough even when a clear distinction is made between them and their mechanisms are fully understood. Unfortunately, as anyone who has worked with diabetic patients can testify, the problem is compounded by an almost universal confusion between ketoacidosis and hypoglycemia. Most patients lump the two together under the common heading of "diabetic coma." Repeated explanations based on physiology, use of graphic material as much as possible, clear and practical instructions on how to respond in each situation, and infinite patience are the miniumum requirements for managing this confusion.

Neurologic Responses to Hypoglycemia

Cerebral Responses. As blood sugar falls below normal, the CNS responds in two distinct fashions: first, with impairment of higher cerebral functions and soon thereafter with an "alarm" response in vegetative functions.

Patients most commonly describe the symptoms of mild or early insulin reactions as fuzziness in the head, trouble with thinking or concentrating, shakiness, light-headedness, and giddiness. These changes occur when the cerebral cortex is deprived of its main energy supply. This part of the brain is apparently the most sensitive to the loss of glucose.

Almost as common but usually inapparent to the patient are changes in personality and behavior during insulin reactions. As with alcohol and other agents that affect cerebral function, these changes in personality vary with the person, the situation, the rapidity of onset, and other unknown factors. They range from silly, manic, inappropriate behavior through withdrawal, sullenness, or truculence, to grumpy, irritable, suspicious, or, in the extreme, paranoid and even, rarely, violent behavior. It is no wonder that, particularly when combined with difficulties in motor function such as trouble walking and slurred speech, patients who are well into insulin reactions may closely resemble people who have been drinking alcohol. It is for this reason that diabetic identification cards and jewelry indicate that such findings in the bearer may represent hypoglycemia rather than drunkenness.

The major lesson to be learned from this discussion is that *any patient taking insulin whose behavior or personality becomes inappropriate or uncharacteristic for him should be suspected of having an insulin reaction and treated accordingly.* The index of suspicion should be particularly high if such changes are episodic, occur at a time when the particular form of insulin used is expected to have its maximum activity, and are accompanied by consistently negative urine tests for sugar.

A major source of anxiety for many diabetics who are taking insulin is concern for unrecognized hypoglycemia during sleep, leading to possible brain damage, such that they may "never wake up." Many patients who are having insulin reactions are wakened by the reaction, so it is possible to be realistically reassuring about this. However, some patients seem not to waken consistently and must rely on the presence or availability of a family member or partner to detect and treat nocturnal reactions.

Although the manifestations of cerebral cortical dysfunction from hypoglycemia are usually diffuse rather than focal, some patients develop focal signs or symptoms such as aphasia, vertigo, localized weakness, and even focal seizures with their insulin reactions. Such focal changes usually occur when there is prior focal damage to the specific area of the cortex, as from a previous stroke or head injury. Occasionally, these focal symptoms occur without any obvious predisposing factor, which makes for an extremely confusing diagnostic puzzle.

Vegetative Responses. Closely following the cortical changes is a series of vegetative neurologic responses. The primary response is discharge from the centers that control adrenergic autonomic impulses, with the resultant release of norepinephrine throughout the body and epinephrine from the adrenals. The resultant tachycardia, pallor, sweating, and tremor are characteristic of hypoglycemia and usually serve as important early warning signs by which many patients recognize an oncoming reaction. This adrenergic discharge is part of a larger stress response that includes release of large quantities of the "counterregulatory" hormones, such as glucocorticoids, growth hormone, and glucagon, which attempt to drive the blood sugar back up, primarily by stimulating hepatic glycogen breakdown.

Other vegetative signs and symptoms may occur during hypoglycemic reactions but are less constant. Despite myths to the contrary, hunger is not a prominent feature of insulin reactions in most patients (although it does sometimes occur), headache may be seen, and the stress response may on occasion trigger secondary sequences of symptoms, including angina or pulmonary edema in patients with fragile cardiovascular disease.

Ultimately, as hypoglycemia persists and worsens, consciousness is progressively impaired, leading to stupor, then coma. The vegetative centers controlling fundamental systems of respiration, blood pressure maintenance, and so forth are the most resistant to hypoglycemia and will continue to function even when most other cerebral functions are lost.

The more profound the hypoglycemia and the longer it lasts, the greater the chance of transient or even permanent cerebral damage after blood sugar is restored. There does not seem to be a clear duration threshold for such damage, but severe hypoglycemia lasting more than 15 to 30 minutes not uncommonly results in at least some symptoms that persist for a time after glucose is given.

Pathophysiology

The minute-to-minute dependence of the brain on glucose supplied by the circulation results, as we have noted, from the inability of the brain to burn long-chain free fatty acids, the lack of glucose stored as glycogen within the adult brain, and the unavailability of ketones under fed or postabsorptive conditions.

There is little doubt that when blood sugar falls abruptly, the brain recognizes its energy deficiency once the serum level goes much below about 45 mg/dl. The exact level at which symptoms occur varies widely from person to person, however, and it is not uncommon for levels as low as 30 to 35 mg/dl to occur, as during glucose tolerance tests, with no symptoms whatsoever.[36]

More controversial is the question of whether symptoms develop in response to a rapidly falling blood sugar even before it has gone below the usual lower limit of normal. Because certain physiological responses, such as growth hormone release, occur with declining but still normal blood sugars, it is likely that symptoms may occur on this basis, but the stimulus of a falling level is probably less strong and consistent than reduction below an absolute threshold. However, the brain seems to adapt at least partially to lowered blood sugar levels, particularly if the decline is slow and chronic. It is not unusual for patients with extremely low blood sugars, as occurs in patients with insulin-secreting tumors, to exhibit perfectly normal cerebral function in the face of blood sugars that are persistently below the normal range.

Diagnosis

In principle, the diagnosis of hypoglycemia should be relatively simple and clear-cut. Because of the extreme *nonspecificity* of its manifestations and the extraordinary *biologic variation* in response to a low blood sugar, the diagnosis, in actual practice, is often subtle and complex. A serum sugar found to be below 25 mg/dl may always be held responsible for accompanying symptoms. Even in the range from 25 to 45 mg/dl, however, symptoms may not always be attributable to the hypoglycemia (particularly in spontaneous or reactive hypoglycemia), and between 45 to 65 mg/dl the relationship becomes even more difficult to prove.[37, 38]

Making a reasonably secure diagnosis of *symptomatic hypoglycemia* therefore depends on three elements:

- Documentation by an independent observer that symptoms are occurring, at a time when the blood sugar can be determined
- Correlation of the symptoms with a blood sugar level that is either absolutely low or declining very rapidly
- Prompt reversal of the symptoms upon administration of glucose, with a correlated rise in blood sugar level

In the absence of any of these three criteria, the diagnosis, although it may be strongly suspected, is less certain. It is therefore of prime importance that a blood sugar level be drawn (or determined by glucose oxidase strip at the bedside) if at all possible *prior* to administration of glucose. Although blood sugar is easily measured in the hospital, it is much less feasible in outpatients, in whom the diagnosis often rests on suspicion plus the response to glucose.

Urine sugars are an unreliable indicator of hypoglycemia because the bladder urine represents an "integral" sample of blood sugar levels over time. The sample voided just before or after an insulin reaction may well contain glucose from a prior glucose peak several hours previously, thus giving a *false-positive* impression. However, uniformly negative urine tests are consistent with the diagnosis and help increase its likelihood.

Management

The treatment of insulin reactions is always glucose. If the patient can swallow, the glucose is most conveniently given as a glucose- or sucrose-containing drink because in this form it probably gets through the stomach and into the absorbing intestine in the fastest possible time. Addition of several teaspoons of sugar to a small volume of liquid produces excessive sweetness that is nicely masked by the tartness of the traditional "O.J." (orange juice) therapy. If the patient is too groggy, stuporous, or uncooperative to drink, 30 to 50 ml of 50% glucose solution is given intravenously from a syringe over several minutes. If this route or dosage is unavailable, 1 mg of glucagon given subcutaneously or intramuscularly will reverse the symptoms by inducing a rapid breakdown and release of glucose into the bloodstream from hepatic glycogen stores.

The amount of glucose needed to reverse an insulin reaction acutely is not large. The blood sugar can be raised from 20 to 120 mg/dl with less than 15 g (3 teaspoons) of glucose in an average-sized adult. Glucose in almost any oral form will serve. Starch, as in crackers and cookies, is broken down to free glucose once through the stomach and absorbed so rapidly that blood sugar rises virtually as fast as with free glucose or sucrose.

As an extension of their fears that they might "never wake up" from nocturnal insulin reaction, patients are frequently concerned about what to do if they do not respond to the initial therapy. They must be reassured that if the first bolus of glucose consumed does not seem to work, the sensible thing to do is to take in more: Insulin reactions are *always* reversible with enough glucose. The response to oral glucose, of course, takes time, perhaps 5 to 15 minutes, whereas the response to intravenous glucose should occur within 1 or 2 minutes at most.

Failure to respond fully in the appropriate time indicates either that not enough glucose has been given, that the diagnosis is incorrect, or that the hypoglycemia has been long and severe enough to produce persistent, although not necessarily permanent, cerebral dysfunction.

Prevention

Occasional insulin reactions can and do happen in even the most stable insulin-requiring diabetic. As long as they are mild, they can usually be tolerated without difficulty and are not cause for alarm or for changes in regimen. Frequently, the precipitating event is clear: a skipped meal, an unusually strenuous bout of exercise.

When reactions are relatively frequent, recurrent, or severe, however, it is a different matter entirely. Unless the reactions are prevented, the patient may be functionally disabled—always terrified that one is about to occur, unwilling or unable to drive a car, overeating to prevent them from happening, and so forth.

The search for causes and for corrective measures is

a complex and individual matter for each patient, but it is usually rewarded by the discovery of one of several underlying mechanisms at fault. Perhaps the most common and most important mechanism is an atypical response to the usual intermediate-acting insulin that serves as the mainstay of therapy in most diabetics. Such "early" and "late responders" are quire common and frequently not recognized as such.[39] When the nature of their response pattern is properly defined, some relatively simple adjustments in insulin regimen often virtually eliminate both insulin reactions and excessive spill.

A related problem is the patient whose urine glucose appears to be getting progressively worse, particularly in the morning, despite higher and higher insulin doses. Such a paradoxical response may be a clue to undetected nocturnal insulin reactions, followed by a counterregulatory response of such intensity that the blood sugar overshoots, leading to the increasing spill by the next day, the so-called Somogyi effect.

A second mechanism must be sought when a previously stable, reaction-free patient begins to experience hypoglycemic episodes. Certain biological explanations must, of course, be excluded, including increased insulin sensitivity due to weight loss, the onset of azotemia, and so forth. More often than not, such a physiological phenomenon is not discovered, and a meticulous search for problems with insulin dosage or administration should then be undertaken.

Murphy's Law applies to insulin excesses as well as to deficiencies, and *nothing* should be taken for granted. One must thoroughly investigate every detail of insulin therapy, including insulin purchase, appearance, unitage of insulin and syringes, injection sites, injection technique, and especially any recent change in any part of the regimen should be explored in detective fashion, looking for flaws and inconsistencies. Prescription errors, mismatched syringe and insulin unitages, use of new injection sites, and other errors as yet unheard of may very well emerge.

Finally, the administration or withdrawal of other drugs may be the precipitating event for recurrent insulin reactions.

Alcohol is by far the worse offender. Not only do patients often eat less when they have a few drinks but also alcohol shuts off gluconeogenesis by interfering with intermediate biochemical steps within the liver. When combined with injected insulin, this combination not infrequently leads to hypoglycemia, which may be difficult to distinguish clinically because of concurrent inebriation.

Salicylates in large doses can reduce blood sugar and again, in combination with insulin, can produce hypoglycemia when either drug alone would not do so in the doses employed.

Because *glucocorticoids* used therapeutically cause

insulin resistance, insulin doses are often raised to meet the increased insulin demand. If the steroids are then tapered without appropriate downward adjustments in insulin dose, frequent reactions may supervene.

These are the major but by no means the only examples of drug–insulin interactions relevant to hypoglycemic episodes. It must not be forgotten, moreover, that oral hypoglycemic agents (sulfonylureas), which are still used in a great many patients, also can produce severe and long-lasting hypoglycemia.

Typically, patients who experience such episodes tend to be elderly and undernourished with impaired renal or hepatic function. Virtually any patient on oral agents may become hypoglycemic, especially in the presence of another potentiating agent such as phenylbutazone, salicylates, or, above all, alcohol.[40]

Hypoglycemia in diabetics

- Is frequently confused with ketoacidosis by patients and their families
- Produces a wide range of signs and symptoms, from personality change to confusion to coma
- Should be documented by correlation of blood sugar with symptoms whenever possible
- Responds promptly to glucose administration
- May be precipitated in insulin-dependent patients by many factors, including inappropriate insulin regimen, errors in insulin administration, exercise, and ingestion of alcohol and other drugs

---

REFERENCES

1. Garrow JS: Energy Balance and Obesity in Man, 2nd ed. New York, Elsevier/North Holland Biomedical Press, 1978
2. Cahill G: Starvation in man. N Engl J Med 282:668–675, 1970
3. Daniel PM, Pratt OE, Spargo E: The metabolic homeostatic role of muscle and its function as a store of protein. Lancet 2:446–448, 1979
4. Service FJ, Nelson RL: Characteristics of glycemic stability. Diabetes Care 3:58–62, 1980
5. Cahill G: Op cit.
6. Fajans S, Floyd JC: Fasting hypoglycemia in adults. N Engl J Med 294:766–772, 1976
7. Service FJ, Nelson RL: Op cit.
8. Kreisberg RA: Diabetic ketoacidosis: New concepts and trends in pathogenesis and treatment. Ann Intern Med 88:681–695, 1978
9. Kandel G, Aberman A: Selected developments in the understanding of diabetic ketoacidosis. Can Med Assoc J 128:392–397, 1983
10. Foster DW, McGarry JD: The metabolic derangements and treatment of diabetic ketoacidosis. N Engl J Med 309:159–169, 1983
11. Daughaday WH: Diabetic acidosis. In Williams RH (ed): Diabetes, pp 516–548. New York, Paul Hoeber, 1960

12. Fulop M, Tannenbaum H, Dreyer N: Ketotic hyperosmolar coma. Lancet 2:635–639, 1973
13. Cooperman M, Davidoff F, Spark R et al: Clinical studies in alcoholic ketoacidosis. Diabetes 23:433–439, 1974
14. Daughaday WH: Op cit.
15. Alberti KGMM, Hockaday TDR: Rapid blood ketone body estimation in the diagnosis of diabetic ketoacidosis. Br Med J 211:565–568, 1972
16. Daughaday WH: Op cit.
17. Editorial: Crystalloid infusions in diabetic ketoacidosis. Lancet 2:308–309, 1982
18. Hillman KM: Resuscitation in diabetic ketoacidosis. Crit Care Med 11:53–54, 1983
19. Clements RS Jr, Vourganti G: Fatal diabetic ketoacidosis: Major causes and approaches to their prevention. Diabetes Care 1:314–325, 1978
20. Ibid.
21. Brown RH, Rossini AA, Calloway CV et al: Caveat on fluid replacement in hyperglycemic, hyperosmolar nonketotic coma. Diabetes Care 1:305–307, 1978
22. Clements RS, Blumenthal SA, Morrison AD et al: Increased cerebrospinal-fluid pressure during treatment of diabetic ketosis. Lancet 2:671–675, 1971
23. Barrett EJ, DeFronzo RA, Bevilacqua A et al: Insulin resistance in diabetic ketoacidosis. Diabetes 31:923–938, 1982
24. Fisher JN, Shahshahani MN, Kitabchi A: Diabetic ketoacidosis: Low-dose insulin therapy by various routes. N Engl J Med 297:238–240, 1977
25. Madison L: Low-dose insulin: A plea for caution. N. Engl J Med 294:393–394, 1976
26. Androgue HJ, Madias NE: Changes in plasma potassium concentration during acute acid-base disturbances. Am J Med 71:456–467, 1981
27. Fulop M: Serum potassium in lactic acidosis and ketoacidosis. N Engl J Med 300:1087–1089, 1979
28. Fisher JN, Kitabchi A: A randomized study of phosphate therapy in the treatment of diabetic ketoacidosis. J Clin Endocrinol Metab 57:177–180, 1983
29. Lever E, Jaspan AE: Sodium bicarbonate therapy in severe diabetic ketoacidosis. Am J Med 75:263–268, 1983
30. Garella S, Dana CL, Chazan JA: Severity of metabolic acidosis as a determinant of bicarbonate requirements. N Engl J Med 289:121–126, 1973
31. Daughaday WH: Op cit.
32. Miller LV, Goldstein J: More efficient care of diabetic patients in a county hospital setting. N Engl J Med 286:1388–1391, 1972
33. Bavli S, Gordon EE: Experimental diabetic hyperosmolar syndrome in rats. Diabetes 20:92–95, 1971
34. Cooperman M, Davidoff F, Spark R et al: Op cit.
35. Lentz RD, Brown DM: Treatment of severe hypophosphatemia. Ann Intern Med 89:941–944, 1978
36. Hofeldt FD: Reactive hypoglycemia. Metabolism 24:1193–1208, 1975
37. Fajans S, Floyd JC: Op cit.
38. Hofeldt FD: Op cit.
39. Marler E, Bressler R, Styron C: The use of insulin in unstable diabetes mellitus. South Med J 57:1447–1451, 1964
40. Seltzer HS: Severe drug-induced hypoglycemia: A review. Compr Ther 5:21–29, 1975

36
Poison and Drug Overdose

Deborah A. Moisan*

The daily emergence of new chemicals and drugs and the consequences of their use, misuse, and abuse present special challenges for nurses practicing in critical care environments. In the past, acute poisonings went largely unrecognized in nursing. This is no longer the case. Present societal exposure to numerous compounds makes it imperative that health professionals have some basic knowledge of toxicologic emergencies and the subsequent care necessary to maintain life in these situations.

Poisoning is no longer an obscure ailment but has become something that physicians and nurses can treat. Community physicians and nurses are encouraged to keep poisoned patients in their own hospitals and under their own care. The poison center provides the specific consultative expertise so that the physicans and nurses can successfully treat a patient. The incidence of poisoning within the United States is estimated at 2 to 5 million/year, with this number steadily increasing. Approximately 5000 of these cases result in death. Although all age groups are affected, children account for 85% of human accidental poisonings. The remaining 15% includes adolescents and adults involved in intentional (suicide/abuse), accidental, or industrial exposure.

The mortality rate among poisoned patients steadily dropped from 2.6% in 1972 with the establishment of regional poison centers to 0.3% in 1981. This change in mortality is a direct result of better emergency de-

*The author of this chapter wishes to acknowledge the assistance of Dr. Barry Rumack from the Rocky Mountain Poison Center, who provided continual updating of information on improved care of the poisoned client, and Mary Ellen McManus, who was coauthor of the corresponding chapter in the previous edition of this text.

partment care, improved intensive care techniques, and consultation as to specific treatment with the poison centers. Although the majority of poison center calls involve children, adults attempting suicide will most often be seen and cared for in a critical care environment. The intent of this chapter is to present *basic* guidelines for assessment and therapeutic management of the acutely poisoned patient, followed by discussions of selected commonly observed poisonings, their basic clinical course, and their general management.

ASSESSMENT

When a person presents with poisoning or drug overdose, it can be an assessment and management dilemma, a dilemma that begins with the history taking.

Frequently, neither the person nor his family is able to give an accurate account of the circumstances surrounding the exposure. Sometimes the person, family member, or friend feels guilty about the incident and gives incomplete information. Or, as a result of the drug's effects, the person may arrive comatose or delirious, thus leaving the history surrounding the exposure an enigma.

Three areas of information are needed:

• General history
• Basic exposure information
• Possible first aid that might have been given

General History. Included in the history are name, age, weight, address, phone number, and health history. An initial recording of weight is indicated because the toxicity of many agents can be predicted on a per kilogram basis. The address and phone number are important if both the patient and family are unable to provide a verbal history. A relative may have access to the residence and can explore possible sources of poisoning. The health history is most useful because illnesses and medication regimens can influence the severity of the poisoning.

History of the Overdose or Exposure. The product's name, ingredients, amount, route, and time of exposure are vital to poison treatment. Although the majority of acutely poisoned patients in the critical care unit involve intentional ingestion, other routes of exposure include inhalation, ocular, dermal, and parenteral exposure, and envenomation through bites and stings. Knowing the approximate time of the exposure will determine when and what treatment is indicated. When used concomitantly, alcohol can potentiate the initial poison. Thus, multiple substance exposure must be anticipated.

Evaluate Severity

Is life in

- Immediate danger
- Potential danger
- No immediate danger

Information about the Initial First Aid. It is always wise to question what was done as first aid by family, paramedics, or emergency room personnel. Surprisingly, initial measures are overlooked in the haste to admit the person to the critical care unit.

If verbal history and clinical status conflict or if history is lacking, laboratory analysis of blood, urine, and emesis may help one make the diagnosis. Again, the time post exposure is important to note because some drugs do not peak in the system for several hours, and a toxic level could be missed if analysis is performed too soon.

Many times, the patient plus the poisoning create a large range of potential problems, and the poisoned person will arrive in the unit with varying degrees of clinical emergencies. The initial assessment of the core systems is at least as important as the history and sometimes more crucial. Emergency support measures to maintain life must take priority.

Initial Physical Assessment and Intervention. Initial evaluation of the patient's immediate danger

and timely intervention form the basic management of any poisoned patient. Care consists of the following steps:

1. Assess, establish, and manage the airway. *There is no contraindication to breathing.* Assess level of consciousness. It is essential to intubate the patient if the gag reflex is lost, if seizures are present, or if the patient has lost consciousness. Frequent suctioning may be neccessary (see Chap. 15).
2. Assess for and control bleeding. Prevent and treat shock with whole blood or fluids if necessary. Fluids should be given cautiously and only to hydrate the person in order to prevent pulmonary edema.
3. Assess for any associated injuries or other disease processes.
4. Assess, establish, and manage acid-base and electrolyte status.
5. Assess cardiac status. Cardiac monitoring is essential in a comatose patient. Many overdoses predispose the patient to cardiac irregularities and dysrhythmias (see Chap. 8).
6. Nalaxone (Narcan) is never harmful. It is a pure narcotic antagonist with little, if any, other antagonist activity. In suspected narcotic overdose, one may need to give 10 to 20 times the usual recommended dose to reverse the narcotic effects. Naloxone can be repeated frequently because the half-life is relatively short—approximately 60 minutes. When given to patients who have not recently ingested narcotics, it has little or no pharmacologic activity.
7. Glucose administration may be warranted.

Most poisoned patients require this supportive care in combination with a poison protocol.

MANAGEMENT OF THE ACUTELY POISONED PATIENT

Only after the patient has been sufficiently stabilized and supportive care has been established can further measures to prevent absorption or to enhance excretion be carried out.

Prevention of Absorption

Although there are several treatments that prevent or minimize absorption, the poison, the amount, the route, and the time of exposure all will contribute to the decision as to which methods are best.

Ocular Exposure. For an ocular exposure, a lukewarm water or saline irrigation must be done as soon as possible. The eye should be flooded from a large glass that is held 5 to 8 cm (2 to 3 inches) from the eye. The washing should be continued for 15 minutes. One should hold the eye open but have the patient blink the eye open and closed. A lukewarm shower also may be used. One must be sure to use *low* pressure.

Decontamination. If there is the slightest suspicion of an insecticide or pesticide exposure, the first consideration should be a thorough decontamination of the skin. After all the person's clothes have been removed and placed in a plastic bag so that further contamination to others in the area is prevented, three separate showers should be given:

• Soap washing
• Rubbing alcohol washing
• Soap washing

By performing such washings, one can remove 90% of an organophosphate or carbamate insecticide even 6 hours after the exposure. A gasoline or chlorine bleach exposure can result in serious burns, and a 20-minute skin decontamination with soap and water should be performed.

Dilution. For all ingested poisonings, dilutions can be done safely at home or enroute to the hospital. The recommended diluents are milk and water. These can be beneficially used unless the patient is experiencing a seizure, has lost the gag reflex, or is unconscious. The amount recommended is 15 ml/kg body weight to a maximum amount of 200 to 300 ml. Fruit juices, vinegar, and oils are contraindicated, especially if the substance ingested is an acid or alkaline. When fruit juice or vinegar is given, it can cause an exothermic heat reaction. This reaction can lead to further burning and damage of the esophagus.

Emetics. A constant dilemma facing the emergency personnel is when to vomit or not to vomit. Vomiting is contraindicated in a patient who has lost the gag reflex, has seizures, has lost consciousness, or has oropharyngeal burns. The use of emetics in a hydrocarbon exposure will be discussed later in this chapter.

Syrup of Ipecac. Administration of syrup of ipecac (not ipecac elixir) is the preferred method of gastric emptying. The recommended dose of ipecac for children is 15 ml orally, which can be repeated one time if necessary. The recommended dose for adults is 30 ml. It should be followed with 15 ml/kg of clear fluids to a maximum of 200 to 300 ml. The child should be kept ambulatory. If no emesis results in 15 to 30 minutes, one repeat dose may be given. Fluids should be given after each consecutive emesis until the emesis is clear because the person may need to vomit three or four times. Once the emesis is clear, the person should be kept to NPO (not allowed to eat or drink) for 1½ hours. This will stop the emesis.

Apomorphine, Salt, and Mustard Powder. Other emetics are not recommended. Apomorphine depresses the central nervous system and creates respiratory depression. Other emetics such as salt water have produced fatalities, and the therapeutic/toxic ratio for such substances as mustard power and copper sulfate may be too narrow to judge.

Lavage. Gastric lavage has been considered the standard method of emptying the stomach for many years. Emesis is now preferred to gastric lavage because of the frequent poor recovery of the poison or drug. This may be due to the *inadequate size* of the bore in the lavage tube. If a No. 16 or No. 18 French nasogastric tube is used in an adult, no intact pieces will be recovered. A No. 36 French tube is recommended.

Gastric lavages are indicated when the patient is comatose, is having seizures, or has no gag reflex or when a decrease in consciousness is expected. The airway should be cleared, a cuffed endotracheal tube inserted for airway protection, and the patient placed in a left lateral head-down position. Again, to obtain maximum efficacy, one must use a large bore lavage tube.

Repeated washings should be conducted until the returns are clear — 10 to 15 washings. For each washing, 100 to 200 ml of fluids are used for an adult and 10 to 15 ml/kg to a maximum of 200 ml for a child. Lukewarm water or normal saline is recommended, and it is important to recover any lavage fluid that is instilled. At the completion of the lavage, the tube should be kept in the stomach for activated charcoal or a cathartic instillation, if needed. When there is no further need for the tube, it should be pinched off and removed. One must remember to keep suction close at hand for the possibility of aspiration!

Absorbant. Activated charcoal is an inert ingredient with tremendous absorbant properties. There is no contraindication to giving it, but it is not recommended in cases of poisoning with a strong alkaline or acid. At the very least, it will act as a gastrointestinal marker, which will be a tell-tale sign of a cleared gastrointestinal tract. Because it absorbs syrup of ipecac, the two should not be given together. Activated charcoal should be given only after the emesis is clear and the patient has been NPO for 1 hour.

In theory, the recommended dose is five to ten times the amount of the toxin ingested. In practice, the adult dose is 30 to 100 g (approximately 10 to 30 tablespoons). It can be premixed with water to form a thick soup or catsuplike consistency, and, when the bottle is tightly sealed, it can be stored indefinitely. Evidence

TABLE 36-1
CHARCOAL-ABSORBED DRUGS

Alcohol	Mercuric chloride
Amphetamines	Morphine
Aspirin	Opium
Barbiturates	Oxalates
Camphor	Parathion
Chloroquine ipecac	Phenothiazine
Chlorpromazine	Propoxyphene
Digitalis	Quinine
Ethchlorvynol	Salicylates
Glutethimide	Strychnine
Malathion	

TABLE 36-2
EFFECTIVE ANTAGONISTS FOR SPECIFIC INTOXICATIONS

Intoxications	*Antagonists*
Carbon monoxide	Oxygen
Cyanide	Amyl nitrite
	Sodium nitrite
	Sodium thiosulfate
Nitrites	Methylene blue
Organophosphates	Atropine
	Protopam (2-PAM)
Narcotics	Naloxone (Narcan)
Anticholinergics or tricyclic anti-depressants	Physostigmine
Acetaminophen	N-acetylcysteine (Mucomyst) (investigational)
Ethylene glycol and methanol	Ethanol

suggests that activated charcoal, either alone or in combination with a cathartic, is at least as effective in preventing absorption of certain drugs as gastric emptying. Drugs that are well-absorbed by charcoal are listed in Table 36-1.

Cathartics.   To prevent further absorption and to speed elimination, one should use a saline cathartic. It is preferred to oil base cathartics because a saline cathartic does not leave the patient at risk to aspiration pneumonitis. Saline cathartics such as magnesium sulfate, magnesium citrate, and sodium sulfate provide safe and effective intestinal evacuation. Administered orally or by nasogastric tube, the dosage is as follows:

- Magnesium Sulfate: adults — 30 g with a maximum of 100 g in 24 hours; children — 250 mg/kg
- Magnesium Citrate: Adults — 4 ml/kg up to 300 ml/kg; children — 200 ml/kg
- Sodium Sulfate: adults — 30 g with a maximum of 100 g in 24 hours; children — 250 mg/kg

Enhancement of Excretion

The pharmacologic characteristics of a drug greatly influence the severity and the length of clinical course of the acutely poisoned patient. These properties — absorption rate, body distribution, and elimination rate — are taken into consideration when methods that will enhance a drug's excretion from the body are being chosen.

Forced Diuresis.   Forced diuresis is beneficial for severe poisoning in which the drug is primarily excreted in the urine in its active form. If this method is used, one must monitor carefully to ensure that cerebral edema does not occur. Some drugs are best excreted when urine is made alkaline; others are best excreted when the urine is made acidic. Frequently, pH testing and electrolyte monitoring are indicated if these methods are employed.

Hemodialysis and Peritoneal Dialysis.   Hemodialysis and peritoneal dialysis are used as supportive care when more conservative methods (gastric emptying, charcoal, cathartics, antagonists) have failed (see Chap. 20). If a drug or poison is highly bound to the body's tissues or widely distributed throughout the body, attempts to dialyze the drug will be futile. Therefore, one may need to consult a pharmacologist to determine a drug's characteristics. The rate of removal of a dialyzable substance is usually five to ten times greater with hemodialysis than with peritoneal dialysis. However, peritoneal dialysis is easier to perform and can be initiated more rapidly.

ANTAGONISTS
Myths of the Universal Antidote

"The universal antidote," with which you may be familiar, *should be considered useless!* It consists of the following:

2 parts burnt toast = activated charcoal
1 part milk of magnesia = cathartic
1 part strong tea = tannic acid

Burnt toast is burnt carbohydrate and not activated charcoal. Milk of magnesia is not as effective as saline cathartics, and a sufficient amount of tannic acid would cause liver impairment.

Table 36-2 lists the only recognized effective antagonists for specific intoxicants. Caution must be taken with dosage and route of administration because if given incorrectly, some antagonists will cause further complications.

Text continued on page 640.

TABLE 36-3
COMMONLY OBSERVED POISONINGS

Substance/Examples	Symptoms	Laboratory Work	Treatment	Comments
Benzodiazepines Diazepam (Valium) Chlordiazepoxide (Librium) Flurazepam (Dalmane) Lorazepam (Ativan) Clorazepate (Tranxene) Oxazepam (Serax)	Lethargy, stage 1 coma Hypotension Tachycardia Decreasing bowel sounds Decreasing respirations Dilated pupils may be present Dry mouth may be noted Ataxia Slurred speech	Plasma screen Urine	Ipecac/lavage/charcoal/cathartic Ventilatory support Fluids for hypotension, vasopressor if necessary Treatment of withdrawal Forced diuresis: ineffective Hemodialysis: ineffective	Benzodiazepines exhibit central nervous system depressant effects. Because of the long half-life, these drugs may cause prolonged drowsiness in the overdose situation. No documented fatalities have occurred from the ingestion of these agents alone, but frequently they are involved in the multiple overdose, most notable with alcohol. Ingestions of 500 to 1500 mg have occurred with only minor toxicity. Physical dependence can occur with chronic ingestion; therefore, withdrawal may be anticipated if a person arrives with an acute oral benzodiazepine overdose.
Amphetamines Diet pills Illicit drugs (MDA, STP, DMT)	Restlessness, seizures Coma Cardiac arrhythmias Hypotenion Hypertension Tachycardia Acute cardiomyopathy may be noted following IV abuse Delusions Paranoia Aggressive behavior	Urine for amphetamines	Ipecac/lavage/charcoal/cathartic Forced acid diuresis for severe overdose IV diazepam for seizures Oral chlorpromazine for hypertension Fluids for hypotension Suicide precautions Acid diuresis should be used only in severe cases to enhance urinary excretion but should be avoided in the presence of rhabdomyolysis because this would precipitate renal failure.	Amphetamines have a stimulant effect on both central and peripheral nervous systems and also have analeptic properties. The response is variable, and dependency can occur with chronic abuse. Clinical effects are easily seen within an hour of ingestion, and death occurs from cardiac arrhythmias and circulatory collapse. Because of the rapid excretion of these drugs, treatment of acute intoxication is achieved in 24 to 36 hours. The withdrawal for chronic abusers requires psychiatric intervention because these persons are often suicidally depressed. Withdrawal should take place over 2 to 3 weeks because rapid withdrawal will lead to seizures.

(Continued)

TABLE 36-3
Continued

Substance/Examples	Symptoms	Laboratory Work	Treatment	Comments

Methanol
Antifreeze
Windshield washer solvent
Varnish
Sterno
Wood alcohol
	Three major types:
	1. CNS depression, malaise, headache, dizziness
	2. High anion gap metabolic acidosis
	  a. Plasma HCO_3^- markedly decreases
	  b. Urine *p*H often drops to 5
	3. Ophthalmic
	  a. Transient visual abnormalities, blurred and/or double vision, changes in color perception, constricted visual fields, spots, sharply reduced visual acuity
	  b. Temporary ocular defects
	    (1) Peripapillary edema
	    (2) Hyperemia of optic disc
	    (3) Dimished pupillary light reactions
	    (4) Central scotoma
	  c. Permanent ocular defects
	    (1) Pallor of optic disc
	    (2) Attenuation
	    (3) Sheathing of retinal arterioles
	    (4) Decreased visual acuity
	    (5) Defects involving nerve fibers
	    (6) Permanent blindness
		Blood methanol
		Arterial blood gases
		While on drip: glucose, blood alcohol
			Ipecac/lavage/charcoal/cathartic
			Correct acidosis with sodium bicarbonate 0.5 to 1.0 mEq/kg
			Correct potassium depletion
			Ethanol drip if there are symptoms or if blood methanol is greater than 20 mg/dl
			Hemodialysis for marked acidosis or blood methanol 50 mg/dl
			Do *not* stop drip if patient is dialyzed
				Methanol is an alcohol commonly found in antifreeze, windshield washer fluid, and Sterno. After rapid absorption by ingestion, inhalation, and dermal exposure, it undergoes hepatic metabolism for formaldehyde and formic acid, both of which are much more toxic than methanol itself. These two end products produce severe acidosis and blindness, with the onset of symptoms in several hours to several days. The administration of intravenous alcohol (ETOH) is the treatment of choice. Alcohol competes with methanol at the enzyme site in the liver, blocking the formation of toxic metabolites and allowing methanol to be excreted unchanged. The drip must be continued for 2 to 3 days or until the blood methanol level is less than 20 mg/dl and acidosis is corrected.

Ethylene Glycol Antifreeze solvents	Acidosis Persistent vomiting Lethargy, coma Seizures Renal tubular necrosis Myocardial failure	Blood ethylene glycol Arterial blood gases Urine for crystals While on drip: glucose, blood alcohol	Ipecac/lavage/charcoal/cathartic ETOH drip Hemodialysis for uncorrected acidosis Monitor renal function Bicarbonate for correction of acidosis Treatment of seizures if necessary with diazepam	Ethylene glycol is an alcohol found primarily in antifreeze and solvents and is rapidly absorbed upon ingestion. Hepatic metabolism produces organic acids, which cause severe acidosis, and oxalic acid (crystals), which leads to renal tubular necrosis. As with methanol, the administration of intravenous

alcohol will compete with ethylene glycol at the enzyme site and prevent the formation of toxic metabolites. The alcohol drip should continue 1 to 3 days until acidosis disappears and crystaluria resolves.

Pharmacology
1. Liver breaks down parent compound to its more toxic metabolites at peak levels 6° to 12° post ingestion.
2. Accumulation of aldehydes interferes with
   a. Oxidative phosphorylation
   b. Cellular respiration
   c. Glucose metabolism
3. Accumulation of oxalate and glycolic acid causes
   a. Severe renal damage
   b. Acidosis
   c. Death

	Signs/Symptoms	Laboratory	Treatment	Comments
Propoxyphene Darvon Darvon compound Darvocet N-100	Seizures Pinpoint pupils Coma Respiratory arrest Hypotension Cardiac arrhythmias	Arterial blood gases Propoxyphene levels are not clinically useful	Lavage with protected airway/charcoal/cathartic Naloxone hydrochloride (Narcan) 0.4 to 0.8 mg IV (may bolus with 5 to 10 amps if no initial response) Diazepam (Valium) for seizures unresponsive to naloxone hydrochloride (Narcan) Maintenance of fluids Monitoring of patients in ICU for at least 24 hours or until patient is persistently alert	Propoxyphene is a weak synthetic narcotic found in a variety of preparations and acts directly on the CNS. Its rapid action allows for observable symptoms within 30 minutes of ingestion, and effects may be exhibited for 8 to 12 hours. Because narcotics decrease gastrointestinal motility, pill fragments may be recovered several hours later. A diagnostic clue to propoxyphene overdose is that the person will present with seizures and pinpoint pupils. The propensity toward seizures makes lavage preferable to ipecac. Large amount of naloxone (2 to 20 ampules as a bolus) have been required for reversal of the effects of propoxyphene overdose.

(Continued)

TABLE 36-3
Continued

Substance/Examples	Symptoms	Laboratory Work	Treatment	Comments
Organophosphates Parathion Tepp Dursban Diazinon Malathion Insect sprays Pest strips	1. Muscarinic (secretions) 　a. Increased salivation 　b. Increased lacrimation 　c. Increased urination 　d. Diarrhea 　e. Vomiting 2. Nicotinic (muscles) 　a. Muscle weakness 　b. Respiratory paralysis 3. Central nervous system 　a. Psychotic behavior 　b. Coma	Red blood cell (RBC) cholinesterase	Ingestion: ipecac/lavage/ charcoal/cathartic Dermal: decontamination washings—health care personnel *must* protect themselves from contamination Atropine: 1 to 2 mg IV, repeated 2 to 3 minutes until secretions are dry Treatment of hydrocarbon pneumonitis Protopam (2-PAM) if atropine is ineffective or RBC cholinesterase is 50% of normal	Organophosphates are insecticides that are widely used in agriculture and for home/garden pest control. Well absorbed through ingestion and percutaneously, these agents exhibit their main effects by preventing the breakdown of the neurotransmitter acetylcholine. The enzyme accumulates at nerve synapses and creates a cholinergic crisis, with all symptoms being the result of acetylcholine stimulation. The effecient dermal absorption requires a rigorous skin decontamination. Leather products cannot be decontaminated; therefore, the patient's leather shoes, watchbands, belts, and so forth must be discarded. Atropine blocks the effects of excessive acetylcholine if it persists in high enough concentrations, and the administration of 2000 mg has been required to reverse the symptoms of a severe poisoning. Atropine is not effective for reversing muscular manifestations (respiratory paralysis), and, if this occurs, the additional administration of protopam (2-PAM) may be required. Because many organophosphates are in combination with hydrocarbon propellants, the toxicity of both agents demands attention.

Iron				
Multivitamins with iron Ferrous gluconate Entron Fergon Ferralet plus Ferrous sulfate Mol-Iron Feosol Fer-In-Sol Ferrous fumarate	1. 1st phase: 30 minutes to 2 hours a. Lethargy b. Restlessness c. Hematemesis d. Abdominal pain e. Bloody diarrhea 2. 2nd phase: immediately following period of apparent recovery 3. 3rd phase: 2 to 12 hours after the first phase a. Onset of shock b. Refractory acidosis c. Cyanosis d. Fever 4. 4th phase: 2 to 4 days a. Possible hepatic necrosis	STAT: serum iron, total iron binding capacity Flat plate of abdomen Typing and crossmatching for blood Electrolytes	Life support by correction of shock with fluids or blood and administration of electrolytes as indicated Ipecac if not contraindicated Lavage: sodium bicarbonate or Fleet Phosphate Enema Solution Deferoxamine for severe symptoms or if serum iron is greater than 350 mg/dl	Iron is found in a number of preparations, including multivitamins with iron and prenatal vitamins. Iron has a direct effect on the gastrointestinal mucosa. In less than 2 hours there can be severe hemorrhagic necrosis with large losses of blood and fluid. The plasma iron concentration and total iron-binding capacity may vary and are regulated by hemoglobin synthesis. In children, iron preparations have been fatal. Careful calculations must be made of the amount of elemental iron ingested.
Acetaminophen Tylenol Datril Liquiprin Nyquil	Toxicity mainly to liver. (Death related to hepatic failure occurs in 10% of serious ingestions.) *Phase I* (up to 24 hours post ingestion): anorexia, nausea, vomiting, diaphoresis, malaise *Phase II* (after 24 hours): RUQ pain secondary to hepatic damage, which occurs in first 24 hours; abnormal blood chemistries with increased liver function tests and total bilirubin *Phase III* (3–5 days): characterized by sequelae of hepatic necrosis; coagulation defects, jaundice, renal failure, myocardial pathology, hepatic encephalopathy *Phase IV:* recovery	Serum glutamic-oxaloacetic transaminase (SGOT), serum glutamic-pyruvic transaminase (SGPT) Blood urea nitrogen (BUN) every 24 hours Total bilirubin Prothrombin time (PT) Acetaminophen level 4 hours post ingestion and repeated in 4 to 8 hours (4-hr toxic level equals 150 µg/ml)	Acetaminophen only: lavage Mixed: charcoal and cathartic lavage after 1 hour Induce emesis, if appropriate Cathartics Supportive care Avoid steriods, epinephrine, analeptics Criteria for use of acetylcysteine (Mucomyst) 1. 7.5 g or more by history; 140 mg/kg for children under 12 years 2. Within 24 hours: time of ingestion within 2 hours must be known 3. Final determinant: plasma level above 150 mcg/ml 4 hours post ingestion Dosage of acetylcysteine (Mucomyst) 1. Loading dose 140 mg/kg PO of 20% × 1 2. Maintenance doses: 70 mg/kg PO of 20% × 17 doses every 4 hours 3. If patient vomits the dose within 1 hour repeat dose. If the patient vomits after 1 hour go to next dose. For persistent vomiting use NG or MA tube.	Acetaminophen is an antipyretic and analgesic used commonly by those who cannot or would prefer not to take aspirin. Because it is so common, acetaminophen is often confused with aspirin. One needs to be cautious about identifying which medication was taken when there is an accidental or intentional overdose. Acetaminophen overdose is considered to be an acute ingestion of 7.5 g or more. There are no unique signs or symptoms in the first 24 hours following the exposure that would make the diagnosis definite. Persons present with general symptoms commonly seen with medical problems as well as with overdose. Treatment with acetylcysteine must be initiated within 16 hours. If not, acute hepatocellular necrosis will result, and 1 out of 10 cases of massive overdose will cause death. It should be

(Continued)

TABLE 36-3
Continued

Substance/Examples	Symptoms	Laboratory Work	Treatment	Comments
			4. Diluent: Use only Coke, Pepsi, Fresca, orange juice, or grapefruit juice. When using 20% Mucomyst, dilute 3 parts to 1 part Mucomyst. Miscellaneous 1. Pregnancy test if patient is child-bearing age 2. Diet and activity as tolerated; Acetylcysteine 1° ac (before meals) and 2° pc (after meals) 3. Avoidance of medications, if possible	noted here that those patients who die from severe Darvocet-N ingestions most likely expire from propoxyphene effects rather than from the effects of acetaminophen.
Hydrocarbons Aliphatic (straight chain): gasoline, kerosene, fuel oil	Aspiration pneumonitis CNS depression Cyanosis Tachycardia Hyperpyrexia Dermal irritation Eye: transient corneal epithelial injury	Arterial blood gases Chest roentgenogram, repeated in 12 to 24 hours Renal studies Hepatic studies	Different compounds result in many varied symptoms. Check the specific management. Induce emesis for A large amount A small amount with GI symptoms An aromatic hydrocarbon A halogenated hydrocarbon A hydrocarbon with a toxic additive like a heavy metal or a pesticide If a patient is comatose or seizing, protect the airway and lavage. Do not induce emesis for mineral seal oil, signal oil of furniture polish. Check for symptoms of aspiration (cough, congestion, fever) up to 12 hours. If symptomatic, send in for chest radiograph, repeated at 6 to 8 hours. Supportive care should be given for an aspiration pneumonitis. Steriods are not useful. Antibiotics are to be used only if indicated.	Hydrocarbons are substances with various numbers of carbon atoms and are found in numerous products. Their toxicity largely depends on their viscosity and votility, with main clinical effects on the pulmonary bed. Hydrocarbons of low viscosity are easily aspirated, are spread quickly over lung surfaces, and cause a chemical pneumonitis within 8 to 12 hours. Thicker hydrocarbons do not spread easily and therefore have a lower degree of toxicity. Some hydrocarbons have systemic toxicity associated with them and can cause CNS depression and renal and hepatic damage. When a hydrocarbon causes systemic symptoms or when it is in combination with other ingredients that have systemic toxicity, it is best to remove it from the stomach. Ipecac is highly preferred, and contrary to earlier beliefs, aspiration occurs on

ingestion and not in the process of inducing emesis. Lavage, however, increases the chance of aspiration because hydrocarbons cling to the tube and on withdrawal more easily enter the trachea. When treating aspiration, the use of steroids is contraindicated. They inhibit the natural immunosuppressive response of the cell. The following hydrocarbons are not considered toxic. With frank aspiration they may cause a low-grade lipoid pneumonia.

1. Asphalt and tar
2. Lubricants: motor oil, transmission oil, cutting oil, household oil, heavy greases
3. Mineral oil or liquid petroleum: laxatives, baby oil, white petroleum, sun tan oil

Cathartics MgSO$_4$—children, 250 mg/kg; adults, 30 g

Aromatic (containing a benzene ring): benzene, toluene, xylene. Found in glues and nail polish removers. Toxic effects produced chiefly by inhalation of vapors

Burning sensation in the mucous membranes of the mouth and esophagus
Nausea and vomiting
Cough, hoarseness, chest pain: bronchial, laryngeal irritation
CNS excitation followed by depression: euphoria, HA, giddiness, vertigo, ataxia, convulsions, coma
Dermal: skin irritation
Eye: corneal burns

Fluorinated: Freons. Commonly used as refrigerants and as propellants in aerosols.

Bronchial constriction and lung irritation
Decreased contractility of the heart
Sniffing from a bag produces hypoxia due to replacement of O$_2$
Arrhythmias, which are difficult to reverse

Chlorinated: Perchloroethylene (dry cleaning agent), trichloroethylene, polyvinyl chloride,

CNS depressant
renal and hepatic damage

(Continued)

635

TABLE 36-3
Continued

Substance/Examples	Symptoms	Laboratory Work	Treatment	Comments
different types of insecticides, methylene chloride, trichoroethane, carbon tetrachloride				
Salicylates Aspirin Alka Seltzer, Midol, Aspergum Cold and allergy preparations: Congesprin Enteric coated, rectal suppositories Oil of wintergreen (methyl salicylates: 1 ml = 1.46 g salicylates) Pepto Bismol (bismuth subsalicylate) Sunscreens (homomethyl salicylate): Coppertone Linaments Other salt forms: sodium salicylate, calcium carbasprin, magnesium salicylate	Gastrointestinal: nausea, vomiting, gastric irritation Metabolic: hyperthermia, hyperglycemia, hypoglycemia (children) hyponatremia, hypernatremia, hypokalemia, acidemia, alkalemia Respiratory: hyperpnea, hyperventilation, pulmonary edema Neurologic: tinnitus, confusion, coma, seizures Renal: altered renal function, oliguria Hepatic: hepatitis, altered liver function studies Hematologic: hypoprothrombinemia, hemorrhagic disorders Acute toxicity 1. Therapeutic or less than 150 mg/kg: Nausea, vomiting, gastritis, tinnitus 2. 150–300 mg/kg: Mild to severe hyperpnea, lethargy and/or excitability, neurologic disturbances 3. 300–500 mg/kg: Life-threatening cardiorespiratory complications, metabolic acidosis, seizures, coma, death 4. Greater than 500 mg/kg: Potentially lethal toxic reaction Chronic toxicity 1. A chronic ingestion of greater than 100 mg/kg/24 hours over 2 or more days	Done Nomogram 1. Not applicable in chronic salicylism. 2. Symptomatic patient with low level may indicate chronic use or continuous absorption from bolus. 3. Absorption of enteric coated tablets is erratic and a lag of up to 28 hours may occur before peak levels. Ferric chloride Test 1. 1:1 mixture of urine with 105 ferric chloride will turn violet to purple if salicylates are present. (Heat urine briefly to remove diacetic acid prior to tests).	Supportive care 1. Establishment of respiration 2. Cardiac monitoring 3. External cooling 4. Hydration 5. Monitoring of electrolytes and correction of acid-base imbalances Prevention of Absorption 1. Emesis or lavage 2. Charcoal (adults, 60–100 g; children, 30–60 g) 3. Cathartic: magnesium sulfate (adults, 30 g; children, 250 mg/kg) Enhancement of excretion 1. Maintain urine flow at 3–6 ml/kg/hr 2. Alkalinize urine with 35–50 mEq/liter of sodium bicarbonate and 40 mEq/liter potassium chloride to get pH of 7.5–8.5 (change in urine pH from 7.5–8.5 increases excretion 20 ×). Follow-up procedures for salicylates 1. If ingestion is 100 mg/kg or less, no treatment is necessary. 2. If ingestion is 100–150 mg/kg, administer cathartic. 3. If ingestion is 150–300 mg/kg, induce vomiting and cathart. 4. If ingestion is greater than 300 mg/kg, induce vomiting or lavage, administer charcoal and cathartic, and draw 6 hour	Salicylates are used as antipyretic, analgesic, anti-inflammatory, and antirheumatoid medications. Absorption is erratic, and a lag of up to 28 hours can occur. Salicylates obey a zero order of kinetics; that is, doubling the dose may more than double the plasma level. Half-life may be increasingly prolonged. A plasma level before 6 hours after ingestion is useless. In children, chronic ingestions cause hypoglycemia, but hyperglycemia is more common with overdose in adults. Salicylates interrupt prothrombin production and inhibit platelet function and other clotting factors. Pharmacology 1. Large doses decrease gastric motility. May form bolus in stomach, which will provide a source for further absorption. 2. Obey zero order kinetics; i.e., doubling the dose more than doubles plasma level, increased half life (15–30 hours). 3. Uncouple oxidative phosphorylation, resulting in heat formation and increased cardiac output. 4. Hypoglycemia may occur

Agent / Source	Clinical Features	Laboratory	Treatment
	5. Hyperglycemia can occur (more common in adults). 6. Hyperthermia can occur 7. Direct respiratory stimulant, producing tachypnea 15–20 minutes post ingestion, resulting in respiratory alkalosis. 8. Replacement of respiratory alkalosis with severe acidosis is common in children. 9. Produce clotting disorders.	...post ingestion salicylate level is thought to be associated with toxicity. 2. Clinical findings, not blood levels of salicylate, are more useful as an indicator of the severity of the intoxication.	
Carbon Monoxide Incomplete combustion of carbon containing fuels 1. Exhaust from autos or any gas engines 2. Charcoal 3. Poorly ventilated wood/coal stoves 4. Propane, kerosene heaters 5. Furnaces Methylene chloride commonly found in paint, varnish removers.	Carbon monoxide is an odorless and tasteless gas. It is found in the exhaust of automobiles, in the emissions of backyard barbecue devices, after the inhalation of methylene chloride, and when gas burns incompletely. Carbon monoxide is not found in natural gas but can be contained in the gas produced from coal. It has a strong affinity to and combines quickly with hemoglobin to produce carboxyhemoglobin. In persons with a compromised cardiovascular system, 15% saturation of carboxyhemoglobin or greater can produce a heart attack. Pharmacology 1. Carbon monoxide binds rapidly, specifically, and avidly with hemoglobin to form carboxyhemoglobin. 2. Affinity of CO for hemoglobin is over 200 times that of oxygen. 3. Reduces the carrying capacity of blood for oxygen. 4. Inhibits unloading of oxygen in all tissues of the body.	See Table 36–4 Carboxyhemoglobin LDH, CPK, transaminase, SGOT Arterial blood gases CT scan, if indicated EKG Chest film	Remove the patient to fresh air. Establish airway. Administer 100% oxygen by face mask. Carboxyhemoglobin level. Seizures: IV diazepam. EKG monitor for 24 hours if patient is unconscious or symptomatic or has a high COHB level. Cerebral edema: dexamethasone. Limit fluids to 2/3–3/4 of normal maintenance. Admit any patient found unconscious or with a level above 25%. Watch for delayed CNS effects 48–72 hours later. Hyperbaric chamber for severe cases.

(Continued)

TABLE 36-3
Continued

Substance/Examples	Symptoms	Laboratory Work	Treatment	Comments
				5. Results in hypoxia, with main effect on the brain and heart.
				Kinetics
				1. Absorption: rapidly absorbed by lungs
				2. Elimination: lungs
				3. Half-life
				a. Room air: 5–6 hours
				b. 100% oxygen through a tightly fitted mask: 40–90 minutes.
				c. Hyperbaric oxygen (3 atmospheres of pressure) less than 30 minutes
Barbiturates				Barbiturates are of two basic types: short-acting and long-acting. They are used as anticonvulsants, sedatives, and hypnotics. The effects seem to be primarily due to the interference with impulse transmission to the cerebral cortex—CNS depression. They have no analgestic properties. They are metabolized in the liver. Short-acting barbiturates have little excretion in the kidney, whereas long-acting barbiturates are primarily cleared in the kidney in overdosage. The drug is generally highly protein bound. Addiction is frequently a possibility.
Short-acting	CNS depression: respiratory/ cardiac arrests	Plasma levels, repeated	Establish airway	
1. Pentobarbital (Nembutal)	Coma	Electrolytes	Prevent absorption: ipecac/ lavage/charcoal/cathartic	
2. Secobarbital (Seconal)	Hypotension		Charcoal perfusion, forced diuresis, and hemodialysis not effective	
	Hypoxia		Diazepam for seizures	
	Hypothermia			
	Bullae			
	Withdrawal symptoms			
	1. Tremors			
	2. Nausea			
	3. Anorexia			
	4. Vomiting			
	5. Muscular weakness			
	6. Convulsions			
Long-acting	Same as short-acting barbiturates	Plasma levels, repeated	Establish respirations	
1. Phenobarbital (Luminal)	Varying degrees of coma and CNS depression: respiratory/ cardiac arrest	Electrolytes	Prevent absorption: ipecac/ lavage/charcoal/cathartic	
2. Metharbital (Gemonil)	Aspiration pneumonia	Urine pH	Forced alkaline diuresis (hemodialysis if unresponsive)	
3. Primidone (Mysoline) (15% converted to phenobarbital)				

Cyclic Antidepressants

Amitriptyline (Elavil, Triavil Endep)
Imipramine (Tofranil, Presamine, SK-Pramine)
Desipramine (Norpramine)
Nortriptyline (Aventyl, Pamelor)
Trimipramine
Doxepin (Sinequan)
Amoxapine (Ascendin) (May have different toxicity than prototype).
Protriptyline (Vivactil)
Tetracyclics such as maprotoline (Ludiomil).

Mild
1. Lethargy
2. Tachycardia
3. Urinary retention
4. Dry mouth

Severe
1. Coma
2. Respiratory depression
3. Convulsions
4. Mycolonus
5. Hypotension
6. Cardiac conduction delays
7. Ventricular arrythmias

Toxic range
1. It is generally unreliable to calculate mg/kg of ingestion for possible toxicity.
2. Any adult with a history of 8–10 tablets ingested may be at risk for serious toxicity.
3. Children are more sensitive to toxicity.

Presence of drug can be detected in urine and gastric contents.
Serum levels are usually not helpful in patient management (therapeutic or overdose).
QRS duration (12-lead EKG) of more than 0.10 seconds suggests cardiac toxicity.

Airway support
Anticonvulsants: phenytoin/ diazepam
Prevention of absorption
Multiple dose charcoal
Norepinephrine probably pressor of choice for hypotension
Physostigmine may be indicated for seizures, severe hallucinations, hypertension, and arrythmias when in the presence of anticholinergic symptoms *unresponsive* to standard anticonvulsants and antiarrhythmic agents.
Alkalinization: sodium bicarbonate as needed to achieve a physiologic blood *p*H of (7.40–7.45). Monitor blood gases to guide therapy.
Enhanced excretion by diuresis and/or hemodialysis is ineffective.
Hemoperfusion is of unknown clinical value.
Admit and cardiac monitor 48 hours if symptomatic. Do not discharge until patient remains asymptomatic and arrhythmia-free for at least 24 hours.
Children are frequently more sensitive to antidepressants and may demonstrate symptoms at lower doses. All suspected antidepressant ingestions in children warrant an ER evaluation for prevention of absorption and cardiac monitor.

Hypotension/shock: fluids first, then vasopressors
Bullae: burn treatment
Seizures: diazepam

Cyclic antidepressants are used in the treatment of endogenous depression. The cyclic antidepressants are rapidly absorbed from the gastrointestinal tract. They are highly lipid- and protein-bound, which is very important to remember when treating this type of overdose. Cyclic antidepressants have both central and peripheral effects resulting from the blockage of the re-uptake of norepinephrine, an atropinelike anticholinergic effect, and a direct myocardial depressant effect. The major cause of mortality is cardiotoxicity.

Pharmacology
1. Rapid absorption
2. Protein-bound
3. Large volume of distribution
4. Half-life 12–36 hours
5. Tertiary and secondary amines.

Cyclic antidepressant overdose: mechanism of toxicity
1. Anticholinergic effect
2. Blockage of re-uptake of norepinephrine
3. Direct myocardial depression (quinidine-like effect)
4. Alpha blockade resulting in hypotension.

TABLE 36-4
SYPMTOMS OF CARBON MONOXIDE POISONING

CO in Atmosphere	Duration of Exposure	Saturation of Blood	Symptoms
Up to 0.01% 0.01%–0.02%	Indefinite Indefinite	0%–10%} 10%–20%}	Tightness across forehead; slight headache; dilation of cutaneous vessels
0.02%–0.03%	5–6 hours	20%–30%	Headache; throbbing in temples
0.04%–0.06%	4–5 hours	30%–40%	Severe headache; weakness and dizziness; nausea and vomiting; collapse. Pathognomonic cherry-red color to lips, mucous membranes and skin; leucocytosis
0.07%–0.10%	3–4 hours	40%–50%	As above, plus increased tendency to collapse and syncope; increased pulse and respiratory rate
0.11%–0.15%	1.5–3 hours	50%–60%	Increased pulse and respiratory rate, syncope, Cheyne-Stokes respiration; coma with intermittent convulsions
0.16%–0.30%	1–1.5 hours	60%–70%	Coma with intermittent convulsions; depressed heart action respirations; death possible
0.50%–1%	1–2 minutes	70%–80%	Weak pulse; depressed respirations; respiratory failure and death

Note: In patients with cardiovascular disease, a carboxyhemoglobin level of 15% or greater can precipitate a heart attack or a stroke. (Rumack BH [ed]: Poisondex, Englewood, CO, Micromedex, 1983)

COMMONLY OBSERVED POISONINGS

Symptoms and treatment related to poisoning by various substances are give in Table 36-3. Symptoms of carbon monoxide poisoning are listed in Table 36-4.

BIBLIOGRAPHY

Bayer MJ, Rumack BH (eds): Poisonings and Overdoses. Curr Top Emerg Med 1, No. 3, 1979

Curtis RA et al: Efficacy of ipecac and activated charcoal/cathartic. Arch Intern Med 144: 48–52, 1981

Kulig K, Rumack BH: Hydrocarbon ingestion. Curr Top Emerg Med 3, No. 4, 1981

Peterson RG, Rumack BH: Treating acute acetaminophen poisoning with acetylcystine. J.A.M.A. 237:2406–2407, 1977

Rumack BH, Peterson RC, Koch GG et al: Acetaminophen overdose. 662 cases with evaluation of oral acetylcysteine treatment. Arch Intern Med 141:380–385, 1981

Rumack BH (ed): Poisondex. Englewood, CO, Micromedex, 1983

Rumack BH, Sullivan JB: Management of the Acutely Poisoned Patient. The Rocky Mountain Poison Center, September, 1979

Snodgrass W, Rumack BH, Peterson RG et al: Salicylate toxicity following therapeutic doses in young children. Clin Toxicol 18:247–259, 1981

Temple AR: Acute and chronic effects of aspirin toxicity and their treatment. Arch Intern Med 141:364–369, 1981

Zimmerman SS, Truxal B: Carbon monoxide poisoning. Pediatrics 68, No. 2, 215–224, 1981

37
Burns

Margaret A. Marcinek

Burn injury is a serious problem in the United States. According to the National Fire Data Center, the United States ranks first in per capita fire deaths and property loss among the major industrialized nations and has a rate nearly double that of second-ranked Canada.

People who suffer burn injury present one of the most challenging health care crises. A person who at one moment is well can rapidly become a victim of extensive burns. Concomitant with the dramatic physiological alterations is the emotional impact of burn injury, which affects both the victim and his family. Major advances have occurred in burn therapy since the early 1960s: The prognosis has changed from *expecting death* to *expecting life*.

Comprehensive nursing care given once burn injury occurs is vital to the prevention of death and disability. It is essential that nurses have a clear understanding of the interrelated changes in all body systems following burn injury as well as an appreciation of the emotional impact of the injury on the patient and family. Only with such a comprehensive knowledge base can the nurse provide the therapeutic interventions necessary in all stages of recovery.

CLASSIFICATIONS OF BURN INJURY

Burn Depth

The nurse must have an understanding of the basic anatomy and physiology of the skin to appreciate the classification of the various degrees of burn injury (Fig. 37-1). The skin is the largest organ of the body, and it performs several complex functions. It is the body's first line of defense against invasion by microorganisms and environmental radiation. It prevents loss of body fluids, controls body temperature, functions as an excretory and sensory organ, produces vitamin D, and influences body image.

Damage to the skin is frequently described according to the depth of injury and is defined in terms of partial-thickness and full-thickness injuries, which correspond to the various layers of the skin (Table 37-1).

Partial-Thickness Burns

Partial-thickness burns are differentiated into superficial and deep partial-thickness burns.

Superficial partial thickness burns damage the epidermis, which is the thin layer of epithelial cells that are continuously being replaced. This keratinized layer provides a protective wall between the host and the environment. A sunburn is a familiar example of a superficial partial-thickness injury. It feels painful at first and later itches owing to the stimulation of sensory receptors. Because the epithelial cells of the epidermis are continuously being replaced, this type of injury will heal spontaneously without scarring.

A deep partial-thickness injury (*i.e.,* a second-degree burn) will involve varying degrees of the dermal layer. The dermis contains structures essential to normal skin function: sweat and sebacious glands, sensory and motor nerves, capillaries, and hair follicles. A deep partial-thickness burn will be pinkish-red and painful and it will form blisters and subcutaneous edema. Depending on the depth, these wounds will heal spontaneously in 3 to 35 days as the epidermal elements germinate and migrate until the epidermal surface is

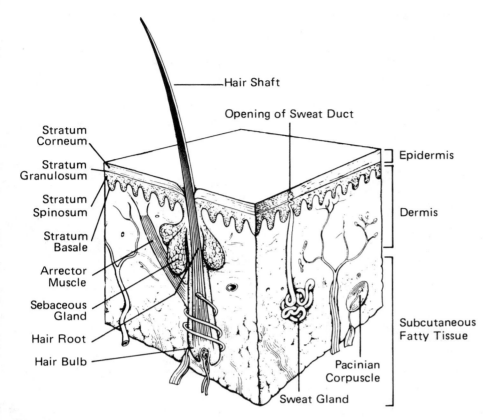

FIGURE 37-1
A three-dimensional view of the skin.

restored. If the wound becomes infected or traumatized or if the blood supply is compromised, these burns will develop into full-thickness burns.

Full-Thickness Burns (Third-Degree Burns)

Full-thickness burns (*i.e.,* third-degree burns) expose the fat layer composed of adipose tissue, which is poorly vascularized. This layer contains the roots of the sweat glands and hair follicles. All epidermal elements are destroyed. These burns may appear white, red, brown, or black. Redened areas do not blanch in response to pressure because the underlying blood supply has been interrupted. Brownish streaks are evidence of thrombosed blood vessels.

These burns are completely anesthetic because the sensory receptors have been totally destroyed. In addition, they may appear sunken because of the loss of underlying fat and muscle.

The small wound (<4 cm) may be allowed to heal by granulation and migration of healthy epithelium from the wound margins. Extensive open full-thickness wounds leave the patient highly susceptible to overwhelming infection and malnutrition. Wound closure by skin grafting restores the integrity of the skin.

Causative Agent

Burns may also be classified according to the agent causing the injury:

- Thermal — scald, contact, and flame injuries
- Electrical
- Chemical
- Radiation

The extent and depth of burn injury are related to the intensity and duration of exposure to the causative agent.

Severity of Burn

Part of the confusion concerning the statistical incidence of burn injury stems from the confusion surrounding its definition. A burn injury may range from a small blister to massive third-degree burns. Recognizing the need for a clear description of terms, the American Burn Association (ABA) developed the Injury Severity Grading System, which is used to determine the magnitude of the burn injury and to provide optimal criteria for hospital resources for patient care. The

TABLE 37-1
CHARACTERISTICS OF VARIOUS DEPTHS OF BURNS

Depth	Tissues	Usual Cause	Characteristics	Pain Sensations

First-Degree
Superficial
   partial-thickness
	Epidermis
	Part of dermis
		Sun
		Minor flash
			Dry
			No blisters
			Pinkish-red
			Blanches with
			   pressure
				Painful
				Itching
				Hyperesthetic

Second-Degree Deep partial- thickness	Epidermis Dermis	Flash Hot liquids	Moist Pinkish-red Blisters Subcutaneous edema	Pain Hyperesthetic
Third-Degree Full-thickness	Epidermis Dermis Subcutaneous tissue	Flame	Dry Skin color: red, white, brown, black No blanching Brown streaks Sunken appearance	Little pain Anesthetic

Fourth-degree
All tissues
	All of above plus
	   muscle and bone
		Sustained flame
		   or electrical
			Charred block
			Cracked
			Edema
			Immobility of area
				Little pain

magnitude of burn injury has been categorized into minor, moderate, and major burns.

Minor Burn Injury

A *minor burn injury* is a partial-thickness injury of less than 15% total body surface area (TBSA) in adults or 10% TBSA in children or a full-thickness injury of less than 2% TBSA that is not associated with any complications. Patients with these injuries may be treated in a hospital emergency room and followed on an outpatient basis, but they must be seen every 48 hours until the risk of infection decreases and wound healing is underway.

Moderate Uncomplicated Burn Injury

A *moderate uncomplicated burn injury* is a partial-thickness injury of 15% to 25% TBSA in adults or 10% to 20% TBSA in children or a full-thickness injury of less than 10% TBSA that is not associated with complications. These patients can be treated in an average hospital with appropriate facilities and personnel.

Major Burn Injury

A *major burn injury* is any of the following:

• a partial-thickness injury of more than 25% TBSA in adults or 20% in children;
• a full-thickness injury of 10% or greater TBSA;

• a burn involving the hands, face, eyes, ears, feet and perineum;
• an inhalation injury;
• an electrical injury;
• a burn associated with extenuating problems, such as a soft tissue injury, fractures, other trauma, or pre-existing health problems.

Patients with these injuries should be cared for in a burn unit or a burn center.

NURSING MANAGEMENT OF THE BURN PATIENT

The burn patient goes through phases of recovery. Each phase has specific problems, and nursing care must be directed toward enabling the patient to resolve these problems effectively. The phases of recovery following burn injury can be categorized as the emergent period, the acute phase, and rehabilitation.

The emergent period may be defined as the time required to resolve the immediate problem resulting from the burn injury. It may last from 1 to 5 days and will terminate with the onset of a spontaneous diuresis, the classic hallmark that the capillaries have regained their integrity and can mobilize third-space fluid. Intelligent emergent care not only aids in minimizing later complications but also contributes greatly to the patients chances of survival.

Following the emergent period, attention is directed toward prevention of infection. The acute phase, then, is primarily concerned with wound management.

The rehabilitation phase is directed toward achievement of nutritional requirements and prevention of scarring and contractures.

Throughout the entire process of recovery, the nurse must be keenly aware of the psychosocial implications of burn injury for the patient and the family.

The Emergent Period

Prompt, accurate assessment and management of the burn victim are essential to recovery. With inadequate or poorly monitored resuscitation efforts, many burn patients develop serious complications and die of their injuries during the emergent period.

The Emergency Department

The major clinical problems, nursing diagnoses, and goals of nursing intervention for the burn patient in the emergency department are listed in Table 37-2.

Stop the burning process. The first priority is to remove the source of heat and stop the burning process. Smoldering clothing, constricting clothing, belts, and jewelry should be removed before swelling begins. Clothing and jewelry retain heat and may cause the burns to progress into deeper tissues.

Maintain Adequate Ventilation. Signs and symptoms of upper and/or lower airway obstruction must be accurately assessed and closely monitored throughout the entire emergent period.

A decreased arterial oxygenation is often seen early following burn injury. Although the reason for this decrease is not known, the restoration of cardiac output improves oxygenation. It is important to note that this decreased oxygenation may be due to poor tissue perfusion and shock rather than to airway obstruction. Thus, a falling arterial PO_2 may indicate either an airway obstruction or a declining left heart output.

Often, the burn victim has been trapped in a burning building and has inhaled significant amounts of carbon monoxide. The patient may arrive at the hospital disoriented and possibly combative. The burned and unburned skin may or may not reveal a cherry red color. Significant carbon monoxide poisoning is indicated by elevated carboxyhemoglobin levels. Carbon monoxide poisoning should always be suspected in a patient who is restless, hypoxic, and confused, even though several hours may have elapsed since the incident. The treatment is administration of 100% oxygen.

Upper airway obstruction may occur with or without smoke inhalation. The immediate cause of respiratory distress is often laryngeal edema or spasm and the accumulation of mucus. Because actual signs of obstruc-

TABLE 37-2
NURSING MANAGEMENT OF THE BURN VICTIM: EMERGENCY DEPARTMENT

Nursing Diagnosis/ Clinical Problem	Patient Outcome	Goals of Nursing Intervention
Impairment of skin integrity due to burn injury (potential)	The patient will experience minimum tissue damage.	Minimize tissue damage: Stop the burning process.
Impaired gas exchange due to upper airway obstruction, lower airway obstruction, carbon monoxide poisoning, or inhalation injury	The patient will experience adequate ventilation and gas exchange.	Maintain adequate ventilation: Initiate CPR if indicated; maintain a patent airway; decrease edema; improve oxygenation.
Decreased cardiac output due to hypovolemic shock	The patient will experience hemodynamic stability.	Maintain hemodynamic stability with fluid resuscitation therapy.
Impairment of skin integrity due to burn injury (actual)	The patient will experience early and accurate assessment of burn and concomitant injuries.	Assess the burn injury. Assess for concomitant injury. Prevent hypothermia. Prevent infection by instituting infection control measures.
Pain due to burn injury	The patient will be as comfortable as possible.	Maintain comfort as possible.

TABLE 37-3
FINDINGS THAT SUGGEST POSTBURN INHALATION INJURY

Singed nasal hairs
Burns of the oral or pharyngeal mucous membranes
Burns in the perioral area or neck
Coughing up of soot or change in voice
History of being burned in a confined area

Note: Skin color changes, radiographic changes, and chest signs may be absent despite severe pulmonary damage.

tion may not become apparent for several hours, it is necessary to monitor the patient continuously for hoarseness, drooling, or inability to handle secretions. Hoarseness indicates a significant decrease in the diameter of the airway. The edema may continue to develop for 72 hours, and endotracheal intubation or tracheostomy may be indicated. Because airway obstruction due to laryngeal edema subsides within 3 to 5 days, endotracheal or nasotracheal intubation is preferable to a tracheostomy. Supportive measures during this time include frequent suctioning, indirect laryngoscopy to aid in mucus removal and to permit evaluation of the extent of involvement, analgesics to reduce pain and hyperventilation, and humidified oxygen to prevent mucosal dehydration and drying of secretions.

Circumferential full-thickness burns of the chest limit thoracic movement, and the patient may have increasing symptoms of respiratory distress. Because the tight eschar prevents adequate chest expansion, arterial oxygenation levels fall. An escharotomy allows the chest to expand and thereby alleviates respiratory distress.

Upper airway obstruction may proceed to total airway obstruction; thus, early recognition is extremely important.

If the mechanism of injury was a flame burn, smoke inhalation must be suspected. Table 37-3 represents findings that suggest inhalation injury.

Inhalation injury usually appears within the first 24 to 48 hours post burn and is secondary to the inhalation of combustible products; it is not the result of thermal injury because most heat is dissipated at the level of the distal trachea. Most commonly, especially in closed-space injuries, inhalation of the products of incomplete combustion results in a chemical pneumonitis. Inflammatory changes occur during the first 24 hours post burn: The pulmonary tree becomes irritated and edematous. However, changes may not become apparent until the second 24 hours. Pulmonary edema is a possibility anytime from the first few hours to 7 days following the injury. Symptomatology of inhalation injury may include rales, rhonchi, stridor, hacking cough, and labored or rapid breathing. The patient may be irrational or even unconscious, depending on the degree of hypoxia. Serial arterial blood gases will show a falling PO_2. Usually, the admission chest film will appear normal because changes are not reflected until 24 to 48 hours post burn. A sputum specimen should be obtained for culture and sensitivity studies. Laryngoscopy and bronchoscopy may be of value in determining the presence of extramucosal carbonaceous material (the most reliable sign of inhalation injury) and the state of the mucosa (blistering, edema, erythema), which may have an effect on bronchospasm, atelectasis, hypoxemia, and pulmonary edema.

The goals in treating inhalation injury are as follows:

• Improvement of oxygenation
• Decrease interstitial edema and airway occlusion

Humidified oxygen is administered to prevent drying and sloughing of the mucosa. Intubation and mechanical ventilation should be instituted if indicated. Bronchodilators and mucolytic agents may be used. Steroids are thought to aid in decreasing bronchospasm and the inflammatory edema of the small bronchi, in maintaining surfactant, and in preventing atelectasis. However, some researchers question the value of steroid therapy in these patients.

The patient should be placed in a high-Fowler position, encouraged to cough and deep breathe every hour, repositioned every 1 to 2 hours, given chest physiotherapy, and suctioned as needed. Respiratory parameters should be closely monitored, and extreme attention should be paid to the patient's breath sounds and vital signs so that fluid overload can be detected as early as possible (in the absence of a Swan-Ganz catheter). Serial ABGs and chest films allow one to evaluate the effectiveness of the interventions.

Bronchopneumonia may be superimposed on other respiratory problems at any time, and it may be hematogenous or airborne. Airborne bronchopneumonia is the most common type, with an onset occurring soon after the injury. It is often associated with a lower-airway injury or aspiration. Hematogenous, or miliary, pneumonia begins as a bacterial abcess secondary to another septic source, usually the burn wound. The time of the onset is usually 2 weeks after injury.

Maintain Hemodynamic Stability. The major burn victim presents in the emergency department in a state of hypovolemic shock. Burn shock results from the loss of fluids and electrolytes from all three body compartments: plasma from the vascular compartment, sodium from the vascular and interstitial compartments, and potassium from the intracellular compartment. However, burn shock is primarily caused by the rapid shift of plasma fluid from the vascular compartment, across the heat-damaged capillaries, into the interstitial areas (resulting in edema), and/or to the surface of the burned area. The burn shock is proportional to the extent and depth of injury. The loss is mainly plasma fluid rather than whole blood; however, in deep extensive burns, the red cell mass is usually lowered because of hemolysis due to heat from the burn, depression of red cell formation, edema of the wound, and altered iron and globin metabolism. Damaged red blood cells within the damaged capillaries may sludge, which could lead to thrombosis and significantly affect oxygen carrying capacity.

The loss of plasma fluid begins almost immediately following injury and reaches a peak within the first few hours. Burn shock, therefore, is mainly a problem of the first 24 to 36 hours after injury, and if correct treatment and nursing care are instituted promptly, it is rarely a problem after 48 hours.

Figure 37-2 summarizes the fluid shift that occurs in burn shock. It is important to note that the fluid largely remains in the body as interstitial edema.

The initial compensatory mechanism that occurs in relation to fluid loss is selective vasoconstriction. Simultaneously, the protein concentration in the blood vessels draws fluid from interstitial spaces in unburned areas of the body into the vascular system in an attempt to offset some of the lost volume. The blood pressure may appear normal at first, but if fluid replacement is inadequate and plasma protein loss ensues, hypovolemic shock soon occurs.

The loss of fluid from the intravascular space results in a thickened, sluggish flow of the remaining circulatory blood volume. The effects reach to all body systems. (Fig. 37-3).

This slowing of circulation allows bacteria and cellular material to settle to the lower portion of the blood vessels, especially in the capillaries, resulting in

FIGURE 37-2
Fluid shifts in burn shock. (Reprinted with permission of Macmillan Company from Patterns of Shock by Katherine J. Bordicks. Copyright © 1980 by Katherine J. Bordicks.)

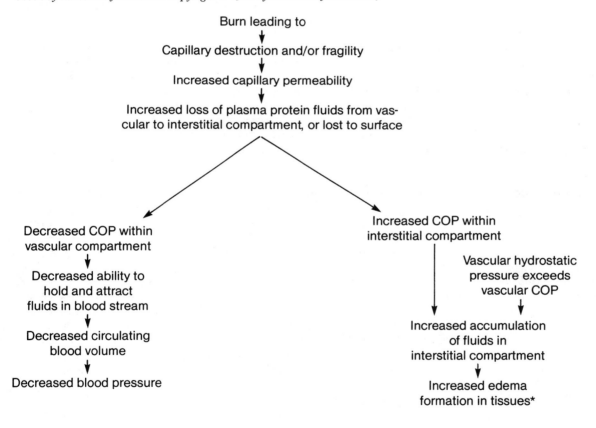

* Wound edema progresses during the acute phase. As much as 10 liters or more of plasmalike fluid may accumulate in the tissues and, therefore, be unavailable to the circulatory system.

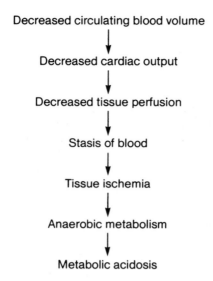

Decreased circulating blood volume

↓

Decreased cardiac output

↓

Decreased tissue perfusion

↓

Stasis of blood

↓

Tissue ischemia

↓

Anaerobic metabolism

↓

Metabolic acidosis

FIGURE 37-3
Effects of decreased blood volume.

sludging. The inactivity of a patient on bed rest further contributes to this state.

The antigen-antibody reaction to burned tissue adds to the circulatory congestion by the clumping or agglutination of cells. Coagulation problems occur as a result of the release of thromboplastin by the injury itself and the release of fibrinogen from injured platelets. If thrombi occur, they may cause ischemia of the affected part and lead to necrosis. Because this is a widespread occurrence, any organ in the body—heart, lung, liver, kidney, brain—may be involved, and organ failure can occur. The increased coagulation process may also develop into disseminated intravascular coagulation.

Blood Cell Count. In relation to blood cells (CBC), the leukocyte count is initially high because of the hemoconcentration. If leukocytosis persists after 1 week, it usually indicates infection by a gram-positive organism, often *Staphylococcus aureus.* The erythrocyte count in severe burns is decreased, and the patient is anemic. Some of the red cells are hemolyzed by the effects of the heat as they pass through the burned area at the time of the injury. Other red cells are simply trapped in engorged capillaries. Thus, they are unavailable to the general body. Anemia is also due to bleeding at the burn site that occurs initially when the wound is sustained and later as debridement is performed.

Electrolyte Alterations. Electrolyte concentrations are altered not only from the leaking process but also from direct injury to burned cells. Chemical changes are due to shifts in the composition of various fluids as they move from one body compartment to another.

Electrolyte studies at first show an increase in serum potassium because of intracellular potassium release due to cell injury. The intracellular potassium is replaced by sodium, and therefore normal cellular function is impaired. After approximately 48 hours, the capillary walls have healed sufficiently to stop the fluid shift from the vascular tree. Fluid is then drawn back into the blood vessels, edema subsides, the plasma volume expands, and diuresis begins. At this time, large amounts of potassium are lost, and replacement may be necessary. In severe burns, one must carefully monitor the alterations in potassium levels to avoid cardiac failure in the patient. The plasma level of both sodium and chloride is normal or slightly elevated at first but increases rapidly as excessive interstitial fluid is reabsorbed. The blood urea nitrogen (BUN) may be elevated if excessive protein catabolism occurred. Blood glucose levels may be temporarily increased as a result of the action of epinephrine, which is released in reaction to the stress of the burn injury. The epinephrine acts on amino acids to produce glucose (gluconeogenesis), which the patient requires to meet the body's demands during stress.

Cardiac Function. The sudden precipitous fall in cardiac output does not parallel the gradual reduction in blood volume. Research indicates the presence of a myocardial depressant factor in extensive burns. Poor perfusion of coronary arteries, hypothermia, and acidosis also contribute to the decreased cardiac output. With adequate fluid therapy, the cardiac output will return to normal within 24 to 36 hours.

Because of cardiovascular instability, the burn victim in the emergency room requires an intravenous line adequate to deliver fluids at a high flow rate, even if it necessitates placing a subclavian catheter through burned tissue. Ringer's lactate solution is most often recommended to start fluid resuscitation. A Foley catheter should be inserted and urine output monitored hourly. Urine specimens should be sent for urinalysis, culture, and sensitivity studies. Baseline bloodwork should include coagulation studies, CBC, SMA-12, and creatinine phosphokinase for an index of muscle damage (particularly important in electrical injuries). If possible, the patient should be weighed to get an accurate baseline weight. This will help one monitor fluid status, which is most important during the emergent period.

Assess the Burn Wound. The extent and depth of the burn as well as the time and circumstances surrounding the burn injury are vital data that must be communicated to the burn facility prior to the patient's transfer.

In order to assess the severity of the wound, one must consider several factors:

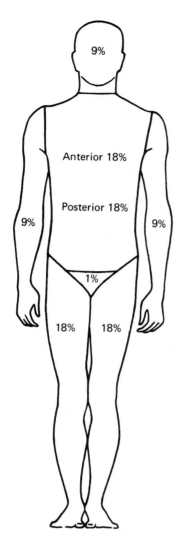

FIGURE 37-4
The "Rule of Nines" method for determining percentage of body area with burn injury.

- The percentage of body surface area (BSA) burned
- The depth of the burn
- The anatomic location of the burn
- The age of the person
- Past medical history
- Concomitant injury

Burn Area Size. Several possible rules are available for estimating the extent of a burn in percentages of the total body surface. The "rule of nines" divides the body parts into multiples of 9% (Fig. 37-4). The head is considered to account for 9% of total body area, each arm for 9%, each leg 18%, the anterior trunk for 18%, the posterior trunk for 18%, and the perineum for 1%, making a total of 100%. It is important to remember that burns may either be circumferential or involve only one surface of a body part: A circumferential burn of an arm is 9%, whereas if only the anterior surface were burned, the value would be 4.5%.

Although the rule of nines is the most commonly used method of estimating burn area size, Berkow's method is more accurate, particularly for infants and children, because it accounts for proportionate growth. The nurse can estimate the extent of small scattered burns by comparing the size of her hand to the victim's hand. Allowing for differences, she will find that the palmar surface of an adult's hand equals approximately 1% of an adult's total body surface. The chart from the National Burn Institute (Fig. 37-5) demonstrates how the nurse uses Berkow's method and assesses the color, characteristics, and pain sensations of the burn in order to assess whether it is first-, second-, or third-degree.

Burn Depth. Burn classifications are based on the tissues involved (as discussed previously) or classified as first-, second-, third-, and fourth-degree burns (see Table 37-1).

Anatomical Location. The location of the burn is important to healing and general rehabilitation. Burns of the face, head, neck, hands, feet, and genitalia create particular problems. Although they may be limited in surface area, these burns usually require hospitalization of the injured person and special care because they are important areas where rapid, unifected healing with minimal scarring is desired. Facial burns may involve edema and present problems with airway management. Burns of the head that involve the external ear and burns of the hands that involve the distal phalanges are particularly difficult to heal because these structures are primarily composed of cartilage, which lacks a good blood supply. Perineal burns are difficult, if not impossible, to keep from becoming infected. Edema also can be a problem, and the patients need to be catheterized as soon as possible.

If burns in any of these special areas do not heal well, serious psychosocial and economic problems related to appearance, self-concept, manual dexterity, and locomotion can occur.

Victim's Age. Although burns occur in all age groups, the incidence is higher at both ends of the age continuum. Persons under 2 years and over 60 years of age have a higher mortality than other age groups with burns of similar severity. A child under 2 years of age is more susceptible to infection because of his immature immune response. The older person may have degenerative processes that complicate his recovery and that may be aggravated by the stress of the burn. As a general rule, children with burns of 10% or more and all

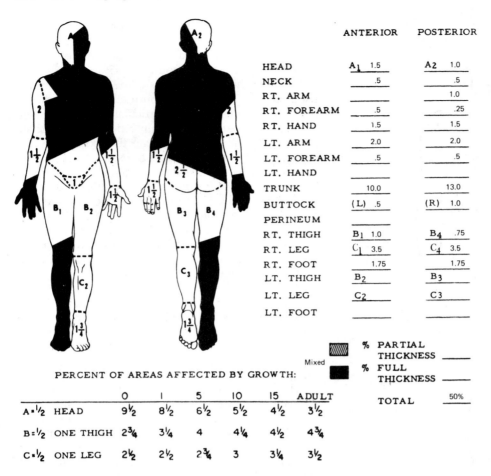

	ANTERIOR	POSTERIOR
HEAD	A_1 1.5	A_2 1.0
NECK	.5	.5
RT. ARM		1.0
RT. FOREARM	.5	.25
RT. HAND	1.5	1.5
LT. ARM	2.0	2.0
LT. FOREARM	.5	.5
LT. HAND		
TRUNK	10.0	13.0
BUTTOCK	(L) .5	(R) 1.0
PERINEUM		
RT. THIGH	B_1 1.0	B_4 .75
RT. LEG	C_1 3.5	C_4 3.5
RT. FOOT	1.75	1.75
LT. THIGH	B_2	B_3
LT. LEG	C_2	C_3
LT. FOOT		

% PARTIAL THICKNESS _____
% FULL THICKNESS _____
TOTAL 50%

PERCENT OF AREAS AFFECTED BY GROWTH:

Mixed

	0	1	5	10	15	ADULT
A = ½ HEAD	9½	8½	6½	5½	4½	3½
B = ½ ONE THIGH	2¾	3¼	4	4¼	4½	4¾
C = ½ ONE LEG	2½	2½	2¾	3	3¼	3½

FIGURE 37-5
Burn Evaluation Chart—estimation of percentage of body burns. (Crozer-Chester Medical Center)

adults whose injuries account for 12% to 15% or more of total body surface will require hospitalization.

Past Medical History. It is important to determine whether the victim has a disease that compromises his ability to manage fluid shifts and resist infection (*i.e.,* diabetes mellitus, congestive heart failure, cirrhosis) or if he has renal, respiratory, or gastrointestinal problems. Some problems, such as diabetes and renal failure, may become acute during the burn process. If inhalation injury has occurred in the presence of cardiopulmonary disease (*i.e.,* CHF, emphysema), the respiratory status is tremendously compromised.

Concomitant Injuries. It is important to obtain a brief history from the victim and check for concurrent injuries. Burn victims are usually awake and alert, so any changes in neurologic status usually indicates other injury, such as anoxia, head injury, drug use or intoxication, hypoglycemia, or myocardial infarction. Burn

wounds do not bleed; therefore, any external bleeding indicates lacerations of deeper structures. Extremities should be assessed for fractures.

Institute Infection Control to Prevent Further Contamination. The burn wound may be cleansed gently with saline, then covered with sterile sheets and then blankets to prevent hypothermia. If the patient is to be transferred to a burn facility, it is not necessary to begin topical antibacterial therapy and dressings in the emergency room.

Pain Control. The victim should be covered with a nonadherent, nonfuzzy cover. The nurse can add additional blankets as needed to provide warmth and to prevent hypothermia. Burn victims chill easily because they have lost their skin's protection against temperature changes. Covers also guard the wound against contamination and ease the pain caused by air currents. One may apply cool, sterile water or saline to the burn to ease the pain; however, it is important to guard against hypothermia and tissue damage. Ice or ice water should not be used because extreme cold can cause further tissue damage.

The Burn Unit

The major problems, stated as nursing diagnoses, and related goals for this phase of the emergent period are outlined in Table 37-4. During the emergent period, the primary goal of treatment is the establishment and maintenance of an adequate intravascular volume and tissue perfusion wihtout overloading.

Immediately, the patient requires rapid administration of large amounts of intravenous fluids for control of burn shock from fluid shift. Regardless of etiology, the shock syndrome remains the same. A marked reduction of blood flow through tissues results in cellular hypoxia, which leads to tissue death.

The hypotension, reduced blood flow, and hypoxia stimulate compensatory mechanisms in the body; for example, stimulation of the aortic and carotid pressor receptors increases pulse rate and selective vasoconstriction. These pressure receptors will maintain normal blood pressure until approximately 20% of the blood volume has been lost. The adrenal glands re-lease epinephrine, which augments the aforementioned responses, and the patient becomes restless and anxious. Respirations increase in rate and depth in order to promote venous return and cardiac filling. Changes in circulatory hydrostatic and osmotic pressures, due to decreased volume, pull fluids from the interstitial spaces into the blood vessels. It is easily seen why, in a severe burn, rapid fluid replacement is necessary to prevent the shock process from continuing. Fluid resuscitation is the primary intervention in the emergent phase, the goals of which are as follows:

- Correction of antecedent fluid, electrolyte, and protein deficits
- Replacement of continuing losses and maintenance of fluid balance
- Prevention of excessive edema formation

The basic fluid therapy is ordered by the physician, but the amount infused each hour is based on nursing judgement within established protocols. Most often, intravenous infusion is titrated to maintain a urine output of 30 to 50 ml/hour in an adult. Numerous formulas have been developed for fluid resuscitation, each with advantages and disadvantages. They differ primarily in terms of recommended volume adminis-

---

TABLE 37-4
NURSING MANAGEMENT OF THE BURN VICTIM: EMERGENT PERIOD

Nursing Diagnosis/ Clinical Problem	Patient Outcome	Goals of Nursing Intervention
Fluid volume deficit due to plasma loss, fluid shift, third spacing	The patient will experience fluid-electrolyte balance.	Establish and maintain adequate fluid-electrolyte balance through fluid resuscitation therapy.
Decreased tissue perfusion due to edema, thrombosis, and eschar formation	The patient will experience adequate tissue perfusion to all body parts.	Establish and maintain tissue perfusion through fluid resuscitation therapy.
Alteration in tissue perfusion due to edema, thrombosis, and eschar formation	The patient will experience adequate tissue perfusion in burned area.	Prevent edema and ischemia. Monitor tissue perfusion.
Alteration in gastrointestinal function due to injury, stress, and paralytic ileus (potential)	The patient will experience adequate function of the gastrointestinal tract.	Monitor for distention, bleeding, nausea, and vomiting, and bowel sounds.
Potential for infection due to burn injury, invasive procedures, immobility, stress	The patient will experience wound healing without infection.	Promote optimal wound healing and prevent infections by proper wound management. Monitor for pneumonia and sepsis. Administer prophylactic medications as indicated (*i.e.,* tetanus toxoid, penicillin).
Ineffective individual coping due to fear, pain, anxiety (potential)	The patient will be able to express anxiety, fears, and concerns; demonstrate effective coping behaviors; accept burn injury.	Provide emotional support, explanations, and reassurance; encourage verbalization of fears; help patient regain self-control.
Ineffective family coping due to fear, anxiety, lack of knowledge (potential)	The family will be able to express anxiety, fears, misconceptions; demonstrate effective coping behaviors; accept patient's burn injury.	Provide emotional support, guidance, and counseling.

TABLE 37-5
FORMULAS FOR FLUID REPLACEMENT/RESUSCITATION

	First 24 hours			Second 24 hours		
	Electrolyte	Colloid	Glucose in water	Electrolyte	Colloid	Glucose in water
Burn budget of F. D. Moore	1000–4000 ml lactated Ringer's and 1200 ml 0.5N saline	7.5% of body weight	1500–5000 ml	1000–4000 ml lactated Ringer's and 1200 ml 0.5N saline	2.5% of body weight	1500–5000 ml
Evans	Normal saline, 1 ml/kg/% burn	1.0 ml/kg/% burn	2000 ml	One half of first–24-hour requirement	One half of first-hour requirement	2000 ml
Brooke	Lactated Ringer's, 1.5 ml/kg/% burn	0.5 ml/kg/% burn	2000 ml	One half to three quarters of first–24-hour requirement	One half to three quarters of first–24-hour requirement	2000 ml
Parkland	Lactated Ringer's, 4 ml/kg/% burn				20%–60% of calculated plasma volume	
Hypertonic sodium solution	Volume to maintain urine output at 30 ml/hour (fluid contains 250 mEq Na/liter)			One third of salt solution orally, up to 3500 ml limit		
Modified Brooke	Lactated Ringer's, 2 ml/kg/% burn				0.3–0.5 ml/kg/% burn	Goal: Maintain adequate urinary output

(From Pruitt BA: Fluid and electrolyte replacement in the burned patient. Surg Clin North Am 58:1291, 1978)

TABLE 37-6
CLINICAL MANIFESTATIONS OF ADEQUATE FLUID REPLACEMENT

Blood pressure	Normal to high ranges
Pulse rate	<120
CVP	<12 cm H_2O
PCWP	<18 torr
Urinary output	30–70 ml/hour
Lungs	Clear
Sensorium	Clear
GI tract	Absence of nausea and paralytic ileus

tration and salt content. (Table 37-5). In general, rigorous replacement of lost crystalloid and colloid solutions must be made. Free water, given as 5% dextrose/water with or without added electrolytes, is regulated so that insensible fluid loss is covered. Ringer's lactate is used as the crystalloid solution because it is a balanced salt solution that closely approximates the composition of extracellular fluid. In addition, it has large molecules, which serve to expand the circulating plasma volume. It is important to remember that formulas are simply guides. The exact amount of fluid administered should be based on the clinical response of the patient.

The following example may help illustrate the very large amounts of fluid required. The Baxter, or Parkland, formula for a patient weighing 75 kg who received burns over 50% of his body would be stated as follows:

$$4 \text{ ml} \times 75 \text{ kg} \times 50\% = 15{,}000 \text{ ml}$$

Of this, 7500 ml is to be administered during the first 8-hour period, and 3750 ml is to be administered in the second and third 8-hour periods. Thus, avoidance of fluid overload and pulmonary edema is extremely difficult when it is necesary to infuse fluids so rapidly. Consequently, one may give digoxin to severely burned patients to create maximal function of the left ventricle and to minimize the chances of transient increases in left atrial pressure. Isoproterenol infusions may be used for symptoms of decreased cardiac output.

Adequacy of fluid replacement is judged clinically for adults by a urinary output of 30 to 70 ml/hour, pulse rate below 120, blood pressure in normal to high ranges, central venous pressure (CVP) readings less than 12 cm H_2O or a pulmonary capillary wedge pressure (PCWP) reading below 18 torr, clear sensorium and clear lung sounds, and the absence of intestinal symptoms such as nausea and paralytic ileus (Table 37-6). Patients are usually weighed daily: A gain of 15% of admission weight may be expected. Intake and output must be meticulously monitored.

Because early intravascular dehydration causes hemoconcentration and oliguria, a high myoglobin or hemoglobin load may be reflected by a dark "sludgy" urine. Mannitol, an osmotic diuretic, is the drug of choice in this situation. The urine output is maintained at a higher rate to "flush" the kidney tubules. All other diuretics should be avoided because they only deplete an already compromised intravascular volume, aggravating the shock state.

The onset of spontaneous diuresis is a hallmark indicating the end of the emergent period. Infusion rates can be decreased by 25% for 1 hour if the urine output is satisfactory and can be maintained for 2 hours, then the reduction can be repeated. It is essential that urinary outputs be maintained in normal limits (50 to 70 ml/hour). Early renal failure is the result of decreased cardiac output and decreased renal perfusion. Without adequate volume therapy, the urinary output is minimal. As volume is replaced, the renal blood flow improves and the urinary volume increases. Complications in renal function are usually the result of inadequate fluid and electrolyte replacement. Other causes include DIC, myocardial depression, delayed resuscitation, respiratory injury, and renal failure.

Tissue Perfusion. Once fluid therapy has been instituted, a second area of concern during the emergent period is tissue perfusion. With tissue injury, vessels are damaged and thrombosed. Adjacent intact vessels soon dilate, and platelets and leukocytes adhere to the vascular endothelium, resulting in eschar formation. The underlying tissues swell, but the area of a circumferential full-thickness burn is inelastic and remains contracted. The area acts like a tourniquet. An unyielding eschar contributes to a compromised vascular state with ischemic necrosis, which may eventually necessitate amputation. It is vital, therefore, that the nurse monitor tissue perfusion hourly by checking for capillary refill, neurologic changes, temperature and color of the skin, and the presence of peripheral pulses. An ultrasonic flowmeter is often useful in assessing for peripheral pulses. Extremities should be elevated and put through passive range of motion. Although elevation decreases the edema, *escharotomy* is often necessary. An escharotomy is an incision through the entire thickness of the eschar that allows underlying viable edematous tissues to expand, thereby restoring adequate tissue perfusion. In the case of a deeper wound, the fascia is incised during a procedure called a *fasciotomy*.

These procedures involve minimal blood loss and may be performed at the bedside with a scalpel or with electrocautery. The escharotomy site is covered with a topical agent because viable tissue is exposed, and a light dressing may be applied.

Pain Control. Assessment of pain in the burn patient requires careful thought. Thermally injured victims with partial-thickness injury suffer a great deal of pain because the nerve endings are exposed. Even the slightest air current across sensitive tissues will cause extreme discomfort. Patients with massive injury, however, may have little pain because the nerve endings are destroyed in full-thickness injury (see Table 37-1). Coverage of the wound with a sterile sheet or a topical antimicrobial agent will decrease the air currents and significantly decrease pain. Calm, knowledgeable administration of care with explanations when appropriate will reduce anxiety. The importance of astute observation and intelligent interpretation of signs and symptoms cannot be overemphasized because the restlessness of a burn patient may be due to pain or hypoxia. Small, frequent intravenous doses of narcotics are usually effective in controlling pain. Intramuscular injections should be avoided. These medications will be sequestered in the muscle with virtually no therapeutic effect until the patient becomes hemodynamically stable and adequate tissue perfusion is achieved. At this time, the intramuscular medications would flood the vascular system, with the total circulating dose unknown.

Gastrointestinal Tract Management. Soon after injury, blood flow to the gastrointestinal tract diminishes because of selective vasoconstriction. Compounded with loss of potassium from cell injury, paralytic ileus and gastric dilitation may occur. The patient should remain NPO (*i.e.,* receiving nothing by mouth) and a nasogastric tube should by inserted if distention or nausea occurs. Initial drainage may contain some blood; close observation is indicated to ensure that the quantity of blood subsides. The most common life-threatening gastrointestinal complication for the burn victim is Curling's ulcer. Prophylactic antacid therapy has significantly reduced the incidence of bleeding.

Infection Prophylaxis. Tetanus toxoid should be administered intramuscularly to combat possible anaerobic infection. In many institutions, tetanus hyperimmune globin also is administered. Penicillin prophylaxis is often adminstered for the first 5 days for protection against overwhelming streptococcal infection, to which innumerable burn victims have succumbed in the past.

Psychological Support. Providing psychological support for the newly admitted burn patient and his family is not the least of the many tasks facing the critical care nurse. The patient is most often awake and alert although anxious and overwhelmed by the suddenness and magnitude of his injuries. The overriding concern of the patient and his family at this time is whether he will live or die. This should be handled as gently, tactfully, and honestly as possible. This may be the all-important basis for establishing a trusting relationship for the long months of rehabilitation ahead.

Burn patients are under severe, long-term stress, and they nearly always develop personality variants. Four of the most common are

• Depression
• Regression
• Paranoia
• Schizophrenia

Often, burn patients become depressed and withdrawn, asking to be left alone and to not be made uncomfortable. The nurse should respond by making certain *expectations* clear. For example, she may expect the patient to feed himself, go to the bathroom, or do as much for himself as his physical condition permits. This communicates to the patient that his condition is not hopeless; he is expected to recover.

The best way to handle regression in a burn patient is to acknowledge it. First, the nurse must accept the fact that the patient is unable to cope on an adult level, that he is unstable emotionally as well as physically. Second, the nurse must devise ways to help the patient cope on an appropriate level. She can accomplish this by following a regular schedule so that the patient knows what is expected of him, by rewarding him for adult behavior, and by returning control to the patient by permitting him as much choice as possible in his care.

It is not uncommon for severely burned patients to transfer their fears to a specific caregiver (physician, nurse, therapist) and to complain that they are being treated unjustly or unkindly. If the situation becomes severe, the staff member may need to be reassigned to another patient.

Hallucinations, confusion, and combativeness are common in severely burned patients for physical as well as mental reasons. Exhaustion, pain, and medications may distort reality and produce schizophrenic behavior.

All four of the listed personality variants are temporary. The schizophrenia and paranoia almost always disappear by the time the patient is discharged from the hospital. The regression and depression may continue into the rehabilitation period.

The emergent period is a traumatic time for the family as well. With high anxiety levels and lack of knowledge of burn care, the family approaches the burn unit with fear, hesitancy, and sometimes hysteria. The physical appearance of the patient and the high-technology atmosphere of the burn unit are indeed frightening. Preparing the family for the initial visit by explaining what to expect and escorting them to the bedside is extremely important. Visitors are often overwhelmed on the first visit and often stand silently with feelings of anxiety and helplessness growing. It may be helpful for the nurse to suggest that the family members leave and return when they feel stronger.

Although the patient tends to concentrate on the present, the family members look to the future and want to know what to expect. Information about the patient's condition and treatments should be shared with them. The trusting relationship that was initially established provides a strong base for patient and family teaching and rehabilitation in the months to follow.

The Acute Phase

Once the patient's general condition has stabilized, attention can be directed toward the burn itself. The purposes of topical burn care are to promote healing, to control infection, and to help alleviate pain. (Table 37-7).

The most significant complication in the acute phase of injury is sepsis, which may arise from burn wound sepsis, pneumonia, suppurative thrombophlebitis, urinary tract infection, infection elsewhere in the body, invasive procedures, and invasive monitoring devices. The burn wound is the most frequent source of infection and may be caused by a variety of organisms. Early after the injury, the organisms tend to be gram-positive; after the first week, the organisms tend to be gram-negative.

Septic shock, seen mostly in patients with extensive full-thickness burns, is caused by invading bacteria from the wound entering the bloodstream. Clinically, the patient should show a fever, but the range of temperature elevation is extremely variable. The usual febrile reaction is altered when great heat losses from fluid loss are occurring. Other symptoms are a rapid yet regular pulse (140 to 170: sinus tachycardia), decreased blood pressure, oliguria, paralytic ileus, petechiae, frank bleeding from wounds, and disorientation (Table 37-8).

TABLE 37-7
NURSING MANAGEMENT OF THE BURN VICTIM: ACUTE PHASE

Nursing Diagnosis/ Clinical Problem	Patient Outcomes	Goals of Nursing Intervention
Impairment of skin integrity due to burn injury	The patient will experience wound healing without infection.	Promote healing and prevent infection by effective burn wound management. Prevent sepsis. Monitor for early signs of septic shock.
Alteration in gas exchange due to pneumonia (potential)	The patient will experience adequate ventilation and gas exchange.	Maintain respiratory function and maintain arterial oxygenation.

TABLE 37-8
SYMPTOMS OF SEPTIC SHOCK

Temperature (varies)
Pulse (140 to 170 – sinus tachycardia)
Decreased blood pressure
Paralytic ileus
Petechiae
Frank bleeding from wounds
Disorientation

Topical Burn Care

Debridement, grafting, and various topical agents are used to promote healing, prevent infection, and alleviate pain. *Hydrotherapy and mechanical debridement* are important procedures in preparing the wound for surgical debridement and skin grafting. At least daily, the nurse places the patient in a tub for the purpose of loosening exudates, cleansing and assessing the wound, and providing range of motion exercises. Bath solutions vary and may contain salt, water, betadine solutions, and bleach. The wounds are gently washed, and loose eschar is debrided. Because the baths are usually quite painful, patients may receive an analgesic 20 to 30 minutes before tubbing.

Surgical Debridement and Skin Grafting. Surgical debridement is the actual excision of the eschar under anesthesia. The wound is excised down to viable, bleeding tissue.

Skin grafting is the permanent closure of the wound with the patient's own skin (split thickness). Donor skin is harvested from an unburned area, and the resulting wound is similar to a partial-thickness burn. Bleeding is controlled, and the site is covered with an agent such as pigskin or scarlet red. Donor sites should be inspected frequently for signs of infection and should heal completely in 7 to 10 days.

The split-thickness graft can be applied in several ways:

- *Sheet grafts,* in which the harvested skin is placed on the recipient site in sheets. The graft must be inspected frequently for collections of fluid under the graft, which must be rolled or aspirated.
- *Mesh grafts,* in which the harvested skin is slit to allow it to expand, and then placed on the burn site. This allows for greater coverage and drainage.
- *Postage stamp grafts,* in which the harvested skin is cut into small pieces and placed on the wound to allow for drainage between grafts. This is used on a poorly granulated bed or on an irregularly shaped area.

Nursing management of the grafted area includes immobilization for the first 3 to 4 days in order to permit formation of new blood vessels that anastomose to the graft. The nurse should carefully roll the grafted site with a cotton-tipped applicator to remove fluid and to allow the graft to adhere and survive. The graft may be covered with a xeroform dressing or left open to air.

Epithelialization should occur by the fourth day. On the fourth or fifth day post grafting, the patient is taken to hydrotherapy for gentle cleansing. Topical agents can then be applied.

Topical Agents

The ideal topical agent for burn care would promote epithelialization, completely sterilize the wound,

CHOICES IN TOPICAL TREATMENT

1st Degree {
- No dressing
- Dry dressing (to protect from injury and infection)
- Xeroform (to remove outer dead layer of skin — débridement)
- Mercurochrome (has drying effect and stimulates epithelialization)
- Polymyxin B with Bacitracin (used mainly on the face and ears)

2nd Degree {
- Scarlet Red (used on donor sites)
- Silvadene (most popular topical)
- Betadine (used if wound is too soupy from bacterial growth with use of Silvadene)
- Pig skin and amniotic membrane (promote epithelialization, substitute covering for clean granulation tissue, reduce size of open wound to decrease the % of burn, used over new grafts and donor sites)
- Neomycin (used to prepare granulation bed for grafting)
- Synthetic membranes (Opsite, Biobrane, and Hydron — used for the same purposes as pig skin)

3rd Degree {
- Dakin's solution and Third's solution (used to clean up a dirty wound)
- Furacin (wide-spectrum antibacterial)
- Silver Nitrate
- Gentamicin (active against *Pseudomonas*)
- Travase and Elase (enzymatic débridement)
- Sulfamylon (used primarily on electrial burns — deep penetration into eschar)
- Autograft (best covering 0.008 – 0.02 of an inch)
- Cadaver

FIGURE 37-6
Topical treatment of burns. (Gaston S, Schumann L: Burn wound management. Critical Care Update. October, 1980)

have no side effects, and serve as a second skin. Unfortunately, it has not yet been developed. The best agent for each burn depends on the type of burn, the area of the body, the bacterial count, the stage of the burn, and its effectiveness on this specific wound. Figure 37-6 depicts practical choices in topical treatment.

Ointments and Creams. These substances generally penetrate the burn wound well, require less occlusive dressing, and often can be left open to air. The best agents are water-soluble because they will not hold in heat and macerate the wound. The nurse may apply the agent directly to the eschar using a sterile glove and then leave the wound open to air or apply the agent to gauze that is then placed on the burn surface. Silver sulfadiazine (Silvadene) is the most commonly used topical agent.

Soaks. These can be used at various stages of wound care. They are useful for debriding a dirty wound and preparing a granulation bed. They also may be used to keep freshly grafted areas moist and to decrease bacterial growth. Solutions used vary, including Dakin's solution, Betadine, Furacin, silver nitrate, gentamycin, Third's solution, and neomycin. Soaks may be applied in two different ways:

- Wet to dry: Gauze soaks are applied directly to the wound and allowed to dry. When the dressing is changed, debris will be removed. These are changed two to six times daily.
- Soaks: Gauze soaks are applied to the wound in several layers. The dressing is kept wet by irrigation or frequent changing. The patient must be monitored for hypothermia.

Biological Dressings. These dressings serve as temporary skins. They are used on clean partial thickness wounds, on donor sites, and on granulating wounds in preparation for grafting. Because these dressings act as the patient's own skin, they reduce pain, heat and water loss from the wound, and bacterial contamination and stimulate epithelialization. These dressings are applied directly to the wound and may be left open to air or covered with a sterile dressing or a topical ointment. They may be changed daily or left in place for up to 1 week. Biological dressings include amniotic membranes, cadaver skin, and pigskin.

Enzymatic Debridement. Enzymatic debridement is one method used to remove eschar without damaging viable tissue. Prior to application of the agent, the wound must be cleansed and debrided of any loose necrotic tissue. Travase and elase are the most commonly used enzymatic debriding agents.

REHABILITATION

Patients who have sustained extensive burns will obviously require many months for recovery and rehabilitation. Physical and psychological rehabilitation measures are begun in the critical care unit and continued through the entire recovery period.

Physical Rehabilitation

Two very important physical measures are nutrition and prevention of scarring and contractures (Table 37-9).

Nutrition

The severely burned patient may need as much as 50 to 80 calories/kg of body weight to meet his metabolic requirements. This includes 2 to 3 g of protein/kg and supplementary vitamins. If anemia is present, vitamins B and C and iron are especially important. As an example of the huge caloric intake needed, a patient weighing 75 kg would require 3750 to 6000 calories/day. Even though the patient is usually started cautiously, a difficult cycle may be created as intake increases. Although he needs a large intake, he is not hungry, feels full, and may have diarrhea. Prevention of excessive weight loss in adults and allowances for growth in children also must be considered, and nutritional formulas may be added to their diets.

Augmentation of the caloric value of oral intake may be accomplished with intralipid therapy. There is some controversy over *hyperalimentation* in burn care. The tendency is to reserve it for patients who have extensive injuries and who cannot tolerate other means of feeding. Major arguments against it are the possibility of infection and the number of other procedures it necessitates.

Avoidance of Scarring and Contractures

Once regarded as inevitable, hypertrophic scarring and joint contractures are now largely preventable. Preventive measures start when the person is admitted to the hospital and continue for at least 12 months or until the scar is fully mature.

These preventive measures, positioning the body and helping the patient perform range of motion exercises, are not new to the nurse. Positioning the body with extremities extended is extremely important. Although tightly flexed positions are preferred by patients for comfort, they will result in severe contractures. Range of motion exercises should be carried out with each dressing change or more often if indicated. Special splints are used to maintain arms, legs, and hands in extended yet functional positions. Later, when the wounds have healed sufficiently, the person is custom-fitted for special pressure garments. The garment, by continuous uniform pressure over the entire area of the burn, prevents hypertrophic scarring and must be worn 24 hours a day for approximately 1 year. The smooth elastic garment forms a shield that permits the person to wear normal clothing and resume ordinary activities much sooner.

Psychological Rehabilitation

Psychological care of the burned patient is extremely difficult; he may, in the course of his therapy, run the full gamut of behavioral responses. Early in the care, a combination of physical pain and emotional disturbances may lead to abnormal behavior, as previously discussed. Guilt may be particularly severe if the patient feels that his carelessness was the cause of injuries to himself or others, especially if others died as a result of the accident.

TABLE 37-9
NURSING MANAGEMENT OF THE BURN VICTIM: REHABILITATION

Nursing Diagnosis/ Clinical Problem	*Patient Outcome*	*Goals of Nursing Intervention*
Alteration in nutrition (less than body requirements) due to burn injury	The patient will demonstrate an understanding of nutritional requirements; demonstrate adequate nutritional intake to meet increased caloric needs.	Provide nutrition adequate for wound healing and maintain nitrogen balance.
Disturbance in self-concept due to sequelae of burn injury	The patient will experience as little scarring and contractures as possible; demonstrate acceptance of burn injury; demonstrate positive coping behaviors.	Prevent or minimize scarring and contractures. Provide supportive measures that allow the patient time to assimilate burn injury. Assist the patient in developing effective coping behaviors.

If burns involve the face, eyes, or hands, additional emotional support will be needed because damage to these structures will have a long-term effect on the patient's life and livelihood.

A consistent, truthful team approach that includes the patient and his family is necessary. Supportive measures that will allow the patient time to assimilate what has happened to him and to grow in his ability to cope are as follows:

- Staff should be stabilized as much as possible so that caregivers can maximize their familiarity with the patient's needs and so that a sense of identification between patient and nurse is established.
- Family members can be very helpful if incorporated into the overall plan of care and instructed in selected procedures.
- Diversional therapy (*i.e.,* reading, watching television, listening to music) should be encouraged as soon as possible.
- Occupational therapy should be started as soon as the patient is able to participate.

In addition to the emotional support of the patient, support for the nursing staff is advisable. Faced with long and arduous care of these patients, where progress is slow and setbacks are common, staff quickly develop ''burnout'' unless some of their emotional reactions and problems can be aired and solved (see Chap. 38).

SUMMARY

The skin serves multiple physiological functions that render it indispensible to life. When a large area of skin surface is destroyed, severe systemic reactions occur.

The burn victim goes through phases of recovery, each with its own special problems. The emergent phase begins with the burn injury and lasts until diuresis occurs (1 to 5 days). The major problems for the patient at this time are maintenance of an airway and adequate tissue perfusion. After diuresis, the victim enters the acute phase, during which his major problem is sepsis. Burn wound management is essential during this phase. Rehabilitation focuses on adequate nutrition and prevention of scarring and contractures. Psychological support is essential throughout the entire experience. A firm, compassionate team approach is essential throughout recovery.

BIBLIOGRAPHY

Bordicks K: Patterns of Schock. New York, Macmillan, 1980

Diehl P: Burns, In Hudak C, Gallo B, Lohr T (eds): Critical Care Nursing, 3rd ed. Philadelphia, JB Lippincott, 1982

Finlayson L: Emergent care of the burn patient. Critical Care Update, October, 1980, pp 18–22

Fire in the United States. United States Department of Commerce, United States Fire Administration, National Fire Data Center, 1978

Fitzgerald RF: Pre-hospital care of burned patients. Crit Care 1:13, 1981

Fonger L: Emergency: First aid for burns. Nursing 12:71–73, 1982

Gaston S, Schumann L: Burn wound management. Critical Care Update October, 1980, pp 5–17

Jones CA, Feller I: Burns: What to do during the first crucial hours. Nursing 7:22, 1977

Kenner CV: Burn injury. Critical Care Nursing: Body-Mind-Spirit. Boston, Little, Brown, 1981

Kenner C, Manning S: Emergency care of the burn patient. Critical Care Update October, 1980, pp 24–33

Moylan JA, Chun CK: Inhalation injury—an increasing problem. Ann Surg 188:34, 1978

Pruitt BA: Progressive pulmonary insufficiency and other complications of thermal injury. Trauma 15:369, 1975

Richards KE: Emotional consequences of severe burns. Nursing September, 10:49, 1980

Stein JM, Stein ED: Safe transfer of civilian burn causualties. JAMA 238:489, 1977

Wooldridge-King M: Nursing considerations of the burned patient during the emergent period. Heart Lung 11, No. 4:353–361, 1982

Section III

Professional Practice Issues in the Critical Care Unit

38
Effects of the Critical Care Unit on the Nurse

Patricia D. Barry

Critical care unit (CCU) nurses have been the subject of numerous articles dealing with the stress of working with critically ill patients. They probably have been the focus of more articles than any other nurse subpopulation. There are many reasons why this is so. One of the main ones is that critical care units are places in which the forces of life and death are in constant battle. Nurses and physicians are the main defenders of the patient—but it is the nurses who are in constant attendance. Accordingly, they are continually charged with the responsibility of maintaining the patient's homeostasis.

CCU NURSE STRESS: REVIEW OF THE LITERATURE

Many of the early articles about CCU nursing stress were authored by psychiatrists and psychologists.[1-6] These articles were based on informal contacts and on individual and group discussions with the nurses by the authors who were usually psychiatrist leaders of the nurse support groups. Authors of these reports discussed the stress of working in CCUs from a psychological perspective and recommended that psychiatric liaison nurse support groups could relieve some of the stress that was generated by working in such units. The most commonly identified stressors were the losses nurses experience in working with critically ill patients; the workload, which is heavy, unpredictable, and tedious at different times; communication conflicts; and the environmental stimuli within the unit.

Formal research on the specific factors that CCU nurses found most stressful did not begin until the mid 1970s.[7-11] These studies were authored by a variety of mental health clinicians, including psychiatrists, psychologists, social workers, and nurses. The development of nursing research on CCU stressors was concomitant with the acquisition of research skills by increasing numbers of nurses with advanced degrees.

The study of nursing stress by nurses is a positive trend in understanding the adverse effects of the CCU on nurses. It seems safe to say that a profession is more than the scientific body of knowledge that it utilizes: It also socializes its members so that they acquire qualities and dynamics that may be unique to that profession. These factors can contribute to nurses' stress response and may be best articulated by other nurses who understand their importance and effects. This chapter will examine the different types of stressors experienced by CCU nurses. It will also review the most recent trend in CCU nursing stress research—identifying the personality factors that may be helpful in coping with the CCU—as a way of better understanding the potentially adverse effects on the nurse and what can be done about them.

THE SOCIALIZATION OF CCU NURSES

Nurses in CCUs often feel a special sense of pride in themselves. The level of work that they perform and the knowledge that they require to do their jobs well are known to be the most complex of any staff nursing positions in the hospital. Accompanying this justified self-pride and positive professional self-image is another self-expectation that many critical care nurses experience: to be calm and cool under pressure. This calmness has been commented on by several authors.[12-16]

It is interesting that it is frequently the nurses themselves who impose this expectation on themselves. Physicians (whom, it should be noted, have the opportunity to go into and out of the CCU, rather than remaining for assigned tours of duty) frequently remark on the nurses' apparent ability to tolerate the very high level of stress that exists there. Many doctors believe that the environment is difficult to tolerate for any period of time.[17] This implies that physicians would find it difficult to remain for several-hour periods and still maintain an outward calm. Patients and families react well and are calmed themselves by a cool, professional nurse demeanor. Importantly, they are also comforted by nurses who are able to become emotionally involved with them and occasionally "let go" of the professional demeanor and demonstrate their caring.

If physicians, patients, and families all are willing to accept the need for the nurse to be human and occasionally slip out of the cool, professional role, why, then, do so many CCU nurses impose this rigid expectation on themselves?

STRESSORS IN THE CCU

Unquestionably, the most important reasons that CCU nurses set such high expectations for themselves is that they view this as a way of maintaining emotional equilibrium. This is the greatest coping defense that most nurses use in dealing with the constant pressures of the CCU. Before explaining and discussing the need for coping abilities in nurses, it is important to accurately present the variety of stresses on the intensive care nurse.

Most nurses would immediately identify the unpredictability of the CCU environment as a leading stressor. Other stressors are the "incessant repetitive routine . . . ; every step must be charted . . . ; floating in nurses from elsewhere . . . ; frequent situations of acute crisis . . . ; physical dangers (inadequate protection from x-rays, needles, isolation patients, and those who are delirious; lifting heavy, unresponsive patients) . . . ; distraught relatives . . . ; (constant sounds of) moaning, crying, screaming, buzzing and beeping monitors, gurgling suction pumps, and whooshing respirators . . ."[18] Another very important stress on the nurse, and one that should not be underestimated, is also described by Hay and Oken: Everywhere there are human bodies, many of them wasted, mutilated, or discolored. There are exposed genitalia and excretions of feces, blood, chest mucus, vomitus, and urine. Some patients' dressings are soaked with purulent discharge or serous or bloody drainage.

STOP READING

Think back to your *honest* reaction as you read each of the stressors in the preceding section. Be honest with yourself.

TAKE A BIG BREATH AND LET IT OUT SLOWLY

Now, pretend that you are on a beautiful, green hillside that slopes gently downward to a sandy beach. There are large, crashing waves that you can see and hear. The sun is shining. You are lying under a graceful old maple tree that protects you from the sun. A breeze is gently blowing your hair. Beautiful! Right? Now, slowly reread the list of stressors and let yourself *feel* a response. You may feel nothing as you read some of them. For others you may feel disgust, anxiety, or boredom. Are you able to detect a difference between your first set of responses and your second set? If not, it is possible that the coping strategies that you have unconsciously developed have resulted in an emotional detachment that is causing you to miss many of the good and positive aspects of life in and *out* of the CCU. It is very difficult to deaden one's response to negative emotional experiences without concurrently deadening it to pleasure and joy. What a high cost! What causes it to happen?

A common personality trait in many nurses is selflessness. This trait is nurtured and praised by nursing educators and administrators. When people are selfless they deny their own physical or emotional needs in the service of others. A nurse who legitimately refuses to work a double shift, float to another unit, or take on extra assignments because of chronic understaffing is usually not as popular with supervisors as one who denies her own needs and acquiesces immediately.

Because in the past selflessness has been a desired trait in nurses and because the selfless nurse has received far more approval from peers and supervisors than the outspoken nurse who tries to assert her rights, many nurses have been socialized into denying their own needs, their own feelings—their own humanness!

Remember that nowhere on earth are people born knowing how to deny their own needs and feelings. Instead they have *learned* to deny them. The most important motivation in this process is the need for approval.

Think for a moment: If it is true that physicians, patients, and families are all able to recognize the nurse's humanness and accept that, on occasion, the professional, calm, cool exterior shell can safely slide away, revealing the real person who is underneath, why then do we hold on so tightly to the cover and try to stifle our own humanness?

If we are looking for approval, to whom are we looking? Nursing peers and supervisors are the obvious answer—the easy answer! The tough answer is to admit that we do it to ourselves. Sometimes nurses are their own severest critics. If they fail in their own, sometimes impossible self-expectations, the result is guilt.

Many nurses were taught that it is not good to feel grief, fear, disgust, or love when working intimately with other human beings. Despite their own humanness they were taught that it was not "professional" to feel such emotions about patients. When a person feels something he was taught not to feel, the result is guilt. Because guilt is an unpleasant feeling, the mind (the ego, specifically) helps defend the person so that the guilt will not occur. Repression is a defense or coping mechanism that buries the original feelings of grief, fear, and so forth so that they are no longer felt. It is important to know, however, that the memories of the experiences that *normally* cause such feelings remain stored in our unconscious memories. The repression does not get rid of those memories.

The *constant* burying of these feelings is *not* normal. Remember that the nursing educators and supervisors who have taught that it is "professional" to bury them have been socialized by other nurses. Theirs is a harmful approach. It will not change until they themselves are socialized into a more humane approach and become kinder to themselves as well as to other nurses.

BURNOUT

The result of constant denial of self is probably one of the most important, yet underrecognized, dynamics of burnout. Critical care nurses, because of the highly stressful nature of their work, are "at risk" for burnout. Burnout is the result of working in a stressful environment. The worker eventually feels resigned, ineffective, and hopeless about working in such an environment. The result of burnout is that the employee either leaves the job or remains in the position functioning ineffectively. Burnout is an energyless state.

There are other important causes of burnout. Alvin Toffler, in *Future Shock,* suggests that we live in a highly technologic environment in which there is rapid change occurring at a faster and faster rate.[19] The result is that the knowledge needed by critical care nurses and the complexity of patients they care for are constantly increasing, imposing even greater stress in an already stressful milieu.

If nurse : patient ratios were improved to be proportionate to the increasing complexity of care, nurses would be able to adapt to the stress of the CCU more readily. If this does not happen, chronic understaffing will result. The effects of chronic understaffing are many. Frustration occurs when nurses are consistently under pressure and repeatedly feel that they are not giving the full kind of care that their patients need. This type of frustration ultimately leads to burnout.

Burnout is causing ever-increasing numbers of nurses to leave nursing. As a result, the problem of burnout is receiving more attention in both the professional and lay sectors. As nurses, it is important for us to understand the causes of burnout. Certainly the aforementioned root problems have always been there. Until the 1970s, if nurses were victims of burnout because of overwork or because of repression of self, they frequently remained in their positions, but in a diminished state. Today, however, nurses are responding to a different current in society.

The feminist movement, with its strong emphasis on selfhood, has made women increasingly aware of their right to experience their lives fully. The essential goal of this movement is improvement in the quality of life for all women. It attempts to make them aware of the traditional role that they have filled in society and to present alternatives that they may then choose or reject. Nursing is a predominately female profession. Its members, whether men or women, strongly represent the most traditional female qualities of caring, nurturing, and selflessness.

The women's movement has created more of an awareness in women that they are "givers." In her book, Jean Baker Miller quoted a woman who said, "I can't give anymore, but I don't feel allowed to stop."[20] Insightful women have begun to realize that the permission to stop has to come *first* from the giver — not from the takers. After all, why would anyone who is receiving good things tell the giver to stop?

This giving-taking relationship has been the traditional relationship between nurse and hospital. Intelligent nurses who value themselves as people are beginning to call a halt to this "hospital-takes-all" approach. A new dynamic is being observed in nurses that is probably directly related to their raised consciousness as women. In the past they became burned-out, resigned, and ineffective caregivers as a result of difficult working conditions. Today, it is far more common for nurses to feel angry and frustrated by these conditions. They leave their positions rather than allowing their selfhood and their own needs to diminish.

In most cases, their anger and frustration are justifiable, and they have few options other than leaving. Frequently, however, when they move to other positions, the cycle repeats itself. It is possible that after several of these moves the nurse may still become burned-out. After all, the resiliency of any human being eventually has a breaking point.

Hopeless? No! There are many alternatives. The important point is that the alternatives must be considered before the breaking point is in view. Baker says, "Clearly, women need to allow themselves to take, openly, as well as give."[21] The amount of energy necessary to create this change of thinking in nurses can be likened to pulling teeth—from a whale! Or stopping a 50-ton locomotive as it is hurtling down a hill! Nurses have always been givers. It is why they entered nursing. It is okay to give. It is beautiful to give. But it is also okay and beautiful to be a full human being and to value one's own worth. Judeo-Christian teaching has frequently been the basis of giving to others. It is important to note, however, that the most basic rule is "love thy neighbor as thyself." This rule assumes that we first love ourselves, and that we should love others as much as—not more than—we love ourselves! This may come as a surprise to many nurses who have traditionally valued the needs of others much more than their own.

ASSERTIVENESS: A HELP OR A HINDRANCE?

One of the catchwords of the feminist movement is "assertiveness." This movement has encouraged women to become more assertive. For many women who favor the traditional feminine characteristics, the word *assertiveness* has some negative implications. It is possible that this is due to a lack of distinction between the behavioral characteristics of assertiveness and those of aggressiveness. The differences between being aggressive, being assertive, and being passive, or nonassertive, are presented in Table 38-1.

The difference between the passive person and the assertive person is that the passive person is "done unto" by another who has no awareness of the passive person's needs or desires. Passive people seem more like nonpersons. Actually, they usually put their faith in others to know what they need, usually with unexpressed expectations (also called a *hidden agenda*). When the others fail them in any way there are usually two outcomes:

1. They further submerge their "selves" and needs. The implied meaning is "I have no worth."
2. They feel resentment. "Why did they do this to me?" Actually, the agency or other person had no idea of the unexpressed needs.

Assertive persons, however, are always aware of their own needs and the treatment that they are entitled to as human beings. They express these needs when appropriate. When their rights are openly violated, they speak up and express their feelings. Assertive persons are not offensive and do not infringe on the rights of other people or institutions. They place value on their own thoughts and beliefs. They place value on themselves.

Aggressive persons are offensive people. They impose their beliefs on others, expecting them to agree, and become angry when the others do not acquiesce. They actually deny others the right to their own thoughts or opinions.

THINKING VS. FEELING: WHICH IS IN CONTROL?

Learning to distinguish our thoughts from our feelings will help us change from passive to assertive. For example, if a person feels guilty, he has a gut reaction inside. Guilt is a *feeling*. A person can't think guilt; he feels it. Accordingly, if he thinks that Gerald Ford was a good president, he cannot *feel* that Ford was a good

TABLE 38-1
ASSERTIVENESS VS. PASSIVITY AND AGGRESSIVENESS

	Characteristics	*Feelings in Self*	*Reactions of Others*
Assertive	Open Honest Does not impinge on others' beliefs	At peace inside Good self-esteem Respects others' rights	Respect
Passive	Weak Yielding Self-denying Hidden bargaining Deceptive about real feelings	Uncertain Tries to please others Resentful	Pity Uncertainty Unconcern Annoyance
Aggressive	Quarrelsome Bold Degrades others Bulldozes over others' opinions, beliefs, and feelings	Anger Contempt for others Extreme self-pride Anxious when aggressiveness is out of control	Indignance Displeasure Hurt Disgust

president. He may think that it is time to paint his house; he cannot *feel* that it is time to paint his house.

In the beginning of the chapter guilt was briefly discussed. Guilt is a strong feeling. It is not pleasant to feel guilty. Most people go to any lengths to avoid feeling guilty. As a result, guilt is a very strong motivator. For most nurses, it is a troublesome and frequent companion in the working place. There are so many things nurses *think* they have to do. When they are unable to accomplish all of them, even though the limitations are beyond their control, they *feel* guilty. In order to avoid feeling guilty they frequently push themselves harder and harder.

Nurses' work, similar to women's work, is "never done." It is impossible to make a finite list of things to be done within an 8-hour shift. For example, once the absolutely required tasks are accomplished and charted, you could still give Mrs. Jones, the woman with the postcardiotomy infection in isolation, some more time; she seemed depressed today. Or, you could update some nursing care plans; they've been neglected because the unit was so busy.

Even when nurses push themselves to do more and more, the end result is still guilt—and sometimes resentment. Remember this very important point. No one can make you feel guilty. No one! Institutions and other people can make demands on you, but only you can allow yourself to feel guilty. You *let* yourself feel guilty. Your intellect—the thinking, knowing side of you—is the greatest ally you have in overcoming unnecessary guilt. It must be consciously willed into action.

I will give you an exaggerated, nonnursing example of this. If a mother buys her youngster four electronic games for his birthday and the child demands to know why he did not receive five, the mother can either *think* to herself, "How ungrateful; I did far more than was necessary," or she may *feel* guilty. The child did not make her feel guilty. She allowed his statement to cause her guilt feelings. By not consciously guarding ourselves against guilt-inducing statements or expectations of others, we become victims of guilt.

In working with nurses I have repeatedly found that feelings of guilt are the greatest cause of nurses' inability to break away from passivity. It is necessary to understand how to suppress unnecessary guilt before we can learn to be assertive, full, actualized persons.

WILL THE REAL YOU PLEASE STAND UP?

Another concept that is important in the process of being comfortable with assertiveness is one that is explained by Bowen as the *pseudo* self and the *solid* self.[22] The pseudo self is the side of us we allow others to know. Some people are all pseudo self. They are to

their family members, friends, patients, and physicians exactly what those people need them to be. Their own needs, desires, and so forth are submerged to meet the expectations of others.

The solid self is the real you. Many nurses have a difficult time identifying the real self. It has almost entirely been given away to meet the demands of others. The real self must be dug up and reinflated. It's still there. It can return and be bigger and better than it ever was. It requires hard work and concentration and a strong imposition of intellect to break the chains of passivity. It requires control over feelings that can quickly undermine the best intentions. The greatest challenge to your success will be the same family, friends, patients, and physicians who have previously been very successful at "pulling your strings." Being assertive means speaking up for what you need, what you think, and what you believe in. It means knowing your real self.

COPING: KEEPING IT ALL TOGETHER

Coping is a popular word that is being used during the stress-conscious era of the 1980s and appears frequently in articles about the response of CCU nurses to their environment.[23-26] It could be helpful to make certain that the concept of coping is understood before proceeding. Coping is "a combination of conscious strategies that have worked successfully in the past that join with unconscious defense mechanisms in order to reduce the level of stress that a person is experiencing."[27]

It is very important to remember that coping consists of the *automatic* use of defense mechanisms by the ego. These automatic mechanisms (*e.g.,* denial, avoidance, and repression) are used whenever the ego senses a threat to the self. It is also important to remember that an event that is perceived as threatening to one person may not be to another. The following case study is an example:

CASE STUDY

Evelyn, Joan, and Carol are working nights in the coronary intensive care unit. Evelyn has worked there for 12 years. Joan and Carol were hired as new graduates 6 months ago. Joan is an astute nurse who learns quickly but is not yet fully confident in all situations. Carol is currently on probation because her head nurse has found her to be lacking in both assessment and problem-solving skills. During the night a patient developed a severe episode of tachycardia. Within 5 minutes another patient arrested. The perception and responses of the three nurses were as follows:

Evelyn is skilled in all aspects of emergency cardiac assessment and intervention. She is alert and fully monitoring the initial patient's condition. When the other patient arrested she rapidly assessed the condition of the two patients, gave orders to Joan to assume care of the first and moved to call the code and resuscitate the second. Her ego has become so accustomed to these events that it automatically switches on the cognitive or thinking mode and switches off her emotional response. If her emotions prevailed, she would react with anxiety. Moderate to high levels of anxiety markedly lower a person's problem-solving abilities. Joan, when thinking in advance about emergency situations in the CCU, experiences many symptoms of anxiety, such as increased heart and breathing rates and cold perspiration. During the critical situation just described, however, she maintained full control and awareness of herself and felt little anxiety. Her emotional response was repressed by her ego.

As the double emergencies began, Carol reacted to them by "freezing." Her ego shut out her initial anxiety about the situation by denial. With Evelyn and Joan pushing her to action she quickly began to work with them but was highly anxious. Her ego was not repressing her anxiety.

In the situation just described, each of the three nurses experienced the emergency in a different way. *No two human beings ever perceive the same event in the same way.* This is because every person is born with a basic temperament.[28] This inborn set of basic personality traits is then affected by the environment in which the child is raised.

The ego evolves as a response to the surroundings of the child. It determines what is good, bad, harmless, or threatening during the first several years of life.[29] It develops consistent patterns of defenses against situations that it decides are harmful. Depending on the types of experiences the child encounters and the capacity of the ego to defend him from feelings of anxiety, he will perceive a situation as stressful or not stressful.[30, 31]

Coping is actually a complex process that involves a usually consistent response in each person. For example, a person who copes well in one type of stressful situation will usually cope well in all situations. The exceptions are when a person is profoundly fatigued; has had a previous similar experience in which coping failed, so that another similar event causes a burst of anxiety; or has experienced a number of stressful incidents over a brief period of time, so that the new stressor is like "the straw that broke the camel's back."[32]

COPING STYLES OF CCU NURSES

The most recent literature on CCU stress has begun to focus on the way that CCU nurses perceive their working environment and the manner in which they adapt to it.[33-37] Because there has been so much emphasis on CCU nursing stress, CCU nursing turnover, and so on, the following question is being asked: Are there particular coping abilities or certain personality styles that are helpful for CCU nurses to have in order to adapt successfully to a stressful environment?

Maloney and Bartz approached this question by studying the personality and coping characteristics of nurses in intensive care and non–intensive care settings. They examined a number of factors in order to determine whether there were differences between the two groups of nurses. Their findings showed that the intensive care nurses differed significantly in a number of ways.[38]

Power. The CCU nurses generally felt less powerful and more controlled by the environment than the non-CCU staff. This is a realistic finding of adaptation in view of the emergency and unpredictable nature of the CCU setting.

Detachment. The CCU nurses were found to be more detached than their non-CCU counterparts. It was suggested by the authors that this quality helped the nurses cope with the perceptual bombardment present in the CCU. The capacity for detachment is based on use of the defense mechanisms of denial, repression, intellectualization, and similar defenses that reduce the level of anxiety that a person might normally feel in a threatening situation.

Adventurousness and Challenge. These qualities were found to be present more often in CCU nurses than in non-CCU nurses and are believed to contribute toward their attraction to the CCU environment and their capacity to experience satisfaction in it.

In an earlier study,[39] Maloney had compared the coping capacity of CCU nurses with that of non-CCU nurses by examining the ways that both groups experienced anxiety. It was found that CCU nurses experience less anxiety in both normal and new situations than do non-CCU nurses. This information can lead to speculation that CCU nurses have a stronger capacity to use defense mechanisms in anxiety reduction. One can further wonder whether persons who are not attracted to CCU settings are motivated by the desire to avoid excessive anxiety.

Another finding of the study revealed that non-CCU nurses had higher scores on somatic complaints, personal and family problems, and work load dissatisfaction. The generalized conclusion is that CCU nurses have a stronger capacity for coping and adaptation than do nurses attracted to non-CCU settings.

STRESS FACTORS IDENTIFIED BY CCU NURSES

A previous section presented the factors that physicians identified as being the most stressful for nurses in critical care. Now it is time to learn the factors that nurses themselves have identified as the most stressful and then to examine the ways in which they can be alleviated or eliminated. It is important for nurses to remember that these adverse effects will not be lessened by nursing or hospital administrators or by physicians. Changes that improve the physical and emotional states of CCU nurses must be initiated by the nurses themselves. By understanding the underlying causes of burnout and the value of assertiveness in combating burnout and by instituting personal change and accepting their own authenticity, nurses can improve their working environment.

Huckabay and Jagla surveyed CCU nurses from six hospitals.[40] The nurses identifed the factors that they found most stressful in the CCU environment. The authors ranked them in order of their stressfulness, as indicated in the following chart:

Rank Order of Sixteen Components of Stressful Factors in the CCU

1. Workload and amount of physical work
2. Death of a patient
3. Communication problems between staff and nursing office
4. Communication problems between staff and physicians
5. Meeting the needs of the family
6. Numerous pieces of equipment and their failure
7. Noise level in the CCU
8. Physical setup of the CCU
9. Number of rapid decisions that must be made in the CCU
10. Amount of knowledge needed to work in the CCU
11. Physical injury to the nurse
12. Communication problems between staff members
13. Meeting the psychological needs of the patient
14. Communication problems between the staff and other departments in the hospital
15. Cardiac arrest
16. Patient teaching

At first glance, the possibility of lessening any of these factors may seem to be beyond the control of the nurse. It takes firm resolve and energy to *think* that changes can occur, rather than *feeling* hopeless about being able to change anything in the environment.

Let us review the list. In the first five items, those identified as *most* stressful, there is really only one that is beyond the control of the nurse—the death of a patient (although some nurses impose such high expectations on themselves that they view the death of a patient as something that they *should* have been able to prevent). The remaining four items are ones that the nursing staff in a CCU, if unified, can do something about. The key word is *unified*. If the nursing group is

splintered by hopelessness, competitiveness, or disparate views, their potential strength in negotiating the changes that would lessen these stress factors will never be realized.

The next five items (6 to 10) all are built into the CCU environment. They cannot realistically be changed. The stress that nurses feel as a result of them can be lessened, however, and suggestions will follow later. The last six items (11 to 16) contain only one item, cardiac arrest, that is beyond the control of the group.

Six items on the list can be directly attributed to understaffing—a chronic problem in many CCUs. If nurses consistently tolerate an understaffed environment without protest, it is understandable that hospital and nursing administrations will not improve the nurse : patient ratio. Many staff nurses complain loudly among themselves yet passively leave the job of persuading hospital administrators of the need for better staffing to head nurses, supervisors, and nursing administrators. Who better to stand up for their needs and proclaim the results of understaffing than the nurses who are victimized? It is rarely the patients who are victimized. Most nurses selflessly accept the chronically heavy workload in the CCU in order to save their patients' lives.

If the thought of making such demands on an institution leaves you feeling weak and asking, "How dare I even think such things?" review the first five basic rights for women in the health professions written by Melodie Chenevert.[41]

1. You have the right to be treated with respect.
2. You have the right to a reasonable workload.
3. You have the right to an equitable wage.
4. You have the right to determine your own priorities.
5. You have the right to ask for what you want.

GROUP MEETINGS

If chronic understaffing is eliminated, six of the sixteen stress factors that affect CCU nurses will be decreased. The remaining factors can be addressed and usually lessened in a group setting.

Mohl and others speculated that factors other than the primary task of delivering specialized care to patients could contribute to the stress of CCU nurses.[42] They studied the work attitudes and level of stress reported by the staff members of two non–intensive care units and two intensive care units. The results of the study indicated that the nature of the work in the CCU does, indeed, affect the nurses' level of stress. More importantly, however, this study also showed that factors within the unit and nursing organization social system have a significant effect on nurses' stress levels. These include the following:

- Support and respect from nursing supervisors
- Acceptance by staff and supervisors that mutual support in the form of informed one-on-one and formal support groups are important stress reducers
- Staff nurse/unit cohesiveness that includes the head nurse

A recommendation unanimously presented by authors who have addressed the problem of stress in the CCU nurse is to have the CCU nursing staff meet regularly with an objective outsider who is trained in individual and group dynamics.[43-48] The ideal leader is one who is schooled in *liaison psychiatry,* which is based on the study of the effects of stress on the individual and on the social systems to which he belongs: the family, working environment, hospital, and so on. Other successful leaders reported in the literature have been psychiatrists and nurse clinicians from the field of general psychiatry, social workers, and hospital chaplains trained in group process.

These are professionals employed by the hospital who usually are willing to give an extra hour of their time to this type of group. The request for such a group should come from the nursing staff. Meetings should be held once a week, at a regularly scheduled time, when the largest number of staff members can attend. A quiet meeting place adjacent to or in the CCU should be used.

The discussion group is used to address any CCU-related issue. The time is nonstructured, with the nurses raising the issues to be discussed. In the beginning weeks of the group, these issues frequently are centered around the emotional management of problem patients or families. Once the staff members feel trusting of themselves and their leader, they frequently discuss some of their own psychological reactions to specific incidents, such as the hopelessness of weaning a specific patient from a respirator, grief about the death of a long-term CCU patient, anger about house staff who are not there when needed, frustration with an insensitive nursing administration, or helplessness in dealing with the spouse of a dying 30-year-old patient.

Critical care nurses invest large amounts of energy and time in the care of one or two patients a day. It is inevitable that they will lose these patients, either by discharge from the unit or by death. When patients die, their nurses are left with many emotions: grief, sadness, depression, guilt, and anger. Without a safe place to talk about these repetitive losses, nurses may unconsciously repress or deny their feelings in order to survive emotionally. Two other coping mechanisms that they use are avoidance and withdrawal.[49]

Although avoidance and withdrawal are two different coping mechanisms, they have the same result. They occur when nurses consciously or unconsciously become numb to their own feelings and the emotional needs of patients and families. Another name for this phenomenon is *professional distancing.*[50]

As a result, nurses care for the physical needs of patients but hold back from an emotional commitment. This helps them avoid the intolerable grief that occurs when the people they care for are repeatedly lost to them.

In a liaison group meeting, these feelings of grief and loss can be talked about in a supportive setting. The nurses' needs for rigid defenses against these feelings are eventually decreased. When it is safe for them to feel their own honest feelings once again, they usually become more aware of the emotional needs of patients and their families. Their care becomes humanistic rather than technical.

Another issue that can cause conflict in the staff and also be alleviated is intrastaff conflict. CCU staff nurses are bright, ambitious, and highly motivated. When they are working in close contact with others like themselves in a stress-filled environment, competition, staff schisms, or conflicts can result. Ideally, they should be resolved quickly.[51] Without an available forum this is not easily accomplished.

Another problem in the CCU is nurse-doctor relationships. Eisendrath and Dunkel suggest that this may be a masked male-female issue. "This is particularly so when, despite a broader base of experience with critically ill patients, the nurse has to defer to a junior house officer with less relevant background."[52]

In addition, a problem that causes much resentment in nurses is that some doctors consistently avoid family members who need to ask questions or need reassurance.[53] When these concerns are discussed in a liaison group and the anger is vented, nurses can learn better ways of discussing these issues directly with the doctors rather than allowing resentment to grow.

STRESS: IS THERE ANY WAY TO MAKE IT BETTER?

The final section of this chapter will include suggestions for reducing stress during off-duty hours and recommendations that can also alleviate stress during working hours in the CCU. It is important to understand that the body's normal physiological reaction to stress was designed to help cavemen fight or flee from danger. In today's CCU, the nurse's response to stress causes a strong increase in tension and an increase in physical activity to help with the increased workload. There is an excess of energy available, however. When a nurse finishes work and feels tense, it is frequently a result of this unexpended energy.

Because of the sedentary trend in our society, many people live with chronic tenseness. The proliferation of tranquilizer and alcohol usage attests to the uncom-

Recommended Changes for Reducing Stress

1. Institute 4-day work weeks with 10-hour shifts.[54]
2. Employ a full-time physician as permanent CCU director.[55]
   a. A competent physician would always be available, especially during emergencies.
   b. He or she would supervise and teach house staff as they rotate into the unit.
3. Schedule automatic rotations out of the CCU every 3 months for 2 weeks. These should be to an adjacent clinical area, preferably the step-down unit to which CCU patients are routinely discharged.[56]
4. Allow nurses time to visit their "special" patients who are discharged from the CCU to other hospital units.
5. Schedule a senior staff nurse on the day shift with a light patient assignment. She can assist and teach the less experienced nursing staff.[57]
6. Pay CCU nurses an extra wage increment — especially when chronic understaffing occurs.[58]
7. Upgrade the nurse : patient ratio in direct proportion to increased technology.[59]
8. Allow 6 weeks for a comprehensive orientation and training period for new CCU nurses.[60]
9. Require orderlies or other non-CCU personnel to prepare the body of a deceased patient for the morgue.[61]

In construction of new CCUs hospitals should
1. Allow larger space between patient beds.[62]
2. Ideally, build small rooms for one or two patients or install permanent partitions between patient units.[63]
3. Build nurses' lounge out of view of patients, in the center of the CCU.
4. Install windows in the unit. Install clocks within sight of patient.
   a. These are important orienting cues for patients *and* nurses.
   b. If patients are less disoriented, the stress on the nurse will be less.
5. Seek advice from CCU nurses in the architectural design.
6. Install extra amounts of sound-deadening material.

---

fortable levels of tenseness in people. The best way to reduce physical and mental tension is by physical exercise. One mile of jogging or brisk walking every day will return the body's equilibrium to normal. Many people are pleasantly surprised to discover that their emotional state also improves when they begin a regular exercise program. Their depression, anxiety, or fatigue is lessened and gradually disappears.

The relationship between physical tension and emotional disequilibrium is not fully understood. It is known, however, that adrenalin and the other catecholamines, which are the biochemical stimulators of the stress response, are also an integral part of the limbic system — the anatomical part of the brain that is the center of emotions. When adrenalin and the other neurotransmitters return to normal levels as a result of physical exercise, it is possible that the response of the limbic system is to regain emotional equilibrium as well.

If there is mental stress about specific patients, sadness about losing a special patient, or discouragement about the working environment, the best solution is to become involved in an activity that causes you to mentally "focus in" on something else. This could be an academic course or something like an arts and crafts class — anything that requires intense concentration. The mental stress – reducing should always be accompanied by physical stress – reduction activities, such as walking or jogging, as already mentioned.

The stress that occurs as a result of working in a CCU can also, ideally, be alleviated by changes within the CCU. These changes will not be instituted by nursing or hospital administrators unless there is the impetus of strong recommendations by the CCU nursing staff. A list of such recommendations follows:

REFERENCES

1. Cassem N, Hackett T: Sources of tension for the CCU nurse. Am J Nurs 72, No. 8:1426–1430, 1972
2. Gardam J: Nursing stresses in the intensive care unit. JAMA 208:2337–2338, 1969
3. Gardam J: Observations on intensive care units. Superv Nurse 3, No. 7:27–28, 33–42, 44, 1972
4. Gentry W, Foster S, Froeling S: Psychologic response to situational stress in intensive and non-intensive nursing. Heart Lung 1:793–796, 1972
5. Kornfeld D: Psychiatric problems of an intensive care unit. Med Clin North Am 55, No. 9:1353–1363, 1971
6. Koumans A: Psychiatric consultation in an intensive care unit. JAMA 194:633–637, 1965
7. Esteban A, Ballestros P, Caballero J: Psychological evaluation of intensive care nurses. Crit Care Med 11, No. 8:616–620, 1983
8. Jacobsen S: Stressful situations for neonatal intensive care nurses. J Maternal Child Nurs 3:144, 1978
9. Maloney J, Bartz C: Stress-tolerant people: Intensive care nurses compared with non-intensive care nurses. Heart Lung 12, No. 4:389–394, 1983
10. Mohl P, Denny N, Mote T, Coldwater C: Hospital unit stressors that affect nurses: Primary task vs. social factors. Psychosomatics 23, No. 4:366–374, 1982
11. Nichols K, Springford V, Searle J: An investigation of distress and discontent in various types of nursing. J Adv Nurs 6:311, 1981
12. Alberts M: Doctor-nurse communication. RN 39, No. 5:ICCU-6, 1976
13. Gardner D, Parzen Z, Stewart N: The nurse's dilemma: Me-

diating stress in critical care units. Heart Lung 9, No. 1:103–106, 1980

14. Hay D, Oken D: The psychological stresses of intensive care nursing. Psychosom Med 34, No. 2:109–118, 1972

15. Nadelson T: The psychiatrist in the surgical intensive care unit. RN 39, No. 7:ICCU/CCU-6, 7, 1976

16. Simon N, Whitely S: Psychiatric consultation with MICU nurses: The consultation conference as a working group. Heart Lung 6, No. 3:497–504, 1977

17. Ibid.

18. Hay D, Oken D: Op cit

19. Toffler A: Future Shock, pp 19–47. New York, Bantam Books, 1970

20. Miller J: Toward a New Psychology of Women, pp 50–51. Boston, Beacon Press, 1976

21. Ibid, p 51

22. Bowen M: Theory in the practice of psychotherapy. In Guerin P (ed): Family Therapy: Theory and Practice, pp 42–90. New York, Gardner Press, 1976

23. Blackburn S: The neonatal ICU: A high-risk environment. Am J Nurs 82, No. 11:1708–1712, 1982

24. Caldwell T, Weiner M: Stresses and coping in ICU nursing: A review. Gen Hosp Psychiatry 3:119, 1981

25. Gentry W, Parkes K: Psychologic stress in intensive care unit and non–intensive care unit nursing: A review of the past decade. Heart Lung 11:42–47, 1982

26. Stehle J: The findings revisited. Nurs Res 30, No. 3:182–186, 1981

27. Barry P: Psychosocial Nursing Assessment and Intervention, p 327. Philadelphia, JB Lippincott, 1984

28. Chess T, Chess S: Temperament and Development. New York, Brunner/Mazel, 1977

29. Blanck G, Blanck R: Ego Psychology II: Psychoanalytic Developmental Psychology. New York, Columbia University Press, 1979

30. Horowitz M: Stress Response Syndromes. New York, Jason Aronson, 1976

31. Lazarus R: Cognitive and coping processes in emotion. In Monat A, Lazarus R (eds): Stress and Coping: An Anthology. New York, Columbia University Press, 1977

32. Barry P: Op cit, pp 175–182

33. Esteban A, Ballestros P, Caballero J: Op cit

34. Jacobsen S: Op cit

35. Maloney J, Bartz C: Op cit

36. Mohl P, Denny N, Mote T, Coldwater C: Op cit

37. Nichols K, Springford V, Searle J: Op cit

38. Maloney J, Bartz C: Op cit

39. Maloney J: Job stress and its consequences on a group of intensive and non–intensive care nurses. Adv Nurs Sci 4:31, 1982

40. Huckaby L, Jagla B: Nurses' stress factors in the intensive care unit. J Nurs Admin 2:21–26, 1979

41. Chenevert M: Special Techniques in Assertiveness Training for Women in the Health Professions, p 20. St Louis, CV Mosby, 1978

42. Mohl P, Denny N, Mote T, Coldwater C: Op cit

43. Baldwin A: Mental health consultation in the intensive care unit: Toward a greater balance and precision of attribution. J Psychiatr Nurs 2:17–21, 1978

44. Cassem N, Hackett T: The setting of intensive care. In Hackett T, Cassem N (eds): Massachusetts General Hospital Handbook of General Psychiatry, pp 319–341. St Louis, CV Mosby, 1978

45. Eisendrath S, Dunkel J: Psychological issues in intensive care unit staff. Heart Lung 8, No. 4:751–758, 1979

46. Gowan N: The perceptual world of the intensive care unit: An overview of some environmental considerations in the helping relationship. Heart Lung 8, No. 2:340–344, 1979

47. Melia K: The intensive care unit: A stress situation? Nurs Times 73, No. 5:17–20, 1977

48. West N: Stresses associated with ICUs affect patients, families, staff. Hospitals 49, No. 24:62–63, 1975

49. Eisendrath S, Dunkel J: Op cit, p 755

50. Barry P: Op cit

51. Hay D, Oken D: Op cit

52. Eisendrath S, Dunkel J: Op cit, p 755

53. Gardner D, Parzen Z, Stewart N: Op cit

54. Nelson J: Intensive stress. Nurs Mirror 146, No. 3:20, 1978

55. Hay D, Oken D: Op cit

56. Melia K: Op cit

57. Nelson J: Op cit

58. Ibid.

59. Huckaby L, Jagla B: Op cit

60. Gardner D, Parzen Z, Stewart N: Op cit

61. Melia K: Op cit

62. Nelson J: Op cit

63. Gowan N: Op cit

39
Critical Care Nursing: Applied Legal Principles

Sarah Dillian Cohn

Legal issues involving the critical care area have been highly publicized and are of increasing concern to health care providers, hospitals, and the public. Our society seems to be more litiginous than ever; thus, the number of malpractice suits that name or involve nurses is increasing. Issues such as refusal and termination of treatment have been widely discussed and written about; even legislatures have acted—so-called living will statutes have been enacted in many jurisdictions.

This chapter will begin with a discussion of principles of negligence as they apply to the critical care nurse (CCN). It will then proceed to identify and address certain current legal issues most applicable to the CCN.

NURSING NEGLIGENCE IN THE CRITICAL CARE AREA

There are few reported cases of negligence by nurses in a critical care area. This does not mean that cases necessarily are rare; instead, the hospital may be the only named defendant (as the employer of the nurse), the case may be settled in advance of trial, or a judgment simply may not be appealed. The incidents in many reported nurse malpractice cases, however, could have taken place in a critical care area and can serve as examples of potential CCN negligence.

When a malpractice case is presented, the legal principles are the same as those applicable to non–critical care nurses. They are not difficult to understand, and an awareness of them can reinforce some of the fundamental requirements of competent nursing practice.

Common elements of a malpractice suit are as follows:

Elements of a Malpractice Suit: The 4 Ds

Duty
Dereliction of Duty
Direct causation
Damages

DUTY AND DERELICTION OF DUTY

A nurse who cares for a patient has a duty to that patient to use reasonable care. Failure to do so is negligence, for which the patient may recover monetary damages. Generally, the law does not require a critical care nurse or any other health care professional to have been perfect or always to have made the correct decision. Instead, the standard is what a reasonably prudent CCN would have done under the same or similar circumstances. Thus, if a reasonable, prudent CCN would have avoided the problem, the defendant nurse will be held to be negligent. However, if the reasonable CCN would have acted as the defendant did, no negligence exists, and there will be no recovery of damages despite the plaintiff's very real and substantial injuries.[1] This standard permits variation among cases regarding the education and experience of the nurse and the equipment and personnel available at the time of the incident.

The plaintiff must prove the standard of care as it existed at the time of the incident, and this proof is often one of the most difficult parts of the case. The standard must be established by an expert witness. For example, the generalist nurse would be competent to explain injection technique and sites; however, if the case involves the reading of an ECG, the expert must be a nurse who is competent in that clinical area. Her testimony will be based on such items as written standards or position statements from relevant professional organizations, the current literature, job descriptions and hospital policies and procedures. The defendant nurse may also use experts in an effort to show that the standard of care is different from the one that the plaintiff has demonstrated.

Once the duty is established, a breach of that duty is required—that is, the nurse must have been negligent. Negligence is found or refuted by a comparison of the nurse's conduct with the standard of care. Generally, negligence is either ordinary or gross. Ordinary negligence implies professional carelessness, whereas gross negligence suggests that the nurse willfully and consciously ignored a known risk of harm to the patient. Most cases involve ordinary negligence, but gross negligence may be present if a nurse harmed a patient while she was under the influence of drugs or alcohol.

CAUSATION AND DAMAGE

There must be a causal relationship between what the CCN did or failed to do and the damages suffered by the patient. Thus, a negligent medication error that occurred near the time of the patient's death either may have had nothing to do with the death or may have caused it; expert testimony on the cause of death would be critical in this case because the nurse, even if negligent, will not be liable if her actions did not contribute to the patient's suffering or death. Generally, however, the law interprets damages broadly. Any physical injury is sufficient to award monetary damages. Small injuries merit small compensation, whereas larger injuries merit larger amounts. If there have been physical injuries, compensation for emotional distress may also be paid; in a few states under some circumstances, compensation for emotional anguish may be awarded even in the absence of physical injury.

A merely undersirable event or outcome does not constitute negligence. Not every fall from a hospital bed is a result of some negligent act of the part of a health care provider. The facts surrounding the event must be examined in light of the applicable standard of care. Further, the plaintiff must prove all four elements of the action to the jury. In summary, the plaintiff (the patient) must prove "upon a preponderance of the evidence" that the nurse breached a duty and caused harm.

CCN NEGLIGENCE AND CASE LAW

The following recent cases will illustrate the legal and professional principles that are applicable in malpractice cases. There are numerous allegations that are commonly made against members of the nursing staff. One is failure to monitor the patient's condition properly, as illustrated in the first case:

CASE 1

A 4-month-old boy was admitted for correction of a congenital trachea condition and underwent a tracheotomy. The surgery was uneventful, and he was last examined by the surgeon in the CCU at 11:00 P.M. The physician left orders and went home. At that time, the infant's condition was satisfactory and he had no manifestations of postoperative complications. At 3:55 A.M., he stopped breathing and suffered devastating and irreversible brain damage when the resuscitation team was unable quickly to restore respirations or a heartbeat. The cause of the arrest was a massive pneumothorax from the gradual accumulation of trapped air beneath the skin (subcutaneous emphysema), which had entered the body at the site of tracheotomy and had subsequently worked down until it broke through the surface of the lung. Expert testimony determined that the infant had exhibited signs and symptoms of the complication for almost 2 hours before the arrest occurred. The jury found the hospital liable for the negligence of the nurses and the resident.[2]

The infant in the preceding case was a fresh postoperative patient, and the standard of care required diligence in observing his condition. This included the prompt recognition and treatment of complications. In essence, the court held that even though the complication itself might be unavoidable, the failure to recognize it and treat it constituted negligence. This principle also applies in other circumstances. A patient had surgery for acute gallbladder disease. He fell from his bed during his first postoperative night. Twenty-four hours after the fall, he went into shock, and the drug Levophed was ordered. He had infusions running into both arms, but they were discontinued when they infiltrated. An IV was begun in the patient's leg, infiltrated, and caused a permanent partial disability. Evidence at the trial determined that the infusion containing the Levophed had been infusing into the tissues for a period of 2 hours. The court found the evidence sufficient to warrant a finding of negligence for failing to detect the situation within a reasonable time.[3] Infiltration of intravenous fluids is fairly common, and tissue necrosis is an acknowledged and not unusual complication with the administration of Levophed. Generally, the courts have held that as long as the drug is indicated by the patient's condition and the patient has constant attention during the infusion, the occurrence of tissue necrosis is an unavoidable side effect, and damages will not be awarded.[4]

Failure to record observations can lead to the conclusion that the patient was improperly monitored, as illustrated in the following case.

CASE 2

A 6-year-old boy was admitted after he was struck by an automobile while he was riding his bicycle. In addition to sustaining several other injuries, the boy had a fractured left leg, which was placed in traction on the day of admission (May 7). That night, the nurse who was observing the patient wrote several entries in the nurse's notes suggesting that the circulation in the affected leg was good. The next day, the left leg circulation remained adequate at least until 11:00 P.M., when the patient was last examined by a physician. By 6:00 A.M., the circulation was seriously compromised. Nurse's notes for that night contain no information about circulation in the leg, although the nurse wrote that the boy was medicated for pain and that he was unable to sleep. Ultimately, it was necessary to amputate the patient's left leg. The court held that the failure by the nurse "who was on duty during the crucial period to make any entry of observations that she made concerning the circulation in [the patient's] foot . . . could very well have led the jury to infer than no such observations were made between 11:00 P.M. and 6:00 A.M., when the nurse wrote that the left foot was cold, had no feeling, and was dusky. The case was remanded for trial on the hospital's liability (as the nurse's employer) in this case.[5]

Another common malpractice allegation is that the nurse failed to notify the physician of abnormalities in the patient's condition or history. This is illustrated in the next case.

CASE 3

The Ramsey family lived in a rural county in Maryland. In May, 1974, the parents brought their infant sons (ages 1 and 2 years) to the emergency room of a hospital when each developed a rash and a high fever. While there, Mrs. Ramsey told the nurse on duty that she had removed two ticks from one of the boys; the nurse did not tell the examining physician of that history. The physician testified that he asked the parents about exposure to ticks and was told nothing. The children were treated as if they had measles for several days, and one died. The second was subsequently treated for, and recovered from, Rocky Mountain spotted fever; an autopsy on the younger child revealed that he had died of the same disease. Because of the rarity of the disease in Maryland and the atypical nature of the children's symptoms, the physicians involved were held not liable. However, the emergency room nurse was found negligent because she had not recorded or communicated significant medical data and because expert testimony indicated that this failure was a contributing cause of the death of one child and of serious illness in the other.[6]

Finally, medication and transfusion errors have frequently been the subject of malpractice actions. The next case is an example:

CASE 4

A 3-month-old infant was afflicted with congenital heart disease and was admitted to the hospital. The physician ordered "elixir pediatric digoxin (Lanoxin) 2.5 ml (0.125mg) q6h × 3 then once daily." Later in the hospitalization an order stated, "Give 3.0 ml Lanoxin today for 1 dose only." The route of administration was not indicated on either order. A nursing supervisor assisting on the unit that day administered 3 ml of Lanoxin in its injectable form, a lethal overdose. Medical testimony revealed that 3 ml of Lanoxin in its elixir form and administered orally would not have harmed the child. The infant died 75 minutes after receiving the intramuscular injection. The physician was found negligent in failing to denote the intended route of administration when the same dose was fatal by one route and therapeutic by another. The nurse was also negligent because she was in doubt about the medication order and did not call the prescribing physician. Furthermore, the nurse was unfamiliar with the drug and did not know that it was available for administration in an oral form as well as an injectable form.[7]

VICARIOUS LIABILITY

Potential liability exists for both the hospital and the health care provider. The hospital, as a corporation, may be liable for an equipment failure or for failure to provide a competent medical and nursing staff in a CCU. It will also be liable as an employer for the negligence of its physician and nursing employees. Those staff members will also be independently liable for the injuries that were directly and proximately caused by poor decision-making skills or for theory and skill incompetency.

The doctrine of respondeat superior ("let the master answer") is the major legal theory under which hospitals are responsible for the negligence of their employees. Thus, as long as the nurse acts within the scope of her employment, the hospital will be liable as well; it will not be liable if the nurse acts outside the scope of her employment.

Because the hospital is also liable, hospitals carry professional liability insurance for the activities of their employees. Generally, a hospital will defend a nurse named in a malpractice case. However, some critical care nurses choose to carry their own personal malpractice insurance. Personal insurance is important if the CCN feels, for example, that the hospital liability coverage may be inadequate.

PROTOCOLS

When the critical care nurse is required to perform medical acts and is not under the direct and immediate supervision of a delegating physician, the activities must be based on established protocols. These protocols should be created by the medical and nursing departments and should be reviewed for compliance with state nurse practice acts. They must be frequently reviewed so that health care professionals can determine whether these protocols reflect current medical and nursing standards of care. It is likely that, in the event of a malpractice suit, one may introduce the critical care protocols and procedures as evidence to help establish the applicable standard of care. Although it is important that protocols provide direction, excessive detail may restrict the flexibility that a CCN needs to select a proper course of action.

THE QUESTIONABLE MEDICAL ORDER

In addition to protocols, a policy statement should exist (in procedures or by directive) that indicates the manner of resolving the issue of the "questionable" medical order. This is important for all medical orders, but particularly for those given for critically ill patients because of the unusual doses of medication that are frequently ordered. The nurse who questions a particular order should express her specific reasons for concern to the physician who has written the order. This initial approach frequently results in an explanation of the order and a medical justification for the order in the patient's medical record. If this approach is unsuccessful, many hospitals require that the attending physician or the nursing supervisor be notified; others have a policy that states that the chief of service may be consulted about "questionable" orders. If these options are unavailable or are unsuccessful, a CCN or any other nurse may refuse to give a medication.

It is important for the critical care nurse to realize that an order that is patently wrong may harm the patient if it is followed; a secondary result may be liability for both the physician and the nurse (and the hospital, her employer) if the patient suffers harm as a direct result.

INADEQUATE STAFFING

One of the most important factors that sets the critical care nurse apart from a generalist medical and surgical nurse is the critical care nurse's knowledge of scientific theories and nursing skills that are unique to a critical care setting and necessary to meet the needs of critically ill patients. The nurse functioning in a CCU, for example, must be competent to make immediate nursing judgments and to act on those decisions. A nurse who does not possess the theory and skills required of a critical care nurse should be rendering critical care. If a generalist nurse is floated to a CCU, she should inform her nursing supervisor that she lacks the necessary critical care skills. The nurse should make it clear that she can carry out only nursing care activities in which she is competent. The CCU staff should also

know of the skills of the generalist nurse and should delegate only those activities in which the floated nurse is competent. It is reasonable to expect that any hospital that has a CCU or an emergency room will take precautionary measures to assure that it is adequately staffed. Increasingly, nurses are regarding the adequacy of staff as a professional practice issue and are bringing this issue to the attention of hospital watch administration.

DEFECTIVE EQUIPMENT

There is a duty not to use equipment that is patently defective. If the equipment suddenly ceased to do what it was intended to do, made unusual noises, or had a history of malfunction and was not repaired, the hospital may be liable for damage caused by it, and a nurse also may be liable if she knew or should have known of these problems and used the equipment anyway. The following case involved liability for defective equipment:

CASE 5

A woman who had a complex pancreatic condition was being transferred from one hospital room to another. The room was a short distance from one hospital room to another. The room was a short distance from her old room, and during the transfer she experienced severe respiratory distress. It was known that she had previously experienced respiratory difficulty. When the nurses reached the new room and attempted to attach the oxygen supply to the wall outlets, they discovered that the oxygen plugs did not fit into the outlets. The patient expired before emergency oxygen could be obtained. The court held that the cause of death was attributable to the negligence of the hospital as a corporation for its failure to standardize the outlets and the oxygen plugs. There was no liability on the part of the nurses. If the facts had been that the woman was experiencing respiratory problems before the transfer was begun or that the rooms were separated by a great distance, there may have been a duty to have the woman transferred with portable oxygen or to delay the transfer until her status improved.[8]

CONSENT

Both surgical and medical procedures are frequently required by patients who are being cared for in critical care settings. In some institutions consent forms are used, whereas in others the patient's consent is documented in the medical record notes. In general, it is the responsibility of the physician to obtain consent for treatment from the patient or the family, but a CCN may be asked to sign a consent form as a witness. Unless there is a statute stating otherwise, a witness who signs the form is simply able to testify that the signature is not a forgery. The witness is not required to state that legal consent has been obtained.[9]

ISSUES THAT INVOLVE LIFE SUPPORT MEASURES

There are several basic issues involving refusal and termination of treatment that may involve the CCN. No code orders, living wills, and withdrawal of life support measures are only three. As the discussions will indicate, these are complex topics for which only an overview can be provided.

No-Code Orders

It has been reported that cardiopulmonary resuscitation (CPR) takes place in 30% of patients who die at a major Boston hospital.[10] However, CPR is not appropriate for all patients who experience a cardiac arrest because it is highly invasive and may constitute a "positive violation of an individual's right to die with dignity."[11] Furthermore, CPR may not be indicated in cases in which the illness is terminal and irreversible and in which the patient will gain no benefit.

Prestigious authorities (*e.g.,* the President's Commission for the Study of Ethical Problems in Medicine and Biomedical and Behavioral Research) have recommended that hospitals have an explicit policy on the practice of writing and implementing DNR [do not resuscitate] orders."[12] Several hospital[13] and medical society[14] have published DNR policies.

Whether or not to resuscitate any particular patient is a decision that is made by the attending physician, the patient, and his family, although critical care nurses and other nurses often have substantial input into the decision. Generally, however, the consent of a competent patient should be required when a DNR order is written. When the patient is incompetent, the physician and family members make the decision. Of course, the situation may be more complex, and the physician and the family or patient may disagree. The President's Commission has published advisory tables regarding the cardiopulmonary resuscitation of both competent and incompetent patients that take into account the patient's preference and the likelihood that CPR would benefit the patient.[15]

Once the DNR decision has been made, the order should be written, signed, and dated by the responsible physician. It should be reviewed periodically; hospital policies may require review every 24 to 72 hours.[16] More informal methods of designating those patients in whom CPR is not to be undertaken may lead to errors when an arrest occurs. For example, the wrong patient may be allowed to die.

If an arrest occurs in an emergency room or in another situation in which a formal DNR decision has not been made and written the presumption of the medical and nursing staffs should be in favor of life, and a code should be called. A "slow code" (a case in which the nurse takes excessive time to call or the team takes its time responding) should never be permitted — either CPR is indicated or it is not.

Courts are beginning to be involved in no-code decisions. In 1978, a Massachusetts appellate court ruled that an attending physician may lawfully write a no-code order for an incompetent patient for whom there was no life-saving or life-prolonging treatment.[17] More recently, a New York grand jury investigated a hospital that indicated DNR decisions using purple dots stuck to nursing cards that were discarded after the death of the patient. The grand jury found that the dot system "virtually eliminated professional accountability, invited clerical error and discouraged physicians from obtaining informed consent from the patient or his family."[18] Nurses from the hospital complained that the decals could be stuck to the wrong patient's card; one card had two dots affixed to it.

Living Wills

A living will is a directive from a competent patient to family and medical personnel about the treatment he wishes to receive when he is incompetent and unable to make decisions for himself.[19] In general, a living will is not needed when a patient is competent and can communicate; under these circumstances treatment can be refused when it is offered.

At least 16 United States jurisdictions (Table 39-1) have so-called natural death, or living will, statues, although provisions of these laws vary. Usually, however, a person who is 18 years of age or older can execute a living will. It must be written, signed and witnessed. Because many statutes bar medical personnel who are attending the patient or who are employed by the facility in which the patient is hospitalized from

TABLE 39-1
JURISDICTIONS THAT HAVE LIVING WILL STATUTES*

Alabama	Mississippi
Arizona	Montana
Arkansas	Nevada
California	New Hampshire
Colorado	New Mexico
Connecticut	North Carolina
Delaware	Oklahoma
District of Columbia	Oregon
Georgia	Tennessee
Idaho	Texas
Illinois	Utah
Indiana	Vermont
Iowa	Virginia
Kansas	Washington
Louisiana	West Virginia
Maine	Wisconsin
Maryland	Wyoming

*As of September, 1984. To confirm this information, contact the Society for the Right to Die at (212) 246-6973.

being witnesses, a CCN should not witness a document for her patient. The directive should be reviewed and resigned by the patient annually.

Even in states with living will statutes, the directive may not be binding on the physician. However, in a few states, it is unprofessional conduct for a physician to refuse to comply with the directive, although he may transfer the patient to the care of another physician. In all states with statutes, personnel and facilities that comply in good faith with the directive are immune from civil and criminal prosecution.

In states without statutes, it is likely that a recent living will would be taken as evidence of what the patient would have wanted had he been competent when the decision was presented. Athough there have been no cases concerning a written living will, there was one in New York involving a patient who had expressed his wishes orally about life-sustaining measures:

CASE 6

Brother Fox was an 83-year-old member of a religious order who became permanently comatose during hernia surgery. After hospital officials and physicians refused to cease respirator therapy, Brother Fox's order began court proceedings. New York's highest court, the Court of Appeals, ruled (after the death of the priest) that Brother Fox's oral, solemn statement of his wishes (made to members of his order after the Karen Ann Quinlan case had occurred, see further on) were sufficient to authorize termination of treatment.[20]

When a patient or family member reveals the existence of a written living will, a copy should be placed in the medical record, and the attending physician should be notified. If the patient is competent, attempts should be made to clarify the meaning of terminology in the directive; these discussions should be well documented in the medical record. This is necessary to enable nursing and medical personnel to understand exactly what treatment the patient wishes to avoid.[21]

The vast majority of states have statutes that permit the appointment of a proxy to act when a person becomes incompetent. These are called *durable power of attorney acts,* and, although they were not originally intended to delegate health care decisions, some authorities feel that language contained in these acts is broad enough to authorize health care decision-making.[22] California has become the first state to pass a special durable power of attorney for health care act. Some of its provisions are described subsequently. When reviewing them, the critical care nurse must remember that each durable power of attorney law is different and that it is important to understand the law in the jurisdiction in which it applied.

The California statute permits a patient to designate another as his "attorney in fact" to make certain health care decisions on his behalf. The power to make health care decisions may include consent, refusal of consent, or withdrawal of consent to any care or treatment of a mental or physical condition. The document may limit the powers of the attorney in fact, and the statute does not permit him to consent to certain treatments (*e.g.,* sterilization and committment to a mental health facility).

To be effective, a durable power of attorney in California must be executed as required by statute: Two witnesses are required. Generally, the power expires after 7 years, but it may be revoked at any time by oral or written notification of the attorney in fact or the health care provider. Treatment authorized by the attorney in fact may not be administered over the objection of the patient.[23]

Withdrawal of Life Support Measures

What constitutes life support, when these measures must be used and when they may be terminated have been issues raised in many court cases. However, the law in these areas is still developing and will continue to do so as each jurisdiction creates its own guidelines.

Given the regularity with which life support decisions must be made in health care facilities, it is remarkable that it was not until 1976 that the first case, In Re Quinlan,[24] focused national attention on the "right to die" controversy. The cases have concerned minors and adults, competent patients and incompetent ones, afflicted with a disease or condition that would eventually be terminal. States have not been consistent in their decisions, even when the situations are arguably similar. For example, the New Jersey court in the case of Karen Ann Quinlan, a 21-year-old woman in a persistent vegetative state, held that the decision about treatment is in the hands of the patient's guardian in consultation with the hospital ethics committee.[25] Massachusetts, however, has rejected the New Jersey approach in favor of judicial review of decisions made by physicians and family members.[26] The President's Commission for the Study of Ethical Problems in Medicine and Biomedical and Behavioral Research has stated that judicial review of these decisions should be reserved for occasions when "adjudication is clearly required by state law or when concerned parties have disagreements that they cannot resolve over matters of substantial import."[27]

The Florida case of Satz v. Perlmutter involved a competent patient and his right to refuse treatment and is described subsequently:

CASE 7

Abe Perlmutter was 73 years old, suffered from amyotrophic lateral sclerosis, and was dependent on respirator therapy. He was conscious, competent, and able to speak, although he found speech difficult and painful. He had expressed his suffering and had attempted to disconnect his respirator himself. State officials argued that anyone who helped him disconnect his respirator would be guilty of aiding suicide. The Florida Supreme Court ruled that disconnection of the respirator was not suicide because Mr. Perlmutter's condition was not self-inflicted.[28]

The following New Jersey case concerns whether or not it is necessary to provide patients with fluids and nutrition if they cannot feed themselves:

CASE 8

In re Conroy involves an 84-year-old nursing home patient who suffered from severe organic brain syndrome. Her guardian, a nephew, petitioned the court to permit removal of her nasogastric tube, on which she was dependent. The trial court held that the tube could be removed.[29] An appeals court has held removal of the tube improper because the bodily invasion suffered by the patient as a result of the treatment was small and death by dehydration and starvation would be painful.[30] Although the patient has died, the New Jersey Supreme Court held in 1985 that treatment (including artificial feeding and hydration) for nursing home residents may be terminated under certain circumstances and set forth the procedures to be followed. This decision is restricted to nursing home residents who were once competent and who will probably die within approximately 1 year, even with treatment.[31]

Another case involved the criminal liability of physicians who order termination of treatment:

CASE 9

Clarence Herbert was 55 years old when he had a cardiac arrest in the recovery room after elective surgery for closure of a colostomy. Three days later, he was deeply comatose and unlikely to recover; the respirator was removed with the consent of the family. Mr. Herbert then began to breathe on his own. Two days later, IVs and the nasogastric tube were removed. Mr. Herbert died 7 days later from dehydration and pneumonia.[32] Two physicians were charged with murder for terminating IV feeding. Finding that the physicians did not have a legal duty to continue life-sustaining treatment that is futile or ineffective, a California appellate court ordered the criminal charges dropped.[33]

In most states, problems of terminating treatment need not be resolved in court. Decisions regarding treatment or nontreatment that meet accepted medical standards and with which the patient concurs are made virtually every day in every health care setting. When the patient is incompetent to decide, generally family members may do so although they may not refuse therapy that will benefit the patient. Finally, a distinction should be made between termination of treatment and termination of care: Even patients who will not be treated for their terminal condition require competent and sensitive nursing and medical care so that their final days can be as comfortable as possible. The families of these patients may also require information along with sensitive emotion support: The need for good nursing care does not end with the decision "not to treat."

Brain Death

In 1968, the Harvard criteria established standards for determining brain death (see Chap. 22). The criteria have been found quite reliable. In fact, no case has "yet been found that met these criteria and regained any brain functions despite continuation of respirator support."[34] Some states adopted the Harvard criteria by statute, whereas other states enacted legislation defining brain death in broader, less restrictive terms.

The President's Commission for the Study of Ethical Problems in Medicine and Biomedical and Behavioral Research published *Defining Death* in July, 1981. The Commission has recommended a uniform statute defining death; it has recommended that the statute address "general physiological standards rather than medical criteria and tests, which will change with advances in biomedical knowledge and refinements in technique."[35]

A patient who is brain dead is legally dead and there is no legal duty to continue to treat him. It is not necessary to obtain court approval to discontinue life support on a patient who is brain dead. Furthermore, although it may be desirable to obtain family permission to discontinue treatment of a brain dead patient, there is no legal requirement. However, prior to terminating life support, physicians and nurses should be sure that organs are not intended for transplant purposes.[36]

SUMMARY

The legal responsibility of the registered nurse in the CCU does not differ from that of the registered nurse in any work setting. Five principles to which the registered nurse adheres for the protection of both patient and practitioner are as follows:

- A registered nurse performs only those functions for which she has been prepared by education and experience.
- A registered nurse performs these functions competently.
- A registered nurse delegates responsibility only to personnel whose competence has been evaluated and found acceptable.
- A registered nurse takes appropriate measures as indicated by her observations of the patient.
- A registered nurse is familiar with policies of the employing agency.

REFERENCES

1. Holder AR: Medical Malpractice Law, 2d ed, p 43. New York. John Wiley & Sons, 1978
2. Variety Children's Hospital, Inc v. Perkins et al: 382 So2d 331, Florida, 1980
3. North Shore Hospital v. Luzi: 194 So2d 63, Florida, 1967
4. Holder AR: Op cit, p 158
5. Collins v. Westlake Community Hospital: 312 NE2d 614, Illinois, 1974
6. Ramsey v. Physicians Memorial Hospital, Inc et al: 373 A2d 26, Maryland, 1977
7. Norton v. Argonaut Insurance Company et al: 144 So2d 249, Louisiana, 1962
8. Bellaire General Hospital v. Campbell: 510 SW2d 94, Texas, 1974
9. Holder AR: What commitment is made by a witness to a consent form? IRB 1:7, 1979
10. Bedell SE, Delbanco TL, Cook EF, Epstein FH: Survival after cardiopulmonary resuscitation in the hospital. N Engl J Med 309:569, 1983
11. Matter of Dinnerstein: 380 NE2d 134, Massachusetts, 1978
12. President's commission: Deciding to Forego Life-Sustaining Treatment, p 248, March, 1983
13. Doudera AE, Peters JD (eds): Legal and Ethical Aspects of Treating Critically and Terminally Ill Patients (Appendices B–E). Ann Arbor, MI, Health Administration Press, 1982
14. Parrella GS: No Code? Conn Med 47:49, 1983
15. President's Commission: Op cit, pp 244–247
16. Greenlaw J: Orders not to resuscitate: Dilemma for acute care as well as long term care facilities. Law Med Health Care 10:30, 1982
17. Manner of Dinnerstein: Op cit
18. Panel Accuses Hospital of Hiding Denial of Care. New York, New York Times, March 21, 1984
19. Cohn S: The living will from the nurse's perspective. Law Med Health Care 11:121, 1983
20. In re Eichner (Fox), 420 NE2d 64, New York, 1981
21. Eisendrath SJ, Jonsen A: The living will: Help or hindrance? J Am Med Assoc 249:2054, 1983
22. President's Commission: Op cit, pp 145–147
23. California Civil Code, sections 2430–2443
24. In re Quinlan, 70 NJ 10, 355 A2d 647, New Jersey, 1976
25. Ibid
26. Superintendent of Belchertown State School v. Saikewicz: 373 Mass. 728, 370 NE2d 417, Massachusetts, 1977
27. President's Commission: Op cit, p 6
28. Satz v. Perlmutter: 379 So2d 359, Florida, 1980
29. In the Matter of Claire C Conroy: 457 A2d 1232, New Jersey Superior Court, 1983
30. In re Conroy, 464 A2d, 303, New Jersey, 1983
31. In the Matter of Claire C. Conroy. Slip Opinion 98 NJ:321, A2d, 1985
32. Steinbock B: The removal of Mr. Herbert's feeding tube. The Hastings Center Report 13:13, 1983
33. Barber v. Superior Court of California for the County of Los Angeles: 195 Cal Rptr 484, California Appellate Court, 1983
34. President's Commission for the Study of Ethical Problems in Medicine and Biomedical and Behavioral Research: Defining Death, p 25, July, 1981
35. Ibid, p 1
36. Robertson J: The Rights of the Critically Ill, p 121, New York, Bantom Books, 1983

40
Planning for the Training and Development of the Critical Care Nursing Staff

Naomi Domer Medearis

Would you believe . . .

> . . . A new nurse starts the first day of orientation in critical care with the instruction, "For the moment, read this (critical care protocol). I'll get back to you as soon as things are less hectic"?

It happens!

> . . . On a Cor Zero, the nurses are immobilized by high levels of anxiety because they lack sufficient "hands on experience" to feel confident of their life-supporting skills?

It happens!

> . . . A critical care unit (CCU) staff becomes overwhelmed by the constant flow of crises, and there is no plan to handle the stress, anxiety, and exhaustion generated by these day-in, day-out situations?

It happens!

> . . . A clinical specialist accepts the educator role in the CCU and has little or no preparation for developing problem-centered and people-centered programs for the staff?

It happens!

Perhaps you can identify with these situations or have similar incidents of your own. Situations like these demand new ways of training and developing staff.

WHAT IS AHEAD IN THE 1980s?

Alvin Toffler gave a preview of the future in his book *The Third Wave.* He identifies some of the changes we face as individuals and as members of organizations in the decades prior to the year 2000 — changes that hold crucial implications for health care systems and CCUs! He emphasizes that one faces the task of integrating the stresses and strains created in the work setting with the multiplicity of pressures experienced in his personal life. Add to these daily living circumstances the complexity and uncertainty of issues and conflicts on the local, national, and international scenes, and the task becomes more complex. New individual and organizational approaches are necessary for survival and growth.

The integration of personal- and work-life goals for achieving a sense of wholeness is a key goal for all our lives, according to Lippitt.[1] When our personal-, social-, and work-life goals are out of balance, our effectiveness and sense of wholeness are affected. This poses a dilemma for organizations. The effective integration of organization, service unit, and individual goals and values challenges health care administration as never before. The quality of one's work life depends on how well organizations respond to these demands. In a health care system in which delivery of service depends almost exclusively on individuals, new ways of dealing with human resources are essential.

Today's health care professionals are people who (1) hold different perceptions of the work ethic; (2) look to the organization to provide support for personal and professional growth needs; and (3) look to administration for structured opportunities to share not only their competencies but also their beliefs, concerns, and ideas. Such expectations call for innovative, appropriate, and economically feasible strategies for developing hospital personnel.

One health care area in which the impact of work and life stresses culminates is the CCU. There the staff sees some of the ravages of individual responses to life situations. Survival in this highly accelerated, ever-changing environment challenges every critical care staff member. Increasingly, hospitals are focusing on redefining the role of the educational arm of their professional staff. Organizational development and staff development are emerging as the new frontier in education programs. The health care field is beginning to respond in cost-effective ways. Training *does* occur whether it is planned or unplanned! Both cost money!

In a *Wall Street Journal* interview, Peter Drucker stated

> Let's make no mistake about it. Training is a cost! Every industry must measure its ability to cover the costs of its basic resources, its people, its physical plan and capital. . . . Believing you can hire people who fully understand their jobs, your company, and how to competently do your business without expending any training and development effort is like looking for a free lunch. Training is a necessary expense.

Developing people is "where it is at."[2]

DECENTRALIZED EDUCATION FOR CLINICAL UNITS

The impact of many forces within and outside the hospital points to decentralization training as an educational strategy to manage change. Included in these forces are (1) increased emphasis of hospitals on critical care, (2) the establishment of standards for special care units by the Joint Commission on Accreditation of Hospitals, (3) the professional certification program of the American Association of Critical Care Nursing, and (4) the legal prerequisite for contact hours in continuing education. Thus, education has become an important issue and program in the management of CCUs.

Critical care nurses look for hospital systems that offer educational/staff development programs, that are committed to maintaining high levels of competency, that provide opportunities for personal and professional growth, and that work to prevent burnout of professionals. A viable staff development program becomes an important criterion in the recruitment, retention, and promotion of the professional nurse in special care units.

The proliferation of technical specialties, new drugs, sophisticated equipment, and medical procedures creates high levels of anxiety and frustration among the people who need to function as *inter*dependent team members. In most professional disciplines, people are trained to function *in*dependently. As a result, professionals, performing services for the patient, do not know how to deal with one another and to collaborate in working with the patient. Tailoring

educational programs to set goals, clarify roles, and share perceptions and expectations *can* be accomplished through decentralization of education and staff development. The beginning point is orientation that is designed around the training and experience the nurse brings to the job, the level of competency demonstrated, and the particular needs the nurse has to become a member of the critical care social system.

Thirteen hospitals participated in a research study focusing on the purpose, organization, and plan for orientation and continuing education.[3] The results supported decentralization in clinical services such as critical care. Decentralization does not exclude critical care nurses from participating in *relevant* in-service and orientation programs offered by the education department of nursing service. Most important, decentralization needs solid support from administration as opposed to token compliance, relevant in-service as opposed to one-shot traditional sessions, and accountability for results as opposed to numbers and mere program visibility on paper. In return, administration will expect bottom-line results — quality assurance, stable staff, quality work-life, achievement of goals, and demonstration of critical care cost-effective education. Learn to document results!

PROGRAM-PLANNING FOR CRITICAL CARE EDUCATION

To survive organizational politics and interfaces, a well-planned decentralized educational program is essential. An effective approach to program development is diagrammed in Figure 40-1. Five components constitute the model: philosophy, needs, objectives, implementation, and evaluation.

Philosophy

First, a statement of philosophy should set forth the beliefs and values of staff education and development for critical care personnel as well as the concepts and beliefs about the quality of care and the competencies of staff. It should also include statements identifying its organizational functions and its importance in achieving the organizational goals.

Examples of philosophical statements are as follows:

> We believe that a quality staff education program is essential if the hospital's goals for quality assurance in patient care and cost-effective operations are to be realized.
>
> We believe the hospital has a responsibility to support staff education by providing adequate manpower, budget, space, materials, and opportunities for personal and professional growth.

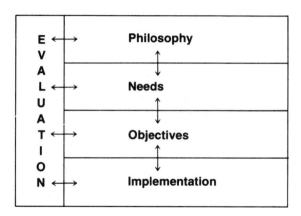

FIGURE 40-1
Program planning model.

We believe each employee has a right to be oriented to the unit; to be able to use current professional skills on-the-job; to participate in continuing education programs; and to receive recognition in merit/performance appraisal programs for demonstrating increased competency based on achievement of professional goals.

We believe the quality of work-life and the genuine concern for humanizing the work setting will humanize patient care and guarantee quality care.

Needs

Educational needs occur at all levels — patient and family, individual staff members, multidisciplinary critical care committee members, and administration. Consideration of needs from all levels makes need assessment a complex and difficult task.

Determining the needs and then categorizing them will facilitate identification of essential program areas. Programs from the identified areas will become the service one delivers as nurse educator.

One method for identifying needs consists of (1) description of the current condition (the situation as it is now); (2) description of the desired condition (the way you would like for it to be); and (3) definition of the knowledge, attitudes, and skills necessary to bring about the desired condition. The following example illustrates all these steps.

The *current condition* might be described as follows:

> A "buddy," or preceptor, is assigned to orient and train new nurses. The buddy was selected because she was perceived to be competent and a good role model. The methods used are primarily demonstration, imitation, and provision of some information on procedures and protocols. The new nurse is assigned one patient, and the buddy has her regular patient load. The teaching is done on the job.

Several problems become evident with this method of orienting new staff nurses:

> . . . Some buddies resent add-on responsibilities because they are still expected to carry a full assignment. There is no recognition or monetary reward for this additional work.
>
> . . . Some see training as an encroachment on the quality of care they hold themselves accountable for with their own patients. This condition creates frustration or dissatisfaction with self and the job. Some feelings are communicated directly or indirectly to the new nurse, who then reacts to the value conflict that her buddy is experiencing.
>
> . . . Sometimes these reactions are norm setters for the new nurse — she learns to stay out of the way, keep a low profile, live with fear and anxiety about her ability to perform, and use trial and error as the way to learn.
>
> . . . The high turnover, less commitment to learning, resistance to change, low self-concept, and lack of job satisfaction make the cost of unplanned training or training by assumption ("a nurse knows . . .") very costly and increase the probability of early burnout.

The *desired condition* might be described as follows:

> A buddy, or preceptor, will have an opportunity to discuss with the nurse educator what is involved in becoming a buddy. The buddy will willingly decide to accept the responsibility and will contract for training and assistance with the nurse educator. Assistance will include negotiating for a realistic patient load during the intensive part of the training of new staff people. The buddy will receive systematic training and feedback using the principles and concepts of adult education. The co-learner model will become the model not only for staff education but also for patient and family education.

Creation of the desired condition by preparing the buddy to accept and successfully carry out the teaching-learning assignment might include the following knowledge, attitudes, and skills.

Knowledge the buddy needs:

- An understanding of the differences between adult education and traditional education principles and practice
- Characteristics of the adult learner
- An understanding of the co-learner role and how it works
- Dynamics of learner involvement
- Insight as to how the holistic approach to the learner facilitates learning and increases self-concept

Attitudes the buddy needs:

- Positive reinforcement, not constructive criticism
- Expectations that the new nurse will succeed
- Sharing of responsibility
- Positive attitudes for positive results

Skills the buddy needs:

- Contracting (*i.e.,* negotiating)
- Active listening
- Problem-solving
- Interpersonal
- Writing ability for the teaching-learning plan:
- Learning needs (skills inventory)
- Learning objectives
- Methods to be used
- Skills evaluation
- Organization and planning of time
- Selection of clinical experiences

This example highlights the need for a program to train buddies or preceptors who are resource people in staff education. Before plans for such a program are launched, however, the need for it must be screened against the statements of philosophy that have been approved and accepted by administration. Then one determines priorities by seeing where the proposed program fits with what is already being done. Not everything that needs to be done can be done at once. Educational programs are built around *survival needs first.*

Another approach is determination of *deficiency needs.* These are needs that may be met by improving working conditions, elevating salary, and changing policies. Then, the *inherent growth needs* should be identified. These are needs that may be met by acknowledging achievement and providing advancement. This approach will create an environment that supports a "quality-of-life" philosophy and that helps staff achieve a balance between personal and professional goals. (For specific techniques for needs assessment, see discussion of step 1 in the training cycle shown in Fig. 40-2.)

The next component, objectives, is based on meeting the identified needs and making the statement of philosophy a dynamic power.

Objectives

Objectives are statements that describe the goal or outcomes of the educational program. These objectives are broad statements that can serve as guidelines for the structure of several different programs. Objectives provide constraints so that resources can be channeled effectively and efficiently and provide the framework for fixing responsibility and accountability for the educational activities of the unit.

Examples of program objectives are as follows:

> Given adequate support and resources, develop educational programs that enable CCU staff to perform their roles effectively, efficiently, and with personal satisfaction.

Given information and learning activities, each critical care nurse will develop a self-directed learning contract with the nurse educator to achieve relevant continuing education that will (1) meet relicensure requirements and (2) achieve professional goals.

Each program objective must be screened through the statements of philosophy and needs, not only *prior* to implementation but also on a regular basis *after* implementation. This process permits evaluation to take place at each stage of program development. It also provides necessary checks and balances so that the unit can respond to changes and evaluations of the programs.

Implementation

The structure for implementation is a master plan with clearly stated policies and procedures and with specifically identified program areas.

There may be no precedent, with suggested policies, procedures, and programs, for initiating this plan. Even so, one is needed for the nurse educator who is responsible for staff education. Otherwise, she will find it impossible to be accountable for anything that is ill defined, ambiguous in nature, or unstructured. Perhaps you, the reader, are the nurse educator. If so, you can ensure your own need to be successful and satisfied with your work by using your competence and exercising your leadership, and by being motivated by your own beliefs you can build your expertise and interpersonal relationships. You can be assertive through the way in which you get your peers, supervisors, and medical colleagues involved in creating the master plan. Most important, you will want to work with a mentor. As you acquire sensitivity to consensus decision-making and to timing (not moving too fast for those involved), you will need to separate rejection of ideas from rejection of self and from being discouraged and disillusioned.

To begin building the master plan structure, clearly stated policies are needed. *Policies* serve as guidelines for the administration of the staff educational programs. Thus, some areas to explore are as follows:

- Educational leave—paid or unpaid
- Reimbursement for travel, lodging, or mileage incurred for approved education
- Recognition through promotion, merit increases, and performance appraisals of increased competence resulting from training and development opportunities
- Prerequisites for enrolling in core programs and advanced programs
- Requirements for participation in planning and conducting in-service programs

Policies are tested and evaluated as they are used. Criteria for testing their practicality and effectiveness include evaluating them against the philosophy, needs assessment, and objectives previously developed and implementing the program requests and situations that evolve.

Examples of policy statements follow:

Each employee in the CCU will be expected to complete 12 contact hours of continuing education as a regular part of her work schedule each year, based on anniversary date.

New employees will complete 40 hours of scheduled core orientation during the first 3 months of employment. Upon satisfactory completion of the probationary period, the new employee may apply for the critical care advanced course after 6 months of demonstrated increased competency.

Each professional nurse in critical care will develop a self-directed learning plan that will include (1) a statement of objectives, (2) proposed activities to be carried out, (3) possible resources to be used, (4) validation process to determine degree of achieving objectives, and (5) a contract with nurse educator, colleague, or self to carry out the plan, meet deadlines, and set checkpoints for progress reports.[4]

Procedures are systematic and ensure some degree of uniformity in implementing certain aspects of the master plan. They are necessary to clarify the way things are to be done, such as applying for educational leave, preparing budget and justifying new programs, scheduling space for in-service, keeping records of completed training, and documenting increased competency for merit review.

The following is an example of a procedure:

Purpose
• An educational calendar will be set to log continuing education requests for training outside the hospital.
Procedure
• Requests should be entered 3 weeks prior to the scheduled event.
• Each person is responsible for entering requests on the calendar.
• Educational requests will be determined on a first-come basis.
• Exceptions to this procedure will be discussed with the nurse educator or critical care supervisor.
• Prior to attending the event, the nurse will schedule a conference with the nurse educator to review expectations and how the program relates to personal and professional goals.
• After the event, the nurse will share with the nurse educator how the learning experience will be used in the work situation. This will be done 1 week after the scheduled event.

Procedures need to be screened against policies to validate their feasibility and relevance and then screened with staff and others involved in the process.

If procedures are cumbersome — they present obstacles rather than gateways to learning — they will need to be reviewed, revised, or eliminated.

Program areas included in the master plan will be the broad areas one expects to develop. Individual modules, units, and independent programs within each area are discussed in the following section. The broad areas will include some or all of the following, depending on the philosophy, needs, objectives, policies, and procedures of staff education:

Examples of program areas are as follows:

Orientation programs
    Introduction to unit, unit goals, and personnel
    Introduction to role as interdependent practitioner
    Unit skills module based on skills inventory
On-the-job training
    Individualized training (*i.e.,* buddy system)
    Modules — specific basic skills for new graduate
            specific skills for general nursing R.N.
            advanced skills for critical care nurse
In-service education
    On-going, regular training sessions to update staff in other areas as well as critical care
    Satisfaction of relicensure requirements
Staff development
    Interpersonal competence
    Leadership development
    Preparation for advancement
    Lateral development for mastery of critical care specialties
    Certification in American Association of Critical Care Nurses
Organizational development
    Increasing effectiveness of unit
    Role clarification and team-building
    Creative problem-solving and conflict resolution
    Planning for and implementing significant change

The last three program areas hold special significance for the nurse educator. Today's professionals set high standards for themselves and look for ways to balance their work with their personal and social lives. These program areas prepare people for the changes, improve the quality of life and effectiveness of the unit, and prevent burnout by anticipating growth needs and reducing frustration, fear, and anxiety in a prime time — the 8-hour shift.

The nurse educator generates the leadership; however, the responsibility of program development is shared with each person on the staff and with all others who have a stake in a quality care unit.

Evaluation

You will note that in the model (see Fig. 40-1), the evaluation component is a two-way feedback system. The process of evaluation constantly checks the interaction and relationship of the other four components.

For instance, in order to justify certain programs, one checks the proposed objectives against the statements of philosophy, the statements of need, and the various policies and procedures to validate the "fit." The same is true of any change—the feedback process is built in to evaluate and validate the feasibility of change.

An example of an evaluation follows:

> *Situation*
> • The state law has been changed and so have the number of contact hours for certification.
> • The staff requests more than the approved number of hours of regularly scheduled work time devoted to continuing education.
>
> The policy would have to be evaluated with the new data and its impact on the staff. This does not necessarily mean that the policy will be changed. It does mean the policy would be reviewed and evaluated for its effectiveness.

An increasingly common practice of many organizations is to set aside several days (weekends, usually) to go to a local retreat site and evaluate the elements of the program planning model and set new goals and objectives for the following year. It is very important to know where you are going and even more important to know if you really got there!

In summary, developing a staff program around this planning model gives one a foundation on which to build various educational programs. Administrative decisions regarding the program would be made within this structure. Creating the master plan, with each type of training and development program, brings the model together. The ongoing process of evaluating each component in the model with the other components ensures a viable plan and one that is structurally sound.

Assessing Feasibility

If you are the one responsible for critical care and education is decentralized, you may need to assess the feasibility of this new role. The following will enable you to look at your total job with particular emphasis on the teaching-learning role.

1. List the functions you are accountable for. By writing a detailed list, you will develop a concrete picture of what you do.
2. Next, rank-order these functions according to your own priorities. Perhaps this will be difficult to do, for most everything you do will be of equal importance. However, do number them. In so doing, you lay the foundation for the next important step.
3. Critically evaluate each of these functions. Should you delegate, discontinue, reschedule, reorganize the function or retain the function as it is? This evaluation may provide data for reallocating your time and some job functions so that you can assume new training functions.
4. Now, on your priority listing of responsibilities, insert training and staff development functions in a realistic position. By doing this, you crystallize intent to create new job functions and willingness to allocate time and effort to do so.
5. Evaluate the personal resources you bring to this new role of educator. Write down the teaching you are already doing. Find answers to questions, such as "What help do I give new employees and floats? How do I introduce new ideas, procedures, equipment, and supplies? After attending an educational event, how do I share the information? Do I work side by side with my staff in a crisis situation, and what does my staff learn from me? How do I use the time when census is low? What do employees learn in the periodic performance appraisals?"

Have you found that you are doing many of these? You may want to add questions that occurred to you and more completely analyze the teaching and learning that is going on in your unit at the present time. The process of disciplining yourself to write down what you do will help you to

• Determine the training currently occurring
• Recognize and build on the teaching you are already doing
• Clarify those areas that you may want to change

Now, following the pattern used in assessing your own resources, list the administrative resources available to you, especially those that will provide needed support for launching your educational program. Your answers to the following questions may help:

• What is the attitude of nursing service toward experimenting with new ideas, new functions, new programs?
• What position does nursing administration take when plans do not work out?
• What can you expect from the multidisciplinary committee on critical care?
• What kind of financial support would administration provide, such as additional coverage, compensatory time, overtime pay for educational program attendance, underwriting the costs for outside consultants and courses?
• What hospital space is provided for staff conferences and how available is it?

Next, assess the resources that the education department offers. What support will the director give a decentralized in-service program? What materials are available? What unique resources are available within the hospital and community?

As a result of the resource assessment, you will have a basis for deciding whether or not decentralization or nurse educator is for you. If it shows promise, you are ready to study the characteristics of decentralized programming—programming tailored for adult learners.

CHARACTERISTICS OF DECENTRALIZED CLINICAL EDUCATION

The most unique characteristics of clinically based education are its flexibility, spontaneity, timing, relevance, conscious exploitation of daily situations for learning, active involvement of everyone present, and supportive nonjudgmental climate. The following brief description of each may illustrate the dynamic nature of a small, interdependent staff, personally involved in meeting their own learning goals and the general goals of the unit.

Flexibility implies that even though there are thoughtfully developed plans to meet long-term goals, changes can be made when unexpected developments occur that offer excellent learning opportunities. It allows freedom to change the master plan and to alter priorities based on current situations and needs. If the staff can be comfortable with the freedom to deviate from scheduled plans and then exercise this freedom, flexibility to meet staff's needs becomes evident.

Spontaneity helps the staff learn from daily, on-the-spot situations as they occur. Out of these situations grows the opportunity to acquire insights, identify new knowledge, and recognize new skills. Staff will develop a sensitivity for the inherent learning that is to be found in the moment. This quality spawns unexpected opportunities to learn. It makes learning fun!

A *sense of timing* is essential in planning programs and designing individualized staff development. Developing a "feeling for the pulse of what is happening" in the unit allows you to feed-in either programmed or spontaneous learning experiences and to use time more effectively.

Relevance of potential learning is validated by identifying basic issues such as

• How the information will be used
• Why it should be offered
• What changes will be required
• What changes individuals will need to make
• What results can be expected
• What risks and payoffs can be anticipated

Taking time to articulate these issues will pinpoint their relevance to patient service and to the goals of the unit.

To *exploit daily situations for learning,* one selects a situation on the basis of frequency and uniqueness of the experience. Another criterion is the opportunity for all those involved to see the same occurrence and share their different perceptions and how they experienced it. From this, you can create new procedures, anticipate similar problems, and check out the understanding for future events. It also affords an opportunity to demonstrate role and task relationships.

Active involvement of the total person is vital in the teaching-learning process. Research shows that people remember

• 10% of what they read
• 20% of what they hear
• 30% of what they see
• 50% of what they see and hear
• 80% of what they say
• 90% of what they say as they do a thing[5]

These facts encourage new methods and techniques in staff training and development.

A *nonjudgmental climate* in the clinical unit supports a creative educational program. For staff who want to grow personally and professionally while working, such a climate allows moderate risk-taking, acceptance of responsibility for experimentation, and accountability for results. It thus facilitates understanding and acceptance of team relationships and individual differences. *The emphasis is not on what is right or wrong but on what is the most effective way to accomplish the task.* This attitude is the most significant one to develop when a new training program, based on staff involvement, is undertaken.

The preceding paragraphs describe the characteristics separately, but in a well-conceived program these features are blended, balanced, and counterbalanced. You can measure your degree of effectiveness by the degree to which you have integrated these components.

NEW ROLE: CO-LEARNER

Probably the most exciting part of this new role is the fact that there is little precedent for it. Part of the reason is the recent major shift in emphasis from "teaching" to "learning." Becoming a learning specialist in the CCU offers a unique opportunity to develop the role as you live it.

The eminent psychologist Carl Rogers points out that as a teacher he discovered he couldn't teach anyone anything. He believes the *student learns what he wants and needs to learn.* This fact imposes a significant change in the role of the traditional teacher. Rogers believes his role as teacher is to help the student learn. To do this, the teacher needs to assume a new role of co-learner and learn many things about the learner, from the learner, and with the learner.

All members of the staff will enter into a co-learner relationship in the teaching-learning process. The learner role for staff will change from listening passively to the teacher to being actively involved in and responsible for what they want and need to learn and when they need to learn it.

Two important pieces of research have influenced the present approach to adult education. One is the impact of the adult stages of development, as popularly described in Gail Sheehey's *Passages,* and the other is the concept of life-long learning based on the work of Allen Tough.[6]

Because employees are adults, they need to be thought of as adults who want to learn to be effective and successful in their work. Powell and Aker point this out in the following:

> Adults do not need, nor do they wish, to be overly directed or controlled in their learning experiences. They are self-directed, autonomous human beings, and desire a strong sense of dignity and individual worth. Nothing will offend this sense of dignity more than to have an individual throw bits of information at them, like raw chunks of meat, and demand that they accept them.
>
> The adult is a learner; as such, the responsibility for learning should be placed upon him. He will choose, if allowed, what he learns and how he learns it, and will also decide the rate and speed at which he learns best. He will need helpful advice and suggestions, however, as to how he should best continue his self-directed learning . . . and this is where the teacher comes in, as a helpful aide who is prepared, not to answer the student's every question, or to solve his problem, but to help him develop the skills to solve his own problems. *The teacher should not attempt to play God.* Her adult students are as mature as she, and in certain ways probably more so. With a deep interest in the student the teacher can help him find his own way, but find his own way he must.*

The teacher, as co-learner, does assume part of the responsibility for the teaching-learning process. This responsibility centers around planning and organizing learning activities for the satisfaction of the learner's needs by having "the right resources and materials, at the right time and in the right place" so that the learner can learn when ready.

If you embrace this concept of teacher, you will probably have to unlearn many preconceived ideas. However, the excitement of sharing responsibility for learning with your fellow professionals will bring its own rewards.

Characteristics of effective co-learners include

- Considerable time for planning
- Individualized instruction made practical in terms of interests, needs, wants, and aspirations of staff

* Powell T, Aker GF: Teaching and learning in adult basic education. Mimeographed, Department of Adult Education, Florida State University, Florida

- High degree of flexibility
- Acceptance of "people as they are" and "where they are"
- Use of a wide variety of methods and techniques
- Role model for learner behavior and resource behavior
- Holistic approach to each person—recognition of the intellectual, emotional, physical, social, and spiritual attributes of the learner that strongly influence the learning process

Planning is certainly needed in order to develop unit, staff, and individual goals; to determine which method, technique, or material will facilitate the achievement of objectives; and to develop criteria for evaluating progress and change. Much of planning, however, is shared with staff members, as are the instructional responsibilities. A sensitive teacher constantly adjusts and changes the plan as new opportunities are presented and as feedback is obtained from the staff.

Many techniques and methods are available. Choice is governed by the learning need and the situation.

- Presentation techniques: lecturettes, videotape, dialogue, interview, group interview, demonstration, slides, dramatization, cassette tapes, exhibits, trips, reading
- Discussion techniques: guided discussion, article or book-based discussion, problem-solving discussion, group-centered discussion
- Simulation techniques: role-playing, role rehearsal, critical-incident process, case method, games, participative cases, sociodrama
- Organizational development techniques: goal-setting, role clarification, negotiating, group process, sharing, support groups, experiential exercises
- Nonverbal exercises
- Skill-practice techniques: exercises, drills, coaching

Allow yourself to be a learner and develop a repertoire of techniques by experimenting. Keep in mind the objective, match it with a technique, and then evaluate its effectiveness. Certain techniques are more effective in bringing about behavioral and attitudinal changes than others. So, if you have a choice, choose the one that involves your staff in active participation.

DYNAMICS OF STAFF INVOLVEMENT

If you can trigger creativity, enhance curiosity, encourage new interests, and stimulate the desire for learning and self-fulfillment, while reducing fear of failure and resistance to change, you will effectively perform your tasks and fulfill your role as an adult educator.

Powell and Aker offer several principles to make the

Principles of Adult Learning

1. *Adults learn better when they are actively involved in the learning process.* The more they participate through discussion groups and in other group techniques and the more responsibility they are given for what happens in a learning situation, the more effectively they will progress.

2. *Adults can learn materials that apply to their daily work more quickly than they can learn irrelevant materials.* Adults will be receptive to new information only if they are sure it is useful to them immediately.

3. *Adults will accept new ideas more quickly if these ideas support previous beliefs.* Adults come to learning situations with a well-fixed set of values and beliefs, regardless of whether or not they verbalize them. They tend to reject information that attacks or destroys their beliefs.

4. *Adults' needs and backgrounds must be understood and integrated into their learning experiences as much as possible. Out of feelings of inadequacy, many adults believe they cannot learn.* This belief will be evident in their attitude toward learning situations and toward themselves. Before they are placed in a learning situation, adults should first feel encouraged enough to attempt to learn; otherwise they are likely to fail before they begin.

5. *To the extent possible, adults should be allowed to pursue their own areas of interest at their own rate and to find answers to questions on their own.* Regardless of how they may react to an authoritarian learning atmosphere, adults are not likely to grasp knowledge that is forced on them. A teacher should act as a resource person, available to guide or discuss a problem with the learner. The teacher should *not* have all the answers or even pretend to have them.

6. *Adults, because of possible unhappy past experiences, should be prepared for learning so it will be a pleasant, rather than an unpleasant, experience.* Drill and repetition of material will not help them to learn. It will only make them dislike the learning experience even more than they did before.

7. *Adult learners should be rewarded immediately for success and should never feel as if they are being punished for making a mistake.* When rewarded, they will want to continue the experience. If punished, they are apt to reject the entire situation either by leaving it physically or by refusing to become involved.

8. *Adults learn in a series of "plateaus"; that is, they do well for a while, then level off in performance, but they will move on again if they have not become discouraged.* This is a natural process, and adults should understand that it is, so that they will not give up.

9. *Adults should always know why they are learning and toward what goal they are aiming.* They should understand what steps are necessary to reach a particular learning goal, and in what order they should come. If adults become confused about where they are going or why they are going there, they will lose interest in going any place.*

* Powell T, Aker GF: Teaching and Learning in Adult Basic Education. Mimeographed. Tallahassee, FL, Florida State University, 1971

---

job easier. These are listed in the chart titled "Principles of Adult Learning" (see further on).

In summary, the decentralization of education and staff development in the CCU offers an opportunity to experiment with innovative ways of meeting the learning needs and to achieve a higher quality of nursing service for patients. The characteristics of a decentralized training program provide a framework upon which one can create the new co-learner role. The risks in undertaking this task should be moderate, but the rewards should be great.

THE PROCESS OF STAFF TRAINING AND DEVELOPMENT

The preceding section focused on the overall, general educational plan for decentralization. The following section focuses on a practical and systematic approach to the process of designing specific programs within the broad program areas of orientation, in-service, on-the-job, continuing education, and self-directed learning projects.

One needs to keep in mind the purposes of training and staff development:

- *Training's* primary purposes are the discovery, development, and change of people's behaviors and attitudes to improve job performance.
- *Staff development's* primary purposes include those of training and meeting some of the staff members' need for self-worth and satisfaction through work.

Careful thought to the blending and balancing of these two is crucial if one is to achieve the ultimate goals of improving quality of work life for staff and providing quality, effective care for the patient and the family.

Industrial Systems

To provide some background for your orientation, we will consider the contributions of progressive industrial management in integrating organizational and individual goals. Researchers attempted to discover the key to releasing motivational energy of employees toward achieving the company's objectives. The findings showed that management's concentrated effort and the employees' willingness to participate resulted in collaborative planning in job and staff development. Over a period of time the results of these cooperative efforts lowered operating costs and turnover, facilitated produce development and new marketing and management techniques, and increased profits—the bottom line!

Health Systems

In shifting from industrial to health care systems and to hospitals in particular, the problem of tapping the full potential of people resources is of genuine concern. With cost containment, fewer people will be expected to do more work and do it more effectively and efficiently. With the pressure to deliver higher quality health care, control costs, and more fully use staff, hospitals must look for alternatives to the narrowly conceived industrial assembly-line way of delivering health services. The product in health care is not a *thing*; it is individualized total care for the patient.

With the multiple numbers of professional specialties and skilled technicians, the challenge to integrate persons who come with special education and varied work experiences is somewhat overwhelming. To this complex situation add the fact that these people come initially with a desire to use their special expertise and with the need to keep growing in their occupational life as well as their personal life. It appears that the key to genuine motivation rests within the employee and is released when the need to keep growing is met.

The Training Cycle

The training cycle is the process model offered as a means to release motivational energy to facilitate the planning of realistic and needed training that can be made manageable and measurable (Fig. 40-2). Becoming familiar with the model enhances development of individual units of instruction within broad general areas. It can be used for one's own personal and professional learning plan or as a guide for working and planning with each staff member. Moreover, it will provide a continuing framework for recycling as new needs emerge. The training cycle involves seven steps:

1. Identify and validate individual and group needs.
2. Set learning objectives for performance and growth.
3. Plan and contract to achieve learning objectives.
4. Select resources.
5. Manage learning activities.
6. Evaluate objectives, performance, and learning plans.
7. Recycle.

If you have made an assessment of personal resources, you may now be aware of how good you feel as a teacher and of the value of more active staff involvement in planning the training. Such an initial awareness is shown in the model in a kind of free form. It represents consciousness of a need but lacks validation necessary to determine whether or not it is a viable learning need.

Step 1. Identify and Validate Individual Needs

In the determination of training needs, the best source of information will be the people with whom one works and by whom patient care is provided. As might be anticipated, different needs will come from each shift and from persons who "float" or "relieve" on days off. Remember, all persons involved in critical care have relevant training needs, including physicians, clergy, and ward clerks.

Data on needs can be obtained in many ways. Following are four that may be familiar: interviewing, observation, periodic performance evaluations, and planned and unplanned changes. Several methods usually are employed and result in a *data base* of "conscious needs."

Interviewing. Individuals in the CCU can be interviewed either formally or informally and either on a one-to-one basis or in a group. Preparation prior to interviewing will facilitate gathering specific data and guide the discussion. The use of some open-ended questions will permit free-flowing input from participants. Examples of open-ended questions are

• What do you like best about your job?
• What do you like least?
• If you could, how would you change working in the unit?
• What problems bother you the most?
• How could training for the unit be improved?
• What plans do you have to earn contact hours for relicensure?

Actively listening to what is said and being aware of what is not said will help identify the needs. Taking notes verbatim while interviewing and then summarizing with the same words will assist in validating them with the person or persons involved. Or, the interviewer can ask the participants to prioritize the needs. Validation of need and priority will help in overall planning.

Observation. Observation during the training cycle involves guided observations of job performance and of interactions with patients, ancillary personnel, and one another. It also includes observation of contacts with persons who provide direct services to the patients but who are not part of the critical care staff. These perceptions will provide the criteria for deter-

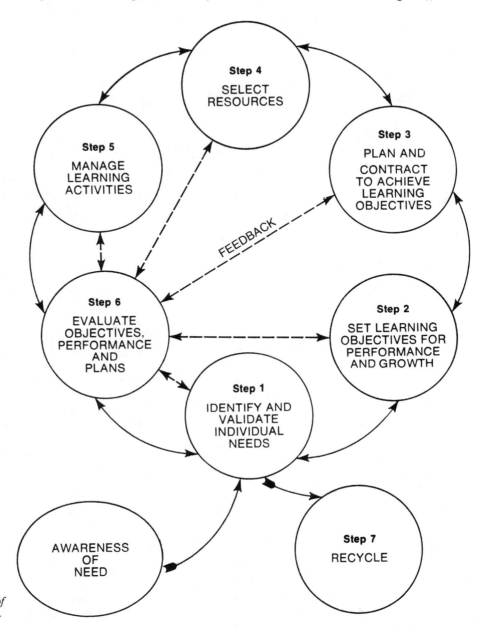

FIGURE 40-2
Training cycle: relationship of components; feedback system.

mining the required level of competence for effective performance. Therefore, observations must be based on criteria set and shared prior to making the observations. The skills inventory for critical care would be a logical starting point. The quality assurance standards would be another. The observational data will reveal skill deficiencies as well as unconscious needs (needs not revealed in the interviews but evident in behavior and attitude). To validate one's perceptions, feedback to each person is necessary.

Periodic Performance Evaluation Data. This information may indicate needs and resources that both employee and educator are aware of. In some cases,

reports may cover several evaluation periods and reflect changes in the performance level. In studying this data, consider the evaluator and his perceptions and biases and the abilities, skills, and attitudes that each employee demonstrates toward self, job, and others. Currently, most performance evaluations are based on goals set by the employee, the degree of achievement, and the way in which they were achieved.

A suggestion from Malcolm Knowles might help pinpoint how the educational needs, which the data produced, are defined.[7] He states that a need is "the gap between present level of competency and a higher level required for effective performance" as defined by the organization, the individual, or society. His con-

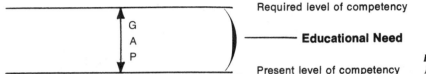

FIGURE 40-3
Definition of an educational need.

cept is illustrated in Figure 40-3. Writing statements to describe clearly the two levels of competency will make need identification easier. An example follows:

Reduced level of competency (standard)	The primary nurse will talk with patient's family in the waiting room a minimum of two times a shift.
Possible educational need	G A P
Present level of competency	The primary nurse has not talked with the families of patients because she is "too busy"

Gap: determine the reasons for failure to meet the standard. For example, does the nurse have difficulty managing time, is she uncomfortable with interpersonal relationships with families in crisis, or does she not accept the standard? Is it a training need?

To answer this question, a profile of each nurse's experience and some well-designed open-ended questions will help identify or validate whether or not there really is an educational need.

Planned Change. This is more easily handled than unplanned change. People are constantly in need of obtaining pertinent information, clarification of expectations, and knowledge of the skills and competencies necessary to manage the variety of changes that are occurring effectively. Thus, the responsibility of preparing people for change whenever possible is included in the educational package. An example follows:

> The installation of new computers at the nursing station will provide information needed for physicians' decisions. Getting staff ready for the change by providing information about the reasons for change, the new equipment, the advantages and disadvantages, and the changes in staff work prepares people for the learning that will follow and will, it is hoped, lower the resistance to change.

It is important to lower the resistance before it has a strong basis. The job will be easier for those who know the staff's concerns and who have time to work with them in indentifying alternatives, modifications, and suggestions that will involve them in finally accepting and implementing the change.

In the case of *unplanned change,* recognition of the fact that some people would rather not do something than fail at unfamiliar tasks is essential. Coaching them as they perform different tasks will help them meet their need to be successful. By taking the time to individualize training, one not only builds commitment to the change, but also strengthens the co-learner role with them.

Validation. To "check out and make sure the need is real" becomes the issue of validation. Validation requires that data sources are sought that will verify the reality and the extent of the need. It supports the fact that the *gap,* or educational need, exists and justifies further consideration. The best source of validation and the one most frequently overlooked is the person for whom the training is being planned—the learner. Sources such as supervisors, administrators, researchers, and consultants also provide verification. In many instances, their input is essential; however, learners not only must be aware of the need to increase competency but also must want to do it for their own reasons. Therefore the learner provides one of the soundest answers.

Knowles phrases it this way:

> The more concretely an individual can identify his aspirations and assess his present level of competencies in relation to them—the more exactly he can define his educational needs—the more intensely will he be motivated to learn. And the more congruent the needs of the individual are with the aspirations of the organization . . . [and vice versa] the more likely will effective learning take place.[8]

Assuming the need identified and validated is an educational need, the capabilities of the unit and staff form the first criterion of whether or not the need can be met. The probability that training needs can best be met in the unit is a basic assumption. To increase the level of competency on the job, the reality situation offered by the unit provides the best learning laboratory. If the need is more long-range, staff development may be the logical approach. This may involve feasible programs outside the unit, such as a core critical care course.

The final consideration is determining the priority of needs that result from the assessment. It is wise to involve the staff in helping to establish priorities. If the first need undertaken is "bite size" and the chances of meeting it are good, one probably has a winning combination to move to the next step in the process.

Step 2. Set Individual Learning Objectives for Performance and Growth

The second step is setting goals and objectives so that training and staff development efforts will have direction and achieve positive results. *Goals* will be identified as long-term targets and will be broad in scope. For instance, an educational goal might be stated:

> To involve each staff member in planning and implementing the in-service program for the unit.

Another might be stated:

> To provide more effective nursing care in the unit by increasing the level of competency of each person in meeting not only the physical needs but also the psychosocial needs of critical care patients and their families.

Although these examples are explicitly stated and provide guidelines on which a training program can be structured, more specific objectives (short-range targets) are needed to ensure understanding and measurable achievement of goals.

These more specific learning objectives are stated in behavioral terms that describe outcomes, or results.[9] By writing behavioral objectives, the learner has a clearer idea of what is expected, and both educator and learner can measure the results. Use of active verbs (*e.g.,* "perform," "demonstrate," "master," "use") sharpens statements of objectives. Writing objectives helps in determining content and learning experiences. They keep one on target.

Short-term objectives usually include the following characteristics:

- They represent behaviors that are observable by others.
- They are specific, limited in scope, and include certain conditions, such as time and method.
- They are measurable.

There are three types of objectives that will need to be considered if improved performance and growth are expected outcomes.

- *Cognitive* objectives: information
- *Affective* objectives: attitudes, self-concept
- *Psychomotor* objectives: skills

An example of a psychomotor learning objective follows:

> Given instruction on the use of monitoring equipment (information) by the head nurse, within 5 days (time) a new staff nurse will be able to prepare a patient and properly attach equipment (result/outcome).

When initiating the idea of having staff write personal objectives to increase their effectiveness and job satisfaction, one will find that a warm-up to the idea is necessary. At first it may be difficult. Determining objectives may be a new skill, and the staff will need training to do it successfully. Also, they may feel threatened by the idea because it represents a change and it fixes responsibility on them to achieve their objectives. To involve staff from the very beginning, one might find it helpful to raise questions that stimulate their active involvement:

- What would I be doing differently if I were to set a goal?
- How might someone else know that I have changed my style in interacting with patients and their families?
- What will I need to know and do to reach my goal?
- What can I do for myself?
- What help will I need from others? Who specifically?

After each person identifies goals, co-workers can review and critique them. In the process of sharing, staff can sharpen one another's goals by asking questions. This helps determine what kind of goal is being set. Is it a "must" (a survival) goal? Is it a "want" (it would be nice) goal? Is it attainable? Is it an ideal goal that could never be attained and yet would set direction for the maker? Is it a maintenance goal? Or is it a growth goal that combines elements of the ideal and achievable reality?

With feedback, each staff member will clarify the goal, making it more specific, more realistic, more measurable, and more attainable. This process makes it possible for a person to request feedback from co-workers and to assess progress. Another outcome of this process is the building of a mutual support group, and this kind of positive reinforcement is essential in high-stress areas.

After setting the goals, it is necessary to develop a plan to achieve individual goals. Thus, objectives, or mini-goals, are defined. Each person identifies the barriers or blocks that stand in the way of attaining the goal. Along with this, each person is encouraged to identify all of his personal assets or strengths. After listing the blocks and assets, each person writes objectives to deal with each block. These objectives become short-term and consist of the small steps one takes toward the desired outcome.

Example of translating a barrier into a short-term objective:

> *Barrier:* When I'm not sure what to do next, I procrastinate.
> *Objective:* I will list all of the information I need and ask for assistance to begin moving toward my goal

This process helps each person understand how functional objectives can be in generating action that is aimed directly at the target.

The step of goal-objective formation is probably the most difficult of all, but it is essential and can never be overlooked. As staff become more comfortable with working together in planning the initial steps, goals and objectives may change. It should be remembered that this element of change is implicit when working with the concept of process.

Step 3. Plan and Contract to Achieve Learning Objectives

In order to reach objectives, staff will need assistance in developing a plan of action that will zero in on the forces that slow down learning. Kurt Lewin's force-field analysis provides a model that is useful for effective planning.

There is a natural resistance to change, and the removal of this resistance is essential if the desired learning is to take place. Honest acknowledgment of resistance to learning and acceptance of it as a normal phenomenon will remove some of it. This strategy helps the learner identify the reasons for resisting, and this awareness will make it easier to move toward building on the assets, abilities, and strengths that support new learning.

Encourage learners to identify the specific resources they can use to weaken, reduce, or overcome these blocks and free energy to accomplish their objectives. Help them identify the driving forces—those things that tend to propel them into action and move them toward the learning objective. These forces provide the motivation. When a person capitalizes on these and applies personal resources to offset the resistance, that individual is ready to develop a plan.

Work with each person in determining what is to be done, when it is to be done, how it is to be done, why it is to be done, what the payoffs are, what the risks are, and what degree of success is anticipated. Help each one assign specific responsibilities to himself and to other resource people that were identified. Help clarify the self-assignment of responsibilities—things the person holds himself accountable for. Encourage specific information on the person's expectations of others, including the educator.

A contract, or working agreement, is an effective device for achieving and supporting goals and objectives. The contract is not formal. It evolves as staff and learners openly discuss expectations of one another in terms of what needs to be done to achieve learning objectives. For instance, in assigning responsibilities, dialogue clarifies what is needed, why a particular resource is best, and who does what and when. To clarify the assignment, the persons involved should discuss reasonable checkpoints and set deadlines. This prac-

tice provides specific data for mutually shared expectations. This agreement provides the mechanism for checking progress, the status of assignments, and problems as well as an opportunity to renegotiate if indicated.

If one keeps in mind a strategy that will help staff understand and accept the tension between their desire to grow and their desire to remain the same, their movement through the process of *unlearning, learning,* and *relearning* will be greatly assisted.

Adults resist unlearning things that have worked for them in the past and that were adequate for the situation. In the process of giving up familiar ways, adults will accept the necessity of learning new ways if they increase competence. However, learning is not enough: Adults need to internalize the learning—make it a regular part of their behavior. Thus they need the opportunity and time to relearn, or "refreeze" the new behavior so that it becomes their typical response to a situation. Follow-up with coaching provides positive reinforcement that speeds up the refreezing process. One might find it helpful to make notes on a daily schedule as a reminder to do the follow-up because it may require only observation to measure the internalization of new behaviors.

Risks and payoffs, two basic factors, are powerful and influence the learning process. Because learning imposes change, it is important to make sure that the risk is a moderate one. Moderate risks result in a fair degree of safety and a good chance for success. Knowing the degree of risk that they are taking enables staff to accept responsibility for learning. (A nonjudgmental climate supports risk-taking.)

Equally important are the payoffs. Because frequently these are taken for granted, plan very carefully for genuine payoffs. An open discussion of "both sides of the coin" of the learning experience—risks and payoffs—will make it much easier for learners to buy into an experience. It will allow co-workers to give support during the learning process, and learners will have a gauge to anticipate the results of changed behavior as they strive for increased competency and self-fulfillment. Self-fulfillment is one of the most valued regards.

One further point: Adults want immediate payoffs in return for learning new things. They want to be able to use the learning *now,* not at some indefinite future time. Being able to use the learning effectively and feeling competent about it is the most effective immediate payoff. Documented goal achievement through the learning objectives provides information for merit increases—another concrete payoff.

Step 4. Select Resources

After the action plan has been developed, and even as it is taking shape, the identification of appropriate learning resources follows. Look for situations, people, and materials that will enhance learning opportunities.

Situations offer unique resources. For example

- *Participative learning as a resource.* Unstructured learning groups provide rich resource material for learning about "people things." Task groups are useful for integrating theory inputs into operational objectives.
- *The learner as a resource for planning and implementing programs.* The creative and practical forces generated by employees who accept the role of learner release resources that can be obtained only from such involvement.
- *Daily living experiences as a resource for learning.* When employees accept role playing and role training as a way of improving their competency, daily happenings in the unit provide the content for the learning situations. These offer a rare potential for reality-checking attitudes, values, and habitual responses to situations. They afford employees the opportunity to try on different behaviors—to expand their behavioral repertoire for meeting common experiences. As resources, these are among the most stimulating and exciting.
- *Spontaneity as a resource in learning.* When spontaneity is present, learning is precious, stimulating, and fun. How does one develop spontaneity, make room for it, and capitalize on it? Spontaneity develops in a supportive, nonevaluative climate. Some norms that govern behavior in the critical care unit may inhibit the development of spontaneity.
- *Conflict as a resource for learning.* From genuine differences in values, expectations, techniques, roles, and priorities comes the grist for conflict. Working through these differences provides another viable resource for learning. Here the issue is how to develop a climate in which people can learn from conflict, to create a norm where conflict is legitimatized or sanctioned, and to set ground rules so that the conflict can be resolved. Probably one of the most effective resources for learning is found in the differentness of people and their perceptions that can openly be dealt with.
- *Failure as a resource for learning.* If the staff within the unit can be desensitized so that persons who believe they have failed can learn from the experience, failure can become a motivational force. Role training helps the learner find new ways to approach the problem. The question, "How would you do it differently?" may help the learner develop spontaneous responses that can be capitalized on later.

Resource People. Selecting competent resource people requires careful planning. Criteria for this selection are threefold:

- The resource person's ability to adapt professional knowledge, expertise, and vocabulary to staff's background and experience
- The person's ability to adapt expertise to the objectives. Unless the resource person has been given a well-developed set of objectives prior to the session, the information will be based on his own perception of what is needed. This may subvert achieving the learning objectives.
- The resource's ability to listen to and respect the knowledge and experience that staff members bring to the session. The assessment of this quality places a special responsibility on the educator. If the resource person believes in and communicates respect for the staff and their work and builds on this, he will be an acceptable resource person. Therefore, take time prior to the session to share this information.

Resource people will need well-prepared answers to questions like these:

- Why me? What do you want from me?
- How do I fit in with the overall educational program?
- What are the people like that you want me to work with?
- What will they want to know?
- What do you expect to happen when the session is over?

These or similar questions need to be answered for staff members involved in in-service and staff development programs. They, too, provide a reservoir of resources that needs to be tapped. To tap such resources, however, people will need to know honestly what is in it for them. In other words, what's the payoff for being a resource person? If they can see a payoff, they will be motivated to learn and to become involved. They will accept the change that learning creates and demands. For instance, why would a staff member take on the responsibility of becoming a preceptor or buddy in the orientation program?

Materials. With the help of the in-service educator, in-service educators in your community, manufacturer's representatives, and learning laboratories in schools of nursing, it is possible to locate excellent materials to use in group sessions or for individual work. Materials can range from programmed instruction units to reading materials for personal use or group discussion. Also, setting the expectations for staff to bring in items such as articles, cartoons, and news items enriches resources and underscores mutual responsibility.

Software (flip charts, markers, masking tape, mockups, posters, workbooks) creates a variety for pacing learning.

In summary, select the resource for achieving specific learning objectives and keep in mind the work situation, the timing, and the learners. Accommodating all these elements becomes an art, so allow time to develop this particular ability.

Step 5. Manage Learning Activities

Once the potential resources have been selected, the next step in the process model is managing the activities in such a way that both learning and unit objectives are achieved. To gear learning to the work cycle in a practical and realistic manner demands artistry in juggling the components that shape an effective and satisfying learning experience. These components include time, place, materials, equipment, situations, and human resources. One may have to settle for something less than the ideal educational setting and schedule learning in conjunction with work in progress. As these functions become more complimentary, less time and energy will be used in their integration.

Readiness of the Learner. To manage opportunities for individual learning, become thoroughly familiar with the level of performance of each staff member and his learning objectives. The skills inventory and nurse's experience data provide a baseline for determining content. Interaction observations and skill behaviors will provide data on readiness. Readiness to learn is important — physically, intellectually, and psychologically. Recognizing this, timing then becomes the vital element. Sometimes training will be scheduled for a specific time; at other times it can be done in the process of the day's activities on an unscheduled basis. The educator's responsibility is to see that training happens when the learner is prepared and ready to learn and that appropriate techniques are used.

A long enough period of time for learning is necessary to capitalize on the learning potential of staff. Consider the fact that each time the learners experience a new behavior, they are in effect relearning it in each new situation. When it becomes evident that a new behavior has been well integrated into performance, taper off any coaching or special attention.

Situation. Tune in to the daily experiences within the CCU that offer content for learning — such readiness and spontaneity facilitates learning. Getting people together and orienting them to the situation require presence of mind and quick action. At first this practice will be awkward. But as staff members become comfortable with it, this cooperative effort can be directed or suggested by any person. Being sensitive to feedback (verbal and nonverbal) allows adjusting the teaching to the activity's progress. This flexibility in style of managing the situation and oneself will increase the potential for learning. It also increases the potential for using unique resources.

Content. Several cautions for managing content may save time and effort. So often the tendency is to tell learners *what you want them to know,* and rarely to take time to *find out what they already know — or even need to know.* The usual response of the learners in this situation is mixed; they feel put down, or they are bored and tune out the instructor. Thus a guideline might be to take time to find out "who knows what" and build from there. This behavior is compatible with seeing one's own self as a co-learner.

When it is necessary to provide a considerable amount of information, organize it into segments or modules that can be grasped by the learner. An overload of information with little or no breathing space between segments is discouraging. Prepare information in lecturette formats. Research on listening cites the traps that listeners fall into when listening to long lectures.[10] Twenty minutes is suggested as an effective block of time for content. Follow this with learner involvement techniques so that some internalization of content takes place and retention is enforced. Pacing facilitates absorption of information.

When extensive content in a particular sequence is indicated, look at the potential resources within the staff as presenters. If sharing responsibilities for content is expected, staff can prepare specific information in collaboration with the planner. In this way it decreases the exposure of the educator as "teaching resource" and increases the versatility of the unit's resources. This approach to managing content allows one more time to manage the overall CCU and directs the resources toward both unit goals and individual growth goals.

Human Resources. This subject is covered rather extensively in step 4. However, a point that bears repeating is this: Take time to carefully prepare all resources — regardless of whether they are outside or from within the hospital.

A great deal of the success and effectiveness of the resource depends on how the following have been managed: scheduling, objectives of the session, information announcing the session, rationale for the content and method of presentation, plan to involve the learners and the preparation of the learners, and the setting for holding the session.

Attention to these details creates a climate that supports the teaching-learning activities and the people involved.

Place, Material, Time, and Equipment. One asset of the CCU not to be overlooked is its dual function as a treatment area and as a learning area. This fact simplifies some of the management problems of providing an educational facility. The standard equipment and materials used serve the needs of both patient and staff-learner. As one begins to blend the service of nursing care to patients with on-the-spot teaching, there will also begin to develop a keen appreciation of the versatility, efficiency, and capacity of the CCU.

Space for in-service sessions and team meetings poses a problem. Explore space adjacent to the unit such as classrooms, conference rooms, and board rooms. Usually, if sessions are scheduled in advance, the space can be reserved. Ask the multidisciplinary staff for the unit to assist in locating space.

The most difficult problem will be finding time for educational activities. Give up the idea that numbers mean good in-service. If the people attending can use the information, training, or discussion, the time will be spent profitably. Because the census in critical care varies, scheduling learning activities poses a real challenge! Several ideas may help stretch the imagination to discover feasible alternatives.

- What about having several "packaged" programs available so that they can be pulled out when the census is low? Working on current performance problems is another agenda.
- What about overlapping schedules at the end of one shift and the beginning of the next shift?
- What about taping sessions and planning discussion guides to go with them?
- What about occasionally conducting a special in-service during each shift?
- How about rotating staff so that everyone scheduled for the day shift has the opportunity to work with a preceptor, or attend scheduled in-service that is especially pertinent to what they want to learn?
- How about getting ideas from the staff to determine best time for all shifts and regular floats?
- How about working out a plan with another department? One example in a hospital was set up by the operating room (OR) staff. The OR scheduled surgery one hour later than usual on Friday mornings so that prime time could be devoted to in-service, team-building, and creative problem-solving. The surgeons supported the plan. Could you hitchhike on such a schedule? Would someone care for patients in the unit while others would be free for training?

Step 6. Evaluate Objectives, Performance, and the Learning Plan
The next step is to evaluate the learning, which means measuring the degree of change in performance of persons involved in the training activities. It also means measuring the achievement of the learner's own objectives. Observing these changes in terms of overt behavior and guided observations over a period of time will result in the evaluation of the employee's ability to integrate new learning into job performance.

Another form of evaluating learning is open staff meetings. This allows staff to give feedback on the significance of the learning and how they have been able to use what they have learned. In this process, evaluation can be made of staff effectiveness. Successes, failures, conflicts, creative solutions—all these are part of the evaluation process and contribute information essential to ongoing needs and new objectives for the next sequence of learning activities.

The action plan can be evaluated for how effectively the driving and restraining forces were identified and handled. Learner resources can be evaluated for how effectively they overcame the blocks to learning. Working agreements and deadlines can be reviewed for how well the contract contributed to objective achievement.

Grist for evaluation includes organization of the learning activities in terms of the working situation, readiness of learners, preparation of resource people, materials used, and timing.

Perhaps the most difficult element to measure will be the *results.* Results that are "winners" give data that support long-term effects such as lower turnover, effective patient care on a cost basis, and a high level of staff competence in less time than the former training plan.

Factors for documenting costs for training and development include some of the following. The list offers possible data for justifying budget and results of training and development.[11]

- Planning time (percentage of salary for time spent by each member of the planning team, or number of hours spent by each member multiplied by the hourly salary rate, and fees for consultants)
- Staff time (percentage of salary for time spent by each member engaged in planning and production and in gathering materials or the number of hours spent by each person multiplied by the hourly salary rate)
- Supplies and materials
- Outside services for preparing or purchasing materials
- Construction or renovation of facilities
- Equipment
- Installation of equipment
- Testing, evaluation, redesign, reproduction of resources (including personnel time and costs of materials and services)
- In-service education for others who might participate in the in-service

- Overhead (utilities, furniture, room, or building costs)
- Miscellaneous (office supplies, telephone, travel, and other items)
- Documenting the amount of time spent directly on creating the overall education program in addition to the other functions performed with staff and patients will give one some experience in tracking supportive data.

A great deal of time and effort are already being expended in the unit on informal teaching, learning from imitation, and learning from mistakes. Gathering data for a period of time on the current level of performance and then data to support the new overall education program will help justify adequate budget.

To facilitate gathering data, use resources such as the hospital's personnel director, in-service educator, and cost accountant. There may be a researcher on the hospital staff who could help design effective evaluation tools. If not, local colleges and universities have resource people who design such evaluations. Graduate students in schools of nursing look for real research projects, and professors welcome opportunities to place students in primary research situations.

Use feedback from everyone involved in the learning activities. Data from these resources will provide viable information to use in moving into the recycling process, which is step 7.

Step 7. Recycle
The last step starts the process all over again. Based on validation of new needs and unmet needs that emerge from the process and on changes that have evolved during the intervening time, recycling educational programs begins again.

All the steps in the process model involve other people, and in the final analysis, the process model is also a participative model offering the greatest potential for working with peers and professionals.

CONCLUSION

After reading this chapter and reflecting on how people learn to cope with the significant changes in their personal and professional lives and to realize self-fulfillment and satisfaction as a result, where can they go?

Where Can I Go?*

If this is not a place where tears are understood,
Where can I go to cry?

If this is not a place where my spirits can take wing,
Where do I go to fly?

If this is not a place where my questions can be asked,
Where do I go to seek?

If this is not a place where my feelings can be heard,
Where do I go to speak?

If this is not a place where you'll accept me as I am,
Where can I go to be?

If this is not a place I can try, and learn, and grow,
Where can I just be me?

If this is not a place where tears are understood,
Where can I go to cry?

* (Modified from a song by Ken Medina, "Where Can I Go?" by OD Network Newsletter, May, 1978; reproduced with special permission, Training and Development Journal, American Society for Training and Development, Madison WI, May, 1980)

REFERENCES

1. Lippitt GL: Integrating personal and professional development. Training and Development Journal 34, No. 5:34, 1980
2. Drucker P: Learning from foreign management. New York, Wall Street Journal, June 4, 1980
3. Decentralized staff faculty: Innovations in in-service. Tempe, Arizona, Arizona State University, 1975
4. Knowles M: The Adult Learner: A Neglected Species, 2nd ed. Houston, Gulf Publishing, 1978
5. Special survey/research project conducted by the Industrial Audiovisual Association. Lecture, Colorado State University, Fort Collins, Co. 1973
6. Tough A: The Adult's Learning Project, 2nd ed. Toronto, Ontario Institute for Studies in Education, 1979
7. Knowles M: The Modern Practice of Adult Education: From Pedagogy to Androgogy. New York, Cambridge Press, 1980
8. Ibid
9. Mager R: Preparing Instructional Objectives. Belmont, Fearon Publishers, 1963
10. Nichols RG, Stevens L: Are You Listening? New York, McGraw-Hill, 1957
11. Kemp JE: Instructional Design, 2nd ed. Belmont, Fearon Publishers, 1977

BIBLIOGRAPHY

Cross KP: Adults as Learners. San Francisco, Jossey-Bass, 1981
Hoyt KB: Getting to work—Can productivity and humanistic values be integrated in the American workplace? Training and Development Journal 38, No. 9:71, 1984
Houle CO: Patterns of Learning. San Francisco, Jossey-Bass, 1984
Jackson CN: Training's role in the process of planned change. Training and Development Journal 39, No. 2:70, 1985
Juechter, WM: Wellness: Addressing the "whole" person. Training and Development Journal 36, No. 5:112, 1982
Karp HB: Working with resistance. Journal of Training and Development Journal 38 No. 3:69, 1984
Kindler HS: Time out for stress management training. Training and Development Journal 38, No. 6:64, 1984
Kram K: Improving the mentoring process. Training and Development Journal 39, No. 4:40, 1985
Moore ER: Competency-based evaluation. Training and Development Journal 38, No. 11:92, 1984
Parry SB, Reich LR: An uneasy look at behavior modeling. Training and Development Journal 38, No. 3:57, 1984

Rosen RH: The picture of health in the work place. Training and Development Journal 38, No. 8:24, 1984

Short RR: Managing unlearning: How to keep education from blocking learning. Training and Development Journal 35, No. 7:37, 1981

Smith RM: Learning how to learn: Applied theory for adults. New York, Cambridge Press, 1982

Strauch R: Training the whole person. Training and Development Journal 38, No. 11:82, 1984

Tjosvold D: The dynamics of positive power. Training and Development Journal 38, No. 6:72, 1984

Index

Page numbers followed by *f* indicate illustrations; *t* following a page number indicates tabular material.